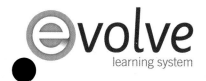  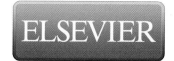
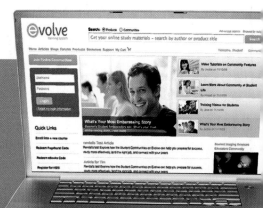

NURSING CARE OF CHILDREN

Principles & Practice

FOURTH EDITION

SUSAN ROWEN JAMES, PhD, RN
Professor
Curry College Division of Nursing
Milton, Massachusetts

KRISTINE ANN NELSON, MN, RN
Assistant Professor of Nursing
Tarrant County College
Trinity River East Campus Center for Health Care Professions
Fort Worth, Texas

JEAN WEILER ASHWILL, MSN, RN
Assistant Dean, Undergraduate Student Services
College of Nursing
University of Texas at Arlington
Arlington, Texas

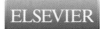

ELSEVIER
SAUNDERS

3251 Riverport Lane
St. Louis, Missouri 63043

NURSING CARE OF CHILDREN: PRINCIPLES AND PRACTICE   ISBN: 978-1-4557-0366-1

Library of Congress Cataloging-in-Publication Data

Nursing care of children : principles & practice.—4th ed. / [edited by] Susan Rowen James, Kristine Ann Nelson, Jean Weiler Ashwill.
      p. ; cm.
  Includes bibliographical references and index.
  ISBN 978-1-4557-0366-1 (pbk. : alk. paper)
  I. James, Susan Rowen, 1946-   II. Nelson, Kristine Ann.   III. Ashwill, Jean Weiler.
  [DNLM: 1. Pediatric Nursing—methods. 2. Adolescent. 3. Child. 4. Infant. 5. Nursing Process. WY 159]
      618.92′00231—dc23   2011044713

Content Manager: Michelle Hayden
Content Development Specialist: Heather Bays
Publishing Services Manager: Jeffrey Patterson
Senior Project Manager: Mary G. Stueck
Design Direction: Paula Catalano

L ast digit is the print number: 10   9   8   7   6   5   4

Printed in the United States of America

Mary Jane Piskor Ashe, RN, MN
Clinical Instructor
Smart Hospital;
College of Nursing
University of Texas at Arlington
Arlington, Texas

Jamie Bankston, RN, MS
Director of Clinical Education
Cook Children's Medical Center
Fort Worth, Texas

Jacqueline Carroll, RN MSN CPNP
Assistant Professor
Curry College Division of Nursing
Milton, Massachusetts

Joe Don Cavender, RN, MSN, CPNP-PC
Pediatric Nurse Practitioner
Director of Advanced Practice Services
Children's Medical Center of Dallas
Dallas, Texas

Sheryl Cifrino, RN, DNP, MA
Associate Professor
Curry College Division of Nursing
Milton, Massachusetts

Melissa A. Saffarrans LeMoine, RN, MSN, CPNP
Pediatric Nurse Practitioner
Nephrology, Dialysis, and Transplant Services
Cook Children's Health Care System
Fort Worth, Texas

Renee C.B. Manworren, PhD, APRN, PCNS-BC
Nurse Scientist
Division of Pain and Palliative Medicine
Connecticut Children's Medical Center;
Assistant Professor of Pediatrics
University of Connecticut School of Medicine
Hartford, Connecticut

Gwendolyn T. Martin, RN, MS, CNS, CPST-I
Assistant Professor of Nursing
Tarrant County College
Department of Nursing
Fort Worth, Texas

Lindy Moake, RN, MSN, PCCNP
Clinical Manager of Advanced Practice Services
Heart Center
Children's Medical Center of Dallas
Dallas, Texas;
Clinical Faculty
University of Texas at Arlington
Arlington, Texas

Patricia Newcomb, RN, PhD, CPNP
Director
Genomics Translational Research Laboratory
College of Nursing
University of Texas at Arlington
Arlington, Texas

Eileen O'Connell, PhD, RN
Associate Professor
Curry College Division of Nursing
Milton, Massachusetts

Fiona E. Paul, RN, DNP, CPNP
Pediatric Nurse Practitioner
Children's Hospital of Boston;
Harvard Medical School
Boston, Massachusetts

Meagan Rogers, RN, MSN, CPEN
Clinical Educator
Emergency Department
Children's Medical Center at Legacy
Dallas, Texas

Jennifer Roye, RN, MSN, CPNP
Clinical Coordinator
Academic Partnership BSN Program
College of Nursing
University of Texas at Arlington
Arlington, Texas

Ann Smith, PhD, CPNP, CNE
Coordinator, Nurse Residency
Cook Children's Medical Center
Fort Worth, Texas

PowerPoint Presentations and Pediatric Skills
Susan Golden, RN, MSN
Nursing Program Director
Department of Nursing
Eastern New Mexico University, Roswell
Roswell, New Mexico

Test Bank
Mary L. Dowell, PhD, RN, BC
Assistant Professor
Nursing Department
San Antonio College;
LVN-ADN Program Coordinator
Kerrville Distance Site
Kerrville, Texas

Corine K. Carlson, RN, MS
Associate Professor
Luther College
Decorah, Iowa

Hobie Etta Feagai, EdD, MSN, FNP-BC, APRN-Rx
Associate Professor of Nursing
Hawai'i Pacific University
College of Nursing & Health Sciences
Kaneohe, Hawai'i

Erica Fooshee, RN, MSN, CNE, CPN
Program Manager, Nursing
Western Governors University
Salt Lake City, Utah

Susan Golden, RN, MSN
Nursing Program Director
Department of Nursing
Eastern New Mexico University at Roswell
Roswell, New Mexico

Cynthia Gordy, RN, MSN
Clinical Nursing Instructor
Indian Hills Community College
Centerville, Iowa

Vivian Kuawogai, RN, MSN
Associate Professor of Nursing
Prince George's Community College
Largo, Maryland

Renee C.B. Manworren, PhD, APRN, PCNS-BC
Nurse Scientist
Division of Pain and Palliative Medicine
Connecticut Children's Medical Center;
Assistant Professor of Pediatrics
University of Connecticut School of Medicine
Hartford, Connecticut

Claudia Perry, RN, BSN, MBA
Nursing Instructor
Clovis Community College
Clovis, New Mexico

Ann Petersen-Smith, PhD, RN, CPNP-AC
Assistant Professor
PNP Option Coordinator
Division of Women, Children, and Family Health
University of Colorado
College of Nursing
Anschutz Medical Campus
Aurora, Colorado

Jill Pitts, RNC, MSN
Assistant Professor
Associate Degree Nursing
South Plains College
Levelland, Texas

Janice Ramirez, MSN, RN BC, CRRN, CNE
RN Instructor
North Idaho College
Coeur d'Alene, Idaho

Cheryl C. Rodgers, PhD, RN, CPNP, CPON
Pediatric Nurse Practitioner
Texas Children's Hospital;
Clinical Instructor
Baylor College of Medicine
Houston, Texas

Chris Shanks
Vancouver Island University
Department of Nursing
Nanaimo, British Columbia
Canada

Jana Wiscaver Thompson, MNSc, RN
Clinical Assistant Professor
Department of Nursing
University of Arkansas for Medical Sciences
Little Rock, Arkansas

NCLEX Review Questions

Colleen W. Bible, MSN, RN
Nursing Faculty
Division of Health Sciences—Nursing
Technical College of the Lowcountry
Beaufort, South Carolina

TEACH for Nurses

Betty Hamlisch, RN, BSN, MS
Health Fducation
Professor Emerita
Tompkins Cortland Community College
Dryden, New York

Test Bank

Nan Riedé, MSN, RN, CPN
Assistant Professor
Baptist College of Health Sciences
Memphis, Tennessee

PREFACE

Children are precious gifts. Two of the most satisfying nursing roles are being a resource to children and families as they develop their own unique identities and comforting them in times of illness and stress. Holding a child, talking softly, or entering into imaginary play—all are parts of nursing children. Hugging or sitting quietly with a parent, explaining a procedure or a disease, or providing reassurance through quiet, competent care can literally change the way a parent views the child's experience of illness.

High-quality nursing care of children combines compassion with the most up-to-date clinical knowledge grounded in basic theoretical principles of nursing care. This fourth edition of *Nursing Care of Children: Principles & Practice* emphasizes using evidence as the basis for the care nurses provide daily to pediatric patients and their families. This scientific base is demonstrated in the narrative and features in which the nursing process is applied. Physiologic and pathophysiologic processes are presented in a format that assists the student to understand why health problems occur and how to derive appropriate nursing care. Current references provide students with the latest information that applies to the clinical area. National standards and guidelines, such as those from the American Nurses Association and the Society of Pediatric Nurses, have been incorporated where applicable. There is an enhanced focus on quality and safety to assist students with achievement of the Quality and Safety Education for Nurses (QSEN) competencies.

This text addresses contemporary changes in health care, recognizing that health care costs have led to shorter hospital stays and a shift to health care provided in the community and the home. The fourth edition of *Nursing Care of Children* includes a strong focus on the growing and changing roles of nurses caring for children in varied settings. To expand and enhance its community emphasis, the text incorporates the recently released *Healthy People 2020* national objectives. In addition, adaptation of principles to the home, community, and school settings is illustrated throughout and has been increased in this edition.

The text's emphasis on health and wellness is found in a comprehensive unit covering growth and development, with anticipatory guidance for families. This unit is organized around the recommended schedule of well-child visits as described by the American Academy of Pediatrics. *Health Promotion* boxes assist students with information needed to understand developmental milestones, health promotion activities, and anticipatory guidance for infants and children of specific ages and developmental levels.

Legal and ethical issues add to the complexity of practice for today's nurse. The first chapter of our book discusses the ethical and legal obligations of nurses who work with children and how to meet these obligations while providing optimum client care. Issues such as including children in research, what constitutes a mature minor, and the care of technology-dependent children are discussed where applicable throughout the book.

Contemporary nursing students have time demands from work, family, and community activities in addition to their nursing education. A significant number of students use English as a second language. With those realities in mind, we have written a text to effectively convey essential information that focuses on critical elements and that is concise without unnecessarily complex language. Important items are highlighted within each chapter and defined in a comprehensive glossary for ready access as the student studies. Teaching guidelines in the form of *Patient-Centered Teaching* boxes and other material are written in language that will assist students to teach parents and children about home care, self-care, preventive care, and follow-up care.

In keeping with the focus of incorporating Evidence-Based Practice as a thread throughout most nursing curricula, this edition includes Evidence-Based Practice boxes, which facilitate critical thinking about how evidence could be used by nurses to make clinical practice decisions.

CONCEPTS

Several conceptual threads are interwoven throughout the text.

Family

The nurse must care for the child within the context of the family. In this text, emphasis is placed on the importance of focusing on the family when caring for children of all ages and in many different settings. Changing family structure and diversity in types of families are considered. Special sections are devoted to the needs of siblings.

Growth and Development Within the Concept of Health Promotion

Concepts of health promotion and anticipatory guidance are organized around a developmental framework. A chapter on general health promotion for developing children describes the various developmental assessment areas: parameters of growth, factors influencing growth and development, developmental milestones, play; nutrition; immunizations; and safety. Each of the subsequent growth and development chapters discusses these areas as they apply to the infant, child, or adolescent of a specific age or developmental level. Each chapter also provides a review of physical and psychosocial changes unique to that age-group and emphasizes the nurse's role with children of specific ages and at varying developmental levels.

Child Advocacy

Legal and ethical responsibilities of nurses are identified and explained in such areas as violence, abuse, neglect, drug abuse, and access to health care.

Communication

Communicating appropriately with children can be a challenge. The fourth edition includes special *Communication Cues* and describes techniques to enhance therapeutic communication with children and families. An entire chapter is devoted to communicating with children and families.

Culture

Cultural variety characterizes nursing practice today as the lines between individual nations become more blurred. The nurse must assess for unique cultural needs of children and their families and incorporate them into care, promoting acceptance of nursing interventions. Cultural influences are examined in many ways in our text, and principles of culturally sensitive care are incorporated throughout as an important thread.

TEXT ORGANIZATION

Similar to the third edition, the text uses an objective-oriented approach that makes it easy for students to understand and retain important material. Nursing care sections are organized around the nursing process to facilitate learning using a problem-solving method. The text begins with an overview of contemporary nursing of children, including general principles of care. Comprehensive growth and development chapters follow. Principles for adapting care of well children to those requiring admission to an emergency or hospital setting precede the final chapters, which cover care of children with specific health alterations. Narrative coverage of important childhood disorders is consistently organized in a nursing process format, again with NANDA diagnoses, expected outcomes, and evaluation questions. Less common disorders are grouped and discussed in tables in each body system chapter.

FEATURES

Visual appeal characterizes many features in the text. Beautiful full-color illustrations and photographs convey clinical information and also capture the essence of nursing care of children. Illustrations reinforce knowledge of growth and development, explain pathophysiology, make learning procedures easier, show manifestations of diseases and disorders, and provide models of interactions with patients and families.

Clinical Reference Pages

This edition continues the popular Clinical Reference pages, which are a resource for the student when reviewing basic anatomy and physiology and differences between children and adults as they pertain to the body system being discussed. They also include diagnostic studies, laboratory values, and nursing care associated with these procedures.

Critical Thinking Exercises

Critical thinking is encouraged in multiple ways throughout *Nursing Care of Children*, but specific Critical Thinking Exercises are included in most chapters in the text. These present scenarios of real-life situations or issues and ask the student to solve nursing care problems that are not always obvious. Answers are given on the Evolve website, so the students can check solutions to these problems.

Drug Guide Boxes

Drug information is generally presented through Drug Guide boxes. Drug guides for specific, commonly used medications provide the student nurse with detailed information.

Health Promotion Boxes

Health Promotion boxes summarize needed information to perform a comprehensive assessment of well infants and children at various ages. Organized around the American Academy of Pediatrics' recommended schedule for well-child visits, examples are given of questions designed to elicit developmental and behavioral information from parent and child. These boxes also include what the student might expect to see for health screening or immunization and review specific topics for anticipatory guidance.

Key Concepts

Key Concepts summarize important points of each chapter. They provide a general review for the material just presented to help the student identify areas in which more study is needed.

Learning Objectives

Learning Objectives provide direction for the reader to understand what is important to glean from the chapter. Many objectives ask that the learner use critical thinking and apply the nursing process—two crucial components of professional nursing.

Nursing Process

Although all steps of the nursing process are used consistently in nursing process sections, nursing process appears in two different formats throughout the text. The different formats show the student that there is more than one way to communicate nursing process. Nursing process can be applied to care of children with the most common childhood conditions through an in-text discussion that demonstrates how the process relates to a typical child with a specific condition. Nursing process for children with more complex nursing problems is illustrated through the use of a care plan format, which encompasses focused assessment, nursing diagnoses, expected outcomes, interventions, rationales, and evaluation criteria. This format helps the nursing instructor teach students how to individualize care for their specific clients based on a generic plan of care.

Pathophysiology Boxes

Pathophysiology boxes give the student a brief overview of how various illnesses occur. The boxes provide a scientific basis for understanding the therapeutic management of the illness and its nursing care.

Patient-Centered Teaching

Because teaching is an essential part of nursing care, we give students teaching guidelines for common client needs in terms that most lay people can understand. Patient-Centered Teaching boxes provide sample answers for questions that children or parents are most likely to ask.

Procedure Boxes

Clinical skills are presented in Procedure boxes throughout the text. The text includes two chapters that describe step-by-step general and medication procedures used when caring for children. Many of these procedures have been expanded to include home adaptations.

Safety Alerts and Nursing Quality Alerts

Safety Alert boxes provide critical information needed to deliver safe nursing care. Nursing Quality Alert boxes contain condensed knowledge on ways students can enhance and improve the care they provide to children and families.

ACKNOWLEDGMENTS

We would first like to thank our families and friends who supported us in this endeavor by understanding when we were unavailable and encouraging us when we were overwhelmed.

We express our sincere appreciation to the clinicians (listed on p. vi), experts in their fields, who contributed to the book. They provided the up-to-date clinical information needed in a teaching text. Thank you is also extended to the reviewers, who very conscientiously made suggestions to improve the text.

Both Emily McKinney and Sharon Murray, who, along with us, are authors and editors of the combined book, *Maternal-Child Nursing*, provided input that helped us focus on needed improvements for this edition. Their suggestions are always invaluable. Heather Bays, developmental editor, worked with us to make our vision for an improved text a reality. Her untiring work on our behalf has kept the project moving forward, despite having to manage some unavoidable and difficult obstacles. She and Michele Hayden, our Managing Editor, have used their excellent problem-solving skills every step of the way. Mary Stueck, project manager, saw to it that the production process proceeded in a timely fashion and responded quickly to our editing and production concerns.

Finally, as educators we are teaching but also learning from our students. Some of the new features in *Nursing Care of Children:* *Principles & Practice*, fourth edition, have their origin in wonderful feedback given by our students about their learning needs. We hope that this edition supports and strengthens students' ability and desire to learn about this exciting and ever-changing specialty of ours.

Susan Rowen James, PhD, RN
Kristine Ann Nelson, MN, RN
Jean Weiler Ashwill, MSN, RN

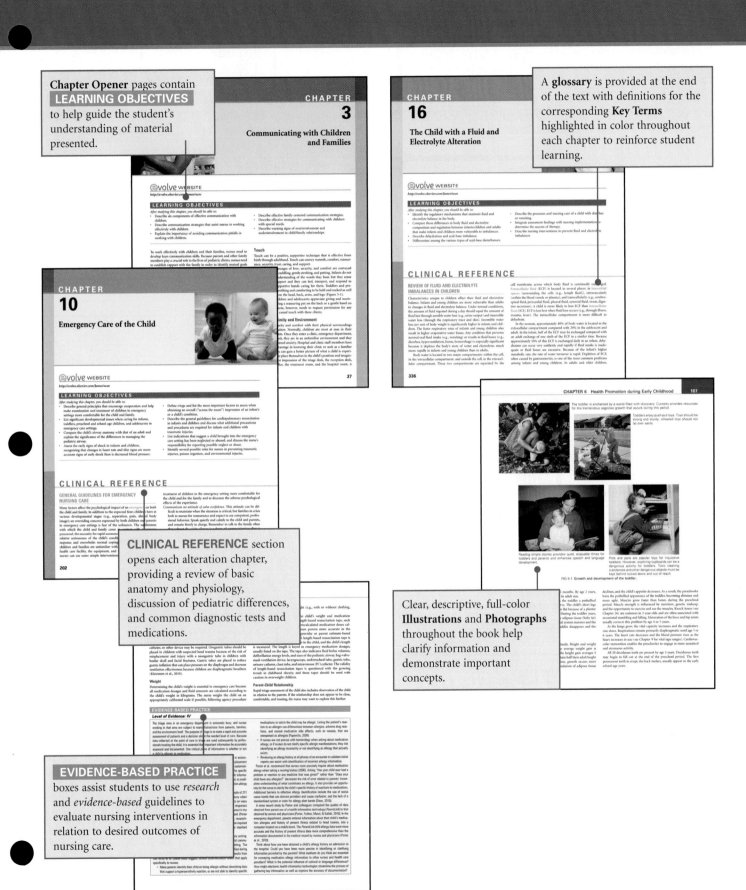

Chapter Opener pages contain **LEARNING OBJECTIVES** to help guide the student's understanding of material presented.

A **glossary** is provided at the end of the text with definitions for the corresponding **Key Terms** highlighted in color throughout each chapter to reinforce student learning.

CLINICAL REFERENCE section opens each alteration chapter, providing a review of basic anatomy and physiology, discussion of pediatric differences, and common diagnostic tests and medications.

Clear, descriptive, full-color **Illustrations** and **Photographs** throughout the book help clarify information and demonstrate important concepts.

EVIDENCE-BASED PRACTICE boxes assist students to use *research* and *evidence-based* guidelines to evaluate nursing interventions in relation to desired outcomes of nursing care.

Marginal Notes are placed throughout the text to highlight additional exercises and resources found on the Evolve website.

PROCEDURE boxes provide clear, step-by-step instructions for common nursing tasks to assist students in clinical practice.

PATHOPHYSIOLOGY boxes describe how disease conditions develop, presenting a scientific basis for understanding the therapeutic management and nursing care of an illness.

Safety Alerts and **Nursing Quality Alerts** highlight vital information that is crucial to delivering safe and effective nursing care.

PATIENT-CENTERED TEACHING boxes guide the student in answering questions commonly asked and teaching the parents and child about self-care.

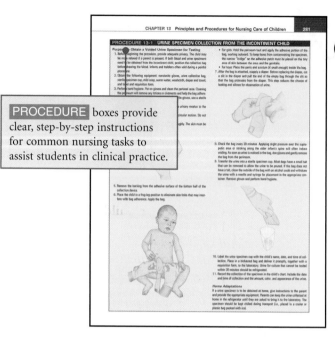
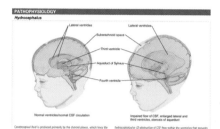
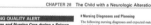

CONTENTS

UNIT IV CARING FOR CHILDREN WITH HEALTH PROBLEMS

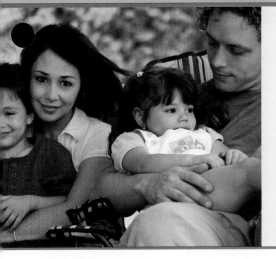

Introduction to Nursing Care of Children

evolve WEBSITE

http://evolve.elsevier.com/James/ncoc

LEARNING OBJECTIVES

After studying this chapter, you should be able to:

- Describe the historical background of children's health care.
- Identify trends that led to the development of family-centered care of children.
- Describe issues that affect child health nursing, including cost containment, outcomes management, home care, and advances in technology.
- Discuss trends in infant and childhood mortality rates.
- Identify some of the effects of poverty and violence on children and families.
- Apply theories and principles of ethics to ethical dilemmas.
- Discuss ethical conflicts that the nurse may encounter in pediatric nursing practice.

- Relate how major social issues, such as poverty and access to health care, affect children's health.
- Describe the legal basis for nursing practice.
- Identify measures used to defend malpractice claims.
- Explain roles the nurse may assume in pediatric nursing practice.
- Explain the roles of nurses with advanced education for pediatric nursing practice.
- Describe the steps of the nursing process and relate them to nursing care of children.
- Explain issues surrounding the use of complementary and alternative therapies.
- Discuss the importance of nursing research in clinical practice.

PRINCIPLES OF CARING FOR CHILDREN

To better understand contemporary child health nursing, the nurse needs to understand the history of this field, trends and issues affecting contemporary practice, and the ethical and legal frameworks within which pediatric nursing care is provided.

HISTORICAL PERSPECTIVES

The nursing care of children has been influenced by multiple historical and social factors. Children have not always enjoyed the valued position that they hold in most families today. Historically, in times of economic or social instability, children have been viewed as expendable. In societies in which the struggle for survival is the central issue and only the strongest survive, the needs of children are secondary. The well-being of children in the past depended on the economic and cultural conditions of the society. At times parents have viewed their children as property, and children have been bought and sold, beaten, and, in some cultures, sacrificed in religious ceremonies. At times, infanticide has been a routine practice. Conversely, in other instances,

children have been highly valued and their birth considered a blessing. Viewed by society as miniature adults, children in the past received the same remedies as adults and during illness were cared for at home by family members, just as adults were.

Societal Changes

On the North American continent, as European settlements expanded during the seventeenth and eighteenth centuries, children were valued as assets to the community because of the desire to increase the population and share the work. Public schools were established, and the courts began to view children as minors and protect them accordingly. Devastating epidemics of smallpox, diphtheria, scarlet fever, and measles took their toll on children in the eighteenth century. Children often died of these virulent diseases within 1 day.

The high mortality rate in children led some physicians to examine common child-care practices. In 1748 William Cadogan's "Essay Upon Nursing" discouraged unhealthy child-care practices, such as swaddling infants in three or four layers of clothing and feeding them thin gruel within hours after birth. Instead, Cadogan urged mothers to breastfeed their infants and identified certain practices that were

TABLE 1-1 FEDERAL PROJECTS FOR MATERNAL-CHILD CARE

PROGRAM	PURPOSE
Title V of Social Security Act	Provides funds for maternal and child health programs
National Institute of Health and Human Development	Supports research and education of personnel needed for maternal and child health programs
Title V Amendment of Public Health Service Act	Established the Maternal and Infant Care (MIC) project to provide comprehensive prenatal and infant care in public clinics
Title XIX of Medicaid program	Provides funds to facilitate access to care by pregnant women and young children
Head Start program	Provides educational opportunities for low-income children of preschool age
Women, Infants, and Children (WIC) program	Provides supplemental food and nutrition information
Temporary Assistance to Needy Families (TANF)	Provides temporary money for basic living costs of poor children and their families, with eligibility requirements and time limits varying among states; tribal programs available for Native Americans Replaces Aid to Families with Dependent Children (AFDC)
Healthy Start program	Enhances community development of culturally appropriate strategies designed to decrease infant mortality and causes of low birth weights
Individuals with Disabilities Education Act (PL 94-142)	Provides for free and appropriate education of all disabled children
National School Lunch/Breakfast program	Provides nutritionally appropriate free or reduced-price meals to students from low-income families

thought to contribute to childhood illness. Unfortunately, despite the efforts of Cadogan and others, child-care practices were slow to change. Later in the eighteenth century, the health of children improved with certain advances such as inoculation against smallpox.

In the nineteenth century, with the flood of immigrants to eastern American cities, infectious diseases flourished as a result of crowded living conditions; inadequate and unsanitary food; and harsh working conditions for men, women, and children. It was common for children to work 12- to 14-hour days in factories, and their earnings were essential to the survival of the family. The most serious child health problems during the nineteenth century were caused by poverty and overcrowding. Infants were fed contaminated milk, sometimes from tuberculosis-infected cows. Milk was carried to the cities and purchased by mothers with no means to refrigerate it. Infectious diarrhea was a common cause of infant death.

During the late nineteenth century, conditions began to improve for children and families. Lillian Wald initiated public health nursing at Henry Street Settlement House in New York City, where nurses taught mothers in their homes. In 1889 a milk distribution center opened in New York City to provide uncontaminated milk to sick infants.

Hygiene and Hospitalization

The discoveries of scientists such as Pasteur, Lister, and Koch, who established that bacteria caused many diseases, supported the use of hygienic practices in hospitals and foundling homes. Hospitals began to require personnel to wear uniforms and limit contact among children in the wards. In an effort to prevent infection, hospital wards were closed to visitors. Because parental visits were noted to cause distress, particularly when parents had to leave, parental visitation was considered emotionally stressful to hospitalized children. In an effort to prevent such emotional distress and the spread of infection, parents were prohibited from visiting children in the hospital. Because hospital care focused on preventing disease transmission and curing physical diseases, the emotional health of hospitalized children received little attention.

During the twentieth century, as knowledge about nutrition, sanitation, bacteriology, pharmacology, medication, and psychology increased, dramatic changes in child health occurred. In the 1940s and 1950s medications such as penicillin and corticosteroids and

vaccines against many communicable diseases saved the lives of tens of thousands of children. Technologic advances in the 1970s and 1980s, which led to more children surviving conditions that had previously been fatal (e.g., cystic fibrosis), resulted in an increasing number of children living with chronic disabilities. An increase in societal concern for children brought about the development of federally supported programs designed to meet their needs, such as school lunch programs, the Special Supplemental Nutrition Program for Women, Infants, and Children (WIC), and Medicaid (Table 1-1), under which the Early and Periodic Screening, Diagnosis, and Treatment program was implemented.

Development of Family-Centered Child Care

Family-centered child health care developed from the recognition that the emotional needs of hospitalized children usually were unmet. Parents were not involved in the direct care of their children. Children were often unprepared for procedures and tests, and visiting was severely controlled and even discouraged.

Family-centered care is based on a philosophy that recognizes and respects the pivotal role of the family in the lives of both well and ill children. It strives to support families in their natural caregiving roles and promotes healthy patterns of living at home and in the community. Finally, parents and professionals are viewed as equals in a partnership committed to excellence at all levels of health care.

Most health care settings have a family-centered philosophy in which families are given choices, provide input, and are given information that is understandable by them. The family is respected, and its strengths are recognized.

The Association for the Care of Children's Health (ACCH), an interdisciplinary organization, was founded in 1965 to provide a forum for sharing experiences and common problems and to foster growth in children who must undergo hospitalization. Today the organization has broadened its focus on child health care to include the community and the home.

Through the efforts of ACCH and other organizations, increasing attention has been paid to the psychological and emotional effects of hospitalization during childhood. In response to greater knowledge about the emotional effects of illness and hospitalization, hospital policies and health care services for children have changed. Twenty-four-hour parental and sibling visitation policies and home care services have become common. The psychological preparation of children for hospitalization and surgery has become standard nursing practice. Many hospitals have established child life programs to help children and their families cope with the stress of illness. Shorter hospital stays, home care, and day surgery also have helped minimize the emotional effects of hospitalization and illness on children.

CURRENT TRENDS IN CHILD HEALTH CARE

During recent years the government, insurance companies, hospitals, and health care providers have made a concerted effort to reform health care delivery in the United States and to control rising health care costs. This trend has involved a change in where and how money is spent. In the past, most of the health care budget was spent in acute care settings, where the facility charged for services after the services were provided. Because hospitals were paid for whatever materials and services they provided, they had no incentive to be efficient or cost conscious. More recently, the focus has been on health promotion, the provision of care designed to keep people healthy and prevent illness.

In late 2010 the U.S. Department of Health and Human Services (USDHHS) launched *Healthy People 2020*, a comprehensive, nationwide health promotion and disease prevention agenda that builds on groundwork initiated 30 years ago. Developed with input from widely diverse constituencies, *Healthy People 2020* expands on goals and objectives developed for *Healthy People 2010*. While a major focus of *Healthy People 2010* was reducing disparities and increasing access to care, *Healthy People 2020* re-emphasizes that goal and expands it to address "determinants of health," or those factors that contribute to keeping people healthy and achieving high quality of life (USDHHS, 2010b).

Many of the national health objectives in *Healthy People 2020* are applicable to children and families. In fact, among the thirteen new and additional topic areas, two, Adolescent Health and Early and Middle Childhood, are specifically directed to the health of children and adolescents. Benchmarks that will evaluate progress toward achieving the *Healthy People 2020* objectives are called "Foundation Health Measures" and these include general health status, health-related quality of life and well-being, determinants of health, and presence of disparities (USDHHS, 2010b). National data measuring the objectives are gathered from federal and state departments and from voluntary private, nongovernmental organizations.

The focus of nursing care of children has changed as national attention to health promotion and disease prevention has increased. Even acutely ill children have only brief hospital stays because increased technology has facilitated parents' ability to care for children in the home or community setting. Most acute illnesses are managed in ambulatory settings, leaving hospital admission for the extremely acutely ill or children with complex medical needs. Nursing care for hospitalized children has become more specialized, and much nursing care is provided in community settings such as schools and outpatient clinics.

The current practice of child health nursing requires nurses to understand the importance of adapting procedures to the specific needs of children and families and to think critically about children's developmental differences. For example, why do infants and children become so acutely ill so quickly? Is there a smaller margin of safety when administering fluids or medications to children? Other adaptations are directed toward issues such as protecting children, providing for their activity, assessing nonverbal behaviors, planning and carrying out nursing care, and teaching home care to children and families. Table 1-2 presents principles of caring for children.

SELECTED *HEALTHY PEOPLE 2020* OBJECTIVES*

AHS-1	Increase the proportion of persons with health insurance.
AHS-5.2	Increase the proportion of children and youth ages 17 and under who have a specific source of ongoing care.
AH-6	Reduce the proportion of individuals who are unable to obtain or delay in obtaining necessary medical care, dental care, or prescription medicines.
DH-20	Increase the proportion of children with disabilities, birth through age 2 years, who receive early intervention services in home or community-based settings.
EMC-1	Increase the proportion of parents who use positive parenting and communicate with their doctors or other health care professionals about positive parenting.
ECBP-1&2	Increase the proportion of preschool, elementary, middle, and senior high schools that provide comprehensive school health education to prevent health problems in the following areas: unintentional injury; violence; suicide; tobacco use and addiction; alcohol or other drug use; unintended pregnancy, HIV/AIDS, and STD infection; unhealthy dietary patterns; and inadequate physical activity.
ECBP-11	(Developmental) Increase the proportion of local health departments that have established culturally appropriate and linguistically competent community health promotion and disease prevention programs.
EH-8	Reduce blood lead levels in children.
IID-7	Achieve and maintain effective vaccination coverage levels for universally recommended vaccines among young children.
IVP-1	Reduce fatal and nonfatal injuries (includes: motor vehicle crashes, poisoning, falls, suffocation, sports-related, firearm, homicide and self-harm).
IVP-42	Reduce children's exposure to violence.
NWS-10	Reduce the proportion of children and adolescents who are considered obese.
OH-8	Increase the proportion of low-income children and adolescents who received any preventive dental service during the past year.
PA-4	Increase the proportion of the Nation's public and private schools that require daily physical education for all students.

*Abbreviations refer to specific topic areas.

Cost Containment

Recently, the government, insurance companies, hospitals, and health care providers have made a concerted effort to reform health care delivery in the United States and control rising costs. This trend has involved a change in where and how money is spent.

One way in which those paying for health care have attempted to control costs is by shifting to a *prospective* form of payment. In this arrangement clients no longer pay whatever charges the hospital decides on for service provided. Instead, a fixed amount of money is agreed to in advance for necessary services for specifically diagnosed conditions. Any of several strategies have been used to contain the cost of services.

Diagnosis-Related Groups

Diagnosis-related groups (DRGs) are a method of classifying related medical diagnoses based on the amount of resources that are generally required by the client. This method became a standard in 1987, when

TABLE 1-2   NURSING OF CHILDREN: PRINCIPLES OF CARE

PRINCIPLE	DESCRIPTION
Growth and development	The nurse applies growth and development principles to meet the child's physical and emotional needs. Involves understanding the principles of maturation, physiologic immaturity, and response to illness. Nursing care is tailored to the child's chronologic age and developmental level.
Health promotion	Guides the child and family toward independent responsibility for health. Anticipatory guidance is education that facilitates health promotion by providing developmentally appropriate information about nutrition, exercise, safety, play, and wellness issues such as immunizations and injury prevention.
Family focus	Family-centered care is at the core of nursing of children because of the intimate relationship between the child and family in areas of support, love, security, values, beliefs, attitudes, and health practices. Because the family is a partner in the child's care, the nurse provides information for appropriate decision making, assesses family needs, and refers the family to appropriate resources within the community.
Child advocacy	Includes specific responsibilities as child advocates in the areas of health promotion, violence, abuse, neglect, drug abuse, infant morbidity and mortality, and access to care. Nurses exercise legal and ethical responsibilities cautiously, being aware of their accountability.
Communication	Nurses use a variety of techniques to communicate with children and families in a developmentally appropriate manner. Includes use of play and other developmentally appropriate verbal and nonverbal communication techniques for effective communication.
Concepts applied across age groups	Integration of the principles of pediatric nursing care across many disorders and with all age-groups. Recognizes that with any health encounter, children may have needs related to play and activity, chronicity, nutrition, safety, illness, and family. Knowing pathophysiologic human development, family theory, and evidence-based principles enhances nursing care.

the federal government set the amount of money that would be paid by Medicare for each DRG. If the facility delivers more services or has greater costs than what it will be reimbursed for by Medicare, the facility must absorb the excess costs. Conversely, if the facility delivers the care at less cost than the payment for that DRG, the facility keeps the remaining money. Health care facilities working under this arrangement benefit financially if they can reduce the client's length of stay and thereby reduce the costs for service. Although the DRG system originally applied only to Medicare clients, most states have adopted the system for Medicaid payments, and most insurance companies use a similar system.

Managed Care

Health insurance companies also examined the cost of health care and instituted a health care delivery system that has been called *managed care*. Examples of managed care organizations are health maintenance organizations (HMOs), point of service plans (POSs), and preferred provider organizations (PPOs). HMOs provide relatively comprehensive health services for people enrolled in the organization for a set fee or premium. Similarly, PPOs are groups of health care providers who agree to provide health services to a specific group of clients at a discounted cost. When the client needs medical treatment, managed care includes strategies such as payment arrangements and preadmission or pretreatment authorization to control costs.

Managed care, provided appropriately, can increase access to a full range of health care providers and services for children, but it must be closely monitored. Nurses serve as advocates in the areas of preventive, acute, and chronic care for children. The teaching time lines for preventive and home care have been shortened drastically, and the call to "begin teaching the moment the child enters the health care system" has taken on a new meaning. Parents, the child, and other caregivers are being asked to do procedures at home that were once done by professionals in a hospital setting. Systems must be in place to monitor adherence, understanding, and the total care of a child. Assessment and communication skills need to be keen, and the nurse must be able to work with specialists in other disciplines.

Capitated Care

Capitation may be incorporated into any type of managed care plan. In a pure capitated care plan, the employer (or government) pays a set amount of money each year to a network of primary care providers. This amount might be adjusted for age and sex of the client group. In exchange for access to a guaranteed client base, the primary care providers agree to provide general health care and to pay for all aspects of the client's care, including laboratory work, specialist visits, and hospital care.

Capitated plans are of interest to employers as well as the government because they allow a predictable amount of money to be budgeted for health care. Clients do not have unexpected financial burdens from illness. However, clients lose most of their freedom of choice regarding who will provide their care. Providers can lose money (1) if they refer too many clients to specialists, who may have no restrictions on their fees, (2) if they order too many diagnostic tests, or (3) if their administrative costs are too high. Some health care providers and consumers fear that cost constraints might affect treatment decisions.

Effects of Cost Containment

Prospective payment plans have had major effects on infant care, primarily in relation to the length of stay. Mothers who have a normal vaginal birth are typically discharged from the hospital at 48 hours after birth and 96 hours for cesarean births, unless the woman and her health care provider choose an earlier discharge time. This leaves little time for nurses to adequately teach new parents newborn care and to assess infants for subtle health issues. Nurses find providing adequate information about infant care is especially difficult when the mother is still recovering from childbirth. Problems with earlier discharge of mother and infant often require readmission and more expensive treatment than might have been needed if the problem had been identified early.

Another concern in regard to cost containment is that some children with chronic health conditions have been denied care or denied insurance coverage because of pre-existing conditions. Denying care can exacerbate a child's condition, resulting in greater cost for the health care system, not to mention greater emotional cost for the child and family.

Despite efforts to contain costs related to the provision of health care in the United States, the percentage of the total government expenditures for services (Gross Domestic Product) allocated to health care was 17.6% in 2009, markedly higher than many similar developed countries (Centers for Medicare and Medicaid, 2011; Kaiser Family Foundation, 2011). This percentage has nearly doubled since 1980 and, without true health care reform, is expected to continue to increase.

In March, 2010, the *Patient Protection and Affordable Care Act* was signed into law. Designed to reign in health care costs while increasing access to the underserved, provisions of this law are to be phased in over the course of four years (USDHHS, 2011b). In general improved access will occur through access to affordable insurance coverage for all citizens. Persons who do not have access to insurance coverage through employer provided insurance plans will be able to purchase insurance through an insurance exchange, which will offer a variety of coverage options at competitive rates (USDHHS, 2011b). Several of the provisions of this law specifically address the needs of children and families. They include the following (USDHHS, 2011b):

- Prohibiting insurance companies from denying care based on pre-existing conditions for children younger than 19 years old.
- Keeping young adults on their family's health insurance plan until age 26 years.
- Coordinated management for children and other individuals with chronic diseases.
- Expanding the number of community health centers
- Increasing access to preventive health care.
- Providing for home visits to pregnant women and newborns.
- Supporting states to expand Medicaid coverage.
- Providing additional funding for the Children's Health Insurance Program (CHIP).

An additional provision of the *Affordable Care Act* is the creation of Accountable Care Organizations (ACO). These are groups of hospitals, physicians' offices, community agencies and any agency that provides health care to patients. Enhancing patient-centered care, the ACO collaborates on all aspects of coordination, safety, and quality for individuals within the organization. The ACO will reduce duplication of services, decrease fragmentation of care, and give more control to patients and families (USDHHS, 2011a).

Cost containment measures have also altered traditional ways of providing patient-centered care. There is an increased focus on ensuring quality and safety through such approaches as case management, use of clinical practice guidelines and evidence-based nursing care, and outcomes management.

Case Management

Case management is a practice model that uses a systematic approach to identify specific clients, determine eligibility for care, arrange access to appropriate resources and services, and provide continuity of care through a collaborative model (Lyon & Grow, 2011). In this model, a case manager or case coordinator, who focuses on both quality and cost outcomes, coordinates the services needed by the client and family. Inherent to case management is the coordination of care by all members of the health care team. The guidelines established in 1995 by the Joint Commission require an interdisciplinary, collaborative approach to patient care. This concept is at the core of case management. Nurses who provide case management evaluate patient and family needs, establish needs documentation to support reimbursement, and may be part of long-term care planning in the home or a rehabilitation facility.

Evidence-Based Nursing Care

The Agency for Healthcare Research and Quality (AHRQ), a branch of the U.S. Public Health Service, actively sponsors research in health issues facing children. From research generated through this agency as well as others, evidence can be accumulated to guide the best clinical practices. Focus of research from AHRQ is primarily on access to care for children and adolescents. This includes such topics as: timeliness of care (care is provided as soon as necessary), patient-centeredness (quality of communication with providers), coordination of care for children with chronic illnesses, access to a medical home, and safe medication delivery systems (AHRQ, 2011). Effectiveness of health care also is a priority for research funding; this focus area includes immunizations, preventive vision care, preventive dental care, weight monitoring, and mental health and substance abuse monitoring (AHRQ, 2011). Clinical practice guidelines are an important tool in developing parameters for safe, effective, and evidence-based care for children and families. AHRQ has developed several guidelines related to adult and child care, as have other organizations and professional groups concerned with children's health. Important children's health issues, which include quality and safety improvements, enhanced primary care, access to quality care, and specific illnesses, are addressed in available practice guidelines. For detailed information see the website at www.ahcpr.gov or www.guidelines.gov.

The Institute of Medicine (IOM) (2011) has published standards for developing practice guidelines to maximize the consistency within and among guidelines, regardless of guideline developers. The IOM recommends inclusion of important information and process steps in every guideline. This includes ensuring diversity of members of a clinical guideline group; full disclosure of conflict of interest; in-depth systematic reviews to inform recommendations; providing a rationale, quality of evidence, and strength of recommendation for each recommendation made by the guideline committee; and external review of recommendations for validity (IOM). Standardization of clinical practice guidelines will strengthen evidence-based care, especially for guidelines developed by nurses or professional nursing organizations.

Outcomes Management

The determination to lower health care costs while maintaining the quality of care has led to a clinical practice model called *outcomes management*. This is a systematic method to identify outcomes and to focus care on interventions that will accomplish the stated outcomes for children with specific issues, such as the child with asthma.

Nurse Sensitive Indicators. In response to recent efforts to address both quality and safety issues in health care, various government and privately funded groups have sponsored research to identify patient care outcomes that are particularly dependent on the quality and quantity of nursing care provided. These outcomes, called *nurse sensitive indicators,* are based on empirical data collected by such organizations as the AHRQ and the National Quality Forum (NQF), and represent outcomes that improve with optimal nursing care (American Nurses' Association [ANA], 2011; Lacey, Smith, & Cox, 2008). The following are in the process of development and delineation for pediatric nurses: adequate pain assessment, peripheral intravenous infiltration, pressure ulcer, catheter-related bloodstream infection, smoking cessation for adolescents, and obesity (ANA, 2011; Lacey, Smith, & Cox, 2008). Nurses need to use evidence-based intervention to improve these patient outcomes.

Variances. Deviations, or *variances,* may occur in either the time line or in the expected outcomes. A variance is the difference between what was expected and what actually happened. A variance may be positive or negative. A positive variance occurs when a child progresses faster than expected and is discharged sooner than planned. A negative variance occurs when progress is slower than expected, outcomes are not met within the designated time frame, and the length of stay is prolonged.

Clinical Pathways. One planning tool used by the health care team to identify and meet stated outcomes is the *clinical pathway*. Other names for clinical pathways include *critical* or *clinical paths, care paths, care maps, collaborative plans of care, anticipated recovery paths,* and *multidisciplinary action plans.* Clinical pathways are standardized, interdisciplinary plans of care devised for clients with a particular health problem. The purpose, as in managed care and case management, is to provide quality care while controlling costs. Clinical pathways identify client outcomes, specify time lines to achieve those outcomes, direct appropriate interventions and sequencing of interventions, include interventions from a variety of disciplines, promote collaboration, and involve a comprehensive approach to care. Home health agencies use clinical pathways, which may be developed in collaboration with hospital staff.

Clinical pathways may be used in various ways. For instance, they may be used for change of shift reports to indicate information about length of stay, individual needs, and priorities of the shift for each child. They also may be used for documentation of the child's nursing care plan and his or her progress in meeting the desired outcomes. Many pathways are particularly helpful in identifying families that need follow-up care.

Students' Use of Clinical Pathways. Clinical pathways are guidelines for care. Although a pathway provides insight into the scheduling of assessments and care, it is not meant to teach nursing skills and procedures. One purpose of this text is to provide ample information so that students can use clinical pathways in a clinical setting. This involves teaching *why* and *how* to perform assessments and to interpret the significance of the data obtained. Moreover, the text emphasizes ways of providing information, care, and comfort for children and their families as they progress along a clinical pathway.

HOME CARE

Home nursing care has experienced dramatic growth since 1990. Advances in portable and wireless technology, such as infusion pumps for administering intravenous nutrition or subcutaneous medications and various monitoring devices, such as telemonitors, allow nurses, and often clients or family, to perform procedures and maintain equipment in the home. Consumers often prefer home care because of decreased stress on the family when the child is able to remain at home rather than be separated from the family support system because of the need for hospitalization. Optimal home care also can reduce re-admission to the hospital for children with chronic conditions.

Home care services may be provided in the form of telephone calls, home visits, information lines, and lactation consultations, among others. Online and wireless technology allows nurses to evaluate data transmitted from home. Infants with congenital anomalies, such as cleft palate, may need care that is adapted to their condition. Moreover, increasing numbers of technology-dependent infants and children are now cared for at home. The numbers include those needing ventilator assistance, total parenteral nutrition, intravenous medications, apnea monitoring, and other device-associated nursing care.

Nurses must be able to function independently within established protocols and must be confident of their clinical skills when providing home care. They should be proficient at interviewing, counseling, and teaching. They often assume a leadership role in coordinating all the services a family may require, and they frequently supervise the work of other care providers.

COMMUNITY CARE

A model for community care of children is the school-based health center. School-based health centers provide comprehensive primary health care services in the most accessible environment. Students can be evaluated, diagnosed, and treated on site. Services offered include primary preventive care, including health assessments, anticipatory guidance, vision and hearing screenings, and immunizations; acute care; prescription services; and mental health and counseling services. Some school-based health centers are sponsored by hospitals, local health departments, and community health centers. Many are used in off hours to provide health care to uninsured adults and adolescents.

The role of the school nurse as a care provider has expanded rapidly and school nurses are considered to be primary care providers who function as a "safety net" for children (Robert Wood Johnson Foundation, 2010). In addition to the health promotion activities described previously, school nurses provide complex nursing care to children with chronic conditions or disabilities, manage life-threatening and traumatic events, assist families to access resources, and address students' health and illness concerns (Robert Wood Johnson Foundation, 2010).

Access to Care

Access to care is an important component when evaluating preventive care and prompt treatment of illness and injuries. Access to health care is strongly associated with having health insurance. The American Academy of Pediatrics (2010) has issued a policy statement that states, "All children must have access to affordable and comprehensive quality care" (p. 1018). This care should be ensured through access to comprehensive health insurance that can be carried to wherever the child and family reside, provide continuous coverage, and allow for free choice of health providers (AAP, 2010).

Having health insurance coverage, usually employer sponsored, often determines whether a person will seek care early in the course of an illness. However, greater restrictions on private insurance are blurring the distinction between private and public health coverage. Many private health plans have restrictions such as prequalifications for procedures, drugs that the plan covers, and services that are covered. People with employer-sponsored health insurance often find that they must change providers each year because the available plans change, a situation that may negatively affect the provider-client relationship. As the *Affordable Care Act* is phased in over the next few years, these issues may be resolved.

Public Health Insurance Programs

Despite improvements in federal and state programs that address children's health needs, the number of uninsured children in the United States was 7.5 million in 2009 (most recent figure reported); this represents 10% of children younger than age 18 years (DeNavas-Walt, Proctor & Smith, 2010) (Figure 1-1). Health insurance coverage varies among children by poverty, age, race, and ethnic origin (DeNavas-Walt, Proctor & Smith, 2010). The proportion of children with health insurance is lowest among Hispanic children compared with white children and lower among poor, near-poor, and middle-income children compared with high-income children (Forum on Child and Family Statistics, 2011). Nearly 23% of children in the United States are underinsured, meaning that their resources are not sufficient to meet their health care needs (Health Resources and Services Administration [HRSA], 2010a).

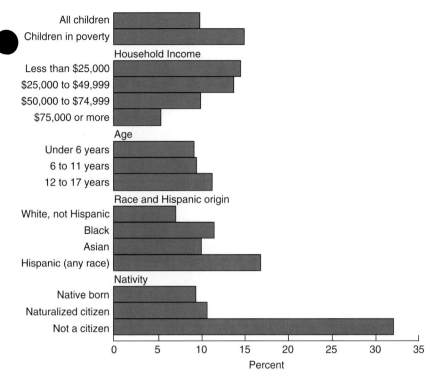

FIG 1-1 Uninsured Children by Poverty Status, Household Income, Age, Race and Hispanic Origin, and Nativity, 2009. Federal surveys now give respondents the option of reporting more than one race. This figure shows data using the race-alone concept (e.g., *Asian* refers to people who reported Asian and no other race). (From DeNavas-Walt, C., Proctor, B.D., Smith, J.C., U.S. Census Bureau. [2010]. *Current population reports: Income, poverty, and health insurance coverage in the United States: 2009*, P60-238, Washington, DC: U.S. Government Printing Office.)

Children in poor and near-poor families are more likely to be uninsured (15.1%) (DeNavas-Walt, Proctor & Smith, 2010), have unmet medical needs, receive delayed medical care, have no usual provider of health care, and have higher rates of emergency room service than children in families that are not poor. Greater than 6% of all children have no usual place of health care (Forum on Child and Family Statistics, 2011).

Public health insurance for children is provided primarily through Medicaid, a federal program that provides health care for certain populations of people living in poverty, or the Children's Health Insurance Program (formerly the State Children's health Insurance Program), a program that provides access for children not poor enough to be eligible for Medicaid but whose household income is less than 200% of poverty level. In 2009, funding was renewed for CHIP through the Children's Health Insurance Program Reauthorization Act (CHIPRA); since that time, the number of children insured by Medicaid and CHIP increased by 2.6 million (USDHHS, 2010a).

Medicaid covered 34.5% of children younger than age 18 years in 2009 (National Center for Health Statistics [NCHS], 2011). Medicaid provides health care for the poor, aged, and disabled, with pregnant women and young children especially targeted. Medicaid is funded by both the federal government and individual state governments. The states administer the program and determine which services are offered. In 2014, a provision of the Affordable Care Act will alter the income requirements for acceptance to Medicaid so that the number of eligible children will be increased (USDHHS, 2011a).

Medicaid can be frustrating for a family. The application process often takes weeks and needs to be renewed regularly with supporting documentation. The family must fill out lengthy, complicated forms, provide documentation of citizenship and income, and then wait for determination of eligibility. Medicaid criteria may deny payment for some services that are routinely provided to those who hold private insurance. There are several barriers to children becoming enrolled and staying in public health insurance programs. These include children losing and regaining eligibility on a regular basis, changes in eligibility requirements, changes in family status, and the complexity of the enrollment process itself (HRSA, 2010b). One proposed approach is to provide continuity of information management using health information technology, with online source of information, online application, and maintaining an accessible database to verify eligibility (HRSA, 2010b).

Preventive Health

Oral health of children in the United States has become a topic of increasing focus. Services available through Medicaid are limited, and many dentists do not accept children who are insured by Medicaid. Racial and ethnic disparities exist in this area of health, with a high percentage of non-Hispanic Black school-age children and Mexican-American children having untreated dental caries as compared to non-Hispanic white children (Forum on Child and Family Statistics, 2011). In addition, maternal periodontal disease is emerging as a contributing factor to prematurity, with its adverse effects on the child's long-term health.

Besides the obvious implication of not having health insurance—the inability to pay for health care during illness—another important effect on children who are not insured exists: They are less likely to receive preventive care such as immunizations and dental care. This places them at increased risk for preventable illnesses and, because preventive health care is a learned behavior, these children are more likely to become adults who are less healthy.

Health Care Assistance Programs

Many programs, some funded privately, others by the government, assist in the care of infants and children. The WIC program, which was established in 1972, provides supplemental food supplies to low-income women who are pregnant or breastfeeding and to their children up to the age of 5 years. WIC has long been heralded as a cost-effective program that not only provides nutritional support but also links families with other services, such as prenatal care and immunizations.

Medicaid's Early and Periodic Screening, Diagnosis, and Treatment program was developed to provide comprehensive health care to Medicaid recipients from birth to 21 years of age. The goal of the program is to prevent health problems before they become severe. This program pays for well-child examinations and for the treatment of any medical problems diagnosed during such checkups.

Public Law 99-457 is part of the Individuals with Disabilities Education Act (IDEA) that provides financial incentives to states to establish comprehensive early intervention services for infants and toddlers with or at risk for developmental disabilities. Services include screening, identification, referral, and treatment. Although this is a federal law and entitlement, each state bases coverage on its own definition of developmental delay. Thus coverage may vary from state to state. Some states provide care for at-risk children.

The Healthy Start program, begun in 1991, is a major initiative to reduce infant deaths in communities with disproportionately high infant mortality rates. Strategies used include reducing the number of high-risk pregnancies, reducing the number of low-birth-weight and preterm births, improving birth-weight–specific survival, and reducing specific causes of postneonatal mortality.

The March of Dimes, long an advocate for improving the health of infants and children, has been conducting a *Prematurity Campaign.* Designed to reduce the devastating toll that prematurity takes on the population, the campaign emphasizes education, research and advocacy. Since 1981, the incidence of prematurity increased 30%, often resulting in permanent health or developmental problems for survivors of early birth. Currently, one in every eight newborns (12.5%) in the United States is born prematurely (March of Dimes, 2011).

STATISTICS ON INFANT AND CHILD HEALTH

Statistics are important sources of information about the health of groups of people. The newest statistics about infant and child health for the United States can be obtained from the National Center for Health Statistics (www.cdc.gov/nchs).

Mortality

Throughout history, infants have had high death rates, especially shortly after birth. Infant mortality rates began to fall when the health of the general population improved, basic principles of sanitation were put into practice, and medical knowledge increased. A further large decrease was a result of the widespread availability of antibiotics, improvements in public health, and better prenatal care in the 1940s and 1950s. Today the infant mortality rate is falling, although the rate of change has slowed. Racial inequality of infant mortality continues, with nonwhite groups having higher mortality rates than white groups.

Infant Mortality

Between 1950 and 1990, the infant mortality rate (death before the age of 1 year) dropped from 29.2 to 9.2 deaths per 1000 live births. Currently, the infant mortality rate is 6.8, which has been relatively stable the past several years (NCHS, 2011) (Figure 1-2). The fall in infant mortality is attributed to the mother's health, increased availability of resources, socioeconomic status, and various public service campaigns. The *Back to Sleep* campaign, for example, has contributed to a reduction of more than 50% in the number of deaths attributed to sudden infant death syndrome in the United States since 1980 (NCHS, 2011).

Racial Disparity for Mortality. Although infant mortality rates in the United States have declined overall, they have declined faster for whites than for non-Hispanic black infants. The mortality rate in 2007 for white infants was 5.6. For black infants the rate was 13.2 (NCHS,

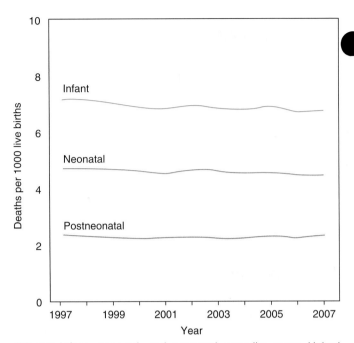

FIG 1-2 Infant, neonatal, and postnatal mortality rates: United States, 1997–2007. (From National Center for Health Statistics. [2011]. *Health, United States, 2010: With Special Feature on Death and Dying,* Hyattsville, MD: U.S. DHHS.)

2011). Much of the racial disparity for infant mortality is attributable to prematurity (born before 37 weeks) and low birth weight (less than 2500 g), both more common among African-American infants. Premature and low-birth-weight infants have a greater risk for short-term and long-term health problems as well as death (March of Dimes, 2011).

Poverty is an important factor. Proportionally more nonwhites than whites are poor in the United States. Poor people are less likely to be in good health, to be well nourished, or to get the health care they need. Obtaining care becomes vital during pregnancy and infancy, and lack of care is reflected in the high mortality rates in all categories.

International Infant Mortality. One would expect that a nation such as the United States would have one of the lowest infant mortality rates when compared with other developed countries. The most recent year for which comparative international data on infant mortality are available is 2006. (Table 1-3) (NCHS, 2011). The estimate of the United States' ranking worldwide is 46th of 223 countries reporting (Central Intelligence Agency, 2011). International rankings are difficult to compare because countries differ in how and when they compute statistics, but the numbers show the need for improvement in the United States. One of the major reasons for the poor U.S. showing is the large racial disparity as described previously (NCHS, 2011).

Childhood Mortality

Death rates for children have significantly declined over the past 20 years. Table 1-4 shows the leading causes of death in children. Although death rates attributed to unintentional injury also have dropped, they are still the leading cause of death in children aged 1 to 19 years. Motor vehicle crashes lead the causes of death from unintentional injury, followed by drowning, fire-related injury, and death by firearm (Forum on Child and Family Statistics, 2011). Homicide has become the third leading cause of death in children ages 1 to 4 years and is the fourth leading cause of death for children 5 to 14 years; homicide remains the

TABLE 1-3	INFANT* MORTALITY RATES FOR SELECTED COUNTRIES (BASED ON 2006 DATA—MOST RECENT COMPLETE DATASET)
Iceland	1.4
Luxembourg	2.5
Japan	2.6
Sweden, Finland	2.8
Norway	3.2
Czech Republic, Portugal	3.3
Austria	3.6
Greece, Ireland, Italy	3.7
Denmark, France, Germany, Spain	3.8
Belgium	4.0
Netherlands, Switzerland	4.4
Australia	4.7
Canada, United Kingdom	5.0
New Zealand	5.2
Hungary	5.7
Poland	6.0
Slovak Republic	6.6
United States	6.7

From National Center for Health Statistics: *Health, United States, 2010: With Special Feature on Death and Dying,* Hyattsville, MD, 2011. Data from The Organisation for Economic Co-operation and Development (OECD) Health Data 2009, incorporating revisions to the annual update. Available from: www.ecosante.org/oecd.htm.
*Under 1 year of age.

TABLE 1-4	LEADING CAUSES OF DEATH AMONG CHILDREN AGES 1 TO 14 YEARS	
		DEATH RATE PER 100,000
Ages 1 to 4 Years		
Unintentional injury		8.5
Congenital malformations		2.8
Homicide		2.3
Cancer		2.0
Heart disease		0.9
Ages 5 to 14 Years		
Unintentional injury		4.1
Cancer		2.2
Congenital malformations		0.9
Homicide		0.8
Heart disease		0.5

From Forum on Child and Family Statistics. (2011). Child injury and mortality: Death rates among children ages 1-14 by gender, race, and Hispanic origin and all causes and all injury causes 1980–2009. In *America's Children: Key National Indicators of Wellbeing 2011.* Retrieved from www.childstats.gov.

second leading cause of death for older adolescents, followed by suicide (NCHS, 2011). Other common causes of death in children include congenital malformations, cancer, and cardiac and respiratory diseases. Self-inflicted injury is a leading cause of death in the adolescent population (Forum on Child and Family Statistics, 2011).

Morbidity

Morbidity describes illness. The morbidity rate is the ratio of sick to well people in a population and is presented as the number of ill people per 1000 population. This term is used in reference to acute and chronic illness as well as disability. Because morbidity statistics are collected and updated less frequently than mortality statistics, presentation of current data in all areas of child health is difficult.

Diseases of the respiratory system, which include bronchitis or bronchiolitis, asthma, and pneumonia, are a major cause of hospitalization for children younger than 18 years (NCHS, 2011). A reported 10% of children in the United States currently have asthma; approximately 5% of these report having one or more acute episodes during the previous year (Forum on Child and Family Statistics, 2011). Other health problems of significant concern include: obesity (19%), activity limitations related to chronic disease (9%), depression (8%), and emotional or behavioral difficulties (5%) (Forum on Child and Family Statistics, 2011). Dental decay is one of the most preventable of chronic diseases in children, yet between 25% and 50% of children in the United States suffer from tooth decay. The prevalence of decay is higher for children living in poverty and those from some racial and ethnic groups (Centers for Disease Control and Prevention [CDC], National Center for Chronic Disease Prevention and Health Promotion, 2011). Statistics regarding morbidity related to particular disorders are presented throughout this text as the disorders are discussed.

The Youth Risk Behavior Surveillance System conducts a national survey of students in grades 9 to 12 every 2 years on the odd year. The CDC (2011) has identified categories of health risk behaviors among youth that contribute to increased morbidity rates: tobacco use; unhealthy dietary behaviors; inadequate physical activity; alcohol and other drug use; sexual risk behaviors and behaviors that result in intentional injuries (violence, suicide) and unintentional injuries (motor vehicle crashes). The YRBSS also monitors obesity and asthma in adolescents.

A link exists between children living in poverty and poorer health outcomes. Children who live in families of higher income and higher education have a better chance of being born healthy and remaining healthy. Access to health care, the health behaviors of parents and siblings, and exposure to environmental risks are among the factors contributing to the disparity in children's health (Forum on Child and Family Statistics, 2011; NCHS, 2011).

Adolescent Births

Adolescent birth rates in the United States decreased markedly over the past 20 years, although they have increased slightly since 2006 in adolescents aged 15 to 19 years old. The current birth rate for adolescent mothers is 42.5 per 1000. In adolescents ages 10 to 14 years, the rate is significantly lower at 0.6 per 1000. The adolescent birth rate is lowest in the Asian/Pacific Islander group and highest in black Hispanic girls (HRSA, 2009).

ETHICAL PERSPECTIVES IN CHILD HEALTH NURSING

Nurses who care for children often struggle with ethical and social dilemmas that affect families. Nurses must know how to approach these issues in a knowledgeable and systematic way.

Ethics and Bioethics

Ethics involves determining the best course of action in a certain situation. Ethical reasoning is the analysis of what is morally right and reasonable. Bioethics is the application of ethics to health care. Ethical

---

BOX 1-1   ANA CODE FOR NURSES

The nurse, in all professional relationships, practices with compassion and respect for the inherent dignity, worth and uniqueness of every individual, unrestricted by considerations of social or economic status, personal attributes, or the nature of health problems.

The nurse's primary commitment is to the patient, whether an individual, family, group, or community.

The nurse promotes, advocates for, and strives to protect the health, safety, and rights of the patient.

The nurse is responsible and accountable for individual nursing practice and determines the appropriate delegation of tasks consistent with the nurse's obligation to provide optimum patient care.

The nurse owes the same duties to self as to others, including the responsibility to preserve integrity and safety, to maintain competence, and to continue personal and professional growth.

The nurse participates in establishing, maintaining, and improving health care environments and conditions of employment conducive to the provision of quality health care and consistent with the values of the profession through individual and collective action.

The nurse participates in the advancement of the profession through contributions to practice, education, administration, and knowledge development.

The nurse collaborates with other health professionals and the public in promoting community, national, and international efforts to meet health needs.

The profession of nursing, as represented by associations and their members, is responsible for articulating nursing values, for maintaining the integrity of the profession and its practice, and for shaping social policy.

Reprinted from American Nurses Association. (2001). *Code for nurses with interpretive statements*. Washington, DC: Author.

---

behavior for nurses is discussed in various codes, such as the American Nurses Association Code for Nurses (Box 1-1). Ethical issues have become more complex as developing technology has allowed more options in health care. These issues are controversial because there is lack of agreement over what is right or best and because moral support is possible for more than one course of action.

Ethical Dilemmas

An ethical dilemma is a situation in which no solution seems completely satisfactory. Opposing courses of action may seem equally desirable, or all possible solutions may seem undesirable. Ethical dilemmas are among the most difficult situations in nursing practice. Finding solutions involves applying ethical theories and principles and determining the burdens and benefits of any course of action.

Ethical Principles

Ethical principles are important in solving ethical dilemmas. Four of the most important principles are beneficence, nonmaleficence, autonomy, and justice (Box 1-2). Although principles guide decision making, in some situations it may be impossible to apply one principle without encountering conflict with another. In such cases, one principle may outweigh another in importance.

For example, treatments designed to do good may also cause some harm. A child who undergoes chemotherapy may see improvement or disappearance of the cancer. However, the chemotherapy that cures the cancer can harm other body organs. In this instance the caregiver and parent need to weigh the principle of beneficence against the principle of nonmaleficence.

BOX 1-2   ETHICAL PRINCIPLES

- *Beneficence.* One is required to do or promote good for others.
- *Nonmaleficence.* One must avoid risking or causing harm to others.
- *Autonomy.* People have the right to self-determination. This includes the right to respect, privacy, and the information necessary to make decisions.
- *Justice.* All people should be treated equally and fairly regardless of disease or social or economic status.

Solving Ethical Dilemmas

Although using a specific approach does not guarantee a right decision, it provides a logical, systematic method for going through the steps of decision making.

Decision making in ethical dilemmas may seem straightforward, but it may not result in answers agreeable to everyone. Many agencies therefore have bioethics committees to formulate policies for ethical situations, provide education, and help make decisions in specific cases. The committees include a variety of professionals such as nurses, physicians, social workers, ethicists, and clergy members. The child and family also participate, if possible. A satisfactory solution to ethical dilemmas is more likely to occur when a variety of people work together.

Ethical dilemmas also may have legal ramifications, so nurses must consider both ethical principles and what is legal in their field and place of practice.

Ethical Concerns in Child Health Nursing

Ethical concerns can arise in many areas of child health care. For example, disclosure of HIV status to HIV positive children who are entering middle school is an issue that brings up ethical differences between pediatric providers and parents (see Chapter 18). Two important areas are cessation of treatment and terminating life support.

Cessation of Treatment

The decision to cease treatment is an ethical situation that is always difficult and seems to be compounded when the client is an infant or child. Children who would have died in the past can now have their lives extended through the use of life support. Parents must be involved in the decision-making process immediately and informed about available options. Laws in some states permit parents to provide advance directives for their minor children. When older children are involved, their views are considered.

In this age of resource allocation, debate centers on how to manage critical care resources. Many believe that these decisions should not be made at the bedside. The American Academy of Pediatrics, in its statement *Ethics and the Care of Critically Ill Infants and Children* (1996), encouraged society to engage in a thorough debate about the economic, cultural, religious, social, and moral consequences of imposing limits on which clients should receive intensive care.

Terminating Life Support

Decisions to terminate life-support systems continue to present gut-wrenching ethical and legal situations to nurses, especially when an infant or child is involved. Contrary to the common belief that such decisions should be determined by what is termed *quality of life,* the legal system plays a major role in this area of health care.

Frequently parents become attached to a primary care nurse and request that the nurse participate in the decision as to whether to terminate life support for their child. A nurse might be faced with such a situation in the neonatal intensive care unit (NICU) with a teenage parent of a premature infant with a congenital defect or in a chronic care oncology unit with a terminally ill child.

In such instances a team conference should be arranged with the parent, primary nurse, physician, and a hospital staff attorney who is knowledgeable about applicable laws in that particular state. Problems may arise when there is a discrepancy among what families, physicians, and nurses think is best.

The issue of when first to discuss with adolescents the idea of cardiopulmonary resuscitation, mechanical ventilation, and do-not-resuscitate (DNR) orders is always sensitive. Adolescents who have reached majority age must give consent if they are of sound mind. In most states, minority status ends at the age of 18 years.

LEGAL ISSUES

The legal foundation for the practice of nursing provides safeguards for health care and sets standards by which nurses can be evaluated. Nurses need to understand how the law applies specifically to them. When nurses do not meet the standards expected, they may be held legally accountable.

Safeguards for Health Care

Three categories of safeguards determine how the law views nursing practice: (1) state nurse practice acts, (2) standards of care set by professional organizations, and (3) rules and policies set by the institution employing the nurse. Additional information about nursing responsibilities is presented later in this chapter.

Nurse Practice Acts

Every state has a **nurse practice act** that determines the scope of practice for registered nurses in that state. Nurse practice acts define what the nurse is and is not allowed to do in caring for clients. Some parts of the law may be very specific, whereas others are stated broadly enough to permit flexibility in the role of nurses. Nurse practice acts vary from state to state, and nurses must be knowledgeable about these laws wherever they practice.

In 1998 the National Council of State Boards of Nursing initiated a nurse licensure compact program. A nurse licensure compact allows a nurse who is licensed in one state to practice nursing in another participating state without having to be licensed in that state. Nurses must comply with the practice regulations in the state in which they practice. Since 1998, 24 states have become participants in the nurse licensure compact program (National Council of State Boards of Nursing, 2011). To learn current status, visit www.ncsbn.org.

Laws relating to nursing practice also delineate methods, called *standard procedures* or *protocols*, by which nurses may assume certain duties commonly considered part of health care practice. The procedures are written by committees of nurses, physicians, and administrators. They specify the nursing qualifications required for practicing the procedures, define the appropriate situations, and list the education required. Standard procedures allow for changing the role of the nurse to meet the needs of the community and to reflect expanding knowledge.

Standards of Care

Courts have generally held that nurses must practice according to established standards and health agency policies, although these standards and policies do not have the force of law. **Standards of care** are set by professional associations and describe the level of care that can be expected from practitioners. The Society of Pediatric Nurses is the primary specialty organization that sets standards for pediatric nurses (www.pedsnurses.org).

Other regulatory bodies, such as the U.S. Occupational Safety and Health Administration (OSHA), the U.S. Food and Drug Administration (FDA), and the Centers for Disease Control and Prevention (CDC), also provide guidelines for practice. Accrediting agencies, such as The Joint Commission and the Community Health Accreditation Program, give their approval after visiting facilities and observing whether standards are being met in practice. Governmental programs such as Medicare, Medicaid, and state health departments require that their standards be met for the facility to receive reimbursement for services.

Agency Policies

Each health care facility sets specific policies, procedures, and protocols that govern nursing care. All nurses should be familiar with those that apply in the facilities in which they work. Nurses are involved in writing evidence-based nursing policies and procedures that apply to their practice and in reviewing or revising them regularly.

Accountability

Nursing accountability involves knowing current laws. Accountability in child health nursing requires special consideration because the nurse must be accountable to the family as well as the child. For example, the Individuals with Disabilities Education Act (PL 94-142), which mandates free and appropriate education for all children with disabilities, provides for school nurses to be part of a team that develops an individual education plan for each child who is eligible for services. In school districts that are reluctant to involve the school nurse as part of the team, nurses may need to advocate for services for the child and family.

Federal as well as state legislative bodies have addressed the issue of child abuse. Considerable variation exists among state laws in the investigative authority and procedures granted to child protective workers. When child abuse is suspected, issues often arise as to whether a health care provider may investigate the home situation and obtain relevant records.

A recent issue pertaining to nursing accountability is inadequate hospital staffing as a result of budget cuts. A nurse has a duty to communicate concerns about staffing levels immediately through established channels. A nurse will not be excused from responsibility (e.g., late medication administration or injury resulting from inadequate supervision of a client), just as a hospital will not be excused for insufficient staffing because of budget cuts.

Accountability also involves competency. If a nurse is not competent to perform a nursing task (e.g., to administer a new chemotherapeutic drug), or if a patient's status worsens to the point at which the care needs are beyond the nurse's competency level (e.g., a child requiring hemodynamic monitoring), the nurse must immediately communicate this fact to the nursing supervisor or physician. The fact that a patient's transfer to the intensive care unit (ICU) was requested but denied because the ICU was at full capacity is an insufficient defense in a charge of nursing negligence. In addition, the fact that a call was placed to a physician but there was no return call is no excuse for harm caused to a child because of delayed treatment. The nurse has an obligation to pursue needed care through the established chain of command at the facility.

Use of Unlicensed Assistive Personnel

In an effort to reduce health care costs, many agencies have increased the use of unlicensed assistive personnel to perform direct client care and have decreased the number of nurses who supervise them. An unlicensed person may be trained to do everything from housekeeping tasks to drawing blood and performing other diagnostic testing to giving medications, all in the same day. This practice raises grave concerns about the quality of care clients receive when the nurse is responsible and accountable for the care of more clients but must rely on unlicensed personnel to perform much of the care formerly provided only by professionals. At the same time, use of an expert nurse for housekeeping and other mundane, but necessary, unit tasks is inefficient and detracts from available time for care. A balanced approach is needed when incorporating unlicensed assistive personnel into an agency's work.

Nurses must be aware of their legal responsibilities in these situations. They must know that the nurse is always responsible for assessments and must make the critical judgments that are necessary to ensure safety. Nurses must know what each unlicensed person caring for children is able to do and must supervise them closely enough to ensure that they perform delegated tasks competently.

One area in which unlicensed assistive personnel may have greater responsibilities is in the school setting. Registered nurses who practice in schools are caring for children with more complex medical and nursing needs, responding to increased requirements for routine health screenings, and dealing with budgetary cuts that result in a nurse caring for children in more than one school. These pressures have led to increased use of unlicensed assistive personnel to provide routine care to children with uncomplicated needs, including medication administration. The American Academy of Pediatrics (2009b) has issued a policy statement that strongly recommends that a nurse be present in every school. If this is not possible, then the school nurse can consider delegating certain responsibilities to properly trained and competent unlicensed assistive personnel. Nurses who consider delegation must be familiar with their state's nurse practice act and appropriate professional standards (Resha, 2010). Prior to delegating, the nurse needs to determine tasks that are appropriate and safe, the complexity of children's needs, and school district policy (AAP, 2009b; Resha, 2010). The nurse needs to work with the school administration to develop a comprehensive school-based policy (e.g., the nurse, not the administrator, decides what responsibilities will be delegated) before any responsibilities are delegated to others. The nurse is also responsible for educating and evaluating the competency of the unlicensed personnel; this includes requiring return demonstrations of procedures and regular onsite supervision (Resha, 2010). Most important is that delegation does not relieve the nurse from regular assessment of the children's responses to all treatments and medications (AAP, 2009b; Resha, 2010).

Malpractice

Negligence is failure to perform the way a reasonable, prudent person of similar background would act in a similar situation. Negligence may consist of doing something that should not be done or failing to do something that should be done.

Malpractice is negligence by professionals, such as nurses or physicians, in the performance of their duties. Nurses may be accused of malpractice if they do not perform according to established standards of care and in the manner of a reasonable, prudent nurse with similar education and experience. Four elements must be present to prove negligence. They are duty, breach of duty, damage, and proximate cause.

Prevention of Malpractice Claims

Malpractice awards have escalated in both number and amount of awards to plaintiffs, resulting in high malpractice insurance for all health care providers. In addition, more health care workers practice

---

> ### ! NURSING QUALITY ALERT
> #### Elements of Negligence
>
> - *Duty.* The nurse must have a duty to act or give care to the client. It must be part of the nurse's responsibility.
> - *Breach of Duty.* A violation of that duty must occur. The nurse fails to conform to established standards for performing that duty.
> - *Damage.* There must be actual injury or harm to the client as a result of the nurse's breach of duty.
> - *Proximate Cause.* The nurse's breach of duty must be proved to be the cause of harm to the client.

defensively, accumulating evidence that they are acting in the client's best interest. For example, nurses must be careful to include detailed data when they chart.

Prevention of claims is sometimes referred to as *risk management* or *quality assurance.* Although it is not possible to prevent all malpractice lawsuits, nurses can help defend themselves against malpractice judgments by following guidelines for informed consent, refusal of care, and documentation; acting as a client advocate; working within accepted standards and the policies and procedures of the facility; and maintaining their level of expertise.

Informed Consent. When clients receive adequate information, in other words, when an agency's emphasis is on transparency, they are less likely to file malpractice suits. Informed consent is an ethical concept that has been enacted into law. Clients and families have the right to decide whether to accept or reject treatment options as part of their right to function autonomously. To make wise decisions they need full information about treatments offered. Without proper informed consent, assault and battery charges can result.

The law mandates what procedures require informed consent and what to inform about as "risks" specific to each procedure. Nurses must be familiar with those procedures requiring consent.

> ### ! NURSING QUALITY ALERT
> #### Requirements of Informed Consent
>
> - Competence to consent
> - Full disclosure of information
> - Understanding of information
> - Consent is voluntary

Competence. Certain requirements must be met before consent can be considered informed. The first requirement is that the person giving the consent be competent, or able to think through a situation and make rational decisions. A person who is comatose or severely mentally retarded is incapable of making such decisions. Minors are not allowed to give consent; however, children should have procedures explained to them in terms appropriate for their age. In most states, minority status for informed consent ends at the age of 18 years.

Most states allow some exceptions for parental consent in cases involving emancipated minors. An *emancipated minor* is a minor child who has the legal competency of an adult because of circumstances involving marriage, divorce, parenting of a child, living independently without parents, or enlistment in the armed services. Legal counsel may be consulted to verify the status of the emancipated minor for consent purposes.

Most states allow minors to obtain treatment for drug or alcohol abuse or sexually transmitted diseases and to have access to birth control without parental consent. At present, laws governing adolescent abortion vary widely from state to state.

Full disclosure. The second requirement is that of full disclosure of information, including the treatment's purpose and the expected results. The risks, side effects, and benefits as well as other treatment options must be explained to parents and children. They must also be informed as to what would happen if no treatment were chosen.

For example, the National Childhood Vaccine Injury Act mandates that explanations about the risks of communicable diseases and the risks and benefits associated with immunizations should be given to all parents to enable them to make informed decisions about their child's health care. Parents need to know the common side effects and what to do in an emergency if any occur. The law stipulates that children injured by the vaccine must go through the administrative compensation system (funds from an excise tax levied on the vaccines) and reject an award before attempting to sue in a civil suit either the manufacturer or the person who gave the vaccine. Furthermore, the law mandates certain record-keeping and reporting requirements for nurses.

Understanding of information. The parent or legal guardian of a child must comprehend information about proposed treatment. Health professionals need to explain the facts in terms the person can understand. Nurses must be advocates when they find that a parent does not fully understand a treatment or has questions about it. If it is a minor point, the nurse may be able to explain it. Otherwise the nurse must inform the provider so that the parent's misunderstandings can be clarified.

Throughout hospitalization and discharge preparations, considerations should be given to those who do not understand the prevailing language and to the hearing impaired. Foreign language and sign language interpreters must be obtained when indicated. Provision for those who cannot read any language or adults with a low education level must be considered as well.

Voluntary consent. Parents and children should be allowed to make choices voluntarily without undue influence or coercion from others. Although others can give information, the parent or legal guardian of a child makes the decision. Families should not feel pressured to choose in a certain way or feel that their future care depends on their decision.

Children cannot legally consent for treatment or participation in research. However, they should be given the opportunity to give voluntary assent for research participation. Assent involves the principles of competence and full disclosure. Children should be given information in a developmentally appropriate format. Clients 18 years and older must provide full consent. When seeking assent from children, the nurse considers both the child's age and development. In general, when children have reached 14 years old, they are competent to understand ramifications of treatment or participation in research; some children are competent at a somewhat younger age (Masty & Fisher, 2008). Other factors to consider are the child's physical and emotional condition and behaviors, cognitive ability, history of family shared decision making, anxiety level, and disease context (Masty & Fisher, 2008). In some states, the child's dissent to participate in research is legally binding, so nurses need to be aware of the legal issues in the states in which they practice. The Committee on Pediatric Emergency Medicine has issued a policy regarding consent for emergency medical services for children and adolescents. The policy recommends that every effort be made to secure consent from a parent or legal guardian, but emergency treatment should not be denied if there are problems obtaining the consent (American Academy of Pediatrics Committee on Pediatric Emergency Medicine, 2011).

Refusal of Care

Sometimes parents or children decline treatment, including hospitalization, offered by health care workers. They may refuse treatment when they believe that the benefits of treatment do not outweigh the burdens of the treatment or the quality of life they can expect after that treatment. Parents have the right to refuse care, and they can withdraw agreement to treatment at any time. When a person makes this decision, a number of steps should be taken.

First, the physician or nurse should establish that the parent and child understand the treatment and the results of refusal. The physician, if unaware of the decision, should be notified by the nurse. The nurse documents on the chart the refusal, explanations given to the parent, and notification of the physician. If the treatment is considered vital to the child's well-being, the physician discusses the need with the parent and documents the discussion. Opinions by other physicians may be offered as well.

Parents may be asked to sign a form indicating that they understand the possible results of rejecting treatment. This measure is to prevent a later lawsuit in which a parent claims lack of knowledge of the possible results of a decision. If there is no ethical dilemma, the client's decision stands.

When parents refuse to give consent for what is deemed necessary treatment of a child, the state may be petitioned to intervene. The court may place the child in the temporary custody of the government or a private agency. The nurse may be asked to witness such a transaction when physicians act in cases of emergencies, such as a lifesaving blood transfusion for a child despite parental objections based on religious beliefs.

Adoption

Nurses may care for infants involved in adoptions. The nurse may need to consult with the birth parents, adoptive parents, social workers, obstetrician, or pediatrician to determine the various rights of the child, birth parents, and adoptive parents (e.g., in matters concerning visitation rights, informed consent, or discharge planning).

In open adoptions, the birth mother may opt to room in with the infant during hospitalization. The birth mother and adoptive parents typically have had contact before the delivery and have an informal agreement regarding shared responsibility for the infant. The birth parent may even participate in discharge planning because she may have extended rights to visit the child after adoption.

Issues may develop as to the state of mind of the birth mother at the time of relinquishing parental rights (which cannot occur until after birth, unlike the relinquishment of the birth father's rights). State laws vary as to the legal time period necessary (1 day to several weeks after the birth of the child) before a birth mother can lawfully relinquish her rights to the child.

Some state laws allow the birth mother to relinquish her rights immediately after birth. In such cases, the nurse has the responsibility of protecting the birth mother and child to ensure that the birth mother is not coerced into making a decision while under the effects of medication. Factual documentation of such circumstances may be requested if the birth mother later asserts her rights to the child, claiming "undue influence" or "coercion."

Birth fathers have the same rights as the birth mother. Unless the birth father relinquishes his legal rights to the child, he may later assert his rights to the child after attachment has occurred with the adoptive parents. This situation may occur if the birth mother denies knowledge of the father's identity.

Documentation

Documentation, whether on paper or electronic, is the best evidence that a standard of care has been maintained. All information recorded about a child should reflect that standard of care. This information includes both electronic and written nurses' notes, flow sheets, and any other data in the child's record. In many instances, notations on hospital records are the only proof that care has been given. Expert witnesses, often registered nurses in the appropriate specialty, will search for evidence that the standard of care at the time of the incident was met. If not found in case documents, the expert witness must conclude that what should have been done was not done. When documentation is not present, juries tend to assume that care was not given. Although documentation is not listed as a step in the nursing process, it is an integral part of the process.

Documentation must be specific and complete. Nurses are unlikely to be able to recall situations that happened years ago and must rely on their documentation to explain their care if sued. Documentation must show that the standards of care and facility policies and procedures in effect at the time of the incident were met. Documentation must demonstrate that the child was appropriately assessed, that continuing monitoring of problems was provided, that problems were identified and correct interventions were instituted, and that changes in the child's condition were reported to the primary care provider. If the nurse believes that the primary care provider has responded inappropriately, the nurse must refer the provider response through the appropriate chain of command for the facility and must document the notification.

Documenting Discharge Teaching. Because of brief hospital stays, discharge teaching is essential to ensure that parents know how to care for their child at home. Nurses must document the teaching they perform as well as the parents' and child's understanding, if appropriate, of that teaching. The nurse should also note the need for reinforcement and how that reinforcement was provided. If follow-up home care is planned, teaching can be continued at home and documented on forms by the home care nurse.

Documenting Incidents. A type of documentation used in risk management is the *incident report,* often called a *quality assurance, occurrence,* or *variance report.* The nurse completes a report when something occurs that might result in legal action, such as in injury to a child or a departure from the expectations in a situation. The report warns the agency's legal department that there may be a problem. It also helps identify whether changing processes within the system might reduce the risk for similar incidents in the future. Incident reports are not a part of the child's chart and should not be referred to on the chart. Documentation of the incident on the chart should be restricted to the same type of factual information about the child's condition that would be recorded in any other situation.

The analysis of medical error from a systems perspective is called a *root cause* analysis. The process involves identifying errors or near misses as soon as they occur, asking relevant questions about the factors that might have contributed to the error, analyzing the contributing causes, and developing interventions to prevent a similar error from occurring in the future. A root cause analysis is not intended to be punitive if an error was made. Instead, root cause analysis is used as a tool to prevent future error or near misses.

The Nurse as Child and Family Advocate

Malpractice suits may be brought if nurses fail in their role of child and family advocate. Nurses are ethically and legally bound to act as the child's advocate. This means that the nurse must act in the child's best interests at all times. When nurses believe that the child's best interests are not being served, they are obligated to seek help for the child from appropriate sources. This usually involves taking the problem through the chain of command established at the facility. The nurse consults a supervisor and the child's physician. If the results are not satisfactory, the nurse continues through administrative channels to the director of nurses, hospital administrator, and chief of the medical staff, if necessary. All nurses should know the chain of command for their workplaces.

Nurses must be advocates for health promotion and illness prevention for vulnerable groups such as children. Nurses can participate in groups dedicated to the welfare of children and families, such as professional nursing societies, parent support groups, religious organizations, and voluntary organizations. Through involvement with health care planning on a political or legislative level and by working as consumer advocates, nurses can initiate changes for better quality health care.

Maintaining Expertise

Maintaining expertise is another way for nurses and other health professionals to prevent malpractice liability. To ensure that nurses maintain their expertise to provide safe care, most states require proof of continuing education for renewal of nursing licenses. Nursing knowledge changes rapidly, and it is essential that all nurses keep current. Incorporating new information learned by attending classes or conferences and reading nursing journals can help nurses perform the way a reasonably prudent peer would perform. Journals provide information from nursing research that may be important in updating nursing practice. It is important for all nurses to analyze research articles to determine whether changes in pediatric care are indicated.

Employers often provide continuing education classes for their nurses. Many workshops and seminars are available on a wide variety of nursing subjects. Membership in professional organizations, such as state branches of the American Nurses Association or specialty organizations such as the Society of Pediatric Nurses, gives nurses access to new information through publications as well as nursing conferences and other educational offerings.

Maintaining expertise may be a concern when nurses "float" or are required to work with children who have needs different from those of their usual clients. In these situations, the employer must provide orientation and education so that the nurse can perform care safely in new areas. Nurses who work outside their usual areas of expertise must assess their own skills and avoid performing tasks or taking on responsibilities in areas in which they are not competent. Many nurses learn to provide care in two or three different areas and are floated only to those areas. This system meets the need for flexible staffing while providing safe care.

SOCIAL ISSUES

Nurses are exposed to many social issues that influence health care and often have legal or ethical implications. Some of the issues that affect child health care include poverty, homelessness, access to care, and allocation of funds.

Poverty

Poverty is an underlying factor in problems such as inadequate access to health care and homelessness and is a major predictor for unmet health needs in children and adults. The percentage of children in the United States who are living in poverty (21%) has increased with the downturn in the national economy. Children younger than 5 years are more often found in families with incomes below the poverty line than are older children. Children in female-headed households are more likely to be living in poverty and the poverty rate is three times higher in black and Hispanic households than in white non-Hispanic households (Forum on Child and Family Statistics, 2011).

Poverty affects the ability to access health care for any age-group and decreases opportunities linked with health promotion. Nurses can play a role in helping to meet the health care needs of infants and children by recognizing the adverse effect of poverty on health and identifying poverty as a practice concern. Several of the *Healthy People 2020* goals (USDHHS, 2010b) have implications for pediatric nurses:

- To reduce the infant mortality rate to no more than 6.0 per 1000 live births and the childhood mortality rate to 25.7 per 100,000 for children 1 to 4 years old and 12.3 per 100,000 for children 5 to 9 years old and to similarly reduce the rate of adolescent deaths
- To reduce the incidence of low birth weight to no more than 7.8% (from 8.2% in 2007) of live births and the incidence of very low birth weight to 1.4% of live births
- Reduce preterm births to 11.4%
- To achieve and maintain effective vaccination coverage levels for universally recommended vaccines in children from 19 to 35 months of age and increase routine vaccination coverage for adolescents
- To reduce, eliminate or maintain elimination of cases of vaccine-preventable diseases To increase to 100% the proportion of people with health insurance

Poverty tends to breed poverty. In low-income families children may leave the educational system early, making them less likely to learn skills necessary to obtain good jobs. The cycle of poverty (Figure 1-3) may continue from one generation to another as a result of hopelessness and apathy.

Homelessness

Homeless families make up over 40% of the homeless population (Forum on Child and Family Statistics, 2011; National Coalition for the Homeless, 2009). This percentage is increasing due to multiple factors that include the national economic downturn, job loss, shortage of affordable housing, decrease in government assistance programs, family violence, and poverty (National Coalition for the Homeless, 2009). Some homeless women are substance abusers and others are fleeing domestic violence. Homeless children are poorly nourished, are more susceptible to illness, may be exposed to violence, experience school absences with subsequent learning difficulties, and are at risk for depression and other emotional consequences (National Coalition for the Homeless, 2009).

Pregnancy and birth, especially among teenagers, are important contributors to homelessness. Adolescent mothers are more likely to be single mothers and poor. Pregnancy interferes with a woman's ability to work and may decrease her income to the point at which she loses her housing. Without child care or a home address, she may have less chance of obtaining and keeping employment. In addition, her children are more likely to be sick because of inadequate food and shelter. Without money to pay for insurance or early health care, there is an increased chance that children will need hospitalization (Little, Gorman, Dzendoletas, & Moravac, 2007).

Federal funding has provided assistance with shelter and health care for homeless people. The homeless, however, have the same difficulties in obtaining health care as other poor people because of lack of transportation, inconvenient hours, and lack of continuity of care.

Allocation of Health Care Resources

Expenditures for health care in the United States in 2009 totaled $2.5 trillion, which represents 17.6% of the total expenditures on services and goods in the United States and a 4% increase from the previous year (Centers for Medicare and Medicaid, 2011). These expenditures are expected to continue to increase, as the population of baby boomers, born from 1946 through 1964, is expected to need more health care dollars as it ages.

Reforming health care delivery and financing is a complex area of national concern. How to provide care for the poor, the uninsured or underinsured, and those with long-term care needs are some areas that must be addressed. In addition, major acute care facilities often deal with greater financial burdens because of the growing numbers of uninsured clients presenting for treatment who are often very ill or severely injured. Escalating liability costs are another drain on health care dollars, leading some states to enact legislation that places a cap on awards for damages in malpractice cases.

Care versus Cure

One problem to be addressed is whether the focus of health care should be on preventive and caring measures or on cure of disease. Medicine has traditionally centered more on treatment and cure than on prevention and care. Yet prevention not only avoids suffering but also is less expensive than treating diseases once they are diagnosed.

The focus on cure has resulted in technologic advances that have enabled some people to live longer, healthier lives. Financial resources are limited, however, and the costs of expensive technology needs to be balanced against the benefits obtained. Indeed, the cost of one organ transplant would pay for the prenatal care of many low-income mothers, possibly preventing the births of many low-birth-weight infants who may suffer disability throughout life.

In addition, quality-of-life issues are important in regard to technology. Neonatal nurseries are able to keep very-low-birth-weight babies alive because of advances in knowledge. Some of these infants go on to lead normal or near-normal lives. Others gain time but not quality of life. Families and health care professionals face difficult decisions about when to treat, when to terminate treatment, and when suffering outweighs the benefits.

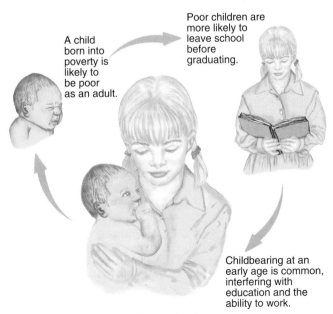

A child born into poverty is likely to be poor as an adult.

Poor children are more likely to leave school before graduating.

Childbearing at an early age is common, interfering with education and the ability to work.

FIG 1-3 The cycle of poverty.

Health Care Rationing

Modern technology has had a great impact on health care rationing. Some might argue that such rationing does not exist, but it occurs when some people have no access to care and there is not enough money for all people to share equally in the technology available. Health care also is rationed when it is more freely given to those who have money to pay for it than to those who do not.

Many questions will need answers as the costs of health care increase faster than the funds available. Is health care a fundamental right? Should a certain level of care be guaranteed to all citizens? What is that basic level of care? Should the cost of treatment and its effectiveness be considered when one is deciding how much government or third-party payers will cover? Nurses will be instrumental in finding solutions to these vital questions.

Violence

In today's society, women and children are the victims and sometimes the perpetrators of violence. Violence is not only a social problem but also a health problem. Acts of violence can include child abuse, domestic abuse, and murder. Children who live in an environment of violence feel helpless and ineffective. These children have difficulty sleeping and show increased anxiety and fearfulness. They may perpetuate the violence they see in their homes when they are adults because they have known nothing else in family relationships.

Although violent crimes among children have decreased over the past decade, violence in schools continues to rise, and for many children it is a daily stressor. Experts in the field of education have cited socioeconomic disparity, language barriers, diverse cultural upbringing, lack of supervision and behavioral feedback, domestic violence, and changes within the family as possible causes for the increased violence. Traditional approaches to aggressive behavior in the school, such as suspension, detention, and being sent to the principal's office, have been ineffective in changing behavior and serve only to exclude the student from education, leading to an increased dropout rate. Nurses need to educate themselves on the issue of violence and work with schools and parents to combat the problem. In addition, they should not ignore the child who is afraid to go to school or is having other school-related problems.

Children and adolescents are also exposed to violence via television, movies, video games, and youth-oriented music. Nurses should make this issue a part of anticipatory guidance. The American Academy of Pediatrics (2009a)encourages parents to monitor their children's media exposure and limit their children's screen time (TV, computer, video games) to no more than 1 to 2 hours per day. The AAP (2009a) also recommends that parents remove televisions and computers from children's bedrooms, limit viewing of programs and video games that have sexual or violent content, view television programs with children and discuss these, and educate children and adolescents about media literacy.

The AAP (2009a) suggests that clinicians ask parents and children about media exposure at every well visit. Providers also need to be concerned about adolescents who display aggressive or acting-out behaviors, such as lying, stealing, temper outbursts, vandalism, excessive fighting, and destructiveness. It further recommends that health care providers promote the responsibility of every family to create a gun-safe home environment. This includes asking about the presence of guns in the home at every well visit and counseling children, parents, and relatives on the importance of firearm safety and the dangers of having a gun, especially a handgun.

Nurses working with children should ask them about violence in their school, home, or neighborhood, and whether they have had any personal experience with violent behavior. In some cases it may be necessary to contact parents, human resource departments, police, or other authorities to protect children and adolescents who are either in violent situations or at risk for violence.

THE PROFESSIONAL NURSE

As nursing care changed from the category-specific care of the child to family-centered care, pediatric nursing entered a new era of autonomy and independence. Nurses today must be able to communicate with and teach effectively children of many ages and levels of development and education. They must be able to think critically, have appropriate clinical judgment, and use the nursing process to develop a plan of care that meets the unique needs of each child and family. They are expected to incorporate evidence-based nursing to solve problems, to answer clinical questions related to high-quality patient-centered care, and to practice interdisciplinary collaboration with other health care providers.

The Role of the Professional Nurse

The professional nurse has a responsibility to provide the highest quality care to every child and family. The American Nurses Association (ANA) Code of Ethics for Nurses (see Box 1-1) provides guidelines for ethical and professional behavior. The code emphasizes a nurse's accountability to children and families, the community, and the profession. The nurse should understand the implications of this code and strive to practice accordingly. Professional nurses have a legal obligation to know and understand the standard of care imposed on them. It is critical that nurses maintain competence and a current knowledge base in their areas of practice.

Standards of practice describe the level of performance expected of a professional nurse as determined by an authority in the practice. Nurses who care for children in all clinical settings can use the ANA/Society of Pediatric Nurses (SPN) Standards of Care and Standards of Professional Performance for Pediatric Nurses and the SPN/ANA Guide to Family Centered Care as guides for practice. Other standards of practice for specific clinical areas, such as pediatric oncology nursing or emergency nursing, are available from nursing specialty groups.

As health care continues to move to family-centered and community-based health services, all nurses should expect to care for children, adolescents, and their families. Under the leadership of the Child and Family Expert Panel of the American Academy of Nursing, representatives from 10 pediatric and subspecialty organizations met to identify the commonalities of practice across all areas of pediatric practice and produced the document *Health Care Quality and Outcome Guidelines for Nursing of Children and Families.* The guidelines set forth in the document can serve as a framework for practice when caring for children and their families. Educators and administrators in health care should find them useful when planning programs (Betz, 2005).

Pediatric nurses function in a variety of roles, including those of care provider, teacher, collaborator, researcher, advocate, and manager.

Care Provider

The nurse provides direct patient-centered care to infants, children, and their families in times of illness, injury, recovery, and wellness. Nursing care is based on the nursing process. The nurse obtains health histories, assesses child and family needs, monitors growth and development, performs health-screening procedures, develops comprehensive plans of care, provides treatment and care, makes referrals, and evaluates the effects of care. Nursing of children is especially based on an understanding of the child's developmental stage and is aimed at meeting the child's physical and emotional needs at that level. Developing a therapeutic relationship with and providing support to children and their families are essential components of nursing care. Pediatric nurses practice family-centered care, embracing diversity in family structures and cultural backgrounds. These nurses strive to empower families, encouraging them to participate in their self-care and the care of their child.

Teacher

Education is an essential role of today's nurse. Nurses who care for children prepare them for procedures, hospitalization, or surgery, using knowledge of growth and development to teach children at various levels of understanding. Families need information as well as emotional support so that they can cope with the anxiety and uncertainty of a child's illness. Nurses teach family members how to provide care, watch for important signs, and increase the child's comfort. They also work with new parents and parents of ill children so that the parents are prepared to assume responsibility for care at home after the child has been discharged from the hospital.

Education is essential to promote health. The nurse applies principles of teaching and learning to change the behavior of family members. Nurses motivate children and families to take charge of and make responsible decisions about their own health. For teaching to be effective, it must incorporate the family's values and health beliefs.

Nurses caring for children and families play an important role in preventing illness and injury through education and anticipatory guidance. Teaching about immunizations, safety, dental care, socialization, and discipline is a necessary component of care. Nurses offer guidance to parents with regard to child-rearing practices and preventing potential problems. They also answer questions about growth and development and assist families in understanding their children. Teaching often involves providing emotional support and counseling to children and families.

Factors that influence learning at any age include the following:
- *Developmental level.* Teenage parents often have very different concerns than older parents. Grandparents who must assume long-term care of a child often need information that may not have existed when their own child was the same age. Developmental level also influences whether a person learns best by reading printed material, using computer-based materials, watching videos, participating in group discussions, play, or other means. When teaching children, teaching must be adapted to the child's developmental level rather than the child's chronological age.
- *Language.* The ability to understand the language in which teaching is done determines how much the family learns. Families for whom English is not the primary language may not understand idioms, nuances, slang terms, informal use of words, or medical words. An interpreter for the deaf may be necessary for the client who is hearing impaired.
- *Culture.* People tend to forget or disregard content with which they disagree. The nurse's teaching can be most effective if cultural considerations are weighed and incorporated into the education.
- *Previous experiences.* Parents who have other children may need less education about infant and child care. They may, however, have additional concerns about meeting the needs of several children and about sibling rivalry.
- *Physical environment.* The nurse must consider privacy when discussing sensitive issues such as adolescent sexuality or domestic violence. A group discussion, however, may prompt

participants to ask questions of concern to all members of the group.
- *Organization and skill of the teacher.* The teacher must determine the objectives of the teaching, develop a plan to meet the objectives, and gather all materials before teaching. The nurse must determine the best way to present the material for the intended audience. A summary of the information is helpful when concluding a teaching session.

Collaborator

Nurses collaborate with other members of the health care team, often coordinating and managing the child's care. Care is improved by an interdisciplinary approach as nurses work together with dietitians, social workers, physicians, and others.

Managing the transition from a hospital or any other acute-care setting to the child's home or another facility involves discharge planning and collaboration with other health care professionals. The trend toward home care makes collaboration increasingly important. The nurse needs to be knowledgeable about community resources, appropriate home care agencies for the type of family or problem, and financial resources. Cooperation and communication are essential because parents and caregivers of children are encouraged to participate in their care.

Researcher

Nurses contribute to their profession's knowledge base by systematically investigating theoretic or practice issues in nursing. Nursing does much more than simply "borrow" scientific knowledge from medicine and basic sciences. Nursing generates and answers its own questions based on evidence within its unique subject area. The responsibility for providing evidence-based, patient-centered care is not limited to nurses with graduate degrees. It is important that all nurses appraise and apply appropriate research findings to their practice, rather than basing care decisions merely on intuition or tradition.

Evidence-based practice is no longer just an ideal but an expectation of nursing practice. Nurses can contribute to the body of professional knowledge by demonstrating an awareness of the value of nursing research and assisting in problem identification and data collection. Nurses should keep their knowledge current by networking and sharing research findings at conferences, by publishing, and by evaluating research journal articles.

Advocate

An advocate is one who speaks on behalf of another. Care can become impersonal as the health care environment becomes more complex. The wishes and needs of children and families are sometimes discounted or ignored in the effort to treat and to cure. As the health professional who is closest to the child and family, the nurse is in an ideal position to humanize care and to intercede on their behalf. As an advocate the nurse considers the family's wishes and preferences in planning and implementing care. The nurse informs families of treatments and procedures, ensuring that the families are involved directly in decisions and activities related to their care. The nurse must be sensitive to families' values, beliefs, and customs.

Nurses need to be advocates for health promotion for vulnerable groups. Nurses can promote the rights of children and families by participating in groups dedicated to their welfare, such as professional nursing societies, support groups, religious organizations, and voluntary organizations. Through involvement with health care planning on a political or legislative level and by working as consumer advocates, nurses can initiate changes for better quality health care. Nurses possess unique knowledge and skills and can make valuable contributions in developing health care strategies to ensure that all children and families receive optimal care.

Manager of Care

Because of shorter stays in acute care facilities, nurses often are unable to provide total direct care. Instead they delegate concrete tasks, such as giving a bath or taking vital signs, to others. As a result, nurses spend more time teaching and supervising unlicensed assistive personnel, planning and coordinating care, and collaborating with other professionals and agencies. Nurses are expected to understand the financial effects of cost-containment strategies and to contribute to their institutions' economic viability. At the same time they must continue to act as advocates and to maintain a standard of care.

ADVANCED ROLES FOR PEDIATRIC NURSES

The increasing complexity of care and a focus on cost containment, error reduction, and quality of care have led to a greater need for nurses with advanced educational preparation. Pediatric nurses who have obtained advanced education may practice as nurse practitioners, clinical nurse specialists, or clinical nurse leaders (CNL®). They may also practice in administrative, education, or research roles. Preparation for these roles usually involves obtaining a master's or doctoral degree.

Nurse Practitioners

Nurse practitioners are advanced practice nurses who work according to protocols and provide many primary care services that were once provided only by physicians. Most nurse practitioners collaborate with a physician, but, depending on their scope of practice and their individual state's board of nursing mandates, they may work independently and prescribe medications. Nurse practitioners provide care for children and families in a variety of settings (primary-care facilities, schools, acute-care facilities, rehabilitation centers). They may address occupational health, women's health, family health, and the health of the elderly or the very young.

Pediatric nurse practitioners use advanced skills to assess and treat well and ill children according to established protocols. The health care services they provide range from physical examinations and anticipatory guidance to the treatment of common illnesses and injuries. It is becoming more common for newborn nurseries and some children's hospital specialty units to be staffed by neonatal or pediatric nurse practitioners.

School nurse practitioners receive education and training that is similar to that of pediatric nurse practitioners. However, because of the setting in which they practice, the school nurse practitioners receive advanced education in managing chronic illness, disability, and mental health problems in a school setting, as well as developing skills required to communicate effectively with students, teachers, school administrators, and community health care providers. School nurse practitioners expand the traditional role of the school nurse by providing on-site treatment of acute care problems and providing extensive well-child examinations and services.

Clinical Nurse Specialists

Clinical specialists are registered nurses who, through study and supervised practice at the graduate level (master's or doctorate), have become expert in the care children and families. Four major subroles have been identified for clinical nurse specialists: expert practitioner, educator, researcher, and consultant. These professionals often function as role models, advocates, and change agents. Unlike nurse practitioners, clinical nurse specialists have an acute care focus.

Clinical Nurse Leaders

As newly defined by the American Association of Colleges of Nursing (2011), the Clinical Nurse Leader is a master's prepared generalist whose focus is on quality, safety, and optimal patient outcomes at point of care. All CNLs receive the same basic preparation in a master's program, which includes advanced pathophysiology, pharmacology, and health assessment, among other courses that prepare them to assume leadership roles within their specific practice settings. Extensive practicum experiences assist them with assessing quality and safety at the micro- and macrosystems levels in order to improve direct patient care. A certification examination is available. CNLs work in a variety of pediatric settings, providing safe and optimal care to children and families.

Implications of Changing Roles for Nurses

As nursing care has changed, so also have the roles of pediatric nurses with both basic and advanced preparation. Nurses now work in a variety of areas. Although they previously worked almost exclusively in the hospital setting, many now provide home care and community-based care. Some of the settings for care children and families include:

- Acute-care settings: general hospital units, intensive care units, surgical units, postanesthesia care units, emergency care facilities, and onboard emergency transport craft
- Clinics and physicians' offices
- Home health agencies
- Schools
- Rehabilitation centers and long-term care facilities
- Summer camps and daycare centers
- Hospice programs and respite care programs
- Psychiatric centers

THE NURSING PROCESS IN PEDIATRIC CARE

The nursing process is the foundation for all nursing. The nursing process is a problem-solving process used to provide unique, individualized, and patient-centered nursing care. Underlying successful use of the nursing process are techniques of therapeutic communication and exercise of appropriate clinical judgment using critical thinking.

Therapeutic Communication

Therapeutic communication is a skill nurses require to carry out the many facets of providing patient-centered care. Therapeutic communication, unlike social communication, is purposeful, goal directed, and focused. Although it may seem simple, therapeutic communication requires conscious effort and considerable practice. Fluency in therapeutic communication relies on active listening, being aware of nonverbal messages, incorporating cultural communication differences, and focusing on specific child and family needs.

Critical Thinking

Nursing process also relies on the nurse's expertise in clinical judgment. Critical thinking, as a component of clinical judgment, underlies the nursing process steps (Huckabay, 2009). Unlike undirected thinking, which is random and unfocused, critical thinking is controlled, purposeful, directed toward solving problems and achieving outcomes based on evidence. Critical thinking involves thorough reflection and analysis of one's own thought processes. The critical thinker examines and questions assumptions (Alfaro-LeFevre, 2009). Critical thinking improves clinical judgment by reducing habits that result in poor decision making and increases the ability to apply knowledge to clinical situations. It reduces the risk for decision making based on emotion, fatigue, or anxiety. Critical thinking begins when nurses realize that it is not enough to accumulate a fund of knowledge from texts and lectures. They must also be able to *apply* the knowledge to specific clinical situations to provide the most effective patient-centered care.

Steps of the Nursing Process

The nursing process consists of five distinct steps: (1) assessment, (2) nursing diagnosis, (3) planning, (4) implementation of the plan (interventions), and (5) evaluation. Despite the apparent complexity of the process, the nurse soon learns to use the steps of the nursing process in order when caring for children and families.

Pediatric nursing, including care of a newborn, presents a challenge for many nursing students. Whereas use of the nursing process when caring for adults may involve only the patient, in caring for infants and children it must involve their family as well. Therefore it is common for planning and interventions to state what the parent is expected to do or to specify interventions such as teaching a parent. The involvement of a third party (the family) may be different to the nursing student who has applied the nursing process only to care of adults in the past.

Assessment

Nursing assessment is the systematic collection of relevant data to determine the child's and family's current health status, coping patterns, needs, and problems. The data collected include not only physiologic data but also psychological, social, and cultural data relevant to life processes. Nurses must assess the belief systems, available support, perceptions, and plans of other family members in an effort to provide the best nursing care.

During the assessment phase, three activities take place: collecting data, grouping findings, and writing the nursing diagnoses. Data can be collected through interview, physical examination, observation, review of records, and diagnostic reports, as well as through collaboration with other health care workers and the family. Two levels of nursing assessment are used to collect comprehensive data: (1) screening, or database, assessment; and (2) focused assessments.

Screening Assessment. The screening, or database, assessment is usually performed during the initial contact with the child and family. Its purpose is to gather information about all aspects of the child's health. This information, called *baseline data,* describes the child's health status before interventions begin. It forms the basis for identifying both strengths and problems. An example of baseline data would be the child's immunization and developmental history.

A variety of methods may be used to organize the assessment. For example, information may be grouped according to body systems. Assessment can also be organized around nursing models that are based on nursing theory, such as Roy's adaptation model, Gordon's functional health patterns, NANDA International's human response patterns, or Orem's self-care deficit theory.

Focused Assessment. A focused assessment is used to gather information that is specifically related to an actual health problem or a problem that the child or family is at risk for acquiring. A focused assessment is often performed at the beginning of a shift and centers on areas relevant to the child's diagnosis and current status. For example, the nurse would perform a focused assessment of the respiratory system several times during the child's hospitalization for the child with acute asthma.

Nursing Diagnosis

The data gathered during assessment must be analyzed to identify problems or potential problems. Data are validated and grouped in a process of critical thinking so that cues and inferences can be determined. The nurse identifies the child and family's responses to actual or potential health problems and to normal life processes. The nursing diagnosis provides a basis for nursing accountability for interventions and outcomes.

There are three types of nursing diagnoses. An *actual nursing diagnosis* describes a human response to a health condition or life process affecting an individual, family, or community. It is supported by defining characteristics (manifestations, signs, and symptoms) that can be clustered in patterns of related cues or inferences. *Risk nursing diagnoses* describe human responses to health conditions or life processes that may develop in a vulnerable individual, family, or community. They are supported by risk factors that contribute to increased vulnerability. *Wellness nursing diagnoses* describe human responses to levels of wellness in an individual, family, or community that have a potential for enhancement to a higher state.

Each nursing diagnosis is a concise term or phrase that represents a pattern of related cues or signs and symptoms. One problem that nurses often encounter is writing nursing diagnoses that nursing actions cannot address. For example, a medical diagnosis, such as pyloric stenosis, cannot be treated by a nurse. It is appropriate, however, to say that there are nursing actions that can decrease the fluid volume deficit associated with pyloric stenosis.

A nursing diagnosis consists of two sections joined by the phrase "related to." The statement begins with the response to the current problem and then describes the causative factor or factors. An example is Interrupted Family Processes related to *the diagnosis of a child with cancer.* The causative factors can be physiologic, psychological, sociocultural, environmental, or spiritual. They assist the nurse in identifying nursing interventions as planning takes place.

Planning

The nurse next plans care for problems that were identified during assessment and are reflected in the nursing diagnoses. During this step nurses set priorities, develop goals or outcomes that state what is to be accomplished by a certain time, and plan interventions to accomplish those goals.

Setting Priorities. Setting priorities includes (1) determining what problems need immediate attention (i.e., life-threatening problems) and taking immediate action; (2) determining whether there are problems that call for a physician's orders for diagnosis, monitoring, or treatment; and (3) identifying actual nursing diagnoses, which take precedence over at-risk diagnoses. For children with many health and psychosocial problems, a realistic number of nursing diagnoses must be chosen.

Establishing Goals and Expected Outcomes. Although the terms *goals* and *outcome criteria* are sometimes used interchangeably, they are different. Generally, broad goals do not state the specific outcome criteria and are less measurable than outcome statements. If broad goals are developed, they should be linked to more specific and measurable outcome criteria. For example, if the goal is that the parents will demonstrate effective parenting by discharge, *outcome criteria* that serve as evidence might be steps in that process such as prompt, consistent responses to infant signals and competence in bathing, feeding, and comforting the infant.

Certain rules should be followed when writing outcomes.

- Outcomes should be stated in client terms. This wording identifies who is expected to achieve the goal (the infant or child, or family).
- Measurable verbs must be used. For example, "identify," "demonstrate," "express," "walk," "relate," and "list" are verbs that are observable and measurable. Examples of verbs that are difficult to measure are "understand," "appreciate," "feel," "accept," "know," and "experience."
- A time frame is necessary. When is the person expected to perform the action? After teaching? Before discharge? By 1 day after hospitalization?
- Goals and outcomes must be realistic and attainable by nursing interventions only.
- Goals and outcomes are worked out in collaboration with the child and family to ensure their participation in the plan of care.

Implementation

Implementation is the action phase of the nursing process. Once the goals and desired outcomes are developed, it is necessary to select nursing interventions that will help the child and family meet the established outcomes. During this phase the nurse is constantly evaluating and reassessing to determine that the interventions remain appropriate. As the child's condition changes, so does the plan of care.

The type of nursing interventions implemented depends on whether the nursing diagnosis was an actual, risk, or wellness diagnosis. Nursing interventions for actual nursing diagnoses are aimed at reducing or eliminating the causes or related factors. Interventions for risk nursing diagnoses are aimed at (1) monitoring for onset of the problem, (2) reducing or eliminating risk factors, and (3) preventing the problem. For a wellness nursing diagnosis, interventions focus on supporting the child's or family's coping mechanisms and promoting a higher level of wellness.

Nursing interventions in care plans or protocols are most easily implemented if they are specific and spell out exactly what should be done. A well-written nursing intervention is specific: "Provide 5 mL of fluid (water or juice of choice) at least every 10 minutes while the child is awake." Vague interventions, such as "keep the child hydrated," do not provide specific steps to follow.

Evaluation

The evaluation determines how well the plan worked or how well the goals or outcomes were met. To evaluate, the nurse must assess the child's or family's status and compare the current status with the goals or outcome criteria that were developed during the planning step. The nurse then judges how well the child or family is progressing toward goal achievement, and makes a decision. Should the plan be continued? Modified? Abandoned? Are the problems resolved or the causes diminished? Is another nursing diagnosis more relevant?

The nursing process is dynamic, and evaluation frequently results in expanded assessment and additional or modified nursing diagnoses and interventions. Nurses are cautioned not to view lack of goal achievement as a failure. Instead it is simply time to reassess and begin the process anew.

Collaborative Problems

In addition to nursing diagnoses, which describe problems that respond to independent nursing functions, nurses must also deal with problems that are beyond the scope of independent nursing practice.

These are sometimes termed *collaborative problems*—physiologic complications that usually occur in association with a specific pathologic condition or treatment.

Nurses monitor to detect the onset of the complication and collaborate with physicians to manage changes in status. Both physician- and nursing-prescribed interventions are necessary to minimize complications (Carpenito-Moyet, 2008).

Planning. It is inappropriate to identify patient-centered goals for a collaborative problem because the goals cannot be achieved by independent nursing action. Collaborative problems should reflect the nurse's responsibility in situations requiring physician-prescribed interventions. The nurse's responsibility includes (Carpenito-Moyet, 2008):

- Monitoring for signs of complications
- Managing the complications with nursing- and physician-prescribed interventions

Interventions. Nursing interventions for collaborative problems include (1) performing frequent assessments to monitor the child's or family's status and detect signs and symptoms of complications; (2) communicating with the physician when signs and symptoms of complications are noted; (3) performing physician-prescribed interventions, including standing orders and protocols, to prevent or correct the complication; and (4) performing nursing interventions described in the standards of care or policy and procedure manuals.

Evaluation. Although client-centered goals or outcomes are not developed for collaborative problems, the nurse collects data, compares the data with established norms, and judges whether the data are within normal limits. If the data are not within normal limits, the nurse consults the physician for additional direction and implements physician-prescribed interventions as well as nursing interventions.

COMPLEMENTARY AND ALTERNATIVE MEDICINE

Today's nurse will likely encounter clients who use complementary and alternative medicine (CAM). Complementary and alternative medicine can be defined as those systems, practices, interventions, therapies, applications, theories, or claims that are currently not an integral part of the dominant or conventional medical system in North America (National Center for Complementary and Alternative Medicine, 2010). The therapies may be used instead of conventional medical therapy (alternative therapy) or in addition to conventional medical therapy (complementary therapy). Integrative medicine combines conventional medical therapies with CAM therapies that have substantial evidence as to their safety and effectiveness.

A major concern in the use of CAM is safety. Those who use these techniques may delay needed care by a conventional health care provider, or they may take herbal remedies or other substances that are toxic when combined with conventional medications or when taken in excess. Adverse effects of CAM therapies may be unknown for children. Safety and effectiveness of botanical or vitamin therapies are often unregulated. Thus people may take in variable amounts of active ingredients from these substances. Some may not consider these therapies to be medicine and may not report them to their conventional health care provider, setting the stage for interactions between conventional medications and CAM therapies that have pharmacologic properties. Many people may not consider some of these therapies "alternative" at all because the therapy is mainstream in their culture.

Nurses may find that their professional values do not conflict with many of the CAM therapies. Nursing as a profession supports a self-care and preventive approach to health care in which the individual bears much of the responsibility for his or her health. Nursing practice has traditionally emphasized a holistic, or body-mind-spirit, model of health that fits with CAM. Nurses already practice CAM therapies such as therapeutic touch fairly often. The rising interest in CAM provides an opportunity for nurses to participate in research related to the legitimacy of these treatment modalities.

The National Center for Complementary and Alternative Medicine, a division of the National Institutes of Health, has a website (www.nccam.nih.gov) for information and classification of the therapies.

NURSING RESEARCH AND EVIDENCE-BASED PRACTICE

As nursing and the health care system change, nurses will be challenged to demonstrate that what they do improves child outcomes and is cost-effective. To meet this challenge nurses must participate in research and use evidence that is based on current research to improve patient-centered care. With the establishment of the National Institute of Nursing Research as a member of the National Institutes of Health (www.nih.gov/ninr), nurses now have an infrastructure in place to ensure that nursing research is supported and that a group of well-prepared nurse researchers will be educated.

The amount of clinically based nursing research conducted is increasing rapidly as nurse researchers strive to develop an independent body of knowledge that demonstrates the value of nursing interventions. The challenge is to move the knowledge acquired by nurse researchers into the clinical area. One way of doing this is through using the principles of evidence-based nursing practice.

Evidence-based practice to improve patient outcomes is a combination of asking an appropriate clinical question; acquiring, appraising and using the highest level of published research; clinical expertise; and patient values and preferences (Melnyk & Fineout-Overholt, 2011). When considering a change in practice, nurses need to take into account both evidence level and evidence quality (rigor, consistency, and sufficiency) of research to determine the strength of evidence (Melnyk & Fineout-Overholt, 2011). To accomplish this effectively, nurses need to be familiar with what constitutes the highest levels of evidence. Evidence level is based on the research design of a study or studies. There are several different approaches to categorizing levels of evidence for nursing, although all are very similar. Table 1-5 summarizes one approach.

Although the area of outcomes research in nursing is expanding, there are not many randomized controlled trials (RCTs) that have been conducted and published by nurses. Nurses can, however, consider

TABLE 1-5	**LEVELS OF EVIDENCE**
EVIDENCE LEVEL	**DESCRIPTION**
I	Evidence from a systematic review or meta-analysis of all relevant RCTs
II	Evidence obtained from well-designed RCTs
III	Evidence obtained from well-designed controlled trials without randomization
IV	Evidence from well-designed case-control and cohort studies
V	Evidence from systematic reviews of descriptive and qualitative studies
VI	Evidence from single descriptive or qualitative studies
VII	Evidence from the opinion of authorities and/or reports of expert committees

Reprinted with permission from Melnyk, B. & Fineout-Overholt, E. (2011). *Evidence-based practice in nursing and healthcare* (2nd ed., p. 12). Philadelphia: Wolters Kluwer/Lippincott Williams & Wilkins.

using high-quality evidence presented in integrative, or systematic, reviews (reviews of collected research on a particular health issue) conducted by a variety of health professionals that includes nurses. One source of high-quality systematic reviews is the *Cochrane Database of Systematic Reviews*; another, as mentioned previously, is the National Guideline Clearinghouse. Nurses should not exclude descriptive or qualitative studies from consideration of a practice change because often, these studies provide more in-depth information about a particular clinical issue.

Finally, practice change should not be made without including the nurse's expertise and abilities to assess what can or cannot be effective for patient outcomes. In some instances, it is not practical or cost effective to make a particular practice change. Nurses should also strongly consider whether a practice change will be acceptable to patients; if the change is not accepted, patients will not incorporate it into their self-care (Melnyk & Fineout-Overholt, 2011).

Although students and inexperienced nurses may not directly participate in research projects, they must learn how useful knowledge obtained by the research team is to their practice. Professional, peer-reviewed journals are the best sources of new information that can help nurses provide improved care and demonstrate that what they do makes a difference in outcomes.

▮ KEY CONCEPTS

- Technologic advances, increasing knowledge, government involvement, and consumer demands have affected changes in child health care in the United States.
- Family-centered child health care, based on the principle that families can make decisions about health care if they have adequate information, has greatly increased the autonomy of families and the responsibility of pediatric nurses.
- Provision of appropriate health care to children relies on adequate health care access, which has been influenced by government and health insurers' responses to efforts to control the costs of health care.

- Infant mortality rates have declined dramatically in the past 50 years; however, the United States continues to rank well below other developed nations, and infant mortality rates still vary widely across ethnic groups. Unintentional injuries are the leading cause of death in children aged 1 to 19 years.
- Poverty is a major social issue that leads to questions about allocation of health care resources, access to care, government programs to increase health care to indigent women and children, and health care rationing.
- Pediatric nurses encounter both ethical and legal issues in their practice and should become familiar with information sources and

standards to assist them with solving ethical dilemmas and adhering to legal regulations.

- Pediatric nurses function in a variety of roles in multiple practice settings, which include acute care, clinics, physicians' offices, home health agencies, schools, rehabilitation centers, summer camps, daycare centers, and hospices.
- The steps of the nursing process, which is integrally related to critical thinking, include assessment (screening and focused), analysis that may result in nursing diagnoses, planning, implementation, and evaluation. The nursing process results in individualized, high-quality, and safe care for children and families.
- Nurses must consider the effect of complementary and alternative therapies when assessing the child and planning care.
- Becoming competent in the collection and application of best evidence for specific care of common problems in nursing practice is now part of the role of every nurse. Relying on traditional care methods rather than determining if evidence supports the methods is no longer sufficient.

REFERENCES

Agency for Healthcare Research and Quality. (2011). AHRQ Publication No. 11-0005-2-EF:*Child and adolescent health care: Selected findings from the 2010 National Healthcare Quality and Disparities Report.* Retrieved from www.ahrq.gov.

Alfaro-LeFevre, R. (2009). *Critical thinking and clinical judgment* (4th ed.). St. Louis: Elsevier.

American Academy of Pediatrics Committee on Child Health Financing. (2010). Principles of health care financing. *Pediatrics, 126,* 1018-1021.

American Academy of Pediatrics Committee on Pediatric Emergency Medicine. (2011). Policy statement: Consent for emergency medical services for children and adolescents. *Pediatrics, 126,* 427-433.

American Academy of Pediatrics, Council on Communications and the Media. (2009a). Policy statement: Media violence. *Pediatrics, 124,* 1995-1503.

American Academy of Pediatrics, Council on School Health. (2009b). Policy statement: Guidelines for the administration of medication in school. *Pediatrics, 124,* 1244-1254.

American Nurses' Association. (2011). *Nursing sensitive indicators.* Retrieved from www.nursingworld.org.

American Association of Colleges of Nursing. (2011). *Defining the clinical nurse leader (CNL®) role.* Retrieved from www.aacn.niche.edu.

Betz, C. (2005). Health care quality and outcome guidelines for nursing of children and families. *Journal of Pediatric Nursing, 20*(3), 149-152.

Carpenito-Moyet, L. (2008). *Handbook of nursing diagnosis* (12th ed.). Philadelphia: Lippincott.

Center for Medicare and Medicaid. (2011). *NHE fact sheet.* Retrieved from www.cms.gov.

Centers for Disease Control and Prevention. (2011). *YRBSS in brief.* Retrieved from www.cdc.gov.

Centers for Disease Control and Prevention, National Center for Chronic Disease Prevention and Health Promotion. (2011). *Oral health: Preventing cavities, gum disease, tooth loss, and oral cancers—at a glance, 2010.* Retrieved from www.cdc.gov.

DeNavas-Walt, C., Proctor, B., & Smith, J. (2010). *Income, poverty and health insurance coverage in the U.S., 2009.* Retrieved from www.census.gov.

Forum on Child and Family Statistics. (2011). *America's children: Key national indicators of well-being, 2011.* Retrieved from www.childstats.gov.

Health Resources and Services Administration. (2009). *Adolescent childbearing.* Retrieved from www.hrsa.gov.

Health Resources and Services Administration. (2010a, August). *Almost one quarter of U.S. children are underinsured.* Retrieved from www.hrsa.gov.

Health Resources and Services Administration. (2010b). *Facilitating children's enrollment and retention in public insurance programs using IT.* Retrieved from www.hrsa.gov.

Huckabay, L. (2009). Clinical reasoned judgment and the nursing process. *Nursing Forum, 44,* 72-78.

Institute of Medicine (IOM). (2011). *Clinical practice guidelines we can trust.* Retrieved from www.iom.edu/cpgstandards.

Kaiser Family Foundation. (2011, April). *Health care spending in the United States and selected OECD countries.* Retrieved from www.kff.org.

Lacey, S., Smith, J., & Cox, K. (2008). *Patient safety and quality: An evidence-based handbook for nurses* (Chapter 15). Retrieved from www.ahrq.gov.

Little, M., Gorman, A., Dzendoletas, D., & Moravac, C. (2007). Caring for the most vulnerable: A collaborative approach to supporting pregnant homeless youth. *Nursing & Women's Health, 11*(5), 458-466.

Lyon, F., & Grow, K. (2011). Case management. In M. Nies & M. McEwen (Eds.). *Community/public health nursing: Promoting the health of populations* (5th ed., pp.152-162). St. Louis: Elsevier.

March of Dimes. (2011). *The serious problem of premature birth.* Retrieved from www.marchofdimes.com.

Masty, J. & Fisher, C. (2008). A goodness-of-fit approach to informed consent for pediatric intervention research. *Ethics and Behavior, 18,* 139-160.

Melnyk, B. & Fineout-Overholt, E. (2011). *Evidence-based practice in nursing and healthcare* (2nd ed., p. 12). Philadelphia: Wolters Kluwer/Lippincott Williams & Wilkins.

National Center for Complementary and Alternative Medicine. (2010). *What is complementary and alternative medicine?* Retrieved from www.nccam.nih.gov.

National Center for Health Statistics (NCHS). (2011). *Health, United States, 2010 with special feature on death and dying.* Hyattsville, Md.: Author.

National Coalition for the Homeless. (2009). *Homeless families with children.* Retrieved from www.nationalhomeless.org.

National Council of State Boards of Nursing. (2011). *Nurse Licensure Compact (NLC).* Retrieved from www.ncsbn.org.

Resha, C. (2010). Delegation in the school setting: Is it a safe practice? *Online Journal of Issues in Nursing, 15*(2), 5.

Robert Wood Johnson Foundation. (2010, August). Unlocking the potential of school nursing: Keeping children healthy, in school, and ready to learn. *Charting Nursing's Future, 14,* 1-8.

United States Department of Health and Human Services. (2010a). *Children's Health Insurance Program Reauthorization Act: One year later, connecting kids to coverage.* Retrieved from www.insurekidsnow.gov.

United States Department of Health and Human Services. (2010b). *Healthy People 2020.* Retrieved from www.healthypeople.gov.

United States Department of Health and Human Services. (2011a). *Accountable care organizations: Improving care coordination for people with Medicare.* Retrieved from www.healthcare.gov.

United States Department of Health and Human Services. (2011b). Understanding the Affordable Care Act. Retrieved from www.healthcare.gov.

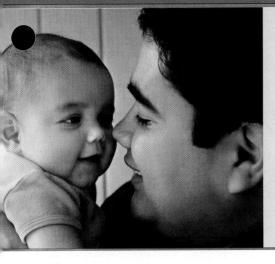

Family-Centered Nursing Care

LEARNING OBJECTIVES

After studying this chapter, you should be able to:

- Explain how important families are for the provision of effective nursing care to children.
- Describe different family structures and their effect on family functioning.
- Differentiate between healthy and dysfunctional families.
- List internal and external coping behaviors used by families when they face a crisis.
- Compare Western cultural values with values of other cultural groups.

- Describe the effect of cultural diversity on nursing practice.
- Describe common styles of parenting that nurses may encounter.
- Explain how variables in parents and children may affect their relationship.
- Discuss the use of discipline in a child's socialization.
- Evaluate the effects of an ill child on the family.

No factor influences a person as profoundly as the family. Families protect and promote children's growth, development, health, and well-being until the children reach maturity. A healthy family provides children and adults with love, affection, and a sense of belonging and nurtures feelings of self-esteem and self-worth. Children need stable families to grow into happy, functioning adults. Family relationships continue to be important during adulthood. Family relationships influence, positively or negatively, people's relationships with others. Family influence continues into the next generation as a person selects a mate, forms a new family, and often rears children.

For nurses in pediatric practice, the whole family is the client. The nurse cares for the child in the context of a dynamic family system rather than caring for just an infant or a child. The nurse is responsible for supporting families and encouraging healthy coping patterns during periods of normal growth and development or illness.

FAMILY-CENTERED CARE

In 1998 the fourth Report of the Pew Health Professions Committee identified 21 competencies for the twenty-first century health professional. One of the competencies is to practice relationship-centered care with individuals and families. In 2003, family-centered care was adopted as a philosophy of care for pediatric nursing (Society of

Pediatric Nurses, 2003). Family-centered care can be defined as an innovative approach to the planning, delivery and evaluation of health care that is grounded in a mutually beneficial partnership among patients, families, and health care professionals (O'Malley, Brown, & Krug, 2008). The American Academy of Pediatrics (AAP) Committee on Hospital Care (2003) noted that family-centered care is grounded in collaboration among patients, families, physicians, nurses, and other professionals for the planning, delivery, and evaluation of health care as well as in the education of health care professionals. The level to which this concept is implemented varies among practitioners. Some of the identified roadblocks are lack of skills in communication, role negotiation, and developing relationships. Other issues that interfere with the full implementation of family-centered care are lack of time, fear of losing one's role, and lack of support from the health care system and other disciplines (Harrison, 2010). Clearly, there is a need for increased education in this area, based on research, to help nurses and other health care professionals implement this concept.

Family Structure

Family structures in the United States are changing. The number of families with children that are headed by a married couple has declined, and the number of single-parent families has increased. In addition, roles have changed within the family. Whereas the role of the provider was once almost exclusively assigned to the father, both parents now may be providers, and many fathers are active in nurturing and disciplining their children.

Types of Families

Families are sometimes categorized into three types: traditional, nontraditional, and high risk. Nontraditional and high-risk families often need care that differs from the care needed by traditional families. Different family structures can produce varying stressors. For example, the single-parent family has as many demands placed on it for resources, such as time and money, as the two-parent family. Only one parent, however, is able to meet these demands.

Traditional Families

Traditional families (also called nuclear families) are headed by two parents who view parenting as the major priority in their lives and whose energies may not be depleted by stressful conditions such as poverty, illness, and substance abuse. Traditional families can be single-income or dual-income families. Generally, traditional families are motivated to learn all they can about pregnancy, childbirth, and parenting (Figure 2-1). Today a family structure composed of two married parents and their children represents 70% of families with children, up 3% from when last reported in 2007. Twenty-six percent of children live with one parent and the remaining 4 percent with no parents (Forum on Child and Family Statistics, 2010).

Single-income families in which one parent, usually the father, is the sole provider are a minority among households in the United States. Most two-parent families depend on two incomes, either to make ends meet or to provide nonessentials that they could not afford on one income. One or both parents may travel as a work responsibility. Dependence on two incomes has created a great deal of stress on parents, subjecting them to many of the same problems that single-parent families face. For instance, reliable, competent child care is a major issue that has increased the stress traditional families experience. A high consumer debt load gives them less cushion for financial setbacks such as job loss. Having the time and flexibility to attend to the requirements of both their careers and their children may be difficult for parents in these families.

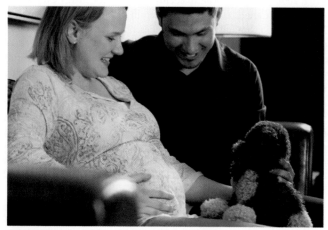

FIG 2-1 Traditional, two-parent families typically have the resources to prepare for childbirth and the needs of infants. (Copyright Getty Images, 2011.)

Nontraditional Families

The growing number of nontraditional families, designated as "complex households" by the U.S. Census Bureau, includes single-parent families, blended families, adoptive families, unmarried couples with children, multigenerational families, and homosexual parent families (Figure 2-2).

Single-Parent Families. Millions of families are now headed by a single parent, most often the mother, who must function as homemaker and caregiver and also is often the major provider for the family's financial needs. Factors contributing to this demographic include divorce, widowhood, and childbirth or adoption among unmarried women. Among the 26% of children who live with one parent, 79% live with their mothers (Forum on Child and Family Statistics, 2010).

Single parents may feel overwhelmed by the prospect of assuming all child-rearing responsibilities and may be less prepared for illness or loss of a job than two-parent families.

Blended Families. Blended families are formed when single, divorced, or widowed parents bring children from a previous union into their new relationship. Many times the couple desires children with each other, creating a contemporary family structure commonly described as "yours, mine, and ours." These families must overcome differences in parenting styles and values to form a cohesive blended family. Differing expectations of children's behavior and development as well as differing beliefs about discipline often cause family conflict. Financial difficulties can result if one parent is obligated to pay child support from a previous relationship. Older children may resent the introduction of a stepmother or stepfather into the family system. This can cause tension between the biologic parent, the children, and the stepmother or stepfather.

Adoptive Families. People who adopt a child may have problems that biologic parents do not face. Biologic parents have the long period of gestation and the gradual changes of pregnancy to help them adjust emotionally and socially to the birth of a child. An adoptive family, both parents and siblings, is expected to make these same adjustments suddenly when the adopted child arrives. Adoptive parents may add pressure to themselves by having an unrealistically high standard for themselves as parents. Additional issues with adoptive families include possible lack of knowledge of the child's health history, the difficulty assimilating if the child is adopted from another country, and the question of when and how to tell the child about being adopted. Adoptive parents and biologic parents need information, support, and guidance to prepare them to care for the infant or child and maintain their own relationships.

Multigenerational Families. The multigenerational or extended family consists of members from three or more generations living under one roof. Older adult parents may live with their adult children, or in some cases adult children return to their parents' home, either because they are unable to support themselves or because they want the additional support that the grandparents provide for the grandchildren. The latter arrangement has given rise to the term *boomerang* families. Extended families are vulnerable to generational conflicts and may need education and referral to counselors to prevent disintegration of the family unit.

Grandparents or other older family members, because of the inability of the parents to care for their children, now head a growing number of households with children. Fifty-two percent of children who do not live with either parent live with a grandparent (Forum on Child and Family Statistics, 2010). The strain of raising children a second time may cause tremendous physical, financial, and emotional stress.

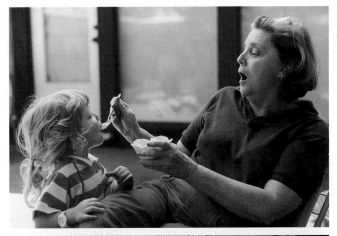

Busy parents may rely on grandparents for child care or for an additional measure of love and attention for their children. Some grandparents raise grandchildren because of their own children's inability to do so.

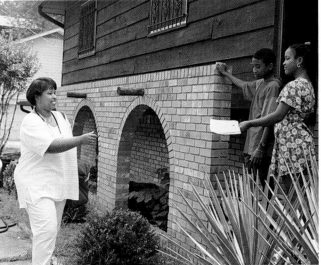

A single parent often experiences financial and time constraints. Children in single-parent families are often given more responsibility to care for themselves and younger siblings.

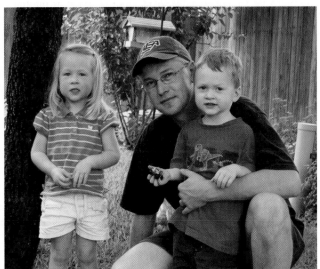

Fathers are the primary child-care providers in a growing number of families. Fathers who are not the primary caregivers often participate more actively in caring for their children than the fathers of previous generations.

FIG 2-2 A nurse caring for a child needs to know the child's family structure and the identity of the child's primary caregiver. This background becomes the context in which the nurse provides care. If family support is a concern, the nurse can provide information about local community resources. For example, in some communities, after-school programs and "warm lines" can help children with schoolwork and alleviate loneliness and fear.

Same-Sex Parent Families. Families headed by same-sex parents have increasingly become more common in the United States. The children in such families may be the offspring of previous heterosexual unions, or they may be adopted children or children conceived by an artificial reproductive technique such as in vitro fertilization. The couple may face many challenges from a community that is unaccustomed to alternative lifestyles. The children's adaptation depends on the parents' psychological adjustment, the degree of participation and support from the absent biologic parent, and the level of community support.

Communal Families. Communal families are groups of people who have chosen to live together as extended family groups. Their relationship to one another is motivated by social value or financial necessity rather than by kinship. Their values are often spiritually based and may be more liberal than those of the traditional family. Traditional family roles may not exist in a communal family.

Characteristics of Healthy Families

In general, healthy families are able to adapt to changes that occur in the family unit. Pregnancy and parenthood create some of the most powerful changes that a family experiences.

Healthy families exhibit the following common characteristics, which provide a framework for assessing how all families function (Cooley, 2009):

- Members of healthy families communicate openly with one another to express their concerns and needs.
- Healthy family members remain flexible in their roles, with roles changing to meet changing family needs.
- Adults in healthy families agree on the basic principles of parenting so that minimal discord exists about concepts such as discipline and sleep schedules.
- Healthy families are adaptable and are not overwhelmed by life changes.

- Members of healthy families volunteer assistance without waiting to be asked.
- Family members spend time together regularly but facilitate autonomy.
- Healthy families seek appropriate resources for support when needed.
- Healthy families transmit cultural values and expectations to children.

Factors that Interfere with Family Functioning

Factors that may interfere with the family's ability to provide for the needs of its members include lack of financial resources, absence of adequate family support, birth of an infant who needs specialized care, an ill child, unhealthy habits such as smoking and abuse of other substances, and inability to make mature decisions that are necessary to provide care for the children. Needs of aging members at the time children are going through adolescence or the expenses of college add pressure on middle-aged parents, often called the "sandwich generation."

High-Risk Families

All families encounter stressors, but some factors add to the usual stress experienced by a family. The nurse needs to consider the additional needs of the family with a higher risk for being dysfunctional. Examples of high-risk families are those experiencing marital conflict and divorce, those with adolescent parents, those affected by violence against one or more of the family members, those involved with substance abuse, and those with a chronically ill child.

Marital Conflict and Divorce

Although divorce is traumatic to children, research has shown that living in a home filled with conflict is also detrimental (Sobolewski & Amato, 2007). Divorce can be the outcome of many years of unresolved family conflict. It can result in continuing conflict over child custody, visitation, and child support; changes in housing, lifestyle, cultural expectations, friends, and extended family relationships; diminished self-esteem; and changes in the physical, emotional, or spiritual health of children and other family members.

Divorce is loss that needs to be grieved. The conflict and divorce may affect children, and young children may be unable to verbalize their distress. Nurses can help children through the grieving process with age-appropriate activities such as therapeutic play (see Chapter 11). Principles of active listening (see Chapter 3) are valuable for adults as well as children to help them express their feelings. Nurses can also help newly divorced or separated parents through listening, encouragement, and referrals to support groups or counselors.

Adolescent Parenting

The teenage birth rate in the United States fell by more than one third from 1991 through 2005 but increased by 5% over the next 2 years. Current data show another downward trend, reaching a historic low of 39.1 per 1000 teen births. Adolescent birth rates vary by race; however, there has been a steady decline in teen birth rates for all racial and ethnic groups. The birth rate for Hispanic teenagers showed the largest decline of all race and ethnicity groups. From 2008 to 2009, the rated declined by 11% (National Center for Health Statistics, 2011).

Teenage parenting often has a negative effect on the health and social outcomes of the entire family. Adolescent girls are at increased risk for a number of pregnancy complications, such as preterm birth, low birth weight, and death during infancy (Ventura & Hamilton,

2011). Those who become parents during adolescence are unlikely to attain a high level of education and, as a result, are more likely to be poor and often homeless. An adolescent father often does not contribute to the economic or psychological support of his child. Moreover, the cycle of teen parenting and economic hardship is more likely to be continued because children of adolescent parents are themselves more likely to become teenage parents.

Violence

Violence is a constant stressor in some families. Violence can occur in any family of any socioeconomic or educational status. Children endure the psychological pain of seeing their mother victimized by the man who is supposed to love and care for her. In addition, because of the role models they see in the adults, children in violent families may repeat the cycle of violence when they are adults and become abusers or victims of violence themselves.

Abuse of the child may be physical, sexual, or emotional or may take the form of neglect (see Chapter 29). Often one child in the family is the target of abuse or neglect, whereas others are given proper care. As in adult abuse, children who witness abuse are more likely to repeat that behavior when they are parents themselves, because they have not learned constructive ways to deal with stress or to discipline children.

Substance Abuse

Parents who abuse drugs or alcohol may neglect their children because obtaining and using the substance(s) may have a stronger pull on the parents than does care of their children. Parental substance abuse interrupts a child's normal growth and development. The parent's ability to meet the needs of the child are severely compromised, increasing the child's risk for emotional and health problems (Children of Alcoholics Foundation, 2011).

The child may be the substance abuser in the home. The drug habit can lead a child into unhealthy friendships and may result in criminal activity to maintain the habit. School achievement is likely to plummet, and the older adolescent may drop out of school. Children as well as adults can die as a result of their drug activity, either directly from the drugs or from associated criminal activity or risk-taking behaviors.

Child with Special Needs

When a child is born with a birth defect or has an illness that requires special care, the family is under additional stress (see Chapters 12 and 30). In most cases their initial reactions of shock and disbelief gradually resolve into acceptance of the child's limitations. However, the parents' grieving may be long term as they repeatedly see other children doing things that their child cannot and perhaps will not ever do.

These families often suffer financial hardship. Health insurance benefits may quickly reach their maximum. Even if the child has public assistance for health care costs, the family often experiences a fall in income because one parent must remain home with the sick child rather than work outside the home.

Strains on the marriage and the parents' relationships with their other children are inevitable under these circumstances. Parents have little time or energy left to nurture their relationship with each other, and divorce may add yet another strain to the family. Siblings may resent the parental time and attention required for care of the ill child yet feel guilty if they express their resentment.

The outlook is not always pessimistic in these families, however. If the family learns skills to cope with the added demands imposed on it by this situation, the potential exists for growth in maturity, compassion, and strength of character.

HEALTHY VERSUS DYSFUNCTIONAL FAMILIES

Family conflict is unavoidable. It is a natural result of a perceived unequal exchange or an imbalance in the use of resources by individual members. Conflict should not be viewed as bad or disruptive; the management of the conflict, not the conflict itself, may be problematic. Conflict can produce growth and improve family functioning if the outcome is resolution as opposed to dissolution or continued conflict. The following three ingredients are required to resolve conflict:

1. Open communication
2. Accurate perceptions about the nature and degree of conflict
3. Constructive efforts to resolve the conflict, such as willingness to consider the view of the other, consider alternate solutions, and compromise

Dysfunctional families have problems in any one or a combination of these areas. They tend to become trapped in patterns in which they maintain conflicts rather than resolve them. The conflicts create stress, and the family must cope with the resultant stress.

Coping with Stress

If the family is considered a balanced system that has internal and external interrelationships, stressors are viewed as forces that change the balance in the system. Stressful events are neither positive nor negative, but rather neutral until they are interpreted by the individual. Positive as well as negative events can cause stress (Smith, Hamon, Ingoldsby, Miller 2009). For example, the birth of a child is usually a joyful event, but it can also be stressful.

Some families are able to mobilize their strengths and resources, thus effectively adapting to the stressors. Other families fall apart. A *family crisis* is a state or period of disorganization that affects the foundation of the family (Smith et al., 2009).

Coping Strategies

Nurses can help families cope with stress by helping each family identify its strengths and resources. Friedman, Bowden, and Jones (2003) identified family coping strategies as internal and external. Box 2-1 identifies family coping strategies and further defines *internal strategies* as family relationship strategies, cognitive strategies, and communication strategies. *External strategies* focus on maintaining active community linkages and using social support systems and spiritual strategies. Some families adjust quickly to extreme crises, whereas other families become chaotic with relatively minor crises. Family functional patterns that existed before a crisis are probably the best indicators of how the family will respond to it.

CULTURAL INFLUENCES ON PEDIATRIC NURSING

Culture is the sum of the beliefs and values that are learned, shared, and transmitted from generation to generation by a particular group. Cultural values guide the thinking, decisions, and actions of the group, particularly regarding pivotal events such as birth, sexual maturity, and death. *Ethnicity* is the condition of belonging to a particular group that shares race, language and dialect, religious faiths, traditions, values, and symbols as well as food preferences, literature, and folklore. Cultural beliefs and values vary among different groups and nurses must be aware that individuals often believe their cultural values and patterns of behavior are superior to those of other groups. This belief, termed ethnocentrism, forms the basis

---

BOX 2-1   COPING STRATEGIES OF FAMILIES

Internal Coping Strategies
Relationship Strategies
- Family group reliance
- Greater sharing together
- Role flexibility

Cognitive Strategies
- Normalizing
- Controlling the meaning of the problem by reframing and passive appraisal
- Joint problem solving
- Gaining of information and knowledge

Communication Strategies
- Being open and honest
- Use of humor and laughter

External Coping Strategies
Community Strategy
- Maintaining active linkages with the community

Social Support Strategies
- Extended family
- Friends
- Neighbors
- Self-help groups
- Formal social supports

Spiritual Strategies
- Seeking advice of clergy
- Becoming more involved in religious activities
- Having faith in God
- Prayer

Reprinted from Friedman, M., Bowden, V., & Jones, E. (2003). *Family nursing: Theory, research, and practice* (5th ed.). Upper Saddle River, NJ: Prentice-Hall.

---

for many conflicts that occur when people from different cultural groups have frequent contact.

Nurses must be aware that culture is composed of visible and invisible layers that could be said to resemble an iceberg (Figure 2-3). The observable behaviors can be compared with the visible tip of the iceberg. The history, beliefs, values, and religion are not observed but are the hidden foundation on which behaviors are based and can be likened to the large, submerged part of the iceberg. To comprehend cultural behavior fully, one must seek knowledge of the hidden beliefs that behaviors express. One must also have the desire or motivation to engage in the process of becoming culturally competent to be effective in caring for diverse populations.

Nurses must first understand their own culture and biases and then begin to acquire the knowledge and understanding of other cultures. Applying the knowledge completes the process (Galanti, 2008).

Religious beliefs often have a strong influence on families as they face the crisis of illness. Specific beliefs about the causes, treatment, and cure of illness are important for the nurse to know to empower the family as they deal with the immediate crisis. Table 2-1 describes how some religious beliefs affect health care.

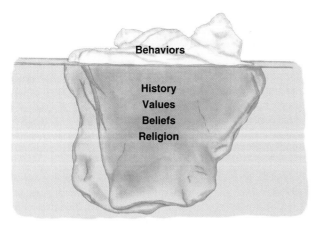

FIG 2-3 Visible and hidden layers of culture are like the visible and submerged parts of an iceberg. Many cultural differences are hidden below the surface.

Implications of Cultural Diversity for Nurses

Many immigrants and refugees are relatively young, so nurses in most localities will provide care for families in culturally diverse circumstances. To provide effective care, nurses must be aware that culture is among the most significant factors that influence parenthood, health and illness, and aging. Many health care workers' knowledge of other cultures and how to care for children and families in a culturally sensitive manner is limited. The following discussion summarizes the characteristics of family roles, health care beliefs and practices, and communication styles of some cultural groups. These descriptions are merely generalizations. Each family is unique and should be assessed and evaluated individually.

Western Cultural Beliefs

Nursing practice in the United States is based largely on Western beliefs. Nurses need to recognize that these beliefs may differ significantly from those of other societies and that the differences may cause a great deal of conflict.

Leininger (1978) identified the following seven dominant Western cultural values; these values continue to greatly influence the thinking and action of nurses in the United States but may not be shared by their clients:

1. *Democracy* is a cultural value not shared by families who believe that elders or other higher authorities in the group make decisions. Fatalism, or a belief that events and results are predestined, may also affect health care decisions.
2. *Individualism* conflicts with the values of many cultural groups in which individual goals are subordinated to the greater good of the group.
3. *Cleanliness* is an American "obsession" viewed with amazement by many people of other cultures.
4. *Preoccupation with time,* which is measured by health care professionals in minutes and hours, is a major source of conflict with those who mark time by different standards, such as seasons or body needs.
5. *Reliance on machines and equipment* may intimidate families who are not comfortable with technology.
6. *The belief that optimal health is a right* is in direct conflict with beliefs in many cultures in the world in which health is not a major emphasis or even an expectation.

7. *Admiration of self-sufficiency and financial success* may conflict with the beliefs of other societies that place less value on wealth and more value on less tangible things such as spirituality.

Cultural Influences on the Care of People from Specific Groups

To provide the best care for all clients, the nurse should know common cultural beliefs and practices that influence nursing care. Because communication is an essential component of nursing assessment and teaching, the nurse must understand cultural influences that may form barriers to communicating with people from another culture.

Asians and Pacific Islanders

"Asian" refers to populations with origins in many areas, such as the Far East, Southeast Asia, and the Indian subcontinent, including Vietnam, China, Japan, and the Philippines. "Pacific Islander" refers to the original peoples of Hawaii, Guam, Samoa, and other Pacific islands. Their roots are in their ethnic viewpoint as well as their country of origin. They are not a homogeneous group, but differ in language, culture, and length of residence in the United States. Asians and Pacific Islanders constitute 4.8% of the U.S. population (United States Census Bureau, 2011).

In the Asian culture the family is highly valued and often consists of many generations that remain close to one another. The elders of the family are highly respected. Self-sufficiency and self-control are highly valued. Asian-Americans place a high value on "face," or honor, and may be unwilling to do anything that causes another to "lose face." When medication or therapy is recommended, they seldom say no. They may accept the prescription or medication sample but not take the medicine, or they may agree to undergo a procedure but not keep the appointment. Stoicism may make pain assessment difficult. Herbal medicines and practices such as acupressure and music therapy may play an important part in healing for this culture.

Besides the national languages of Vietnam, Cambodia, and Laos, numerous languages are spoken within subgroups in each country. People from Southeast Asia speak softly and avoid prolonged eye contact, which they consider rude. Even people who have been in the United States for many years often do not feel competent in English. The nurse should avoid "yes" or "no" questions and have the parent or child demonstrate understanding of any patient teaching (Galanti, 2008).

Families of some hospitalized Pacific Islander clients are involved in their direct care, which may include direct provision of food. Some individuals consult traditional healers. Education related to obesity, diabetes, and hypertension is quite often needed (D'Avanzo, 2008).

Hispanics

Hispanics, also called *Latinos,* include those whose origins are Mexico, Central and South America, Cuba, and Puerto Rico. They are a very diverse group. This group is growing rapidly in the United States, accounting for 14% of the total population in 2005, compared with 16.3% in 2010 (United States Census Bureau, 2011).

Men are usually the head of household and considered strong (macho). Women are the homemakers. Hispanics usually have a close extended family and place a high value on children. Family is valued above work and other aspects of life.

Hispanics tend to be polite and gracious in conversation. Preliminary social interaction is particularly important, and Hispanics may be insulted if a problem is addressed directly without time first being taken for "small talk." This is counter to the value of "getting to the

TABLE 2-1 RELIGIOUS BELIEFS AFFECTING HEALTH CARE

RELIGION AND BASIC BELIEFS	PRACTICES

Christianity

Christianity is generally accepted to be the largest religious group in the world. There are three major branches of Christianity and a number of religious traditions considered to be Christian. These traditions have much in common relative to beliefs and practices. Belief in Jesus Christ as the son of God and the Messiah comprises the central core of Christianity. Christians believe that it is through Jesus' death and resurrection that salvation can be attained. They also believe that they are expected to follow the example of Jesus in daily living. Study of biblical scripture; practicing faith, good works, and sacramental rites (e.g., baptism, communion, and others); and prayer are common among most Christian faiths.

Christian Science

Based on scientific system of healing.

Beliefs derived from both the Bible and the book *Science, and Health with Key to Scriptures.**

Prayer is the basis for spiritual, physical, emotional, and mental healing, as opposed to medical intervention (Christian Science, 2011).

Healing is divinely natural, not miraculous.

Birth: Use physician or midwife during childbirth. No baptism ceremony.

Dietary practices: Alcohol and tobacco are considered drugs and are not used. Coffee and tea also may be declined.

Death: Autopsy and donation of organs are usually declined.

Health care: May refuse medical treatment. View health in a spiritual framework. Seek exemption from immunizations but obey legal requirements. When Christian Science believer is hospitalized, parent or client may request that a Christian Science practitioner be notified.

Jehovah's Witness

Expected to preach house to house about the good news of God.

Bible is doctrinal authority.

No distinction is made between clergy and laity.

Baptism: No infant baptism. Adult baptism by immersion.

Dietary practices: Use of tobacco and alcohol discouraged.

Death: Autopsy decided by persons involved. Burial and cremation acceptable.

Birth control and abortion: Use of birth control is a personal decision. Abortion opposed on basis of Exodus 21:22-23.

Health care: Blood transfusions not allowed. May accept alternatives to transfusions, such as use of non-blood plasma expanders, careful surgical technique to minimize blood loss, and use of autologous transfusions. Nurses should check an unconscious client for identification that states that the person does not want a transfusion. Jehovah's Witnesses are prepared to die rather than break God's law. Respect the health care given by physicians, but look to God and His laws as the final authority for their decisions.

The Church of Jesus Christ of Latter-Day Saints (Mormon)

Restorationism: True church of Christ ended with the first generation of apostles but was restored with the founding of Mormon Church.

Articles of faith: Mormon doctrine states that individuals are saved if they are obedient to God's divine ordinances (faith, repentance, baptism by immersion and laying on of hands).

Holy Communion: Hospitalized client may desire to have a member of the church's clergy administer the sacrament.

Scripture: Word of God can be found in the Bible, Book of Mormon, Doctrine and Covenants, Pearl of Great Price, and current revelations.

Christ will return to rule in Zion, located in America.

Baptism: By immersion. Considered essential for the living and the dead. If a child older than 8 years is very ill, whether baptized or unbaptized, a member of the church's clergy should be called.

Anointing of the sick: Mormons frequently are anointed and given a blessing before going to the hospital and after admission by laying on of hands.

Dietary practices: Tobacco and caffeine are not used. Mormons eat meat (limited) but encourage the intake of fruits, grains, and herbs.

Death: Prefer burial of the body. A church elder should be notified to assist the family.

Birth control and abortion: Abortion is opposed unless the life of the mother is in danger. Only natural methods of birth control are recommended. Other means are used only when the physical or emotional health of the mother is at stake.

Other practices: Believe in the healing power of laying on of hands. Cleanliness is important. Believe in healthy living and adhere to health care requirements. Families are of great importance, so visiting should be encouraged. The church maintains a welfare system to assist those in need.

Adapted from Carson, V.B. (1989). *Spiritual dimensions of nursing practice* (pp. 100-102). Philadelphia: Saunders; Betz, C.L., Hunsberger, M., & Wright, S. (1994). *Family-centered nursing care of children* (2nd ed., pp. 2230-2236). Philadelphia: Saunders; Taylor, E.J. (2002). *Spiritual care: nursing theory, research, and practice.* Upper Saddle River, NJ: Prentice-Hall; Spector, R.E. (2004). *Cultural diversity in health and illness* (6th ed.). Upper Saddle River, NJ: Prentice-Hall; Graham, L., & Cates, J. (2006). Health care and sequestered cultures: A perspective from the old order Amish. *Journal of Nursing and Health, 12*(3), 60-66.

*Eddy, M. B. G. (1875). *Science and Health with Key to Scriptures.* Boston: Christian Science Board of Directors.

Continued

TABLE 2-1 RELIGIOUS BELIEFS AFFECTING HEALTH CARE—cont'd

RELIGION AND BASIC BELIEFS	PRACTICES
Roman Catholicism Belief that the Word of God is handed down to successive generations through scripture and tradition, and is interpreted by the magisterium (the Pope and bishops). Pope has final doctrinal authority for followers of the Catholic faith, which includes interpreting important doctrinal issues related to personal practice and health care.	*Baptism:* Infant baptism by affusion (sprinkling of water on head) or total immersion. Original sin is believed to be "washed away." If death is imminent or a fetus is aborted, anyone can perform the baptism by sprinkling water on the forehead, saying "I baptize thee in the name of the Father, Son, and Holy Spirit." *Anointing of the Sick:* Encouraged for anyone who is ill or injured. Always done if prognosis is poor. *Dietary practices:* Fasting and abstinence from meat optional during Lent. Fasting required for all, except children, elders, and those who are ill, on Ash Wednesday and Good Friday. Avoidance of meat on Ash Wednesday and on Fridays during Lent strongly encouraged. *Death:* Organ donation permitted. *Birth control and abortion:* Abortion is opposed. Only natural methods of birth control are recommended.
Amish Christians who practice their religion and beliefs within the context of strong community ties. Focused on salvation and a happy life after death. Powerful bishops make health care decisions for the community. Problems solved with prayer and discussion. Primarily agrarian; eschew many modern conveniences.	*Baptism:* Late teen/early adult. Must marry within the church. *Death:* Do not normally use extraordinary measures to prolong life. *Other practices:* May have a language issue (modified German or Dutch) and need an interpreter. At increased risk for genetic disorders; refuse contraception or prenatal testing. May appear stoical or impassive—personally humble. Reject health insurance; rely on the Church and community to pay for health care needs. Use holistic and herbal remedies, but accept Western medical approaches.
Hinduism Belief in reincarnation and that the soul persists even though the body changes, dies, and is reborn. Salvation occurs when the cycle of death and reincarnation ends. Nonviolent approach to living. Congregation worship is not customary; worship is through private shrines in the home. Disease is viewed holistically, but Karma (cause and effect) may be blamed.	*Circumcision* is observed by ritual. *Dietary practices:* Dietary restrictions vary according to sect; vegetarianism is not uncommon. *Death:* Death rituals specify practices and who can touch corpse. Family must be consulted, as family members often provide ritualistic care. *Other practices:* May use ayurvedic medicine—an approach to restoring balance through herbal and other remedies. Same-sex health providers may be requested.
Islam Belief in one God that humans can approach directly in prayer. Based on the teachings of Muhammad. Five Pillars of Islam. Compulsory prayers are said at dawn, noon, afternoon, after sunset, and after nightfall.	*Dietary practices:* Prohibit eating pork and using alcohol. Fast during Ramadan (ninth month of Muslim year). *Death:* Oppose autopsy and organ donation. Death ritual prescribes the handling of corpse by only family and friends. Burial occurs as soon as possible.
Judaism Beliefs are based on the Old Testament, the Torah, and the Talmud, the oral and written laws of faith. Belief in one God who is approached directly. Believe Messiah is still to come. Believe Jews are God's chosen people.	*Circumcision:* A symbol of God's covenant with Israel. Done on eighth day after birth. *Bar Mitzvah/Bat Mitzvah:* Ceremonial rite of passage for boys and girls into adulthood and taking personal responsibility for adherence to Jewish laws and rituals. *Death:* Remains are washed according to Jewish rite by members of a group called the Khevra Kadisha. This group of men and women prepare the body for burial and protect it until burial occurs. Burial occurs as soon as possible after death.

point" for many whites in the United States and may cause frustration for the client as well as the health care worker.

Religion and health are strongly associated. The *curandero*, a folk healer, may be consulted for health care before an American health care worker is consulted. Hispanics have great respect for health care providers; however, undocumented Hispanics may fear that a health care worker will disclose their illegal status (Purnell & Paulanka, 2003).

African-Americans

African-Americans constitute 12.6% of the U.S. population (United States Census Bureau, 2011). African-Americans are often part of a close extended family, although many heads of household are single women. They have a sense of loyalty to their people and community, but sometimes distrust the majority group.

Not all black people in the United States were born in this country, however. Natives of Africa and other countries are often found in both health care provider and client populations within the United States.

The African-American minister is highly influential, and religious rituals such as prayer are frequently used. Illness may be seen as the will of God.

American Indians and Alaska Natives

The terms American Indian and Alaska Native refer to people who have origins in any of the original peoples of North and South America and who maintain tribal affiliation or community attachment. This group makes up 0.9% of the total U.S. population (United States Census Bureau, 2011). Many who consider themselves Native Americans are of mixed race. The largest American Indian tribal groups are Cherokee, Navajo, Latin American Indian, Sioux, Chippewa, and Choctaw. The largest tribe among Alaska Natives are the Yupik (United States Census Bureau, 2011).

Native Americans may consider a willful child to be strong and a docile child to be weak. They have close family relationships, and respect for their elders is the norm. Although each American Indian nation or tribe has its own belief system regarding health, the overall traditional belief is that health reflects living in total harmony with nature and disease is associated with the religious aspect of society, because supernatural powers are associated with the causing and curing of disease (Spector, 2009). Native Americans may highly respect a medicine man, whom they believe to be given power by supernatural forces. The use of herbs and rituals is part of the medicine man's curative practice.

Middle Easterners

Middle Eastern immigrants come from several countries, including Lebanon, Syria, Saudi Arabia, Egypt, Turkey, Iran, and Palestine. Islam is the dominant, and often the official, religion in these countries; its followers are known as *Muslims*. The man is typically the head of the household in Muslim families. Islam requires believers to kneel and pray five times a day, at dawn, noon, during the afternoon, after sunset, and after nightfall. Muslims do not eat pork and do not use alcohol. Many are vegetarians. Other dietary standards vary according to the branch of Islam and may include standards such as how the acceptable animal is slaughtered for food.

Muslim women often prefer a female health care provider because of laws of modesty. Many Muslim women cover the head, arms to the wrists, and legs to the ankles although there are many variations in the acceptable degree of coverage. Ritual cleansing before leaving the home or hospital room may be required before the woman dresses in her required modest apparel.

Communication in these countries is elaborate, and obtaining health information may be difficult because Islam dictates that family affairs be kept within the family. Personal information is shared only with friends, and the health assessment must be done gradually. When interpreters are used, they should be of the same country and religion, if possible, because of regional differences and hostilities. Because Islamic society tends to be paternalistic, asking the husband's permission or opinion when family members need health care is helpful.

Cross-Cultural Health Beliefs

More than 100 different ethnocultural groups reside in the United States, and numerous traditional health beliefs are observed among these groups. For example, definitions of health are often culturally based. People of Asian origin may view health as the balance of yin and yang. Those of African or Haitian origin may define health as harmony with nature. Those from Mexico, Central and South America, and Puerto Rico often see health as a balance of hot and cold.

Traditional Methods of Preventing Illness

The traditional methods of preventing illness rest in a person's ability to understand the cause of a given illness in his or her culture. These causes may include the following:

- Agents such as hexes, spells, and the evil eye, which may strike a person (often a child) and cause injury, illness, or misfortune
- Phenomena such as soul loss and accidental provocation of envy, jealousy, or hate of a friend or acquaintance
- Environmental factors such as bad air, and natural events such as a solar eclipse

Practices to prevent illness developed from beliefs about the cause of illness. People must avoid those known to transmit hexes and spells. Elaborate methods are used to prevent inciting envy or jealousy of others and to avoid the evil eye. Protective or religious objects, such as amulets with magic powers or consecrated religious objects (talismans), are frequently worn or carried to prevent illness. Numerous food taboos and traditional combinations are prescribed in traditional belief systems to prevent illness. For instance, people from many ethnic backgrounds eat raw garlic to prevent illness.

Traditional Practices to Maintain Health

A variety of traditional practices are used to maintain health. Mental and spiritual health is maintained by activities such as silence, meditation, and prayer. Many people view illness as punishment for breaking a religious code and adhere strictly to religious morals and practices to maintain health.

Traditional Practices to Restore Health

Traditional practices to restore health sometimes conflict with Western medical practice. Some of the most common practices include the use of natural substances, such as herbs and plants, to treat illness. Religious charms, holy words, or traditional healers may be tried before an individual seeks a medical opinion. Wearing religious medals, carrying prayer cards, and performing sacrifices are other practices used to treat illness.

Homeopathic care, often referred to as "complementary medicine" or "alternative medicine," is becoming more common in health care settings. Acupuncture, massage therapy, and chiropractic medicine are examples of homeopathic care (Spector, 2009).

A variety of substances may be ingested for the treatment of illnesses. The nurse should try to identify what the child is taking and determine whether the active ingredient may alter the effects of prescribed medication.

Practices such as *dermabrasion,* the rubbing or irritation of the skin to relieve discomfort, are common among people of some cultures. The most frequently seen form is *coining,* in which an area is covered with an ointment and the edge of a coin is rubbed over the area. All dermabrasion methods leave marks resembling bruises or burns on the skin and may be mistaken for signs of physical abuse.

Cultural Assessment

All health care professionals must develop skill in performing a cultural assessment so they can understand the meanings of health and illness to the cultural groups they encounter. When assessing a woman, child, or family from a cultural perspective, the nurse considers the following:

- Ethnic affiliation
- Major values, practices, customs, and beliefs related to pregnancy and birth, parenting, and aging
- Language barriers and communication styles
- Family, newborn, and child-rearing practices
- Religious and spiritual beliefs; changes or exemptions during illness, pregnancy, or after birth
- Nutrition and food patterns
- Ethnic health care practices, such as how time is marked and views of life and death
- Health promotion practices
- How health care professionals can be most helpful

After such an assessment, plans for care should show respect for cultural differences and traditional healing practices. A guiding principle for nurses should be one of acceptance of nontraditional methods of health care as long as the practice does not cause harm. In some instances, cultural practices may actually cause unintentional harm; in these circumstances the nurse may need to consult other professionals familiar with the particular cultural practice to provide appropriate care and information for the family. Additional cultural information is presented throughout this book relating to specific areas in child health care.

PARENTING

Parenting implies the commitment of an individual or individuals to provide for the physical and psychosocial needs of a child. Many believe that parenting is the most difficult and yet rewarding experience an individual can have. Many parents assume this important job with little education in parenting or child rearing. If the parents themselves have had parents that are positive role models and if they seek appropriate resources for parenting, the transition to parenting is easier. Nurses are in a good position to provide parents with information on effective parenting skills through many venues, such as formal classes, anticipatory guidance at well-child checkups, and role modeling.

Parenting Styles

Baumrind (1991) described three major parenting styles, which have been generally accepted by experts in child and family development. *Parenting style,* which is the general climate in which a parent socializes a child, differs from *parenting practices,* the specific behavioral guidance parents offer children across the age span. Although the characteristics of parenting styles are described later in their general categories, many specialists in child development acknowledge that characteristics of several parenting styles may be present in parents. In addition, researchers recognize that parenting styles may work in different ways in different cultures.

Authoritarian parents have rules. They expect obedience from the child without any questioning about the reasons behind the rule. They also expect the child to accept the family beliefs and principles without question. Give and take is discouraged.

Children raised with this style of parenting can be shy and withdrawn because of a lack of self-confidence. If the parents are somewhat affectionate, the child may be sensitive, submissive, honest, and dependable. If affection has been withheld, however, the child may exhibit rebellious, antisocial behavior.

Authoritative parents tend to show respect for the opinions of each of their children by allowing them to be different. Although the household has rules, the parents permit discussion if the children do not understand or agree with the rules. The parents emphasize that even though they (the parents) are the ultimate authority, some negotiation and compromise may take place. This style of parenting tends to result in children who have high self-esteem and are independent, inquisitive, happy, assertive, and highly interactive.

Permissive parents have little or no control over the behavior of their children. If any rules exist in the home, they are inconsistent and unclear. Underlying reasons for rules may be given, but the children are generally allowed to decide whether they will follow the rules and to what extent. Limits are not set, and discipline is inconsistent. The children learn that they can get away with any behavior. Role reversal occurs: The children are more like the parents, and the parents are like the children.

Children who come from this type of home are typically disrespectful, disobedient, aggressive, irresponsible, and defiant. They tend to be insecure because of a lack of guidelines to direct their behavior. They are searching for true limits but not finding them. These children tend to be creative and spontaneous.

Regardless of the primary parenting style, parenting is more effective when parents are able to adjust their parenting techniques according to each child's developmental level and when parents are involved and interested in their children's activities and friends.

Parent-Child Relationship Factors

Relationships between parents and children are bidirectional, with the parents' behavior affecting the child and the child's behavior affecting the parenting. The parents' age, experience, and self-confidence affect the quality of the parent-child relationship, the stability of the marital relationship, and the interplay between the child's individualism and the parents' expectations of the child.

Parental Characteristics

Parenting is multidimensional. Parents have an obligation to nurture and care for their children and to provide a moral education through example (Richards, 2010). Parent personality type, personal history of parenting as a child, abilities and competencies, parental skills and expectations, personal health, quality of marital relationship, and relationship quality with others all play a part in determining how a person parents. Parenting behaviors that promote the development of social-emotional, cognitive, and language development are warmth, responsiveness, encouragement, and communication (Roggman, Boyce, & Innocenti, 2008).

In addition, parents who have had previous experience with children, whether through younger siblings, a career, or raising other children, bring an element of experience to the art of parenting. Self-confidence and age also can be factors in a person's ability to parent. How an individual was parented has a major effect on how he or she will assume the role. The strength of the parents' relationship also affects their parenting skills, as does the presence or absence of support systems. Support can come from the family or community. Peer groups can provide an arena for parents to share experiences and solve problems. Parents with more experience are often an important resource for new parents.

Characteristics of the Child

Characteristics that may affect the parent-child relationship include the child's physical appearance, sex, and temperament. At birth the infant's physical appearance may not meet the parents' expectations, or the infant may resemble a disliked relative. As a result, the parent may subconsciously reject the child. If the parents desired a baby of a particular sex, they may be disappointed. If parents are not given the opportunity to talk about this disappointment, they may reject the infant.

Temperament and Parental Expectations

Temperament can be described as the way individuals behave or their behavioral style. Several researchers have studied temperament. Chess and Thomas (1996) developed the following three temperament categories, which are based on nine characteristics of temperament they identified in children (Box 2-2).

1. *Easy:* These children are even tempered, predictable, and regular in their habits. They react positively to new stimuli.
2. *Difficult:* These children are highly active, irritable, moody, and irregular in their habits. They adapt slowly to new stimuli and often express intense negative emotions.
3. *Slow to warm up:* These children are inactive, moody, and moderately irregular in their habits. They adapt slowly to new stimuli and express mildly intense negative emotions.

Some objection to the term *difficult* has been raised because it tends to have a negative connotation. That is the term established in temperament research, however, and parents should recognize that a "difficult" child is quite normal. As is true for other characteristics, such as appearance, the parent-child relationship is likely to have less conflict if the child's temperament meets the parents' expectations.

DISCIPLINE

Children's behavior challenges most parents. The manner in which parents respond to a child's behavior has a profound effect on the child's self-esteem and future interactions with others. Children learn to view themselves in the same way that the parent views them. Thus if parents view their children as wild, the children begin to view

themselves as wild, and soon their actions consistently reinforce their self-image. In this way the children will not disappoint the parents. This pattern is called a *self-fulfilling prophecy* and is a cyclic process.

Discipline is designed to teach a child how to function effectively within society. It is the foundation for self-discipline. A parent's primary goal should be to help the child feel lovable and capable. This goal is best accomplished by the parent's setting limits to enhance a sense of security until the child can incorporate the family's values and is capable of self-discipline.

When a child is in the health care system, the nurse has the opportunity to aid in the socialization of the child to some degree. Scholer, Hudnut-Beumler, and Dietrich (2010) suggest that while parents look to physicians and nurses to provide information about child discipline, time spent assisting parents in this area is not routine in pediatric primary care. In a Level II randomized controlled study, Scholer and colleagues (2010) demonstrated that even a brief intervention in a primary care setting, designed to raise awareness of how to effectively discipline children significantly assisted parents to develop positive disciplinary approaches. Through both formal instruction and informal role modeling, the nurse can help the parent learn how to discipline a child effectively. Box 2-3 lists ways in which a parent or nurse can facilitate children's socialization and increase their self-esteem.

Dealing with Misbehavior

A child's *misbehavior* may be defined as behavior outside the norms of acceptance within the family. Misbehavior stretches the limits of tolerance in all parents, even the most patient. A parent's response to the child's misbehavior can have minor consequences such as short-term frustration or major consequences such as child abuse. To prevent these negative consequences, the nurse can help teach parents various strategies for effective discipline. Whenever disciplinary strategies are used, the parent needs to consider the individual child's developmental level. In addition, discipline should be consistent, the parent should not "give in" to manipulation or tantrums, and the child's feelings should be acknowledged (AAP, 2011). The following are three essential components of effective discipline (AAP Committee on Psychosocial Aspects of Child and Family Health, 1998, reaffirmed 2004):

1. Maintaining a positive, supportive, loving relationship between the parents and the child
2. Using positive reinforcement and encouragement to promote cooperation and desired behaviors
3. Removing reinforcement or applying punishment to reduce or eliminate undesired behaviors

---

BOX 2-2 CHARACTERISTICS OF TEMPERAMENT IN CHILDREN

1. *Level of activity:* The intensity and frequency of motion during playing, eating, bathing, dressing, or sleeping
2. *Rhythmicity:* Regularity of biologic functions (e.g., sleep patterns, eating patterns, elimination patterns)
3. *Approach/withdrawal:* The initial response of a child to a new stimulus, such as an unfamiliar person, unfamiliar food, or new toys
4. *Adaptability:* Ease or difficulty in adjustment to a new stimulus
5. *Intensity of response:* The amount of energy with which the child responds to a new stimulus
6. *Threshold of responsiveness:* The amount or intensity of stimulation necessary to evoke a response
7. *Mood:* Frequency of cheerfulness, pleasantness, and friendly behavior versus unhappiness, unpleasantness, and unfriendly behavior
8. *Distractibility:* How easily the child's attention can be diverted from an activity by external stimuli
9. *Attention span/persistence:* How long the child pursues an activity and continues despite frustration and obstacles

Adapted from Chess, S., & Thomas, A. (1996). *Temperament: Theory and practice.* New York: Brunner-Mazel.

BOX 2-3 EFFECTIVE DISCIPLINE FOR POSITIVE SOCIALIZATION AND SELF-ESTEEM

- Attend promptly to an infant's and young child's needs.
- Provide structure and consistency for young children.
- Give positive attention for positive behavior; use praise when deserved.
- Listen.
- Set aside time every day for one-on-one attention.
- Demonstrate appreciation of the child's unique characteristics.
- Encourage choices and decision making, and allow the child to experience consequences of mistakes.
- Model respect for others.
- Provide unconditional love.

Punishment is used to eliminate a behavior and can be in the form of a verbal reprimand or physical action to emphasize a point. The AAP discourages the use of spanking and other forms of physical punishment (AAP, 2011).

Redirection

Redirection is a simple and effective method in which the parent removes the problem and distracts the child with an alternative activity or object. This method is helpful with infants through preadolescents.

Reasoning

Reasoning involves explaining why a behavior is not permitted. Younger children lack the cognitive skills and developmental abilities to comprehend reasoning fully. For example, a 4-year-old may better understand the consequence that he will have to spend time in his room if he breaks his brother's toy than the concept of respecting the property of others.

When this technique is used with older children, the behavior should be the object of focus, not the child. The child should not be made to feel guilt and shame, because these feelings are counterproductive and can damage the child's self-esteem. The parent can focus on the behavior most effectively by using "I" rather than "you" messages.

A "you" message criticizes children and uses guilt in an attempt to get them to change their behavior. An example of a "you" message is "Don't take your little sister's toys away and make her cry. You're being a bad boy!" By contrast, an "I" message focuses on the misbehavior by explaining its effect on others. An example of an "I" message is, "Your little sister cries when you take her toys away because she doesn't know that you will give them back to her."

Time-Out

Time-out is a method of removing the attention given to a child who is misbehaving. It involves placing the child in a nonstimulating environment where the parent can observe unobtrusively. For example, a chair could be placed facing a wall in a hall or nearby room. The child is told to sit on the chair for a predetermined time, usually 1 minute per year of age. If the child cries or fights, the timing is not begun until the child is quiet. The use of a kitchen timer with a bell is effective because the child knows when the time begins and when it has elapsed and the child can get up. After the child has calmed and the time is completed, discussion of the behavior that prompted the time-out at a level appropriate to the child's age may be helpful.

Consequences

The consequences technique helps children learn the direct result of their misbehavior and can be used with toddlers through adolescents. If children must deal with the consequences of their behavior and the consequences are meaningful to them, they are less likely to repeat the behavior. Consequences fall into the following three categories:

1. *Natural:* Consequences that occur spontaneously. For example, a child loses a favorite toy after leaving it outside and the parent does not replace it.
2. *Logical:* Consequences that are directly related to the misbehavior. For example, when two children are fighting over a toy, the parent removes the toy from both of them for a day.
3. *Unrelated:* Consequences that are purposely imposed. For example, a child comes in late for dinner and, as a consequence, is not allowed to watch TV that evening.

Some parents have difficulty allowing their children to face the consequences of their actions. When parents choose to deny their child this experience, the child loses an important opportunity to teach responsibility for one's actions.

Behavior Modification

The behavior modification technique of discipline rewards positive behavior and ignores negative behavior. This technique requires parents to choose selected behaviors, preferably only one at a time, that they desire to stop. They choose others that they want to encourage. The basic technique is useful for any age from toddlerhood through adolescence. For a young child, the selected positive behaviors are marked on a chart and explained to the child. For an older child, a contract can be written. The negative behaviors are kept in mind by the parents but are not recorded where the child can see them. A system of rewards is established. Stickers or stars on a chart for young children and tokens for older children are effective ways to record the behaviors. Children should receive a predetermined reward (e.g., a movie, book, or outing, but not food) after they successfully perform the behavior a set number of times. This system should continue for several months until the behavior becomes a habit for the child. Then the external reward should be gradually withdrawn. The child develops internal gratification for successful behavior rather than relying on external reinforcement. Children gain a sense of mastery and actually enjoy the process, often viewing it as a game.

⚡ SAFETY ALERT

Avoiding the Use of Corporal Punishment as Discipline

Corporal punishment can lead to child abuse if the disciplinarian loses control. It can also lead to false accusations of child abuse by either the child or other adults. Because of the high cost and low benefit of this form of punishment, parents should avoid its use.

Negative behaviors are simply ignored. If the parent refuses to give the child attention for the behavior, the child soon gives up that strategy. Consistency is the key to success for this technique, and many parents find this method difficult to enforce. Parents need to be warned that children frequently test the seriousness of this attempt by increasing their negative behavior soon after the parents begin ignoring it. If this technique is to be successful, the parents need to ignore the negative behavior every time.

Corporal Punishment

Corporal punishment usually takes the form of spanking. It is highly controversial and should be discouraged. Corporal punishment has many undesirable results, which include physical aggression toward others and the belief that causing pain to others is acceptable (AAP, 2011). Adults who were spanked as children are more likely than those who were not spanked to experience depression, use substances, and commit domestic violence (AAP, 2011). Use of spanking as discipline can result in loss of control and child injury.

Because of the negative consequences of spanking and because it is no more effective than other methods of discipline, the AAP (2011) recommends that parents be encouraged and helped to develop methods of discipline other than spanking.

NURSING PROCESS AND THE FAMILY

Family Assessment

When assessing family health, the nurse first must determine the structure of the family. The structure is the actual physical composition of the family, the family's environment, and the occupations and education of its members. Diagrams can assist with this process. A *genogram*, also known as a *pedigree*, which illustrates family relationships and health issues, looks like a family tree with three generations of family members represented. An *ecomap* is a pictorial representation of the family structure and relationships with factors in the external environment.

Next the nurse needs to determine how well the family is fulfilling its five major functions as described by Friedman, Bowden, & Jones (2003):

1. *Affective function (personality maintenance function):* to meet the psychological needs of family members—trust, nurturing, intimacy, belonging, bonding, identity, separateness and connectedness, need-response patterns, and the therapeutic role of the individuals in the family.
2. *Socialization function (social placement):* to guide children to be productive members of society and transmit cultural beliefs to the next generation.
3. *Reproductive function:* to ensure family continuity and societal survival.
4. *Economic function:* to provide and effectively allocate economic resources.
5. *Health care function:* to provide the physical necessities of life (e.g., food, clothing, shelter, health care), to recognize illness in family members and provide care, and to foster a healthy lifestyle or environment based on preventive medical and dental health practices.

Health problems can arise from structural problems, such as too few or too many people sharing the same living quarters. If too few people are present, children may be left unattended; too many people may lead to overcrowding, stress, and the spread of communicable diseases. Environmental problems include impure drinking water, inadequate sewage facilities, damaged electric wiring and outlets, and inadequate sleeping conditions. Other environmental factors, such as rodents, crime, and noise, can affect health. Occupation and education can affect health through lack of adequate supervision of children; inability to purchase physical necessities, such as food; inability to purchase health insurance; and stress from employment dissatisfaction.

❓ CRITICAL THINKING EXERCISE 2-1

Create a genogram of your family. Can you identify health issues and trends from looking at the genogram? What are the implications for nursing care?

Nursing Diagnosis and Planning

After using the various tools to assess the child's family completely, the nurse identifies the appropriate nursing diagnoses. These will differ according to the specific family assessment data. The following general nursing diagnoses can be used for families:

- Risk for Caregiver Role Strain
- Compromised Family Coping
- Interrupted Family Processes
- Impaired Parenting
- Risk for Impaired Attachment
- Ineffective Family Therapeutic Regimen Management
- Social Isolation

Other diagnoses may also be appropriate. The expected outcomes for each diagnosis would be specifically tailored to the family's needs.

Intervention and Evaluation

Interventions also are specific for the child and family, but most family interventions are directed toward enhancing positive coping strategies and directing the family to appropriate resources. The nurse adapts general family interventions to each family's unique needs but in particular helps the family to do the following:

- Identify and mobilize internal and external strengths
- Access appropriate resources in the extended family and community
- Recognize and enhance positive communication patterns
- Decide on a consistent discipline approach and access parenting programs if needed
- Maintain comforting cultural and religious traditions and sources of healing
- Engage in joint problem solving
- Acquire new knowledge by providing information about a specific health problem or issue
- Become empowered
- Allocate sufficient privacy, space, and time for leisure activities
- Promote health for all family members during times of crisis

Once families have participated in needed intervention, evaluation criteria are tailored to the specific intervention and individualized for the family.

KEY CONCEPTS

- Traditional families may be single-income or dual-income families. Two-income families are much more common at present.
- Nontraditional family structures (single-parent, blended, adoptive, multigenerational [extended], and same-sex parent families) may require nursing care that is different from that required by traditional families.
- High-risk families have additional stressors that affect their functioning. Examples are families headed by adolescents; families affected by marital discord or divorce, violence, or substance abuse; and families with a severely or chronically ill member.
- All families experience stress; how the family deals with stress is the important factor.

- Identifying healthy versus dysfunctional family patterns can help the nurse implement effective strategies to care for the child and the family.
- Clients during health and illness are cared for within the framework of their families and their cultures.
- Traditional cultural beliefs may be used to prevent illness, maintain health, and restore health.
- Differing cultural beliefs and expectations between the health care provider and the family can create conflict.
- The nurse can help parents learn effective discipline methods by teaching and role modeling.
- Assessing the structure and function of the family is a basic part of caring for any child.

REFERENCES

American Academy of Pediatrics. (2011, May). *Disciplining your child*. Retrieved from www.healthychildren.org.

American Academy of Pediatrics Committee on Hospital Care. (2003). Family-centered care and the pediatrician's role. *Pediatrics, 112*(3), 691-696.

American Academy of Pediatrics Committee on Psychosocial Aspects of Child and Family Health. (1998). Guidance for effective discipline. *Pediatrics, 101*(4), 723-728. Policy reaffirmed in 2004.

Baumrind, D. (1991). Effective parenting during the early adolescent transition. In P. Cowan & M. Hetherington (Eds.), *Family transitions (Chapter 5)*. Hillsdale, NJ: Lawrence Erlbaum.

Carson, V. B. (1989). *Spiritual dimensions of nursing practice*. Philadelphia: Elsevier.

Chess, S., & Thomas, A. (1996). *Temperament theory and practice*. New York: Brunner-Mazel.

Children of Alcoholics Foundation. (2011). *Effects of parental substance abuse on children and families*. Retrieved from www.coaf.org/professonals/effects%20.htm.

Christian Science. (2011). *About Christian Science: Core beliefs*. Retrieved from www.christianscience.com.

Cooley, M. (2009). A family perspective in community/public health nursing. In F. Maurer & C. Smith (Eds.), *Community/Public Health Nursing* (4th ed., p. 340). St. Louis: Elsevier.

D'Avanzo, C. E. (2008). *Mosby's pocket guide to cultural health assessment* (4th ed.). St. Louis: Mosby.

Forum on Child and Family Statistics. (2010). *America's children in brief: Key national indicators of well-being, 2010*. Washington, DC: U.S. Government Printing Office.

Friedman, M. M., Bowden, V. R., & Jones, E. G. (2003). *Family nursing: Theory, research and practice* (5th ed., pp. 593-594). Upper Saddle River, NJ: Prentice-Hall.

Galanti, G. A. (2008). *Caring for patients from different cultures*. Philadelphia: University of Pennsylvania Press.

Harrison, T. M. (2010). Family-centered pediatric nursing care: State of the science. *Journal of Pediatric Nursing, 25*, 335-343.

Leininger, M. (1978). *Transcultural nursing: Concepts, theories, practices*. New York: Wiley.

National Center for Health Statistics. (2011). *Data Brief: U.S. Teenage birth rate resumes decline*. Retrieved from www.cdc.gov/nchs/data/databriefs/db58.htm.

O'Malley, P. J., Brown, K., & Krug, S. E. (2008). Patient and family-centered care of children in the emergency department. *Pediatrics, 122*(2), e511-e512.

Purnell, L. D., & Paulanka, B. J. (2003). *Transcultural health care: A culturally competent approach* (2nd ed.). Philadelphia: F.A. Davis.

Richards, N. (2010). *The ethics of parenthood*. New York, Oxford Press.

Roggman, L. A., Boyce, L. K., & Innocenti, M. S. (2008). *Developmental parenting*. Baltimore, MD: Paul H Brookes Publishing Co.

Scholer, S., Hudmut-Beumler, J., & Dietrich, M. (2010). A brief primary care intervention helps parents develop plans to discipline. *Pediatrics, 125*, e242-e249.

Smith, S. R., Hamon, R. R., Ingoldsby, B. B., & Miller, J. E. (2009). *Exploring family theories*. New York: Oxford University Press.

Sobolewski, F., & Amato, P. (2007). Parents' discord and divorce, parent-child relationships and subjective well-being in early adulthood: Is feeling close to two parents always better than feeling close to one? *Social Forces, 85*(3), 1105-1124.

Society of Pediatric Nurses. (2003). *Family centered care: Putting it into action. SPN/ANA Guide to Family-Centered Care*. Washington, DC.: Society of Pediatric Nurses/American Nurses Association.

Spector, R. E. (2009). *Cultural diversity in health and illness* (7th ed.). Upper Saddle River, NJ: Prentice-Hall.

United States Census Bureau. (2011). *2010 Census Briefs*. Retrieved from www.2010.census.gov/2010census/data.

Ventura, M. A., & Hamilton, B. E. (2011). *U.S. teenage birth rate resumes decline*. Centers for Disease Control and Prevention. NCHS Data Brief. Retrieved from www.cdc.gov/nchs/data/databriefs/db58.

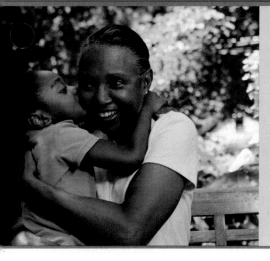

Communicating with Children and Families

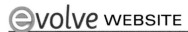 **WEBSITE**

http://evolve.elsevier.com/James/ncoc

LEARNING OBJECTIVES

After studying this chapter, you should be able to:

- Describe six components of effective communication with children.
- Describe communication strategies that assist nurses in working effectively with children.
- Explain the importance of avoiding communication pitfalls in working with children.

- Describe effective family-centered communication strategies.
- Describe effective strategies for communicating with children with special needs.
- Describe warning signs of overinvolvement and underinvolvement in child/family relationships.

To work effectively with children and their families, nurses need to develop keen communication skills. Because parents and other family members play a crucial role in the lives of pediatric clients, nurses need to establish rapport with the family in order to identify mutual goals and facilitate positive outcomes. An awareness of body language, eye contact, and tone of voice must accompany good verbal communication skills when one is listening to children and their families. The same awareness helps nurses assess their own communication styles.

COMPONENTS OF EFFECTIVE COMMUNICATION

Communication is much more than words going from one person's mouth to another person's ears. In addition to the words themselves, the tone and quality of voice, eye contact, physical proximity, visual cues, and overall body language convey messages. These nonverbal communications are often undervalued. Research has shown that verbal content makes up only 7% of a message, whereas body language accounts for 55% and paralanguage (intonation, pauses, sighs) represents the remaining 38% (Topper, 2004). In choosing communication techniques to be used with children and families, the nurse considers cultural differences, particularly with regard to touch and personal space (see Chapter 2). Communication provides an important linkage between parents and providers that is based on honesty, caring, respect, and a direct approach (Fisher & Broome, 2011). Good communication is key to the identification of health issues, adherence to a treatment plan, and improved psychological and behavioral outcomes (Levetown & Committee on Bioethics, 2008).

Touch

Touch can be a positive, supportive technique that is effective from birth through adulthood. Touch can convey warmth, comfort, reassurance, security, trust, caring, and support.

In infancy, messages of love, security, and comfort are conveyed through holding, cuddling, gentle stroking, and patting. Infants do not have cognitive understanding of the words they hear, but they sense the emotional support and they can feel, interpret, and respond to gentle, loving, supportive hands caring for them. Toddlers and preschoolers find it soothing and comforting to be held and rocked as well as stroked gently on the head, back, arms, and legs (Figure 3-1).

School-age children and adolescents appreciate giving and receiving hugs and getting a reassuring pat on the back or a gentle hand on the hand. The nurse, however, needs to request permission for any contact beyond a casual touch with these clients.

Physical Proximity and Environment

Children's familiarity and comfort with their physical surroundings affect communication. Normally, children are most at ease in their home environments. Once they enter a clinic, emergency department, or patient care unit, they are in an unfamiliar environment and they experience heightened anxiety. Hospital and clinic staff members have a tremendous advantage in knowing their clinic or unit as a familiar workplace. Nurses can gain a better picture of what a child is experiencing by trying to place themselves in the child's position and imagining the child's first impression of the triage desk, the reception desk, the admitting office, the treatment room, and the hospital room. A

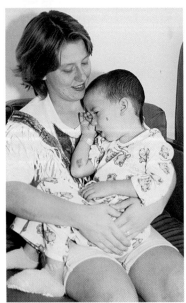

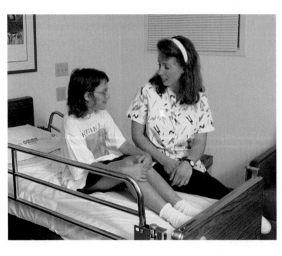

A child can communicate more easily with a nurse who is at eye level and at a comfortable conversational distance. The nurse may need to squat or even sit on the floor to talk with very young children.

Touch is a powerful means of communicating. Toddlers and preschoolers often find touch in the form of cuddling and stroking to be soothing. Even older children who prize their independence find that a parent's hug or pat on the back helps them feel more secure.

FIG 3-1 Communication with children is enhanced by direct eye contact and by body language that conveys attentiveness and openness.

child's perspective is probably very different from an adult's. Creating a supportive, inviting environment for children includes the use of child-size furniture, colorful banners and posters, developmentally appropriate toys, and art displayed at a child's eye level.

Individuals have different comfort zones for physical distance. The nurse should be aware of differences and should move cautiously when meeting new children and families, respecting each individual's personal space. For example, standing over the child and family can be intimidating. Instead, the nurse should bring a chair and sit near the child and family. This action puts the nurse at eye level. If a chair is not accessible, the nurse may stoop or squat. The important part is to be at eye level while remaining at a comfortable distance for the child and family (Figure 3-2).

The nurse should not overlook privacy or underestimate its importance. A room should be available for conducting private conversations away from roommates or family members and visitors. Privacy is particularly critical in working with adolescents, who typically will not discuss sensitive topics with parents present. The nurse's skill and ease with parents of adolescents will increase the adolescents' trust in the nurse. Nurses need to avoid hallway conversations, particularly outside a child's room, because children and parents may overhear only some words or phrases and misinterpret the meaning. Overhearing may lead to unnecessary stress and mistrust between the health care providers and the child or family.

Listening

Messages given must be received for communication to be complete. Therefore, listening is an essential component of the communication process. By practicing active listening skills, nurses can be effective listeners. Active listening skills are as follows.

Attentiveness

The nurse should be intentional about giving the speaker undivided attention. Eliminating distractions whenever possible is important. For example, the nurse should maintain eye contact, close the room door,

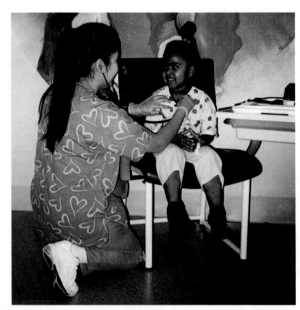

FIG 3-2 For effective communication, the nurse needs to be at the child's eye level. (Courtesy Pat Spier, RN-C. In Leifer, G. [2011]: *Introduction to maternity & pediatric nursing*, [6th ed.], St. Louis: Elsevier.)

and eliminate potential distractions (e.g., TV, computer, video games, smartphones).

Clarification through Reflection

Using similar words, the nurse expresses to the speaker what was heard and understood about the content of the message. For example, when the child or family member says, "I hate the food that comes on my tray," a reflective response would be, "When you say you are unhappy with the food you've been given, what can we do to change that?" As the conversation progresses, the nurse can move the child through a dialogue that identifies those nutritional foods the child would eat.

Empathy

The nurse identifies and acknowledges feelings expressed in the message. For example, if a child is crying after a procedure, the nurse might say, "I know it is uncomfortable to have this procedure. It is okay to cry. You did a great job holding still."

Impartiality

To understand and avoid prejudicing what is heard with personal bias, the nurse listens with an open mind. For example, if a young adolescent shares that she is sexually active and is mainly concerned about sexually transmissible infections, the nurse remains a supportive listener. The nurse can then provide her with educational materials and resources as well as discuss the possible outcomes of her actions in a manner that is open and not judgmental, regardless of the nurse's personal values and beliefs.

During shift report, descriptions of family must be shared objectively and impartially. Otherwise, perceptions of families may negatively affect how colleagues approach and interact with families.

To enhance the effectiveness of communication and maximize normal language patterns that contribute to language development, the nurse focuses on talking with children rather than to them and develops conversations with children.

The nurse must be prepared to listen with the eyes as well as the ears. Information will not always be audible, so the nurse must be alert to subtle cues in body language and physical closeness. Only then can one fully understand the messages of children. For example, when the nurse enters the room to complete an initial assessment of a 4-year-old child and observes the child turning away and beginning to suck her thumb, the child is communicating about her basic security and comfort level, although she has not said a word.

! NURSING QUALITY ALERT

Tips to Enhance Listening and Communication Skills

- Children understand more clearly than they can speak.
- To develop conversations with children, ask open-ended questions rather than questions requiring yes-or-no responses.
- Comprehension is increased when the nurse uses different methods to present and share information.
- Use "people-first" language (e.g., "Sally in 428 has cystic fibrosis" instead of "The CF patient in 428 is Sally.")

Visual Communication

Eye contact is a communication connector. Making eye contact helps confirm attention and interest between the individuals communicating. Direct eye contact may be uncomfortable, however, for people in some cultures, so the nurse needs to be sensitive to responses when making eye contact.

Clothing, physical appearance, and objects being held are visual communicators. Children may react to an individual's presence on the basis of a white lab coat, a bushy beard, or a syringe or video game in the hand. The nurse needs to think ahead and anticipate visual stimuli a child may find startling and those that may be pleasing and to make appropriate adjustments when possible. For example, it is a routine practice for nurses to bring a medication in a syringe for insertion into an intravenous (IV) line. Unless the purpose of the syringe is immediately explained, children might immediately assume they are about to receive an injection.

Some children, and some adults, are visual learners. They learn best when they can see or read instructions, demonstrations, diagrams, or information. Using various methods of presenting and sharing information will increase comprehension for such children.

Concepts can be presented more vividly by using photographs, videotapes, dolls, computer programs, charts, or graphs than by using written or spoken words alone. The nurse needs to select teaching tools and materials that appropriately match the child's growth and developmental level.

Tone of Voice

The spoken word comes to mind most often when communication is the topic. Communication, however, consists of not only what is said but also the way it is said. The tone and quality of voice often communicate more than the words themselves.

Because infants' cognitive understanding of words is limited, their understanding is based on tone and quality of voice. A soft, smooth voice is more comforting and soothing to infants than a loud, startling, harsh voice. Infants can sense from the tone of voice whether the caregiver is angry or happy, frustrated or calm. The nurse can assess how aware of and sensitive to these messages infants are by observing their body language. Infants are relaxed when they hear a calm, happy caregiver and tense and rigid when they hear an angry, frustrated caregiver.

Children can detect anger, frustration, joy, and other feelings that voices convey, even when the accompanying words are incongruent. This incongruity can be very confusing for children. The nurse should strive to make words and their intended meanings match.

Verbal communication extends beyond actual words. All audible sounds convey meaning. An infant's primary mode of audible communication is crying. Crying is a cue to check basic needs, including hunger, pain, discomfort (e.g., wet diaper), and temperature. Cooing and babbling, also heard during the first year of life, generally convey messages of comfort and contentment. As children develop and mature, they have larger vocabularies to express their ideas, thoughts, and feelings.

The choice of words is critical in verbal communication. The nurse needs to avoid talking down to children but should not expect them to understand adult words and phrases. Technical health care terms should be used selectively, and jargon should be avoided (see Table 3-4).

Body Language

From the gentle caress of holding an infant to sitting and listening intently to an adolescent's story, body language is a factor in communication. An open body stance and positioning invite communication and interaction, whereas a closed body stance and positioning impede communication and interaction.

Using an open body posture improves the nurse's understanding of children and the children's understanding of the nurse. Nurses need to learn to read children's body language and should become more aware of their own body language. Table 3-1 compares open and closed body postures.

Timing

Recognizing the appropriate time to communicate information is a developed skill. A distraught child whose parents have just left for work is not ready for a diabetic teaching session. The session will be much more productive and the information better understood if the child has a chance to make the transition. The convenience of a schedule should be secondary to meeting a child's needs.

FAMILY-CENTERED COMMUNICATION

Any discussion about effective ways to communicate with children must also include a discussion of effective communication with families. Family-centered care emphasizes that the family is intimately involved in the care of the child. Parents need to be supported while sustaining their parental role during their child's hospitalization (Sanjari, Shirazi, Heidari, et al., 2009). Family-centered care is achieved when health care professionals can create partnerships with families, recognizing that the family is essential to the child and that the family has the right to participate fully in planning, implementing, and evaluating the child's plan of care.

Commitment to family-centered care means that the nurse respects the family's diversity. Children and parents live in a variety of family structures. An expanded definition of family is required in the twenty-first century, because the term no longer refers to only the intact, nuclear family in which parents raise their biologic children. Contemporary family structures include adolescent parents; extended families with aunts, uncles, or cousins parenting; multigenerational families with grandparents parenting; blended families with stepparents and stepsiblings; gay or lesbian parents; foster parents; group homes; and homeless children. The nurse should be prepared to identify the foundational strengths in all family structures (see Chapter 2). Family-centered care also means that the nurse truly believes that the child's care and recovery are greatly enhanced when the family fully participates in the child's care (Figure 3-3).

! NURSING QUALITY ALERT

Communicating with Families

- Include all involved family members. One essential step toward achieving a family-centered care environment is to develop open lines of communication with the family.
- Encourage families to write down their questions.
- Remain nonjudgmental.
- Give families both verbal and nonverbal signals that send a message of availability and openness.
- Respect and encourage feedback from families.
- Families come in various shapes, sizes, colors, and generations.
- Avoid assumptions about core family beliefs and values.
- Respect family diversity.

Establishing Rapport

Critical to establishing rapport with families is the nurse's ability to convey genuine respect and concern during the first encounter. A nonjudgmental approach and a willingness to assist family members in effectively caring for their child demonstrate the nurse's interest in their well-being.

Availability and Openness to Questions

A nurse who does not take time to see how a child and family are doing—such as a nurse who leaves a room immediately after a treatment or administration of a medication—will not encourage or invite families to ask questions. Families want and need unrushed and uninterrupted time with the nurse. Sometimes this time can be made

TABLE 3-1	OPEN AND CLOSED BODY POSTURES	
OPEN	**CLOSED**
Leaning toward other person	Leaning away from other person
Arms loose at sides	Arms folded across chest
Frequent eye contact	No eye contact
Hands moving freely	Hands on hips
Soft stance, body swaying slightly	Rigid stance
Head up	Head bowed
Calm, slow movements	Constant motion, squirming
Smiling, friendly facial cues	Frowning, negative facial cues
Conversing at eye level	Conversing at a level that requires the child to move to listen

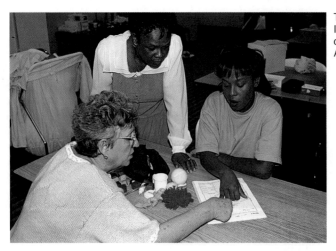

This nurse practitioner has learned Spanish to communicate better with her many Spanish-speaking clients. Speaking with family members in their own language encourages the family to remain in the health care system. The nurse is also using eye contact and has positioned herself at the mother's eye level. (Courtesy Parkland Health and Hospital System Community Oriented Primary Care Clinic, Dallas.)

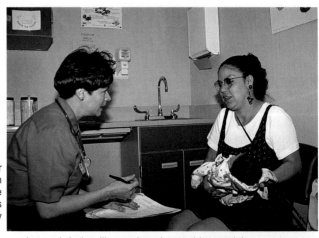

The nurse explains a child's test results to his mother and grandmother. Including all important family members in the child's health care reflects commitment to family-centered care. (Courtesy University of Texas at Arlington College of Nursing.)

FIG 3-3 The child's continuing health care, both preventive and during illness, is enhanced by participation of the family.

available only by purposefully scheduling it into the day. Encouraging families to write down their questions will enable them to take full advantage of their time with the nurse.

The nurse might encourage effective use of time by saying, "I know you have a lot of questions and are very anxious to learn more about your son's condition. I have another patient who has an immediate need, but I will be available in 10 minutes to meet with you. In the meantime, here is a parent handbook that gives general information about seizures. Please feel free to review it and write down any questions that we can discuss when I return."

Family Education and Empowerment

Educating parents about their child's condition, ensuring their continued involvement in planning and evaluating the plan of care, and teaching them the skills to participate empower the family. Families need support as they gain confidence in their skills, and they need guidance to assist them as they navigate through the health care experience. Communication is enhanced when families feel competent and confident in their abilities.

Effective Management of Conflict

When conflict occurs, it should be addressed in an expedient manner to prevent further breakdown in communication. Box 3-1 suggests strategies for managing conflict, and Table 3-2 highlights the importance of choosing words carefully to make families feel welcome and to further facilitate family-centered care.

Feedback from Children and Families

The nurse needs to be alert for both verbal and nonverbal cues. Routinely checking with family members about their experiences, satisfaction with communications, teaching sessions, and health care goals is an effective way to ensure that health care providers obtain appropriate feedback. To enhance the delivery of care, the nurse should explain how this feedback will be used. The nurse should listen and observe carefully to make sure that what family members are saying is truly what they are feeling.

Transparent communication between parents and nurses is integral to providing family-centered care (McCann, Young, Watson, et al, 2008). For example, while one nurse was teaching the mother of a 2-year-old child who was recently diagnosed with type 1 diabetes mellitus, the mother reported that, although she was her child's primary caregiver, the child's grandmother frequently cared for the child while the mother was at work. The nurse therefore notified the other team members and altered the teaching plan for diabetes care to include the child's grandmother.

Spirituality

Children have rich spiritual lives, although they do not use the same vocabulary as adults to describe them. Spiritual care is a vital coping resource for many children. In order to provide holistic care to children, it is important to assess the child's beliefs and faith (Neuman, 2011). Supporting children's existing faith and spiritual practices is recommended. Children can be assisted in maintaining their rituals, whether they are bedtime prayers, songs, or blessings at meals. Nurses can provide spiritual care in ways that offer hope, encouragement, comfort, and respect. A resource to pursue in many hospital or health care settings is the pastoral care or chaplain's department.

BOX 3-1 STRATEGIES FOR MANAGING CONFLICT

- *Understand the parents' perspective (walk in their shoes).* Imagine yourself as the parent of a child in a hospital where your values and beliefs are exposed and scrutinized. Try to understand the parents' perspective better by encouraging them to share it.
- *Determine a common goal and stay focused on it.* Determine the agreed-on result, and work toward it. By staying focused on a common goal, the parties involved are more likely to find workable strategies to achieve the identified goal.
- *Seek win-win solutions.* Conflict should not be about who is right and who is wrong. Effective conflict management focuses on finding a solution whereby both parties "win." By establishing a common goal, both parties win when this goal is achieved.
- *Listen actively.* Critical to resolving situations of conflict is the ability to listen and understand what the other person is saying and feeling. In active listening, the receiver actively and empathically listens to gain a better understanding of the actual and the implied message.
- *Openly express your feelings.* Talking about feelings is much more constructive than acting them out. The nurse might say, "I am very concerned about Jamie's safety when you leave his side rails down."
- *Avoid blaming.* Each party owns part of the problem. Pointing fingers and blaming others will not solve the problem. Instead, identify the part of the problem that each party owns and work together to resolve it. Seek **win-win solutions.**
- *Summarize the decision.* At the end of any discussion, summarize what has been decided and identify who is responsible for follow-up. This process ensures that everyone is clear about the decision and facilitates accountability for implementing solutions.

TABLE 3-2 CHOOSING WORDS CAREFULLY

POOR WORDS	RATIONALE	BETTER WORDS	RATIONALE
Policies allowed or not permitted	Convey attitude that hospital personnel have authority over parents in matters concerning their children	*Guidelines, working together, welcome*	Convey openness and appreciation for position and importance of families
Noncompliant, uncooperative, difficult (when referring to parents and other family members)	Imply that health care providers make decisions and give instructions that families must follow without input	*Partners, colleagues, joint decision makers, experts about their child*	Acknowledge that families bring important information and insight and that families and professionals form a team
Dysfunctional, in denial, overprotective, uninvolved, uncaring (labeling families)	Pronounce judgment that may not incorporate full understanding of family's situation, reactions, or perspective	*Coping (describing family's reactions with care and respect)*	Remain open to reaching a more complete and appreciative understanding of families over time

TRANSCULTURAL COMMUNICATION: BRIDGING THE GAP

Conflict can arise when the nurse comes from a cultural background that is different from that of the child and family. Such differences could influence the approach to care. As the demographics in the United States continue to change, health care professionals will be challenged to become more transcultural in their approach to clients if the professionals want to continue to be effective in their relationships with children and families. Health care professionals need to be aware of their own values and beliefs and need to recognize how these influence their interactions with others. They also need to be aware of and respect the child's and family's values and beliefs. In working with children and families, the initial nursing assessment should address values, beliefs, and traditions. The nurse can then consider ways in which culture might affect communication style, methods of decision making, cultural adaptations for nursing intervention, and other behaviors related to health care practices.

During the initial interview, the nurse ascertains the following information related to the child and family:

Decision-making practices: Are decisions made by individuals or collectively as a group?

Child-rearing practices: Who are the primary caregivers? What are their disciplinary practices?

Family support: What is the family structure? To whom do the patient and family turn for support?

Communication practices: How is the information communicated to the rest of the family?

Health and illness practices: Do family members seek professional help or rely on other resources for treatment and advice?

Once this information is obtained, the nurse can use it to individualize the treatment plan and approach for the child's and family's needs. For example, if the parents of a child with an Orthodox Jewish religious background request a kosher diet, the nurse facilitates the routine delivery of kosher meals and communicates the family's wishes to the rest of the team members so that they can also respect the family's customs. If the family of a child who has a severe brain injury requests the services of a healer, the nurse enables the family to arrange the visit. Coordinating the child's daily schedule to provide an uninterrupted visit with the healer is one aspect of family-centered care. When the nurse communicates the family's cultural preferences to other members of the health care team, communication and holistic care are enhanced.

THERAPEUTIC RELATIONSHIPS: DEVELOPING AND MAINTAINING TRUST

Trust is important in establishing and maintaining therapeutic relationships with families. Trust promotes a sense of partnership between nurses and families. Becoming overly involved with the child or family can inhibit a healthy relationship. Because nurses are caring, nurturing people and the profession demands that nurses sometimes become intimately involved in other people's lives, maintaining the balance between appropriate involvement and professional separation is quite challenging. Box 3-2 delineates behaviors that may indicate overinvolvement. Box 3-3 identifies behaviors that may indicate professional separation or underinvolvement. Whether nurses become too emotionally involved or find themselves at the other end of the spectrum, being underinvolved, they lose effectiveness as objective professional resources.

Family members may display feelings of incompetence, fear, and loss of control by expressing anger, withdrawal, or dissatisfaction. Most

---

BOX 3-2 WARNING SIGNS OF OVERINVOLVEMENT

- Buying gifts for individual children or families
- Giving out one's home phone number
- Competing with other staff for the child's or family's affection
- Inviting the child or family to social gatherings
- Accepting invitations to family gatherings (e.g., birthday parties, weddings)
- Visiting or spending time with the child or family during off-duty time
- Revealing personal information
- Lending or borrowing money
- Making decisions for the family about the child's care

BOX 3-3 WARNING SIGNS OF UNDERINVOLVEMENT

- Avoiding the child or family
- Calling in sick so as not to take assignment of a specific child
- Asking to trade assignments for a specific child
- Spending less time with a particular child

---

important in working with these families is to promote the parents' feelings of competence through education and empowerment. The nurse keeps parents well informed of the child's care through frequent phone calls and actively involves them in decision making. Teaching parents skills necessary to care for their child promotes confidence, enhances self-esteem, and fosters independence.

Nurses must be able to recognize their own personal and professional needs. Being aware of the motives for one's own actions will greatly enhance the nurse's ability to understand the needs of children and families and to give families the tools to manage care effectively.

! NURSING QUALITY ALERT

Maintaining a Therapeutic Relationship

Maintaining professional boundaries requires that the nurse constantly be aware of the fine line between empathy and overinvolvement.

NURSING CARE FOR COMMUNICATING WITH CHILDREN AND FAMILIES

▪ Assessment

A comprehensive needs assessment of the child and family elicits information about problem-solving skills, cultural needs, coping behaviors, and the child's routines. Any assessment requires the nurse to obtain information from the child and the family.

The nurse might say, "Mrs. Jiminez, I value your input as well as your child's. Hearing Ramon explain his understanding of his diabetic dietary restrictions in his own words will help us gain better insight into how best to manage his care. Let's take a few minutes to hear from Ramon, and then we can talk about your perspective."

Assessment enables the nurse to develop better insight by gathering information from multiple perspectives and facilitates the development of a more comprehensive plan of care. A thorough assessment of the child's communication skills presumes that the nurse understands developmental milestones and can relate comprehension and communication skills to the child's cognitive and emotional development and language abilities. During the initial assessment of the child and family, the nurse should also describe routines and provide information about what the child and family can expect during their visit.

The family's level of health literacy is an important component of a communication assessment. Because of language, educational, or other barriers, some family members may not understand medical or health terminology in ways nurses might expect. Consequences, such as not adhering to medication or recommended treatment routines, can result from miscommunication related to low health literacy (Jones & Sanchez-Jones, 2008). Assessment data that might suggest poor health literacy in family members include avoidance of reading or filling out hospital forms, providing incorrect information about the child, and not appearing curious about the child's health status (Jones & Sanchez-Jones, 2008). Providing instructions and explanations in language the caregiver understands as well as having the caregiver repeat or demonstrate back the instructions can increase understanding and adherence (Colby, 2009). In addition, health care professionals should use only trained translators to help explain procedures, treatments, and other health-related information to patients and families with limited English competency. In these instances, the use of untrained translators, such as children or other family members, is unacceptable (Levetown & Committee on Bioethics, 2008).

▉ Nursing Diagnosis and Planning

The nursing assessment may suggest diagnoses that affect communication but that arise from the child's encounter with the health care system. Other diagnoses are related to the child's and family's communication abilities.

- Anxiety related to potential or actual separation from parents (e.g., a 4-year-old girl who becomes withdrawn and unable to cooperate with an office hearing test when separated from her mother).

Expected Outcomes. The child verbalizes the cause of the anxiety and more readily communicates with the health care professional. The child exhibits posture, facial expressions, and gestures that reflect decreased distress.

- Fear related to a perceived threat to the child's well-being and inadequate understanding of procedures or treatments (e.g., a 7-year-old boy scheduled for tonsillectomy who wonders where his throat will be cut to remove his tonsils).

Expected Outcomes. The child talks about fears and accurately describes the procedure or treatment.

- Hopelessness related to a deteriorating health status (e.g., an 11-year-old child in isolation with prolonged illness and uncertain prognosis).

Expected Outcomes. The child verbalizes feelings and participates in care. The child makes positive statements, maintains eye contact during interactions, and has appetite and sleep patterns that are appropriate for the child's age and physical health.

- Powerlessness related to limits to autonomy (e.g., a 3-year-old child with a C6 spinal fracture as a result of a motor vehicle trauma).

Expected Outcomes. The child expresses frustrations and anger and begins to make choices in areas that are controllable. The child asks appropriate questions about care and treatment.

- Impaired verbal communication related to physiologic barriers or cultural and language differences (e.g., a 17-year-old adolescent who has had her jaw wired subsequent to orthodontic surgery).

Expected Outcomes. The adolescent effectively uses alternative communication methods. The child and family who speak and

understand a different language appropriately communicate through an interpreter.

CRITICAL THINKING EXERCISE 3-1

The nurse caring for an 8-year-old boy observes him lying in his bed with his back facing the door. He is crying, although he quickly wipes his eyes when he sees the nurse at the door. He has been hospitalized because of leukemia. He lives in a small community 350 miles from the hospital. His parents visit on the weekends.

1. Identify two things that might be upsetting the child.
2. What strategies could you use to encourage the child to talk about his feelings related to the problems you have identified?

▉ Interventions

Nurses working with children should determine the best communication approach for each child individually on the basis of the child's age and developmental abilities. Table 3-3 presents an overview of developmental milestones related to communication skills in children and some approaches to facilitate successful interactions. Other interventions that facilitate communication between the nurse and children include play, storytelling, and strategies for enhancing self-esteem.

▉ **Play.** Play can greatly facilitate communicating with children. Approaching children at their developmental level with familiar forms of play increases their comfort and allows the nurse to be seen in a more positive, less threatening role.

Because play is an everyday part of children's lives and a method they use to communicate, they are less likely to be inhibited when participating in play interactions. Through play, children may express thoughts and feelings they may be unable to verbalize (see Chapters 5 through 8 for normal play activities and Chapter 11 for therapeutic play).

▉ **Storytelling.** Storytelling is an innovative and creative communication strategy. It is also a skill that can be acquired and refined through practice. Familiarity with stories and frequent practice in storytelling increase a nurse's confidence and competence as a storyteller. Storytelling can be a routine part of a nurse's day. Its purposes range from establishing rapport to approaching uncomfortable topics, such as loss, death, fear, grief, and anger. In storytelling, there is a teller and a listener. In individual situations, the child may be the teller or the listener, although in a shared story, adult and child may each take a turn in both roles (Box 3-4).

▉ **Explaining Procedures and Treatments.** Preparation before a procedure, which includes explaining the reasons for the procedure and the expected sequence of events and outcomes, can greatly reduce a child's fears and anxieties. Preparation enables the child to experience some

BOX 3-4 STORYTELLING STRATEGIES

- Capture a story on paper or on videotape as told by a child or group of children.
- Tell a "yarn story" with two or more people. A long piece of yarn with knots tied at varied intervals is slid loosely through the hands of the teller until a knot is felt, at which time the yarn is passed to the next person, who continues the story.
- Initiate a game of sentence completion, either oral or written, with sentences beginning "If I were in charge of the hospital ... ," "I wish ... ," "When I get home I will ... ," or "My family ..."
- Read stories with themes related to issues a child is facing. The children's section of the local public library is an excellent resource.

TABLE 3-3 DEVELOPMENTAL MILESTONES AND THEIR RELATIONSHIP TO COMMUNICATION APPROACHES

DEVELOPMENT	LANGUAGE DEVELOPMENT	EMOTIONAL DEVELOPMENT	COGNITIVE DEVELOPMENT	SUGGESTED COMMUNICATION APPROACH
Infants (0-12 mo) Infants experience world through senses of hearing, seeing, smelling, tasting, and touching.	Crying, babbling, cooing. Single-word production. Able to name some simple objects.	Dependent on others; high need for cuddling and security. Responsive to environment (e.g., sounds, visual stimuli). Distinguish between happy and angry voices and between familiar and strange voices. Beginning to experience separation anxiety.	Interactions largely reflexive. Beginning to see repetition of activities and movements. Beginning to initiate interactions intentionally. Short attention span (1-2 min).	Use calm, soft, soothing voice. Be responsive to cries. Engage in turn-taking vocalizations (adult imitates baby sounds). Talk and read regularly to infants. Prepare infant as you are about to perform care; talk to infant about what you are about to do. Use slow approach and allow child time to get to know you.
Toddlers (1-2 yr) Toddlers experience world through senses of hearing, seeing, smelling, tasting, and touching.	Two-word combinations emerge. Participate in turn taking in communication (speaker/listener). "No" becomes favorite word. Able to use gestures and verbalize simple wants and needs.	Strong need for security objects. Separation/stranger anxiety heightened. Participate in parallel play. Thrive on routines. Beginning development of independence: "Want to do myself." Still very dependent on significant adults.	Experiment with objects. Participate in active exploration. Begin to experiment with variations on activities. Begin to identify cause-and-effect relationships. Short attention span (3-5 min).	Learn toddler's words for common items, and use them in conversations. Describe activities and procedures as they are about to be done. Use picture books. Use play for demonstrations. Be responsive to child's receptivity toward you and approach cautiously. Preparation should occur immediately before event.
Preschool Children (3-5 yr) Preschool children use words they do not fully understand; they also do not accurately understand many words used by others.	Further development and expansion of word combination (able to speak in full sentences). Growth in correct grammatical usage. Use pronouns. Clearer articulation of sounds. Vocabulary rapidly expanding; may know words without understanding meaning.	Like to imitate activities and make choices. Strive for independence but need adult support and encouragement. Demonstrate purposeful attention-seeking behaviors. Learn cooperation and turn taking in game playing. Need clearly set limits and boundaries.	Begin developing concepts of time, space, and quantity. Magical thinking prominent. World seen only from child's perspective. Short attention span (5-10 min).	Seek opportunities to offer choices. Use play to explain procedures and activities. Speak in simple sentences, and explore relative concepts. Use picture and story books, puppets. Describe activities and procedures as they are about to be done. Be concise; limit length of explanations (5 min). Engage in preparatory activities 1-3 hr before the event.

TABLE 3-3 **DEVELOPMENTAL MILESTONES AND THEIR RELATIONSHIP TO COMMUNICATION APPROACHES—cont'd**

DEVELOPMENT	LANGUAGE DEVELOPMENT	EMOTIONAL DEVELOPMENT	COGNITIVE DEVELOPMENT	SUGGESTED COMMUNICATION APPROACH
School-Age Children (6-11 yr)				
School-age children communicate thoughts and appreciate viewpoints of others. Words with multiple meanings and words describing things they have not experienced are not thoroughly understood.	Expanding vocabulary enables child to describe concepts, thoughts, and feelings. Development of conversational skills.	Interact well with others. Understand rules to games. Very interested in learning. Build close friendships. Beginning to accept responsibility for own actions. Competition emerges. Still dependent on adults to meet needs.	Able to grasp concepts of classification, conversation. Concrete thinking emerges. Become very oriented to "rules." Able to process information in serial format. Lengthened attention span (10-30 min).	Use photographs, books, diagrams, charts, videos to explain. Make explanations sequential. Engage in conversations that encourage critical thinking. Establish limits and set consequences. Use medical play techniques. Introduce preparatory materials 1-5 days in advance of the event.
Adolescents (12 yr and older)				
Adolescents are able to create theories and generate many explanations for situations. They are beginning to communicate like adults.	Able to verbalize and comprehend most adult concepts.	Beginning to accept responsibility for own actions. Perception of "imaginary audiences." (see Chapter 8) Need independence. Competitive drive. Strong need for group identification. Frequently have small group of very close friends. Question authority. Strong need for privacy.	Able to think logically and abstractly. Attention span up to 60 min.	Engage in conversations about adolescent's interests. Use photographs, books, diagrams, charts, and videos to explain. Use collaborative approach, and foster and support independence. Introduce preparatory materials up to 1 wk in advance of the event. Respect privacy needs.

mastery over events, gives the child time to develop effective coping behaviors, and fosters trust in those caring for the child. Adequate preparation is the key to helping a child have a successful, positive health care experience.

In general, the younger the child, the closer in time to the event the child should be prepared for it. For example, a 3-year-old child will generally be very anxious and therefore should be prepared immediately before, whereas teenagers would benefit from a longer preparation time so that they can develop strategies for dealing with the situation. Table 3-3 gives age-related attention span guidelines.

Key elements for communicating complete and accurate information are as follows (Gaynard, Wolfer, Goldberger, et al., 1998):

- *Learn the procedure.* To explain a procedure adequately, the nurse must understand what is involved. What pieces of equipment will be used? Where will the procedure take place? Essentially, the nurse needs to learn what the child can expect to happen during the procedure.
- *Determine what information to share with the child and family.* The preparation should include information only about what the child will experience or perceive directly. Consultation with the family will allow the nurse to learn words and terminology used by the child. Table 3-4 offers other concrete suggestions of appropriate language for nurses to use in working with children.

- *Provide sensory information.* Inviting children to see, hear, feel, taste, smell, and experience similar sensations during the preparation will greatly enhance their preparedness and diminish their anxieties. For example, in preparing a child for an IV line insertion, the nurse can show the child the catheter or explain the purpose of the tourniquet and allow the child to put it on or to put it on the arm of a doll, if the child so desires. The nurse should let the child smell an alcohol swab and feel its coolness when applied to the skin. Showing the child the treatment room and inviting the child to sit on the treatment table where the procedure will be performed are effective ways to convey information.
- *Explain the sequence of events.* Preparation includes a description of the sequence in which events will occur. Recognizing the procedure as a series of sequential steps allows children to anticipate appropriately and gives them a sense of control and a better understanding of the number of steps to expect before the procedure is over.
- *Explain how long the procedure will last.* Whenever possible, the nurse should invite the child to have simulated play experiences. Inviting the child to perform the procedure on a doll or stuffed animal is often effective and gives the child a real sense of time and firsthand experience with the sequence of events. If a concrete demonstration is not possible, the nurse should explain

TABLE 3-4   CONSIDERATIONS IN CHOOSING LANGUAGE

POTENTIALLY AMBIGUOUS	CONCRETE EXPLANATION
"The doctor will give you some dye." *To make me die?*	"The doctor will put some medicine in the tube that will help her see your _____ more clearly."
Dressing, dressing change *Why are they going to undress me?* *Do I have to change my clothes?*	Bandages; clean, new bandages.
Stool collection *Why do they want to collect little chairs?*	Use child's familiar term, such as "poop," "BM," or "doody."
Urine *You're in?*	Use child's familiar term, such as "pee."
Shot *When people get shot, they're really badly hurt.*	Describe giving medicine through a (small, tiny) needle.
CAT scan *Will there be cats?*	Describe in simple terms, and explain what the letters of the common name stand for.
PICU *Pick you?*	Explain as above.
ICU *I see you?*	Explain as above.
IV *Ivy?*	Explain as above.
Stretcher *Stretch her? Stretch whom?*	Bed on wheels.
Special; funny (words that are usually positive descriptors) *It doesn't look/feel special to me.*	Odd, different, unusual, strange.
Gas, sleeping gas *Is someone going to pour gasoline into the mask?*	"A medicine, called an anesthetic, is a kind of air you will breathe through a mask like this to help you sleep during your operation so you won't feel anything. It is a different kind of sleep." (Explain differences.)
"The doctor will put you to sleep." *Like my cat was put to sleep? It never came back.*	"The doctor will give you medicine that will help you go into a very deep sleep. You won't feel anything until the operation is over. Then the doctor will stop giving you the medicine, so you can wake up."
"Move you to the floor." *Why are they going to put me on the ground?*	Unit, ward. (Explain why the child is being transferred, and where.)
OR (or treatment room) table *People aren't supposed to get up on tables.*	A narrow bed.
"Take a picture." (X-ray, CT, and MRI machines are far larger than a familiar camera, move differently, and do not yield a familiar end product.)	"A picture of your insides." (Describe appearance, sounds, and movement of the equipment.)
"Flush your IV." *Flush it down the toilet?*	Explain.

Words can be experienced as "hard" or "soft" according to how much they increase the perceived threat of a situation. For example, consider the following word choices:

HARDER	SOFTER
"This part will hurt."	"It (you) may feel (or feel very) sore, achy, scratchy, tight, snug, full, or (other manageable, descriptive term)."
"The medicine will burn."	(Words such as scratch, poke, or sting might be familiar for some children and frightening to others.)
"The room will be very cold."	"Some children say they feel very warm." "Some children say they feel very cold."
"The medicine will taste (or smell) bad."	"The medicine may taste (or smell) different from anything you have tasted before. After you take it, will you tell me how it was for you?"
"Cut," "open you up," "slice," "make a hole."	"The doctor will make an opening."
"As big as _____" (e.g., size of an incision or of a catheter).	(Use concrete comparisons, such as "your little finger" or "a paper clip" if the opening will indeed be small.) "Smaller than _____."
"As long as _____" (e.g., for duration of a procedure).	"For less time than it takes you to _____."

NOTE: Words or phrases that are helpful to one child may be threatening for another. Health care providers must listen carefully and be sensitive to the child's use of and response to language.

Modified with permission of The Child Life Council, Inc., 11820 Parklawn Dr., Rockville, MD 20852-2529; from Gaynard, L., Wolfer, J., Goldberger, J., et al. (1998). *Psychosocial care of children in hospitals: A clinical practice manual from ACCH Child Life Research Project.* Rockville, Md.: The Child Life Council, Inc.

TABLE 3-4 CONSIDERATIONS IN CHOOSING LANGUAGE—cont'd

HARDER	SOFTER
"As much as _____." (These are open-ended and "extending" expressions.)	"Less than _____." (These expressions help confine, familiarize, and imply the manageability of an event or of equipment.)

The unfamiliar usage or complexity of some common medical words or expressions can be confusing and frightening.

POTENTIALLY AMBIGUOUS	CONCRETE EXPLANATION
"Take your vitals" (or "your vital signs")	"Measure your temperature," "see how warm your body is," "see how fast and strongly your heart is working." (Nothing is "taken" from the child.)
Electrodes, leads	"Sticky like a Band-Aid, with a small wet spot in the center, and small strings that attach to the snap (monitor electrodes); paste like wet sand, with strings with tiny metal cups that stick to the paste (electroencephalogram [EEG] electrodes). The paste washes off easily afterward; the strings go into a box that will make a picture of how your heart (or brain) is working." (Show child electrodes and leads before using. Let child handle them and apply them to a doll or to self.)
"Hang your (IV) medication."	"We will bring in a new medicine in a bag and attach it to the little tube already in your arm. The needle goes into the tube, not into your arm, so you won't feel it."
N.P.O.	"Nothing to eat. Your stomach needs to be empty." (Explain why.) "You can eat and drink again as soon as _____." (Explain with concrete descriptions.)
Anesthesia	"The doctor will give you medicine—you may hear it called 'anesthesia.' It will help you go into a very deep sleep. You will not feel anything at all. The doctor knows just the right amount of medicine to give you so you will stay asleep through your operation. When the operation is over, the doctor stops giving you that medicine and helps you wake up."

the timing in terms that the child can understand; for example, the nurse might say, "The procedure will last as long as it takes to sing your favorite song."

- *Monitor accuracy of information (feedback).* Feedback can be used to modify or reinforce future preparation sessions. Feedback also allows the nurse to correct any misunderstandings the child may have and provides an opportunity for the child to process verbally and express feelings about the experience.

Open, honest communication about treatments and procedures and attentiveness to the learning needs of the child will greatly facilitate achievement of the treatment goals.

Because nonadherence to treatment protocols can be a problem in some families, it is essential that the nurse ensure that children and family members can describe the treatment plan. Using a variety of written, verbal, interactive, and visual materials can improve comprehension and adherence. For psychomotor skill development, return demonstration is important. Reinforcement with written materials in the family's chosen language or at the family's assessed literacy level provides a ready reference for the family after the child's discharge (Jones & Sanchez-Jones, 2008).

■ **Strategies for Enhancing Self-Esteem.** Communication practices play an important role in the development of children's self-esteem and confidence. Nurses are in an excellent position to model communication practices that enhance self-esteem. Table 3-5 compares helpful and harmful communication practices.

The words adults choose, their tone of voice, and the place and timing of message delivery all influence the child's interpretation of the message. The interpretation may be positive, negative, or neutral.

To enhance the child's self-esteem, adults should strive for positive language.

Providing children with developmentally appropriate information about their condition and any treatments they may be receiving enhances their control over the hospitalization experience and increases feelings of self-esteem (Marshall, 2008). If adolescents are to "have a voice" in decision making about their care, they must receive information that is thorough, developmentally appropriate, and understandable (Levetown & Committee on Bioethics, 2008).

■ Evaluation

Although evaluation is traditionally thought of as a closure activity, evaluation should be a continuous activity throughout the nursing process. Keep expected outcomes visible, and assess whether they are being realized. Are the outcomes attainable? Could the wrong nursing diagnosis have been made? Adjust the plan of care as needed.

COMMUNICATING WITH CHILDREN WITH SPECIAL NEEDS

The opportunity to interact with children who have special communication needs presents an exciting challenge for nurses. To identify successful alternative methods of communication, the nurse needs to learn particular techniques for working with children and families. Alternative methods of communicating are critical. Children need to express their wants and needs accurately. Through adequate **preparation** and reassurance, the nurse can offer the child comfort

TABLE 3-5 SELF-ESTEEM IN CHILDREN: COMMUNICATION PRACTICES

TECHNIQUES TO ENHANCE SELF-ESTEEM	PRACTICES THAT HARM SELF-ESTEEM
Praise efforts and accomplishments.	Criticize efforts and accomplishments.
Use active listening skills.	Be too busy to listen.
Encourage expression of feelings.	Tell children how they should feel.
Acknowledge feelings.	Give no support for dealing with feelings.
Use developmentally based discipline.	Use physical punishment.
Use "I" statements.	Use "you" statements.
Be nonjudgmental.	Judge the child.
Set clearly defined limits, and reinforce them.	Set no known limits or boundaries.
Share quality time together.	Give time grudgingly.
Be honest.	Be dishonest.
Describe behaviors observed when praising and disciplining.	Use coercion and power as discipline.
Compliment the child.	Belittle, blame, or shame the child.
Smile.	Use sarcastic, caustic, or cruel "humor."
Touch and hug the child.	Avoid coming near the child, even when the child is open to touching, holding, or hugging. Touch and hold only when performing a task.
Rock the child.	Avoid comforting through rocking.

and understanding. Successfully meeting this challenge is a rewarding experience for the nurse and a positive, supportive experience for the child and family.

The Child with a Visual Impairment

For the child with a visual impairment, the nurse can do the following:

- Obtain a thorough assessment of the child's self-help skills and abilities (i.e., toileting, bathing, dressing, feeding, mobility).
- Orient the child to the surroundings. Walk the child around the room and unit several times, indicating landmarks (e.g., doors, closets, bedside tables, windows) while guiding the child by the hand or by the way the child prefers. Explain sounds that the child may frequently hear (e.g., monitors, alarms, nurse call bells).
- Encourage a family member to stay with the child. This person can facilitate communication and greatly enhance the child's comfort in this unfamiliar environment.
- Keep furniture and other items in the same, consistent place. Consistency aids in the child's orientation to the room, fosters independence, and promotes safety.
- Keep the nurse call bell in the same place and within the child's reach.
- Identify yourself when entering the room, and tell the child when you are departing.
- Carefully and fully explain all procedures.
- Allow the child to handle equipment as the procedure is explained.

! NURSING QUALITY ALERT

Communicating with Children with Special Needs

In working with children with special needs, the nurse must carefully assess each child's physical, mental, and developmental abilities and determine the most effective methods of communication.

The Child with a Hearing Impairment

For the child with a hearing impairment, the nurse can do the following:

- Thoroughly assess the child's self-help skills and abilities.
- Identify the family's method of communication and, if possible, adopt it.
- Encourage a family member to stay with the child at all times to decrease the stress of hospitalization and facilitate communication.
- If sign language is used, learn the most frequently used signs and use them whenever able. Keep a chart of signs near the child's bed.
- Develop a communication board with pictures of most commonly used items or needs (e.g., television, cup, toothbrush, toilet, shower).
- Determine whether the child uses a hearing aid. If so, make sure that the batteries are working and that the hearing aid is clean and intact.
- When entering the room, do so cautiously and gently touch the child before speaking.
- Always face the child when speaking. If the child is a lip reader, face-to-face visibility will greatly enhance the child's ability to understand.
- Do not shout or exaggerate speech. This behavior distorts the face and can be very confusing. Rather, speak in a normal tone and at a regular pace.
- Remember that nonverbal communication can speak as loud as, if not louder than, speech (e.g., a frown or worried face can say more than words).
- When performing a procedure that requires standing behind the child, such as when giving an enema or assisting with a spinal tap, have another person stand in front of the child and explain the procedure as it is being performed.
- Whenever possible, use play strategies to help communicate and demonstrate procedures (see Table 3-3).

The Child Who Speaks Another Language

For the child who speaks another language, the nurse can do the following:

- Thoroughly assess the child's abilities in speaking and understanding both languages.
- Identify an interpreter, perhaps another adult family member, friend of the family, or other individual with proficiency in both languages to be used for communication not related to health care. Other children should not be used as interpreters.
- Use an interpreter whenever possible but always when explaining procedures, determining understanding, teaching new skills, and assessing needs.
- Use a communication board with the names of items printed in both languages.
- Learn the words and names of commonly used items in the child's language, and use them whenever possible. Using the familiar language not only aids in communication but also

demonstrates sincere interest in learning the language and respect for the culture.

- Learn as much about the child's culture as possible and develop plans of care that demonstrate respect for the culture. Sincere attempts to learn to communicate with the child and family demonstrate the nurse's concern for their well-being.
- Use play strategies whenever possible. Play seems to be a universal language.

The Child with Other Communication Issues

For the child who has more severe communication issues, the nurse can do the following:

- Thoroughly assess the child's self-help skills and abilities. Determine the child's and family's methods of communicating and adopt them as much as possible.
- Encourage parents to stay with the child to decrease anxiety and foster communication.
- Determine whether the child uses sign language or augmented communication devices. Use a communication board if appropriate.
- Be attentive to and maximize the child's nonverbal communication. Facial grimaces, frowns, smiles, and nods are effective means of communicating responses and expressing likes and dislikes.
- If appropriate, encourage the child to use writing boards (dry erase or chalk; or pads of paper) to write needs, wants, questions, and concerns.

The Child with a Profound Neurologic Impairment

Because hearing, vision, and language abilities are often hard to determine in the child who is profoundly neurologically impaired, the nurse should assume that the child can hear, see, and comprehend something of what is said. A friendly tone of voice that conveys warmth and respect should be used. For the child with a profound neurologic impairment, the nurse can do the following:

- Address the child when entering and exiting the room. Gently touch the child while saying the child's name.
- Speak softly, calmly, and slowly to allow the child time to process what you are saying.
- While in the room with the child, talk to the child. Do not talk as if the child were not there.
  💬 The nurse might say, "Jenny, I am going to wash your arm now," or "Jenny, now I am going to take your temperature by putting the thermometer under your arm." Identifying an assistant, the nurse might say, "Jenny, Kristi, another nurse, is here to help me lift you into your chair."
- Talk to the child about activities and objects in the room, things that the child might see, hear, smell, touch, taste, or sense.
  💬 For example, the nurse might say, "It is a sunny day today; can you feel the warm sun shining on you through the window?"
- When asking the child questions, allow the child adequate time to respond. Be careful to ask questions only of children who are capable of responding.
- Ascertain the child's ability to respond to simple questions. Some children can respond to yes-or-no questions by squeezing a hand or blinking their eyes (once for yes and twice for no).
- Be extremely attentive to any signs or gestures (e.g., facial grimaces, smiling, eye movements) that may convey responses to likes or dislikes. Signs or gestures may be the child's only means of communicating.
- As with all children with special communication needs, thoroughly document and communicate to others who interact with the child any special techniques that work. Providing information will greatly enhance continuity and more fully facilitate the child's ability to communicate.

▌ KEY CONCEPTS

- Components of effective communication with children involve verbal and nonverbal interactions. Essential components include touch, physical proximity, environment, listening, eye contact, visual cues, pace of speech and tone of voice, and overall body language.
- The best communication approach for an individual child should be determined on the basis of the child's age, developmental abilities, and cultural preferences. Strategies include play and storytelling, explaining procedures and treatments, and modeling communication practices that enhance self-esteem.
- Communication pitfalls, such as using jargon, talking down to children or beyond their developmental level, and avoiding or denying a problem, can lead to a breakdown in the relationship between the nurse and the child and family.
- Family-centered communication strategies include establishing rapport, identifying needs, establishing expectations, being available and open to questions, family education, empowerment, obtaining feedback from children and families, promoting effective conflict management, learning techniques for transcultural communication, and maintaining professional boundaries.
- In working with children with special needs, the nurse should carefully assess each child's physical, mental, and developmental abilities and determine the most effective methods of communication.

REFERENCES

Colby, B. (2009). Repeat back to me: A program to improve understanding. *Journal of Pediatric Nursing, 24*(2), e6. Retrieved from www.pediatricnursing.org.

Fisher, M., & Broome, M. (2011). Parent-provider communication during hospitalization. *Journal of Pediatric Nursing, 26,* 58-69.

Gaynard, L., Wolfer, J., Goldberger, J., et al. (1998). *Psychosocial care of children in hospitals: A clinical practice manual from ACCH Child Life Research Project.* Rockville, MD: The Child Life Council, Inc.

Jones, J., & Sanchez-Jones, T. (2008). Health literacy and communication. In C. Williams (Ed.), *Therapeutic interaction in nursing.* Boston: Jones & Bartlett.

Levetown, M. & Committee on Bioethics (2008). Communicating with children and families: From everyday interactions to skill in conveying distressing information. *Pediatrics, 121,* e1441-e1460. Retrieved from www.pediatrics.org.

Marshall, L. (2008). Communicating with children. In C. Williams (Ed.), *Therapeutic intervention in nursing.* Boston: Jones & Bartlett.

McCann, D., Young, J., Watson, K., et al. (2008). Effectiveness of a tool to improve role negotiation and communication between parents and nurses. *Paediatric Nursing, 20,* 14-19.

Neuman, M. (2011). Addressing children's beliefs through Fowler's Stages of Faith. *Journal of Pediatric Nursing, 26,* 44-50.

Sanjari, M., Shirazi, F., Heidari, S., et al. (2009). Nursing support for parents of hospitalized children. *Issues in Comprehensive Pediatric Nursing, 32,* 120-130.

Topper, E. F. (2004). Working knowledge: It's not what you say, but how you say it. *American Libraries, 35,* 76.

Health Promotion for
the Developing Child

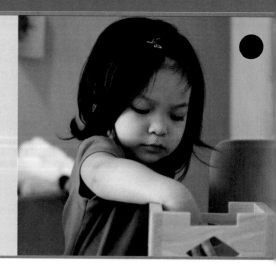

evolve WEBSITE

http://evolve.elsevier.com/James/ncoc

LEARNING OBJECTIVES

After studying this chapter, you should be able to:

- Define terms related to growth and development.
- Discuss principles of growth and development.
- Describe various factors, including genetics and genomics, that affect growth and development.
- Discuss the following theorists' ideas about growth and development: Piaget, Freud, Erikson, and Kohlberg.
- Discuss theories of language development.
- Identify methods used to assess growth and development.

- Describe the classifications and social aspects of play.
- Explain how play enhances growth and development.
- Identify health-promoting activities that are essential for the normal growth and development of infants and children.
- Discuss recommendations for scheduled vaccines.
- Discuss the components of a nutritional assessment.
- Discuss the etiology and prevention of childhood injuries.

Humans grow and change dramatically during childhood and adolescence. Normal growth and development proceed in an orderly, predictable pattern that establishes a basis for assessing an individual's abilities and potential. Nurses provide health care teaching and anticipatory guidance about the growth and development of children in many settings, such as newborn nurseries, emergency departments, community clinics and health centers, and pediatric inpatient units.

OVERVIEW OF GROWTH AND DEVELOPMENT

Nurses are frequently the members of the health care team whom parents approach. Parents are often concerned that their children are not progressing normally. Nurses can reassure parents about normal variations in development and can also identify problems early so that developmental delays can be addressed as soon as possible. Nurses who work with ill children must have a clear understanding of how children differ from adults and from each other at various stages. This awareness is essential to allow nurses to create developmentally appropriate plans of care to meet the needs of their young clients.

Definition of Terms

Although the terms *growth* and *development* often are used together and interchangeably, they have distinct definitions and meanings. Growth generally refers to an increase in the physical size of a whole

or any of its parts or an increase in the number and size of cells. Growth can be measured easily and accurately. For example, any observer can see that an infant grows rapidly during the first year of life. This growth can be measured readily by determining changes in weight and length. The difference in size between a newborn and a 12-month-old infant is an obvious sign of the remarkable growth that occurs during the first year of life.

Development is a more complex and subtle concept. Development is generally considered to be a continuous, orderly series of conditions leading to activities, new motives for activities, and patterns of behavior.

Another definition of development is an increase in function and complexity that occurs through growth, maturation, and **learning**—in other words, an increase in capabilities. The process of language acquisition provides an example of development. The use of language becomes increasingly complex as the child matures. At 10 to 12 months of age, a child uses single words to communicate simple desires and needs. By age 4 to 5 years, complete and complex sentences are used to relate elaborate tales. Language development can be measured by determining vocabulary, articulation skill, and word use.

Maturity and learning also affect development. *Maturation* is the physical change in the complexity of body structures that enables a child to function at increasingly higher levels. Maturity is programmed genetically and may occur as a result of several changes. For example, maturation of the central nervous system depends on changes that occur throughout the body, such as an increase in the number of neurons, myelinization of nerve fibers, lengthening of muscles, and overall weight gain.

Learning involves changes in behavior that occur as a result of both maturation and experience with the environment. Predictable patterns are observed in learning, and these patterns are sequential, orderly, and progressive. For example, when learning to walk, babies first learn to control their heads, then to roll over, next to sit, then to crawl, and finally to walk. The child's muscle mass and nervous system must grow and mature as well.

These examples show how complex and interrelated the processes of growth, development, maturation, and learning are. Children must be monitored carefully to ensure that these complicated events and activities unfold normally. Wide variations occur as children grow and develop. Each child has a unique rate and pattern of development, although parameters are used to identify abnormalities. Nurses must be familiar with normal parameters so that delays can be detected early. The earlier that delays are discovered and intervention initiated, the less dramatic their effect will be.

Stages of Growth and Development

To simplify analysis and discussion of the complex processes and theories related to growth and development, researchers and theorists have identified stages or age-groupings. These stages serve as reference points in describing various features of growth and development (Table 4-1). Chapters 5 through 8 discuss the physical growth and

TABLE 4-1	STAGES OF GROWTH AND DEVELOPMENT

The following stages and age-groupings refer to stages of childhood growth and development:

Newborn	Birth to 1 month
Infancy	1 month to 1 year
Toddlerhood	1 to 3 years
Preschool age	3 to 6 years
School age	6 to 11 or 12 years

cognitive, emotional, language, and motor development specific to each stage.

Parameters of Growth

Statistical data derived from research studies of large groups of children provide health care professionals with information about how children normally grow. Throughout infancy, childhood, and adolescence, growth occurs in bursts separated by periods when growth is stable or consistent.

Weight, length (or height), and head circumference are parameters that are used to monitor growth. They should be measured at regular intervals during infancy and childhood. The weight of the average term newborn infant is approximately $7\frac{1}{2}$ pounds (3.4 kg). Male infants are usually slightly heavier than female infants. Usually, the birth weight doubles by 6 months of age and triples by 1 year of age. Between 2 and 3 years of age, the birth weight quadruples. Slow, steady weight gain during childhood is followed by a growth spurt during adolescence.

The average newborn infant is approximately 20 inches (50 cm) long, with an average increase of approximately 1 inch (2.5 cm) per month for the first 6 months, followed by an increase of approximately $\frac{1}{2}$ inch (1.2 cm) per month for the remainder of the first year. The child gains 3 inches (7.6 cm) per year from age 1 through 7 years and then 2 inches (5 cm) per year from age 8 through 15 years. Boys generally add more height during adolescence than do girls. Body proportion changes are shown in Figure 4-1.

Head circumference indicates brain growth. The normal occipital-frontal circumference of the term newborn head is 13 to 15 inches (32 to 38 cm). Average head growth occurs according to the following pattern: 4.8 inches (12 cm) during the first year, 1 inch (2.54 cm) during the second year; $\frac{1}{2}$ inch (1.27 cm) per year from 3 to 5 years, and $\frac{1}{2}$ inch (1.2 cm) per year from 5 years until puberty. The average adult head circumference is approximately 21 inches (53 cm).

Dentition, the eruption of teeth, also follows a sequential pattern. Primary dentition usually begins to emerge at approximately 6 to 8 months. Most children have 20 teeth by age $2\frac{1}{2}$ years. Permanent teeth, 32 in all, erupt beginning at approximately age 6 years, accompanied by the loss of primary teeth (see Chapter 9). Although some parents place importance on eruption of the teeth as a sign of maturation, dentition is not related to the level or rate of development.

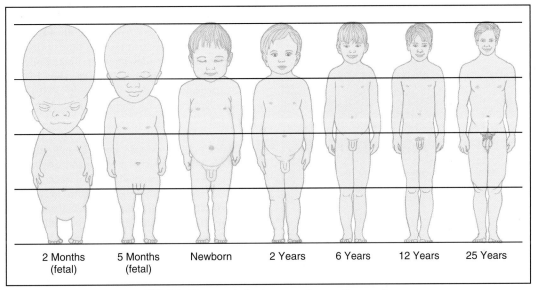

| 2 Months (fetal) | 5 Months (fetal) | Newborn | 2 Years | 6 Years | 12 Years | 25 Years |

FIG 4-1 Changes in body proportions with growth.

PRINCIPLES OF GROWTH AND DEVELOPMENT

Patterns of Growth and Development

Growth and development are directional and follow predictable patterns (Box 4-1 and Box 4-2). The first direction of growth is cephalocaudal, or proceeding from head to tail (or toe). This means that structures and functions originating in the head develop before those in the lower parts of the body. At birth the head is large, a full one fourth of the entire body length, the trunk is long, and the arms are longer than the legs. As the child matures, the body proportions gradually change; by adulthood the legs have increased in size from approximately 38% to 50% of the total body length (see Figure 4-1).

Directional growth and development are illustrated further by myelinization of the nerves, which begins in the brain and spreads downward as the child matures (see Box 4-1). Growth of the myelin sheath and other nerve structures contributes to cephalocaudal development, which is illustrated by an infant's ability to raise the head before being able to sit and to sit before being able to stand.

A second directional aspect of growth and development is proximodistal, which means progression from the center outward, or from the midline to the periphery. The growth and branching pattern of the respiratory tract illustrates this concept. The trachea, which is the central structure of the respiratory tree, forms in the embryo by 24 days of gestation. Branching and growth outward occur in the bronchi, bronchioles, and alveoli throughout fetal life and infancy. Alveoli, which are the most distal structures of the system, continue to grow and develop in number and function until middle childhood.

Growth and development follow patterns, one of which is general to specific. As a child matures, activities become less generalized and more focused. For example, a neonate's response to pain is usually a whole-body response, with flailing of the arms and legs even if the pain is in the abdomen. As the child matures, the pain response becomes more localized to the stimulus. An older child with abdominal pain guards the abdomen.

Another pattern is the progression of functions from simple to complex. This pattern is easily observed in language development. A toddler's first sentences are formed simply, using only a noun and a verb. By age 5 years, the child constructs detailed stories using many complex modifiers.

The rate of growth is not constant as the child matures. *Growth spurts,* alternating with periods of slow or stagnant growth, are observed throughout childhood. Spurts are frequently seen as the child prepares to master a significant developmental task, such as walking. An increase in growth around a child's first birthday may promote the neuromuscular maturation needed for taking the first steps.

All facets of development (cognitive, motor, social/emotional, language) normally proceed according to these patterns. Knowledge of these concepts is useful when determining how a child's development is progressing and when comparing a child's development with normal patterns.

Mastery of developmental tasks is not static or permanent, and developmental stages do not always correlate with chronologic age. Children progress through developmental stages at varying rates within normal limits and may master developmental tasks only to regress to earlier levels when ill or stressed. Also, people can struggle repeatedly with particular developmental tasks throughout life, although they have achieved more advanced levels of development.

Critical Periods

After birth, critical or sensitive periods exist for optimal growth and development. Similar to times during embryologic and fetal life, in which certain organs are formed and are particularly vulnerable to injury, critical periods are blocks of time during which children are ready to master specific developmental tasks. Children can master tasks outside these critical periods, but some tasks are learned more easily during particular periods.

Many factors affect a child's sensitive learning periods, such as injury, illness, and malnutrition. For example, the sensitive period for learning to walk seems to be during the latter part of the first year and the beginning of the second year. Children seem to be driven by an irresistible urge to practice walking and display great pride as they succeed. If a child is immobilized, for instance, for the treatment of an orthopedic condition from age 10 months to 18 months, the child may have difficulty learning to walk. The child can learn to walk, but the task may be more difficult than for other children.

Factors Influencing Growth and Development
Genetics

One factor that greatly influences a child's growth and development is genetics. Genetic potential is affected by many factors. Environment

---

BOX 4-1	PATTERNS OF GROWTH AND DEVELOPMENT

Although heredity determines each individual's growth rate, the normal pace of growth for all children falls into four distinct patterns:

1. A rapid pace from birth to 2 years
2. A slower pace from 2 years to puberty
3. A rapid pace from puberty to approximately 15 years
4. A sharp decline from 16 years to approximately 24 years, when full adult size is reached

---

BOX 4-2	DIRECTIONAL PATTERNS OF GROWTH AND DEVELOPMENT

Cephalocaudal Pattern (Head to Toe)
Examples
 Head initially grows fastest (fetus), then trunk (infant), and then legs (child).
 Infant can raise the head before sitting and can sit before standing.

Cephalocaudal (head to toe)

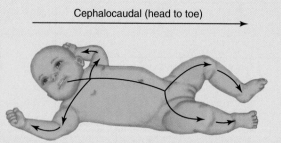

Proximodistal (from the center outward)

Proximodistal Pattern (from the Center Outward)
Examples
 In the respiratory system, the trachea develops first in the embryo, followed by branching and growth outward of the bronchi, bronchioles, and alveoli in the fetus and infant.
 Motor control of the arms comes before control of the hands, and hand control comes before finger control.

influences how and to what extent particular genetic traits are manifested. Genetics is discussed in greater depth later in this chapter.

Environment

The environment, both physical and psychosocial, is a significant determinant of growth and developmental outcomes before and after birth. Prenatal exposures, which include maternal smoking, alcohol intake, chemical exposures, and disease such as diabetes, can adversely affect the developing fetus. Socioeconomic status, mainly poverty, also has a significant effect on the developing child. Imported toys and other equipment for children can pose environmental hazards, particularly if they have multiple small pieces or components with high concentrations of lead or leaded paint.

Scientists suggest that factors in children's physical environment increasingly influence their health status (AAP, 2011). Children are vulnerable to environmental exposures for the following reasons (AAP, 2011; United States Environmental Protection Agency [EPA], 2006; Veal, Lowry, & Belmont, 2007):

- Immature and rapidly developing tissue in multiple body systems increases the risk for injury from exposure to lower-level environmental toxins.
- Increased metabolic rate and growth, which necessitate a higher intake in relation to body mass of food and liquids, result in a higher concentration of ingested toxins.
- More rapid respirations increase inhalation of air pollutants.

- Developmental behaviors, such as mouthing or playing outdoors, increase the risk for hazardous ingestion from hand-to-mouth transfer.
- Environmental toxins can be passed to an infant through breast milk.

Nurses can assist parents in preventing environmental injury by teaching them how to avoid the most common sources of environmental exposure. Anticipatory guidance about avoiding sun exposure, secondhand smoke or other air pollutants, lead in the home environment and in toys, mercury in foods, use of pesticides in gardens and playground equipment, pet insecticides (e.g., flea and tick collars), and radon will provide parents with the information they need to reduce risk. As with communicable disease, teaching about the importance of hand hygiene is paramount.

During well visits, nurses can perform a brief or expanded environmental health screening. Figure 4-2 provides an example of an environmental history. There are thousands of synthetic chemicals to which children are exposed, with very few having federal guidelines for exposure limits (Veal et al., 2007). The American Academy of Pediatrics (2011) has expressed heightened concern that toxic chemicals in the environment are not being regulated to the extent needed to protect children and pregnant women, and this position has been supported by the American Nurses' Association, the American Medical Association, and the American Public Health Association. The AAP (2011) recommends revisions to the Toxic Substances Control Act that

Where does your child live and spend most of his/her time?	_____
What are the age, condition, and location of your home?	_____
Does anyone in the family smoke?	❏ Yes ❏ No ❏ Not sure
Do you have a carbon monoxide detector?	❏ Yes ❏ No ❏ Not sure
Do you have any indoor furry pets?	❏ Yes ❏ No ❏ Not sure
What type of heating/air system does your home have? ❏ Radiator ❏ Forced air ❏ Gas stove ❏ Wood stove ❏ Other_____	
What is the source of your drinking water? ❏ Well water ❏ City water ❏ Bottled water	
Is your child protected from excessive sun exposure?	❏ Yes ❏ No ❏ Not sure
Is your child exposed to any toxic chemicals of which you are aware?	❏ Yes ❏ No ❏ Not sure
What are the occupations of all adults in the household?	_____
Have you tested your home for radon?	❏ Yes ❏ No ❏ Not sure
Does your child watch TV, or use a computer or video game system more than two hours a day?	❏ Yes ❏ No ❏ Not sure
How many times a week does your child have unstructured, free play outside for at least 60 minutes?	_____
Do you have any other questions or concerns about your child's home environment or symptoms that may be a result of his or her environment?	_____

National Environmental Education Foundation
Knowledge to live by

Health & Environment

FIG 4-2 Pediatric environmental history (0-18 years of age). (Reprinted with permission from The National Environmental Education and Training Foundation: www.neefusa.org/pdf/PedEnvHistoryForm_complete.pdf.)

would base decisions about toxic chemical exposures on a "reasonable concern" for harm, especially their potential for harm to children and pregnant women (p. 988), Among other recommendations, the AAP (2011) recommends increased funding for evidence-based research to examine the effects of chemicals exposures on children.

Nurses can access, and can refer parents to, several online resources, including the Environmental Protection Agency (www.epa.gov/children), Pediatric Environmental Health Specialty Units (PEHU) (www.aoec.org), Tools for Schools program (www.epa.gov/schools), and Tox Town (www.toxtown.nlm.nih.gov), among others. Nurses can advise parents to be aware of toy and equipment recalls and to suggest that parents examine toys carefully before purchasing them.

Culture

Culture is the way of life of a people, including their habits, beliefs, language, and values. It is a significant factor influencing children as they grow toward adulthood.

When gathering data, nurses need to recognize how the common family structures and traditional values of various groups affect children's performance on assessment tests. The child's cultural and ethnic background must be considered when assessing growth and development. Standard growth curves and developmental tests do not necessarily reflect the normal growth and development of children of different cultural groups. Growth curves for children of various racial and cultural backgrounds are increasingly available. Nurse researchers and others conduct studies to determine the effectiveness of measurement tools for culturally diverse populations. In addition, culturally sensitive instruments are being developed to gather data to determine appropriate nursing interventions. To provide quality care to all children, nurses must consider the effect of culture on children and families (see Chapter 2).

Nutrition

Because children are growing constantly and need a continuous supply of **nutrients,** nutrition plays an important role throughout childhood. Children need more nutritious food in proportion to size than adults do. Children's food patterns have changed over the years. Children are drinking more low fat or skim milk; however, children over the age of 3 years consistently do not drink enough milk. Instead, they consume juices or other drinks that contain sugar (Peckenpaugh, 2010). Today's children often eat meals outside the home, with 10% of young children having one or more meals in a daycare setting, away from parental supervision (Peckenpaugh, 2010). Nutrition is discussed in more depth later in this chapter.

Health Status

Overall health status plays an important part in the growth and development of children. At the cellular level, inherited or acquired disease can affect the delivery of nutrients, hormones, or oxygen to organs and also can affect organ growth and function. Disease states that affect growth and development include digestive or malabsorptive disorders, heart defects, and metabolic diseases.

Family

A child is an inseparable part of a family. Family relationships and influences substantially determine how children grow and progress. Because of the special bond and influence of the family on the child, there can be no separation of child from family in the health care setting. For example, to diminish anxiety in a child, nurses sometimes attempt to reduce parental anxiety, which may then reduce the stress on the child. Nursing care of children involves nursing care of the whole family and requires skill in dealing with both adults and children.

Nurses might reduce parental anxiety about an ill child by saying, "Your child is in the best place possible here at the hospital. You brought him in at just the right time so that we can help him."

Family structures are in a constant state of change, and these dynamic states influence how children develop. Within the family, relationships change because of marriage, birth, divorce, death, and new roles and responsibilities. Societal forces outside the family, such as economics, population shifts, and migration, change how children are raised. These forces cause changes in family structures and the outcomes of child rearing, which must be considered when planning nursing care for children. The family is discussed in Chapter 2.

Parental Attitudes. Parental attitudes affect growth and development. Growth and development continue throughout life, and parents have stage-related needs and tasks that affect their children. Superimposed on these developmental issues are other factors influencing parental attitudes: educational level, childhood experiences, financial pressures, marital status, and available support systems. Parental attitudes are also affected by the child's temperament, or the child's unique way of relating to the world. Different temperaments affect parenting practices and have a bearing on whether a child's unique personality traits develop into assets or problems.

Child-Rearing Philosophies. Child-rearing philosophies, shaped by myriad life events, influence how children grow and develop. For example, well-educated, well-read parents often provide their children with extra stimulation and opportunities for learning beginning at a young age. This enrichment includes extra parental attention and interaction—not necessarily expensive toys. Generally, development progresses best when children have access to enriched opportunities for learning.

Other parents may not recognize the value of providing a rich learning environment at home, may not have time, or may not appreciate this type of parenting. Children of these parents may not progress at the same rate as those raised in a more enriching atmosphere.

A significant point for parents to remember is that children must be ready to learn. If motor and neurologic structures are not mature, an overzealous approach for accomplishing a task related to those structures can be frustrating for both child and parent. For example, a child who is 6 months old will not be able to walk alone no matter how much time and effort the parent expends. However, at 12 to 14 months, a child usually is ready to begin walking and will do so with ease if given opportunities to practice.

THEORIES OF GROWTH AND DEVELOPMENT

Many theorists have attempted to organize and classify the complex phenomena of growth and development. No single theory can adequately explain the wondrous journey from infancy to adulthood. However, each theorist contributes a piece of the puzzle. Theories are not facts but merely attempts to explain human behavior. Table 4-2 compares and contrasts theories discussed in the text. The chapters on each age-group provide further discussion of these theories.

Piaget's Theory of Cognitive Development

Jean Piaget (1896–1980), a Swiss theorist, made major contributions to the study of how children learn. His complex theory provides a framework for understanding how thinking during childhood progresses and differs from adult thinking. Like other developmental

TABLE 4-2 THEORIES OF GROWTH AND DEVELOPMENT

	PIAGET'S PERIODS OF COGNITIVE DEVELOPMENT	FREUD'S STAGES OF PSYCHOSEXUAL DEVELOPMENT	ERIKSON'S STAGES OF PSYCHOSOCIAL DEVELOPMENT	KOHLBERG'S STAGES OF MORAL DEVELOPMENT
Infancy	**Period 1 (Birth-2 yr): Sensorimotor Period** Reflexive behavior is used to adapt to the environment; egocentric view of the world; development of object permanence.	**Oral Stage** Mouth is a sensory organ; infant takes in and explores during oral passive substage (first half of infancy); infant strikes out with teeth during oral aggressive substage (latter half of infancy).	**Trust vs. Mistrust** Development of a sense that the self is good and the world is good when consistent, predictable, reliable care is received; characterized by hope.	**Premorality or Preconventional Morality, Stage 0 (0-2 yr): Naivete and Egocentrism** No moral sensitivity; decisions are made on the basis of what pleases the child; infants like or love what helps them and dislike what hurts them; no awareness of the effect of their actions on others. "Good is what I like and want."
Toddlerhood	**Period 2 (2-7 yr): Preoperational Thought** Thinking remains egocentric, becomes magical, and is dominated by perception.	**Anal Stage** Major focus of sexual interest is anus; control of body functions is major feature.	**Autonomy vs. Shame and Doubt** Development of sense of control over the self and body functions; exerts self; characterized by will.	**Premorality or Preconventional Morality, Stage 1 (2-3 yr): Punishment-Obedience Orientation** Right or wrong is determined by physical consequences: "If I get caught and punished for doing it, it is wrong. If I am not caught or punished, then it must be right."
Preschool Age		**Phallic or Oedipal/Electra Stage** Genitals become focus of sexual curiosity; superego (conscience) develops; feelings of guilt emerge.	**Initiative vs. Guilt** Development of a can-do attitude about the self; behavior becomes goal-directed, competitive, and imaginative; initiation into gender role; characterized by purpose.	**Premorality or Preconventional Morality, Stage 2 (4-7 yr): Instrumental Hedonism and Concrete Reciprocity** Child conforms to rules out of self-interest: "I'll do this for you if you do this for me"; behavior is guided by an "eye for an eye" orientation. "If you do something bad to me, then it's OK if I do something bad to you."
School Age	**Period 3 (7-11 yr): Concrete Operations** Thinking becomes more systematic and logical, but concrete objects and activities are needed.	**Latency Stage** Sexual feelings are firmly repressed by the superego; period of relative calm.	**Industry vs. Inferiority** Mastering of useful skills and tools of the culture; learning how to play and work with peers; characterized by competence.	**Morality of Conventional Role Conformity, Stage 3 (7-10 yr): Good-Boy or Good-Girl Orientation** Morality is based on avoiding disapproval or disturbing the conscience; child is becoming socially sensitive.
				Morality of Conventional Role Conformity, Stage 4 (begins at about 10-12 yr): Law and Order Orientation Right takes on a religious or metaphysical quality. Child wants to show respect for authority, and maintain social order; obeys rules for their own sake.
Adolescence	**Period 4 (11 yr-Adulthood): Formal Operations** New ideas can be created; situations can be analyzed; use of abstract and futuristic thinking; understands logical consequences of behavior.	**Puberty or Genital Stage** Stimulated by increasing hormone levels; sexual energy wells up in full force, resulting in personal and family turmoil.	**Identity vs. Role Confusion** Begins to develop a sense of "I"; this process is lifelong; peers become of paramount importance; child gains independence from parents; characterized by faith in self.	**Morality of Self-Accepted Moral Principles, Stage 5: Social Contract Orientation** Right is determined by what is best for the majority; exceptions to rules can be made if a person's welfare is violated; the end no longer justifies the means; laws are for mutual good and mutual cooperation.

Continued

TABLE 4-2 THEORIES OF GROWTH AND DEVELOPMENT—cont'd

	PIAGET'S PERIODS OF COGNITIVE DEVELOPMENT	FREUD'S STAGES OF PSYCHOSEXUAL DEVELOPMENT	ERIKSON'S STAGES OF PSYCHOSOCIAL DEVELOPMENT	KOHLBERG'S STAGES OF MORAL DEVELOPMENT
Adulthood			**Intimacy vs. Isolation** Development of the ability to lose the self in genuine mutuality with another; characterized by love.	
			Generativity vs. Stagnation Production of ideas and materials through work; creation of children; characterized by care.	**Morality of Self-Accepted Moral Principles, Stage 6: Personal Principle Orientation** Achieved only by the morally mature individual; few people reach this level; these people do what they think is right, regardless of others' opinions, legal sanctions, or personal sacrifice; actions are guided by internal standards; integrity is of utmost importance; may be willing to die for their beliefs.
			Ego Integrity vs. Despair Realization that there is order and purpose to life; characterized by wisdom.	**Morality of Self-Accepted Moral Principles, Stage 7: Universal Principle Orientation** This stage is achieved by only a rare few; Mother Teresa, Gandhi, and Socrates are examples; these individuals transcend the teachings of organized religion and perceive themselves as part of the cosmic order, understand the reason for their existence, and live for their beliefs.

theorists, Piaget postulated that, as children develop intellectually, they pass through progressive stages (Piaget, 1962, 1967). The ages assigned to these periods are only averages.

During the *sensorimotor* period of development, infant thinking seems to involve the entire body. Reflexive behavior is gradually replaced by more complex activities. The world becomes increasingly solid through the development of the concept of *object permanence,* which is the awareness that objects continue to exist even when they disappear from sight. By the end of this stage, the infant shows some evidence of reasoning.

During the *period of preoperational thought,* language becomes increasingly useful. Judgments are dominated by perception and are illogical, and thinking is characterized, especially during the early part of this stage, by egocentrism. In other words, children are unable to think about another person's viewpoint and believe that everyone perceives situations as they do. *Magical thinking* (the belief that events occur because of wishing) and *animism* (the perception that all objects have life and feeling) characterize this period.

At the end of the preoperational stage, the child shifts from egocentric thinking and begins to be able to look at the world from another person's view. This shifting enables the child to move into the *period of concrete operations,* where the child is no longer bound by perceptions and can distinguish fact from fantasy. The concept of time becomes increasingly clear during this stage, although far past and far

future events remain obscure. Although reasoning powers increase rapidly during this stage, the child cannot deal with abstractions or with socialized thinking.

Normally, adolescents progress to the *period of formal operations.* In this period the adolescent proceeds from concrete to abstract and symbolic and from self-centered to other centered. Adolescents can develop hypotheses and then systematically deduce the best strategies for solving a particular problem because they use a formal operations cognitive style. Not all adolescents, however, reach this landmark at a consistent age, and at any given time, an adolescent may or may not exhibit characteristics of formal operations (Kuhn, 2008).

Nursing Implications of Piaget's Theory

Although other developmental theorists have disputed Piaget's theories, especially the ages at which cognitive changes occur, his work provides a basis for learning about and understanding cognitive development. Piaget's theory is especially significant to nurses as they develop teaching plans of care for children. Piaget believed that learning should be geared to the child's level of understanding and that the child should be an active participant in the learning process. For health teaching to be effective, nurses must understand the different cognitive abilities of children at various ages. Nurses also must know how to engage children in the learning process with developmentally appropriate activities. Because illness and hospitalization are often frightening to children, especially toddlers and preschoolers, nurses must understand the cognitive basis of fears related to treatment and be able to intervene appropriately (see Chapter 11).

Understanding cognitive development that occurs at various ages and developmental levels also has implications for children's health literacy (Borzekowski, 2009). With health related messages so obvious in the media and so accessible on the Internet, it is important that children begin to think about health, evaluate health messages and become involved in their own health promotion (Borzekowski, 2009).

Freud's Theory of Psychosexual Development

Sigmund Freud (1856–1939) developed theories to explain psychosexual development. His theories were in vogue for many years and provided a basis for other theories. Freud postulated that early childhood experiences provide unconscious motivation for actions later in life (Freud, 1960). According to Freudian theory, certain parts of the body assume psychological significance as foci of sexual energy. These areas shift from one part of the body to another as the child moves through different stages of development. Freud's work may help to explain normal behavior that parents may confuse with abnormal behavior, and it also may provide a good foundation for sex education.

Freud believed that during infancy sexual behavior seems to focus around the mouth, the most erogenous area of the infant body (oral stage). Infants derive pleasure from sucking and exploring objects by placing them in their mouths. During early childhood, when toilet training becomes a major developmental task, sensations seem to shift away from the mouth and toward the anus (anal stage). Psychoanalysts see this period as a time of holding on and letting go. A sense of control or autonomy develops as the child masters body functions.

During the preschool years, interest in the genitalia begins (phallic stage). Children are curious about anatomic differences, childbirth, and sexuality. Children at this age often ask many questions, freely exhibit their own sexual organs, and want to peek at those of others. Children often masturbate, sometimes causing parents great concern. Although it is not universal, a phenomenon described by Freud as the Oedipus complex in boys and the Electra complex in girls is seen in preschool children. This possessiveness of the child for the opposite-sex parent, marked by aggressiveness toward the same-sex parent, is considered normal behavior, as is a heightened interest in sex. To resolve these disturbing sexual feelings, the preschooler identifies with or becomes more like the same-sex parent. The superego (an inner voice that reprimands and evokes guilt) also develops. The superego is similar to a conscience (Freud, 1960).

Freud describes the school-age period as the latency stage, when sexuality plays a less prominent role in the everyday life of the child. Best friends and same-sex peer groups are influential in the school-age child's life. Younger school-age children often refuse to play with children of the opposite sex, whereas prepubertal children begin to desire the companionship of opposite-sex friends.

During adolescence, interest in sex again flourishes as children search for identity (genital stage). Under the influence of fluctuating hormone levels, dramatic physical changes, and shifting social relationships, the adolescent develops a more adult view of sexuality. Cognitive skills, particularly in young adolescents, are not fully developed, however, and decisions are made often based on the adolescent's emotional state, rather than on critical reasoning (Cromer, 2011). This can lead to questionable judgments about sexual matters and questions or confusion about sexual feelings and behaviors (A. Freud, 1974).

Nursing Implications of Freud's Theory

Both children and parents may have questions and concerns about normal sexual development and sex education. Nurses need to understand normal sexual growth and development to help parents and children form healthy attitudes about sex and create an accepting climate in which adolescents may talk about sexual concerns.

Erikson's Psychosocial Theory

Erik H. Erikson (1902–1994), inspired by the work of Sigmund Freud, proposed a popular theory about child development. He viewed development as a lifelong series of conflicts affected by social and cultural factors. Each conflict must be resolved for the child and adult to progress emotionally. How individuals address the conflicts varies widely. According to Erikson, however, unsuccessful resolution leaves the individual emotionally disabled (Erikson, 1963).

Each of eight stages of development has a specific central conflict or developmental task. These eight tasks are described in terms of a positive or negative resolution. The actual resolution of a specific conflict lies somewhere along a continuum between a perfect positive and a perfect negative.

The first developmental task is the establishment of trust. The basic quality of trust provides a foundation for the personality. If an infant's physical and emotional needs are met in a timely manner through warm and nurturing interactions with a consistent caregiver, the infant begins to sense that the world is trustworthy. The infant begins to develop trust in others and a sense of being worthy of love. Through successful achievement of a sense of trust, the infant can move on to subsequent developmental stages.

According to Erikson, unsuccessful resolution of this first developmental task results in a sense of mistrust. If needs are consistently unmet, acute tension begins to appear in children. During infancy, signs of unmet needs include restlessness, fretfulness, whining, crying, clinging, physical tenseness, and physical dysfunctions such as vomiting, diarrhea, and sleep disturbances. All children exhibit these signs at times. If these behaviors become personality characteristics, however, unsuccessful resolution of this stage is suspected.

The toddler's developmental task is to acquire a sense of autonomy rather than a sense of shame and doubt. A positive resolution of this task is accomplished by the ability to control the body and body functions, especially elimination. Success at this stage does not mean that the toddler, even as an adult, will exhibit autonomous behavior in all life situations. In certain circumstances, feelings of shame and self-doubt are normal and may be adaptive.

Erikson's theory describes each developmental stage, with crises related to individual stages emerging at specific times and in a particular order. Likewise, each stage is built on the resolution of previous developmental tasks. During each conflict, however, the child spends some energy and time resolving earlier conflicts (Erikson, 1963).

Nursing Implications of Erikson's Theory

In stressful situations, such as hospitalization, children, even those with healthy personalities, evoke defense mechanisms that protect them against undue anxiety. Regression, a behavior used frequently by children, is a reactivation of behavior more appropriate to an earlier stage of development. This defense mechanism is illustrated by a 6-year-old boy who reverts to sucking his thumb and wetting his pants under increased stress, such as illness or the birth of a sibling. Nurses can educate parents about regression and encourage them to offer their children support, not ridicule. They can provide constructive suggestions for stress management and reassure parents that regression normally subsides as anxiety decreases.

Erikson's main contribution to the study of human development lies in his outline of a universal sequence of phases of psychosocial development. His work is especially relevant to nursing because it provides a theoretic basis for much of the emotional care that is given to children. The stages are further discussed in the chapters on each age-group.

Kohlberg's Theory of Moral Development

Lawrence Kohlberg (1927–1987), a psychologist and philosopher, described a stage theory of moral development that closely parallels Piaget's stages of cognitive development. He discussed moral development as a complicated process involving the acceptance of the values and rules of society in a way that shapes behavior. This cognitive-developmental theory postulates that, although knowing what behaviors are right and wrong is important, it is much less important than understanding and appreciating why the behaviors should or should not be exhibited (Kohlberg, 1964).

Guilt, an internal expression of self-criticism and a feeling of remorse, is an emotion closely tied to moral reasoning. Most children 12 years old or older react to misbehavior with guilt. Guilt helps them realize when their moral judgment fails.

Building on Piaget's work, Kohlberg studied boys and girls from middle- and lower-class families in the United States and other countries. He interviewed them by presenting scenarios with moral dilemmas and asking them to make a judgment. His focus was not on the answer but on the reasoning behind the judgment (Kohlberg, 1964). He then classified the responses into a series of levels and stages.

During the *Premorality* (preconventional morality) level, which has three substages (see Table 4-2), the child demonstrates acceptable behavior because of fear of punishment from a superior force, such as a parent. At this stage of cognitive and moral development, children cannot reason as mature members of society. They view the world in a selfish, egocentric way, with no real understanding of right or wrong. They view morality as external to themselves, and their behavior reflects what others tell them to do, rather than an internal drive to do what is right. In other words, they have an external locus of control. A child who thinks "I will not steal money from my sister because my mother will spank me" illustrates premorality.

During the *Morality of Conventional Role Conformity* (conventional morality) level, which is primarily during the school-age years, the child conforms to rules to please others. The child still has an external locus of control, but a concern for social order begins to emerge and replace the more egocentric thinking of the earlier stage. The child has an increased awareness of others' feelings. In the child's view, good behavior is that which those in authority will approve. If behavior is not acceptable, the child feels guilty.

Two stages, stage 3 and stage 4, characterize this level (see Table 4-2). This level of moral reasoning develops as the child shifts the focus of living from the family to peer groups and society as a whole. As the child's cognitive capacities increase, an internal sense of right and wrong emerges and the individual is said to have developed an internal locus of control. Along with this internal locus of control comes the ability to consider circumstances when judging behavior.

Level 3, *Morality of Self-Accepted Moral Principles* (postconventional morality), begins in adolescence, when abstract thinking abilities develop. The person focuses on individual rights and principles of conscience during this stage. There is an internal locus of control. Concern about what is best for all is uppermost, and persons step back from their own viewpoint to consider what rights and values must be upheld for the good of all. Some individuals never reach this point. Within this level is stage 5, in which conformity occurs because individuals have basic rights and society needs to be improved. The adolescent in this stage gives as well as takes and does not expect to get something without paying for it. In stage 6, conformity is based on universal principles of justice and occurs to avoid self-condemnation (Colby, Kohlberg, & Kauffman, 1987; Kohlberg, 1964).

Only a few morally mature individuals achieve stage 6. These people, committed to a moral ideal, live and die for their principles.

Kohlberg believes that children proceed from one stage to the next in a sequence that does not vary, although some people may never reach the highest levels. Even though children are raised in different cultures and with different experiences, he believes that all children progress according to his description.

Nursing Implications of Kohlberg's Theory

To provide anticipatory guidance to parents about expectations and discipline of their children, nurses must be aware of how moral development progresses. Parents are often distraught because their young children apparently do not understand right and wrong. For example, a 6-year-old girl who takes money from her mother's purse does not show remorse or seem to recognize that stealing is wrong. In fact, she is more concerned about her punishment than about her misdeed. With an understanding of normal moral development, the nurse can reassure the concerned parents that the child is showing age-appropriate behavior.

THEORIES OF LANGUAGE DEVELOPMENT

Human language has a number of characteristics that are not shared with other species of animals that communicate with each other. Human language has meaning, provides a mechanism for thought, and permits tremendous creativity.

Because language is such a complex process and involves such a vast number of neuromuscular structures, brain growth and differentiation must reach a certain level of maturity before a child can speak. Language development, which closely parallels cognitive development, is discussed by most cognitive theorists as they explain the maturation of thinking abilities. The process of how language develops remains a mystery, however.

Passive, or *receptive*, language is the ability to understand the spoken word. *Expressive* language is the ability to produce meaningful vocalizations. In most people, the areas in the brain responsible for expressive language are close to motor centers in the left cerebral area that control muscle movement of the mouth, tongue, and hands. Humans use a variety of facial and hand movements as well as words to convey ideas.

Crying is the infant's first method of communication. These vocalizations quickly become distinct and individual and accurately convey such states as hunger, diaper discomfort, pain, loneliness, and boredom. Vowel sounds appear first, as early as 2 weeks of age, followed by consonants at approximately 5 months of age.

By age 2 years, children have a vocabulary of roughly 300 words and can construct simple sentences. By age 4 years, children have gained a sense of correct grammar and articulation, but several consonants, including "*l*" and "*r*," remain difficult to pronounce. For example, the sentence "The red and blue bird flew up to the tree" might be pronounced by the preschooler as "The wed and boo bud fwew up to the twee!"

The language of school-age children is less concrete and much more articulate than that of the preschooler. School-age children learn and understand language construction, use more sophisticated terminology, use varied meanings for words, and can write and express ideas in paragraphs and essays (Feigelman, 2011).

Infants learn much of their language from their parents. Children who are raised in homes where verbalization is encouraged and modeled tend to display advanced language skills. Also, in infancy, receptive ability (the understanding of language) is more developed than expressive skill (the actual articulation of words). This tendency, which persists throughout life, is important to realize when caring for children. In clinical situations, nurses must communicate what is happening to their young clients by use of simple, age-appropriate words, although the child may not verbalize understanding.

Nurses and other health providers need to assess a young child's language development at each well visit. Parent concern or positive family history of language problems, combined with clinical assessment of language development, can identify children who may be at risk for disorders associated with altered expressive or receptive language (Schum, 2007). Language development is discussed in more depth in chapters on each age-group and in Chapter 31.

GENETIC AND GENOMIC INFLUENCES ON GROWTH AND DEVELOPMENT

Heredity, the transmission of genetic characteristics from parent to offspring, is a significant determinant of growth and development. At the completion of the Human Genome Project in 2003, the entire sequence of the 3 billion chemical base pairs in human DNA was determined and 20,000-25,000 genes had been identified. Since then, thousands of disease-associated genetic variants have been identified. These discoveries have opened a frontier in biomedical research that is being pioneered today. Advances in genetics and genomics have moved forward so rapidly that *personalized medicine*, individualized treatment based on a person's genotype, is becoming a reality. This means that pediatric nurses must master a set of genetic/genomic competencies that has expanded to be more relevant to the rapidly changing options that patients will now have.

Nurses need a working knowledge of how genetic traits are transmitted, how common chromosomal abnormalities occur, how genetic factors influence complex conditions, and how genotype affects response to drugs. Pediatric nurses are particularly likely to care for individuals with *monogenic* disorders and must understand the impact of these conditions on children and families. Alert and skilled nurses can provide early assessment, identification, and referral to appropriate professionals for genetic evaluation and counseling. A significant nursing role is offering families support in coping with known genetic abnormalities. Informed nurses can act as advocates, helping children and families maneuver through the complexities of the health care system. Finally, nurses are in an excellent position to educate families and communities about the causes of birth defects and the prevention of environmentally induced disorders.

Genetics and Genomics

Genetics is the study of how inherited characteristics, or traits, are transmitted through single genes and how genetic material, deoxyribonucleic acid (DNA), affects the physiology of cells. The focus of genetics is single genes studied one at a time. *Genomics* is the study of the entire set of genetic instructions (the genome) in an organism, including the interactions of genes with each other and with the environment.

Structure of Genes and Chromosomes

The transmission of traits from parents to their children is a complex process involving basic structures called *DNA, genes,* and *chromosomes.* DNA is a long molecule that resembles a spiral ladder, or double helix. A pair of nitrogen bases forms each rung of the spiral ladder with alternating sugar (deoxyribose) and phosphate groups forming the sides. Each nitrogen base attaches one of its "ends" to a sugar group. It pairs with another nitrogen base at the other "end" by means of weak hydrogen bonds. There are four nitrogen bases in DNA, which always pair in the following manner: adenine with thymine and guanine with cytosine. Genes are specific sequences of base pairs within a DNA molecule.

Genes. A gene is a segment of DNA that directs (codes for) the production of a specific protein needed for body structure or function. Genes may also code for regulatory molecules that control the process of translating the genetic code into a protein. Humans probably have between 20,000 and 25,000 genes (Clamp et al., 2007; Jorde, 2010).

Genes often have two or more alternate forms (alleles). *Wild*-type alleles are those gene versions that occur most commonly in the population. A polymorphism is a place (locus) on the DNA molecule where the sequence of base pairs is different from the expected sequence. Polymorphisms are relatively common. All humans have polymorphisms in their genomes. If it occurs in a gene or a regulatory sequence, a polymorphism may result in production of a protein that is dysfunctional or deficient. On the other hand, it may have no effect or it might be protective.

There are different types of polymorphisms. The most common polymorphisms are *single nucleotide polymorphisms* or SNPs (pronounced "snip"). A SNP happens when a single base is deleted, inserted, or changed in the DNA sequence. The mutation that causes sickle cell disease is a SNP. In the beta globin gene, substitution of an adenine for a thymine at the 17th base position results in producing an altered version of hemoglobin, which causes red blood cells to assume a rigid, sickled shape under certain kinds of stress.

Chromosomes. Usually DNA exists as threadlike structures floating in an unorganized manner within the nucleus of the cell. At certain stages of cell reproduction DNA becomes highly condensed and organized into structures called chromosomes (Figure 4-3). Chromosomes

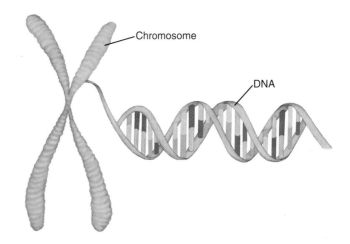

FIG 4-3 Diagrammatic representation of the deoxyribonucleic acid (DNA) helix, which is the building block of genes and chromosomes.

can be seen distinctly under the microscope during the metaphase period of cell division. Technicians photograph or use computer imaging to organize and display the chromosomes from largest to smallest pairs in an image known as a *karyotype*. The karyotype is then analyzed by inspection.

There are normally 46 chromosomes in the nucleus of somatic cells. During cell division chromosomes physically pair. Twenty-two chromosome pairs are called autosomes and are the same in everyone. The 23rd pair makes up the sex chromosomes. Normal females have two X sex chromosomes and normal males have an X and a Y chromosome. Mature sperm or egg cells have half the chromosomes (23) of somatic cells. During germ cell division, one chromosome from each chromosome pair is distributed randomly in daughter cells, resulting in random combinations of maternal and paternal chromosomes. This process of random assortment is one of the primary mechanisms through which human variation occurs. When the ovum and sperm unite at conception, the total number of nuclear chromosomes is restored to 46.

Added or missing chromosomes or structurally abnormal chromosomes are usually harmful. Extra chromosomal material means that extra DNA and, therefore, probably extra genes are present, which may result in an "overdose" of the proteins that the extra genes encode. In a similar fashion, missing or abnormal chromosomal material implies that DNA, and therefore probably some genes that affect function, is missing. This results in an insufficient dose of the proteins that the missing genes encode.

Chromosome analysis is a common procedure during diagnostic evaluation for fetuses, infants, or children with congenital anomalies or intellectual impairment. Cells for chromosomal analysis must be nucleated and alive. Specimens must be obtained and preserved carefully to provide enough living cells for chromosomal analysis. Temperature extremes, blood clotting, or improper preservatives can kill cells and render them useless for analysis. Common cell types used for chromosome analysis include white blood cells, skin fibroblasts, bone marrow cells, and fetal cells from chorionic villi (future placenta) or amniotic fluid.

Alleles. Chromosomes that physically pair during cell division are called homologous chromosomes. Homologous chromosomes have one allele at the same location on each member of the chromosome pair. The paired alleles may be identical (homozygous) or different (heterozygous).

Some alleles occur more frequently in certain groups than they do in the population as a whole. For example, the allele that causes Tay-Sachs disease is carried by about 1 of every 27 Ashkenazi Jews, whose families have their roots in Eastern Europe. Some non-Jewish French-Canadians and Cajun people from Louisiana also have a higher incidence of the disorder. However, an estimated 1 of every 300 people outside these groups carries the mutated allele (Martin, Mark, Triggs-Raine, & Natowicz, 2007). Other disorders that are prevalent in certain ethnic groups are cystic fibrosis (primarily whites of northern European descent) and sickle cell disease (primarily people of African, Mediterranean, Indian, or Middle Eastern descent). The increased frequency of some disease-associated allelic variants in certain racial/ethnic groups is the basis for including race/ethnicity in the health history.

Mutations. Mutations are inheritable changes in the DNA nucleotide sequence or in the structure of chromosomes. Mutations can affect whole chunks of DNA resulting in chromosome abnormalities, or a single base resulting in a SNP, as well as other variations. Mutations occur spontaneously in humans due to errors in DNA replication or exposure to environmental factors, such as radiation or toxic chemicals. Although mutations are often perceived as harmful, they are an important source of human variation.

Principles of Mendelian Inheritance

The fundamental principles of inheritance were discovered by an Augustinian monk, Gregor Mendel, in the mid-19th century. By means of observations of pea plants, Mendel discovered how single traits are inherited. Although advances in contemporary genetics have demonstrated non-Mendelian inheritance patterns, the patterns described by Mendel, termed Mendelian inheritance, remain the major determinants of genetic diseases in children. Mendel's greatest contributions include the principles of segregation, which refers to the separation of paired genes during cell division, and independent assortment, which refers to the random distribution of alleles into gametes during cell division. The characteristic of dominance, in which one allele masks the expression of the other, was also described by Mendel.

Dominant and Recessive Alleles

All humans share the same genes, and each human normally has two copies of each gene. However, all humans do not share the same versions of each gene. Genes have different versions, known as alleles, and some alleles are dominant to others. In the case of a dominant allele, one copy is enough to cause the trait it encodes to be expressed. When an allele is expressed, the trait it encodes becomes observable. It becomes a phenotype.

For example, in the ABO blood system, alleles for group A and group B blood types are dominant. Therefore, a single copy of either of these alleles is enough to be expressed in the person's blood type. If a person's two copies of the gene for blood type contain an allele for blood group A and another allele for blood group O, then the phenotype (the observable trait) will be blood group A because the A allele is dominant to the O allele.

Recessive alleles will only be expressed if two identical copies of the recessive allele are present. The gene for blood group O is recessive. Only if a person receives an allele for blood group O from both parents will laboratory testing identify his or her blood group as O. Some alleles are equally dominant. The person who receives an allele for blood group A from one parent and group B from the other will have type AB blood because both alleles are equally dominant and both are expressed in blood typing.

Dominance and recessiveness are not absolute for all alleles. Some people with a single copy of an abnormal recessive allele (carriers) may have a slightly abnormal level of the gene product (e.g., an enzyme) that can be detected by laboratory methods. These people usually do not have the disease because the normal copy of the allele directs production of enough of the required product to allow normal or near-normal function.

Gene Location

Genes located on autosomes are either autosomal dominant or autosomal recessive, depending on whether one or two identical copies of the allele are needed to produce the trait. Genes located on the X chromosome are paired only in females because males have one X and one Y chromosome. A female with an abnormal recessive gene on one of her X chromosomes usually has a normal gene on the other X chromosome that compensates and maintains relatively normal function. However, the male is at a disadvantage if his only X chromosome has an abnormal gene. He has no compensating normal gene because his other sex chromosome is a Y. The abnormal gene will be expressed in the male because it is unopposed by a normal gene.

Autosomal Dominant Inheritance Pattern

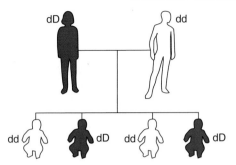

Each child has:
• 50% chance of having the disease
• 50% chance of being normal

No carrier state

No relationship to sex of the child

Examples: Neurofibromatosis
            Blood groups A and B

Key: d = normal gene; D = abnormal, *dominant* gene

Autosomal Recessive Inheritance Pattern

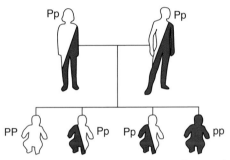

Each child has:
• 25% chance of having the disease
• 50% chance of being a carrier
• 25% chance of being normal

No relationship to sex of the child

Examples: Sickle cell disease
            Cystic fibrosis

Key: P = normal gene; p = abnormal, *recessive* gene

X-Linked Recessive Inheritance Pattern

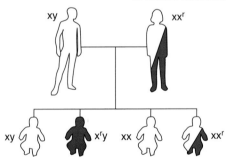

Each *female* child has:
• 50% chance of being a carrier
• 50% chance of being normal

Each *male* child has:
• 50% chance of having the disease
• 50% chance of being normal

Females do not usually have X-linked recessive disorders

Males are not usually carriers

Examples: Hemophilia
            Duchenne muscular dystrophy

Key: xy = normal *male* sex chromosome pattern;
xx = normal *female* sex chromosome pattern;
r = sex-linked *recessive* gene

FIG 4-4 Inheritance pattern and risk.

Mendelian Inheritance Patterns

Three important patterns of inheritance of single alleles are (1) autosomal dominant, (2) autosomal recessive, and (3) X-linked. Figure 4-4 summarizes characteristics and transmission of each pattern. Single-gene traits are traits that are determined by only one gene. Complex traits are determined by multiple interacting genes or interactions between genes and the environment. Complex traits include complex chronic diseases, such as asthma, heart disease, and non-insulin dependent diabetes. Complex, multifactorial diseases are common in adults. In children, the single-gene disorders are of great concern because their manifestations are typically observed in infancy or early childhood and they account for significant allocation of health care resources (Box 4-3).

BOX 4-3 SINGLE-GENE ABNORMALITIES

• A person affected with an autosomal dominant disorder has a 50% risk of transmitting the disorder to each of his or her children.
• Two healthy parents who carry the same abnormal autosomal recessive gene have a 25% risk at each conception of having a child affected with the disorder caused by this gene.
• Parental consanguinity (blood relationship) increases the risk for having a child with an autosomal recessive disorder.
• One copy of an abnormal X-linked recessive gene is enough to produce the disorder in a boy.
• Abnormal genes can arise as new mutations that are then transmitted to future generations.

Single-gene disorders have mathematically predictable rates of occurrence. For example, if a couple has a child with an autosomal recessive disorder, the risk that future children from the same couple will have the disorder is 1:4 (25%) at every conception.

Autosomal Dominant Traits

An autosomal dominant trait is produced by a dominant allele on a non-sex chromosome. The expression of abnormal autosomal dominant alleles may result in multiple and seemingly unrelated effects in the affected person. The gene's effects may vary substantially in severity, leading a family to think that a trait skips a generation. A careful physical examination may reveal subtle evidence of the trait in each generation. Some people may carry the dominant gene but may have no apparent expression of it in their physical makeup.

In some autosomal dominant disorders, such as Huntington's disease, the disease does not manifest until adulthood. The person having the defective gene for Huntington's disease will always have the disease if he or she lives long enough. In other disorders, only a portion of those carrying the gene will ever exhibit the disease. New mutations often account for the introduction of autosomal dominant traits into a family that has no history of the disorder.

The person who is affected with an autosomal dominant disorder is usually heterozygous for the gene—that is, the person has a normal gene on one paired chromosome but has an abnormal gene on the other chromosome in the pair, which overrides the influence of the normal gene. Occasionally, a person is homozygous for the gene, which means that he or she receives two copies of the same abnormal autosomal dominant gene. Such an individual is usually much more severely affected than someone with only one copy.

Autosomal Recessive Traits

An autosomal recessive trait occurs when a person receives two copies of a recessive gene carried on an autosome. Most people carry a few abnormal autosomal recessive genes without problems because a compensating normal gene produces enough of the gene's product for normal function. Because the probability that two unrelated people will share even one of the same abnormal genes is low, the incidence of autosomal recessive diseases is relatively low in the general population.

Situations that increase the likelihood that two parents will share the same abnormal autosomal recessive gene are:
- Consanguinity (blood relationship of the parents)
- Membership in groups that are isolated by culture, geography, religion, or other factors

Many autosomal recessive disorders are severe, and affected persons may not live long enough to reproduce. Two exceptions are phenylketonuria and cystic fibrosis. Improved care of people with these disorders has allowed them to live into their reproductive years. If one member of a couple is affected by the autosomal recessive disorder, all their children will be carriers. Their risk for having similarly affected children is higher as well, depending on the prevalence of the abnormal gene in the general population.

X-Linked Traits

X-linked recessive traits are more common than X-linked dominant ones. Sex differences in the occurrence of X-linked recessive traits and the relationship of affected males to one another distinguish these disorders from autosomal dominant or recessive disorders. Males usually show the full effects of an X-linked recessive disorder because

BOX 4-4	CHROMOSOMAL ABNORMALITIES	
NUMERIC	**STRUCTURAL**
Single chromosome added (trisomy)	Part of a chromosome missing or added
Single chromosome missing (monosomy)	DNA rearrangements within chromosome(s)
One or more added sets of chromosomes (polyploidy)	Part of a chromosome breaks off and becomes attached to another (translocation)
	Fragility of a specific site on a chromosome

their only X chromosome has the abnormal gene on it. Females can show the full disorder when:
- A female has a single X chromosome (Turner syndrome)
- A female child is born to an affected father and a carrier mother

X-linked recessive disorders can be relatively mild, such as color blindness, or they may be severe, such as hemophilia. The disorders may occur with varying degrees of severity.

Chromosomal Abnormalities

Chromosomal abnormalities are common (50% or more) in embryos or fetuses that are spontaneously aborted. Chromosomal abnormalities often cause major defects because they involve many added or missing genes (Box 4-4).

Numerical Abnormalities

Numerical chromosomal abnormalities involve added or missing single chromosomes and multiple sets of chromosomes. Trisomy refers to an additional single chromosome and monosomy indicates deletion of a single chromosome. *Polyploidy* describes abnormalities involving entire sets of chromosomes.

Trisomy. A trisomy exists when each body cell contains an extra copy of one chromosome, bringing the total number to 47. Each chromosome is normal, but there is an extra one in every cell. The most common trisomy is *Down syndrome*, or trisomy 21 (see Chapter 30). In Down syndrome, each body cell has three copies of chromosome 21. Trisomies of chromosomes 13 and 18 are less common and have more severe effects. The incidence of trisomies increases with maternal age, so most women who are 35 years old or older at conception are offered prenatal diagnosis to determine whether the fetus may have Down syndrome or another trisomy.

Monosomy. A monosomy occurs when each body cell has a missing chromosome, with a total number of 45. The only monosomy that is compatible with extended postnatal life is *Turner's syndrome*, or monosomy X. People with Turner's syndrome have a single X chromosome and the female phenotype. Complete absence of an X chromosome is always lethal.

Live-born infants with Turner's syndrome have excess skin around the neck and edema that is most noticeable in the hands and feet. If Turner's syndrome is not identified and treated during infancy or childhood, an affected girl will remain very short and will not have menstrual periods nor will secondary sex characteristics develop. Heart and aortic defects are common. Severe defects are surgically repaired. Children with Turner's syndrome usually have normal intelligence, although they may have difficulty with spatial relationships or solving visual problems, such as reading a map.

Polyploidy. Polyploidy occurs when gametes do not halve their chromosome number during meiosis or when two sperm fertilize an ovum simultaneously. The result is an embryo with one or more extra sets of chromosomes. The total number of chromosomes is a multiple of the haploid number of 23 (69 or 92 total chromosomes). Polyploidy usually results in an early spontaneous abortion but is occasionally seen in a live-born infant.

Structural Abnormalities

The structure of one or more chromosomes may be abnormal. Part of a chromosome may be missing or added, or DNA within the chromosome may be rearranged. Some of these rearrangements are harmless. Others are harmful because important genetic material is lost or duplicated in the structural abnormality, or the position of the genes in relation to other genes is altered so that normal function is not possible.

Another structural abnormality occurs when all or part of a chromosome breaks off and becomes attached to another (translocation). Many people with a chromosomal translocation are clinically normal because their total genetic material is normal, or balanced. If a parent has a balanced translocation, offspring may have normal chromosomes or may have a balanced translocation, too. However, offspring may receive too much or too little chromosomal material and may be spontaneously aborted or suffer birth defects. Balanced or unbalanced chromosomal translocations may occur spontaneously in the child of parents who have no translocation.

Fragile X syndrome is a structural chromosome abnormality that often causes intellectual impairment among males. With this abnormality, a site on the X chromosome is more fragile than normal. Although females can also be affected with fragile X syndrome, males are more severely affected because the female has a second X chromosome that is usually normal. The fragile X syndrome is inherited in an X-linked dominant pattern, with males being most severely affected.

Multifactorial Birth Defects

Multifactorial birth defects result from the interaction of genetic and environmental factors. Gene-environment interactions may influence prenatal and postnatal development positively or negatively. For example, two embryos may have an equal genetic susceptibility for development of a disorder such as spina bifida (open spine), but the disorder will not occur unless an environment favoring its development, such as deficient maternal intake of folic acid, also exists.

Multifactorial birth defects have two characteristics that distinguish them from other types of birth defects. They are typically (1) present and detectable at birth and (2) isolated defects rather than ones that occur with other unrelated abnormalities. A multifactorial defect may *cause* a secondary defect, however. For example, infants with spina bifida often have hydrocephalus because abnormal development of the spine and spinal cord disrupts spinal fluid circulation, allowing it to build up in the brain's ventricular system.

Multifactorial defects represent some of the most common birth defects that a pediatric nurse encounters (Box 4-5). Examples include many heart defects; neural tube defects, such as spina bifida; cleft lip and palate; and developmental dysplasia of the hip. Unlike single-gene traits, multifactorial disorders are not usually associated with one causal gene mutation, nor are they associated with a fixed risk of occurrence or recurrence in a family. Factors that may affect the degree of risk are number of affected close relatives, severity of the disorder in affected family members, sex of the affected child, geographic location, and seasonal variations.

BOX 4-5   MULTIFACTORIAL BIRTH DEFECTS

- Multifactorial defects are some of the most common birth defects encountered in pediatric nursing practice. They result from interactions between genetic susceptibility and environmental factors during prenatal development.
- These are usually single, isolated defects, although the primary defect may cause secondary defects.
- Some occur more often in certain geographic areas.
- A greater risk for occurrence exists for any of the following:
  - Several close relatives have the defect, whether mild or severe
  - One close relative has a severe form of the defect
  - The defect occurs in a child of the less frequently affected gender
- Infants who have several major or minor defects, or both, that are not directly related to each other, probably do not have a multifactorial defect but have another syndrome, such as a chromosomal abnormality.

Exposure to an Adverse Prenatal Environment

Avoiding exposure to harmful influences begins before conception because major organ systems develop early in pregnancy, often before a woman realizes that she is pregnant. Alcohol, substance, or cigarette use requires major lifestyle changes to avoid fetal or infant exposure. *Teratogens* are agents in the fetal environment that either cause or increase the likelihood that a birth defect will occur. Teratogens include certain medications, infectious agents, chemicals or pollutants, and ionizing radiation. Some maternal conditions, such as type I diabetes mellitus, can increase the risk of adverse effects on the fetus.

Genetic Counseling

Genetic counseling provides services to help people understand genetic disorders and the risk that a disorder will occur in their families. Genetic counseling is often available through facilities that provide maternal-fetal medicine services. State departments of mental health and intellectual impairment or rehabilitation services also may provide counseling services. The National Society of Genetic Counselors maintains a database of genetic counselors in the United States, which is searchable by zip code. It is accessible at www.nsgc.org/resourcelink.cfm.

Genetic counseling focuses on the family rather than on an individual. One family member may have a genetic disorder, but study of the entire family is usually needed for accurate counseling. Genetic counselors construct a pictorial representation of the family health history (pedigree), which requires as much information about the health status of family members as possible. This may involve obtaining medical records, including the mother's prenatal and perinatal history, or performing physical examinations or laboratory and other diagnostic studies on numerous family members. Examining photographs, particularly of deceased or unavailable family members, may be helpful. Counseling is impaired if family members are unwilling to provide their medical records or agree to examinations or laboratory studies. Moreover, those who seek counseling may be unwilling to request cooperation from other family members or to share the genetic information they acquire.

Genetic counseling is nondirective; that is, the counselor does not tell the individual or parents what decision to make but educates them about options for dealing with the disorder. Families often interpret the counseling subjectively, however. Some parents may regard a 50% risk of occurrence or recurrence as low, whereas others may think that a 1% risk is unacceptably high. The family's values and beliefs influence whether they seek counseling and what they do with the information that is provided.

Genetic counseling is often a slow process, and despite a comprehensive evaluation, a diagnosis may never be established. Nevertheless, counseling provides families with the best information concerning what is known about the cause and natural course of the disorder, options for caring for an affected child, the likelihood that the disorder will occur in others, the availability of treatment and services (including prenatal diagnosis for future pregnancies), and how to minimize future risk.

Nurses who participate on a genetic counseling team usually are educated in the specifics of genetic disorders and in counseling techniques. These nurses assist women or couples through the process of prenatal diagnosis and support parents as they make decisions after receiving abnormal prenatal diagnostic results. They also help the family deal with the emotional impact of having a child with a birth defect and assist them to access needed services and support.

Expected Genetic Competencies of the Pediatric Nurse

Essential genetic and genomic competencies were established for all registered nurses by 2005 and were endorsed by the Society of Pediatric Nurses. As professionals, all nurses are expected to recognize when personal attitudes toward genetic/genomic science and technologies may affect care that is provided to clients. All nurses are also expected to advocate for client access to desired genetic services and resources. In the practice setting, nurses are expected to identify clients who might benefit from genetic services, facilitate appropriate referrals to genetic specialists, recognize genetic contributions to response to medications, and identify resources for clients seeking genetic information. All nurses should be able to elicit a complete three-generation family health history and construct a pedigree using appropriate symbols and terminology, as well as identify family health history tools that can be used by clients. Nurses are expected to assess client perspectives on genetic issues when relevant and use effective communication skills to enable clients to express their views and wishes in regards to genetic testing or procedures. A complete list of the genetic/genomic competencies established by consensus panel for all registered nurses (Consensus Panel on Genetic/Genomic Nursing Competencies, 2009) is available online.

The full sequence of human genes was completed in April 2003 when the Human Genome Project was completed. That event opened the door to an explosion in new genetic/genomic knowledge. It is critical that pediatric nurses understand basic principles of genetics and be aware of advances in genetic/genomic science relevant to human health in order to communicate information to patients. Information gained from continued progress in genetic/genomic science will allow advances such as:

- Easier, quicker, and less costly types of genetic testing to determine risk for disorders or the actual presence of disorders.
- The ability to base reproductive decisions on more accurate and specific information than has previously been available.
- Early identification of genetic susceptibility to a disorder so that interventions to reduce risk can be instituted.
- Safe use of gene therapy to modify a defective gene.
- Choosing pharmacotherapy and other treatments on the basis of an individual's genetic code or the genetic makeup of tumor cells.

The explosion of knowledge about the genetic basis for disease raises legal and ethical issues for which we do not yet have answers. For instance:

- Genetic information has implications for others in the affected person's family, raising privacy issues.
- Identification of genetic problems could lead to poor self-esteem, guilt, and excessive caution, or, conversely, a reckless lifestyle.
- Presymptomatic identification of a genetically influenced illness could be a source of long-term anxiety.
- Genetic knowledge could affect one's choice of a partner.
- Although federal legislation exists that prohibits discrimination in employment and insurance based on genetics, stigma or other forms of discrimination based on genetic information may occur.
- Ownership of genes through gene patents may affect patient access to specific gene tests and genetic therapies.

ASSESSMENT OF GROWTH

Because growth is an excellent indicator of physical well-being, accurate assessments must be made at regular intervals so that patterns of growth can be determined. Trained individuals using reliably calibrated equipment and proper techniques should perform growth measurement. Methods of obtaining accurate measurements in children are described in Chapter 9. To minimize the chance of error, data should be collected on children under consistent conditions on a routine basis, and values should be recorded and plotted on growth charts immediately.

Standardized growth charts allow an individual child's growth (length/height, weight, head circumference, body mass index [BMI]) to be compared with statistical norms. The most commonly used growth charts for boys and girls ages 2 years to 20 years are those developed by the National Center for Health Statistics. The World Health Organization growth charts are recommended for infants and children younger than 2 years old (see Evolve website).

Because height and weight are the best indicators of growth, these parameters are measured, plotted on growth charts, and monitored over time at each well visit. Brain growth can also be monitored by measuring infant frontal-occipital circumference at intervals and plotting the values on growth charts. It is important to relate head size to weight because larger babies have bigger heads. These measurements are routinely performed during the first 2 years of life.

BMI, which is a function of both height and weight, is an important measure of growth and overall nutritional status in children older than age 2 years. Because childhood overweight and obesity can contribute to health problems later in life, the American Academy of Pediatrics (Barlow, 2007) recommends beginning obesity prevention at birth. Infants and children younger than two-years-old can be screened for overweight using the weight to length measurement; concern is generated when that percentile exceeds the 95th. BMI charts are included in the most recent versions of charts available from the National Center for Health Statistics.

Growth rate is measured in percentiles. The area between any two percentiles is referred to as a *growth channel*. Childhood growth normally progresses according to a pattern along a particular growth channel. Deviations from normal growth patterns may suggest problems. Any change of more than two growth channels indicates a need for more in-depth assessment.

Recognition of abnormal growth patterns is an important nursing function. The earlier that growth disorders are detected, diagnosed, and treated, the better the long-term prognosis.

ASSESSMENT OF DEVELOPMENT

Assessment of development is a more complex process than assessment of growth. To assess developmental progress accurately, nurses and health providers need to gather data from many sources, including observations and interviews, physical examinations, interactions with the child and parents, and various standardized assessment tools.

The American Academy of Pediatrics issued a policy statement in 2006 (reaffirmed in 2010), which calls for providers to do a combination of developmental surveillance and developmental screening throughout a child's infancy and early childhood (AAP, 2006/2010). Developmental surveillance is performed at every well visit and includes eliciting and paying attention to parent concerns, keeping a documented developmental history, identifying protective and risk factors, and direct observation of the child's development (AAP, 2006, p. 419). If surveillance raises a concern, the provider refers the child for more formalized screening. The AAP recommends that providers conduct a formal developmental screening with a sensitive and specific screening instrument when the child is 9 months, 18 months, and 24 to 30 months of age (AAP, 2006/2010). Using formalized screening in addition to routine surveillance can increase appropriate referrals for early intervention (Hix-Small, Marks, Squires, & Nickel, 2007). Although the AAP recommendations were issued initially in 2006, recent mixed (quantitative and qualitative) research using a national sample of 17 pediatric practices found that the percentage of children screened at the appropriate ages is approximately 85% of children, however, the rate of referral for follow-up is far less (King et al., 2010).

Observation is a valuable method most often used to obtain information about a child's **developmental age** (level of functioning). By watching a child during daily activities, such as eating, playing, toileting, and dressing, nurses gather a great deal of assessment data. Observation of the child's problem-solving abilities, communication patterns, interaction skills, and emotional responses can yield valuable information about the child's level of development. Similarly, interviews and physical examinations can provide much information about how the child functions.

In addition to these sources of data, many standardized assessment tools are available for nurses and other health care professionals to use for developmental assessment. Standardized developmental tools should be both sensitive (accurately identifies developmental problems) and specific (accurately identifies those who do not have developmental problems). Additionally, they should be relatively easy to administer or to have the parent complete in a reasonable amount of time. General assessment screening instruments that meet these criteria include the Ages and Stages Questionnaire, the Infant Development Inventory, and the Parents' Evaluations of Developmental Status (PEDS), among others (AAP, 2006/2010). In general, screening tools are organized around major developmental areas (language, cognitive, social, behavioral, and motor). Many are given to parents to complete in the office setting or before the child's appointment. Domain-specific instruments for identifying delays in language/cognitive areas or for screening for autism also are available (Wallis & Smith, 2008).

Developmental assessment should be part of a newborn infant's assessment and of every well-child examination for several reasons. One reason is that parents want to know how their child compares with others and whether development is normal, especially if they had a difficult pregnancy or have other children who are developmentally delayed. Developmental assessment tends to allay fears. Probably the most important reason for assessment is that abnormal development must be discovered early to facilitate optimal outcomes through early intervention.

Denver Developmental Screening Test II (DDST-II)

One, more in-depth, screening tool used for infants and young children is the Denver Developmental Screening Test II (DDST-II). The DDST-II provides a clinical impression of a child's overall development and alerts the user to potential developmental difficulties. It requires training to learn how to administer it properly.

The DDST-II, designed to be used with children between birth and 6 years of age, assesses development on the basis of performance of a series of age-appropriate tasks. There are 125 tasks or items arranged in four functional areas (Frankenburg & Dodds, 1992):

1. Personal-social (getting along with others, caring for personal needs)
2. Fine motor (eye-hand coordination, problem-solving skills)
3. Language (hearing, using, and understanding language)
4. Gross motor (sitting, jumping)

Items for rating the child's behavior are also included at the end of the test.

The test form is arranged with age scales across the top and bottom (see the Evolve website for a sample test form). After calculating the child's chronologic age (age in years), the test administrator draws an age line on the form. Each of the 125 tasks or items is arranged on a shaded bar depicting at which ages 25%, 50%, 75%, and 90% of the children in the research sample completed that particular item. The examiner assesses the child using the items clustered around the age line. The directions must be followed exactly during administration of the test. A score for performance on each item is recorded according to the following scale: pass *(P)*, fail *(F)*, no opportunity *(NO)*, and refusal *(R)*. At the completion of the test, the screener scores test behavior ratings (located at the bottom left of the form).

Interpretation of the test is based first on individual items and then on the test as a whole. Individual items are considered as "advanced, normal, caution, delayed, or no opportunity." Reliability and validity of the test can be altered if the child is not feeling well or is under the influence of medications. Parental presence and input as to whether the child is behaving as usual is desired (Frankenburg & Dodds, 1992).

The results of the test can be used to identify a child's developmental age and how a child compares with others of the same chronologic age. This information can be used to alert health care providers to potential problems. To ensure that the results are accurate, only individuals who are trained to administer the test in a standardized manner should perform testing. Training is obtained through study of the testing manual, review of the accompanying videotape, and supervised practice with children of various ages.

Although the DDST-II is widely used, it is a screening test only, not an intelligence quotient (IQ) test. It is not a definitive predictor of future abilities, and it should not be used to determine diagnostic labels. It is, however, a useful tool for noting problems, validating hunches, monitoring development, and providing referrals.

NURSE'S ROLE IN PROMOTING OPTIMAL GROWTH AND DEVELOPMENT

Nurses are particularly concerned with preventing disease and promoting health. One aspect of preventive care is providing anticipatory guidance or basic information for parents about normal growth and development as their child approaches different ages and developmental levels.

Developmental Assessment

Nursing care for children is not complete without addressing the developmental issues that are unique to each child. Because children grow and change rapidly, the nurse must use knowledge of theories of growth and development to create plans of care for both healthy and ill children. Assessment data are collected from a variety of sources, categorized, and analyzed with a theoretic knowledge base and clinical experience. A list of strengths and problems related to growth and development is generated. Nursing diagnoses are formulated with individualized goals, interventions, and evaluation to address specific problems that are related to, but differ from, physiologic and psychosocial needs.

Interview

During the initial interview, the nurse asks questions about the child's cognitive, language, motor, and emotional development. The parents' emotional state, level of education, and culture must be considered when information is gathered. For example, the nurse might use the following questions and statements when interviewing the parents of a 4-year-old child:

- What does your child like to do at home?
- Does your child know the days of the week?
- Describe your child's typical day.
- Does your child attend preschool? If so, how often?
- Can your child throw a ball, ride a tricycle, climb?
- Can your child draw pictures, color them?
- How effective is your child's use of language?
- How did your child's development progress during infancy and toddlerhood?

The nurse also assesses the child's ability to think through situations and to communicate verbally. In addition, how the child interacts with other children and adults can be a measure of cognitive abilities. The number, type, length, appropriateness, and correct use of words and sentences are also noted. Carefully observing the child in a variety of situations, including play, provides valuable information about cognitive development.

A child's stage of emotional development can be assessed in a number of ways. From Erikson's theory, it is expected that a 4-year-old child's major conflict would be developing a sense of initiative rather than a sense of guilt. If the child is hospitalized, however, regressive behaviors might be exhibited if the anxiety of hospitalization becomes overwhelming. Questions directed to the parents, such as those that follow, could help validate inferences about the child's psychosocial development:

- What types of play activities does your child like best?
- How does your child get along with other children? With adults?
- How does your child usually handle stressful situations?
- What do you do to help your child cope with problems?
- How does your child's ability to cope compare with that of your other children?
- Is the behavior exhibited your child's usual behavior?

The nurse can also obtain valuable information from careful observation of a child who is hospitalized. The nurse should note how the child deals with pain, intrusive procedures, and separation from parents.

Play

Although play is not work in the traditional sense, it is children's work. Play is those tasks, done to amuse oneself, that have behavioral, social, or psychomotor rewards. To adult observers, children's play may appear unorganized, meaningless, and even chaotic. Anyone who watches carefully, however, quickly discovers that play is a rich activity, intricately woven with meaning and purpose. In adulthood, work is any activity during which one uses time and energy to create a product or achieve a goal. Play in childhood is similar to adult work in that it is undertaken by the child to accomplish developmental tasks and master the environment.

Play is also an important part of the developmental process. Play is how children learn about shape, color, cause and effect, and themselves. In addition to cognitive thinking, play helps the child learn social interaction and psychomotor skills. It is a way of communicating joy, fear, sorrow, and anxiety.

Classifications of Play

Piaget (1962) described the following three types of play that relate to periods of sensorimotor, preoperational, and concrete operational functioning. These three types of play are overlapping and are linked to stages of cognitive development.

Sensorimotor, which is also known as *functional* or *practice play*, involves repetitive muscle movements and the introduction of a deliberate complication into the way of doing something. In this type of play the infant plays with objects, making use of their properties (falling, making noises) to produce pleasurable effects (Pellegrini & Smith, 2005).

Symbolic play, as its name suggests, uses games and interactions that represent an issue or concern to be addressed. Garvey (1979) identified three elements of symbolic play: one or more objects, a theme or plan, and roles. As children play, they incorporate some object (a toy syringe), use a theme (getting an injection), and then play the roles each player will have (child, nurse). Because there are no rules in symbolic play, the child can use this play not only to reinforce or learn the good things in life but also to alter those things that are painful.

Games include rules and usually are played by more than one person, although some games can be played by oneself. For example, the card game solitaire is played by one person, as are many video games. Children younger than 4 years of age rarely play games with rules; games are most commonly seen in the school-age child (Piaget, 1962). Games continue throughout life as adults play board games, cards, and sports.

Through games, children learn to play by the rules and to take turns. Board games facilitate this accomplishment. Young children often make up games with unique sets of rules, which may change each time the game is played. Older children have games with specific rules; younger children tend to change the rules.

Social Aspects of Play

As the child develops, increased interaction with people occurs. Certain types of play are associated with, but not limited to, specific age-groups.

Solitary Play. Solitary play is characterized by independent play (Figure 4-5). The child plays alone with toys that are very different from those chosen by other children in the area. This type of play begins in infancy and is common in toddlers because of their limited social, cognitive, and physical skills. It is important for children in all age-groups, however, to have some time to play by themselves.

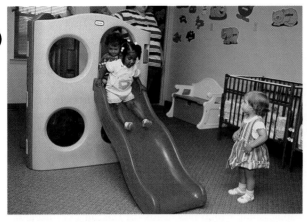

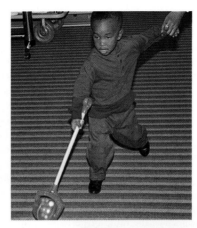

When engaging in solitary play, the child is playing apart from other children and with different types of toys. (Courtesy University of Texas at Arlington School of Nursing.)

The little girl at right demonstrates onlooker play. She is interested in what is going on and observes another girl playing on the slide, but she makes no attempt to join the youngster on the slide.

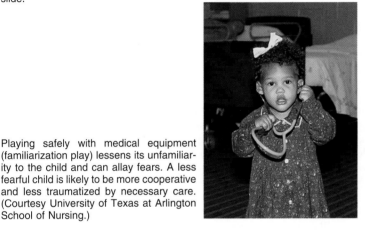

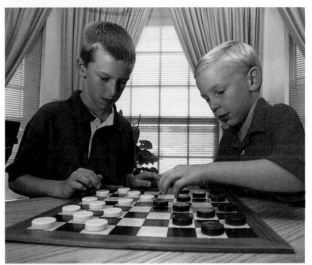

Playing safely with medical equipment (familiarization play) lessens its unfamiliarity to the child and can allay fears. A less fearful child is likely to be more cooperative and less traumatized by necessary care. (Courtesy University of Texas at Arlington School of Nursing.)

Games with rules, such as board games, help children learn boundaries, teamwork, taking turns, and competition. (Courtesy Cook Children's Medical Center, Fort Worth, TX.)

FIG 4-5 Types of play.

Parallel Play. Parallel play is usually associated with toddlers, although it can be found in any age-group. Children play side by side with similar toys, but there is a lack of interactive activity.

Associative Play. Associative play is characterized by group play without group goals. Children in this type of play do not set group rules, and although they may all be playing with the same types of toys and may even trade toys, there is a lack of formal organization. This type of play can begin during toddlerhood and continue into the preschool age.

Cooperative Play. Cooperative play begins in the late preschool years. This type of play is organized and has group goals. There is usually at least one leader, and children are definitely in or out of the group.

Onlooker Play. Onlooker play is present when the child observes others playing. Although the child may ask questions of the players, the child does not attempt to join the play (see Figure 4-5). Onlooker play is usually during the toddler years but can be observed at any age.

Types of Play

Dramatic Play. Dramatic play allows children to act out roles and experiences that may have happened to them, that they fear will happen, or that they have observed in others. This type of play can be spontaneous or guided, and it often includes medical or nursing equipment. It is especially valuable for children who have had or will have multiple procedures or hospitalizations.

Hospitals and clinics with child life specialists on staff usually have a medical play area as part of the activity room. Nurses may provide opportunities for spontaneous and guided dramatic play. The nurse may choose to observe spontaneous play or be an active participant with the child. Occasionally nurses will want to structure the dramatic play to review a specific treatment or procedure. In guided play situations, the nurse directs the focus of the play. Specialized play kits may be developed for specific procedures, such as central line care, casting, bone marrow aspirations, lumbar punctures, and surgery, using supplies related to the hospital or clinic setting.

Familiarization Play. Familiarization play allows children to handle and explore health care materials in nonthreatening and fun ways (see Figure 4-5). This type of play is especially helpful for but not limited to preparing children for procedures and the whole experience of hospitalization.

Examples of familiarization activities include using sponge mouth swabs as painting and gluing tools; making jewelry from bandages, tape, gauze, and lid tops; creating mobiles and collages with health care supplies; making finger puppets with plaster casting material; filling a basin with water and using tubing, syringes without needles, medicine cups, and bulb syringes for water play; decorating beds, wheelchairs, and intravenous poles with health care supplies; and using syringes for painting activities.

Functions of Play

Play enhances the child's growth and development. Play contributes to physical, cognitive, emotional, and social development.

Physical Development and Play. Play aids in the development of both fine and gross motor activity. Children repeat certain body movements purely for pleasure, and these movements in turn aid in the development of body control. For example, an infant will first hit at a rattle, then will attempt to grasp it, and eventually will be able to pick up that same rattle. Next the infant will shake the rattle or perhaps bring it to the mouth.

The parent and child may make a game of repeating sounds such as "ma ma" or "da da," which increases the child's language ability. Repeating rhymes and songs can be a fun way for children to increase their vocabulary. Children love to color on a paper with a crayon and will scribble before being able to draw pictures and to color. This assists the child with eventually learning how to write letters and numerals.

Cognitive Development. Play is a key element in the cognitive development of children. Once a child has learned a general concept, further experiences with that concept expand from that beginning knowledge. Piaget gave the example of an infant learning to swing an object and then subsequently swinging other objects (Piaget, 1962). This could apply, for example, to things to be eaten, read, or ridden. Progression takes place as the child begins to have certain experiences, test beliefs, and understand the surrounding world.

Children can increase their problem-solving abilities through games and puzzles. Pretend play can stimulate several types of learning. Language abilities are strengthened as the child models significant others in role playing. The child must organize thoughts and be able to communicate with others involved in the play scenario. Children who play "house" create elaborate details of what the characters do and say.

Children also increase their understanding of size, shape, and texture through play. They begin to understand relationships as they attempt to put a square peg into a round hole, for example. Books and videos increase a child's vocabulary while increasing understanding of the world.

Emotional Development. Children in an anxiety-producing situation are often helped by role playing. Play can be a way of coping with emotional conflict. Play can be a way to determine what is real and what is not. Children may escape through play into a world of fantasy and make-believe to make sense out of a sometimes senseless world. Play can also increase a child's self-awareness as an event or situation is explored through role playing or symbolic play.

As significant others in children's lives respond to their initiation of play, children begin to learn that they are important and cared for. Whether the child initiates the play or the adult does, when a significant person plays a board game with a child, shares a bike ride, plays baseball, or reads a story, the child gets the message, "You are more important than anything else at this time." This increases the child's self-esteem.

Social Development. The newborn infant cannot distinguish self from others and therefore is narcissistic. As the infant begins to play with others and things, a realization of self and others begins to develop. The infant begins to experience the joy of interacting with others and soon initiates behavior that involves others. Infants discover that when they coo, their mothers coo back. Children will soon expect this response and make a game of playing with their mothers.

Playing make-believe allows the child to try on different roles. When children play "restaurant" or "hospital," they experiment with rules that govern these settings.

Of course, most games, from board games to sports, involve interaction with others. The child learns boundaries, taking turns, teamwork, and competition. Children also learn how to negotiate with different personalities and the feelings associated with winning and losing. They learn to share and to take turns (see Figure 4-5).

Moral Development. When children engage in play with their peers and their families, they begin to learn which behaviors are acceptable and which are not. Quickly they learn that taking turns is rewarded and cheating is not. Group play assists the child in recognizing the importance of teamwork, sharing, and being aware of the feelings of others.

HEALTH PROMOTION

Immunizations

Immunizations are effective in decreasing and, in some cases, eliminating childhood infectious diseases. Naturally occurring smallpox has been virtually eliminated, and the incidence of diphtheria, tetanus, measles, mumps, rubella, varicella, and poliomyelitis has greatly declined in the United States since vaccines against these diseases were introduced. In accordance with recommendations from the Centers for Disease Control and Prevention (CDC) and the American Academy of Pediatrics, children are immunized against 14 communicable diseases before they reach 2 years of age (CDC, 2011d).

Since the introduction of the hepatitis B vaccine, the childhood prevalence of hepatitis B in the United States has decreased 98% (AAP Committee on Infectious Diseases, 2009b). Much of this reduction is due to the decrease in perinatal and household transmission from adults to children.

The incidence of diseases caused by *Haemophilus influenzae* type b (Hib), which can cause meningitis in infants and young children, has been reduced by 99% since the vaccine was introduced in the United States in the late 1980s. The World Health Association reports that Hib infection is virtually nonexistent in industrialized nations. In developing countries, however, Hib is still a leading cause of respiratory deaths in children (World Health Organization, 2011).

Immunization with pneumococcal conjugate vaccine introduced in 2000 has substantially reduced the number of cases of severe disease caused by the bacteria *Streptococcus pneumoniae*. Until recently, infants and children have been vaccinated with PCV7 (Pneumococcal conjugate vaccine, which provides protection from seven different strains of *Streptococcus pneumonia*); PCV13 (protection against six additional strains) became available in 2010 (CDC, 2010).

In response to an increasing incidence of pertussis (whooping cough), particularly among the adolescent population, an adult tetanus, diphtheria, and pertussis vaccine (Tdap) was approved in 2005 (Hall-Baker et al., 2011). Pertussis (whooping cough) has been increasing in incidence in the United States, with nearly 50% of new cases occurring among adolescents (Hall-Baker et al., 2011). The major contributing factor to this phenomenon is presumed to be waning of immunity during midadolescence. Because pertussis can be a serious problem resulting in school absences and health consequences, including possible exposure of underimmunized infants, the CDC (2011a) recommends one dose of Tdap vaccine for children and adolescents. The dose would be administered to 11- and 12-year-old children, so long as they have had the primary diphtheria-tetanus-acellular pertussis (DTaP) series and have not previously received the tetanus-diphtheria (Td) booster, and to older adolescents who have not received the Td booster or for whom 5 years has elapsed since their last Td booster (CDC, 2011a).

Hepatitis A vaccine is recommended for all children at age 1 year (12 to 23 months). The two doses in the series should be administered at least 6 months apart. Children who are not vaccinated by age 2 years can be vaccinated at subsequent visits (CDC, 2011a).

Influenza vaccine is recommended annually prior to the beginning of the flu season for all healthy children. Household contacts of children in these groups, including siblings and caregivers, should also receive the vaccine. If not given previously, any child younger than 9 years needs to receive two doses initially, each dose being 1 month apart (AAP Committee on Infectious Diseases, 2009b).

Meningococcal conjugate vaccine (MCV4) should be administered to all children at age 11 to 12 years, as well as to unvaccinated adolescents at high school entry (15 years). All college freshmen living in dormitories should also be vaccinated. In addition, infants and children between the ages of 9 months to 10 years of age who are considered to be at risk for meningococcal disease (e.g., immunosuppressed, complement deficiency, asplenia) should be immunized (Advisory Committee on Immunization Practices [ACIP], 2011b).

The U.S. Food and Drug Administration has licensed a rotavirus vaccine for use among infants. Depending on the particular vaccine used, the dosage recommendation is for three doses at given to infants at 2, 4, and 6 months of age (RV5), or two doses given at 2 and 4 months of age (RV1) (AAP, 2009a). Rotavirus vaccine is an oral vaccine and should not be given to children older than 8 months of age (AAP, 2009a).

Human papillomavirus (HPV) vaccine is available in both bivalent and quadrivalent forms. The vaccine prevents infection with certain strains of HPV that are known to be associated with later development of cervical cancer. Occasionally, HPV infection can be transmitted perinatally. The Advisory Committee on Immunization Practices (ACIP) recommends immunizing girls at ages 11 to 12 years (ACIP, 2009) with either of the two vaccines. Three doses of the vaccine are given—the second dose 4 weeks after the first, and the third dose 12 weeks or more after the second. The ACIP also recommends routinely vaccinating boys age 11 to 12 years with the quadrivalent vaccine (ACIP, 2011a).

The threat of bioterrorism has generated interest in reintroducing smallpox vaccine. Because children have a high risk for adverse effects from the existing smallpox vaccine, nonemergency vaccination of children younger than 18 years of age is not recommended (CDC, 2007). It is important that adults who have been vaccinated against smallpox be cautious that children not come in contact with the vaccination site until it is completely healed (usually 21 days).

Active and Passive Immunity

Immunizations are effective in preventing illness due to their activation of the body's immune response. *Active immunity* occurs when the body has been exposed to an antigen, either through illness or through immunization, and the immune system creates antibodies against the particular antigen. Active immunity generally confers long-term, and in some cases lifelong, protection against disease. A child acquires *passive immunity* when a serum that contains a disease-specific antibody is transferred to the child via parenteral administration (e.g., intravenous immune globulin) or, in some cases, through placental transfer from mother to infant. Protection from passive immunity is relatively short.

Live or *attenuated* vaccines have had their virulence (potency) diminished so as not to produce a full-blown clinical illness. In response to vaccination, the body produces antibodies and causes immunity to be established (e.g., measles vaccine). Killed or *inactivated* vaccines contain pathogens made inactive by either chemicals or heat. These vaccines also allow the body to produce antibodies but do not cause clinical disease. Inactivated vaccines tend to elicit a limited immune response from the body; therefore, several doses are required (e.g., polio and pertussis).

Toxoids are bacterial toxins that have been made inactive by either chemicals or heat. The toxins cause the body to produce antibodies (e.g., diphtheria and tetanus vaccines).

Immune globulin is made from the pooled blood of many people. Large numbers of donors are used to ensure a broad spectrum of non-specific antibodies. Disease-specific immune globulin vaccines are also available and are obtained from donors known to have high blood titers of the desired antibody (hepatitis B immune globulin [HBIG], rabies immune globulin [RIG]). The disadvantage of human immune globulin is that it offers only temporary passive immunity. Live vaccines must be given on the same day as immune globulin or the two must be separated by 30 days to ensure appropriate immune response from both.

Antitoxins are made from the serum of animals and are used to stimulate production of antibodies in humans. Examples of antitoxins include rabies, snake bite, and spider bite. Animal serums have the disadvantage of being foreign substances, which may cause hypersensitivity reactions; thus a history (including questions about asthma, allergic rhinitis, urticaria, and previous injections of animal serums) and skin sensitivity testing should always precede the administration of an antitoxin.

As all vaccines have the potential to cause anaphylaxis, it is imperative that the nurse ask about allergies and previous reactions before administering any vaccine.

Obstacles to Immunizations

Major reasons identified for low immunization rates during health care visits are presented in Box 4-6. In the 1980s the safety of the pertussis portion of the diphtheria-tetanus-pertussis vaccine was questioned. Some parents elected not to immunize their children, which resulted in an increase in pertussis cases. Medical concern has led to the use in

---

BOX 4-6 BARRIERS TO IMMUNIZATION

- *Complexity of the health care system,* which may lead to a delay in vaccinating children when parents become confused or frustrated with the health care system; special barriers include the following:
  - Appointment-only clinics
  - Excessively long waiting periods
  - Inconvenient scheduling
  - Inaccessible clinic sites
  - The need for formal referral from a primary health care provider
  - Language and cultural barriers
- *Expense* of immunization services
- *Parental misconceptions* about disease severity, vaccine efficiency and safety, complications, and contraindications
- *Inaccurate record keeping* by parents and health care workers
- *Reluctance of the health care worker* to give more than two vaccines during the same visit
- *Lack of public awareness* of the need for immunizations

the United States of the acellular pertussis vaccine, which has fewer side effects.

The media play an important part in the immunization status of children. News programs that highlight the side effects of vaccines, rather than their individual and collective protective effect, create fear and misunderstanding in the public. Health care providers need to address this issue when recommending various immunizations to parents. It is important for nurses to be aware of vaccine controversies and to know how to access appropriate, research-based information. The National Network for Immunization Information, an initiative of the Infectious Diseases Society of America, the Pediatric Infectious Diseases Society, the AAP, and the American Nurses Association, provides up-to-date information about immunization research. It can be accessed on-line at www.immunizationinfo.org.

Informed Consent

The National Childhood Vaccine Injury Act of 1986 requires that the benefits and risks associated with immunizations be discussed with parents before immunizations. The act also requires that families receive vaccine information statements (VISs) before immunization.

All health care providers who administer immunizations are required by federal law to provide general information about immunizations to the child and parents, preferably in the family's native language. This information describes why the vaccine is being given, the benefits and risks, and common side effects. Before providers administer a vaccine, parents should read the federally required information about that vaccine (the VIS) and have the opportunity to ask questions (AAP Committee on Infectious Diseases, 2009b). It is necessary that the parents feel comfortable with the information and with the answers to any questions. It has been shown that VISs do increase the parents' knowledge level and are beneficial. Providing the information before scheduled vaccinations allows parents the time to read all the information. Providers are encouraged to obtain written informed consent for each vaccine administered. If signatures are not obtained, the client's medical record should document that the vaccine information was reviewed.

Immunization Schedule

Each January, recommendations regarding vaccinations in the United States are made by the Advisory Committee on Immunization Practices (ACIP) of the CDC, the AAP Committee on Infectious Diseases, and the American Academy of Family Physicians (AAFP) (CDC, 2011c). All states require immunizations for children enrolled in licensed child-care programs and school. Some states further require immunizations in the upper grades and at the time of college entrance. One group who may be overlooked includes children who receive home schooling. It is of utmost importance therefore that immunization records be traced and that vaccinations be given over the course of the fewest visits possible. State requirements can be obtained from each state health department. Refer to www.aap.org/immunization/izschedule.html to access the current recommendations for immunization of healthy children in the United States.

Children with an Uncertain History of Immunization

When a lapse in immunization occurs, the entire series does not have to be restarted. Children's charts should be flagged to remind health care providers of these children's immunization status. For children of unknown or uncertain immunization status, appropriate immunization should be administered. Readministration of measles, mumps, and rubella (MMR) vaccine, Hib vaccine, inactivated poliovirus

vaccine, or hepatitis B vaccine to someone who is immune has no harmful effects. For children older than 7 years, depending on age, the Td vaccine or Tdap vaccine, rather than the DTaP vaccine, should be administered (CDC, 2011a).

International adoptees, refugees, and exchange students should be immunized according to recommended schedules for healthy infants and children. If written records of prior immunization are not available, the child begins the schedule for children not immunized during infancy. Refer to www.aap.org/immunization/izschedule.html for recommendations for immunizing children who were not immunized during infancy.

When taking an immunization history, the nurse should avoid asking the question, "Are your child's immunizations up to date?" This question will frequently be answered with "yes," but that does not give the nurse sufficient information. The nurse may gain more information by asking, "Can you tell me when and what was the last immunization your child had?"

Administration of Vaccines

The manufacturer's packaging insert for each vaccine includes recommendations for handling, storage, administration site, dosage, and route. Nurses responsible for handling vaccines should be familiar with storage requirements to minimize the risk of vaccine failures. When multidose vials are used, sterile technique should be used to prevent contamination. To ensure safe administration, the vaccines should be given by the recommended route. The deltoid muscle can be used in children ages 18 months and older; for younger children and infants, the anterolateral thigh is used. Vaccines given intramuscularly need to be injected deep into the muscle mass to avoid irritation and possible necrosis.

More than one immunization may be administered at the same age or time. Some vaccines may be given as combined vaccine; several combination vaccines have been approved for use in the United States. When more than one injection is to be given, vaccines should be administered with separate syringes, not mixed into one, unless using a manufactured and approved combined vaccine. They should be given at different sites (preferably in different thighs), and the site used for each vaccine should be recorded to identify possible reactions. For infants and young children, to minimize the stress of vaccine administration, two nurses can give the vaccines simultaneously at different sites. The nurse should also record the lot number for each vaccine given. Box 4-7 lists nursing responsibilities associated with administering vaccines.

Precautions and Contraindications

The main purpose of vaccination is to achieve immunity with the fewest possible side effects (Box 4-8). Most vaccines have no side effects; when side effects occur, they are usually mild. Fever and local irritation are not uncommon after administration of the DTaP vaccine, and fever and rash can occur 1 to 2 weeks after administration of live-virus vaccine.

Some severe side effects have been reported, however. These events are usually not predictable. Because cases have been reported of development of paralytic polio in healthy children after administration of oral polio vaccine, the AAP and the CDC now recommend a full schedule of inactivated polio vaccine. Reactions to the MMR vaccine have included anaphylactic reactions, both in children with and in those without a history of egg allergy. This has prompted consideration of other possible causative agents. For instance, the MMR vaccine contains neomycin, which may be the cause of the sensitivity.

BOX 4-7　NURSING RESPONSIBILITY IN ADMINISTERING VACCINES

- Know the recommended immunization schedule and the recommended alternative schedule for those with lapsed immunizations or unknown immunization history.
- Acquire up-to-date information because recommendations are revised frequently.
- Assess the family's beliefs and values to assist in the education of the family as to the rationale for immunizations, the risks and side effects, and the risks of nonimmunization.
- Take a careful history to determine possible contraindications or precautions and report any pertinent information to the practitioner. Educate the family as to the rationale for any contraindications.
- Some vaccines are combination vaccines (e.g., Pediarix—diphtheria, tetanus, pertussis, hepatitis B, and polio). Other vaccines should not be mixed. Check manufacturer's recommendations.
- Administer vaccines according to the manufacturer's recommended sites.
- Use hand hygiene before vaccine administration and between children.
- Review with the parents common side effects and the signs of potentially severe reactions that warrant contacting the practitioner.
- Instruct the parents that they may administer age-appropriate doses of acetaminophen every 6 hours for 24 hours if the child has discomfort related to vaccine administration.
- For painful or red injection sites, advise the parents to apply cold compresses for the first 24 hours; then use warm or cold compresses as long as needed.
- Give multiple administrations in different sites and record those sites in the medical record.
- Document parental consent in the medical record. Documentation should also include the type of vaccine, date of administration, manufacturer and lot number, expiration date, administration site, any data pertinent to risks and side effects, and the signature and title of the person administering the immunization.

⚡ SAFETY ALERT

Special Considerations Related to Immunizations

- The preferred site for intramuscular administration of vaccines to infants and children is the anterolateral thigh; the deltoid can be used in older children. Subcutaneous injections can be given in the thigh or upper arm.
- For intramuscular (IM) administration, use a needle of sufficient length to penetrate the muscle.
- When giving DTaP, Hib, and hepatitis B vaccines simultaneously, it is advisable to administer the most reactive vaccine (DTaP) in one leg and to inject the others, which cause less reaction, into the other leg.
- Live bacterial or virus vaccines should not be given to immunocompromised children, except under special circumstances.
- Live measles vaccine is produced by chick embryo cell culture, so there is a remote possibility of anaphylactic hypersensitivity in children with egg allergies. Most reactions from the MMR are reactions to other components of the vaccine, so MMR is not usually contraindicated for children with egg hypersensitivity (AAP Committee on Infectious Diseases, 2009b).
- Any immunization may cause an anaphylactic reaction. All offices and clinics must have epinephrine 1:1000 available.

BOX 4-8　COMMON MISCONCEPTIONS ABOUT ADMINISTRATION AND SAFETY OF VACCINES

The following conditions or circumstances are not contraindications to the administration of vaccines:

- Mild acute illness with low-grade fever or mild diarrhea in an otherwise healthy child.
- A reaction to a previous dose of DTaP vaccine with only soreness, redness, or swelling in the immediate vicinity of the injection site.

Before a second dose of any vaccine is given, the nurse needs to ascertain and record whether any side effects or possible reactions occurred after the previous dose of that vaccine. The National Childhood Vaccine Injury Act of 1986 requires health care providers who administer vaccines to maintain permanent vaccination records and to report occurrences of certain adverse events stipulated in the act (Vaccine Adverse Event Reporting System [VAERS]). Anaphylaxis or anaphylactic shock and encephalopathy are examples of two reportable events associated with the tetanus and pertussis vaccines. Providers administering immunizations must be aware of reportable events and comply with the provisions of the act.

Immunocompromised Children

In general, children who are immunologically compromised should not receive live bacterial or viral vaccines (e.g., MMR, varicella vaccine). There are some exceptions related to children with human immunodeficiency virus infection and in some specific instances of children in remission from cancer. Children with human immunodeficiency virus infection who are not severely compromised should receive MMR; varicella vaccine can be given, depending on the CD4+ count (see Chapter 18).

Education

Immunization is a critical component of a child's health care. Knowledge of immunization schedules and an awareness of potential delays will aid the health care provider in identifying children who have not been fully immunized. Health care providers must provide parents with accurate information regarding immunizations because immunizations are the primary and safest means of managing preventable infectious diseases. All children in the United States should have access to appropriate immunization. The State Children's Health Insurance Program (see Chapter 1) and the Vaccines for Children program ensure that there are no financial barriers. Nevertheless, health providers need to be aware that, although immunization rates are increasing through efforts of the federal and state governments, disparities in immunization access for the poor and certain racial or ethnic minorities still exist (CDC, Office of Minority Health, 2007).

Nutrition and Activity

To provide care for infants and children, the nurse must understand the body's nutritional needs. The body is nourished by food. Carbohydrates, fats, proteins, water, vitamins, and minerals are the basic *nutrients* in food. Carbohydrates, fats, and proteins provide energy, which is required by the cells of the body to transport all substances across the cell membrane, to synthesize substances within the cell, and to dispose of waste products.

Carbohydrates

Carbohydrates provide most of the energy needed to maintain a healthy body. They exist in two forms, simple and complex. Complex carbohydrates should make up the majority of calories consumed. Most complex carbohydrates are found in starch from cereal grains, roots, vegetables, and legumes. The more mature the vegetable, the higher the starch content. Foods that are good sources of complex carbohydrates are relatively inexpensive and easily obtained. Insufficient calorie intake causes the body to break down protein and fat for energy and glucose production. Carbohydrates are a food source for many of the essential nutrients, including fiber, vitamins C and E, the majority of B vitamins, potassium, and the majority of trace elements.

Fats

Fats serve as the secondary source of energy by providing 30% or less of daily calorie intake. The Food and Drug Administration requires food manufacturers to list trans fat (i.e., trans fatty acids) on Nutrition Facts and some Supplement Facts panels. Trans fat, like saturated fat and dietary cholesterol, raises the low-density lipoprotein cholesterol. Trans fat can be found in processed foods made with partially hydrogenated vegetable oils such as vegetable shortenings, some margarines, crackers, candies, cookies, snack foods, fried foods, and baked goods. Dietary fat allows the absorption of the fat-soluble vitamins (A, D, E, and K) and adds flavor to foods. The layer of fat beneath the skin plays a role in regulating body temperature. Fat is a component of cell membranes and acts as a protective padding for the internal organs. When excess calories are consumed, dietary fats are stored as excess body fat. The monounsaturated and polyunsaturated fats can raise high-density lipoprotein and decrease low-density lipoprotein cholesterol. For this reason, emphasis should be placed on replacing saturated fats with these fats whenever possible. Most whole grains, breads, pastas, and cereals are naturally low in fat. Families should be taught to choose lean meats, beans, and low-fat dairy products and to limit their intake of processed foods such as crackers, cookies, cakes, and higher-fat snacks.

Proteins

Dietary *protein* is necessary for building and maintaining body tissues. Proteins are involved in homeostasis by working with other elements in the blood to maintain fluid balance. Many vitamins and minerals are bound to protein carriers for transport. Proteins, as antibodies, aid in the regulation of the body's immune system.

Water

Water is essential for life. It transports nutrients to cells and waste products away from cells. It assists in the regulation of body temperature and in chemical reactions. Water lubricates joints and provides form and structure to the cells and the medium for body fluids. Water is found in most foods, including solids. Water requirements can be estimated by a variety of methods. The child's activity level and ambient temperature influence the amount of water needed.

Vitamins and Minerals

Vitamins and *minerals* are necessary in the regulation of metabolic processes. They are present in a wide variety of foods. Vitamins and minerals are added to processed formulas and to other foods such as cereals. Except for Vitamin D supplementation, it is generally not necessary for children to receive supplementation after infancy unless they are at nutritional risk (e.g., have anorexia or a chronic disease).

BOX 4-9   KEY DIETARY RECOMMENDATIONS SPECIFIC TO CHILDREN AND ADOLESCENTS

- Breastfeed infants for a minimum of 4 months; avoid introducing solid foods until 4 to 6 months of age.
- Consume whole-grain products often; at least half the grains should be whole grains.
- Children 1 to 8 years should consume 2 cups per day of milk; use fat-free or low-fat milk or equivalent milk products for children older than 2 years.
- Children 9 years of age and older should consume 3 cups per day of fat-free or low-fat milk or equivalent milk products.
- Limit juice, but provide several servings of fruits and vegetables each day. Use 100% fruit juice and not juice drinks, which contain added sugar.
- Total daily fat intake should not exceed 30% to 35% of calories for children 2 to 3 years of age and 25% to 35% of calories for children and adolescents 4 to 18 years of age. Polyunsaturated and monounsaturated fatty acids, such as fish, nuts, and vegetable oils, should be the primary source of fats.
- Elementary school age children can be taught to read food labels

Data from American Heart Association. (2011). *Dietary recommendations for healthy children.* Retrieved from www.heart.org

---

Dietary Guidelines

The U.S. Department of Health and Human Services and the U.S. Department of Agriculture regularly publishes and updates dietary guidelines, which are used as the basis for a federal nutrition policy. The guidelines recommend that a variety of nutrient-dense foods and beverages within and among the basic food groups be consumed, but foods that contain saturated and *trans* fats, cholesterol, added sugars, salt, and alcohol should be limited (Box 4-9).

The MyPyramid Food Guidance System was developed to provide food-based guidance to help implement the recommendations of the guidelines. Although the food choice and amount recommendations have not changed, the United States Department of Agriculture (USDA) issued the MyPlate system in 2010 (USDA Center for Nutrition Policy and Promotion, 2010) (Figure 4-6). The MyPlate image illustrates the recommended portion of daily nutrients in a way that children, as well as adults, can easily understand. The MyPlate focuses on eating a variety of foods to get the required nutrients and adequate energy. The dietary guidelines suggest consuming half of the daily requirements as fruits and vegetables, limiting saturated fats and sugars, using only lean meats, increasing other sources of protein, such as beans, and using low fat or skim dairy products (USDA & USDHHS, 2011). Other web-based interactive tools and print materials can be accessed at www.choosemyplate.gov.

Energy, Calories, and Servings

Energy is measured in calories. Energy or calorie needs depend on the person's age, sex, height, weight, and level of physical activity. Calorie needs vary during childhood. Infants need sufficient calories to support rapid growth; therefore fat is not restricted in children younger than 2 years. Fat intake should be between 30% and 35% of calories for children 2 to 3 years of age and between 25% and 35% of calories for children and adolescents 4 to 18 years of age, with most fats coming from sources of polyunsaturated and monounsaturated fatty acids, such as fish, nuts, and vegetable oils (American Heart Association [AHA], 2011).

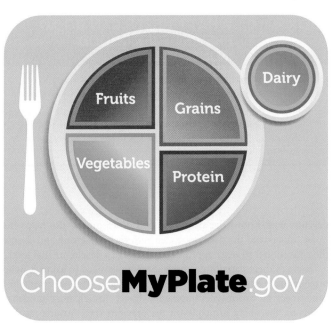

FIG 4-6 **MyPlate.** MyPlate advocates building a healthy plate by making half of your plate fruits and vegetables and the other half grains and protein. Avoiding oversized portions, making half your grains whole grains, and drinking fat-free or low-fat (1%) milk are additional recommendations for a healthy diet. (From U.S. Department of Agriculture: *MyPlate*, Washington, DC, June 2011, The Service, available online at www.choosemyplate.gov.)

Physical Activity

Over the past several decades, children of all ages have become less active and more sedentary. The prevalence of overweight children ages 6 to 11 years has nearly tripled in the past 30 years, going from 7% in 1980 to 20% in 2008 (National Center for Health Statistics, 2010). The rate among adolescents ages 12 to 19 years more than tripled, increasing from 5% to 18% (National Center for Health Statistics, 2010). Physical activity, dietary behavior, and genetics affect weight across all age-groups. Boys who are Mexican American and non-Hispanic black girls have the highest prevalence of obesity (National Center for Health Statistics, 2010).

A person's BMI provides an indication of relative obesity, and this number (a function of weight and height) is being used more frequently to assess for obesity. For children, the BMI percentile for age is a more accurate measurement of overweight and obesity than the adult BMI measurement of >25. The Evolve website contains information about the BMI for children of various ages.

Any health promotion counseling during childhood and adolescence needs to include an emphasis on increasing the child's and parents' daily physical activity. Children particularly enjoy an activity if it is associated with fun and group involvement, and they are more likely to participate in physical exercise if they see their parents exercising as well.

When counseling parents and children about increasing physical activity, the nurse can emphasize the following points (CDC, 2011b & c):

- Children and adolescents should be physically active for at least one hour daily.

- Aerobic exercise should comprise the major component of children's daily exercise, but physical activity should also include muscle-strengthening and bone-strengthening activities.
- Make exercise fun and a habitual activity.
- Encourage students to participate fully in any physical education classes.
- Encourage parents to investigate their community's physical activity programs. City recreation centers, parks, and community YMCAs can provide fun places to engage in physical activities.

Cultural and Religious Influences on Diet

Dietary intake is profoundly affected by both cultural and religious beliefs. An understanding of these patterns will assist the nurse in both the assessment and implementation of nutrition-related behaviors. Hospitalized children who become stressed by being in a new and strange environment do not need the added stress of unfamiliar foods. Information regarding a child's food preferences can be obtained during a dietary history.

A child's religious beliefs may also have an effect on the types of foods eaten and the way in which they are served. Within religious groups there may be a variety of dietary observances. The nurse should assist and encourage the child and the child's family in communicating specific dietary needs.

Assessment of Nutritional Status

A nutritional assessment is an essential component of the health examination of infants and children. This assessment should include anthropometric data, biochemical data, clinical examination, and dietary history. From these data, a plan of care can be developed. In addition, children at risk can be identified and areas of prevention pursued through teaching and further evaluation and follow-up.

Anthropometric Data. Height and head circumference reflect past nutrition or chronic nutritional problems. Weight, skinfold thickness, midarm circumference, and BMI better reflect current nutritional status. The nurse should always be aware of the roles of birth weight and ethnic, familial, and environmental factors when evaluating anthropometric measurements. Infants and children should have anthropometric measurements done during each preventive health care visit.

Clinical Evaluation. The clinical evaluation includes a physical examination and complete history. Special attention is paid to the areas where signs of nutritional deficiencies appear: the skin, hair, teeth, gums, lips, tongue, and eyes. Clinical symptoms usually are not by themselves diagnostic but may suggest conditions, which are then confirmed by biochemical tests and diet histories. More than one deficiency may be present.

Dietary History. Obtaining an accurate history of dietary intake is difficult. The knowledge that what the child is eating is being recorded can influence what the parent feeds the child or what the child eats. Children often cannot remember what they have eaten. If the child or parent is not committed to the process, incomplete information may be obtained. It is still a useful assessment process, however, and should be used. Client teaching includes an understanding of the importance of recording the child's dietary intake and the need for accuracy. Common methods of assessing dietary intake include 24-hour recall, a food frequency questionnaire, and a food diary.

Twenty-four-hour recall. With the 24-hour recall method, the child or parent is asked to recall everything the child has eaten in the past 24 hours. A questionnaire may be used, or the nurse may conduct an interview asking the pertinent questions.

The child or parent may have difficulty remembering the kinds and amounts of food eaten, or the family may have had an atypical day on the previous day or may not feel comfortable relating what was eaten the day being evaluated. How the child or parents see the nurse may influence the response; they may say what they think the interviewer wants to hear. Asking for information in relation to meals eaten as opposed to food groups may increase the accuracy of the assessment.

Food-frequency questionnaire. The food-frequency questionnaire elicits information on the intake of particular foods or food groups on a daily, weekly, or monthly basis. This tool can be used to validate the 24-hour recall data. As for all methods of assessment, this requires the interviewer to be nonjudgmental and objective. Putting the information into a questionnaire may be less threatening to the child and family and will save time.

Food diary. When keeping a food diary, the child or parent records everything consumed during a specified period. Various sources recommend different lengths of time for keeping the diary; 3-day to 7-day records may be used. As in all nursing care, the nurse must evaluate what is a reasonable time to expect the family or child to keep the records. The time, place, and people present when the food was eaten may also be recorded. This provides the nurse with additional information, which may identify trends and other information related to the child's eating behaviors.

Safety

Unintentional injury is the most significant but underrecognized public health threat facing children today. Unintentional injury is the leading cause of death in children. Across age-groups, motor vehicle traffic injuries are the major causes of injury in children and adolescents (Forum on Child and Family Statistics, 2011). (See Chapter 10 for a more detailed discussion of the causes of injury in childhood.)

The number of childhood deaths is staggering, but it is only a fraction of the number of children who are hospitalized and require emergency treatment and who have a permanent disability as a result of injury. The economic burden to society is equally astounding, reaching billions of dollars yearly. What cannot be quantified is the emotional loss, suffering, and pain the child and family must endure once an injury has occurred.

All children are at risk for injury because of their normal curiosity, impulsiveness, and impatience. Everywhere they venture, they are exposed to potentially hazardous situations.

Injury Prevention

Injury prevention is a relatively new focus of health promotion. The term *accident,* with its implied meaning of random chance or lack of responsibility, has been replaced with *injury,* with its implication that injuries have causes that can be modified to prevent or lessen their frequency and severity. Safety education is a critical component of injury prevention. It increases awareness, it attempts to modify human behavior, and it reinforces changes implemented through legal mandates (e.g., seatbelt laws) or product modification (e.g., crib design, airbags).

Nurses need to become proactive in childhood injury prevention by increasing children's and adults' awareness of safety issues (Box 4-10). Nurses who care for children are acutely aware of the devastating effects and complex problems injuries cause. From their experiences, they become well-informed advocates for childhood safety.

Anticipatory Guidance

To be most effective in providing anticipatory safety guidance, nurses must gear educational strategies to the child's level of growth and

---

BOX 4-10   WHAT NURSES CAN DO TO PREVENT CHILDHOOD INJURIES

- Model safety practices in the home, workplace, and community.
- Educate parents and children through anticipatory safety guidance to help reduce needless injuries.
- Support legislative efforts that advocate prevention measures.
- Collaborate with other health care providers to promote safety and injury prevention.

---

development. Knowledge of growth and development also helps the nurse understand the risks associated with each age-group and choose the educational strategy appropriate to a child's developmental level.

Early in their parenting experience, parents need to know how to provide a safe environment for their children and what behaviors they can expect at various developmental levels. Anticipatory guidance builds on the safety principles of the previous stage. Awareness of a child's changing capabilities allows the parent to be more alert and reactive to safety hazards that the child is likely to encounter. This awareness is especially important for first-time parents.

Simply telling parents to "watch your children" or to "child-proof" the home or telling a child to "be careful" has little educational impact. Educational efforts are much more likely to be effective if they focus on specific problems with specific solutions rather than providing broad or vague advice.

⚡ SAFETY ALERT

Relationship Between Safety and Childhood Development

Developmentally, children are vulnerable to injury for the following reasons:
- Children are naturally curious and enjoy exploring their surroundings.
- Children are driven to test and master new skills.
- Children frequently attempt activities before they have developed the cognitive and physical skills required to accomplish the task safely.
- Children often assert themselves and challenge rules.
- Children develop a strong desire for peer approval as they grow older.

Teaching Strategies

Teaching can be formal or informal, simple or elaborate, as long as it provides relevant safety information and coincides with the child's or parents' cognitive abilities. For children younger than 5 or 6 years, it is advisable to incorporate the parents into the teaching process so that the parents can assist with reinforcement or questions the child later has about the safety issue. With younger children, who are easily distracted, the information should be presented in short sessions.

Many local and national organizations have safety information available for distribution. This information can be used to supplement the teaching process. Prepared materials range from pamphlets, booklets, posters, and audiovisual materials to entire teaching programs that can assist in providing injury prevention education to all age-groups. Some programs offer the materials free of cost. Internet information, such as that obtained at www.kidsafe.com, can be extremely helpful to parents.

KEY CONCEPTS

- Growth, development, maturation, language, and learning are complex, interrelated processes that produce complicated series of changes in individuals from conception to death; they are influenced by genetics, the environment, access to care, culture, nutrition, health status, and family structure.

- Developmental theories, such as those developed by Piaget, Erikson, Freud, and Kohlberg, form a basis for understanding the many facets of development.

- A variety of physical and developmental screening tools, administered at regular intervals during infancy and early childhood, provides an overall picture of a child's growth and developmental progress and alerts the nurse to potential growth and developmental delays.

- The 46 human chromosomes are long strands of DNA, each containing up to several thousand individual genes.

- With the exception of those genes located on the X and Y chromosomes in males, genes are inherited in pairs that may be identical or different. Some genes are considered to be dominant and others, recessive.

- Inherited predisposition to disease can occur through Mendelian inheritance patterns, chromosomal abnormalities, or multifactorial influences.

- Pediatric nurses must obtain competencies in genetics and genomics in order to provide appropriate counseling to parents and children.

- Play enhances the child's growth and development through physical, cognitive, emotional, and social interactions with others.

- Personnel who administer immunizations must be aware of recommendations for scheduling, handling, storing, and administering the vaccines. Special attention should be given to the site of administration, dosage, route and previous adverse reactions.

- Components of a nutritional assessment include anthropometric data, biochemical data, clinical examination, and dietary history.

- Many childhood injuries and deaths are predictable and preventable; understanding the developmental milestones of each age-group is important for promoting safety awareness for parents, caregivers, and children.

REFERENCES

Advisory Committee on Immunization Practices [ACIP] Vaccines for Children Program. (2009). *Vaccines to prevent human papillomavirus.* Retrieved from www.cdc.gov.

Advisory Committee on Immunization Practices [ACIP] Vaccines for Children Program. (2011). *Vaccines to prevent meningococcal disease.* Retrieved from www.cdc.gov.

American Academy of Pediatrics. (2006, reaffirmed 2010). Identifying infants and young children with developmental disorders in the medical home: An algorithm for developmental surveillance and screening. *Pediatrics, 118,* 405-420.

American Academy of Pediatrics, Committee on Infectious Diseases. (2009a). Prevention of rotavirus disease: Updated guidelines for use for rotavirus vaccine. *Pediatrics, 123,* 1-9.

American Academy of Pediatrics Committee on Infectious Diseases. (2009b). *Red Book: 2009 Report of the Committee on Infectious Diseases* (28th ed.). Elk Grove Village, Ill.: The Academy.

American Academy of Pediatrics Council on Environmental Health. (2011). Policy statement: Chemical management policy, prioritizing children's health. *Pediatrics, 127,* 983-990.

American Heart Association. (2011). *Dietary recommendations for healthy children.* Retrieved from www.heart.org.

Barlow, S. (2007). Expert committee recommendations regarding the prevention, assessment and treatment of child and adolescent overweight and obesity. *Pediatrics, 120,* S164-S192.

Borzekowski, D. (2009). Considering children and health literacy: A theoretical approach. *Pediatrics, 124*(Supplement 3), S282-S288.

Centers for Disease Control and Prevention. (2007). *Smallpox vaccine: Information for clinicians.* Retrieved from www.bt.cdc.gov.

Centers for Disease Control and Prevention, Office of Minority Health. (2007). *Eliminate disparities in adult and child immunization rates.* Retrieved from www.cdc.gov/omh/Highlights.

Centers for Disease Control and Prevention. (2010). Licensure of a 13-valent pneumococcal conjugate vaccine (PCV13) and recommendations for use among children—Advisory Committee on Immunization Practices (ACIP), 2010. *MMWR Morbidity and Mortality Weekly Report, 59*(9), 258-261.

Centers for Disease Control and Prevention. (2011a). *Catch-up immunization schedule for persons age 4 months through 18 years who start late or who are more than one month behind.* Retrieved from www.cdc.gov.

Centers for Disease Control and Prevention. (2011b). *How much physical activity do children need?* Retrieved from www.cdc.gov.

Centers for Disease Control and Prevention. (2011c). *Making physical activity part of a child's life.* Retrieved from www.cdc.gov.

Centers for Disease Control and Prevention. (2011d). *Recommended immunization schedule for persons aged 0 through 6 years, United States, 2011.* Retrieved from www.cdc.gov.

Clamp, M., Fry, B., Kamal, M., Xie, X., Cuff, J., Lin, M. F., et al. (2007). *Proceedings of the National Academy of Sciences of the United States of America, 104*(49), 19428-19433.

Colby, A., Kohlberg, L., & Kauffman, K. (1987). Theoretical introduction to the measurement of moral judgment. In A. Colby & L. Kohlberg (Eds.), *The measurement of moral judgment (Vol. 1).* Cambridge, England: Cambridge University Press.

Consensus Panel on Genetic/Genomic Nursing Competencies. (2009). *Essentials of genetic and genomic nursing: Competencies, curricula guidelines, and outcome indicators* (2nd ed.). Silver Spring, MD: American Nurses Association. Retrieved from www.genome.gov/Pages/Careers/HealthProfessionalEducation/geneticscompetency.pdf.

Cromer, B. (2011). Adolescent physical and social development. In R. Kliegman, B. Stanton, J. St. Geme, et al (Eds.). *Nelson textbook of pediatrics* (19th ed., pp.649-654).

Erikson, E. H. (1963). *Childhood and society* (2nd ed.). New York: Norton.

Feigelman, S. (2011). Middle childhood. In R. Kliegman, B. Stanton, J. St. Geme, et al. (Eds.). *Nelson textbook of pediatrics* (19th ed., p. 36). Philadelphia: Elsevier.

Forum on Child and Family Statistics. (2011). *America's children: Key national indicators of well-being, 2011.* Retrieved from www.childstats.gov.

Frankenburg, W. K., & Dodds, J. B. (1992). *Denver II screening manual.* Denver: Developmental Materials.

Freud, A. (1974). *Introduction to psychoanalysis.* New York: International Universities Press.

Freud, S. (1960). *The ego and the id* (J. Riviere, Trans.). New York: Norton. (Original work published 1923.)

Garvey, C. (1979). What is play? In P. Chance (Ed.), *Learning through play.* New York: Gardner Press.

Hall-Baker, P. A., Groseclose S. L., Jajosky R. A., et al. (2011). Summary of notifiable diseases—United States, 2009. *MMWR Morbidity and Mortality Weekly Report, 58*(53), 1-100.

Hix-Small, H., Marks, K., Squires, J., & Nickel, R. (2007). Impact of implementing developmental screening at 12 and 24 months in a pediatric practice. *Pediatrics, 120,* 381-389.

Jorde, L. (2010). Genes and genetic diseases. & N. Rote (Eds.). In K. McCance, S. Huether, V. Brashers, & N. Rote (Eds.), *Pathophysiology: The biologic basis for disease in adults and children* (6th ed., pp. 126-143). St. Louis: Elsevier.

King, T., Tandon S. D., Macias M.M., et al. (2010). Implementing developmental screening and referrals: Lessons learned from a national project. *Pediatrics, 125,* 350-360.

Kohlberg, L. (1964). Development of moral character. In M. Hoffman & L. Hoffman (Eds.), *Review of child development research* (Vol. 1). New York: Russell Sage Foundation.

Kuhn, D. (2008). Formal operations from a twenty-first century perspective. *Human Development, 51,* 48-55.

Martin, D. C., Mark, B. L., Triggs-Raine, B. L., & Natowicz, M. R. (2007). Evaluation of the risk for Tay-Sachs disease in individuals of French Canadian ancestry living in New England. *Clinical Chemistry, 53,* 392-398.

National Environmental Education and Training Foundation. (2007). *Pediatric environmental history (0-18 years of age).* Retrieved from www.neetf.org/Health/PEHI.htm.

Peckenpaugh, N. (2010). *Nutrition essentials and diet therapy* (11th ed., pp. 462-513). Philadelphia, PA: Elsevier.

Pellegrini, A. D., & Smith, P. K. (2005). *The nature of play.* New York: Guilford Press.

Piaget, J. (1962). *Play, dreams and imitation childhood.* New York: Norton.

Piaget, J. (1967). *Six psychological studies.* New York: Random House.

Schum, R. L. (2007). Language screening in the pediatric office setting. *Pediatric Clinics of North America, 54,* 425-436.

United States Department of Agriculture, Center for Nutrition Policy and Promotion. (2011). *MyPlate*. Retrieved from www.choosemyplate.gov.

United States Department of Agriculture & United States Department of Health and Human Services. (2011). *Dietary guidelines for Americans, 2010* (7th ed.). Retrieved from www.cnpp.usda.gov.

United States Environmental Protection Agency. (2006). *Children's environmental health 2006 report*. Retrieved from http://yosemite.epa.gov.

Veal, K., Lowry, J., & Belmont, J. (2007). The epidemiology of pediatric environmental exposure. *Pediatric Clinics of North America, 54*(1), 15-31.

Wallis, K., & Smith, S. (2008), Developmental screening in pediatric primary care: The role of nurses. *JSPN, 13,* 130-134.

World Health Organization. (2011). *Invasive Hib disease prevention*. Retrieved from www.who.int.

Health Promotion for the Infant

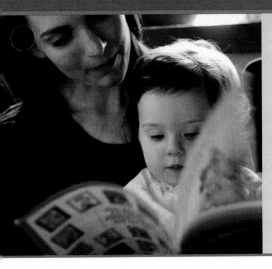

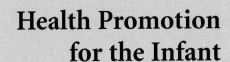
LEARNING OBJECTIVES

After studying this chapter, you should be able to:

• Describe the physiologic changes that occur during infancy.
• Describe the infant's motor, psychosocial, language, and cognitive development.
• Discuss common problems of infancy, such as separation anxiety, sleep problems, irritability, and colic.

• Discuss the importance of immunizations and recommended immunization schedules for infants.
• Provide parents with anticipatory guidance for common concerns during infancy, such as immunizations, nutrition, elimination, dental care, sleep, hygiene, safety, and play.

During no time after birth does a human being grow and change as dramatically as during infancy. Beginning with the newborn period and ending at 1 year, the infancy period, a child grows and develops from a tiny bundle of physiologic needs to a dynamo, capable of locomotion and language and ready to embark on the adventures of the toddler years.

GROWTH AND DEVELOPMENT OF THE INFANT

Although historically adults have considered infants unable to do much more than eat and sleep, it is now well documented that even young infants can organize their experiences in meaningful ways and adapt to changes in the environment. Evidence shows that infants form strong bonds with their caregivers, communicate their needs and wants, and interact socially. By the end of the first year of life, infants can move about independently, elicit responses from adults, communicate through the use of rudimentary language, and solve simple problems.

Infancy is characterized by the need to establish harmony between the self and the world. To achieve this harmony, the infant needs food, warmth, comfort, oral satisfaction, environmental stimulation, and opportunities for self-exploration and self-expression. Competent caregivers satisfy the needs of helpless infants, providing a warm, nurturing relationship so that the children have a sense of trust in the world and in themselves. These challenges make infancy an exciting yet demanding period for both child and parents.

Nurses play an important role in promoting and maintaining health in infants. Although the infant mortality rate in the United States has declined markedly over the past 30 years (see Chapter 1), many infants still die before the first birthday (6.8 per 1000 live births). The leading cause of death in infants younger than 1 year of age is congenital anomalies, followed by conditions related to prematurity or low birth weight (National Center for Health Statistics [NCHS], 2011). Sudden infant death syndrome (SIDS), which for a long time was the second leading cause of infant deaths, is now the third leading cause of death (NCHS, 2011), primarily because of international efforts, such as the *Back to Sleep* campaign. Unintentional injuries rank seventh in this age-group and contribute to mortality and morbidity rates in the infant population (NCHS, 2011). Nurses provide anticipatory guidance for families with infants to reduce morbidity and mortality rates.

During the first year after birth, the infant's development is dramatic as the child grows toward independence. Knowledge of developmental milestones helps caregivers determine whether the baby is growing and maturing as expected. The nurse needs to remember that these markers are averages and that healthy infants often vary. Some infants reach each milestone later than most. Knowledge of normal growth and development helps the nurse promote the safety of children. Nurses teach parents to prepare for the child's safety before the child reaches each milestone.

Providing parents with information about immunizations, feeding, sleep, hygiene, safety, and other common concerns is an important nursing responsibility. Appropriate anticipatory guidance can assist with achieving some of the goals and objectives determined by the U.S. government to be important in improving the overall health of infants. Nurses are in a good position to offer anticipatory guidance on the basis of the infant's growth and achievement of developmental milestones. Table 5-1 summarizes growth and development during infancy.

Physical Growth and Maturation of Body Systems

Growth is an excellent indicator of overall health during infancy. Although growth rates are variable, infants usually double their birth weight by 6 months and triple it by 1 year of age. From an average birth weight of 7½ to 8 pounds (3.4 to 3.6 kg), neonates lose 10% of their body weight shortly after birth but regain birth weight by 2 weeks. During the first 5 to 6 months, the average weight gain is 1½ pounds (0.68 kg) per month. Throughout the next 6 months, the weight increase is approximately 1 pound (0.45 kg) per month. Weight gain in formula-fed infants is slightly greater than in breastfed infants.

During the first 6 months, infants increase their birth length by approximately 1 inch (2.54 cm) per month, slowing to ½ inch (1.27 cm) per month over the next 6 months. By 1 year of age, most infants have increased their birth length by 50%.

The head circumference growth rate during the first year is approximately 4/10 inch (1 cm) per month. Usually the posterior fontanel closes by 2 to 3 months of age, whereas the larger anterior fontanel may remain open until 18 months. Head circumference and fontanel measurements indicate brain growth and are obtained, along with height and weight, at each well-baby visit. Chapter 9 discusses growth-rate monitoring throughout infancy.

HEALTH PROMOTION

Healthy People 2020 *Objectives for Infants*

MICH-20	Increase the proportion of infants who are put to sleep on their back.
MICH-21	Increase the percentage of infants who are breastfed, especially those exclusively breastfed.
MICH-29	Increase the percentage of infants and children who are screened appropriately and referred for autism spectrum disorder and other developmental delays.
AHS-5	Increase the percentage of infants and children who have an ongoing source of medical care.
EH-8	Reduce blood lead levels in infants and children
IID-7	Achieve and maintain effective vaccination coverage levels for universally recommended vaccines among young children.
IVP-11	Reduce deaths caused by unintentional injuries.
IVP-15	Increase use of age-appropriate vehicle restraint systems.
ENT-VSL-1	Increase the proportion of newborns who are screened for hearing loss by no later than age 1 month, have audiologic evaluation by age 3 months, and are enrolled in appropriate intervention services no later than age 6 months.

Modified from U.S. Department of Health and Human Services. (2010). *Healthy People 2020.* Retrieved from www.healthypeople.gov.

TABLE 5-1   SUMMARY OF GROWTH AND DEVELOPMENT: THE INFANT

PHYSICAL	MOTOR	PSYCHOSOCIAL	SENSORY/COGNITIVE	LANGUAGE/COMMUNICATION
1-2 Months				
Fast growth; weight gain of 1½ lb (0.68 kg) per month and height gain of 1 inch (2.54 cm) per month during first 6 months. Upper limbs and head grow faster. Primitive reflexes present; strong suck and gag reflex. Obligate nose breather. Posterior fontanel closes by 2-3 months.	**Gross** May lift head when held against shoulder. Head lag. **Fine** Palmar grasp. *1 month:* Immediately drops object placed in hand. Fist usually clenched (grasp reflex). *2 months:* Holds objects momentarily. Hands often open (grasp reflex fading).	Erikson's stage of trust vs. mistrust. Infant learns that world is good and "I am good." This stage is the foundation for other stages. Child is entirely dependent on parents and other caregivers. Needs should be met in a timely fashion. Touch is important.	Piaget's sensorimotor phase. *1 month:* Notes bright objects if in line of vision. Vision 20/100. Reflexes dominate behavior. *2 months:* Begins to follow objects.	Strong cry. Throaty sounds. Responds to human faces. *6-8 weeks:* Begins to smile in response to stimuli.
3 Months Primitive reflexes fading.	**Gross** Can get hand to mouth. Can lift head off bed when in prone position. Head lag still present but decreasing. **Fine** Holds objects placed in hands. Grasp reflex absent.	Smiles in response to others. Uses sucking to soothe self.	Follows an object with eyes. Plays with fingers.	Babbles, coos. Enjoys making sounds. Responds to voices, watches speaker.

TABLE 5-1   SUMMARY OF GROWTH AND DEVELOPMENT: THE INFANT—cont'd

PHYSICAL	MOTOR	PSYCHOSOCIAL	SENSORY/ COGNITIVE	LANGUAGE/ COMMUNICATION
4-5 Months Can breathe when nose is obstructed. Growth rate declines. Drooling begins in preparation for teething. Moro, tonic neck, and rooting reflexes have disappeared.	**Gross** Plays with feet; puts foot in mouth. Bears weight when held in a standing position. Turns from abdomen to back. **Fine** Begins reaching and grasping with palm. Hits at object, misses.	Mouth is a sensory organ used to explore environment. Attachment is continuing process throughout infancy. Has increased interest in parent, shows trust, knows parent. Shows emotions of fear and anger.	*4 months:* Brings hands together at midline. Vision 20/80. Begins to play with objects. Recognizes familiar faces. Turns head to locate sounds. Shows anticipation and excitement. Memory span is 5-7 minutes. Plays with favorite toys.	Crying becomes differentiated. Babbling is common. *4 months:* Begins consonant sounds: *H, N, G, K, P, B.* *5 months:* Makes vowel sounds: *ee, ah, ooh.*
6-7 Months Weight gain slows to 1 pound (0.45 kg) per month. Length gain of ½ inch (1.27 cm) per month. Birth weight doubles; tooth eruption begins; chewing and biting occur. Maternal iron stores are depleted.	**Gross** Sits, leaning forward on both hands; when supine, lifts head off table. Turns from back to abdomen. **Fine** Transfers objects from one hand to the other. Picks up object well with the whole hand.	Smiles at self in mirror. Plays peek-a-boo. Begins to show stranger anxiety.	Can fixate on small objects. Adjusts posture to see. Responds to name. Exhibits beginning sense of object permanence. Recognizes parent in other clothes, places. Is alert for 1½-2 hours.	Produces vowel sounds and chained syllables. Begins to imitate sounds. Belly laughs. Babbles (one syllable) with pleasure. Calls for help. "Talks" to toys and image in mirror.
8-9 Months Continues to gain weight, length. Patterns of bladder and bowel elimination begin to become more regular.	**Gross** Sits steadily unsupported. Can crawl and pull up. **Fine** Pincer grasp develops. Reaches for toys. Rakes for objects and releases objects.	Stranger anxiety is at its height. Separation anxiety is increasing. Follows parent around the house.	Beginning development of depth perception. Object permanence continues to develop. Uses hands to learn concepts of in and out.	Stringing together of vowels and consonants begins. First few words begin to have meaning (Mama, Dada, bye-bye, baby). Begins to understand and obey simple commands, such as, "Wave bye-bye." Responds to "No!" Shouts for attention.
10-12 Months *12 months:* Birth weight triples; birth length increases by 50%. Head and chest circumference equal. Babinski reflex disappears.	**Gross** Can stand alone. Can walk with one hand held but crawls to get places quickly. **Fine** Releases hold on cup. *10 months:* Finger-feeds self. *12 months:* Feeds self with spoon. Holds crayon to mark on paper. *12 months:* Pincer grasp is complete.	Has mood changes. Quiets self. Is quieted by music. Tenderly cuddles toy.	Vision 20/40. Searches for hidden toy. Explores boxes, inserts objects in container. Symbol recognition is developing (enjoys books).	Can say two or more words. Says "Mama" or "Dada" specifically. Waves bye-bye. Begins to differentiate between words. Enjoys jabbering. Vocalization decreases when walking. Knows own name.

In addition to height and weight, organ systems grow and mature rapidly in the infant. Although body systems are developing rapidly, the infant's organs differ from those of older children and adults in both structure and function. These differences place the infant at risk for problems that might not be expected in older individuals. For example, immature respiratory and immune systems place the infant at risk for a variety of infections, whereas an immature renal system increases risk for fluid and electrolyte imbalances. Knowledge of these differences provides the nurse with important rationales on which to base anticipatory guidance and specific nursing interventions.

Neurologic System

Brain growth and differentiation occur rapidly during the first year of life, and they depend on nutrition and the function of the other organ systems. At birth, the brain accounts for approximately 10% to 12% of body weight. By 1 year of age, the brain has doubled its weight, with a major growth spurt occurring between 15 and 20 weeks of age and another between 30 weeks and 1 year of age. Increases in the number of synapses and expanded myelinization of nerves contribute to maturation of the neurologic system during infancy. Primitive reflexes disappear as the cerebral cortex thickens and motor areas of the brain continue to develop, proceeding in a cephalocaudal pattern: arms first, and then legs (Box 5-1).

Respiratory System

In the first year of life, the lungs increase to three times their weight and six times their volume at birth. In the newborn infant, alveoli number approximately 20 million, increasing to the adult number of 300 million by age 8 years. During infancy, the trachea remains small, supported only by soft cartilage.

The diameter and length of the trachea, bronchi, and bronchioles increase with age. These tiny, collapsible air passages, however, leave infants vulnerable to respiratory difficulties caused by infection or foreign bodies. The eustachian tube is short and relatively horizontal, increasing the risk for middle ear infections.

Cardiovascular System

The cardiovascular system undergoes dramatic changes in the transition from fetal to extrauterine circulation. Fetal shunts close, and pulmonary circulation increases drastically (see Chapter 22). During infancy, the heart doubles in size and weight, the heart rate gradually slows, and blood pressure increases.

Immune System

Transplacental transfer of maternal antibodies supplements the infant's weak response to infection until approximately 3 to 4 months of age. Although the infant begins to produce immunoglobulins (Ig) soon after birth, by 1 year of age the infant has only approximately 60% of the adult IgG level, 75% of the adult IgM level, and 20% of the adult IgA level. Breast milk transmits additional IgA protection. The activity of T lymphocytes also increases after birth. Although the immune system matures during infancy, maximum protection against infection is not achieved until early childhood. This immaturity places the infant at risk for infection.

Gastrointestinal System

The stomach capacity of a neonate is approximately 10 to 20 mL, but with feedings the capacity increases rapidly to approximately 200 mL at 1 year of age. In the gastrointestinal system, enzymes needed for the digestion and absorption of proteins, fats, and carbohydrates mature and increase in concentration. Although the newborn infant's gastrointestinal system is capable of digesting protein and lactase, the ability to digest and absorb fat does not reach adult levels until approximately 6 to 9 months of age.

Renal System

Kidney mass increases threefold during the first year of life. Although the glomeruli enlarge considerably during the first few months, the glomerular filtration rate remains low. Thus the kidney is not effective as a filtration organ or efficient in concentrating urine until after the first year of life. Because of the functional immaturity of the renal system, the infant is at great risk for fluid and electrolyte imbalance.

BOX 5-1 INFANT REFLEXES

Rooting: Stroke or touch the infant's cheek or mouth; the infant should respond by searching for and attempting to suck the examiner's finger.

Sucking: If a nipple or finger is placed in the mouth so that it touches the hard palate, the infant should suck vigorously. This reflex is also indicative of functional gag and swallowing reflexes.

Ciliary: Stroking the eyelashes results in closure of one or both of the eyes.

Doll's eyes: If the infant is placed in a supine position and the head is turned from side to side, the eyes should move to the opposite side.

Moro: Holding the infant in a supine position then displacing the body downward a few centimeters causes the infant to extend, then abduct the extremities, with fingers spread in a symmetrical fashion. This may also elicit a cry.

Tonic neck: When the infant is placed in a supine position, the head is turned to one side with the opposite arm and leg extended and the arm and leg on the same side are flexed. If the head is turned to the other direction, the positioning of the extremities is reversed. This reflex may or may not be present at birth, and its absence is not considered abnormal. This is sometimes called the fencing reflex.

Palmar: If a finger is placed in the palm, the infant should respond by grasping the examiner's finger. The grasp should be symmetrical. If pressure is put on the balls of the feet, the infant should grasp with the toes.

! NURSING QUALITY ALERT
Intake and Output in the Newborn Infant

First 2 days of life
- Intake: 65 mL/kg (30 mL/pound) a day
- Output: 2 to 6 voids

After the first 2 days
- Intake: 100 to 150 mL/kg (45 to 68 mL/pound) a day
- Output: 5 to 25 voids

Motor Development

During the first few months after birth, muscle growth and weight gain allow for increased control of reflexes and more purposeful movement. At 1 month, movement occurs in a random fashion, with the fists tightly clenched. Because the neck musculature is weak and the head is large, infants can lift their heads only briefly. By 2 to 3 months, infants can lift their heads 90 degrees from a prone position and can hold them steadily erect in a sitting position. During this time, active grasping gradually replaces reflexive grasping and increases in frequency as eye-hand coordination improves (see Table 5-1).

The Moro, tonic neck, and rooting reflexes disappear at approximately 3 to 4 months. These primitive reflexes, which are controlled by the midbrain, probably disappear because they are suppressed by growing cortical layers. Head control steadily increases during the third month. By the fourth month, the head remains in a straight line with the body when the infant is pulled to a sitting position. Most infants play with their feet by 4 to 5 months, drawing them up to suck on their toes. Parents need anticipatory guidance about ways to prevent unintentional injury by "baby-proofing" their homes before each motor development milestone is reached.

PATIENT-CENTERED TEACHING

How to "Baby-Proof" the Home

By the time babies reach 6 months of age, they begin to become much more active, curious, and mobile. Although your baby might not be creeping or crawling yet, it is difficult to predict when that will happen. For this reason, you need to be prepared by making sure your house and the toys with which the baby plays are safe. Babies learn through exploring and participating in many different types of experiences. By keeping the baby's environment safe, you can encourage these experiences for your baby.

Be sure to check the following:

- All small or sharp objects or dangerous substances should be out of the baby's reach. Get down to the baby's eye level to be sure. This includes plants and paint chips, which can be poisonous. Be sure to check that any bedside table near the baby's crib is kept clear of ointments, creams, pins, or any other small objects. Be sure to check that small pieces from older siblings' toys are put away. Keep money put away.
- Put plastic fillers in all plugs, and put cabinet and drawer locks on all cabinets and drawers. Doorknob covers are also available that prevent the infant from opening the door.
- Remove front knobs from the stove. Be sure to keep all pot and pan handles turned away from the edge of the stove.
- Remove from lower cabinets and lock away all dangerous or poisonous substances, including such items as pet food, household cleaning agents, cosmetic aids, pesticides, plant fertilizers, paints, matches, medicines, and plastic bags. Be sure to store these products in their original containers. Never give a small child a latex balloon.
- Place a gate on the top and bottom of stairways. Be sure the gate does not have openings that can trap the baby's head, hands, or fingers.
- Remove heavy containers from table tops covered with a tablecloth. Do not hold the baby on your lap while drinking or eating any kind of hot foods.
- Pad furniture with sharp edges. Be sure all windows have screens.
- Keep household hot water temperature at less than 120° F; always test water temperature before bathing the baby. **Never leave a baby unattended near water** (toilet, bathtub, swimming pool, hot tub). Keep water containers or tubs empty when not in use. Be sure there is no direct entrance to a backyard swimming pool through the house.
- Shorten all hanging cords (appliance, window cords, telephone) so they are out of the baby's reach. Be sure pull-toy cords are shorter than 12 inches.
- Have your house tested for sources of lead.
- Never leave your baby unattended or in the care of a young sibling.

The nurse might, for instance, explain, "Infants grow and mature very rapidly, and you will be very busy with a new baby. Now is the time to 'baby-proof' your home before Mary turns over and begins crawling and reaching for objects. By doing this now, you can prevent later injuries and worries."

During the fifth and sixth months, motor development accelerates rapidly. Infants of this age readily reach for and grasp objects. They can bear weight when held in a standing position and can turn from abdomen to back. By 5 months, some infants rock back and forth as a precursor to crawling.

Six-month-old infants can sit alone, leaning forward on their hands (*tripod sitting*). This ability provides them with a wider view of the world and creates new ways to play. Infants of this age can roll from back to abdomen and can raise their heads from the table when supine. At 6 to 7 months, they transfer objects from one hand to the other. In addition, they can grab small objects with the whole hand and insert them into their mouths with lightning speed.

At 6 to 9 months, infants begin to explore the world by crawling. By 9 months, most infants have enough muscle strength and coordination to pull themselves up and cruise around furniture. These new methods of mobility enable the infant to follow a parent or caregiver around the house.

By 6 to 7 months, infants become increasingly adept at pointing to make their demands known. Six-month-old infants grasp objects with all their fingers in a raking motion, but 9-month-olds use their thumbs and forefingers in a fine motor skill called the *pincer grasp*. This grasp provides infants with a useful yet potentially dangerous ability to grab, hold, and insert tiny objects into their mouths.

Nine-month-old infants can wave bye-bye and clap their hands together. They can pick up objects but have difficulty releasing them on request. By 1 year of age, they can extend an object and release it into an offered hand. Most 1-year-old children can balance well enough to walk when holding another person's hand. They often resort to crawling, however, as a more rapid and efficient way to move about.

An increased ability to move about, reach objects, and explore their world places infants at great risk for accidents and injury. Nurses provide information to parents about how quickly infant motor skills develop.

Cognitive Development

Many factors contribute to the way in which infants learn about their world. Besides innate intellectual aptitude and motivation, infants' sensory capabilities, neuromuscular control, and perceptual skills all affect how their cognitive processes unfold during infancy and throughout life. In addition, variables such as the quality and quantity of parental interaction and environmental stimulation contribute to cognitive development.

Cognitive development during the first 2 years of life begins with a profound state of egocentrism. Egocentrism is the child's complete self-absorption and the inability to view the world from anyone else's vantage point (Piaget, 1952). As infants' cognitive capacities expand, they become increasingly aware of the outside world and their separateness from it. Gradually, with maturation and experience, they become capable of differentiating themselves from others and their surroundings.

According to Piaget's theory (1952), cognitive development occurs in stages or periods (see Chapter 4). Infancy is included in the sensorimotor stage (birth to 2 years), during which infants experience the world through their senses and their attempts to control the environment. Learning activities progress from simple reflex behavior to trial-and-error experiments.

During the first month of life, infants are in the first substage, *reflex activity,* of the sensorimotor period. In this substage, behavior such as grasping, sucking, or looking is dominated by reflexes. Piaget believed that infants organize their activity, survive, and adapt to their world by the use of reflexes.

Primary circular reactions dominate the second substage, occurring from age 1 to 4 months. During this substage, reflexes become more organized and new schemata are acquired, usually centering on the infant's body. Sensual activities such as sucking and kicking become less reflexive and more controlled and are repeated because of the stimulation they provide. The baby also begins to recognize objects, especially those that bring pleasure, such as the breast or bottle.

During the third substage, or the stage of *secondary circular reactions,* infants perform actions that are more oriented toward the world outside their own bodies. The 4- to 8-month-old infant in this substage begins to play with objects in the external environment, such as a rattle or stuffed toy. The infant's actions are labeled *secondary* because they are intentional (repeated because of the response that is elicited). For example, a baby in this substage intentionally shakes a rattle to hear the sound.

By age 8 to 12 months, infants in the fourth substage, *coordination of secondary schemata,* begin to relate to objects as if they realize that the objects exist even when they are out of sight. This awareness is referred to as object permanence and is illustrated by a 9-month-old infant seeking a toy after it is hidden under a pillow. In contrast, 6-month-olds can follow the path of a toy that is dropped in front of them; however, they will not look for the dropped toy or protest its disappearance until they are older and have developed the concept of object permanence.

Infants in the fourth substage solve problems differently from how they solve problems in earlier substages. Rather than randomly selecting approaches to problems, they choose actions that were successful in the past. This tendency suggests that they remember and can perform some mental processing. They seem to be able to identify simple causal relationships, and they show definite intentionality. For example, when an 11-month-old child sees a toy that is beyond reach, the child uses the blanket that it is resting on to pull it closer (Flavell, 1964; Piaget, 1952).

Cognitive development in the infant parallels motor development. It appears that motor activity is necessary for cognitive development and that cognitive development is based on interaction with the environment, not simply maturation. Infancy is the period when the child lays the foundation for later cognitive functioning. Nurses can promote the cognitive development of infants by encouraging parents to interact with their infants and provide them with novel, interesting stimuli. At the same time, parents should maintain familiar, routine experiences through which their infants can develop a sense of security about the world. Within this type of environment, infants will thrive and learn.

! NURSING QUALITY ALERT

Possible Signs of Developmental Delays

Lack of eye muscle control after 4 to 6 months suggests a vision impairment and the need for further evaluation.

Lack of a social smile by 8 to 12 weeks requires further evaluation and close follow-up.

Sensory Development
Vision

The size of the eye at birth is approximately one half to three fourths the size of the adult eye. Growth of the eye, including its internal structures, is rapid during the first year. As infants grow and become more interested in the environment, their eyes remain open for longer periods. They show a preference for familiar faces and are increasingly able to fixate on objects. Visual acuity is estimated at approximately 20/100 to 20/150 at birth but improves rapidly during infancy and toddlerhood. Infants show a preference for high-contrast colors, such as black and white and primary colors. Pastel colors are not easily distinguished until about 6 months of age.

Young infants may lack coordination of eye movements and extraocular muscle alignment but should achieve proper coordination by age 4 to 6 months. A persistent lack of eye muscle control beyond age 4 to 6 months needs further evaluation. Depth perception appears to begin at approximately 7 to 9 months and contributes to the infant's new ability to move about independently (see Chapter 31).

Hearing

Hearing seems to be relatively acute, even at birth, as shown by reflexive generalized reactions to noise. With myelinization of the auditory nerve tracts during the first year, responses to sound become increasingly more specialized. By 4 months, infants should turn their eyes and heads toward a sound coming from behind, and by 10 months infants should respond to the sound of their names. The American Academy of Pediatrics (AAP), Joint Committee on Infant Hearing (2007) has recommended that all newborn infants be screened for hearing impairment either as neonates or before 1 month of age and that those infants who fail newborn screening have an audiologic examination to verify hearing loss before age 3 months. The AAP also suggests that infants who demonstrate confirmed hearing loss be eligible for early intervention services and specialized hearing and language services as early as possible, but no later than 6 months of age (AAP, Joint Committee on Infant Hearing, 2007). Newborn hearing screening generally is done before hospital discharge. Rescreening of both ears within 1 month of discharge is recommended for those newborns with questionable results. Additionally, screening should be available to those infants born at home or in an out-of-hospital birthing center (AAP, Joint Committee on Infant Hearing, 2007).

Health providers should assess the risk for hearing deficits at every well-child visit; any child who manifests one or more risks should have diagnostic audiology testing by age 24 to 30 months (Harlor, Bower, & Committee on Practice and Ambulatory Medicine, 2009). Risk factors include, but are not limited to, structural abnormalities of the ear, family history of hearing loss, prenatal or postnatal infections known to contribute to hearing deficit, trauma, persistent otitis media, developmental delay, and parental concern (AAP, Joint Committee on Infant Hearing, 2007). Harlor, Bower, & Committee on Practice and Ambulatory Medicine, (2009) further recommend that referral for more complete testing and intervention be made for any child who fails an objective hearing screening, or whose parent expresses concerns about possible hearing loss.

Language Development

The acquisition of language has its roots in infancy as the child becomes increasingly intrigued with sound, begins to realize that words have meaning, and eventually uses simple sounds to communicate (Box 5-2). Although young infants probably understand tones and inflections of voice rather than words themselves, it is not long before repetition and practice of sounds enable them to understand and

BOX 5-2 LANGUAGE DEVELOPMENT AND DEVELOPMENTAL MILESTONES IN INFANCY

1 to 3 Months
Reflexive smile at first, and then smile becomes more voluntary; sets up a reciprocal smiling cycle with parent. Cooing.

3 to 4 Months
Crying becomes more differentiated. Babbling is common.

4 to 6 Months
Plays with sound, repeating sounds to self. Can identify mother's voice. May squeal in excitement.

6 to 8 Months
Single-consonant babbling occurs. Increasing interest in sound.

8 to 9 Months
Stringing of vowels and consonants together begins. First few words begin to have meaning (Mama, Daddy, bye-bye, baby). Begins to understand and obey simple commands such as "Wave bye-bye."

9 to 12 Months
Vocabulary of two or three words. Gestures are used to communicate. Speech development may slow temporarily when walking begins.

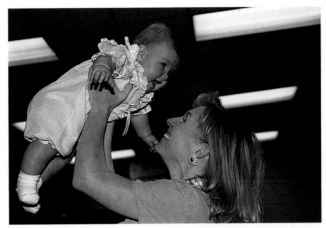

FIG 5-1 This 6-month-old infant responds delightedly to her mother with a true social smile. Such interactive responses between parent and child promote communication and emotional development.

communicate with words. Infants can understand more than they can express.

The social smile develops early in the infant, usually by 3 to 5 weeks of age (Figure 5-1). This powerful communication tool helps to foster attachment and demonstrates that the infant can differentiate between people and objects within the environment. The infant who does not display a social smile by 8 to 12 weeks of age needs further evaluation and close follow-up because of the possibility of developmental delay.

During infancy, connections form within the central nervous system, providing fine motor control of the numerous muscles required for speech. Maturation of the mouth, jaw, and larynx; bone growth; and development of the face help prepare the infant to speak.

Vocalization, or speech, does not appear to be reflexive but rather is a relatively high-level activity similar to conversation. Parents usually elicit vocalization in infants better than other adults can. Language includes understanding word meanings, how to combine words into meaningful sentences and phrases, and social use of conversation. The development of both speech and language can be influenced by environmental cues, such as structures unique to a native language, physical disorders, hearing loss, cognitive impairment, autism spectrum disorders, or learning disabilities such as dyslexia (Schum, 2007).

Although there is great variability, most children begin to make nonmeaningful sounds, such as "ma," "da," or "ah," by 4 to 6 months. The sounds become more meaningful and specific by 9 to 15 months, and by age 1 year the child usually has a vocabulary of several words, such as "mama," "dada," and "bye-bye." Infants who have older siblings or who are raised in verbally rich environments sometimes meet these developmental milestones earlier than other infants.

Psychosocial Development

Most experts agree that infancy is a crucial period during which children develop the foundation of their personalities and their sense of self.

According to Erikson's theory of psychosocial development (1963), infants struggle to establish a sense of basic *trust* rather than a sense of basic mistrust in their world, their caregivers, and themselves. If provided with consistent, satisfying experiences delivered in a timely manner, infants come to rely on the fact that their needs will be met and that, in turn, they will be able to tolerate some degree of frustration and discomfort until those needs are met. This sense of confidence is an early form of trust and provides the foundation for a healthy personality.

On the other hand, if infants' needs are ignored or met in a consistently haphazard, inadequate manner, they have no reason to believe that their needs will be met or that their environment is a safe, secure place. According to Erikson, without consistent satisfaction of needs, the individual develops a basic sense of suspicion or mistrust (Erikson, 1963).

Parallel to this viewpoint is Freudian theory, which regards infancy as the oral stage (Freud, 1974). The mouth is the major focus during this stage. Observation of infants for a few minutes shows that most of their behavior centers on their mouths. Sensory stimulation and pleasure, as well as nourishment, are experienced through their mouths. Sucking is an adaptive behavior that provides comfort and satisfaction while enabling infants to experience and explore their world. Later in infancy, as teething progresses, the mouth becomes an effective tool for aggressive behavior (see Chapter 6).

Parent-Infant Attachment

One of the most important aspects of infant psychosocial development is parent-infant attachment. Attachment is a sense of belonging to or connection with each other. This significant bond between infant and parent is critical to normal development and even survival. Initiated immediately after birth, attachment is strengthened by many mutually satisfying interactions between the parents and the infant throughout the first months of life.

For example, noisy distress in infants signals a need, such as hunger. Parents respond by providing food. In turn, infants respond by quieting and accepting nourishment. The infants derive pleasure from having their hunger satiated and the parents from successfully caring for their children. A basic reciprocal cycle is set in motion in which parents learn to regulate infant feeding, sleep, and activity through a series of interactions. These interactions include rocking, touching, talking, smiling, and singing. The infants respond by quieting, eating, watching, smiling, or sleeping.

Conversely, continuing inability or unwillingness of parents to meet the dependency needs of their infants fosters insecurity and dissatisfaction in the infants. A cycle of dissatisfaction is established in which parents become frustrated as caregivers and have further difficulty providing for the infant's needs.

If parents can adapt to their infant, meet the infant's needs, and provide nurturance, attachment is secure. Psychosocial development can proceed on the basis of a strong foundation of attachment. On the other hand, if parents' personalities and abilities to cope with infant care do not match their infant's needs, the relationship is considered at risk.

Although the establishment of trust depends heavily on the quality of the parental interaction, the infant also needs consistent, satisfying social interactions within a family structure. Family routines can help to provide this consistency. Touch is an important tool that can be used by all family members to convey a sense of caring.

Stranger Anxiety

Another important aspect of psychosocial development is stranger anxiety. By 6 to 7 months, expanding cognitive capacities and strong feelings of attachment enable infants to differentiate between caregivers and strangers and to be wary of the latter. Infants display an obvious preference for parents over other caregivers and other unfamiliar people. Anxiety, demonstrated by crying, clinging, and turning away from the stranger, is manifested when separation occurs. This behavior peaks at approximately 7 to 9 months and again during toddlerhood, when separation may be difficult (see Chapter 6).

Although stressful for parents, stranger anxiety is a normal sign of healthy attachment and occurs because of cognitive development (object permanence). Nurses can reassure parents that, although their infants seem distressed, leaving the infant for short periods does no harm. Separations should be accomplished swiftly, yet with care, love, and emphasis on the parents' return.

HEALTH PROMOTION FOR THE INFANT AND FAMILY

Parents, particularly new parents, often need guidance in caring for their infant. Nurses can provide valuable information about health promotion for the infant. Specific guidance about everyday concerns, such as sleeping, crying, and feeding, can be offered, as well as anticipatory guidance about injury prevention. An important nursing responsibility is to provide parents with information about immunizations and dental care. Nurses can offer support to new parents by identifying strategies for coping with the first few months with an infant. The schedule of well visits corresponds with the schedule recommended by the AAP (see Chapter 4). At each well visit the nurse assesses development, administers appropriate immunizations, and provides anticipatory guidance. The nurse asks the parent a series of general assessment questions (Box 5-3) and then focuses the assessment on the individual infant.

? CRITICAL THINKING EXERCISE 5-1

Mary Brown and her 4-week-old daughter, Tonja, are being seen for a well-baby checkup. Tonja is Mrs. Brown's first child. Mrs. Brown looks very tired and begins to cry when you ask her how she is doing.
1. What are some of the possible causes the nurse should explore?
2. How will you approach exploring these possible causes?
3. What are some of the appropriate nursing measures?

BOX 5-3   CONTINUING ASSESSMENT QUESTIONS

- Nutrition: How much is your child eating, how often, what kinds of foods?
- Elimination: How many wet diapers, stools? Consistency of stools?
- Safety: Use of car restraints? Gun violence? Smoking in the home?
- Hearing/vision: Any concerns?
- Can you tell me about the times you would feel it necessary to call your doctor?
- How is the family adjusting to the baby?
- Are you getting enough time alone and time together?
- Has there been any change in the household or family's lifestyle?
- Are there any financial concerns?
- Are there any other questions or concerns?

Immunization

The importance of childhood immunization against disease cannot be overemphasized. Infants are especially vulnerable to infectious disease because their immune systems are immature. Term neonates are protected from certain infections by transplacental passive immunity from their mothers. Breastfed infants receive additional immunoglobulins against many types of viruses and bacteria. Transplacental immunity is effective only for approximately 3 months, however, and for a variety of reasons many mothers choose not to breastfeed. In any case, this passive immunity does not cover all diseases, and infection in the infant can be devastating. Immunization offers protection that all infants need.

Nurses play an important role in health promotion and disease prevention related to immunization. Nursing responsibilities include assessing current immunization status, removing barriers to receiving immunizations, tracking immunization records, providing parent education, and recognizing contraindications to the receipt of vaccines. Chapter 4 provides detailed information regarding immunizations and their schedule.

Skin Care

Cord care with topical antiseptics prevents umbilical cord infection better than leaving the cord to air dry (Zupan, Garner, & Omari, 2004). Many maternity facilities recommend that routine cord care be performed after each bath and each diaper change. The umbilical stump and the area where it attaches to the abdomen are cleaned with rubbing or isopropyl alcohol; in some instances chlorhexidine powder may be used. The umbilical cord usually falls off about 10 days after birth. Some slight bleeding may be noted. Parents should be taught to recognize the signs and symptoms of umbilical infection (see Patient-Centered Teaching: Care of the Umbilical Cord box).

Seborrheic dermatitis, or cradle cap, is seen in some infants. It appears as thick, yellow, scaly patches that are found on the scalp (most often over the anterior fontanel) but it may also appear on the eyebrows or eyelid. The scales may be removed by warming a small amount of baby oil, applying it to the patches, and allowing it to penetrate the crust. The crusts may then be washed away with baby shampoo. It is important to reassure parents that the condition is temporary and usually disappears by 12 months.

Some infants have *acne neonatorum,* an acne-like condition probably caused by hormonal changes. It generally appears when the infant is approximately 2 to 4 weeks old, and it is self-limiting, disappearing in several weeks to months.

PATIENT-CENTERED TEACHING

Care of the Umbilical Cord

- Call your health provider if you observe:
  - Bleeding
  - Bad odor
  - Redness
  - Drainage
  - The cord does not fall off after 2 weeks
- Do the following:
  - Fold the diaper back below the cord to expose it to the air
  - Change diapers frequently to avoid excessive moisture in the cord area
- Don't:
  - Give tub baths until the cord falls off

The diaper area, including the gluteal folds, should be cleaned and thoroughly dried with each diaper change. Either warm water or baby wipes can be used. Parents should be cautioned not to use commercial baby wipes if any diaper rash is noted. It is important to teach parents to wipe females from front to back and to clean under the scrotum of males.

Feeding and Nutrition

Because infancy is a period of rapid growth, nutritional needs are of special significance. During infancy, eating progresses from a principally reflex activity to relatively sophisticated, yet messy, attempts at self-feeding. Because the infant's gastrointestinal system continues to mature throughout the first year, changes in diet, the introduction of new foods, and even upsets in routines can result in feeding problems.

Parents often have many questions and concerns about nutrition. They are influenced by a variety of sources, including relatives and friends who may not be aware of current scientific practices regarding infant feeding. To provide anticipatory guidance, the nurse must have a clear understanding of gastrointestinal maturation and knowledge about breastfeeding and various infant formulas and foods. Families and cultures vary widely in food preferences and infant feeding practices. The nurse must remain cognizant of these differences when providing anticipatory guidance related to infant nutrition.

! NURSING QUALITY ALERT

Essential Information for Infant Nutrition

Breast milk or commercially prepared iron-fortified formula provides optimal nutrition throughout infancy.

Formula must be prepared according to instructions, and leftover formula should be stored or discarded according to the manufacturer's directions.

Some health care providers discourage the use of powdered formula until the infant is older than 6 weeks.

Factors Influencing Choice of Feeding Method

The AAP strongly recommends exclusive breastfeeding for the first 6 months of life for all infants, including premature and sick newborns, with rare exceptions (Gartner, Morton, Lawrence, and AAP Section on Breastfeeding, 2005). Breast milk provides complete

TABLE 5-2   BENEFITS OF BREASTFEEDING

FOR THE INFANT	FOR THE MOTHER
Allergies are less likely to develop.	Oxytocin release enhances involution of uterus.
Immunologic properties help prevent infections. May have fewer respiratory, ear, and gastrointestinal infections and less risk for SIDS.	Mother loses less blood because of delayed return of menses.
Composition meets infant's specific nutritional needs.	Mother more likely to rest while feeding.
Nutritional and immunologic properties change according to infant's needs.	Mother likely to eat balanced diet that improves healing.
Breast milk easily digested.	Frequent, close contact may enhance bonding.
Protein, fat, and carbohydrate in most suitable proportions.	Convenient: always available, no bottles to prepare, no formula to buy or heat.
No possibility of improper (and potentially dangerous) dilution.	Economical: eliminates cost of formula and bottles.
Breast milk unlikely to be contaminated; not affected by water supply.	Traveling easier: no bottles to prepare, carry, refrigerate, or warm.
Less likely to result in overfeeding.	May reduce the risk of some cancers.
Infant unlikely to have constipation.	

nutrition for infants, and evidence suggests that breastfed infants are less likely to be at risk for later overweight or obesity (Huh, Rifas-Shiman, Taveras et al., 2011). A recent meta-analysis of 18 case control studies provides high level evidence that the odds of a breastfed infant dying of sudden infant death syndrome (SIDS) are far lower than those of infants never given breast milk, and that the protection is even stronger for infants who are exclusively breastfed (Hauck, Thompson, Tanabe, et al., 2011). Mothers who breastfeed need instruction and support as they begin. They are more likely to succeed if they are given practical information (Table 5-2). Many facilities provide lactation consultants or home visits, or nursing staff may call to assess the mother's needs. Significant others are included in teaching to provide a support system for the mother.

Increasing the percentage of infants who are exclusively breastfed is a goal of *Healthy People 2020*. Although 74% of infants in the United States are breastfed at birth, the rate drops to 43.5% for infants in the United States who are breastfed for 6 months, and the percentage goes down to 22% for those who are breastfed for 1 year (United States Department of Health and Human Services [USDHHS], 2010). The percentage of infants who are exclusively breastfed for 6 months is only 14.1%. The goal is to increase the percentage of infants who are breastfed for 6 months to over 60%, and those who are exclusively breastfed for 6 months to 25.5% (USDHHS, 2010). To promote breastfeeding, the United Nations Children's Fund (UNICEF) and the World Health Organization (WHO) advocate that birth facilities become certified as "baby-friendly" hospitals, with policies to actively encourage mothers to breastfeed. Guidelines to becoming certified as a baby-friendly hospital emphasize educating staff and parents about breastfeeding; encouraging early initiation of breastfeeding, demand feedings, and rooming-in; and avoiding use of formula and pacifiers. More information is available at http://babyfriendlyusa.org. The AAP has also recently updated its website on breastfeeding and has information for parents and professionals (www.aap.org/breastfeeding). In 2011, the Surgeon General issued a *Call to Action to Support Breastfeeding;*

HEALTH PROMOTION

⊖ *The Newborn to 1-Month-Old Infant*

Focused Assessment

Ask the parent the following:

- How have you been feeling? Have you made your postpartum checkup appointment?
- How have you and your partner been adjusting to the baby? Do you have other children? How are they adjusting?
- Have you discussed child-rearing philosophies?
- Does anyone in your household smoke cigarettes?
- Does anyone in your household use substances?
- Have you recently been exposed to or had any sexually transmissible disease?
- Have you experienced any periods of sadness or feeling "down"?
- Do you have any concerns about the costs of the baby's care?
- Do you feel that you and the baby are safe?

Developmental Milestones

Personal/social: Looks at parent's face; fixates, tracks, follows to midline; smiles responsively; prefers brightly colored objects

Fine motor: Newborn reflexes present

Language/cognitive: Prefers human female voice: responds to sounds; begins to vocalize

Gross motor: Equal movements; lifts head; lifts head and chin (by 1 month)

Health Maintenance

Physical Measurements

Weight: 7.5 to 8 pounds (3.4 to 3.6 kg) average. Loses 10% of body weight after birth but gains it back by 2 weeks.

Gains ½ ounce a day on average.

Length: Average 20 inches (50 cm). Gains 1 inch (2.5 cm) a month for the first several months.

Head Circumference: 13 to 14 inches (33 to 35.5 cm). Gains average of ½ inch (1.2 cm) per month until 6 months of age. Posterior fontanel closes by 2 to 3 months; anterior by 12 to 18 months.

Immunizations

Thimerosal-free hepatitis B #1 at birth and #2 at 1 to 2 months. Be sure to discuss side effects. Give the parent information about upcoming immunizations.

If planning to use a combination vaccine that contains hepatitis B, wait until 2 months for second hepatitis B.

Health Screening

Phenylketonuria and other metabolic diseases; cystic fibrosis

Hearing screening

Visual inspection for congenital defects

Anticipatory Guidance

Nutrition

Breast milk on demand at least every 2 to 3 hours

Iron-fortified formula 2 to 3 ounces every 3 to 4 hours if not breastfeeding

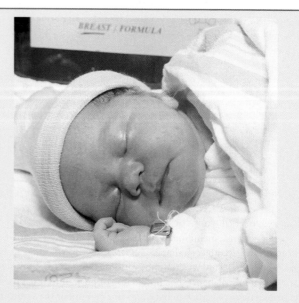

Vitamin D supplement 400 IU/day for breastfed infants and for formula-fed infants if taking less than 1 liter (33 ounces) of formula a day

Place on right side after feeding

Elimination

Six wet diapers

Stools related to feeding method

Dental

Continue prenatal vitamins and calcium if breastfeeding

Sleep

Place on back to sleep in parent's room in a separate crib/cradle/bassinet. Keep loose or soft bedding and toys out of the crib, offer pacifier for nap and bedtime if not breastfeeding.

16 or more hours

By 1 month begin to establish nighttime routine

Hygiene

Sponge bathe until cord falls off

Circumcision care, if applicable

Safety

Be sure crib is safe: Slats <2⅜ inches apart, firm mattress that fits the crib

Eliminate all environmental smoke

Rear-facing approved infant car seat

Fire prevention: Smoke detectors, fire extinguishers

Water temperature <120° F

Cardiopulmonary resuscitation and first aid classes; emergency phone numbers

Violence: Discuss shaking, guns in the home

information can be obtained at http://surgeongeneral.gov/topics/breastfeeding/calltoactiontosupportbreastfeeding.pdf.

Some parents prefer a combination of breastfeeding and bottle feeding. It is best to delay giving formula until lactation has been well established at 3 to 4 weeks of age. Giving breastfeeding infants formula leads to a decrease in breastfeeding frequency and milk production, making successful breastfeeding less likely (Committee on Health Care for Underserved Women, American College of Obstetricians and Gynecologists [ACOG], 2007). However, if the mother chooses to feed both breast milk and formula, the nurse should educate and support her so the infant receives the benefits of breast milk at least part of the time.

Some mothers choose to give a bottle daily or only occasionally, such as when a babysitter is caring for the infant. These mothers feel this allows them to be away from the infant for longer periods of time yet allows the enjoyable closeness with the infant, as well as the physical advantages of breastfeeding, to continue. Mothers may choose to use breast milk or formula for occasional bottle feedings.

Support from Others. The influence of family members is often an important determinant of whether mothers breastfeed. Some women choose not to breastfeed because their partner objects. The opinion of a woman's mother or mother-in-law may also be important. The woman with little support or with active discouragement from her family will probably have a difficult time nursing. Advice from friends who have breastfed may also influence the mother's decision.

Involvement of the fathers in infant care is important for some families and some may feel it is only possible with feedings. Nurses can suggest other infant care measures, such as holding, rocking, and bathing, that fathers can enjoy (AAP, 2011a). Educating family members about the advantages of breastfeeding and how to deal with problems may lead to their encouragement of the breastfeeding mother. Educating fathers about the benefits of breastfeeding as well as techniques for coping with any difficulties that might occur is important. When fathers are knowledgeable and supportive, full breastfeeding is more likely to continue longer (AAP, 2011a). Prenatal classes that include breastfeeding information have been shown to help a woman decide to breastfeed and to successfully persist (Rosen, Krueger, Carney, & Graham, 2008). This can lead to a higher rate of exclusive breastfeeding with less use of formula. It can also increase a woman's satisfaction with the breastfeeding experience. Fathers should also attend the classes so they can provide increased support based on their knowledge (AAP, 2011a).

Encouragement from the woman's health care provider may be a powerful influence in the woman choosing to breastfeed (Newton, 2007). The support the mother receives from the nursing staff plays a significant part in whether she feels comfortable with her chosen feeding method. Those who do not feel confident in their ability to breastfeed before they leave the birth facility are less likely to continue breastfeeding if they encounter difficulties at home.

Peer support also may be important. Trained peer counselors have been effective in helping mothers breastfeed for longer periods without using formula. Peer counseling groups can be particularly helpful because there is a social aspect to them that benefits new mothers as they learn more and become confident about breastfeeding ("Peer counselors," 2011).

Culture. Cultural influences may dictate decisions about how and when a mother feeds her infant. For example, many Mormon women believe that breastfeeding is an important part of motherhood. Muslim women often breastfeed for the infant's first 2 years.

Immigrants to the United States often would breastfeed infants if they were still in their own countries. For example, in Russia women are expected to breastfeed and formula is not available in birth houses (Callister, Getmanenko, Garvrish, et al., 2007). However, immigrants from countries where breastfeeding is the norm may breastfeed for shorter durations or not at all because they lack the support system they had in their own country. Some of these women may think that because formula is available in the hospital and they see American women using formula, it is the preferred method of feeding. They may believe breastfeeding is inferior to formula feeding and that formula will make their infants big and healthy (Hernandez, 2006). Nurses must emphasize the superiority of breastfeeding and encourage these women to continue their cultural tradition of breastfeeding and cultural practices that facilitate it. Nurses should be particularly watchful for ways to help mothers from other cultures who might wish to breastfeed but fail to do so because of lack of support.

Employment. Women should be encouraged to continue breastfeeding when they return to work. Because of the decreased incidence of illness in breastfed infants, the mother is less likely to miss work to take care of a sick infant. This is an advantage for the employer as well as the breastfeeding family.

Unfortunately, returning to work or school is a major cause of discontinuation of breastfeeding. The mother may choose formula from the beginning, plan a short period of breastfeeding before weaning the infant to formula, or use a combination of breastfeeding and bottle feeding with breast milk or formula. Nurses who provide practical information about options, breastfeeding and working, breast pumps, and storage of breast milk help a mother continue breastfeeding for a longer period. Referral to a lactation consultant can provide a mother with continued education and support after she goes home.

Other Factors. Other factors may also influence a woman's decision. Her knowledge and past experience with infant feeding are important. Women who are most likely to breastfeed are Asian or Hispanic and live in the western mountain or Pacific coast regions of the United States. Those with the lowest breastfeeding rates include African-American women who live in the southern region of the United States (Centers for Disease Control and Prevention [CDC], 2011a & 2011b).

Normal Breastfeeding

The pediatric nurse may encounter mothers of newborn infants on the pediatric unit and therefore should have current knowledge of both advantages of breastfeeding and proper breastfeeding techniques.

Advantages. Breast milk contains a more complete protein than cow's milk–based formulas, is more easily digested, and results in more rapid gastric emptying time. For this reason, infants who breastfeed need to eat more frequently than do formula-fed infants. Breastfeeding is convenient, economical, and enhances mother-infant attachment and interaction.

Human milk changes to meet the changing nutrient needs of the infant. Human milk and colostrum contain immunologic and antibacterial components not available in formula. Human milk is higher in lactose, which is converted to monosaccharide galactose, essential for central nervous system development and growth.

The fat content of breast milk is higher in monounsaturated fat, which is more easily digested and absorbed than fat in formulas. The fat content varies during the feeding and the time of day. The milk produced at the end of a feeding (hindmilk) and in the middle of the day has a higher fat content. Because the milk at the beginning of a feeding (foremilk) has less fat content than at the end, it is important that the length of feeding time be sufficient for the infant to derive benefits from the higher-fat hindmilk.

Breast milk does not provide an adequate amount of vitamin D to prevent rickets and other vitamin D–associated conditions. Infants who are exclusively breastfed need vitamin D supplementation to prevent rickets. The AAP (Greer, Sicherer, Burks, & Section on Breast-feeding & Committee on Nutrition, 2008) recommends vitamin D supplementation of 400 International Units/day for all breastfed infants and for formula-fed infants who consume less than 32 ounces of vitamin D–fortified formula a day. In addition to an insufficiency of vitamin D in breast milk, breast milk also lacks iron and zinc. There is some evidence that some infants use up maternal stores of iron before the commonly accepted 6-month benchmark; this increases their risk for iron deficiency (Baker, Greer, & AAP Committee on Nutrition, 2010). The AAP now recommends supplementing the diet of exclusively or partially breastfed infants with 1 mg/kg/day iron, beginning at 4 months of age and ending when the infant is able to take complementary solid foods high in iron (e.g., iron-fortified cereals) (Baker, Greer, & AAP Committee on Nutrition, 2010).

Breastfeeding Techniques. A breastfeeding mother can use one of several positions for feeding (see Patient-Centered Teaching: Guidelines for Breastfeeding). It is important for the infant's head and body to be directly facing the breast in a "tummy to tummy" position at a height that prevents pulling or tension on the nipple. Hand position for feeding is important. Either a "C" position or a "V" position is acceptable. In the "V" position, the mother uses both forefinger and middle finger to lift and support the breast. Because suckling releases *prolactin* (the hormone responsible for milk production), the more frequently the infant feeds, the better the mother's milk supply.

Breastfeeding Concerns. Because they cannot visually observe the amount of milk the infant is receiving, many mothers become concerned that the infant is not receiving enough. The nurse assists the mother to observe the infant swallow during feeding. An infant who is receiving adequate milk will be gaining weight, appear satisfied after feedings, have at least six wet diapers a day (after the first week), and have loose, golden (mustard color and texture) stools.

Although infants are sleepier the few first days after birth, some infants continue this pattern and need some gentle stimulus either to wake for a feeding or to wake up during a feeding. It is best to completely remove the breast from an infant who has fallen asleep while nursing rather than jiggling the breast in the infant's mouth. Excessive sleepiness during feeding in an infant younger than 6 weeks may be cause for further evaluation.

Because movement of the tongue is different between bottle feeding and breastfeeding, it is best to avoid bottle feeding until the mother's milk supply is fully established. Some lactation specialists advise mothers to avoid pacifier use as well. The AAP Task Force on Sudden Infant Death Syndrome (2005), states that evidence suggests that giving an infant a pacifier for nap or night sleep may be protective against SIDS. It recommends that pacifiers be offered to all bottle-fed infants and to breastfed infants older than 1 month (AAP, Task Force on Sudden Infant Death Syndrome, 2005).

EVIDENCE-BASED PRACTICE

The Case for Vitamin D

The American Academy of Pediatrics recommends that all breastfed infants should receive a daily supplement of 400 IU of vitamin D. Infants, children, and adolescents who consume fewer than 32 ounces of vitamin D–fortified infant formula or whole milk (children older than age 1 year) also should receive supplemental vitamin D because they are at risk for vitamin D insufficiency (Misra, Pacaud, Teryk, et al., 2008). The impetus for these recommendations, which are updated from initial recommendations in 2003, was a near-doubling of the reported incidence and prevalence of children diagnosed with rickets in the United States between 1975 and 2003 (Misra et al., 2008). Rickets is a disease that causes malformations in growing bone as a result of decreased bone mineralization; vitamin D is one factor that affects the absorption and use of calcium for bone formation. Because of public health efforts to decrease the prevalence of vitamin D deficiency (e.g., fortifying foods) the prevalence of rickets had markedly decreased; however, the more recent increase in identified cases of rickets has been a matter of concern to health professionals who care for children (Misra et al.). In addition, evidence is increasing that sufficient vitamin D plays a role in the health of other body systems, as demonstrated by the presence of vitamin D receptors in organs of the gastrointestinal, neurologic, endocrine, and immune systems (Misra et al., 2008).

Several studies have suggested that parents of infants and children in the United States have low adherence to vitamin D supplementation recommendations (Misra et al., 2008; Perrine, Sharma, Jefferds, et al., 2010; Taylor, Geyer, & Feldman, 2009). A recent observational (Level VI) study of providers and parents in a northwest American city (Taylor et al., 2009) revealed that overall, parents are not giving breastfed infants vitamin D supplements. This study demonstrated that parents of breastfed infants are significantly more likely to give vitamin D supplements if strongly recommended by a pediatric provider and significantly less likely to give the supplements if they believe that breast milk provides complete nutrition to their child.

Evidence from multiple sources, as described in an in-depth systematic literature review (Level V) by Misra et al. (2008), suggests that vitamin D insufficiency is related to two general issues: (1) the primary natural source of vitamin D is in ultraviolet light from the sun, and (2) infants and children consume inadequate nutritional sources of vitamin D. Use of sunscreen and other protective measures to reduce skin cancer risk from UV rays, along with decreased sun exposure from outdoor play, can decrease the natural synthesis of vitamin D that occurs through the skin. In addition, infants and children with dark skin are more at risk for vitamin D insufficiency if they do not have appropriate vitamin D supplementation because of the UV protection from increased melanin (Misra et al., 2008).

Breast milk is the most nutritionally complete source of nutrition for infants, and exclusive breastfeeding for a minimum of the first 6 to 12 months is recommended by the American Academy of Pediatrics. However, breast milk does not provide a sufficient amount of vitamin D to prevent rickets in exclusively breastfed infants or in infants, children, and adolescents receiving less than 32 ounces of fortified formula or milk a day (Misra et al., 2008). Other nutritional sources of vitamin D include oily fish, cod liver oil, and an assortment of fortified dairy and cereal products, most of which are not appealing to children or adolescents or are consumed in less than recommended amounts.

Because parents rely on health care professionals to provide evidence-based information, think about the following: If a breastfeeding mother were to ask your advice about giving vitamin D supplements to her infant, how might you respond? What is your knowledge about vitamin D?

Misra, M., Pacaud, D., Teryk, A., et al., & Drug and Therapeutics Committee of the Lawson Wilkins Pediatric Endocrine Society. (2008). Vitamin D deficiency in children and its management: Review of current knowledge and recommendations. *Pediatrics, 122*(2), 398-417; Perrine, C., Sharma, A., Jefferds, M., et al. (2010). Adherence to vitamin D recommendations among U.S. infants. *Pediatrics, 125,* 627-632; Taylor, J., Geyer, L., & Feldman, K. (2009). Use of supplemental vitamin D among infants breastfed for prolonged periods. *Pediatrics, 125*(1), 105-111.

PATIENT-CENTERED TEACHING

Guidelines for Breastfeeding

- Wash hands. Wash nipples with warm water, no soap.
- There are three basic positions:
  - *Cradle position:* Cradle your infant in one arm, with the head resting in the bend of your elbows. The infant's mouth is close to the breast. You can be sitting up straight in bed, with pillows supporting your back, or sitting in a chair. Sometimes a pillow may be needed on your lap to elevate the infant to the nipple level.

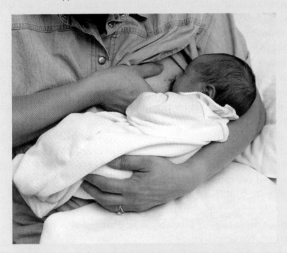

  - *Football hold:* A pillow is needed to be successful with this position. Sit in a chair and place a pillow next to you on the nursing side. The pillow supports the elbow and your infant's buttocks and should bring your infant's head up to the level of your breast.

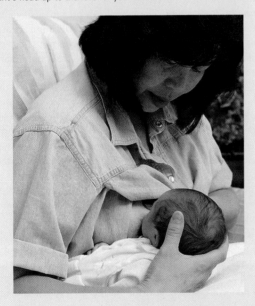

- *Lying-down position:* Lie on your side in bed with your infant lying on the side facing you.

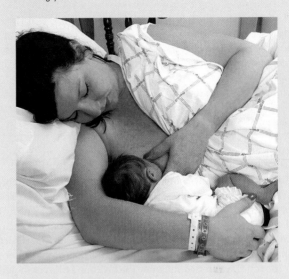

- Hold the breast so the nipple brushes the center of the infant's lips and wait for the infant to open the mouth.
- Your infant's mouth should be opened wide, as with a yawn, and should cover the entire areola, or a large amount of the areola. If necessary, apply pressure to your infant's chin with your index finger to open the infant's mouth wider. Your breast needs to be placed far back into the infant's mouth to drain the breast adequately. Your hand position is important: Hold your hand in a "C" position around your breast with the thumb on top behind the areola and the fingers against the chest wall and supporting the underside of the breast.

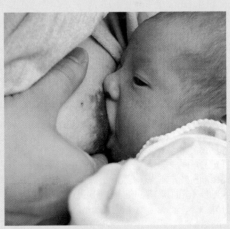

- Both breasts are used in each feeding, usually 10 to 15 minutes on the first side, followed by burping before beginning the second side. The length of time on the second side is related to the quality of the infant's suckling. At the next feeding, your infant starts to feed on the breast used to finish the preceding feeding.
- Break suction by placing your finger in the corner of your infant's mouth and quickly remove your breast.
- The neonate is nursed shortly after birth and approximately every 2 to 3 hours thereafter for a total of 8 to 12 feedings a day.
- Infants should be burped after each breast and at the end of the feeding.
- Nipples often become tender during the first week of nursing but should not become sore. Soreness and prolonged feedings are most often the result of an infant who is not latched onto the breast properly.

BOX 5-4   TIPS FOR STORING BREAST MILK

- Milk may be stored for 24 hours in the refrigerator (colder than 39° F [4° C]), up to 1 month in a freezer compartment that has a separate door from the refrigerator, or up to 6 months in a deep freezer (AAP, 2010).
- Containers, either glass or plastic, used to store breast milk should have a tight cap and should be sterile.
- Freeze in amounts that are likely to be used for one feeding and discard any unused portion. Be sure to mark each container with the date and use the oldest first.
- To thaw breast milk, either thaw in the refrigerator or by holding under cool, running water. Breast milk remains safe if kept in the refrigerator and used within 24 hours of thawing.

Milk Storage. Many mothers choose to pump and store breast milk, either because they have returned to work or want to keep a supply on hand so others may feed the infant. Expressed breast milk is relatively free from bacterial contamination, but it can become contaminated when artificially collected and stored. Hands and collection equipment should be clean and the expressed milk stored appropriately (Box 5-4). Expressed milk not used within 24 hours should be frozen; thawed milk should not be refrozen.

Formula Feeding

Formula given by bottle is a choice selected by many women in the United States. This method is often easier for the mother who must return to work soon after her infant's birth, and it has the advantage of allowing other members of the family to participate in the infant's feeding. Infant formula does not have the immunologic properties and digestibility of human milk, but it does meet the energy and nutrient requirements of infants. If bottle-feeding is chosen as the preferred feeding method, the formula should be iron fortified. The Infant Formula Act of 1980, which was revised in 1986, establishes the standards for infant formulas. It also requires that the label show the quantity of each nutrient contained in the formula. Special formulas are available for low-birth-weight infants, infants with congenital cardiac disease, and for infants allergic to cow's milk–based formulas.

There are some physiologic reasons why some mothers choose to use formula. Infants with galactosemia or whose mothers use illegal drugs, are taking certain prescribed drugs (e.g., antiretrovirals, certain chemotherapeutic agents), or have untreated active tuberculosis should not be breastfed (CDC, 2009). In the United States and other countries where safe water is available and breastfeeding is culturally acceptable, women who are infected with HIV should avoid breastfeeding (AAP, 2009).

Cow's Milk. Cow's milk (whole, skim, 1%, 2%) is not recommended in the first 12 months. Cow's milk contains too little iron, and its high renal solute load and unmodified derivatives can put small infants at risk for dehydration. The tough, hard curd is difficult for infants to digest. In addition, skim milk and reduced-fat milk deprive the infant of needed calories and essential fatty acids. The incidences of allergy and iron deficiency anemia are higher in infants who are given cow's milk than in those who receive breast milk or formula.

Types of Formula. Formula can be purchased in three different forms—ready-to-use, concentrated liquid, and powdered. With the exception of the ready-to-use formula, all need to have water added to obtain the appropriate concentration for feeding. Storage instructions differ, so nurses need to strongly encourage parents to carefully follow the directions for storage of the specific type of formula they are using

for their infant. A variety of bottles and nipples are available; the type chosen is based on parent preference.

Ready-to-use. Ready-to-use formula is available in bottles to which a nipple is added or in cans to be poured directly into a bottle. It should not be diluted. Although expensive, it is practical for traveling, when there is difficulty mixing the formula, or the water supply is in question. An open can should be refrigerated and used within 48 hours.

Concentrated liquid. Explain to the parents how to dilute concentrated liquid formula. Equal parts of formula and water are mixed together in a bottle to provide the amount desired for each feeding. Opened cans should be stored in the refrigerator and used within 48 hours (Janke, 2008).

Powdered formula. Powdered formula is more economical and is particularly useful when a breastfeeding mother plans to give an occasional bottle of formula. Usually one scoop of powder is added to each 2 ounces of warm water in a bottle. Single-portion packets of powder are available for travel. Formula should be well mixed to dissolve the powder and make the solution uniform. New formula should be prepared for each feeding.

Although commercially prepared formulas have many similarities, there are also differences. Some commonly used brands are Enfamil, SMA, Similac, Gerber, and Good Start. There are formulas specifically designed for infants older than 6 months, but it is not necessary to change to a different formula when a child reaches that age. Some formulas are designed for feeding low-birth-weight or ill infants. These include high-calorie formulas and predigested formulas (e.g., Pregestimil, Neutramagen).

Many different types of bottles and nipples are available. Mothers may use glass or plastic bottles or a plastic liner that fits into a rigid container. Some nipples are designed to simulate the human nipple to promote jaw development. Selection of the type of bottles and nipples depends on individual preference.

Formula Preparation. The parent can prepare a single bottle or a 24-hour supply. If the water supply is safe, sterilization is not necessary. If there is any possibility that the water supply is not safe, water should be boiled or sterile, bottled water should be used. Bottles and nipples can be washed in hot, sudsy water using a brush to clean well and then rinsed and allowed to air-dry. Bottles may be washed in a dishwasher, but nipples tend to deteriorate quickly unless washed by hand. Instruct the mother to wash her hands, as well as the top of the can and the can opener. The formula and water are poured into the bottles, which are then capped. Emphasize that the proportion of water and liquid or powdered formula must be adhered to exactly to prevent illness in the infant.

Explain that if safety of the water supply is questionable, sterilization, by aseptic or terminal method, is required. In both methods, all equipment is washed and rinsed well before beginning.

In the aseptic method, equipment needed for the procedure is boiled for 5 minutes in a sterilizer or deep pan. Water for diluting the formula is boiled separately. The bottles are then assembled, using sterilized tongs to avoid contamination by the hands. The formula and boiled water are added, and the bottles are capped and refrigerated until needed.

In the terminal sterilization method, the formula is placed in clean, loosely capped bottles. The bottles are then placed in the sterilizer or pan of water and boiled for 25 minutes. After the bottles cool, the caps are tightened and the bottles refrigerated.

Formula-Feeding Techniques. It should not be assumed that parents know how to bottle feed an infant. The nurse may need to teach them how often and how much to feed, how to hold and cuddle while feeding, when and how to burp, and how to prepare formula. The nurse demonstrates to the mother how to position the infant in a

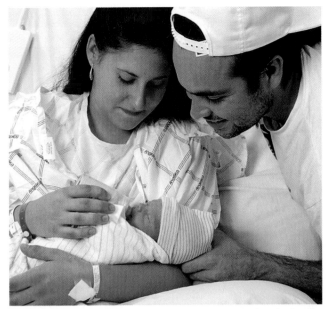

FIG 5-2 This mother holds her infant close during bottle feeding. The bottle is positioned so the nipple is filled with milk at all times. The father offers encouragement.

semiupright position, preferably in a cradle hold (Figure 5-2) to facilitate face-to-face contact.

Instruct the parents to feed the infant every 3 to 4 hours. The infant takes only ½ to 1 ounce per feeding during the first day of life but increases to 2 to 3 ounces per feeding by the third to fifth day. An infant who is satisfied often will go to sleep.

To minimize excessive intake of air during feeding, the bottle should be held so that the nipple is completely filled with formula. Advise the parent to burp the infant frequently, approximately every ½ to 1 ounce. To burp the infant, the parent holds the infant upright, either against the parent's shoulder or sitting on the parent's lap sideways with the child supported. Gentle rubbing of the back usually will elicit a burp.

Caution parents not to prop the bottle. Propping increases the likelihood of choking if regurgitation occurs and eliminates the holding and cuddling that should accompany feeding. Infants who go to sleep with a bottle propped are at risk for aspiration. Pooled milk in the mouth leads to cavities once the teeth are in. Otitis media is more common in infants who sleep with a bottle or who have a propped bottle.

The parent should not try to coax the infant to finish the bottle at each feeding. This action could result in regurgitation and excessive weight gain. Discarding unused formula within an hour prevents feeding the infant formula contaminated by rapidly growing bacteria.

Weaning

Weaning is the replacement of breast or bottle feedings with drinking from a cup. Infants usually have a decreasing interest in the breast or bottle starting between ages 6 and 12 months. This varies from infant to infant, but if solids and a cup have been introduced, the infant will probably begin to indicate a readiness for the cup. Even young infants can be weaned to a regular plastic cup, although they will not be ready to hold the cup themselves until later. Some parents choose to use a sippy cup—a cup with a tight cover that prevents contents from spilling when dropped. When weaning is begun after age 18 months, the infant may resist because of increased attachment to the breast or bottle.

Behaviors that might indicate a readiness to begin weaning include the following:
- Throwing the bottle down
- Chewing on the nipple
- Taking only a few ounces of formula
- Refusing the breast or dawdling

Weaning should not take place during times of change or stress (e.g., illness, starting child care, the arrival of a new baby). Weaning is a gradual process and should start with the replacement of one bottle feeding or breastfeeding at a time. If breastfeeding must be terminated before age 6 months, it should be replaced with bottle feedings to meet the infant's sucking needs. The older infant who has learned to use a cup may not need to use a bottle.

The first bottle feeding or breastfeeding eliminated should be the one in which the infant is least interested. Initially the infant may accept the cup only after drinking some formula from the bottle or milk from the breast. The infant is next offered the cup before the feeding. After several days, another feeding can be eliminated if the infant is not resisting the change. The bedtime feeding is usually the last feeding to be eliminated.

During weaning, the child is giving up time that had been spent being held in the parent's arms. The parent needs to respond to the infant's continued need to be held and cuddled. Infants should not be encouraged to carry bottles or sippy cups around as toys, to take them to bed, or to use them as pacifiers. Infants who indicate sucking needs should be given pacifiers.

Juices

Once the infant is able to take fluids from a cup, the parent can introduce small amounts (no more than 4 to 6 ounces/day) of fruit juice. Fruit juice lacks the fiber present in whole fruit and for that reason, whole fruit is considered more nutritionally acceptable than fruit juice (AAP, 2011c). Fruit juice should be avoided in infants younger than 6 months of age and should not be given to infants at bedtime because it can contribute to tooth decay (AAP, 2011c). Nurses must be aware of the nutritional benefits and limitations of juice; advise parents to give children only 100% fruit juice and not juice drinks, which may contain added sugar.

In infants with a family history of allergies, orange and tomato juice should be delayed until age 1 year. Some prepared foods and dinners contain orange juice and tomato juice. Parents need to be taught to read labels. Juice is not warmed because heating destroys vitamin C. Juices should be kept in a covered container in the refrigerator to prevent the loss of the vitamin.

Water

Sufficient water is provided in breast milk and in prepared formula during early infancy. When solid foods are introduced, it may be necessary to give a small amount of additional water because some foods (e.g., strained meats, high-meat dinners) have a high renal solute load. Additional fluid is necessary when intake is low or the infant has fluid loss because of illness (fever, respiratory disease). Young infants do not need fluoridated water.

Solid Foods

The early introduction of solids may be detrimental to growth because the solids the infant eats cannot be adequately digested related to the immaturity of the gastrointestinal system. In addition, the nutrients in breast or formula milk will not be taken in because the infant's appetite has been satisfied with the less nutritious solids. Evidence suggests that early introduction of solid foods (before 4 months of age) in bottle-fed infants contributes to later overweight and obesity (Huh et al., 2011).

HEALTH PROMOTION

⊖ *The 2-Month-Old Infant*

Focused Assessment

Ask the parent the following:

- How has your family adjusted to the baby?
- Are you able to plan time to give some individual attention to each of your other children?
- Are you getting enough opportunities to continue relationships and activities away from the baby?
- Will you describe your baby's behavior and general mood?
- Did your baby have any reaction to the last immunizations? If so, what happened?

Developmental Milestones

Personal/social: Smiles spontaneously; enjoys interacting with others
Fine motor: Follows past midline; reflexes disappear
Language/cognitive: Vocalizes "ooh" and "ah" sounds; attends to voices
Gross motor: Beginning head control when upright; lifts head 45 degrees onto forearms

Critical Milestones*

Personal/social: Smiles responsively; looks at faces
Fine motor: Follows to midline
Language/cognitive: Vocalizes making cooing or short vowel sounds; responds to a bell
Gross motor: Lifts head; equal movements

Health Maintenance
Physical Measurements

Measure length, weight, and head circumference and plot on growth charts

Immunizations

Diphtheria-tetanus-acellular pertussis (DTaP) #1; inactivated poliovirus (IPV) #1 (may substitute DTaP, hepatitis B, and polio combination vaccine); *Haemophilus influenzae* type b (Hib) #1; pneumococcal #1; rotavirus #1
Discuss potential effects

Health Screening

Hearing screen if not done at birth; hearing risk assessment
Check eyes for strabismus
Assess ability to follow past midline

Anticipatory Guidance
Nutrition

Breastfeed on demand with increasing intervals
Formula, 4 to 6 ounces six times a day
Vitamin D supplement 400 IU/day for breastfed infants and for formula-fed infants if taking less than 1 liter (33 ounces) of formula a day

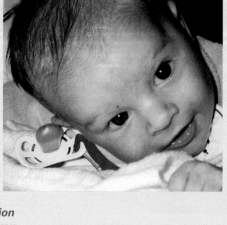

Elimination

Six wet diapers
Stools related to feeding method; may decrease in number

Dental

Continue prenatal vitamins and calcium if breastfeeding
Do not prop baby's bottle

Sleep

Place on back to sleep in parent's room in a separate crib/cradle/bassinet. Keep loose or soft bedding and toys out of the crib, offer pacifier for nap and bedtime if not breastfeeding.
Continue nighttime routine
Play with baby when awake

Hygiene

Bathe several times per week
Watch for diaper rash and seborrheic dermatitis

Safety

Review house and environmental safety and conditions for calling the doctor, posting of emergency numbers near the telephone, car safety, violence, avoidance of exposure to cigarette smoke
Discuss preventing falls and burns from hot liquids

Play

Imitate vocalizations and smile
Sing
Change infant's environment
Encourage rolling over

*Guided by Denver Developmental Screening Test II.

Nutrients supplied by solid foods in the older infant, however, cannot be provided completely by formula or breast milk alone, so solid foods should be introduced beginning no earlier than 4 months and no later than 6 months of age (Greer, Sicherer, Burks, & AAP Committee on Nutrition & Section on Allergy and Immunology, 2008).

The infant goes through a *transitional period,* during which prepared foods are introduced and given together with human milk or formula. Each infant's growth and development vary, and milestones indicate the infant's readiness for solid foods (Box 5-5).

Solids should be introduced one at a time in small amounts (1 teaspoon to 2 tablespoons) for several days before introducing a new food. This is done to avoid confusion should a food intolerance be present. The order of introduction is not critical, but iron-fortified rice cereal is most often recommended as a first food because it is high in iron, is easily digested, and has a low allergenic probability. Other commercially available infant cereals include oatmeal, barley, mixed grain, and cereals with added fruit. When foods are first being introduced, mixed grains and cereals with added fruit should be avoided. A variety

BOX 5-5 READINESS FOR INTRODUCTION OF SOLIDS

Infant can sit.
Birth weight has doubled and infant weighs at least 13 pounds.
Infant can reach for an object and maintain balance.
Infant indicates a desire for food by opening mouth and leaning forward.
Extrusion reflex has disappeared (4 to 5 months).
Infant moves food to back of mouth and swallows during spoon feedings.

of meat, fish, poultry, and eggs can be introduced along with various fruits and vegetables. The focus is on food variety and choices from various food groups (Anderson, Malley, & Snell, 2009). Foods should not be mixed with formula and fed through a nipple with a large hole. This deprives the child of the chewing experience and changes the texture and taste of the food. Pureed foods are given initially, but increases in food texture can occur fairly quickly thereafter (Anderson, Malley, & Snell, 2009).

Several commercially prepared fruits and vegetables are available. In addition, fruits and vegetables can easily be steamed or boiled and then pureed in a blender or food processor at home. It is usually necessary to add a small amount of water during the blending process. The parent should not give an infant home-prepared orange or dark green leafy vegetables because of the elevated nitrate levels, which can cause methemoglobinemia. In addition, infants for whom formula is prepared with well water remain at high risk for nitrate poisoning (Greer, Shannon, AAP Committee on Nutrition, & AAP Committee on Environmental Health, 2005). As with cereals, mixed fruits should be avoided until the infant is older and has tolerated individual foods. The parent should avoid giving the infant mixed meats and vegetables as well; these baby foods may not contain enough meat.

Salt and sugar should not be added to commercial or home-prepared foods. Parents should avoid using canned foods or home-prepared foods that contain large amounts of sugar and salt. Feeding honey to infants under age 12 months has been associated with botulism and should therefore be avoided.

Finger Foods. Between age 8 and 10 months the infant can be introduced to finger foods. At this time the pincer grasp is developing and the infant can pick up foods. The infant will have a palmar grasp before this time and soft foods can be given, but the infant will mainly "play" with the food. This can be a positive experience that enables the infant to feel different textures and increase fine motor skills.

Finger foods should be bite-size pieces of soft food. Arrowroot biscuits, cheese sticks, slices of canned peaches or pears, cut pieces of bananas, and breads can be offered. As children's fine motor skills increase, they may enjoy eating some of the dry cereals, such as Cheerios. Be sure pieces of larger finger foods are not round and are small enough that they will not block the infant's airway, causing a choking hazard. The AAP (Committee on Injury, Violence, and Poison Prevention, 2010) recommends infants not be given such foods as hot dogs, whole grapes, marshmallows, peanut butter, seeds, hard candy, raw carrots, popcorn, and nuts. Encourage the parents to remain with an infant who is eating finger foods.

Snacks. When the infant is on a three-meals-a-day schedule, small snacks are an appropriate addition to the nutritional intake. Because infants have small stomachs, they may not be content to wait until the next meal before eating. Snacks should be nutritious, and parents should resist the urge to give infants a bottle to satisfy their hunger. Some of the safe finger foods previously listed make nutritious snacks. If the infant is not hungry at mealtime, the snack should be given in a smaller portion or eliminated.

Food Allergies

The early introduction of solid foods may be associated with a higher incidence of food allergy in infants determined to be at risk, especially those with a family history of allergy. However, recent evidence—including evidence from a level V integrative literature review—suggests that introduction of a variety of solid foods between 4 and 6 months of age, including foods suspected to be allergenic, does not increase the development of allergy in low-risk infants (Anderson, Malley, & Snell, 2009; Greer et al., 2008). Furthermore, evidence suggests that limiting consumption of allergenic foods during pregnancy and while breastfeeding also has no protective effect (Greer et al., 2008). Therefore, in general, a wide variety of culturally appropriate foods can be introduced, with a focus on foods that are high in iron, protein, and nutrient value. To identify foods to which an infant might react, the parent is taught to introduce one food at a time over 3 to 5 days before introducing another one (Greer et al., 2008).

Some of the more common suspected allergens include cow's milk, egg, soy products, fish, peanuts, chocolate, corn, and wheat. Intolerance of the protein in cow's milk is the most common food allergy during infancy, but this usually does not last past age 3 or 4 years.

Some of the common clinical manifestations of food allergies are abdominal pain, diarrhea, nasal congestion, cough, wheezing, vomiting, and rashes. Many children will outgrow their allergic response to certain foods.

Dental Care

Eruption of the infant's first teeth is a developmental milestone that has great significance for many parents. Deciduous or "baby" teeth usually erupt between 5 and 9 months of age. The first to appear are the lower central incisors, followed by the upper central incisors and then the upper lateral incisors. The next teeth to erupt are usually the lower lateral incisors, first primary molars, canines, and the second primary molars. The average child has six to eight teeth by the first birthday.

Teething

Although sometimes asymptomatic, teething is often signaled by behavior such as night wakening, daytime restlessness, an increase in nonnutritive sucking, excess drooling, and temporary loss of appetite. Some degree of discomfort is normal, but a health care professional should further investigate elevated temperature, irritability, ear tugging, or diarrhea.

To help parents cope with teething, nurses can suggest that they provide cool liquids and hard foods (e.g., dry toast, ice pops, frozen bagels) for chewing. Hard, cold teethers and ice wrapped in cloth may also provide comfort for inflamed gums. Nurses should explain to parents that over-the-counter topical medications for gum pain relief should be used only as directed. Home remedies, such as rubbing the gums with whiskey or aspirin, should be discouraged, but acetaminophen administered as directed for the child's age can relieve discomfort. Although these interventions can be helpful, parents should understand that absolute relief comes only with tooth eruption.

Assessment of Dental Risk

The AAP and the American Academy of Pediatric Dentistry (AAPD) have issued recommendations about prevention and treatment of dental caries in infants and young children (Section on Pediatric Dentistry and Oral Health & Keels, Hale, Thomas et al., 2008; AAPD, 2006). The risk of tooth decay begins in infancy and is higher in families with a history of dental caries, children with special health care needs (especially those involving motor coordination), lower socioeconomic

HEALTH PROMOTION

The 4-Month-Old Infant

Focused Assessment

Ask the parent the following:

- What new activities is your baby doing?
- Is your baby able to settle down to sleep without needing to be consoled?
- Are both parents included in the baby's care?
- Is the mother considering going back to work in the near future?

Developmental Milestones

Personal/social: Loves moving faces; knows parents' voices

Fine motor: Follows an object 180 degrees; binocular vision; bats objects; begins to hold own bottle

Language/cognitive: Initiates conversation by cooing; turns head to locate sounds

Gross motor: Supports weight on feet when standing; pulls to sit without head lag; begins to roll prone to supine

Critical Milestones*

Personal/social: Smiles responsively; smiles spontaneously; stares at own hand

Fine motor: Grasps a rattle; follows past midline; brings hands to middle of body

Language/cognitive: Laughs and squeals out loud; vocalizes; makes "ooh" sounds

Gross motor: Lifts head and chest 45 and 90 degrees when prone; head steady when sitting

Health Maintenance

Physical Measurements

Continue to measure and plot length, weight, and head circumference
Posterior fontanel closed

Immunizations

Diphtheria-tetanus-acellular pertussis (DTaP) #2, inactivated poliovirus (IPV) #2 (may substitute DTaP, hepatitis B, and combination polio vaccine); *Haemophilus influenzae* type b (Hib) #2, pneumococcal #2; rotavirus #2
Review side effects and ask about previous reactions

Health Screening

Assess for strabismus
Hearing risk assessment
No additional screening required

Anticipatory Guidance

Nutrition

Maintain breastfeeding schedule
Formula, 5 to 6 ounces five or six times a day
Bottle supplement if breastfeeding mother has returned to work
Vitamin D supplement 400 IU/day for breastfed infants and for formula-fed infants if taking less than 1 liter (33 ounces) of formula a day
Begin iron supplementation for breastfed and partially breastfed infants (1 mg/kg/day) (Baker, Greer, & The Committee on Nutrition, 2010)

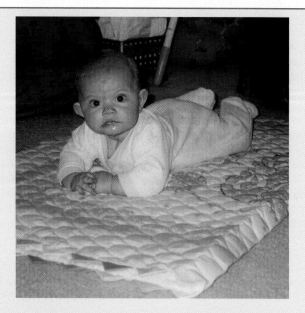

Elimination

Similar to 2-month-old

Dental

May begin drooling in preparation for tooth eruption

Sleep

Place on back to sleep in parent's room in a separate crib/cradle/bassinet. Keep loose or soft bedding and toys out of the crib, offer pacifier for nap and bedtime if not breastfeeding.
Total sleep: 15 to 16 hours
Encourage self-consoling techniques

Hygiene

Continue daily routine of cleanliness

Safety

Review car safety and violence, exposure to cigarette smoke
Discuss choking hazards and management of choking; avoidance of walkers; playpen and swing safety; begin child-proofing

Play

Talk with the baby frequently and from different locations
Respond verbally and smile as infant does; cuddle
Sing; expose to different environmental sounds
Supervised water play
Provide bright rattles, tactile toys, mirror

*Guided by Denver Developmental Screening Test II.

status, children with previous tooth decay, children who snack on sugary foods (including 100% fruit juice) more than three times a day, and those without a dentist (AAPD, 2006). Viewed as an infectious process, mothers with dental caries can transmit bacteria that cause caries to their infants (AAPD, 2006). Taking a dental history from a mother can provide information about an infant's risk, and this should occur as early as the infant's teeth begin to erupt. Infants with observable dental caries should be referred to a dentist as soon as these are observed by the health care provider (Section on Pediatric Dentistry and Oral Health et al., 2008).

The Section on Pediatric Dentistry and Oral Health et al. (2008) recommends that pediatric providers assess infants' and children's oral caries risk periodically throughout infancy and childhood. This should occur, along with dietary counseling on avoiding food sources of sugar, and provision of an appropriate dose of fluoride.

Cleaning Teeth

Because the primary teeth are used for chewing until the permanent teeth erupt and because decay of the primary teeth often results in decay of the permanent teeth, dental care must begin in infancy. The parent can use cotton swabs or a soft washcloth and water to clean the teeth with the infant positioned in the parent's lap or on a changing table. The teeth should be cleaned at least twice a day, and juice should be limited to no more than 4 to 6 ounces a day given at meals (Section on Pediatric Dentistry and Oral Health et al., 2008). Toothpaste should not be used until the child is older and can spit and will not swallow the toothpaste. This is recommended so the infant will not ingest excessive amounts of fluoride. A possible exception is the supervised use of a very small amount of toothpaste (pea-sized quantity) for young children at risk for dental caries. Flossing is recommended to begin as soon as teeth are in direct contact with other teeth (Section on Pediatric Dentistry and Oral Health et al., 2008).

Fluoride Supplementation

To prevent tooth decay in developing teeth, supplemental fluoride has historically been prescribed for infants and children who live in areas where there is no community water fluoridation. In 2010, based on several systematic surveys of published research that looked at the balance of fluoride supplementation with the occurrence of *fluorosis* (excess mineralization of tooth enamel with visible spotting), the American Dental Association changed its fluoride recommendations for infants and children (Rozier, Adair, Graham et al., 2010). The current recommendations state that fluoride supplementation should be based on assessment of risk and the extent to which fluoridated water is available, including the following (Rozier et al., 2010):

- No fluoride supplementation is needed for infants and children determined to be at low risk for dental caries, including those who have access to fluoridated water
- Daily fluoride supplements for at-risk infants and children without access to fluoridated water in the following doses: 6-month to 3-year-olds, 0.25 mg; 3- to 6-year-olds, 0.5 mg; and 6- to 16-year-olds, 1 mg
- Daily fluoride supplements for at-risk children, beginning at age 3 years, who have access to fluoridated water with less than the optimal level of fluoride (<0.7 parts per million) in the following doses: 3- to 6-year-olds, 0.25 mg; and 6- to 16-year-olds, 0.5 mg

Bottle-Mouth Caries

Bottle-mouth caries, or nursing-bottle caries, is a well-described form of tooth decay that can develop in infants and children. The decay pattern usually involves the incisors initially and then spreads to other teeth. Decay may be so serious that tooth loss occurs prematurely. When the infant is allowed to fall asleep with a bottle containing milk or juice, the carbohydrate-rich solution bathes the teeth for a long period and may cause dental caries.

Nurses should discourage parents from giving bedtime bottles of milk or juice to infants. If a nighttime bottle is necessary, plain water is an acceptable substitute for carbohydrate-rich liquids. A pacifier is an acceptable alternative to a nighttime bottle, although the practice of dipping the pacifier in corn syrup or honey to encourage acceptance poses the same problem. An additional danger of the use of honey in infancy is botulism. Pacifier use after age 3 years is a cause for concern and referral to a dentist or orthodontist for possible structural alterations in the oral cavity (Section on Pediatric Dentistry and Oral Health et al., 2008).

Sleep and Rest

Newborn infants may sleep as much as 17 to 20 hours per day. Sleep patterns vary widely, with some infants sleeping only 2 to 3 hours at a time. At approximately 3 to 4 months of age, most infants begin to sleep for longer periods during the night, although some children do not sleep through the night consistently until the second year.

Often one of the most difficult tasks for new parents is the regulation of their infant's sleep-wake cycles. Parents need anticipatory guidance about what to expect regarding sleep and rest. Recent evidence suggests that, beginning at age 1 month, infants begin to regulate their own sleep, sleeping for longer periods of time and returning to sleep without parental intervention after wakening (Henderson, France, Owens, & Blampied, 2010). If self-regulation (sometimes called self-soothing) is facilitated by the parent, infants will sleep through the night (10 PM to 6 AM) at a relatively early age. The keys to this are parental sensitivity to the infant's sleep pattern, establishing a sleep routine by 1 month of age, and allowing the infant to self-soothe (Henderson et al., 2010; Owens, 2011).

It is important to remember that rocking an infant to sleep provides warmth and security for the infant; however, to initiate good sleep habits, the parent should put the infant in the bassinet or crib while the infant is drowsy and before the infant falls completely asleep. Assisting the infant to establish a consistent sleep routine is important during early infancy to avoid problems associated with night waking (Owens, 2011).

Some parents are distressed when an infant or child wakes in the middle of the night crying and are tempted to console by picking the child up. A certain amount of fussiness at bedtime is not unusual; however, placing the infant in the crib or bassinet before the infant is completely asleep facilitates self-consoling behavior. Infants who do not learn to self-console when going to sleep expect the parents to console them should they awaken during the night. This can lead to a situation where neither the infant nor the parents are able to sleep through the night. Prevention is the best approach; however, should the parents express concern about the infant crying at night, the nurse can assist with problem solving. The nurse can advise the parent not to turn on the light in the child's room or pick the child up, but speak softly and reassuringly to the infant until the infant becomes quiet (Owens, 2011). It may take several nights of the infant crying and the parents consoling in this manner to mitigate the problem.

For several years, the AAP has recommended placing all infants on their back to sleep (AAP, Task Force on Sudden Infant Death Syndrome, 2005). In a recent revision of their policy about SIDS, the AAP has issued several other recommendations for preventing SIDS. These include the following recommendations (AAP, Task Force on Sudden Infant Death Syndrome, 2005):

- Putting the infant to sleep for nap or night in the parent's room in a place other than the parent's bed (e.g., cradle, bassinet, crib)
- Ensuring that the mattress surface is firm and that there is no soft or loose bedding (e.g., sheets, blankets, quilts) or toys in the crib
- Avoiding exposing the infant to environmental smoke and avoiding overheating the infant
- Offering the infant a pacifier at nap and bedtime

HEALTH PROMOTION

The 6-Month-Old Infant

Focused Assessment

Ask the parent the following:

- What kind of new activities is your baby doing?
- Have you begun to give your baby solid foods?
- How is any child care working out?
- Have you done anything about child-proofing your home?

Developmental Milestones

Personal/social: Interacts readily and noisily with parents and familiar people; may be cautious with strangers

Fine motor: Rakes objects with the whole hand; begins to transfer; mouths; can hold an object in each hand

Language/cognitive: Begins to imitate sounds (raspberries, clucking, kissing); babbles; says single sounds; beginning object permanence; awareness of time sequence

Gross motor: Tripod sitting unsupported; gets on hands and knees; bears full weight on legs; "swims" when prone

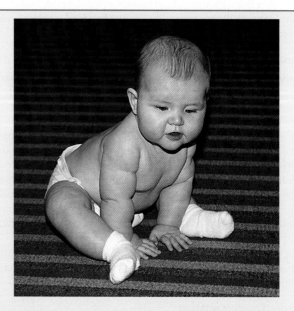

Critical Milestones*

Personal/social: Reaches for toy out of reach; looks at hand; smiles spontaneously

Fine motor: Looks at raisin placed on contrasting surface; reaches out; follows completely side to side

Language/cognitive: Turns to rattle sound made out of vision on each side; squeals; laughs

Gross motor: Rolls over both directions; no head lag; lifts head and chest completely

Health Maintenance

Physical Measurements

Birth weight doubles

Continue to measure and plot length, weight, and head circumference

Immunizations

Diphtheria-tetanus-acellular pertussis (DTaP) #3 (may substitute DTaP, hepatitis B, and polio combination vaccine); *Haemophilus influenzae* type b (Hib) #3; pneumococcal #3; rotavirus #3; inactivated poliovirus (IPV) #3 and hepatitis B #3 may be given between now and 18 months if not in combination vaccine

Influenza vaccine annually; two doses initially, separated by at least 4 weeks

Ask about previous reactions

Review side effects

Health Screening

Initial lead screening risk assessment (see Box 5-6)

Hearing risk assessment

Anticipatory Guidance

Nutrition

Begin introducing solid foods one at a time by spoon; use iron-fortified cereals

Hold infant or place in infant seat for feeding

Begin to offer a cup

Vitamin D supplement 400 IU/day for breastfed infants and for formula-fed infants if taking less than 1 liter (33 ounces) of formula a day

May discontinue iron supplementation for breastfeeding infants consuming sufficient iron-rich solid foods

Elimination

Stools darken and become more formed as the amount of solid food increases

Dental

Tooth eruption begins with lower incisors

May have some pain and low-grade fever (<101° F [38° C])

May be fussy

Clean teeth and gums with wet cloth

Do not put to sleep with a bottle

Assess risk for tooth decay; begin fluoride supplementation only for infants at risk

Sleep

Place on back to sleep (infant may roll over to prone position) in a separate crib. Keep loose or soft bedding and toys out of the crib, offer pacifier for nap and bedtime if not breastfeeding.

Can move to a separate room

Total sleep: 12 to 16 hours each day

Sleeps all night; two or three naps

Maintain sleep routine

Hygiene

Continue daily routine of cleanliness

Clean toys frequently

Safety

Review choking, walkers, violence, exposure to cigarette smoke

Discuss child-proofing, drowning prevention, poison prevention (see Chapter 10)

Play

Expose to different sounds and sights

Begin social games (pat-a-cake, peek-a-boo)

Provide bath toys, rattles, mirror, large ball, soft stuffed animals

Encourage to sit unsupported

Encourage to rock on hands and knees

*Guided by Denver Developmental Screening Test II.

BOX 5-6   LEAD EXPOSURE RISK ASSESSMENT

Do you live in, or does your child spend time in, housing that was built before 1950 that has peeling paint or plaster, or built before 1978 that is being renovated?

Do you live near any sources of environmental lead, such as smelters or places that use leaded gasoline?

Does your child regularly come in contact with a household member who works with lead or lead solder (e.g., plumber, construction worker, stained glass artisan)?

Does your child have a sibling or any other household member who has tested positive for lead exposure or has had lead poisoning?

Has your child recently lived in a foreign country?

Has your infant or child been exposed to any other sources of lead: vinyl miniblinds, imported ceramics, toys, old baby furniture, leaded crystal, or foods that may have been stored in pottery from a foreign country?

Does your infant or child routinely put nonfood items in his or her mouth?

If the infant has any risk factors, a capillary test for lead should be performed. Otherwise, a routine capillary lead screening should be done at the 9-month or 1-year visit.

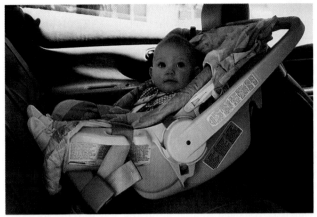

FIG 5-3 The infant rides facing the rear of the vehicle, ideally in the middle of the back seat. The infant seat is secured to the vehicle with the seatbelt, and straps on the car seat adjust to accommodate the growing baby.

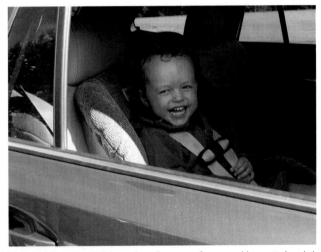

FIG 5-4 After the child reaches 2 years of age and has attained the manufacturer's height and weight recommendations for a rear-facing car seat, the child uses a forward-facing upright car safety seat. The safety straps should be adjusted to provide a snug fit, and the seat should be placed in the back seat of the car, ideally in the middle.

- Not using commercially marketed monitors that state they reduce the risk of SIDS
- Providing opportunities during awake time for "tummy play"

Additional information about SIDS is discussed in Chapter 21.

Safety

The rapidly growing infant becomes mobile seemingly overnight. With newfound mobility comes the potential for unintentional injury. As the infant's musculature strengthens and coordination improves, the infant develops an insatiable desire to explore. Without the cognitive skills needed to differentiate danger from safety, the rolling, crawling, toddling infant is at great risk for injury.

Infants are totally dependent on others for safety and protection. They are especially vulnerable to serious injury because of their relatively large head size. Motor development progresses to the point where infants quickly master new skills to learn more about their environment. They begin impulsively to reach out and move toward interesting objects around them.

Because of an infant's dependence, parents and caregivers are the primary recipients of anticipatory safety guidance. From the first day of life, safety must be considered and incorporated into the infant's world. Providing a safe environment for a rapidly growing infant is challenging. Potential safety hazards multiply as the baby learns to creep, crawl, climb, and explore. Some parents may not have a complete awareness of the safety issues that must be addressed to protect the infant from injury.

Motor Vehicle Safety

Injuries associated with automobile crashes constitute the single greatest threat to an infant's life and health. Restraining seats are the only practical means of reducing this risk.

Infant safety in motor vehicles depends entirely on adults. Parents must be informed that they cannot protect their child from injury in a crash by cradling or holding the infant on their laps. Adults are neither strong enough nor quick enough to prevent the sudden forward motions or to overcome the inertial forces (external forces of motion caused by impact) exerted in a crash. An unrestrained adult is propelled forward, trapping and crushing the infant between the adult's body and the hard surfaces inside the car on impact. The only way to prevent injuries and death to an infant in a car is to use a car safety seat for each trip, no matter how short.

A lifelong practice begins with the newborn infant's first ride home. Getting a child accustomed to using a safety seat at a young age establishes a safety habit and may reduce resistance later (Figure 5-3). All car safety seats should be placed in the rear seat of the vehicle, preferably in the middle, away from the possibility of injury from a side crash (advise parents to consult their automobile operating manual for optimal seat positioning). Newborns and infants should be in a rear-facing seat with a three- or five-point harness until they are 2 years of age or have reached the upper parameters of the manufacturer's recommendation for the specific safety seat (AAP, 2011b). Front-facing seats (Figure 5-4) should be tethered to the tether anchor. LATCH (Lower Anchors and Tethers for Children) systems, which secure the seat without need for the seatbelt, keep the seat tightly anchored to the car. Both car (those made after 2002) and seat must have the LATCH system for it to work without the seatbelt (AAP, 2011b). Children should remain in an approved car safety seat or booster seat until they are approximately 4 feet 9 inches tall (between 8 and 12 years) (AAP, 2011b). Nearly all states have laws regarding at what age a child may begin to use a regulation automobile seatbelt; parents should be aware of the law in the state where they live or plan to travel (state regulations may be accessed through: www.nhtsa.gov).

Some injuries and deaths have been associated with the deployment of airbags. Infants and children younger than 12 years should not be restrained in the front seat of cars equipped with airbags on the passenger side. When deployed, the airbag can severely jolt the car safety seat and harm the infant or child. Both the National Highway Traffic Safety Administration (NHTSA) and the AAP recommend placing all children 12 years and younger in the rear seat with the appropriate restraint (AAP, 2011b; NHTSA, 2011).

Providing a Safe Home Environment

During infancy and early childhood, when children are typically limited to the home environment, safety in and around the home is a top priority. With the exception of injuries and deaths related to motor vehicle crashes, most childhood injuries occur in the home. Major causes of unintentional injury that require visits to an emergency department include contact with sharp objects, bites and stings, cuts, and burns; the leading cause of unintentional injury in infants and children of all age-groups younger than age 14 years, however, is falls (CDC, 2011c). Fire and burn injury, drowning, unintentional firearm injury, and suffocation (e.g., choking, strangulation) are the leading causes of death related to unintentional injury (CDC, 2011d). Parents must also consider safety as a factor when selecting daycare facilities for their child.

Burn Prevention

Infants are especially vulnerable to inflicted burns, particularly scald burns. Infants' limited mobility makes it impossible for them to escape from immersion in hot water. Parents should be instructed to decrease the setting on water heaters to 120° F (48.8° C) to prevent accidental scalds. Infant skin is thin, causing burns to occur faster at lower temperatures than in adults. With water temperature settings of 140° F (60° C), it takes only 3 seconds for the child to suffer serious burns. Lowering the temperature by 20° F causes the same degree of burn injury in 8 to 10 minutes of submersion. An adult should test the water temperature before the infant is bathed to decrease the risk of accidental scald injuries.

Advise parents to avoid smoking, drinking hot liquids, or cooking while holding an infant. As infants begin to crawl around on the floor, open electrical sockets should be covered with appropriate socket protectors. Open stoves or fireplaces are especially intriguing to an exploring infant and should be outfitted with a guard or grid. Avoid use of a steam vaporizer to prevent scald injuries to a curious infant.

Burn injuries in infants can also be caused by a variety of other sources. Exposure to sunlight can result in serious sunburn to their delicate skin. Young infants should not be exposed to sunlight, even for brief periods and on cloudy days; sunscreen should not be used on infants younger than 6 months old (Balk, Council on Environmental Health, & Section on Dermatology, 2011). The best way to prevent the adverse effects of the sun is avoidance. If children are going to be in the sun, they should wear clothing to cover exposed areas of the skin as well as a hat and sunglasses. Parents should be encouraged to apply sunblock and sunscreen (minimum sun protection factor 15) liberally to older infants and children. Sunscreen should be applied 15

to 30 minutes in advance of exposure and be reapplied every 2 hours (Balk & Council on Environmental Health; Section on Dermatology, 2011).

Safe Baby Furnishings

Baby furniture, although seemingly benign, can present lethal hazards to a growing infant. Parents should be aware of safety considerations when planning or decorating the infant's room. Parents need to be aware that older furniture that has been handed down may not meet current safety regulations. In older cribs, the gaps between slats may be large enough to entrap the infant's head, or the paint may contain lead.

Hanging toys or mobiles placed over the crib should be positioned well out of the infant's reach to prevent entanglement and strangulation. Encourage the parent to avoid placing large toys in the crib because an older infant may use them as steps to climb over the side, resulting in a serious fall. Cribs should be positioned away from curtains or blinds to prevent accidental entanglement in dangling cords (see Patient-Centered Teaching: Crib Safety box).

PATIENT-CENTERED TEACHING

Crib Safety

- The distance between slats must be no more than $2\frac{3}{8}$ inches wide to prevent entrapment of the infant's head or body. Mesh-sided cribs should have mesh openings smaller than $\frac{1}{4}$ inch (6 mm).
- The interior of the crib must snugly accommodate a standard-size mattress so that the gap is minimal, less than the width of two adult fingers. Excessive space could allow the infant to become wedged, potentially suffocating.
- Decorative enhancements on the crib are not recommended because they can break apart and be aspirated by the infant. Design cutouts can trap an infant's arm or neck, causing death or serious injury.
- Corner posts or finials that rise above the end panels can snag garments and inadvertently strangle infants.
- The drop side must be impossible for an infant to release. Activating the drop side must take either a strong force (at least 10 pounds) or a distinct action at each locking device. Never leave the drop side down when an infant is in the crib.
- Wood surfaces should be free of splinters, cracks, and lead-based paint.

Preventing Falls

Infants are often placed on surfaces at heights that are convenient for adults, such as on changing tables, counters, or furniture. These surfaces often have no restraining barriers. Infants begin to roll over as early as 2 months, and as they begin to scoot or crawl, fall injuries from these elevations are common. There must be constant adult supervision when an infant is placed at such a height (Figure 5-5). If the parent or nurse must move away from the infant, the adult should either take the infant or, if supplies are close, place a hand on the infant while reaching. At home, parents may choose to place their child on the floor for changing diapers or providing other care.

Falls from infant seats, out of highchairs, or out of strollers are common. Injuries can be prevented with supervision and the use of safety restraining straps to limit the mobility of the infant (see Figure 5-5).

As infants begin to crawl, placing gates at the top and bottom of stairs can prevent falls. Infant walkers are dangerous and are not recommended. They allow infants mobility and the freedom to explore

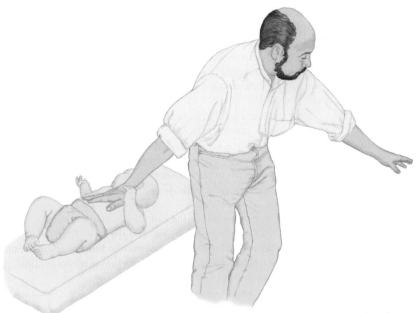

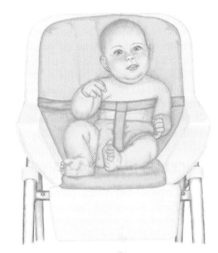

Close supervision and the use of restraining straps can prevent falls from highchairs, a common cause of injuries in children. After the straps are fastened, the highchair tray is secured to the front of the highchair.

Infants begin to roll over by themselves as early as 2 months of age. From the outset, the nurse must warn parents not to leave their infants unattended, even for a second, on the changing table or other high surface.

FIG 5-5 Safety education for parents of infants should emphasize the need for constant supervision and the use of restraining devices to prevent falls.

surroundings before they have developed the ability to interpret heights or protect themselves from falls.

Preventing Asphyxiation

Asphyxiation (suffocation) occurs when air cannot get into or out of the lungs and oxygen supplies are consequently depleted. Carbon dioxide levels then increase, causing life-threatening disruption of cardiac and cerebral functioning. Choking occurs when substances or objects are *aspirated* into the airway or into the branches of the lower airways, causing partial or complete obstruction of the lungs. Strangulation is typically thought of as a constriction of the neck, but it also includes blockage of the nose and mouth by airtight materials, such as plastic. This blockage prevents air exchange. Store all plastic bags or covers out of the infant's reach. Choking is a major concern in the first few months of an infant's life, when aspiration of feedings or vomit can occur easily because of the immature swallowing mechanism. Parents should be taught to position infants on their sides after feedings and to avoid placing small infants in bed with a bottle propped in their mouths.

As infants grow, they begin to explore the world around them by placing anything and everything in their mouths. Size, shape, and consistency are major determinants of whether a food or object is likely to be aspirated by an infant. Food that is round or similar to the size of the airway is especially dangerous. Dangerous foods include sliced hot dogs, hard candy, peanuts, grapes, raisins, and chewing gum, among others. These foods should be avoided until the child is able to chew thoroughly before swallowing. Food should be cut into small pieces, and the child should be supervised while eating. Advise parents to strongly discourage infants and young children from playing, singing, or other activities while eating, to avoid choking. Infants are equally endangered by rattles, pieces of toys, ribbons from stuffed animals, and common household objects such as coins, buttons, pins,

or beads found on the floor or within their reach. Balloons should not be given to infants or young children or used where an infant or young child plays.

Anticipatory guidance for parents includes performing a thorough inspection of the infant's surroundings to remove all potential items that infants could grasp, place in their mouths, and choke on. Parents can be encouraged to crawl through the home to gain a better perspective of the infant's environment. Parents can then substitute safe objects for exploration.

Ornaments or toys with detachable parts are not recommended for infants because of the aspiration risk. The Consumer Product Safety Commission has a long-established toy standard to prevent choking hazards in nonfood products targeted for children younger than 3 years. Parents should take extra care to note the presence of small detachable parts on toys before allowing the infant to play with the items. Although the government regulates the size of parts on infants' toys, older children's toys are not regulated by the same standard. As the infant explores an older sibling's or a playmate's territory, adult supervision is important.

To prevent strangulation injuries, parents should not place a pacifier on a string or cord around the infant's neck, not put an infant to sleep with a bib in place, and not position a crib near blinds or curtain cords. Crib slats should comply with the $2\frac{3}{8}$-inch width requirement to prevent head entrapment.

In addition to inspecting and providing a safe environment for the infant, instruct parents in the appropriate action to take if the infant chokes (see Chapter 10 for a discussion of emergency procedures). The AAP has issued a policy statement that recommends attention to choking prevention at the community level (Committee on Injury, Violence, and Poison Prevention, 2010). These include such recommendations as increasing U.S. Food and Drug Administration (FDA) and Consumer Product Safety Commission surveillance, warning, and recall of dangerous foods and toys, and initiating a choking prevention campaign specifically directed toward the problem in children (AAP Committee on Injury, Violence, and Poison Prevention, 2010).

Preventing Lead Exposure

Although lead poisoning in the United States has decreased markedly since the elimination of lead paint and solder used in homes and leaded gasoline, lead poisoning remains a significant risk, especially in cities where old housing predominates. In addition, paint from old homes can enter the soil and get on children's hands when they are playing. Children inhale lead dust as homes are being renovated. The lead risk assessment begins as the infant begins to be mobile (6 months of age) (AAP, Committee on Environmental Health, 2005). Risk should be assessed at every well visit beginning at the 6-month visit and education or treatment initiated as appropriate (see Box 5-6) (see Chapter 10).

CONCERNS DURING INFANCY

Parents, especially first-time parents, have multiple concerns about their infants. Nurses can intervene to relieve parental anxiety and provide a realistic perspective about normal parental concerns.

Jaundice

Most infants have some physiologic jaundice after the first day of life, characterized by a yellow gold color of the skin. This jaundice is caused by the increased number of erythrocytes (red blood cells) in circulation, the shorter life span of the erythrocytes, and the inability of the immature neonatal liver to conjugate (indirect) bilirubin out of the bloodstream. Because unconjugated bilirubin is bound to albumin, any medications that can interfere with these albumin-binding sites (e.g., phenobarbital) may also interfere with the excretion of bilirubin.

Indirect bilirubin levels usually peak at about 2 to 4 days of age. Their maximum level is usually 5 to 7 mg/dL. After this point, levels should continue to fall. Jaundice appears first on the face and progresses downward; jaundice of the feet represents a markedly elevated bilirubin. For a serum bilirubin more than 15 mg/dL, phototherapy treatment may be considered.

Two types of jaundice have been identified in breastfed infants. The first type is early-onset jaundice, which seems to be related to insufficient intake of breast milk. As with formula-fed infants, this type of jaundice occurs 2 to 4 days after birth and usually resolves within 1 week. Early and frequent breastfeedings appear to decrease the incidence. The second type of jaundice is termed *breast milk jaundice*. This type of jaundice appears at 3 to 5 days of age and may last several weeks. This type of jaundice may be related to certain factors in the breast milk that alter the conjugation or absorption of bilirubin. Treatment approaches include phototherapy or temporarily discontinuing breastfeeding. See Chapter 23 for home care of the infant receiving phototherapy.

Circumcision

Circumcision, the removal of the prepuce (foreskin), a fold of skin that covers the glans penis, is a frequently performed surgical procedure during the newborn period. Although the foreskin can be retracted easily for cleaning in the older child, the prepuce is not usually fully retractable until age 3 years or older. The prepuce should never be forcibly retracted in any infant because trauma and adhesions can result. Circumcision is a controversial procedure, and parents may have questions about whether to choose to have it performed.

The AAP states that, although there are potential benefits of the procedure, data are not sufficient to recommend routine neonatal circumcision (AAP, Task Force on Circumcision, 1999/2005). Circumcision may reduce urinary tract infections, some sexually transmissible infections, inflammation of the glans or prepuce, and cancer of the penis. Other factors may be causative factors in these conditions as well.

Some parents choose circumcision for religious, cultural, or social reasons. Jewish parents may have their infants circumcised on the eighth day after birth as part of a special ceremony. Muslim culture also includes circumcision. Some parents want their son to look like his circumcised father or peers. Others feel circumcision is an expected part of newborn care, and some do not realize that they have a choice in the matter.

Lack of knowledge about the care of the prepuce leads to some circumcisions. Poor hygiene may increase the risk of infections and other problems. Teaching the parents and child the proper care of the uncircumcised penis can prevent surgery and complications related to inadequate cleanliness.

Many parents reject circumcision, and the reasons are as varied as those supporting circumcision. Major reasons include (1) the benefits do not outweigh the risks, (2) belief that it is cosmetic surgery and not necessary, (3) unwillingness to subject the infant to pain, (4) culture, and (5) potential complications.

Only healthy newborn infants should undergo circumcision. Infants with blood dyscrasias may have excessive bleeding if circumcised. For the repair of anatomic abnormalities of the penis, such as hypospadias or epispadias, an intact prepuce may be needed for use in plastic surgery (see Chapter 20).

Circumcision may be performed in the hospital before the infant is discharged or in an outpatient setting during the first week. Circumcision is performed with a scalpel, Gomco clamp, or Hollister Plastibell. Pain control can be achieved through a dorsal penile nerve block, lidocaine infiltration on the prepuce, or topical anesthetic cream (EMLA cream). If a Gomco clamp was used, petrolatum gauze strips or petroleum jelly ointment are placed over the circumcision site and it is covered with gauze to prevent the diaper from sticking to it. Petroleum jelly should not be used with a Plastibell because it might make

---

PATIENT-CENTERED TEACHING

Care for Circumcision

Call the health care provider if your infant:
- Does not urinate within 6 hours after circumcision
- Has swelling of the entire penis
- Bleeds more than tiny drops
- Shows drainage (clear or white)
- Has a fever—rectal temperature 100.4° F (38° C) or higher

Do the following:
- Apply the diaper loosely
- Give sponge baths until circumcision is healed
- Clean penis with clear water
- If Gomco clamp is used, put petroleum gauze dressing on the penis

Don't:
- Clean the penis with alcohol wipes
- Remove the yellowish crusty material that forms on the penis during healing—this represents a normal healing process
- Place a dressing on a Plastibell

HEALTH PROMOTION

⊜ *The 9-Month-Old Infant*

Focused Assessment

Ask the parent the following:

- What kind of new activities is your baby doing?
- How has your baby reacted to solid foods?
- Do you live in a house built before 1978?
- Do you live near sources of environmental lead?
- Do you regularly come in contact with someone who uses lead?
- Do you have a family member who has had lead poisoning?

Developmental Milestones

Personal/social: Stranger wariness; waves bye-bye; plays social games; begins to indicate wants

Fine motor: Beginning pincer grasp; actively searches for out-of-sight objects; bangs toys together

Language/cognitive: Uses consonant and several vowel sounds; beginning to attach meaning to words; understands some symbolic language (blow a kiss); knows own name; says Mama and Dada specifically

Gross motor: Gets to a sitting position; pulls up to stand; creeps and crawls; walks holding on to furniture; may briefly stand alone

Critical Milestones*

Personal/social: Feeds self finger foods; tries to get toys; looks at hands

Fine motor: Transfers; rakes a raisin or Cheerio; picks up and holds a small object in each hand

Language/cognitive: Imitates sounds; says single syllables; begins to put syllables together

Gross motor: No head lag; sits without support; stands holding onto furniture

Health Maintenance
Physical Measurements

Continue to measure and plot length, weight, and head circumference

Immunizations

Hepatitis B #3 (can give between 6 and 18 months); omit if combination vaccine has been used previously

Influenza vaccine annually

Provide information about upcoming measles-mumps-rubella (MMR) and varicella vaccines

Health Screening

Lead risk assessment (routine lead screen at 9 or 12 months, usually in conjunction with hemoglobin and hematocrit)

Hemoglobin or hematocrit (screen at 9 or 12 months)

Formalized developmental screening

Hearing risk assessment

Anticipatory Guidance
Nutrition

Continue to breastfeed on established schedule

Formula, 16 to 32 ounces a day

Vitamin D supplement 400 IU/day for breastfed infants and for formula-fed infants if taking less than 1 liter (33 ounces) of formula a day

Continue iron-fortified cereal

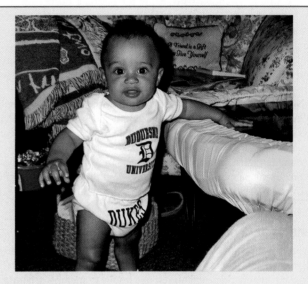

Begin to introduce a variety of soft, mashed or chopped table foods

Encourage cup, rather than bottle

Avoid giving large pieces of food and foods known to be associated with choking

Elimination

Urinary and bowel patterns consistent

Appearance of undigested food in stools

Dental

Four teeth

Brush erupted teeth with soft toothbrush and water

Assess risk for dental caries

Sleep

Night waking diminishes if managed appropriately

Hygiene

More vigilant cleanliness of diaper area as bladder volume increases

Wash infant's hands and face frequently

Keep toys clean

Safety

Review child-proofing, violence, exposure to cigarette smoke

Discuss lowering crib mattress, household and plant poisons, burn prevention, sunscreen use, avoiding sources of lead

Play

Social games

Provide cloth, cardboard, or plastic books

Cuddle, rock, hug

Ball rolling

Pots and pans with wooden spoons

Plastic stacking or nesting containers

Hide-and-seek games with toys

*Guided by Denver Developmental Screening Test II.

the Plastibell slip off too soon. The diaper is attached loosely to prevent pressure.

The wound is checked frequently for bleeding during the first few hours after the procedure. The nurse describes to the parents that spotting of blood can occur but emphasizes that the physician should be notified for more extensive bleeding. The normal yellowish exudate that forms over the site should be described and differentiated from purulent drainage. Signs of complications should be discussed fully.

Noting the first urination after circumcision is important because edema could cause an obstruction; the mother is instructed to call the physician if there is no urinary output within 6 to 8 hours (see Patient-Centered Teaching: Care for Circumcision box on p. 100).

Although nurses usually teach parents of circumcised infants how to care for the penis, they may not think about providing teaching for parents who decide against circumcision. They should include care of the intact penis in the teaching plan for these parents.

Patterns of Crying

Crying is a mode of communication for infants. It is especially challenging for new parents to learn and accurately interpret their individual infant's cry. Some infants respond readily to attempts to comfort them, sleep a great deal, and fit easily into their family's lifestyle. Other infants cry more readily and for longer periods and spend more time in a fretful, restless state than others. These infants often have more colic symptoms and sleep problems. This irritability may be caused by health problems, such as feeding difficulties, infection, or allergies, but often no clear cause emerges. In some cases, the infant's temperament may be the cause.

Nurses can suggest that parents, after ruling out physiologic causes for crying (e.g., hungry, soiled, gassy), console their infants when they cry by holding them, talking softly, or humming. Gently stroking an infant's head, back, and arms may also be soothing. Infant massage techniques and simply "centering" are easily accomplished by positioning the infant's arms and legs toward the midline of the body. Swaddling a new infant is a consoling technique that helps the infant to center.

Specific strategies to diminish infant irritability include activities such as taking the baby for a car ride, carrying the infant in a front pack close to the parent's chest, or swinging the baby in an infant swing. Vertical positioning and constant motion, such as that obtained when walking with the baby carried over the shoulder, are sometimes helpful. The football-carry position, with gentle patting on the back, can also be tried. Sometimes irritable infants need to be left alone to cry for brief periods. If parents choose this strategy, they must be cautioned to limit the crying time and to check the baby frequently.

Few interventions are consistently successful because infant responses may vary. Providing parents with strategies, however, helps decrease their anxiety and increase their feelings of control and competence. As infants grow and develop, they are better able to regulate their sleep-wake cycles. Generally, during the third or fourth month of life, sleep problems and irritability improve.

The Infant with Colic

Colic usually refers to unexplained paroxysmal crying or fussing in infants, which may be characterized by infants pulling up their arms and legs. Periods of crying tend to occur at the same time of day, often in the late afternoon or evening. To be diagnosed with colic, an infant must have the symptoms several times daily for several days a week. Most infants outgrow symptoms of colic by 3 to 4 months of age.

Etiology

The cause of colic is unknown, but several theories have been researched. The possibilities include but are not limited to allergy, cow's milk intolerance, maternal anxiety, familial stress, and too rapid feeding or overfeeding. It is highly likely that more than one factor may be involved. Colic is more common in infants with sensitive temperaments, who seem to need increased attention.

Management

The physician must determine whether, in fact, the infant is crying because of colic and not because of an acute condition such as intussusception, otitis media, or a fracture. Symptoms of milk allergy other than crying should be present before formula changes are made. Many practitioners avoid using medications to treat colic because of their limited success, lack of scientific data, and possible side effects. Savino, Pelle, Palumeri et al. (2007) examined the effect of *Lactobacillus reuteri* on infants with colic and demonstrated that administration of lactobacillus significantly decreased crying in colicky infants as compared to simethicone (Mylicon). Perry, Hunt, & Ernst (2011) included the Savino et al. study in a systematic review of randomized controlled trials of complementary therapies for the treatment of infant colic. They found that fennel extract and sucrose solution were the most effective treatments, and that the use of probiotics and other therapies were not as effective. Herbal remedies should not be used without consulting a health provider first. If parents are using herbs such as chamomile, the nurse should make sure they know the appropriate dose, are aware of possible allergic reactions, and do not administer so much as to interfere with adequate breast milk or formula intake.

Nursing Considerations

Because the etiology of colic and the care of an infant with colic are so individualized, it is important that the nurse obtain a thorough history. The nurse should provide a concerned and caring atmosphere during the assessment and reassure the parents that colic is not related to bad parenting. It should be determined whether any other symptoms are associated with the crying. The infant's eating habits, including whether the infant is breastfed or bottle fed, should be discussed. The nurse should ask the parents whether commonalities are associated with the crying (time of day, associated activities, family members present) and ask what has been tried, what works, and what does not work. If the parents are unsure, they should keep a diary for 48 to 72 hours to determine patterns. The nurse should assess the parents' stress level and support system.

The nurse needs to educate the parents regarding the normal growth and development needs of infants related to sleep and awake times, feeding, soothing, and holding and listen to the parents with an empathic ear. Parents should be encouraged to soothe their infant by rocking and cuddling. Some infants will quiet when given a massage, pacifier, or warm bath. If the parent is busy, a swing may provide a soothing, rhythmic effect. Some of the same strategies for soothing infants may also be effective in quieting infants with colic.

Some infants seem most distressed during high-activity times when the family may be busy preparing meals, doing chores, gathering at the end of the day, and so forth. By assisting parents to see such trends, the nurse can help them establish alternative routines to decrease the infant's stimuli. The parent may choose to feed the infant away from all the activity or to have a later dinner. Each family will be unique, and the nurse's role is to facilitate problem solving.

All families need extra support after the birth of an infant. If the infant has colic, the need increases. During the first few months after

HEALTH PROMOTION

The 12-Month-Old Infant

Focused Assessment

Ask the parent the following:

- Have you and your partner discussed and agreed on approaches to discipline?
- Is your baby able to follow directions and carry out requests?
- Have you assessed the home and environment for sources of lead?

Developmental Milestones

Personal/social: Rolls or throws a ball with another person; explores; drinks from a cup; indicates wants without crying

Fine motor: Actively looks for hidden objects; puts blocks in containers; uses simple toys appropriately

Language/cognitive: Names the appropriate parent; begins to say one to three single words; understands simple requests

Gross motor: Stands alone for increasing lengths of time; stoops and recovers; walks holding onto a hand; may begin to walk alone and climb stairs (on knees)

Critical Milestones*

Personal/social: Plays pat-a-cake; feeds self; works to get a toy

Fine motor: Developed pincer grasp; bangs objects together; picks up two cubes

Language/cognitive: Jabbers; combines syllables; mama/dada is nonspecific

Gross motor: Stands briefly without support; gets to sitting position; pulls to stand

Health Maintenance

Physical Measurements

Continue to measure and plot length, weight, and head circumference

Weight is usually triple birth weight

Length is 50% more than birth length

Immunizations

Measles-mumps-rubella (MMR) #1; varicella vaccine #1 (may use combination MMRV vaccine); pneumococcal and Hib boosters (if not scheduled to be given at 15 months); hepatitis B #3 (if not given previously)

Influenza vaccine annually

Hepatitis A #1

Health Screening

Hemoglobin/hematocrit if not done earlier

Lead screen if not done earlier

Hearing risk assessment

Tuberculosis (TB) screening if at risk

Anticipatory Guidance

Nutrition

May begin whole milk (2 to 3 cups daily)

Offer a variety of table foods from different food groups

Vitamin D supplement 400 IU/day for breastfed infants and for formula-fed infants if taking less than 1 liter (33 ounces) of formula a day

Begins to use table utensils

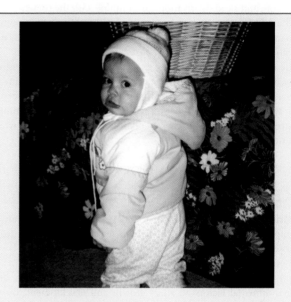

Usually eats three meals and snacks

Avoid giving foods high in salt and sugar

Discuss highchair safety

Elimination

Remains dry for longer periods

Bowel movements decrease in number and become more regular

Dental

Eight teeth

Sleep

Sleeps through the night and has one or two naps

Hygiene

Continue as previously

Safety

Review poisons, burns, violence, exposure to cigarette smoke

Maintain infant in a rear facing car seat

Play

Beginning parallel play

Push-pull toys

Various-size balls

Picture books

Dolls and stuffed animals

"Busy" box

Sandbox

*Guided by Denver Developmental Screening Test II.

the addition of a new baby, demanding work schedules, lack of recovery time from childbirth, the needs of other family members, physical exhaustion, and sleep deprivation can combine with the presence of a fretful infant to create stressful situations for the entire family. Sometimes infant temperament and parental coping styles are not compatible.

The nurse might, for example, explain to new parents, "Parenting is very much a challenge even when parents care about their baby as much as you do. It is difficult at first even to discern what Avery is telling you when she cries. But you will feel more and more comfortable, even see that she has a different cry when she is hungry and when she is tired."

By validating the parents' feelings, the nurse recognizes that the infant's irritability or colic is real, not imagined, and that the infant is a challenge to handle. The nurse can reassure the parents that the infant is healthy, normal, and gaining weight and that the parents are competent in their nurturing role.

The emotional reserves of the parents can be restored through rest and pleasurable activities. Parents may need brief periods of relief from infant care responsibilities. Grandparents or other family members may be able to provide the parents with an evening out or a night of uninterrupted sleep. This direct support can help restore the parents' energy to cope with daily activities and feel more relaxed and confident in their parenting.

KEY CONCEPTS

- During the first year of life, the infant's organs grow and mature at a rapid rate, yet infants' organ systems remain very different from those of older children and adults.
- Physical and neurologic maturation, sensory capabilities, perceptual skills, the quality and quantity of parental interaction, and environmental factors all affect growth and development during infancy.
- Infancy is the period during which children develop the foundation of their personalities, including the sense of trust and strong attachment to others.

- Common problems during infancy, such as separation anxiety, sleep disorders, crying, and colic, cause parents concern and distress. Nurses should be available with information and support to provide anticipatory guidance.
- Nurses play an important role in health promotion and prevention of illness by advising parents both about their concerns and about routine infant care, such as immunizations, nutrition, sleep, dental health, safety, and play.

REFERENCES

American Academy of Pediatric Dentistry. (2006). *Policy on use of a caries risk assessment tool (CAT) for infants, children, and adolescents.* Retrieved from www.aapd.org.

American Academy of Pediatrics. (2011a). *A message for dads.* Retrieved from www.healthychildren.org.

American Academy of Pediatrics. (2011b). *Car safety seats: Information for families for 2011.* Retrieved from www.healthychildren.org.

American Academy of Pediatrics. (2011c). *Where we stand: Fruit juice.* Retrieved from www.healthychildren.org.

American Academy of Pediatrics. (2010). *Storing and preparing expressed breast milk.* Retrieved from www.healthychildren.org.

American Academy of Pediatrics. (2009). *Red book: 2009 Report of the Committee on Infectious Diseases* (28th ed.). Elk Grove Village, IL: Author.

American Academy of Pediatrics, Committee on Environmental Health. (2005). Lead exposure in children: Prevention, detection, and management. *Pediatrics, 116*(4), 1036-1046.

American Academy of Pediatrics, Joint Committee on Infant Hearing. (2007). Year 2007 position statement: Principles and guidelines for early hearing detection and intervention programs. *Pediatrics, 120*(4), 898-921.

American Academy of Pediatrics, Task Force on Circumcision. (1999, reaffirmed 2005). Circumcision policy statement. *Pediatrics, 103*(3), 686-693.

American Academy of Pediatrics, Task Force on Sudden Infant Death Syndrome. (2005). The changing concept of sudden infant death syndrome: Diagnostic coding shifts, controversies regarding the sleeping environment, and new variables to consider in reducing risk. *Pediatrics, 116*, 1245-1255.

Anderson, J., Malley, K., & Snell, R. (2009). Is 6 months still the best for exclusive breastfeeding and introduction of solids? A literature review with consideration to the risk of the development of allergies. *Breastfeeding Review, 17*(2), 23-31.

Baker, R., Greer, F., & Committee on Nutrition American Academy of Pediatrics. (2010). Diagnosis and prevention of iron deficiency and iron-deficiency anemia in infants and young children (0-3 years of age). *Pediatrics, 126*(5), 1040-1050.

Balk, S., & Council on Environmental Health; Section on Dermatology. (2011). Technical report: Ultraviolet radiation: A hazard to children and adolescents. *Pediatrics, 127*(3), e791-e817.

Callister, L., Getmanenko, N., Garvrish, N., et al. (2007). Giving birth: The voices of Russian women. *MCN: The American Journal of Maternal Child Nursing, 32*(1), 18-24.

Centers for Disease Control and Prevention. (2009). *When should a mother avoid breastfeeding?* Retrieved from www.cdc.gov.

Centers for Disease Control and Prevention. (2011a). *Breastfeeding among U.S. children born 2000 to 2008, National Immunization Survey.* Retrieved from www.cdc.gov.

Centers for Disease Control and Prevention. (2011b). *Breastfeeding report card, 2011, United States: Outcomes indicators.* Retrieved from www.cdc.gov.

Centers for Disease Control and Prevention. (2011c). *National estimates of the 10 leading causes of nonfatal injuries treated in hospital emergency departments, United States–2008.* Retrieved from www.cdc.gov.

Centers for Disease Control and Prevention. (2011d). *10 leading causes of injury deaths by age group highlighting unintentional injury deaths, United States—2007.* Retrieved from www.cdc.gov.

Committee on Health Care for Underserved Women, American College of Obstetricians and Gynecologists. (2007). ACOG Committee Opinion No. 361:Breastfeeding: Maternal and infant aspects. *Obstetrics and Gynecology, 109*(2 Pt. 1), 479-480.

Committee on Injury, Violence, and Poison Prevention. (2010). Prevention of choking among children. *Pediatrics, 125*(3), 601-607.

Erikson, E. (1963). *Childhood and society* (2nd ed.). New York: Norton.

Flavell, J. H. (1964). *The developmental psychology of Jean Piaget.* New York: Van Nostrand.

Freud, A. (1974). *Introduction to psychoanalysis.* New York: International Universities Press.

Gartner, L., Morton, J., Lawrence, R., et al.; & American Academy of Pediatrics Section on Breastfeeding. (2005). Breastfeeding and the use of human milk. *Pediatrics, 115*, 496-506.

Greer, F., Sicherer, S., Burks, W., & American Academy of Pediatrics Committee on Nutrition; American Academy of Pediatrics Section on Allergy and Immunology. (2008). Effects of early nutritional interventions on the development of atopic disease in infants and children: The role of maternal dietary restriction, breastfeeding, timing of introduction of complementary foods, and hydrolyzed formulas. *Pediatrics, 121*(1), 183-191.

Greer, F., Shannon, M., & American Academy of Pediatrics Committee on Nutrition; American Academy of Pediatrics Committee on Environmental Health. (2005). Infant methemoglobinemia: The role of dietary nitrate in food and water. *Pediatrics, 116*(3), 784-786.

Harlor, A., Jr., Bower, C., & Committee on Practice and Ambulatory Medicine; Section on Otolaryngology—Head and Neck Surgery. (2009). Hearing assessment in infants and children: Recommendations beyond neonatal screening. *Pediatrics, 124*, 1252-1263.

Hauck, F., Thompson, J., Tanabe, K., et al. (2011). Breastfeeding and reduced risk of sudden infant death syndrome: A meta-analysis. *Pediatrics, 128*, 103-110.

Henderson, J., France, K., Owens, J., Blampied, N. (2010). Sleeping through the night: The consolidation of self-regulated sleep across the first year of life. *Pediatrics, 126*(5), e1081-1087.

Hernandez, I. (2006). Promoting exclusive breastfeeding for Hispanic women. *MCN: The American Journal of Maternal Child Nursing, 31*(5), 318-324.

Huh, S., Rifas-Shiman, S., Taveras, E., et al. (2011). Timing of solid food introduction and risk of obesity in preschool-aged children. *Pediatrics, 127*(3), e544-e551.

Janke, J. (2008). Newborn nutrition. In K. Simpson, & P. Creehan (Eds.), *AWHONN perinatal nursing* (3rd ed., pp. 582-611). Philadelphia: Lippincott, Williams, & Wilkins.

National Center for Health Statistics (NCHS). (2011). *Health, United States, 2010 with special feature on death and dying.* Hyattsville, Md.: Author.

National Highway Traffic Safety Administration. (2011). *Recommendations for all ages.* Retrieved from www.nhtsa.gov.

Newton, E. (2007). Breastfeeding. In S. Gabbe, J. Niebyl, & J. Simpson (Eds.), *Obstetrics: Normal and problem pregnancies* (5th ed., pp. 586-615). New York: Churchill Livingstone.

Owens, J. (2011). Sleep medicine. In R. Kliegman, R. Behrman, B. Stanton, et al. (Eds.), *Nelson textbook of pediatrics* (19th ed., pp. 46-49). Philadelphia: Elsevier Saunders.

Peer counselors double breastfeeding rates. (2011). *Case Management Advisor, 22*(8), 93-94.

Perry, R., Hunt, K., & Ernst, E. (2011). Nutritional supplements and other complementary medicines for infantile colic: A systematic review. *Pediatrics, 127*(4), 720-733.

Piaget, J. (1952). *The origins of intelligence in children.* New York: International Universities Press.

Rosen, I., Krueger, M., Carney, L., & Graham, J. (2008). Prenatal breastfeeding education and breastfeeding outcomes. *MCN: The American Journal of Maternal Child Nursing, 33*(5), 315-319.

Rozier, R., Adair, S., Graham, F., et al. (2010). Evidence-based clinical recommendations on the prescription of dietary fluoride supplements for caries prevention: A report of the American Dental Association Council on Scientific Affairs. *Journal of the American Dental Association, 141*(12), 1480-1489.

Savino, F., Pelle, E., Palumeri, E., et al. (2007). *Lactobacillus reuteri* (American Type Culture Collection Strain 55730) versus simethicone in the treatment of infantile colic: A prospective randomized study. *Pediatrics, 119*(1), e124-e130.

Schum, R. (2007). Language screening in the pediatric office setting. *Pediatric Clinics of North America, 54*(3), 425-436.

Section on Pediatric Dentistry and Oral Health, & Keels, M., Hale, K., Thomas, H., et al. (2008). Preventive oral health intervention for pediatricians. *Pediatrics, 122*(6), 1387-1394.

United States Department of Health and Human Services. (2010). *Healthy People 2020.* Retrieved from www.healthypeople.gov.

Woolf, A. (2003). Herbal remedies and children: Do they work? Are they harmful? *Pediatrics, 112*(1 Pt 2), 240-246.

Zupan, J., Garner, P., & Omari, A. (2004). Topical umbilical cord care at birth. *Cochrane Database of Systematic Reviews,* (3), CD001057.

Health Promotion during Early Childhood

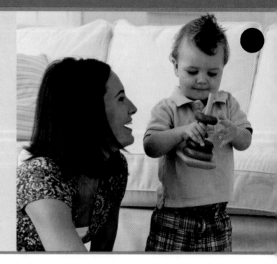

℮volve WEBSITE

http://evolve.elsevier.com/James/ncoc

LEARNING OBJECTIVES

After studying this chapter, you should be able to:

- Describe the physiologic changes and the motor, cognitive, language, and psychosocial development of the toddler and preschooler.
- Provide parents with anticipatory guidance related to the toddler and preschooler.
- Discuss the causes of and identify interventions for common toddler behaviors: temper tantrums, negativism, and ritualism.

- Identify strategies to alleviate a preschool child's fears and sleep problems.
- Discuss strategies for disciplining a toddler and a preschooler.
- Describe signs of a toddler's readiness for toilet training, and offer guidelines to parents.
- Offer parents suggestions for promoting school readiness in the preschool child.

The developmental changes that mark the transition from infancy to early childhood are dramatic. During the toddler years, ages 12 through 36 months, the child begins to venture out independently from a secure base of trust established during the first year. The preschool period, ages 3 through 5 years, is a time of relative tranquility after the tumultuous toddler period.

GROWTH AND DEVELOPMENT DURING EARLY CHILDHOOD

The toddler years are characterized by a struggle for autonomy as the child develops a sense of self separate from the parent. Boundless energy and insatiable curiosity drive the toddler to explore the environment and master new skills (Figure 6-1). The combination of increased motor skills, immaturity, and lack of experience places the toddler at risk for unintentional injury. Toddlers' egocentric and demanding behaviors, often marked by temper tantrums and negativism, have given this age the label the "terrible twos."

The preschooler becomes increasingly independent, mastering many self-care and motor skills and developing greater social and emotional maturity (Figure 6-2). The preschooler is imaginative, creative, and curious. Many parents describe this period as their favorite age as they watch the dramatic transformation of a chubby toddler into an agile, articulate child who is ready to enter the world of peers and school.

The nurse's roles as health care provider, family counselor, and child advocate continue during the toddler and preschool years. Well-child checkups provide the nurse with opportunities for anticipatory guidance related to growth and development, safety, nutrition, and some of the common age-related concerns of parents. The American Academy of Pediatrics [AAP] (2006/2010) recommends that pediatric providers conduct developmental surveillance (assessing developmental milestones and determining risk for developmental delay) at every routine well visit and that formal developmental screening, using a sensitive and specific screening test, be done at the 9-, 18-, and 30 (or 24)- month visits. In addition, an autism-specific screening should be done at the 18-month visit (AAP, 2006/2010). Because parental concerns provide a reliable indicator of possible developmental delay, the nurse should elicit any concerns when taking a developmental history as part of every well-child visit.

Physical Growth and Development
The Toddler

Physical growth slows during the toddler years. The average weight gain is 2.25 kg (5 lb) per year. A child's birth weight has quadrupled by age 2 to 3 years. The rate of increase in height also slows, with the average toddler growing approximately 7.5 cm (3 inches) per year.

The brain grows at a slower rate during this period than during infancy. Head circumference reflects this growth, increasing approximately 3.7 cm ($1\frac{1}{2}$ inches) during the toddler years compared with the

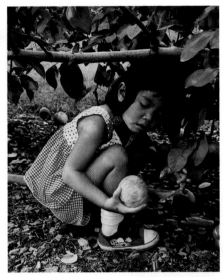

The toddler is enchanted by a world filled with discovery. Curiosity provides resources for the tremendous cognitive growth that occurs during this period.

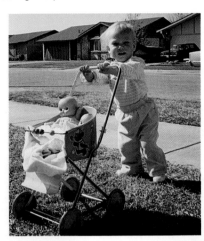

Toddlers enjoy push-pull toys. Toys should be strong and sturdy; wheeled toys should not tip over easily.

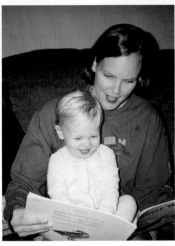

Reading simple stories provides quiet, enjoyable times for toddlers and parents and enhances speech and language development.

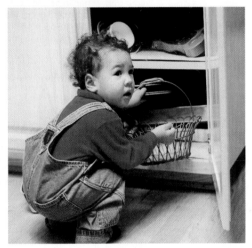

Pots and pans are popular toys for inquisitive toddlers. However, exploring cupboards can be a dangerous activity for toddlers. Toxic cleaning substances and other dangerous objects must be kept behind locked doors and out of reach.

FIG 6-1 Growth and development of the toddler.

growth of 12 cm (4⅘ inches) in the first 12 months. By age 2 years, the head circumference has reached 90% of its adult size.

Immature abdominal musculature gives the toddler a potbellied appearance, with an exaggerated lumbar curve. The child's short legs may appear slightly bowed, and the feet seem flat because of a plantar fat pad that disappears around age 2 years. During the toddler years, muscle tissue gradually replaces much of the adipose tissue (baby fat) present during infancy. As the musculoskeletal system matures and the child walks and runs more, the cherubic toddler disappears and the child grows into a taller, leaner preschooler.

The Preschooler

The preschool child's growth is slow and steady. Height and weight gains are minimal during this period. The average weight gain is approximately 2.25 kg (5 lb) per year, and the height gain averages 5 to 7.5 cm (2 to 3 inches) per year. Children attain half their adult height between ages 2 and 3 years. During this time, growth occurs more rapidly in the legs than in the trunk, accumulation of adipose tissue

declines, and the child's appetite decreases. As a result, the preschooler loses the potbellied appearance of the toddler, becoming slimmer and more agile. Muscles grow faster than bones during the preschool period. Muscle strength is influenced by nutrition, genetic makeup, and the opportunity to exercise and use the muscles. Knock-knees (see Chapter 26) are common in 3-year-olds and are often associated with occasional stumbling and falling. Maturation of the knee and hip joints usually corrects this problem by age 4 or 5 years.

As the lungs grow, the vital capacity increases and the respiratory rate slows. Respirations remain primarily diaphragmatic until age 5 or 6 years. The heart rate decreases and the blood pressure rises as the heart increases in size (see Chapter 9 for vital sign ranges). Cardiovascular maturation enables the preschooler to engage in more sustained and strenuous activity.

All 20 deciduous teeth are present by age 3 years. Deciduous teeth may begin to fall out at the end of the preschool period. The first permanent teeth to erupt, the back molars, usually appear in the early school-age years.

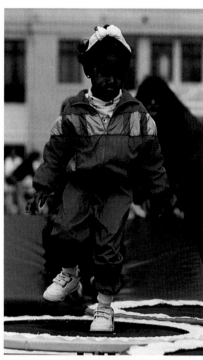

As the brain matures, the preschool child's motor development matures. Opportunities for practice contribute to the development of motor skills. (Courtesy Cook Children's Medical Center, Fort Worth, TX.)

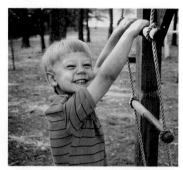

This 4-year-old's motor development has increased to the point that he can jump and climb well. A 4-year-old can also throw a ball overhand and cut on a curved line with scissors.

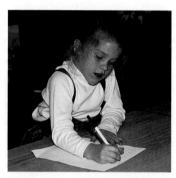

This 5-year-old is printing her name in readable letters. Children of this age can usually skip and can both throw and catch a ball (Courtesy University of Texas at Arlington School of Nursing, Arlington, TX.)

FIG 6-2 Growth and development of the preschooler.

HEALTH PROMOTION

Healthy People 2020 *Objectives for Toddlers and Preschoolers*

EMC-2	Increase the proportion of parents who use positive parenting and communicate with their doctors or other health care professionals about positive parenting.
IID-7	Achieve and maintain effective vaccination coverage levels for universally recommended vaccines among young children (19 to 35 months).
IVP-9	Prevent an increase in the rate of poisoning deaths.
IVP-16	Increase age-appropriate vehicle restraint system use in children.
IVP-23	Prevent an increase in the rate of fall-related deaths.
IVP-25	Reduce drowning deaths.
NWS-11	Prevent inappropriate weight gain in children ages 2 to 5 years.
TU-11	Reduce the proportion of children ages 3 to 11 years exposed to secondhand smoke.

Modified from U.S. Department of Health and Human Services. (2010). *Healthy People 2020*. Retrieved from www.healthypeople.gov.

Motor Development
The Toddler

Learning to walk well is the crowning achievement of the toddler period. The child is in perpetual motion, seemingly compelled to pull up, take a few steps, fall, and repeat the process over and over, oblivious to bumps and bruises. The toddler will repeat this performance hundreds of times until the skill of walking has been perfected.

The age at which children learn to walk varies widely. Most children can walk alone by 15 months. By 18 months of age, toddlers walk well and try to run but fall often. At approximately 15 months of age, many toddlers become avid climbers. Chairs, tables, and bookcases all present irresistible challenges and risks for injury. Parents may have difficulty

keeping the toddler in a crib and may decide to move the child to a regular bed.

Toddlers are also engaged in perfecting fine motor skills. Hand-eye coordination improves with maturity and practice. Mealtimes are still messy. Although most 18-month-olds can hold a cup with both hands and drink from it without much spilling, eating with a spoon is difficult. Most of the food conveyed in a spoon is spilled. Children need a great deal of practice with a spoon before they can feed themselves without spilling. Most toddlers can feed themselves with a spoon by their second birthday if they have been allowed to practice.

At 18 months of age, the toddler enjoys removing clothing. By 24 months, the toddler can put on simple items of clothing but cannot differentiate front from back. Children at this age also can zip large zippers, put on shoes, and wash and dry their hands. Two-year-olds brush their teeth but need help in adequately removing plaque.

The toddler's increasing motor skills allow more independence in all areas of daily life. Feeding, dressing, and play provide opportunities for the child to develop autonomy. Motor development in this age-group is far ahead of development of judgment and perception. This difference in timing of the development of different skills increases the risk for injury.

The Preschooler

Coordination and muscle strength increase rapidly between ages 3 and 5 years. Increases in brain size and nerve myelinization enable the child to perfect fine and gross motor skills.

Motor abilities vary widely among children. Although motor skill is less influenced by environment than other areas of development, such as language, opportunities to practice may contribute to better motor skills. For example, a 4-year-old who often plays catch with a sibling or parent generally finds playing Little League baseball as a 7-year-old easier than a child without a similar experience.

Handedness begins to emerge at approximately 3 years and is usually clearly established by 4 years. The nurse should encourage parents to provide left-handed children with appropriate tools, particularly left-handed scissors. Left-handed children should not be forced to use their right hands because coordination is usually better when they use the dominant side. Hand-eye coordination is usually good enough by age 5 years for a child to hit a nail on the head with a hammer. Increased coordination allows the child to perform many self-care skills and become more independent.

By age 4 or 5 years, the child is independent and can dress, eat, and go to the bathroom without help. Unlike the toddler, who must be restrained to avoid injury, the older preschooler can usually be trusted to heed verbal warnings of danger.

Cognitive and Sensory Development
The Toddler

Toddlers are consumed with curiosity. Their boundless energy and insatiable inquisitiveness provide them with resources for the tremendous cognitive growth that occurs during this period.

Toddlers between ages 12 and 18 months are in Piaget's sensorimotor period (Piaget, 1952) (see Chapter 4). Learning in this stage occurs mainly by trial and error. Toddlers spend most of a busy day experimenting to see what will happen as they dump, fill, empty, and explore every accessible area of their environment. Between 19 and 24 months, the child enters the final stage of the

HEALTH PROMOTION
The 15- to 18-Month-Old Child

Focused Assessment

Ask the parent the following:
- What new activities is your child doing?
- Can your child say single words? Put words together? Understand most of what you say? Communicate needs and wants?
- What kinds of foods does your child eat and how often? Do you have a concern that your child is eating items that are not food? Is your child able to eat with little assistance?
- Is your child walking well? Running? Jumping? Getting up and down the stairs?
- How does your child behave when frustrated? How do you and your partner handle this?
- What kinds of activities do you enjoy doing with your child?

Developmental Milestones

Personal/social: May exhibit negativism, ritualism, and increasing tolerance of separation from parents; undresses; begins temper tantrums when frustrated; may have a transition object; begins to understand gender differences

Fine motor: Turns book pages; begins to imitate vertical and circular strokes; vision 20/50 by 18 months; drinks from a cup by holding it with two hands

Language/cognitive: Increasing receptive language; begins to understand and say "no"; may begin to put two words together; can point to familiar objects; begins to use memory; understands spatial and temporal relations and increased object permanence; has a basic moral understanding (reward and punishment); understands simple directions; by 18 months has a vocabulary of approximately 30 words; holographic speech (uses single words with gestures to express whole ideas)

Gross motor: Walks with increasing confidence and begins to run; climbs stairs first by creeping, then walking with hand held; jumps in place; begins to throw a ball overhand without falling

Critical Milestones*

Personal/social: Begins to imitate; helps in the house; feeds self with increasing skill (still rotates the spoon, if used) and holds a cup

Fine motor: Builds a tower with increasing number of blocks; scribbles; able to put a block in a cup

Language/cognitive: Says 3 to 10 single words; can point to several body parts

Gross motor: Walks well forward and backward; stoops and recovers

Health Maintenance

Physical Measurements

Continue to measure and plot length, weight, and head circumference

Anterior fontanel closed by 18 months

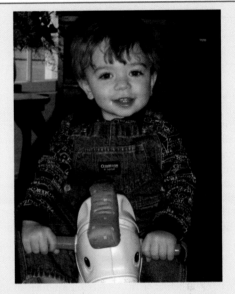

Immunizations

15 months: *Haemophilus influenzae* type b (Hib) #4; measles-mumps-rubella (MMR) #1 (if not given at 1 year); varicella (if not given at 1 year); pneumococcal (if not given at 1 year); hepatitis B #3 (if not given earlier)

18 months: diphtheria–tetanus–acellular pertussis (DTaP) #4; inactivated poliovirus (IPV) #3 (if not given earlier); hepatitis B #3 (if not given earlier)

Influenza vaccine annually

Hepatitis A #2 (6 months after first dose)

Health Screening

Standardized developmental screening

Autism-specific screening

Hearing risk assessment

Anticipatory Guidance

Nutrition

Calorie, protein, and fluid requirements decrease slightly; offer a variety of foods every 2 to 3 hours

Give 2 or 3 cups of whole milk daily for calcium

Vitamin D supplementation 400 international units per day if consuming less than 33 oz/day of milk and vitamin D–fortified foods

Make mealtimes pleasant: use appropriate-size utensils, colorful dinnerware

Child may have fussy eating habits (physiologic anorexia)

Resist giving food as a comfort measure

Do not allow child to walk or play with food in the mouth

*Guided by Denver Developmental Screening Test II.

HEALTH PROMOTION

The 15- to 18-Month-Old Child—cont'd

Elimination

Sphincters become physiologically under voluntary control, but child is usually not ready for toilet training; advise parents to wait but discuss signs of readiness

Dental

Continue to brush with a soft toothbrush twice daily

Parent should floss the child's teeth

Maintain a diet low in sugar

Do not put the child to sleep with a bottle

Dental risk assessment (18 months); refer to dentist if not done earlier

Sleep

Sleep cycles decrease and the child has longer awake periods

Still naps one or two times per day

May resist going to bed; likes a bedtime routine

Hygiene

Begins to participate in self-care (washes face and hands with assistance)

Safety

Review car safety, violence, falls, water safety, toy and toy box safety, bicycle passenger helmet, poisons

Discuss choking, toy safety, firearm access, burn prevention, sun protection

Play

Provide push-pull toys with short strings

Noise-making toys

Dolls and stuffed animals (watch for small parts)

Musical toys

Art supplies: large crayons, finger paints, clay

Large blocks and balls

---

sensorimotor period. Object permanence is firmly established by this age. The child has a beginning ability to use symbols and words when referring to absent people or objects and begins to solve problems mentally rather than by repeating an action over and over. A toddler at this stage is often seen imitating the parent of the same sex performing household tasks (termed *domestic mimicry*). Late in this stage, the child displays *deferred imitation* (e.g., imitating the parent putting on makeup or shaving hours after that parent has left for work). The 18-month-old has a beginning ability to wait, as evidenced by appropriate response of the toddler to a parent or caregiver who says "just a minute." The child's concept of time is still immature, however, and "a minute" may seem like an hour to the toddler.

Toddlers think in terms of the predictable routines of their daily schedule. When talking with the toddler, the nurse should use time orientation in relation to familiar activities. For example, a toddler understands "Your mother will be here after your nap" better than "Your mother will be here at 2 o'clock."

Many hours each day are spent putting objects into holes and smaller objects into each other as the child experiments with sizes, shapes, and spatial relations. Toddlers enjoy opening drawers and doors, exploring the contents of cabinets and closets, and generally wreaking havoc throughout the house, as well as exposing themselves to potential danger.

According to Piaget (1952), the preoperational stage of cognitive development characterizes the second half of early childhood (see Chapter 4). This stage is divided into two phases: the preconceptual phase (2 to 4 years) and the intuitive phase (4 to 7 years). During the preconceptual phase, the child is beginning to use symbolic thought—the ability to allow a mental image (words or ideas) to represent objects or ideas. Mental symbols allow the child to remember the past and describe events that happened in the past. At approximately 24 months, children enter the preconceptual phase, which ends at age 4 years. In this phase, children begin to think and reason at a primitive level. Two-year-olds have a beginning ability to retain mental images. This ability allows them to internalize what they see and experience. Symbols in the form of words can be used to represent ideas. Increasing amounts of play time are spent pretending. A box may become a spaceship or a hat; pebbles may be money or popcorn. The child's rapidly growing vocabulary enhances **symbolic play.** The toddler begins to think about alternative solutions to a problem and can even consider the consequences of an action without carrying it out (touching a hot stove, running too fast on a slippery sidewalk).

The toddler's thinking is immature, limited in its logic, and bound to the present. Egocentrism, animism, irreversibility, magical thinking, and centration characterize the preoperational thought of the toddler (Table 6-1). The predominant words in the toddler's language repertoire are "me," "I," and "mine."

TABLE 6-1   CHARACTERISTICS OF PREOPERATIONAL THINKING

CHARACTERISTIC	EXAMPLE
Egocentrism: Views everything in relation to self. Is unable to consider another's point of view.	Toddler takes a toy away from another child and cannot understand that the other child wants (or has a right to) the toy, too.
Animism: Believes that inert objects are alive and have wills of their own.	Toddler trips over a toy and scolds the toy for hurting her. She believes that the toy hurt her on purpose.
Irreversibility: Cannot see a process in reverse order. Cannot follow a line of reasoning back to its beginning. Cannot hold on to two or more sequential thoughts simultaneously.	If the child takes a toy apart, the child cannot remember the sequence for putting it back together.
	If a child is taken on a walk, the child cannot retrace steps and find the way home.
Magical thought: Believes that magical thought is the cause of events and that wishing something will make it so.	Toddlers often feel extremely powerful and believe that their thoughts cause events to happen.
Centration: Tends to focus on only one aspect of an experience, ignoring other possible alternatives. Focuses on the dominant characteristic of an object, excluding other characteristics.	May have difficulty putting together a puzzle, concentrating on only one detail of a piece (e.g., shape) and ignoring other qualities (e.g., color, detail).
	Cannot follow more than one direction at a time.

HEALTH PROMOTION

The 2-Year-Old Child

Focused Assessment
Ask the parent the following:
- How are you managing any discipline problems your child may be having?
- Do you have any concerns about any daycare arrangements you have?
- Does your child use a bottle or a cup?
- What do you do when your child has a temper tantrum? Do you feel confident about setting behavioral limits?
- How does your child communicate with others?
- What, if anything, have you done to begin toilet training your child?
- What activities do you enjoy doing together?

Developmental Milestones
Personal/social: Imitates household activities and begins to do helpful tasks; uses table utensils without much spilling; drinks from a lidless cup; removes a difficult article of clothing; begins developing sexual identity; is stubborn and negativistic: wants own way in everything; brushes teeth with help; is learning to walk; understands "soon"

Fine motor: Puts blocks into a cup after demonstration; builds tower of four to six blocks; able to imitate a horizontal and circular stroke with a crayon; turns a doorknob; turns book pages one at a time; can unzip and unbutton

Language/cognition: Has an approximately 300-word vocabulary, two-word sentences; points to six body parts and pictures of several familiar objects (e.g., bird, man, dog, horse); understands cause and effect, object permanence, sense of time; follows two-step directions; uses egocentric language (I, me, mine)

Gross motor: Stoops and recovers well; walks forward and backward; climbs stairs holding the railing; runs, jumps, kicks a ball

Critical Milestones*
Personal/social: Removes one article of clothing; feeds a doll; uses a spoon or fork

Fine motor: Holds a pencil and spontaneously scribbles; dumps a raisin out of a bottle on command after demonstration; builds a two-block tower

Language/cognitive: Points to two pictures; says three to six words

Gross motor: Runs; walks up steps; kicks a ball forward

Health Maintenance
Physical Measurements
Gains approximately 2.25 kg (5 lb) per year
Length or height is approximately half eventual adult height
Grows approximately 7.5 cm (3 inches) per year
Compute and plot BMI

Immunizations
Administer any immunizations not given previously according to the recommended schedule
Influenza vaccine annually

Health Screening
Hemoglobin and lead screen
Standardized developmental screening (now or at 30 months)
Autism-specific screening
Fasting lipid screen for child with cardiovascular disease risk factors
Tuberculosis (TB) screening if at risk

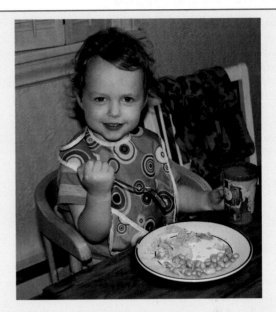

Anticipatory Guidance
Nutrition
May begin low-fat milk
Daily diet: 2 or 3 cups of milk, two servings of protein, three small servings of vegetables, two servings of fruit, and six servings of bread
Modify diet for children with elevated cholesterol (no more than 200 mg cholesterol/day, no more than 30% calories from fat and 7% from saturated fat): egg substitute, low-fat cheeses and meats, added fiber
Decrease added fat and high-calorie, high-fat desserts; increase fruits, vegetables, and carbohydrates
Vitamin D supplementation 400 international units per day if consuming less than 33 oz/day of milk and vitamin D–fortified foods

Elimination
Bowel movements decrease in number and become more regular
Child remains dry for several hours
Begin to think about a positive approach to toilet training

Dental
Sixteen teeth; may use pea-size amount of fluoridated toothpaste, encourage not to swallow
Parent should floss the child's teeth
Schedule first dental visit if not done earlier

Sleep
12 to 14 hr/day
Usually a long afternoon nap
Limit television viewing to no more than 1 hour daily

Hygiene
Girls are prone to vaginal irritation; advise to wipe from front to back; adding ¼ cup vinegar to bath water can relieve irritation
Boys' foreskin begins to retract; retract gently to clean; never force

*Guided by Denver Developmental Screening Test II.

HEALTH PROMOTION

The 2-Year-Old Child—cont'd

Safety

Review toy safety, firearm safety, burn prevention, and other previously discussed subjects

May change to a forward-facing child safety seat

Discuss choking on food, street safety, water safety, outside poisons, playground safety, sun protection

Self-Esteem and Competence

Discuss the following with parent:
- Modeling appropriate social behavior
- Encouraging the child to learn to make choices
- Helping the child to appropriately express emotions

- Spending individual time with the child daily
- Providing consistent and loving limits to help the child learn self-discipline
- Beginning toilet training only when the child is ready (dry for 2 hours, able to pull pants down, can use appropriate toileting words, can indicate the need to use the toilet)

Play

Parallel play; play begins to become imitative and imaginative

Choose toys that are safe and durable: balls, picture books, puzzles with large pieces, sandbox toys, trucks, riding toys, household toys (e.g., broom, mop, carpet sweeper)

The Preschooler

By age 3 years, the brain has reached two thirds of its adult size. Maturation of the central nervous system contributes to the child's increasing cognitive abilities.

The 3-year-old can retain a mental image of a loved one and can periodically "refuel" by thinking about that person. A photograph can help some children cope with separation by bridging the gap between physical presence and mental image. Preschoolers' ability to remember their parents and recognize that their needs can be met even though their parents are not present enhances their ability to tolerate separation.

Because preschoolers still engage in animism, they often endow inanimate objects with lifelike qualities during play. A doll may become a crying baby, or a teddy bear may become a friend who listens sympathetically. Symbolic play is important for emotional development because it allows the child to work through distressing feelings. For this reason, allowing a child to play with medical equipment after a painful procedure can be therapeutic. Four-year-olds who have received injections may be found working out their feelings by giving their dolls "lots of shots."

During the preconceptual phase, reality may be distorted by *transductive reasoning*. The preschool child reasons from particular to particular rather than from particular to general, and vice versa, as adults do. The child cannot understand that relationships exist and cannot view the whole in relation to its parts. The preschool child has difficulty focusing on the important aspects of a situation. To a child, everything is important and interdependent. This type of thinking is called *field dependency*. For example, the preschooler may have difficulty falling asleep at night because the parent did not follow the usual bedtime routine. Objects, routine, and sameness are important to the preschool child. Rituals provide the preschool child with a feeling of control.

The second phase of Piaget's preoperational stage, the intuitive phase, is characterized by centration and lack of reversibility. *Centration* is the tendency to center or focus on one part of a situation and ignore the other parts. The child cannot understand logical relationships and is unable to focus on more than one aspect of a situation at a time. For example, the child may not be able to follow a sequence of directions but will perform well if the directions are given one at a time.

The 4- or 5-year-old shows *irreversibility* in thought (Piaget, 1952). Children this age cannot reverse a process or the order of events. They may be able to take a complex puzzle apart but have difficulty putting it back together. The 4- or 5-year-old also lacks reversibility for mathematical processes. The child may be able to add 3 and 1 and get 4, but reversing the problem ($4 - 1 = 3$) would be too difficult.

The preschool years are a period of rapid learning. The preschool child is curious and wants to know how things work. Preschoolers' thinking is still magical and egocentric (focused on the self). Children at this age tend to understand events only as these events affect them, believing that everyone else has had the same experience. Children seeing their mother in distress may bring her a doll, assuming that it would comfort the mother as it does the child.

Preschool children often think that their thoughts are powerful enough to cause things to happen. They may frighten themselves with some of their ideas, believing that they may become what they imagine they will be. Preschoolers may feel overwhelmed by guilt when a sibling is hospitalized because they believe that their hostile feelings caused the sibling's illness. Likewise, a child of this age may say, "I got sick because I was bad."

Language Development

The Toddler

The acquisition of language is one of the most dramatic developments of early childhood. Although the age at which children begin to talk varies widely, most can communicate verbally by their second birthday. The rate of language development depends on physical maturity and the amount of reinforcement that the child has received. Between 15 and 24 months of age, language ability develops rapidly. Toddlers understand many more words than they can say because receptive language (what the child understands) develops earlier and more quickly than speech. Sometime after 18 months, many children experience a sudden spurt in speech production and comprehension, resulting in a vocabulary of 300 or more words at 24 months. By 2 years of age, roughly 60% to 70% of toddlers' speech should be understandable. Because children age 24 to 30 months are less egocentric and better able to consider another's point of view, they engage in more conversation with others and less monologue.

The standardized developmental screening recommended by the American Academy of Pediatrics (AAP) to occur at age 18 months is designed to identify children with communication delay (AAP, 2006/2010). If language development is not progressing normally, parents should be advised to pursue follow-up care. Children of bilingual families, children who are twins, and children other than firstborns may have slower language development. Because language development depends on adequate hearing, delayed language can be seen in children who have had repeated ear infections or who have undiagnosed hearing loss (see Chapter 31).

Parents can promote language development by talking to their children and incorporating teaching into daily routines. Feeding, bathing, dressing, and going on outings to both new and familiar places offer opportunities for verbal interaction and the practice of growing language skills. The child should be encouraged to express needs rather than have the parent anticipate and provide what the child wants before the child asks for it. Reading simple, entertaining stories with colorful pictures provides quiet, enjoyable times for toddlers and parents and enhances speech and language development.

The Preschooler

A dramatic increase in language skill in the preschool period promotes self-control and increases the child's ability to direct and be directed by others. Children at this age may be heard talking to themselves about things they have heard or been taught.

The preschooler's vocabulary increases rapidly, from 300 words at 2 years of age to more than 2100 words at 5 years. In less than 3 years, the child grows from a toddler who knows only a few words into a child who skillfully uses an extensive vocabulary to describe events, share feelings, and ask questions. Three-year-olds speak in short, telegraphic sentences. They may talk to themselves or to imaginary friends. A delightful characteristic of young preschoolers is the tendency to engage in lengthy monologues, regardless of whether anyone is listening or even present. Such self-talk provides the child with opportunities to practice speech and is often accompanied by symbolic play.

By 4 years old, children talk incessantly and tend to boast and exaggerate. They enjoy rhymes and silly ways to use similar words. Four-year-olds expect more detailed answers to their questions. They may use speech aggressively and may use profanity to gain attention. "Bad" language should be ignored, thus depriving the child of reinforcement of the behavior. When children feel that they gain power over their parents by using bad language, these verbalizations will continue.

Five-year-olds speak in sentences of adult length and use all parts of speech. They usually are proficient storytellers who produce elaborate tales for anyone who will listen. Their tendency to mix fantasy with reality may be perceived by adults as lying. The child of 5 years usually can recite the days of the week and can name the seasons.

Nurses can teach parents strategies to promote their child's language development. It is important for parents to talk with the child and respond to the child's attempts at communication. Reading to the child and making reading materials available can help build vocabulary and promote a lifelong love of reading. Watching educational television programs with their child may augment parents' communication skills with their child. Preschoolers spend a lot of time asking "how" and "why" questions, often taxing parents' patience. Short, simple, honest answers encourage vocabulary building and boost self-esteem.

Psychosocial Development
The Toddler

The toddler is developing a sense of autonomy, giving up the comfort of dependence enjoyed during infancy. If a basic sense of trust was established during the first year, the toddler can venture forward and separate from parents for short periods to explore and experience the world.

According to Erikson (1963), the toddler is struggling with the developmental task of acquiring a sense of autonomy while overcoming a sense of shame and doubt. Toddlers discover that they have a will of their own and that they can control others. Asserting their will and insisting on their own way, however, often lead to conflict with those they love, whereas submissive behavior is rewarded with affection and approval. Toddlers experience conflict because they want to assert their own will but do not want to risk losing the approval of loved ones. If the child continues to practice dependent behavior, doubt related to abilities develops. Toddlers may feel shame for independent impulses, particularly if frequent punishment is associated with their actions.

The toddler learns which behaviors gain approval and which result in censure and punishment. Two-year-olds do not have a conscience but avoid punishment by controlling their behavior. Right and wrong are determined by the consequences of actions.

At approximately 15 months toddlers begin to demonstrate their developing autonomy with two almost universal behaviors: negativism and ritualism.

Negativism. Negativism, one of the most dramatic expressions of independence, is shown in a variety of ways. The toddler's favorite word seems to be "no." Unable to distinguish between requests and directives, the toddler seems to believe that saying "yes" would mean giving up free will. The child often seems to delight in this test of wills with the parent. Negativism may result in screaming, kicking, hitting, biting, or breath-holding. Parents often interpret the child's negative behavior as being bad or stubborn. Nurses can help parents understand their toddler's behavior as an important sign of the child's progress from dependence to autonomy and independence. The nurse should give support and encourage the parents to deal with the toddler's trying behavior with patience and a sense of humor. Although general permissiveness is not recommended, too much pressure and forceful methods of control often lead to defiance, tantrums, and prolonged negative behavior.

Ritualism and the Importance of Routine. Ritualism helps the child venture out and away from the safety of the parents by ensuring uniformity and security. Ritualism allows the toddler to have a sense of control. The child feels more confident with a secure home base. The toddler insists on sameness. Milk may have to be poured into the same cup, parents may have to sit in the same chairs at dinnertime, and a specified routine may have to be followed countless times throughout the day. The child may be unable to go to sleep unless a bedtime ritual is followed exactly (e.g., a drink of water, two stories, prayers, and a teddy bear). The child may experience distress if this routine is not followed exactly the next night. Failure to recognize the importance of such rituals may increase stress and insecurity.

Events such as hospitalization, during which continuity of routine cannot be ensured, are difficult for the toddler. The nurse can decrease the stress of hospitalization by incorporating the child's usual rituals and routines from home into nursing care activities. Keeping hospital routines as similar to those of home as possible and recognizing ritualistic needs give the toddler some sense of control and security and reduce feelings of helplessness and fear. See Chapter 11 for further discussion of the hospitalized child.

Separation Anxiety. Separation anxiety peaks again in the toddler period. Although the concept of object permanence is fully developed in the toddler, children at this stage have difficulty differentiating their own feelings from those of their parents. Although the children experience a strong desire to be independent and leave their mothers, they fear that their mothers also want to leave them. A toddler may strike out independently across the room, only to rush back in tears to the mother, as if the child were frightened and angry with the mother for leaving. For a brief period, the parent may find talking on the telephone without interruption or even going into the bathroom without being

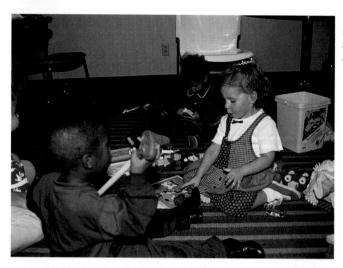

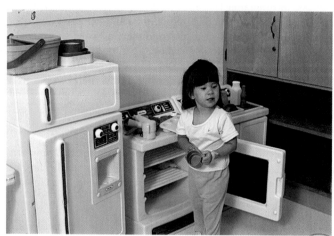

Parallel play occurs when children play side by side with similar toys but no organized group activity occurs. The children play *beside* one another but not *with* one another. (Courtesy University of Texas at Arlington School of Nursing, Arlington, TX.)

Symbolic play consists of activities that children use to express their perception of reality. This little girl is acting out a familiar adult scenario as she manipulates child-size toys that represent kitchen equipment.

FIG 6-3 Types of play.

followed virtually impossible. Leave-taking and brief separations are acceptable to a toddler if they are the toddler's idea, but the parent's departure may cause desperate clinging and crying. Games such as hide-and-seek help the child master fears of separation. Repeating separation under conditions the child can control helps the toddler overcome the anxiety associated with separation. The child learns from experience that loved ones will return after separation.

Being left with a stranger can be stressful. Toddlers should be told honestly and clearly about a separation shortly before it occurs. The parent or nurse should reassure the child that the parent is coming back. When the parent returns, the toddler often shows anger at being left by ignoring the parent or by pretending to be more interested in play than in going home. Parents of hospitalized toddlers are frequently distressed by such behavior when they visit their child (see Chapter 11).

Tolerating brief separations from parents is an important developmental task for the toddler. *Transition objects,* such as a favorite blanket or toy, provide comfort to the toddler in stressful situations, such as separation, illness, and even bedtime. Such objects help children make the transition from dependency to autonomy. Toddlers may become so attached to an object that they can hardly bear to part with it, even for a brief time while it is being laundered.

The nurse can offer support by explaining that the behavior is a normal growth and development milestone and telling the parents that plenty of affection and attention are needed to help the toddler cope with the stress of separation. The nurse counsels parents to leave a toddler only briefly at first and, if possible, to delay extended separations until the toddler can handle them better. The nurse who helps parents understand normal toddler behavior in response to separation helps parents cope with the frustrations of this transition.

Play. Toddlers spend most of their time at play. Play is serious business to the toddler—it is the child's work. Many hours are spent each day in play, perfecting fine and gross motor skills, learning to control inner urges, and gaining self-esteem. Play during this period reflects the egocentric toddler's developmental level. The toddler engages in parallel play, in which children play alongside but not with

other children (Figure 6-3). Little regard is given to the feelings of others. Children engaged in this type of play frequently grab toys away from other children or may hit or fight to obtain a wanted toy. Because toddlers are egocentric, they do not realize that they are hurting the other child and feel no shame for aggressive actions.

Imitation and acting out scenes of everyday life are common as the toddler begins to try out roles and identify with adults. Active, large-muscle play helps the toddler vent frustrations and dissipate excess energy. The nurse can help parents understand how play enhances the toddler's development. The nurse should encourage parents to play with their toddler and provide opportunities for the toddler to play with other children. The nurse teaches parents about child-proofing and checking the house on a daily basis. Toys must be strong, safe, and too large to swallow or place in the ear or nose. Toddlers need supervision at all times. A variety of play materials, which need not be expensive, and a safe play environment enhance the toddler's development (Box 6-1).

Psychosexual Development. At approximately 18 months, toddlers enter Freud's anal stage. Freud (1960) theorized that as children focus on mastery of bowel and bladder functions, their attention is also directed to the genital area. Even before age 2 years, children are aware of their own gender and begin to develop a sense of gender identity. By 2½ or 3 years, toddlers can correctly identify anatomic pictures of boys and girls. Gender identity is not fully established until age 5 years, when the child understands gender as permanent (i.e., that gender does not change with the addition of a wig or a dress) (Kohlberg, 1966).

Children begin to be aware of expected gender role behaviors at an early age. By age 3 years most toddlers show an awareness of gender role stereotypes and tend to imitate the same-gender parent during play. Gender role identification continues throughout the toddler and preschool years as the child incorporates the attitudes, roles, and values of the same-gender parent. Although gender role stereotypes have relaxed somewhat in recent years, children behave according to adult expectations. Children learn behavior by reinforcement and punishment, as well as by imitation. If a boy repeatedly hears that boys do not play with dolls, he will spurn such "girls' toys" and will play

BOX 6-1 AGE-RELATED ACTIVITIES AND TOYS FOR TODDLERS AND PRESCHOOLERS

General Activities
Toddler
- The toddler fills and empties containers, begins dramatic play, has increased use of motor skills, enjoys feeling different textures, explores the home environment, imitates orders, and likes to be read to and to look at books and television programs that are age-appropriate.
- Toys should meet the child's need for activity and inquisitiveness.
- The child also enjoys manipulating small objects such as toy people, cars, and animals.

Preschooler
- Dramatic play is prominent.
- The child likes to run, jump, hop, and, in general, improve motor skills.
- The child likes to build and create things (e.g., sand castles and mud pies).
- Play is simple and imaginative.
- Simple collections begin.

Toys and Specific Types of Play
Toddler
- Continued exploring of the body parts of self and others; mechanical toys; objects of different textures such as clay, sand, finger paints, and bubbles; push-pull toys; large ball; sand and water play; blocks; painting; coloring with large crayons; nesting toys; large puzzles; trucks; dolls.
- Therapeutic play can begin at this age.

Preschooler
- Riding toys, building materials such as sand and blocks, dolls, drawing materials, crayons, cars, puzzles, books, appropriate television and videos, nonsense rhymes, singing games, pretend play as something or somebody, dress-up, finger paints, clay, cutting, pasting, simple board and card games.

with toys that his parents consider masculine to gain their praise and approval. Nurses should be aware of their own biases about gender-typed behaviors and should support the parents in their choice of toys and activities for their child. The nurse can be most helpful by encouraging parents to make traditionally gender-typed toys available to both boys and girls if this approach is consistent with the parents' beliefs. Parents' expectations of appropriate gender role behavior differ according to their cultural backgrounds. In most cultures, boys and girls are treated differently and thus are taught "male" and "female" behaviors.

Parents are often concerned about their toddler's interest in and curiosity about gender differences. Sex play and masturbation are common among toddlers. Nurses can reassure parents that self-exploration or exploration of another toddler's body is normal behavior during early childhood. Parents should respect the child's curiosity as normal without judging the child as "bad." The child should be told that touching private parts is something that is done only in private. When parents discover children involved in sex play, casually telling them to dress and directing them to another activity can limit sex play without producing feelings of shame or anxiety. The nurse should explain to parents that positive attitudes toward sexuality are learned from parents who are comfortable with their own sexuality. As young children learn about their bodies and explore anatomic differences,

they frequently ask questions about where babies come from or why "Brian looks different from Emily." Honest, straightforward answers that use the correct terminology satisfy the toddler's curiosity and lay the foundation for healthy sexual attitudes.

! NURSING QUALITY ALERT
Important Tasks of the Toddler Period

- Recognition of self as a separate person with own will
- Control of impulses and acquisition of socially acceptable ways to communicate wants and needs
- Control of elimination
- Toleration of separation from the parent

The Preschooler

The preschool years are a critical period for the development of socialization. Children need opportunities to play with others to learn communication and social skills. They also need appropriate guidance to learn acceptable behavior.

According to Erikson (1963), the preschooler's developmental task is to achieve a sense of initiative. The preschooler is busy learning how to do things and takes great pride in new accomplishments. If the child acts inappropriately or is repeatedly criticized or punished for attempts to explore and learn, feelings of guilt, anxiety, shame, and fear may result. For example, an adult's comment, "That's nice, but it would look better if you did it this way," may cause the child to feel inferior. Such subtle criticism can make the child reluctant to try new activities. A feeling of inferiority also may develop if adults are always doing things for the child rather than encouraging independence. The child who does not achieve a sense of initiative will feel defeated, angry, and afraid of people and new situations. Nurses can promote healthy psychosocial development in preschoolers and help them gain a sense of initiative by teaching parents the importance of providing the child with opportunities to explore in a safe, stimulating environment. Adults should encourage the preschooler's imagination and creativity and should praise appropriate behavior.

Play. Learning to relate to age mates is another developmental task that is significant during the preschool period. Preschoolers need experience playing with other children to learn how to relate to other people. Three-year-olds are capable of sharing and are more likely to do so than toddlers. Four-year-olds tend to be more argumentative and less generous with playmates. Although this behavior may appear to be a step backward to parents, it is actually a sign of growth because 4-year-olds feel more secure in a group and are testing their roles and communication skills. The 5-year-old enjoys playing with other children and generally can play with another child for longer periods before arguments develop.

Children between ages 3 and 5 years enjoy parallel and associative play. Children also learn to share and cooperate (cooperative play) as they play in small groups. During play, preschoolers learn simple games and rules, language concepts, and social roles. Play is often imitative, dramatic, and creative. Various roles are explored through play as children imitate significant adults. Preschoolers enjoy dress-up clothes, housekeeping toys, doll houses, and other toys that encourage pretending (see Figure 6-3). Tricycles and climbing toys help develop muscles and coordination. Preschoolers also enjoy materials for cutting, pasting, and painting. Such manipulative and creative materials stimulate imagination and fine motor development (see Box 6-1).

Imaginary friends are common near age 3 years. Boundaries between reality and fantasy are blurred at this age, and "pretend" can seem real, especially during play. Imaginary friends serve many purposes. They may take the blame when the child misbehaves, allowing the child to save face when feeling guilty about a certain behavior. Imaginary friends may be companions during lonely times. They may accomplish a task with which the child is struggling or allow the child to practice roles. For example, the child may scold an imaginary friend and administer punishment, just as a parent would. Imaginary friends seem to be more common in highly imaginative and intelligent children.

Psychosexual Development. Sexual identity and body image are developing. Sexual curiosity and explorations are normal. Preschoolers are curious about anatomic differences and seek to investigate them. Preschoolers show interest in the differences between the sexes and often compare their bodies with those of others. Playing doctor and hiding with a friend to investigate anatomic differences are common activities during the preschool period. The nurse can reassure parents that the child is simply learning about his or her body and that the parents can direct the child to another activity. Preschoolers are interested in where they came from and how babies are made. Parents should be encouraged to assess what the child already knows about the subject and to determine why the child is asking the question. The parent should answer questions simply, honestly, and matter-of-factly. The child usually neither wants nor understands detailed explanations.

Parents greatly influence their children's sexual development. Positive signs of physical and emotional intimacy between parents send a positive signal to the child. A warm, accepting, matter-of-fact attitude toward sexual matters promotes a positive, healthy perspective in children. Parents can create an atmosphere of acceptance in the early preschool years when the first questions arise. A parental attitude of "You can ask me anything" can set the stage for healthy interaction from early childhood into adolescence, when parental guidance is so important.

Masturbation is common and may increase in frequency when the child is under stress. Parents often express concern about such behavior. The nurse can help parents handle these situations by explaining that such self-comforting behaviors are normal for this age. If the parent discovers the child masturbating, simple redirection of the child's attention without punishing, shaming, or reprimanding is best. Children should be taught that touching their genitals is not appropriate in public.

At this age, a sense of rivalry with the same-gender parent develops. Preschool boys commonly compete with their fathers for the attention of their mothers. A girl likewise may become "Daddy's girl," often cuddling and flirting with her father while excluding her mother from the relationship. This rivalry is usually resolved early in the school-age period as the child identifies strongly with the same-gender parent and same-gender peers. According to Freudian theory, the oedipal stage is resolved when the child strongly identifies with the parent of the same gender. By the end of the preschool period, the child identifies with and imitates the same-gender parent. In single-parent and nontraditional families the child should have a friendly, stable relationship with an adult relative or friend of the same sex who can serve as a role model. By age 3 years, children know gender differences. They imitate masculine and feminine behaviors in play, and gender identity is well established by 6 years.

Spiritual and Moral Development. Learning the difference between right and wrong (the development of a conscience) is another important task of the preschool period. According to Kohlberg (1964),

children between ages 4 and 7 years are in the second stage of the preconventional level of moral development. In this stage, children obey rules out of self-interest. They tend to believe that if the consequences of an action are personally advantageous, the action is right. An "eye-for-an-eye" orientation guides their behavior.

The preschooler begins to use self-control to resist temptation and tries to "be good" to avoid feelings of guilt. Preschoolers determine right from wrong by the consequences of disobeying their parents' rules. At this age, children have little understanding of the reason for a rule. For example, when asked why hitting another child is wrong, the preschooler might reply, "Because my mother says so." Preschoolers adhere to parents' rules dogmatically, deciding whether to break a rule on the basis of the resulting punishment.

Preschoolers often have difficulty applying rules in different situations. The child may know that hitting a sibling is wrong but may not understand that hitting another child at daycare is also wrong. Because the preschooler is egocentric, understanding another's viewpoint is difficult. The child begins to develop a conscience as a result of consistent rewards for good behavior and punishment for bad behavior.

The preschool child's concept of God is concrete. The family's religious beliefs and customs, such as bedtime prayers, mealtime grace, and Bible stories, are important to preschoolers. Such rituals, practiced in an atmosphere of love, can be deeply meaningful and comforting to children of this age.

HEALTH PROMOTION FOR THE TODDLER OR PRESCHOOLER AND FAMILY

When doing health promotion with parents of children in early childhood, the nurse inquires about areas discussed in Box 5-3 at every visit. These include nutrition (quantity and types of food), elimination, safety (car restraints, gun violence), hearing and vision, family adjustment, and any other concerns.

Nutrition

The rate of growth slows during the toddler and preschool period, as does the child's appetite. This is sometimes referred to as physiologic anorexia. The child's food experiences during this period can have a lasting effect on how food and meals are viewed. The family is the primary influence at this time, although television plays an important role. Children should be discouraged from eating while watching television, and family mealtimes should be encouraged.

Nutritional Requirements

The U.S. Department of Agriculture (USDA) (2011) has issued new nutritional guidelines for the American public and has represented them graphically through the MyPlate icon (see Figure 4-7). Although specific recommendations for children have not yet been released, the USDA states that there is no change in the quantity and variety of foods recommended (USDA, 2011) (see Box 4-9). Children 2 to 8 years of age should consume 2 cups per day of fat-free or low-fat milk or equivalent milk products. Yogurt and cheese are other milk-group sources. Total fat intake should remain between 30% and 35% of calories for children ages 2 to 3 years and between 25% and 35% of calories for children age 4 years and older. Most fats should come from sources of polyunsaturated and monounsaturated fatty acids, such as fish, nuts, and vegetable oils (American Heart Association, 2011). Poultry, fish, and lean meat are good sources of iron. Low-sugar breakfast cereals are sources of iron and vitamins. Snacks of fruits and vegetables assist in meeting the child's nutritional requirements (Box 6-2).

BOX 6-2   NUTRITIOUS SNACKS

- Fresh fruit
- Celery sticks with cheese spread
- Yogurt
- Bagels
- Carrot sticks
- Graham crackers
- Pretzels
- Puddings

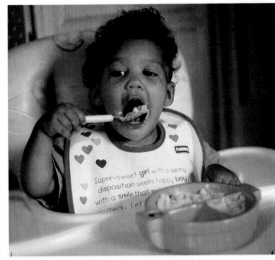

FIG 6-4 By age 1 year, most children are eating the same foods as the rest of the family. Toddlers should be offered three meals and two healthy snacks each day. Most 2-year-olds can drink from a cup and use a spoon well if given the opportunity to practice.

Many similarities exist in the nutritional needs of the toddler and the preschooler. Children this age who eat well-balanced diets should not experience iron deficiency. If milk remains the primary food, however, it will replace foods rich in iron, vitamins, and minerals, such as dark-green leafy vegetables, meats, and legumes. Although giving children a daily multivitamin is not harmful, in general the child who is healthy does not need vitamin supplementation. The exception to this is vitamin D. The AAP recommends vitamin D supplementation (400 IU daily) for children who consume fewer than 33 ounces of milk or fortified dairy products a day (Wagner, Greer, & Section on Breast-feeding and Committee on Nutrition, 2008).

Solid Foods

Children at this age are improving their proficiency in using a spoon and cup. By age 2 years, children can hold a cup in one hand and use a spoon well (Figure 6-4). By age 12 months, most children are eating the same foods as the rest of the family. The child should be offered three meals and two snacks each day.

By age 3 to 4 years, the child begins to use a fork. The child continues to develop fine motor skills and by the end of the preschool period should begin to use a rounded knife for cutting.

One method to determine serving size for children is 1 tablespoon of solid food per year of age. Children may be more likely to try new foods and eat nutritious meals if smaller portions are served. Foods of different textures, colors, consistencies, tastes, and temperatures should be offered. The child should sit in a chair that allows easy access to the food; the dishes should be small, nonbreakable and, when possible, steady enough to prevent spilling. Thick, short-handled spoons and forks and shallow bowls increase the toddler's ability to eat successfully.

Foods that could be aspirated should continue to be avoided during the toddler period. Soft drinks and candy need to be discouraged. Sugar is a source of calories and is naturally present in breast milk as lactose, in fruits as fructose, and in grain products as maltose. A diet with too much sugar, however, can replace other, more nutritious foods and increase tooth decay. Artificial sweeteners and foods that contain artificial sweeteners are not recommended for children younger than 2 years.

Age-Related Nutritional Challenges

Food Jags. The volume of food the child eats may vary from day to day. The child may want the same food at every meal for several days and then suddenly reject the food completely. Children this age may refuse foods because of odor and temperature. They may not like mixing foods and therefore may not eat casseroles. This dislike does not seem to apply to foods such as pizza, spaghetti, and macaroni and cheese. Many children prefer juices to milk and water. Too much milk

is not good, but neither is too much juice, which can replace other foods and their nutrients. For toddlers and preschoolers, juices should be limited to no more than 4 to 6 oz a day (AAP, Committee on Nutrition, 2011d). Parents and older siblings can affect how a child views a food and should be careful about making negative comments about a certain food. Children should be assisted in developing tastes for new foods through role modeling and making the foods available.

Physiologic Anorexia. The nurse teaches parents appropriate ways to approach the child who is experiencing physiologic anorexia. Advise parents not to allow their child to fill up with snacks, milk, and juices. Small portions should be offered so that the child does not feel overwhelmed by the amount of food. Mealtimes should be pleasant and not times to discuss discipline problems or even the child's poor appetite. Children should not be made to sit at the table after the rest of the family has left. This approach will only create a negative association with mealtime. Parents need to maintain a balance between ignoring their child's nutritional intake and making it the focus of their parenting.

The nurse can encourage parents to focus more on their child's weekly nutritional intake, rather than on one day's intake. Frequently children are the best judges of what they need, and they may eat primarily fruit one day and peanut butter the next. Nutritional consumption tends to balance out over a week. Box 6-3 illustrates ways parents can increase their child's nutritional intake.

Obesity Risk. The prevalence of obesity in the United States has risen dramatically among adults, but of particular concern is overweight and obesity in children. In *Healthy People 2020*, the United States Department of Health and Human Services (USDHHS) has specifically addressed the problem of obesity in young children, ages 2 to 5 years (USDHHS, 2010). Stating that 10.7% of 2- to 5-year-olds are identified as obese, objective NWS-10.1 is directed toward reducing obesity in children of this age-group. Strategies designed to approach this important issue include much of what has been discussed previously: increasing fruits and vegetables, increasing the percentage of whole grains, increasing calcium and iron intake, and decreasing solid fats, sodium, and sugar (USDHHS, 2010).

BOX 6-3   INCREASING NUTRITIONAL INTAKE

- Limit to two nutritious snacks per day, and give only at toddler's request.
- Limit to 4 to 6 oz of juice per day.
- Introduce to finger foods at age 8 to 10 months, and continue to make these types of food available.
- Limit to 16 to 24 oz of milk per day.
- Keep mealtimes pleasant.
- Do not force feed.
- Do not feed children who can feed themselves.

The AAP (Daniels, Greer, & the Committee on Nutrition, 2008) recommends screening children at risk for overweight and obesity beginning at age 2 years. This includes plotting a body mass index (BMI). Children with a family history of dyslipidemia or early cardiovascular disease development, and children whose BMI percentile exceeds the definition for overweight (≥85th percentile) or who have high blood pressure, should have a fasting lipid screen (Daniels, Greer, & the Committee on Nutrition, 2008).

Dental Care

Most toddlers have a complete set of 20 deciduous teeth by the time they are 30 months old. Although the exact time of eruption of teeth varies, an approximate rule of thumb to assess the number of teeth is the age of the toddler in months minus six. One tooth usually erupts for each month of age past 6 months up to 30 months of age.

Permanent teeth are calcifying during the toddler period, long before they are visible. Proper care of the deciduous teeth is crucial for the toddler's general health and for the health and alignment of the permanent teeth. Deciduous teeth play an important role in the growth and development of the jaws and face and in speech development. Premature loss of the deciduous teeth complicates eruption of the permanent teeth, often leading to malocclusion. Nurses need to be aware that some parents do not understand the value of preserving primary teeth.

Because toddlers do not have the manual dexterity to remove plaque adequately, parents must be responsible for cleaning their teeth. Children can be encouraged to brush their teeth after the teeth have been thoroughly cleaned by a parent. Because toddlers like to imitate, watching parents brush their teeth can be motivating. A small, soft, nylon-bristle brush works best. Optimal access and visibility are provided if the parent sits on the floor or bed with the child's head in the parent's lap and the child's body perpendicular to the parent's. This position also gives the parent some control of the child's head movement. Fluoride toothpaste is not recommended for young children because they often do not like the taste or, if they do, tend to swallow it. If the child receives fluoride from other sources, such as a fluoridated water supply, an excessive amount of fluoride may be ingested if fluoride toothpaste is swallowed. Ingestion of excessive amounts of fluoride may lead to *fluorosis,* which produces white speckles or brown discoloration of the enamel. Ideally, teeth should be brushed after every meal and especially at bedtime. Flossing between teeth helps remove plaque and should be done daily by the parent after the toddler's teeth are brushed.

Fluoride makes tooth enamel resistant to acid attack, preventing decay. Striking a balance between what is a protective level of fluoride and avoidance of fluorosis has lead the AAP and the American Dental Association to revise recommendations regarding fluoride supplementation (AAP, 2008; Rozier, Adair, Graham et al., 2010). Recommendations currently state that pediatric health care providers should perform an oral risk assessment at regular intervals throughout childhood and provide dietary counseling specifically directed toward preventing tooth decay (AAP, 2008). Supplemental fluoride is prescribed only for children determined to be at risk for dental caries (see Chapter 5 for information about risk assessment) and no access to a community fluoridated water source. For these children, the dose of fluoride supplementation is as follows: 6 months to 3 years, 0.25 mg daily; 3 to 6 years, 0.5 mg daily (Rozier et al., 2010). A diet that is low in sweets and high in nutritious food promotes dental health. Sweets are most likely to cause caries if they are sticky or if they are eaten between meals rather than with meals. The nurse should encourage the parent to offer nutritious snacks, such as fresh fruit, yogurt, or cheese, instead of candy, soda, or cookies.

All infants and children should have a source of dental care by age 1 year (AAP, 2008). Because bacterial organisms contribute to tooth decay, and children can acquire these organisms from their mother, primary preventive interventions need to be implemented as soon as possible in infancy (AAP, 2008). The child should first see the dentist 6 months after the first primary tooth erupts and no later than age 12 months. The first appointment should precede any needed dental work so that the visit is enjoyable and free from discomfort. This visit provides an opportunity for early assessment of the child's dental health as well as for teaching parents good preventive dental health practices, including not sharing eating or drinking utensils with the child.

Because the enamel on primary teeth is thinner than on permanent teeth, preschoolers' teeth are prone to destruction from decay. The distance from the tooth surface to the pulp is shorter as well, so tooth abscesses from caries can occur rapidly. Untreated caries can lead to pain, abscess formation, and poor digestion because of ineffective chewing. Many parents do not realize that the deciduous teeth are important to protect the dental arch. If deciduous teeth are lost early (e.g., because of decay), the remaining teeth may drift out of position, blocking proper eruption of the permanent teeth and leading to malocclusion.

Nurses play an important role in the promotion of dental health by teaching proper tooth cleaning, including the removal of plaque, encouraging a balanced diet limited in sweets, and recommending twice-yearly visits to the dentist. Preschoolers can usually brush their own teeth (Figure 6-5). Short back-and-forth or up-and-down strokes are easiest for the child to manage. Parents should monitor the child's toothbrushing and inspect the child's teeth to be sure that all plaque has been removed. Parents must help with flossing because it requires more manual dexterity than preschoolers have.

Sleep and Rest

During the second year, children require approximately 12 to 14 hours of sleep each day. Most 2-year-olds take one nap each day until the end of the second or third year, when many children give up the habit. Toddlers often resist going to bed, using dawdling or even temper tantrums to postpone separation from loved ones and the exciting events of the day. Firm, consistent limits are needed when toddlers try stalling tactics, such as asking for one more drink of water.

Warning the child a few minutes before it is time for bed may reduce bedtime protests. Winding down with a quiet activity for 30 minutes before bedtime also helps toddlers prepare for sleep. Bedtime offers an opportunity for some snuggle time, when the parent and toddler can read a story and share the events of the day. Children of this age often have trouble relaxing and falling asleep. A warm bath before bedtime promotes relaxation. Bedtime rituals are important

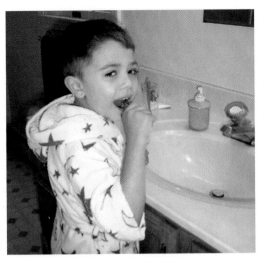

FIG 6-5 Care of the deciduous teeth promotes healthy development of the permanent teeth. Some toddlers and preschoolers enjoy brushing their own teeth, but because toddlers and preschoolers lack the manual dexterity to remove plaque adequately, parents must assume this responsibility.

and should be followed consistently. Transition objects, such as a favorite blanket or stuffed animal, are often an important part of the child's bedtime routine.

Because preschoolers expend so much energy growing and learning, they need adequate rest. The preschooler needs an average of 10 to 12 hours of sleep in a 24-hour period. Some preschoolers do well without a nap during the day, but others still need a nap. Resistance to naps is common at this age. The child usually does not want to leave family or playmates, toys, and exciting activities to go into a darkened room to lie down and rest. A quiet time spent listening to music or looking at a favorite book may help the child relax and get some rest. Insufficient rest during the day may lead to irritability, decreased resistance to infection, and difficulty sleeping at night.

Sleep problems are more common during the preschool years than in any other period of childhood. Because of their active imaginations and immaturity, preschoolers often have nightmares and have trouble falling asleep at night. The boundaries between reality and fantasy are not well defined for children of this age, so monsters and scary creatures that lurk in the preschooler's imagination become real to the child after the light is turned off. Patient and repeated reassurance from a caring parent may be needed. Nightmares—frightening dreams that awaken the child from sleep—are common among preschoolers. A familiar environment and comfort with a hug and verbal reassurance from a parent usually enable the child to return to sleep. Night terrors differ from nightmares. Night terrors occur during deep sleep, and the child remains asleep even though the eyes may be open. The child does not awaken but moans, screams, or cries and does not recognize parents. Efforts to comfort the child may lead to agitation. The child does not remember the episode in the morning, even if awakened during the night terror. Parents should be instructed not to attempt to comfort or awaken the child during a night terror but should allow the child to sleep.

The nurse should assess sleep patterns during well-child visits and address parental concerns. The nurse can reassure parents that resistance to going to bed, fears, and nightmares are normal for children of this age. The nurse should assess the frequency of sleep problems and

parents' reactions to them. If sleep problems occur often and are disruptive to the family, further investigation and intervention may be indicated.

Ritualistic techniques and transition objects that help decrease bedtime resistance in the toddler continue during the preschool period. Avoiding high-carbohydrate snacks and excitement before bedtime promotes relaxation. Children should not be forced to face their fears alone by sleeping in a completely dark room or with the door shut. Parents can search the room to reassure the preschooler that the room is safe. Progressive head-to-toe relaxation is an effective technique for helping preschoolers fall asleep. A set bedtime promotes security and healthy sleep habits.

A child who has slept for a long time at the babysitter's or at daycare may not be ready to sleep again. Communication with the child's daytime caretaker is important to determine whether the child is maintaining a balance of activity, rest, and sleep.

❓ CRITICAL THINKING EXERCISE 6-1

Mr. and Mrs. Thomas have brought 2-year-old Todd to the clinic for his annual physical examination. The parents report that bedtime is a major production almost every night. They state that he cries, comes out of his room, and displays various other behaviors that delay sleep. They wonder if he has a sleep disorder. They relate that, other than an occasional temper tantrum, they do not have any other concerns.

1. What information do you need from the parents to assess the problem?
2. After you have the above information, what advice should you give the Thomases?

Discipline

Effective discipline strategies should involve a comprehensive approach that does not emphasize punishment, but instead promotes the development of self-control in a child (Backlin, Scheindlin, Ip et al., 2007). How a parent uses discipline and the type of discipline used depends on a variety of factors that include the maternal age and cultural background, experiences the parent had with discipline as a child, and the child's age (Backlin et al., 2007). When discipline is used in a positive manner, the child internalizes controls established by parental limits and begins to develop a conscience.

Toddlers need and want discipline to feel secure. They have little control over their behavior and need limits to learn how to behave and how to follow the rules and expectations of society. Toddlers' negativism, intense emotions, and curiosity put them at risk for injury. Because they are usually unaware of the consequences of their actions, vigilance and limits are needed for safety. Toddlers are frightened by a lack of limits and will deliberately test their parents until they are shown how far they can go. Firm discipline promotes the development of autonomy by giving the child a feeling of freedom within bounds.

Toddlers often repeat parental prohibitions to themselves while engaging in a forbidden activity. For example, a toddler may walk over to an electrical outlet, knowing that it is out of bounds, and mumble, "No, no, hurt!" while playing with the outlet. Although remembering the prohibition, the toddler lacks sufficient self-control to prevent the behavior.

Effective discipline techniques for children of this age include a time-out (1 minute per year of age), diversion, and positive reinforcement. Teaching parents how to discipline their child helps avoid problems related to the incorrect use of discipline. Parents must be consistent. Physical punishment, such as spanking, is one of the least effective discipline techniques and is discouraged by the AAP (2011c) (see Chapter 2).

Preschoolers struggle to gain control over their strong inner impulses. To achieve this control, they need limits set on their behavior. When limits are set, the child feels more secure and can explore the environment and try new roles in an atmosphere of freedom and safety. Appropriate limit setting helps the child learn self-confidence, self-control, and moral values. The child must be consistently disciplined for acts that are destructive, socially unacceptable, or morally wrong. Limits must be clearly defined and consistently enforced to be effective. To prevent confusion and anxiety, the consequences of misbehavior should be spelled out in advance and carried out immediately after misbehavior occurs. When the child is disciplined for misbehavior, a simple, truthful explanation of why the behavior was unacceptable should be given.

The focus of the explanation should be on the behavior rather than on the child. For example, "Throwing toys could hurt someone. I don't like to see you doing that" is a better response than "I don't want to be around you when you act like that" or "You're a bad girl for doing that."

Discipline techniques that are effective with preschoolers include the following:

- Time-out (removing the child from a situation for a short period and offering an explanation for the punishment).
- Time-in (frequent, brief, nonverbal, physical contact when the child is acting appropriately). For example, the mother periodically strokes the child's hair or rubs his back when he is quietly playing on the floor near her while she talks on the telephone. The child who receives this type of reinforcement is more likely to continue what he is doing and much less likely to interrupt the mother.
- Offering restricted choices (e.g., "You may drink your juice in the kitchen or you may go into the living room without your juice.").
- Diversion (e.g., "You must stop marking on the wall with crayons. Here, mark on this paper instead.").

PATIENT-CENTERED TEACHING

Guidelines for Disciplining a Toddler

- Discipline must be consistent. Inconsistency is confusing and counterproductive. Consistent follow-through every time is important.
- Discipline must be immediate. Consequences of behavior should occur as soon as possible after the behavior occurs. Threats such as "Just wait until your father gets home!" are confusing and ineffective for a child of this age.
- Discipline must be realistic and age appropriate. Toddlers should not be expected to act like "little ladies" or "little gentlemen."
- Discipline must be related to the incident. Consequences that are logical results of a behavior are most effective.
- Limits must be clearly explained to the child.
- Toddlers must be given time to respond to instructions.
- Withdrawal of love should never be used as punishment. Comforting the child after discipline promotes positive feelings. Love is the key to effective discipline.
- Arguments and extensive explanations should be avoided.
- Praise for good behavior should be used to build self-confidence and self-esteem.
- The toddler must be separated from the behavior: "I love you very much. Hitting your sister needs to stop."

Consistent positive reinforcement for desired behavior is a powerful tool. If the parent does not care or is too busy to enforce rules consistently, the child will not internalize rules and will not feel guilty about breaking them. The child will be unruly and will be unable to follow the rules set by society.

Spending enjoyable time with their children is another way parents can model positive behaviors. Having good times with children increases their self-esteem and reinforces good behavior. Chapter 2 and the Patient-Centered Teaching "Guidelines for Disciplining a Toddler" box present additional discussions of discipline.

Toddler Safety

Understanding the developmental changes a toddler undergoes helps the nurse and parent appreciate why children are more injury prone in this stage of development than at any other time. Constant supervision is challenging for parents but is the most important factor in preventing injuries in this energetic age-group.

Car Safety

Motor vehicle injuries are a significant threat to the toddler. Although toddlers begin to develop more independent behaviors, they are still wholly reliant on an adult for protection while traveling in a car. Toddlers should be secured in a rear-facing, approved car safety seat, placed in the middle of the rear seat until age 2 years or until the child has achieved the weight and height recommendations recommended by the car seat manufacturer (AAP, 2011a). Harness safety straps (used according to manufacturer weight and height guidelines) should be adjusted to provide a snug fit (AAP, 2011a). After age 2 years, toddlers are secured in an upright forward-facing safety seat with a 3- or 5-point harness (AAP, 2011a).

⚡ SAFETY ALERT

Car Safety

Toddlers should be restrained in an upright, forward-facing position in a car safety seat until they outgrow the manufacturer's weight or height recommendations.

Car doors should be locked while the car is in motion to prevent a curious toddler from opening a door.

Until passenger vehicles are equipped with airbags that are safe and effective for children, children younger than 13 years should not ride in a front passenger seat that is equipped with an airbag.

An approved booster seat (high-back seat preferred) may be used for a child who is older than age 4 years or who has exceeded the height and weight recommended by the manufacturer for a forward-facing car safety seat. It raises the child to a level that accommodates the car's seatbelt system. Children usually use a booster seat until they are tall enough to properly wear the seat lap and shoulder belt (height 4 feet, 9 inches and 8 to 12 years old) (AAP, 2011a).

Because children begin to imitate their parents at an early age, the nurse encourages parents to model safe behavior by consistently wearing their seatbelts. As the toddler's cognitive and fine motor skills develop, some children wiggle free of the restraint system despite releases that are designed to be difficult for a child to operate. Parents must insist on adherence despite temper tantrums.

Because of the toddler's short physical stature, adults should visually inspect the area surrounding the automobile before placing it in gear. A toddler near the car may not be visible and can sustain serious crushing injuries if run over by the car or trapped between the car and a stationary object. Toddlers may also dart out on foot into oncoming traffic. Parents need to closely supervise play activities and remain physically close to the toddler to prevent these types of injuries.

Toddlers and infants should never be left unattended in a car, even for a moment. Exposure to extreme heat or cold is dangerous in this age-group. Injuries have occurred when parents have left a car running for various reasons and a curious toddler has disengaged the gears, causing the car to roll and collide with other objects.

Airplane Safety

The lack of regulations to ensure that children younger than 2 years are properly restrained during airplane flights is an ongoing cause for concern. The AAP recommends a mandatory federal requirement for restraint use for children on aircraft (AAP Council on Injury and Poison Prevention, 2001/2009). Both the AAP (2011b) and the Federal Aviation Administration (2011) strongly suggest that infants and children younger than 4 years should be restrained during takeoff and landing, during turbulence, and as much as is feasible during flight. Children should be placed in properly secured age-appropriate safety seats, which have been government approved for both automobile and aircraft, in a similar manner as a car safety seat. The most desirable location of the safety seat is by a window (FAA, 2011). The FAA also has an approved harness restraint system to be used for children weighing between 22 and 44 pounds; parents need to request these restraint systems from the airline on which they are traveling (FAA, 2011).

Fire and Burn Safety

Injuries related to fire and scalds are a significant cause of morbidity and mortality in children ages 1 to 4 years (CDC, 2011b).Toddlers, with their increased mobility and developing fine motor skills, can reach hot water, open fires, or hot objects placed on counters and stoves above their eye level. A child at this age is at increased risk to reach up and pull a hot liquid off a surface or to grab or overturn a container of hot water onto himself or herself. They may pull objects off stoves, pull down cords attached to small appliances, open oven doors, and place electrical cords or frayed wires into their mouths. They may drink liquids that are dangerously hot. The nurse should emphasize to parents to remain in the kitchen when preparing a meal, use the back burners on the stove, and turn pot handles inward and toward the middle of the stove to reduce the toddler's risk of burn injuries. Dangling cords from irons or other small appliances should not be accessible to toddlers. Open fires and heaters are also inviting. Sturdy guards fixed to the wall prevent young children from getting too close to these burn hazards. In addition, curious toddlers are fascinated with matches and lighters, which must be kept out of reach.

Toddlers depend on adults for their protection in the event of a house fire. Anticipatory guidance emphasizes the importance of smoke detectors and escape plans.

Preventing Falls

Toddlers move quickly and climb everywhere. Toddlers can fall from playground equipment, off tricycles, and out of windows. Falls are the leading cause of morbidity from unintentional injury during early childhood (CDC, 2011a). More than 5000 children fall from windows annually and over 50% of children that fall from a window are boys (Harris, Rochette, & Smith, 2011). Falls from above the first floor of a building can result in serious injury, particularly head injury. A chair next to a kitchen counter or table allows the toddler easy access to dangerously high places. Because climbing and exploration are normal aspects of the developmental process, safety education for the parent emphasizes constant supervision and some anticipatory planning, such as moving furniture, installing screen guards, and restricting access to potential climbing hazards.

Water Safety

Toddlers love to play in water. Most drownings occur when a child is left alone in a bathtub or falls into a residential pool. Drowning has become the leading cause of death due to unintentional injury during early childhood (CDC, 2011b) and an increasing number of children are drowning in above-ground swimming pools (Shields, Pollack-Nelson, & Smith, 2011). Even when a child survives a submersion injury, the risk of permanent brain and lung damage is great (see Chapter 10).

The AAP has issued new recommendations to prevent childhood drowning (AAP, 2010). Parents should not leave a child alone in or near a bathtub, pail of water, wading or swimming pool, or any other body of water, even for a moment. A competent swimmer should be within arm's reach when a child is near any swimming area. All swimming pools, whether in-ground or above ground require a "climb-resistant" fence (minimum height of 4 feet) that completely surrounds the pool and remains locked in a way that a young child cannot accidentally open it. Pool drains should be protected by covers that prevent children from being trapped or having long hair caught in the drain. In addition, the AAP (2010) recommends that all children learn to swim, preferably with swimming lessons beginning during early childhood, and that children who do not swim use an approved personal flotation device (PFD) when around or in water.

A toddler can drown in as little as 1 inch of water. Toilet lids need to remain closed. Toddlers can inadvertently fall headfirst into a toilet or bucket, and they lack the upper-body strength and coordination to remove themselves from submersion. Drowning prevention requires constant parental supervision of the toddler. Nurses need to be involved not only with individual counseling about drowning prevention, but also with advocacy at the community or state level for legislation that ensures pool safety.

Preventing Poisoning

Children younger than 6 years are the most common victims of poisoning, with the majority being 1- to 3-year olds (Bronstein, Spyker, Cantilena et al., 2010). The home is the site of exposure in most cases, with poisoning from medication ingestion being the major cause, followed by cosmetics or personal care products and household chemicals (Bronstein et al., 2010). With exploration, everything eventually finds its way to the child's mouth, even if it does not smell or taste good. Small children who are thirsty or hungry will ingest poisons that look or smell inviting.

The nurse can help parents poison-proof the home and teach them the appropriate action to take if an ingestion occurs (see Patient-Centered Teaching: Childhood Poison Prevention box). Calling the American Association of Poison Control Centers'(AAPCC) Help Line (1-800-222-1222) needs to be the first action a parent takes if the child has ingested a poison; the professionals who staff the help line have experience in managing a wide variety of poisoning situations and can assist the parent to intervene immediately (AAPCC, 2011). In partnership with the AAPCC, pediatric health care providers recommend this action, rather than having the parent call the emergency department or their health care provider (AAPCC, 2011). If the child is unconscious, having a seizure, or not breathing, the parent should immediately call 911 or the local emergency number. Medicine should not be called candy, and because young children often mimic their parents, adults should be discouraged from taking medicine in the child's presence. The nurse needs to advise parents to take the same precautions when small children go to a grandparent's home to visit. Child-proof caps slow the child but are not an absolute barrier. Labels with characteristic symbols, such as the skull and crossbones or "Mr. Yuk," help provide visual cues to young children; however, labels are not absolute deterrents for a determined child. The best way to prevent toxic ingestions is by carefully storing all potential poisons in a place that is inaccessible to children. (See Chapters 4 and 10 for information about environmental poisonings.)

PATIENT-CENTERED TEACHING

Childhood Poison Prevention

- Keep all poisons, medicines, cleaners, and toxic substances out of the reach of children. Never discard poisons in a wastebasket.
- Be familiar with poisons commonly found in or near the home, including detergents, drain cleaner, dishwashing soap, furniture polish, cleaning agents, window cleaners, all medicines, vitamins, children's medications, sprays, powders, cosmetics, fingernail preparations, hair care products, sachets, mothballs, rodent poisons, fertilizers, gasoline, antifreeze, paints, glues, insecticides, cigarette butts, plants, and shrubs.
- Store poisons out of reach in areas that are secured with locks or protected by child-resistant safety latches.
- Medicines and all harmful substances should be purchased in child-resistant packages.
- Keep alcoholic beverages out of the reach of your children or locked in a separate cabinet. Do not give sips of alcohol to your children because small amounts can be toxic to young children.
- Children should not be allowed to chew on plants or shrubs.
- Keep ashtrays empty and out of the reach of small children.
- Handbags and overnight luggage of guests in the home often contain medicines or other toxic substances and should be kept out of a child's reach.
- Store poisons or harmful substances in the original container. Do not place toxic substances in food or beverage containers for storage.
- Teach your children to ask an adult before they touch a nonfood substance.
- Poison-proof all areas of the home, especially the kitchen, bathroom, pantry, bedroom, garage, basement, and work areas. Grandparents and other caregivers should be encouraged to do the same.
- Post the telephone number of the local poison control in an area that can be accessed immediately in the event of a poisoning. The Poison Control Centers' Help Line number (1-800-222-1222) will connect to the local poison control number, which is staffed 24 hours a day, 7 days a week. When contacting the poison control center, be able to provide the following information: the substance ingested (have the label on hand for prompt identification of toxic ingredients), time the substance was ingested, and the child's age and weight. Do not administer anything to your child without contacting the poison control center first.

Preschooler Safety

Preschoolers are active and inquisitive. They have greater self-control, but their understanding of danger is not fully developed. Safety becomes even more challenging for the parent because preschoolers are no longer content with their own backyards. Preschoolers are mesmerized by cartoons that depict make-believe situations. They see cartoon characters engaging in daring endeavors and walking away

unharmed. Because of their magical thinking, preschoolers may believe that these feats are possible and may attempt them.

Safety education can now be directed toward the child as well as the parent. Children of this age have a strong sense of rhythm, and songs and rhymes about safety can enhance the learning process. Instruction should be simple, with one concept introduced at a time. Short stories, puppet shows, songs, coloring activities, and role-playing games are all suitable learning activities that help preschoolers learn safety-conscious behaviors.

Car Safety

Preschoolers need to remain in an approved car safety seat until they are 4-years-old or are too tall for the safety seat according to the manufacturer's recommendations (AAP, 2011a). Once a child has outgrown the child car safety seat, use of an approved booster seat, positioned high enough to safely use the lap and shoulder belt, is strongly recommended (Figure 6-6). Although preferable to no restraints at all, standard seatbelts alone can contribute to injury because they fit poorly over the small frame of the preschooler. The standard shoulder harness often crosses the child's face or neck, and the lap belt is positioned across the mid-abdomen rather than across the bony structure of the pelvis. Booster seats are designed to raise the child high enough so that the restraining straps are correctly positioned over the child's smaller body frame.

Parents continue to have primary responsibility for ensuring that a child is safely restrained before the vehicle is started and in motion. Parents must insist that children remain restrained at all times and that seatbelts be used correctly. Although riding in the open bed of a pickup truck or in the cargo area of a van or station wagon may seem fun and relatively harmless, it can be deadly in the event of a crash. Most states require children under a certain age to be restrained in an approved child safety seat at all times while riding in a vehicle.

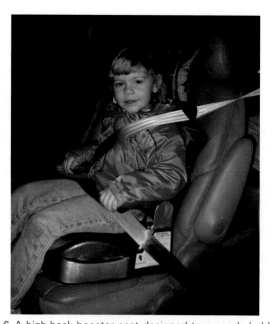

FIG 6-6 A high-back booster seat designed to properly hold a car lap and shoulder belt is strongly recommended for children who have outgrown a child safety seat. Booster seats raise the young child high enough to allow the car seatbelts to be correctly positioned over the child's chest and pelvis. (Photo courtesy M. Hayden.)

Fire and Burn Safety

Preschoolers imitate adults in all types of daily routines and activities. They may attempt household activities before they are able to manage an appliance safely (e.g., stove, iron, oven), increasing the risk of burn injuries. Matches and lighters continue to fascinate preschoolers. With their increased fine motor skills, preschoolers may be able to ignite a flame. Preschoolers should be taught that lighters and matches are adult tools and instructed to tell an adult immediately if they find these items. These actions can prevent burn injuries.

Children younger than 5 years are at the greatest risk for burn deaths in a house fire. They often panic and hide in closets or under beds rather than escape safely. Parents need to practice fire drills with their children to teach them what to do in the event of a house fire. Preschoolers should become familiar with the sounds emitted by smoke alarms and should be taught to crawl under smoke and to check doors for heat.

Preschoolers are at an ideal age to learn what to do if their clothing ignites in flames. Instruct preschoolers to stop immediately if their

---

HEALTH PROMOTION

The 3-Year-Old Child

Focused Assessment
Ask the parent the following:
- How are you managing any discipline problems your child may be having?
- Have you been able to encourage your child to be independent? Does your child's developing independence create anxiety or conflict for you? Is your child in preschool or daycare? How many hours or days?
- How does your child get along with other children the same age?
- How well does your child communicate with others? Do you have any concerns about your child's speech?
- How well is your child doing with toilet training?
- What activities do you enjoy doing together?

Developmental Milestones
Personal/social: Puts on articles of clothing; brushes teeth with help; washes and dries hands using soap and water; notices gender differences and identifies with children of own gender; exhibits sexual curiosity, may begin to masturbate; knows own name and names one or more friends; increasing independence, may start preschool; ritualistic; understands taking turns and sharing but may not be ready to do so; begins to show fears (dark, shadows, animals)

Fine motor: Vision approaches 20/20; builds a tower of at least eight blocks; begins purposeful drawing, can imitate a circle and a cross and draw a person with three parts; feeds self well

Language/cognition: Increasing vocabulary with intelligible speech, although dysfluency is common (thinks faster than can talk); names four familiar objects and begins to describe qualities or actions of objects; knows meaning of common adjectives (sleepy, hungry, hot); begins color identification; uses symbolic language; still egocentric; increased concept of time, space, causality; constantly asks "how" and "why" questions; can count to three; can tell full name, age, and gender

Gross motor: Jumps with both feet up and down and over a short distance; throws a ball overhand; catches a large ball with both hands; balances on each foot for at least 2 seconds; begins to ride a tricycle

Critical Milestones*
Personal/social: Brushes teeth with help, puts on clothing, feeds a doll
Fine motor: Builds a tower of at least four to six cubes
Language/cognition: Points to and names four familiar pictures (cat, horse, bird, dog, man); speech understandable 50% of the time
Gross motor: Throws a ball overhand; jumps; kicks a ball forward

Health Maintenance
Physical Measurements
Continue to plot height, weight, and BMI
Growth rate is similar to that of a 2-year-old

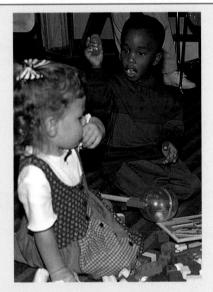

Immunizations
Administer any immunizations not given previously according to the recommended schedule
Influenza vaccine annually

Health Screening
Objective vision screening using an appropriate chart (see Chapter 9)
Objective hearing screening with age-appropriate audiometric equipment
Blood pressure measurement
Hemoglobin, hematocrit, and lead screening
Tuberculosis (TB) screening if at risk
Fasting lipid screen if at risk

Anticipatory Guidance
Nutrition
Similar to that of a 2-year-old
Vitamin D supplementation 400 international units per day if consuming less than 33 oz/day of milk and vitamin D–fortified foods

Elimination
Usually is toilet trained but not at night

Dental
Continue to have the child brush with toothpaste
Parent should floss the child's teeth
Child should see the dentist every 6 months

*Guided by Denver Developmental Screening Test II.

Continued

HEALTH PROMOTION
The 3-Year-Old Child—cont'd

Sleep
Similar to that of a 2-year-old
May relinquish the nap
Consider changing to a full bed if climbing out of the crib
May begin to experience night terrors

Hygiene
Similar to that of a 2-year-old
Remind the child about good handwashing, especially after toileting and before meals

Safety
Review choking on food, street safety, water safety, sun protection, outside poisons, playground safety
Discuss bicycle and tricycle safety, fire safety, car seats (child should be in an approved forward-facing car safety seat until age 4 years or until larger than the manufacturer's recommended size and weight for the particular model)

Self-Esteem and Competence
Model appropriate social behavior
Encourage your child to learn to make choices
Help your child to express emotions appropriately
Spend individual time with your child daily, and encourage your child to talk about the day's events
Provide consistent and loving limits to help your child learn self-discipline

Play
Similar to that of a 2-year-old
Likes imitative toys, large building blocks, musical toys, and riding toys such as large trucks

---

clothes catch on fire and to cover the face and mouth with the hands. They should then drop to the ground and roll to smother the flames. This simple command (stop, drop, roll) can help prevent severe burn injuries. Teaching specific behaviors educates children to remain calm and not to panic.

Firearm Safety

Guns are often kept in the home loaded and readily accessible to young children. Parents should be encouraged to critically evaluate their need for a firearm in the home. Do the potentially devastating risks outweigh any benefits of keeping a weapon in the home? The nurse should talk to all parents about gun safety at every well visit, because even though parents may not keep a gun in the house, children may visit friends whose parents do. Parents who choose to keep a gun in the home should receive anticipatory guidance about injury prevention. Guns kept in the home should always be unloaded, stored with trigger guards in place, securely locked in metal vaults, and inaccessible to all children.

Personal Safety

Preschoolers have an interest in establishing relationships with others as they expand the boundaries of their world. With the child's increasing assertion of independence, parents are less able to provide the constant protection they once did.

Teaching children about personal safety encourages them to develop skills to detect danger and teaches appropriate ways to handle threatening situations. Strangers are often portrayed as evil characters, when in reality their appearance and approach may be nonthreatening and friendly. Distinguishing a stranger from a well-intentioned person is challenging and often difficult for the preschooler. Basic guidelines that a child needs to know about personal safety include saying no, getting away, and telling an adult.

Children need to know how to access emergency help if they need it. Parents should help their children learn to identify safety officials and how to dial 911 or other locally appropriate emergency numbers. Children need to respond to emergency operators with their full name, address, parent's name, and other appropriate information and should

remain on the phone until help arrives. Parents can practice this safety skill with their children to ensure proper reactions in an emergency and help the child understand what constitutes an emergency situation.

Sexual Abuse

Sexual abuse is another threat to personal safety. Preventing sexual abuse begins with teaching children the normal, healthy boundaries of their bodies and what constitutes inappropriate behavior. Often the perpetrators are known and trusted by the child. Abusers frequently intimidate the child into silence with threats of personal harm or suggestions that the child initiated the behavior. Children need to know that no matter how great the threat, if someone is touching their bodies in an inappropriate way, they should always tell an adult. If that adult cannot help them, they should tell as many adults as necessary until the inappropriate behavior is stopped (see Chapter 29).

Selected Issues Related to the Toddler
Toilet Training

Control of elimination is one of the major tasks of toddlerhood. Successful toilet training depends on both the child's and parent's readiness. The parent must be willing to spend the necessary time and emotional energy to encourage the child on a daily basis.

Toilet training is one of the most frustrating and time-consuming tasks that parents face. It can be so frustrating for some that researchers have linked toilet training accidents with many cases of child abuse. Parents who do not understand normal growth and development patterns often have unrealistic expectations and can become frustrated to the point of rage.

The nurse can assist parents by explaining developmental milestones and encouraging parents not to begin training until the child shows signs of readiness. Toilet training proceeds at different times in different cultures. Helping the parent recognize signs of readiness and factors that interfere with toilet training, such as stress, can make the training easier (Box 6-4). The parent may not have the necessary reserves of patience and energy for toilet training during stressful times, such as near the birth of another child or while moving to a new

BOX 6-4 SIGNS OF READINESS FOR TOILET TRAINING

Physical Readiness
- Child can remove own clothing.
- Child is willing to let go of a toy when asked.
- Child is able to sit, squat, and walk well.
- Child has been walking for 1 year.

Psychological Readiness
- Child notices if diaper is wet.
- Child may indicate that diaper needs to be changed by pulling on diaper, squatting, or repeating a word or phrase.
- Child communicates need to go to the bathroom or can get there by self.
- Child wants to please parent by staying dry.

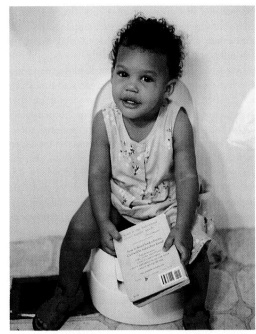

FIG 6-7 No set rules exist for toilet training. The nurse can help parents understand that both physical readiness and psychological readiness are necessary for success.

house. Training may be easier if it is postponed until routines return to normal.

The nurse can assist parents with toilet training the toddler by explaining the importance of maturation to successful toilet training. Parents need to know that both physical readiness and psychological readiness are necessary for toilet training to be successful. Myeliniztion of the spinal cord, which usually occurs between 12 and 18 months, must be complete before the child can voluntarily control bowel and bladder sphincters. The nurse can offer anticipatory guidance to parents by teaching them the signs that the toddler is ready for toilet training. The average toddler is not ready for toilet training to begin until 18 to 24 months of age. Waiting until the child is 24 to 30 months old makes the task considerably easier because toddlers of this age are less negative and usually are more willing to control their sphincters to please their parents. Nurses advise parents to try to be tuned in to their child's individual elimination patterns and responses to facilitate the ease of achieving control (AAP, 2003/2010).

There are no set rules or timetables for toilet training (Figure 6-7). The age at which toilet training is usually begun varies from culture to culture. If the child resists, training may be stopped for 30 to 60 days before it is begun again. Bowel control is usually achieved before bladder control. Some children, however, do achieve daytime bladder control before bowel control, which can be somewhat distressful for parents. Daytime bladder control occurs before nighttime bladder control. A relaxed, child-centered approach, with plenty of praise for each success, is most effective. Punishment and coercive techniques cause feelings of shame and lead to power struggles. The child should not be forced to sit on the toilet for long periods. Successful toilet training is a gradual process, and relapses must be expected. Toileting accidents often occur when children are too busy playing to notice a full bladder until too late. Many children cannot remain completely dry until age 3 years. Parents should respond to accidents with tolerance instead of scolding or shaming the child.

Temper Tantrums

Temper tantrums are a common toddler response to anger and frustration and often result from thwarted attempts at mastery and autonomy. Tantrums may also occur as an emotional release of tension after a long, tiring day. Unable to express anger in more productive ways because of limited language and reasoning abilities, toddlers may react by screaming, kicking, throwing things, or even biting themselves or banging their heads. Tantrums occur more often when toddlers are tired, hungry, bored, or excessively stimulated.

The nurse can help parents by identifying strategies to decrease the frequency of tantrums. Limiting situations that are too much for the child to handle is helpful. Anticipating periods of fatigue, having a snack ready before the child gets too hungry, and offering the toddler choices when possible can minimize temper tantrums. Parental practices such as inconsistency, permissiveness, excessive strictness, and overprotectiveness increase the probability of tantrums.

Toddlers need appropriate and consistent limits. Letting the child know that temper tantrums will not be tolerated gives the child a sense of security. The intensity of a toddler's outburst almost seems to be a plea for someone to stop the behavior. Probably the most effective method for handling tantrums is to isolate safely and then ignore the child. The child should learn that nothing is gained from a tantrum, not even attention. Giving in to the child's demands or scolding the child only increases the behavior. Toddlers stop using tantrums when they do not achieve their goals and as their verbal skills increase. Once the tantrum has subsided and the toddler has regained some self-control, the parent should offer comfort and let the child know that limits are necessary and that the child is loved. Acknowledging the child's angry feelings and rewarding more mature ways of expressing them assist the child in gaining self-control.

Sibling Rivalry

Sharing parents' love and attention is difficult for most toddlers. Often toddlers have intense feelings of jealousy and envy toward a new infant sibling. Toddlers' egocentrism makes understanding that a parent can love more than one child at a time difficult.

Because the infant needs a great deal of time and attention, the toddler's routine is disrupted. The toddler has limited resources to cope with such stress and may react by treating the baby roughly, damaging property, or harming pets. The toddler may exhibit signs of regression by asking for a bottle or pacifier or by using baby talk.

Any changes, such as moving the toddler to a new bedroom or beginning daycare, should be made as far in advance as possible so that the toddler will not feel displaced by abrupt changes when the baby arrives. Many hospitals offer sibling preparation classes. When the mother and infant come home from the hospital, the mother's first concern should be greeting the older sibling. It is helpful if the father or another caregiver carries the newborn, to allow the mother's arms to be free to hug the waiting toddler and express how much she missed her child. A toddler's jealous feelings can become intense when visitors lavish gifts and praise on the baby. Giving an inexpensive gift to the toddler each time the baby receives one can minimize these feelings. Visitors should be encouraged to pay attention to the older child as well as the baby. Parents should anticipate behavior changes, even if the toddler has been prepared for the arrival of a new baby. The parents should be present when the toddler is with the infant to prevent the toddler from inadvertently harming the newborn sibling.

Toddlers should be helped to recognize and identify negative feelings toward a new sibling. Firm limits must be set, however, if the toddler tries to harm the baby. The child may be told "It's okay to feel like you don't like the baby right now, but it's not okay to hurt the baby." Praise should be given for affectionate, cooperative behavior.

PATIENT-CENTERED TEACHING

Strategies to Decrease Sibling Rivalry

- Include the toddler in preparations for the new baby.
- Explain to the toddler what new babies are like.
- Let the child feel the fetus move.
- Read picture books about new siblings.
- Talk about changes that the newborn might create.
- Acknowledge the older child's feelings about these changes.
- Refer to the baby as "ours."

Planned, uninterrupted private time is important to maintain feelings of closeness between parent and toddler. Even 10 or 15 minutes each day while the baby is sleeping is valuable. Allowing the toddler to choose an activity for this time with the parent makes it even more special. This special time should be given to the child each day, regardless of the child's behavior.

Selected Issues Related to the Preschooler

Stuttering

Stuttering, or stammering, is a disturbance in the flow and time patterning of speech. During the preschool years, children often have experiences they want to share but have difficulty putting the words together. Children this age commonly repeat whole words or phrases and interject "uh" and "um" in their speech. As children's communication skills develop, most grow out of their normal developmental dysfluency. Dysfluency may be more frequent during times of excitement when formulating long and complex sentences, or when trying to think of a particular word.

Reactions from others can worsen the dysfluency. Indications for referral include the presence of whole-word or part-word repetitions, sound prolongations, word pauses, facial tension or appearance of discomfort when talking, avoidance of talking, and suspicion of an underlying neurologic or psychological condition (Kliegman, 2011).

Parents can help their child by focusing on the ideas the child is expressing, not on the way the child is speaking. Parents should not complete their child's sentences or draw attention to their child's speech. They should not criticize or correct the child's speech and should advise others to do the same (see Patient-Centered Teaching: How to Help the Child Who Stutters box above, right).

PATIENT-CENTERED TEACHING

How to Help the Child Who Stutters

- Listen closely when your child speaks and refrain from interrupting.
- Speak slowly, and pause frequently. Doing so provides a model for the child and gives the child more time to understand what is being said and to formulate thoughts.
- Designate time every day to listen and talk individually with your child without distractions or competition from other family members.
- Limit the number of questions you ask your child. Do not ask a second question before the first question is answered.
- Observe situations where the child's fluency is increased or decreased, and try to maximize the situations that lead to fluent behavior.
- Look directly at your child when she or he is talking to convey interest in what is being said.
- Recognize that certain environmental factors may have a negative effect on fluency: competition to speak, excitement, time pressure, arguments, fatigue, new situations, unfamiliar listeners.
- Model your behavior to assist other family members communicate with each other and with the child.
- Show your child love and acceptance.

Data from American Speech-Language-Hearing Association. (2001). *Stuttering: Do's and don'ts for parents. Healthtouch on-line for better health.* Retrieved from www.healthtouch.com/bin/EContent_HT/showAllLfts.asp?lftname5ASLHA021&cid=HT and Guitar, B., & Conture, E. (2008). *7 tips for talking with your child.* Retrieved from www.stutteringhelp.org

Preschool and Daycare Programs

A quality daycare program provides an environment in which the child can expand social and play skills as well as manipulate play materials unavailable at home. Working mothers often express guilt and concern about the effect of daycare on their children's emotional well-being and cognitive development. Some concerns about the effect of daycare on the child's development can be minimized by careful selection of the daycare facility.

The nurse is in an excellent position to advise parents about child care. Parents need specific advice about options that are affordable but will not compromise the child's health and development. Parents need to visit the provider or daycare center to evaluate the quality of the program. Areas to evaluate include the attitude and qualifications of the caregivers, as well as operating procedures, costs, child-care and disciplinary practices, meals, safety precautions, sanitary conditions, and the child/staff ratio. The parent should ask to see the center's health policy manual.

The child needs preparation before beginning daycare and information about what to expect in simple, concrete terms. Emphasizing the exciting parts of the experience will help the child view the experience positively. The parent should also explain the reason for separation. Imaginative preschoolers may believe that they are being "sent away" because of some misdeed.

When parents must take their child to a baby-sitter or daycare center, they should give the child an explanation for the separation. A statement such as "I have to work so I can buy food and clothes for the family and toys for you" is not adequate. In response to this explanation, one 3-year-old boy wailed, "But I have enough toys!" More effective would be to explain the separation by saying, "We both have work to do. My work is at my office, and your work is at school."

HEALTH PROMOTION

The 4- and 5-Year-Old Child

Focused Assessment

Ask the parent the following:

- Have you been able to encourage your child to be independent? Does your child's increasing independence create any anxiety or conflict for you?
- Is your child in preschool or daycare? How many hours or days?
- How does your child get along with other children the same age?
- How well does your child communicate with others? Do you have any concerns about your child's speech?
- Has your child's play become more imaginative? Does your child describe any fears?
- Can your child independently manage feeding, cleanliness, toileting, and dressing?
- Have you started giving your child small responsibilities or chores to do around the house?
- What activities do you enjoy doing together?

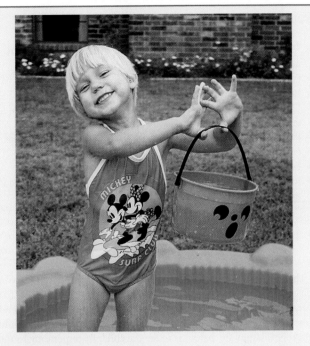

Developmental Milestones

Personal/social: Develops a sense of initiative; learns new skills and games; begins problem solving; develops a positive self-concept; develops a conscience: begins to learn right from wrong and good from bad (based on reward and punishment); learns to understand rules; identifies with parent of same gender, often closely imitating characteristics; aware of gender differences; independence in self-care; sociable and outgoing (might be aggressive or bossy); has an attention span of approximately 20 minutes

Fine motor: Proficient holding a crayon or pencil, draws purposefully; copies circle, cross, square, diamond, and triangle; draws a person with several body parts; drawings resemble familiar objects or people; may begin to write name or numbers; can tie shoelaces

Language/cognitive: Vocabulary of 1500 words; begins to understand concepts of size and time (related to familiar events such as meals and bedtime); understands two opposites (e.g., same/different, hot/cold, big/little); can follow several directions consecutively; uses four-word sentences with prepositions (e.g., on, under, behind); defines five words, counts to five, names four colors; begins to see others' viewpoints; uses magical thinking; very imaginative; can complete an 8- to 10-piece puzzle

Gross motor: Hops on one foot or alternate feet; walks heel to toe (front and back); balances on each foot for longer time; begins to ride bicycle with training wheels; throws and catches a ball; walks downstairs using alternate feet

Critical Milestones*

Personal/social: Puts on a T-shirt; washes and dries hands; names a friend

Fine motor: Imitates a vertical line; wiggles thumbs; builds a tower of eight cubes

Language/cognitive: Knows two adjectives (e.g., tired, hungry, cold); identifies one color; knows the use of two objects (e.g., cup, chair, pencil)

Gross motor: Balances on each foot for 1 second; jumps forward; throws a ball overhand

Health Maintenance

Physical Measurements

Weight increases 2.25 kg (5 lb) per year
Height increases approximately 7.5 cm (3 inches) per year
Compute and plot BMI

Immunizations

Diphtheria–tetanus–acellular pertussis (DTaP) #5; inactivated poliovirus (IPV) #4; measles-mumps-rubella (MMR) #2; varicella #2
Influenza vaccine annually

Health Screening

Hemoglobin and lead screen
Vision
Audiometry
Blood pressure
Fasting lipid screen if at risk
Tuberculosis (TB) screening if at risk

Anticipatory Guidance

Provide information and health teaching to the child as well as the parent

Nutrition

Continue as for a 3-year-old
Provide nutritious snacks (child too often in a hurry to eat at mealtime)
Begin to emphasize table manners
Vitamin D supplementation 400 international units per day if consuming less than 33 oz/day of milk and vitamin D–fortified foods

Elimination

Bowel movements once or twice daily
Urinary output 1000 mL/day
Nighttime control achieved

Dental

Dental examinations every 6 months
Continue brushing and flossing
Child might begin to lose deciduous teeth

Sleep

10 to 12 hours, no nap
May experience night terrors or nightmares

Safety

Review bicycle safety, playground safety, fire safety, poisoning (outside plants), pedestrian safety, automobile safety, sun protection
May change to an approved booster seat if child has outgrown the forward-facing car safety seat
Discuss gun safety, stranger awareness, good touch versus bad touch

*Guided by Denver Developmental Screening Test II.

Continued

HEALTH PROMOTION

The 4- and 5-Year-Old Child—cont'd

Self-Esteem and Competence

Discuss the following with the parent:

- Modeling appropriate social behavior; begin to include participation in religious services
- Encouraging the child to learn to make choices
- Helping the child to express emotions appropriately
- Spending individual time with the child daily and encouraging the child to talk about the day's events
- Providing consistent and loving limits to help the child learn self-discipline
- Encouraging curiosity, and providing formal learning experiences
- Establishing opportunities for the child to do small household chores
- Assessing the child's readiness for kindergarten entrance, and beginning to prepare the child for the school experience

Play

Peak of imaginative play: Misbehavior projected onto inanimate object or imaginary friend; participate in imaginary play; encourage curiosity and creativity

Teach songs and nursery rhymes

Read to the child frequently

Teach basic skills of sports and games

Provide playground equipment, household and garden tools, dress-up clothes, building and construction toys, art supplies, more sophisticated books and puzzles

---

The parent should reassure the child ("I'm really going to miss you today, and I wish you could be with me") and let the child know that separation is painful for the parent as well but is necessary. At the end of the day, when picking up the child, the parent should tell the child be told how happy the parent is to see the child. By responding to the child's feelings, parents can lessen the stress of separation.

Transition objects may help the child adjust to the new environment. Providing the staff with information about the child's interests, home routine, special terms, and names of pets and siblings helps the new caregiver make the child feel more comfortable. Parents should always assure the child that they will return to take the child home at the end of the day.

Preparing the Child for School

Preparation for school begins long before the preschool period. The earliest interactions between parent and infant lay the foundation for school readiness. Probably the most important factor in the development of academic competency is the relationship between parent and child. Parents who are attuned to their child and who structure the environment to provide challenges as well as security facilitate the child's cognitive growth. An interesting environment, combined with parental encouragement and support, maximizes the child's potential.

Parents are the child's first and most important teachers. They structure the child's environment and offer opportunities for learning. Visiting a zoo, fire station, or museum and talking about the experience increase the child's general knowledge and vocabulary. Cooking together, playing simple games, or putting together puzzles also fosters intellectual development. Playing with clay, paint, and scissors promotes fine motor skills and provides opportunity for self-expression. Reading to the child is one of the most valuable activities for promoting school readiness. Listening to stories and discussing them can promote reading readiness. Dramatic play encourages reading readiness by providing opportunities for symbolic thinking and problem solving.

Preschool and daycare programs can supplement the developmental opportunities provided by parents at home. Opportunities to play with other children and learn how to share the attention of an adult are some benefits of a good preschool program. Head Start programs offer low-income children and their families opportunities for

remedial and supportive activities. Kindergarten provides a transition between home and first grade through a structured learning environment. In kindergarten, children prepare for school by learning to cooperate with other children, developing listening skills, and forming a positive attitude toward school.

Nurses can provide parents with strategies designed to promote safety as part of preparation for school. Teaching children about street safety and dealing with strangers and ensuring that children know their home telephone numbers and addresses are important aspects of preparation for school.

Not every 5-year-old is ready for kindergarten. Both chronologic age and developmental maturity should be considered in the assessment of a child's readiness for school (Box 6-5). At this age, boys tend to lag behind girls developmentally by approximately 6 months.

BOX 6-5   CHECKLIST FOR SCHOOL READINESS

- Child is physically healthy and strong enough to enjoy the challenge of going to school and handle the increased stresses involved.
- Child attends to own toileting needs and washes hands independently.
- Child can separate from parent and spend several hours each day in an unfamiliar place with adults and children who are largely unknown at first.
- Child's attention span is long enough that child can sit for a fairly long period and concentrate on one thing at a time, gradually learning to enjoy the practicing and problem-solving activity involved.
- Child can listen to and follow two- or three-part instructions.
- Child can restrict talking to appropriate times.
- Child is able to tolerate the frustration of not receiving immediate attention from the teacher or others; can wait for and take turns.
- Child has some basic hand-eye skills necessary for learning to read and write.
- Child can hold a pencil properly and turn pages one at a time.
- Child knows the alphabet and can recognize some letters visually.
- Child counts to 10.
- Child recognizes the colors of the rainbow.

KEY CONCEPTS

- During the early childhood period, physical growth rate slows (compared with that during infancy) and this leads to a reduced demand for calories and associated decrease in appetite.

- Children's coordination, muscle strength and variety of gross and fine motor activities increase rapidly between ages 3 and 5 years, however, the combination of increased motor skills, immaturity, and lack of experience places the toddler and preschooler at risk for unintentional injury. Anticipatory guidance for the parents about injury prevention is an essential nursing role.

- During early childhood, children's thinking is magical and egocentric. Their relationships with others and understanding of real-world events are affected by these aspects of cognitive development. Negativism and ritualism are behaviors that assist children maintain control over their experiences.

- The preschool years are a critical period for the development of socialization. Children need opportunities to play with others, to learn communication skills, exercise autonomy, and develop ways to get along with others. Preschool children learn to share and cooperate as they play in small groups. Their play is often imitative, dramatic, and creative.

- Gender identity and body image are developing in the preschool period. Sexual curiosity, anatomic explorations, and masturbation are common. The nurse should encourage parents to answer the preschooler's questions simply and honestly. Children should not be shamed or punished for self-comforting behaviors or for investigating gender differences.

- During early childhood children need consistent discipline to learn acceptable behavior and self-control. Appropriate limit setting helps the child learn self-confidence and moral values. Discipline techniques that are effective at this age include time-out, time-in, the use of restricted choices, and diversion.

- Nurses play an important role in health promotion and prevention of illness by advising parents both about their specific concerns and about routine health issues such as ensuring adequate sleep, optimal nutrition, dental care, immunizations, and prevention of injuries.

- Special issues of parental concern that the nurse may need to address during early childhood include toilet training, temper tantrums, sibling rivalry, dysfluency, and readiness for preschool.

REFERENCES AND READINGS

American Academy of Pediatrics. (2003, updated in 2010). *Guide to toilet training*. Retrieved from www.healthychildren.org.

American Academy of Pediatrics. (2008). Preventive oral health intervention for pediatricians. *Pediatrics, 122*(6), 1387-1394.

American Academy of Pediatrics. (2006 reaffirmed in 2010). Identifying infants and young children with developmental disorders in the medical home: An algorithm for developmental surveillance and screening. *Pediatrics, 118*, 405-419.

American Academy of Pediatrics. (2010). Policy statement—prevention of drowning. *Pediatrics, 126*(1), 178-185.

American Academy of Pediatrics. (2011a). *Car safety seats: Information for families for 2011*. Retrieved from www.healthychildren.org.

American Academy of Pediatrics. (2011b). *Travel safety tips*. Retrieved from www.healthychildren.org.

American Academy of Pediatrics. (2011c). *What is the best way to discipline my child?* Retrieved from www.healthychildren.org.

American Academy of Pediatrics. (2011d). *Where we stand: Fruit juice*. Retrieved from www.healthychildren.org.

American Academy of Pediatrics, Council on Injury and Poison Prevention. (2001, reaffirmed 2009). Policy statement: Restraint use on aircraft. *Pediatrics, 108*(5), 1218-1222.

American Association of Poison Control Centers. (2011). *Health care providers and poison centers: A partnership for patients*. Retrieved from www.aapcc.org.

American Heart Association. (2011). *Dietary recommendations for healthy children*. Retrieved from www.heart.org.

Backlin, S., Scheindlin, B., Ip, E., et al. (2007). Determinants of parental discipline practices: A national sample from primary care practices. *Clinical Pediatrics, 46*(1), 64-69.

Bronstein, A., Spyker, D., Cantilena, L., et al. (2010). 2009 annual report of the American Association of Poison Control Centers' National Poison Data System (NPDS): 27th annual report. *Clinical Toxicology, 48*, 979-1178.

Centers for Disease Control and Prevention, Injury and Violence Prevention and Control. (2011a). *National estimates of the 10 leading causes of nonfatal injuries treated in hospital emergency departments, United States—2008*. Retrieved from www.cdc.gov.

Centers for Disease Control and Prevention, Injury and Violence Prevention and Control. (2011b). *Ten leading causes of injury deaths by age group, highlighting unintentional injury deaths, United States, 2007*. Retrieved from www.cdc.gov.

Daniels, S., Greer, F., and the Committee on Nutrition. (2008). Lipid screening and cardiovascular health in childhood. *Pediatrics, 122*(1), 198-208.

Erikson, E.H. (1963). *Childhood and Society* (2nd ed.). New York: Norton.

Federal Aviation Administration. (2011). *Child safety on airplanes*. Retrieved from www.faa.gov.

Freud, S. (1960). *The ego and the id (J. Riviere, Trans.)*. New York: Norton.

Harris, V., Rochette, L., & Smith, G. (2011). *Pediatric injuries attributable to falls from windows in the United States in 1990–2008*. Retrieved from www.aap.org.

Kliegman, R. (2011). Dysfluency (stuttering, stammering). In R. Kliegman, B. Stanton, & J. St. Geme, et al. (Eds.), *Nelson textbook of pediatrics*. (19th ed., p. 122). Philadelphia: Elsevier Saunders.

Kohlberg, L. (1964). Development of moral character. In M. Hoffman & L. Hoffman (Eds.), *Review of child development research*, vol. 1. New York: Russell Sage Foundation.

Kohlberg, L. (1966). A cognitive developmental analysis of children's sex-role concepts and attitudes. In E.E. Macoby (Ed.), *The development of sex differences*. Stanford, Calif.: Stanford University Press.

Piaget, J. (1952). *The origins of intelligence in children*. New York: International Universities Press.

Rozier, G., Adair, S., Graham, F., et al. (2010). Evidence-based clinical recommendations on the prescription of dietary fluoride supplements for caries prevention. A report of the American Dental Association Council on Scientific Affairs. *Journal of the American Dental Association, 141*(12), 1480-1489.

Shields, B., Pollack-Nelson, C., & Smith, G. (2011). Pediatric submersion events in portable above-ground pools in the United States, 2001–2009. *Pediatrics, 128*(1), 45-52.

United States Department of Agriculture. (2011). *Dietary guidelines for Americans, 2010*. Retrieved from www.cnpp.usda.gov/DietaryGuidelines.html.

United States Department of Health and Human Services. (2010). *Healthy People 2020*. Retrieved from www.healthypeople.gov.

Wagner, C., Greer, F., & Section on Breastfeeding and committee on Nutrition. (2008). Prevention of vitamin D deficiency in infants, children, and adolescents. *Pediatrics, 122*(5), 1142-1152.

Health Promotion
for the School-Age Child

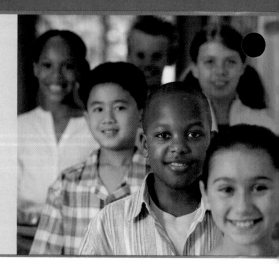

Evolve WEBSITE

http://evolve.elsevier.com/James/ncoc

LEARNING OBJECTIVES

After studying this chapter, you should be able to:

- Describe the school-age child's normal growth and development and assess the child for normal developmental milestones.
- Describe the maturational changes that take place during the school-age period and discuss implications for health care.
- Identify the stages of moral development in the school-age child and discuss implications for effective parenting strategies.

- Discuss the effect school has on the child's development and implications for teachers and parents.
- Discuss anticipatory guidance related to various health and safety issues seen in the school-age child.
- Describe anticipatory guidance that the nurse can offer to decrease children's stress.

Middle childhood, ages 6 to 12 years, is probably one of the healthiest periods of life. Slow, steady physical growth and rapid cognitive and social development characterize this time. During these 6 years, the child's world expands from the tight circle of the family to include children and adults at school, at a worship community, and in the community at large. The child becomes increasingly independent. Peers become important as the child starts school and gradually moves away from the security of home. This period is a time for best friends, sharing, and exploring.

The school years also are a time that can be stressful for a child, and this stress can impede the child's successful achievement of developmental tasks. The *Healthy People 2020* objectives that relate to school-age children include such goals as reducing obesity, improving nutrition, facilitating access to dental and mental health care, increasing physical activity and preventing high-risk behaviors.

GROWTH AND DEVELOPMENT OF THE SCHOOL-AGE CHILD

The school-age child develops a sense of industry (Erikson, 1963) and learns the basic skills needed to function in society. The child develops an appreciation of rules and a conscience. Cognitively, the child grows from the egocentrism of early childhood to more mature thinking. The ability to solve problems and make independent judgments that are based on reason characterizes this new maturity. The child is invested

in the task of middle childhood: learning to do things and do them well. Competence and self-esteem increase with each academic, social, and athletic achievement. The relative stability and security of the school-age period prepare the child to enter the emotional and physical changes of adolescence.

Physical Growth and Development

The school-age years are characterized by slow and steady growth. The physical changes that occur during this period are gradual and subtle. Although growth rates vary among children (Figure 7-1), the average weight gain is 2.5 kg (5½ lb) per year and the average increase in height is approximately 5.5 cm (2 inches) per year. During the early school-age period, boys are approximately 1 inch taller and 2 lb heavier than girls. At around age 10 or 12 years, girls begin to catch up in size as they undergo the preadolescent growth spurt. By age 12 years, girls are 1 inch taller than boys and 2 lb heavier. This growth spurt, which signals the onset of puberty, occurs usually between ages 12 and 14 years and occurs 2 years later in boys than in girls.

Body Systems

School-age children appear thinner and more graceful than preschoolers do. Musculoskeletal growth leads to greater coordination and strength. The muscles are still immature, however, and can be injured from overuse. Growth of the facial bones changes facial proportions. As the facial bones grow, the eustachian tube assumes a more

Video—Muscular Development

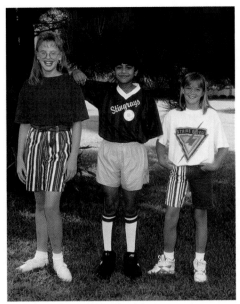

Children of the same age can vary significantly in height and physical development.

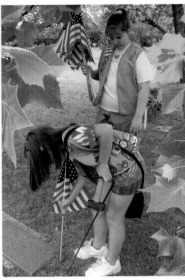

Organizations such as Girl Scouts help foster self-esteem and competence.

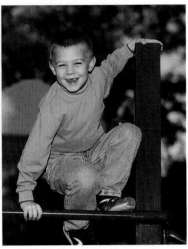

School-age children often have a snaggle-tooth appearance while they are losing their primary teeth.

FIG 7-1 Growth and development of the school-age child.

HEALTH PROMOTION

Healthy People 2020 *Objectives for School-Age Children*

ECBP-2	Increase the proportion of elementary, middle, and senior high schools that provide comprehensive school health education to prevent health problems in the following areas: unintentional injury; violence; suicide; tobacco use and addiction; alcohol or other drug use; unintended pregnancy, HIV/AIDS, and STD infection; unhealthy dietary patterns; and inadequate physical activity.
ECBP-4	Increase the proportion of elementary, middle, and senior high schools that provide school health education to promote personal health and wellness in the following areas: handwashing or hand hygiene; oral health; growth and development; sun safety and skin cancer prevention; benefits of rest and sleep; ways to prevent vision and hearing loss; and the importance of health screenings and checkups.
DH-14	Increase the proportion of children and youth with disabilities who spend at least 80% of their time in regular education programs.
IVP-21	Increase the number of States and the District of Columbia with laws requiring bicycle helmets for bicycle riders (especially for children under age 15 years).
MHMD-6	Increase the proportion of children with mental health problems who receive treatment.
NWS-10	Reduce the proportion of children and adolescents who are overweight or obese.
NWS-17-20	Increase the contribution of number and variety of vegetables, fruits, and whole grains in the population ages 2 years and older; reduce consumption of solid fats (including saturated fats), added sugars, and sodium, and increase the consumption of calcium.
OH-1.2	Reduce the proportion of children aged 6 to 9 years with dental caries experience in their primary and permanent teeth.
OH-9 and OH-12.2	Increase the proportion of school-based health centers with an oral health component that includes dental sealants, dental care, and topical fluoride, and increase the proportion of children aged 6 to 9 years who have received dental sealants on one or more of their permanent first molar teeth.
PA-4	Increase the proportion of the Nation's public and private schools that require daily physical education for all students.
PA-8.2	Increase the proportion of children and adolescents aged 2 years through 12th grade who view television, videos, or play video games for no more than 2 hours a day .

Modified from U.S. Department of Health and Human Services. (2010). *Healthy People 2020*. Retrieved from www.healthypeople.org.

downward and inward position, resulting in fewer ear infections than in the preschool years. Lymphatic tissues continue to grow until about age 9 years; immunoglobulin A and G (IgA, IgG) levels reach adult values at approximately 10 years. Enlarged tonsils and adenoids are common during these years and are not always an indication of illness. Frontal sinuses develop at age 7 years. Growth in brain size is complete by 10 years. The respiratory system also continues to mature. During the school-age years, the lungs and alveoli develop fully and fewer respiratory infections occur.

Dentition

During the school-age years, all 20 primary (deciduous) teeth are lost and are replaced by 28 of the 32 permanent teeth. All permanent teeth, except the third molars, erupt during the school-age period. The order of eruption of permanent teeth and loss of primary teeth is shown in Figure 9-7. The first teeth to be lost are usually the lower central incisors, at around age 6 years. Most first-graders are characterized by a snaggle-tooth appearance (see Figure 7-1), and visits from the "tooth fairy" are important signs of growing up.

Sexual Development

Puberty is a time of dramatic physical change. It includes the growth spurt, development of primary and secondary sexual characteristics, and maturation of the sexual organs. The age at onset of puberty varies widely, and puberty is occurring at an earlier age than previously thought (Biro, Galvez, Greenspan et al., 2010). Onset of puberty is no longer unusual in girls who are 8 or 9 years old. On the average, African-American girls begin puberty 1 year earlier than white girls and by age 8 years, 42.9% of African-American girls, as compared to 18.3% of white girls, demonstrate initial signs of pubertal development (e.g., breast budding) (Biro et al., 2010). The reason for the earlier development among African-American girls is not known; however, recent research suggests that it may be related to food-intake patterns. Puberty begins about 1½ to 2 years later in boys.

Menarche, the onset of menstruation, occurs, on average, during the 12th year, however, with the decrease in the age of puberty onset, the age at menarche is also likely to decrease. Females who are significantly overweight tend to have earlier onset of puberty and menarche. Because puberty is occurring increasingly earlier, many 10- and 11-year-old girls have already had menarche. Wide variations in maturity at this age are a common cause of embarrassment because the school-age child does not want to appear different from peers. Children who mature either early or late may struggle with feelings of self-consciousness and inferiority. Table 8-1 describes the usual sequence of appearance of secondary sex characteristics during the school-age and adolescent periods.

! NURSING QUALITY ALERT

Components of Sex Education

- Basic anatomy and physiology
- Body functions
- Expected changes related to puberty
- Menstruation, nocturnal emissions
- Reproduction
- Teenage pregnancy
- Human immunodeficiency virus (HIV) infection prevention
- Sexually transmissible disease prevention

Because of the earlier onset of puberty, sex-education programs should be introduced in elementary school. Nurses are in an excellent position to serve as resource persons for parents and teachers who are responsible for sex education. Children's questions about sexuality and related issues should be answered honestly and in a matter-of-fact way. If sex education is presented within the context of learning about the human body, with its wonders and mysteries, children are less likely to feel embarrassed and anxious. Regardless of whether sex education is a part of a formal school curriculum, children need accurate information. Basic anatomy and physiology, information about body functions, and the expected changes of puberty should be introduced to children before the onset of puberty. Older school-age children need information about menstruation, nocturnal emissions, and reproduction. Sex education programs must also include information about responsible sexuality and related issues, such as teenage

pregnancy, human immunodeficiency virus (HIV), and other sexually transmissible diseases.

Motor Development

Development of Gross Motor Skills

During the school years, coordination improves. A developed sense of balance and rhythm allows children to ride a two-wheeled bicycle, dance, skip, jump rope, and participate in a variety of sports. As puberty approaches in the late school-age period, children may become more awkward as their bodies grow faster than their ability to compensate.

Importance of Active Play

School-age children spend much of their time in active play, practicing and refining motor skills. They seem to be constantly in motion. Children of this age enjoy active sports and games, as well as crafts and fine motor activities (Box 7-1). Activities requiring balance and strength, such as bicycle riding, tree climbing, and skating, are exciting and fun for the school-age child. Coordination and motor skills improve as the child is given an opportunity to practice.

Children should be encouraged to engage in physical activities. During the school-age years, children learn physical fitness skills that contribute to their health for the rest of their lives. Cardiovascular fitness, strength, and flexibility are improved by physical activity. Popular games such as tag, jump rope, and hide-and-seek provide a release of emotional tension and enhance the development of leader and follower skills.

Team sports, such as soccer and baseball, provide opportunities not only for exercise and refinement of motor skills but also for the development of sportsmanship and teamwork. Nurses should advise parents on ways to prevent sports injuries and how to assess a recreational sports program (see the Patient-Centered Teaching: Assessing an Organized Recreational Sports Program box). Sports activities should be well supervised, and protective gear (e.g., helmets for T-ball, shin guards for soccer) should be mandatory.

Obesity has become a major problem in children in the United States, with 20% of children ages 6 to 11 years being overweight (National Center for Health Statistics, 2011). Time spent watching television, watching movies, or playing computer games often diminishes a child's interest in active play outside. Nurses can help reverse this trend by advising parents to limit their children's television watching time to 2 hours or less per day and to encourage them to engage in more active play. Parents need to provide adequate space for children to run, jump,

---

BOX 7-1   AGE-RELATED ACTIVITIES AND TOYS FOR THE SCHOOL-AGE CHILD

General Activities

Play becomes organized with more direction.

Early school-age child continues dramatic play with increased creativity but loses some spontaneity.

Child is aware of rules when playing games.

Child begins to compete in sports.

Toys and Specific Types of Play

Collections, drawing, construction, dolls, pets, guessing games, complicated puzzles, board games, riddles, physical games, competitive play, reading, bicycle riding, hobbies, sewing, listening to the radio, watching television and videos, cooking.

PATIENT-CENTERED TEACHING

Assessing an Organized Recreational Sports Program

Whenever your child begins playing in an organized recreational sports program, you need to consider the following:

- *Coaches' training:* Coaches not only need to understand how to play a sport and to teach it to young children but also should have undergone a training program in injury prevention and first aid. Check to see that the training emphasizes preventing overuse injuries.
- *Coaches' attitude:* Coaches should have a positive, encouraging manner with children—not critical and demeaning. Check whether the coach emphasizes skill development and plays all the children, regardless of whether required to. Be sure the coach is a good role model on the field and is courteous to referees, other coaches, and the children. Avoid coaches who have a "win at all costs" philosophy.
- *Safety:* Check to see that protective and athletic equipment is used correctly by all children participating in the sport. Facilities and equipment should be well maintained and safe. Be sure your child has enough fluids available and that the child stretches before playing. Children should be divided into teams according to size and maturation level rather than by age. Many sports programs require a preseason physical examination.
- *Enjoyment:* Sports programs can do wonderful things for your child's skill development, confidence, sense of cooperation, and self-esteem. Remember that it is your child playing the sport and not you. Be encouraging and positive, help the child when asked, and cheer the team on in an appropriate manner.

and scuffle. Children should have enough free time to exercise and play. Parents need to role model both good nutrition and exercise.

Preventing Fatigue and Dehydration

Because children enjoy active play and are so full of energy, they often do not recognize fatigue. Six-year-olds in particular will not stop an activity to rest. Parents must learn to recognize signs of fatigue or irritability and enforce rest periods before the child becomes exhausted. Because the child's metabolic rate is higher than an adult's and sweating ability is limited, extremes in temperature while exercising can be dangerous. Dehydration and overheating can pose threats to the child's health. Frequent rest periods and adequate hydration are essential for the child during physical exercise.

Development of Fine Motor Skills

Increased myelinization of the central nervous system is shown by refinement of fine motor skills. Balance and hand-eye coordination improve with maturity and practice. School-age children take pride in activities that require dexterity and fine motor skill, such as model building, playing a musical instrument, and drawing.

Cognitive Development

Thought processes undergo dramatic changes as the child moves from the intuitive thinking of the preschool years to the logical thinking processes of the school-age years. The school-age child gains new knowledge and develops more efficient problem-solving ability and greater flexibility of thinking. The 6-year-old and the 7-year-old remain in the intuitive thought stage (Piaget, 1962) characteristic of the older preschool child. By age 8 years, the child moves into the stage of concrete operations, followed by the stage of formal operations at

around 12 years (Piaget, 1962). See Chapter 4 for a discussion of formal operations and Chapter 30 for a discussion of the child with cognitive deficits, including intellectual and developmental disabilities.

Intuitive Thought Stage

In the intuitive thought stage (6 to 7 years), thinking is based on immediate perceptions of the environment and the child's own viewpoint (Piaget, 1962). Thinking is still characterized by egocentrism, animism, and centration (see Chapter 6). At 6 and 7 years old, children cannot understand another's viewpoint, form hypotheses, or deal with abstract concepts. The child in the intuitive thought stage has difficulty forming categories and often solves problems by random guessing.

Concrete Operations Stage

By age 7 or 8 years, the child enters the stage of concrete operations. Children learn that their point of view is not the only one as they encounter different interpretations of reality and begin to differentiate their own viewpoints from those of peers and adults (Piaget, 1962). This newly developed freedom from egocentrism enables children to think more flexibly and to learn about the environment more accurately. Problem solving becomes more efficient and reliable as the child learns how to form hypotheses. The use of symbolism becomes more sophisticated, and children now can manipulate symbols for things in the way that they once manipulated the things themselves. The child learns the alphabet and how to read. Attention span increases as the child grows older, facilitating classroom learning.

Reversibility. Children in the concrete operations stage grasp the concept of *reversibility.* They can mentally retrace a process, a skill necessary for understanding mathematical problems (5 + 3 = 8 and 8 − 3 = 5). The child can take a toy apart and put it back together or walk to school and find the way back home without getting lost. Reversibility also enables a child to anticipate the results of actions—a valuable tool for problem solving.

The understanding of time gradually develops during the early school-age years. Children can understand and use clock time at around age 8 years. Although 8- or 9-year-old children understand calendar time and memorize dates, they do not master historical time until later.

Conservation. Gradually, the school-age child masters the concept of conservation. The child learns that certain properties of objects do not change simply because their order, form, or appearance has changed. For example, the child who has mastered conservation of mass recognizes that a lump of clay that has been pounded flat is still the same amount of clay as when it was rolled into a ball. The child understands conservation of weight when able to correctly answer the classic nonsense question, "Which weighs more, a pound of feathers or a pound of rocks?" The concept of conservation does not develop all at once. The simpler conservations, such as number and mass, are understood first, and more complex conservations are mastered later. An understanding of conservation of weight develops at 9 or 10 years old, and an understanding of volume is present at 11 or 12 years.

Classification and Logic. Older school-age children are able to classify objects according to characteristics they share, to place things in a logical order, and to recall similarities and differences. This ability is reflected in the school-age child's interest in collections. Children love to collect and classify stamps, stickers, sports cards, shells, dolls, rocks, or anything imaginable. School-age children understand relationships such as larger and smaller, lighter and darker. They can comprehend class inclusion—the concept that objects can belong to more than one classification. For example, a man can be a brother, a father, and a son at the same time.

School-age children move away from magical thinking as they discover that there are logical, physical explanations for most phenomena. The older school-age child is a skeptic, no longer believing in Santa Claus or the Easter Bunny.

Humor. Children in the concrete operations stage have a delightful sense of humor. Around age 8 years, increased mastery of language and the beginning of logic enable children to appreciate a play on words. They laugh at incongruities and love silly jokes, riddles, and puns ("How do you keep a mad elephant from charging? You take away its credit cards!"). Riddle and joke books make ideal gifts for young school-age children. Evidence from multiple disciplines that address the needs of children suggests that children who have a good sense of humor may use it as a positive coping mechanism for stress associated with painful procedures and other situational life events.

Sensory Development
Vision

The eyes are fully developed by age 6 years. Visual acuity, ocular muscle control, peripheral vision, and color discrimination are fully developed by age 7 years. Just before puberty, some children's eyes undergo a growth spurt, resulting in myopia. Children with poor visual acuity usually do not complain of vision problems because the changes occur so gradually that they are difficult to notice. Usual behaviors that parents notice include squinting, moving closer to the television, or complaints of frequent headaches. The young child may never have had 20/20 vision and has nothing with which to compare the imperfect vision. For these reasons, yearly vision screening is important for school-age children.

Hearing

With maturation and growth of the eustachian tube, middle ear infections occur less frequently than in younger children. However, chronic middle ear infections are a problem for a few children, when they result in hearing loss. Annual audiometric screening tests are important to detect hearing loss before unrecognized deficits lead to learning problems (see Chapter 31).

Language Development

Language development continues at a rapid pace during the school-age years. Vocabulary expands, and sentence structure becomes more complex. By age 6 years, the child's vocabulary is approximately 8000 to 14,000 words. There is an increase in the use of culturally specific words at this age. Bilingual children may speak English at school and a different language at home.

Reading effectively improves language skills. Regular trips to the library, where the child can check out books of special interest, can promote a love of reading and enhance school performance. School-age children enjoy being read to as well as reading on their own. Older children enjoy horror stories, mysteries, romances, and adventure stories.

School-age children often go through a period in which they experiment with profanity and "dirty" jokes. Children may imitate parents who use such words as part of their vocabulary.

Psychosocial Development
Development of a Sense of Industry

According to Erikson (1963), the central task of the school-age years is the development of a sense of industry. Ideally, the child is prepared for this task with a secure sense of self as separate from loved ones in the family. The child should have learned to trust others and should have developed a sense of autonomy and initiative during the preceding years. The school-age child replaces fantasy play with "work" at school, crafts, chores, hobbies, and athletics. The child is rewarded with a sense of satisfaction from achieving a skill, as well as with external rewards, such as good grades, trophies, or an allowance. School-age children enjoy undertaking new tasks and carrying them through to completion. Whether it is baking a cake, hitting a home run, or scoring 100 on a math test, purposeful activity leads to a sense of worth and competence. Successful resolution of the task of industry depends on learning to do things and do them well. School-age children learn skills that they will need later to compete in the adult world. A person's fundamental attitude toward work is established during the school-age years.

Fostering Self-Esteem

The negative component of this developmental stage is a sense of inferiority (Erikson, 1963). If a child cannot separate psychologically from the parent or if expectations are set too high for the child to achieve, feelings of inferiority develop. If a child believes that success is unattainable, confidence is lost and the child will not take pleasure in attempting new experiences. Children who have this experience will then have a pervasive feeling of inferiority and incompetence that will affect all aspects of their lives. The child who lacks a sense of industry has a poor foundation for mastering the tasks of adolescence. The reality is that no one can master everything. Every child will feel deficient or inferior at something. The task of the caring parent or teacher is to identify areas in which a child is competent and to build on successful experiences to foster feelings of mastery and success. Nurses can suggest ways in which parents and teachers can promote a sense of self-esteem and competence in school-age children (see the Patient-Centered Teaching: How to Promote Self-Esteem in School-Age Children box).

PATIENT-CENTERED TEACHING

How to Promote Self-Esteem in School-Age Children

- Give your children household responsibilities according to their developmental level and capabilities. Set reasonable rules, and expect the child to follow them.
- Allow your child to solve problems and make responsible choices.
- Give praise for what is praiseworthy. Do not be afraid to encourage your child to do better. Refrain from being critical, but gently point out areas that could be improved.
- Allow your children to make mistakes and encourage them to take responsibility for the consequences of their mistakes.
- Emphasize your child's strengths and help improve weaknesses.
- Do not do your children's homework for them because this will make them think you do not trust them to do a good job; provide assistance and suggestions when asked and praise their best efforts.
- Model appropriate behavior toward others.
- Provide consistent and demonstrative love.

At this age, the approval and esteem of those outside the family, especially peers, become important. Children learn that their parents are not infallible. As they begin to test parents' authority and knowledge, the influence of teachers and other adults is felt more and more. The peer group becomes the school-age child's major socializing influence. Although parents' love, praise, and support are needed, even craved during stressful times, the child begins to prefer activities with friends to activities with the family. As the child becomes more independent, increasing time is spent with friends and away from the family.

The concept of friendship changes as the child matures. At 6 and 7 years old, children form friendships merely on the basis of who lives nearby or who has toys that they enjoy. By the time children are 9 or 10 years old, friendships are based more on emotional bonds, warm feelings, and trust-building experiences. Children learn that friendship is more than just being together. Children at 11 and 12 years are loyal to their friends, often sharing problems and giving emotional support. School-age children tend to form friendships with peers of the same sex. Developing friendships and succeeding in social interactions lead to a sense of industry. Friendships are important for the emotional well-being of school-age children. Friends teach children skills they will use in future relationships.

Children learn a body of rules, sayings, and superstitions as they enter the culture of childhood. Rules are important to children because they provide predictability and offer security. Learning the sayings, jokes, and riddles is an important part of social interaction among peers. Sayings such as "Step on a crack and you'll break your mother's back" or "Finders, keepers; losers, weepers" have been part of the lore of childhood for generations.

Children become sensitive to the norms and values of the peer group because pressure to conform is great. Children often find that it is painful to be different. Peer approval is a strong motivating force and allows the child to risk disapproval from parents.

The school-age years are a time of formal and informal clubs. Informal clubs among 6-, 7-, and 8-year-olds are loosely organized, with fluid membership. Membership changes frequently, and it is based on mutual interests, such as playing ball, riding bicycles, or playing with dolls. Children learn interpersonal skills, such as sharing, cooperation, and tolerance, in these groups.

Clubs among older school-age children tend to be more structured, often characterized by secret codes, rituals, and rigid rules. A club may be formed for the purpose of exclusion, in which children snub another child for some reason.

Formal organizations, such as Boy Scouts, Girl Scouts, Camp Fire USA, and 4-H, organized by adults, also foster self-esteem and competence as children earn ranks and merit badges. Transmission of societal values, such as service to others, duty to God, and good citizenship, is an important goal of these organizations.

Spiritual and Moral Development

Middle childhood years are pivotal in the development of a conscience and the internalization of values. Tremendous strides are made in moral development during these 6 years. Several theorists have described the dramatic growth that occurs during this stage.

Piaget

Piaget (1962) asserted that young school-age children obey rules because powerful, all-knowing adults hand them down. During this stage, children know the rules but not the reasons behind them. Rules are interpreted in a literal way, and the child is unable to adjust rules to fit differing circumstances. The perception of guilt changes as the child matures. Piaget stated that up to about age 8 years, children judge degrees of guilt by the amount of damage done. No distinction is made between accidental and intentional wrongdoing. For example, the child believes that a child who broke five china cups by accident is guiltier than a child who broke one cup on purpose. By age 10 years, children

are able to consider the intent of the action. Older school-age children are more flexible in their decisions and can take into account extenuating circumstances.

Kohlberg

Kohlberg (1964) described moral development in terms of three levels containing six stages (see Chapter 4). According to Kohlberg's theory, children 4 to 7 years old are in stage 2 of the preconventional level, in which right and wrong are determined by physical consequences. The child obeys because of fear of punishment. If the child is not caught or punished for an act, the child does not consider the act wrong. At this stage, children conform to rules out of self-interest or in terms of what others can do in return ("I'll do this for you if you'll do that for me."). Behavior is guided by an eye-for-an-eye philosophy.

Kohlberg describes children between ages 7 and 12 years as being in stage 3 of the conventional level. A "good-boy" or "good-girl" orientation characterizes this stage, in which the child conforms to rules to please others and avoid disapproval. This stage parallels the concrete operations stage of cognitive development. Around age 12 years, children enter stage 4 of the conventional level. There is an orientation toward respecting authority, obeying rules, and maintaining social order. Most religions place the age of accountability at approximately 12 years.

Family Influence

Children manifest antisocial behaviors during middle childhood. Behaviors such as cheating, lying, and stealing are not uncommon. Often, children lie or cheat to get out of an embarrassing situation or to make themselves look more important to their peers. In most cases, these behaviors are minor; however, if they are severe or persistent, the child may need referral for counseling.

Parents and teachers profoundly influence moral development. Parents can teach children the difference between right and wrong most effectively by living according to their values. A father who lectures his child about the importance of honesty gives a mixed message when he brags about fooling his boss or cheating on his income tax return. The moral atmosphere in the home is a critical factor in the child's personality development.

Children learn self-discipline and internalization of values through obedience to external rules. School-age children are legalistic, and they feel loved and secure when they know that firm limits are set on their behavior. They want and expect discipline for wrongdoings. For moral teaching to be effective, parents must be consistent in their expectations of their children and in administering rewards and punishment.

Spirituality and Religion

Spiritually, school-age children become acquainted with the basic content of their faith. Children reared within a religious tradition feel a part of their religion. Although their thinking is still concrete, children begin to use abstract concepts to describe God and are able to comprehend God as a power greater than themselves or their parents. Because school-age children think literally, spiritual concepts take on materialistic and physical expression. Heaven and hell fascinate them. Concern for rules and a maturing conscience may cause a nagging sense of guilt and fear of going to hell. Younger school-age children still tend to associate accidents and illness with punishment for real or imagined wrongdoing. One 6-year-old child hospitalized for an appendectomy said, "God saw all the bad things I did, and He punished me." Reassurance that God does not punish children by making them sick reduces anxiety.

HEALTH PROMOTION FOR THE SCHOOL-AGE CHILD AND FAMILY

It is recommended that during middle childhood children should visit the health care provider at least every 2 years. Many school districts require documentation of a routine physical examination at least once during the elementary school years after the kindergarten visit. If children are participating in organized sports or attending camp, an annual physical examination might be required.

Nutrition during Middle Childhood
Nutritional Requirements

Growth continues at a slow, regular pace, but the school-age child begins to have an increased appetite. Energy needs increase during the later school-age years. Children in this age-group tend to have few eating idiosyncrasies and generally enjoy eating to satisfy appetite and as a social function. Children who developed dislikes for certain foods during earlier periods may continue to refuse those foods. School-age children are influenced by family patterns and the limitations their activities put on them. They may rush through a meal to go out to play or watch a favorite program on television.

Children need to choose a variety of culturally appropriate foods and snacks daily. Dietary recommendations for school-age children include 2½ cups of a variety of vegetables; 1½ cups of a variety of fruits; 5 ounces of grains (half of which should be whole grain); 5 ounces of protein (lean meat, poultry, fish, beans); and 3 cups of fortified nonfat milk or dairy products (U.S. Department of Agriculture, 2011). They need to limit saturated fat intake and processed sugars. Caloric and protein requirements begin to increase at about age 11 years because of the preadolescent growth spurt. The requirements for boys and girls also begin to vary at this age. A gradual increase in food intake will also take place. The nurse should ask children to describe specifically what they eat at meals and for snacks to develop a more comprehensive picture of their eating habits.

When children's nutritional status is assessed, it is important to also assess any body image concerns; be sure to ask children how they feel about the way they look. Eating disorders, although thought to be a problem of adolescence, can begin in the late elementary school years.

Age-Related Nutritional Challenges

During the school years, the child's schedule changes and more time is spent away from home. Most children eat lunch at school, and they usually have a choice of foods. Even if the parent packs a lunch for the child to take to school, there are no guarantees that the child will eat the lunch. Unless specifically prohibited by the school, children sometimes trade foods with other children or they may not eat a particular item. It is also during this period that the child becomes more active in clubs, sports, and other activities that interrupt the normal meal schedule.

The federal government funds the National School Lunch Program, which provides lunches free or at a reduced cost for low-income children. The school lunch program includes approximately one third of the recommended daily dietary allowances for a child. School lunch programs usually follow the dietary guidelines to meet recommended nutritional requirements; however, many school lunches are somewhat high in fat. Some schools also offer breakfast and milk programs. Many schools offer low-nutrient, high-calorie snacks as an add-on to the school lunch or in snack machines available in various locations throughout the school. In some cases, children use their lunch money to buy snacks. Advise parents to communicate with their children about appropriate lunch and snacks in school and to know what is being offered in the school cafeteria.

School-age children usually request a snack after school and in the evening. Encourage parents to provide their children with healthy choices for snacks. By not buying foods high in calories and low in nutrients, the parent can remove the temptation for the child to choose the less healthy foods.

Unpredictable schedules, advertising, easy access to fast food, and peer pressure all have an effect on the foods a child chooses. The child may begin to prefer "junk foods," which do not have much nutritional value. Most of these foods are high in fat and sugar. In addition, school-age children often skip breakfast. The family plays an important role in modeling good eating habits for the child. Schools also have a responsibility to provide nutritious meals for children.

Dental Care

Although the incidence of dental **caries** (tooth decay) has declined in recent years, tooth decay remains a significant health problem among school-age children (American Academy of Pediatrics [AAP], 2008). Unfortunately, many parents and school-age children consider dental hygiene to be of minor importance. Many parents erroneously believe that dental care, even brushing, is not important for primary teeth because they will all fall out anyway. However, premature loss of these deciduous teeth can complicate eruption of permanent teeth and lead to malocclusion.

School-age children are able to assume responsibility for their own dental hygiene. Good oral health habits tend to be carried into the adult years, reducing cavity formation for a lifetime. Thorough brushing with fluoride toothpaste followed by flossing between the teeth should be done after meals and especially before bedtime. Proper brushing and flossing and a well-balanced diet promote healthy gums and prevent cavities. Sugary or sticky between-meal snacks should be limited. Candy that dissolves quickly, such as chocolate, is less cariogenic than sticky candy, which stays in contact with teeth longer. The American Dental Association no longer recommends routine fluoride supplementation for children who are not at risk for tooth decay (Rozier, Adair, Graham, et al., 2010).

Malocclusion

Good *occlusion*, or alignment, of the teeth is important for tooth formation, speech development, and physical appearance. Many school-age children need orthodontic braces to correct malocclusion, a condition in which the teeth are crowded, crooked, or out of alignment. Factors such as heredity, cleft palate, premature loss of primary teeth, and mouth breathing lead to malocclusion. Thumb sucking is not believed to cause malocclusion unless it persists past age 5 or 6 years. However, because of concern about the risk for future malocclusion, the AAP (2008) recommends that children older than 3 years not continue to use a pacifier. Malocclusion becomes particularly noticeable between ages 6 and 12 years, when the permanent teeth are erupting.

Children with braces are at increased risk for dental caries and must be scrupulous about their dental hygiene. School nurses can encourage children who wear braces to brush after every meal and snack, eat a nutritious diet, and visit the dentist at least once every 6 months. Use of a water pick keeps gums healthy and helps remove food particles from around wires and bands.

Braces cause many children to feel self-conscious and may be difficult for a school-age child to accept. However, for some children, orthodontic appliances may be a status symbol. Parental support and encouragement are important to help the child adjust to orthodontic treatment.

Preventing Dental Injuries

During the school-age years, injuries to the teeth can occur easily. Many injuries can be avoided by use of mouth protectors. These resilient shields protect against injuries by cushioning blows that might otherwise damage teeth or lead to jaw fractures (American Dental Association [ADA], 2011). Children should wear a mouth protector when participating in contact sports, bicycle riding, or in-line skating. Custom-made mouth protectors constructed by the dentist are more expensive than stock mouth protectors purchased in stores, but their better fit makes them more comfortable and less likely to interfere with speech and breathing. Wearing a mouth protector is especially important for children with orthodontic braces; they protect against accidental disruption of the appliance as well as soft tissue injury that would occur from the contact between the orthodontic appliance and the interior of the lips and gums (ADA, 2011).

Dental Health Education

Health education curricula need to be designed to foster attitudes and behaviors among children that promote good personal oral hygiene practices and awareness of the risks of dental disease. The school nurse is in an excellent position to educate children about dental health and to detect problems such as untreated caries, inflamed gums, or malocclusion. The nurse should look for signs of smokeless tobacco use (irritation of the gums at the tobacco placement site, gum recession, stained teeth) and should take this opportunity to explain to the child the risks of using tobacco. The use of snuff and chewing tobacco carries multiple dangers, including a greatly increased risk of oral cancer and heart disease.

Sleep and Rest

The number of hours spent sleeping decreases as the child grows older. Children ages 6 and 7 years need about 12 hours of sleep per night. Some children also continue to need an afternoon quiet time or nap to restore energy levels. The 12-year-old needs about 9 to 10 hours of sleep at night. More sleep is needed when the child enters the preadolescent growth spurt. Adequate sleep is important for school performance and physical growth. Inadequate sleep can cause irritability, inability to concentrate, and poor school performance.

To promote rest and sleep, a period of quiet activity just before bedtime is helpful. A leisurely bedtime routine, with adequate time for the child to read, listen to the radio or MP3 player or just daydream, promotes relaxation. Children who do not obtain adequate rest often have difficulty getting up in the morning, creating a family disturbance as they rush to get ready for school, perhaps skipping breakfast or leaving the house in the heat of frustration. A set bedtime and waking time, consistently enforced, promote security and healthful sleep habits. Bedtime offers an ideal opportunity for parent and child to share important events of the day or give a kiss and a hug, unthinkable in front of peers earlier in the day.

Occasionally, school-age children have sleep problems, most commonly sleepwalking and sleep terrors (night terrors). Both conditions occur during deep sleep. Children with night terrors scream and appear excessively frightened; they may be difficult to console during the episode, but the episode is self-limiting, usually lasting less than 30 minutes. Children who walk in their sleep do not respond to their environment and are in danger of injuring themselves. Episodes of both sleep terrors and sleepwalking are frightening to parents, but the child is unlikely to remember the episode on awakening. The nurse can advise a parent to quietly soothe the child during an episode and protect the child from harm. Episodes may increase when the child is under stress.

Discipline

Because school-age children possess a strong sense of justice and believe in the importance of rules, they want and expect limits to be set on their behavior. Firm, consistent limits increase children's sense of security and reinforce the message that an adult cares about them.

HEALTH PROMOTION

The 6- to 8-Year-Old Child

Focused Assessment

Ask the child the following:

- Can you tell me how often and what foods you like to eat? How often do you eat at fast-food restaurants? How do you feel about how much you weigh? Do you think you need to gain or lose any weight?
- What types of physical activities do you like to do? How often and for how long do you do them? Do you have any quiet hobbies that interest you?
- How many hours each day do you watch television, movies, or use the computer (including playing video games)? What is your favorite television program? Do you have a television in your room?
- How often do you brush your teeth, floss, and see the dentist?
- What time do you go to bed at night? What time do you get up in the morning? Do you have any trouble falling asleep, or do you wake up in the middle of the night?
- How often do you have a bowel movement? Are there any problems with urination? (Use the child's familiar terminology if known.) Do you wet the bed? If so, how often?
- What grade in school are you? Are you doing well in school or having any problems? Do you feel safe at school? Do you participate in any before- or after-school programs?
- What kinds of activities do you enjoy doing with your friends?
- How do you get along with other members of your family? Is there a special family member you could talk to if you are having a problem? If so, who?

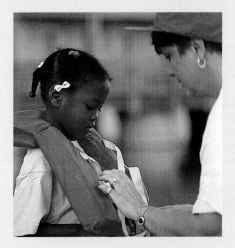

- Do you do any or all of the following: use a seatbelt every time you get in a car; wear a helmet every time you ride a bicycle; wear a helmet and protective pads every time you skate or use a scooter; use sunscreen; swim with a buddy and only when an adult is present; always look both ways before crossing the street; use the right equipment when you play sports; know to avoid strangers and how to call for help if needed?

Continued

HEALTH PROMOTION—cont'd

The 6- to 8-Year-Old Child

- Has anyone ever physically hurt you or touched you in a way that made you uncomfortable?

Ask the parent the following:

- Are there any concerns related to the child's nutrition, body image, physical activity, oral health, sleep, elimination, school, family interactions, self-esteem, and ability to practice safety precautions?
- Is there a gun in the home? If so, is it locked away and the ammunition stored locked in a separate place?
- Do you have a swimming pool? If so, is it fenced on all four sides and not directly accessible from the house?
- Do you have a fire escape plan that you practice regularly?

Developmental Milestones

Personal/social: Develops positive self-esteem through skill acquisition and task completion; peer group becoming the primary socializing force; outgoing and boisterous, "know-it-all," but becomes more reflective and quiet by age 8 years; loves new ideas and places; has a good sense of humor, may tell crude jokes; may be argumentative and use tension-releasing behaviors such as nail biting, hair twisting, wriggling; likes to make things but often does not finish projects; loves family members but worries about them; has a strong sense of fairness and justice—uses rules to define cooperative relationships with others (sees rules as being imposed by others)

Fine motor: Ties shoelaces, buttons and zips clothes, dresses and undresses without help; can print, draw, color well, model clay, and cut with scissors; visual acuity is fully developed

Language/cognitive: Vocabulary expands; understands the different properties of language: play on words, puns, mnemonics, jokes; adapts well to changing physical properties of objects (e.g., conservation, reversibility, identity); improved long-term memory; organizes concepts and classifies in several ways; uses various memory strategies to improve schoolwork

Gross motor: Improved muscle mass and coordination allow for participation in a variety of sports and games

Health Maintenance

Physical Measurements

Average weight gain is 2.5 kg (5½ lb) per year

Average increase in height is approximately 5.5 cm (2 inches) per year

Continue to plot height and weight

Plot BMI and percentile

Note any breast budding or signs of other secondary sex characteristics

Immunizations

If not given earlier, administer measles, mumps, rubella (MMR) #2; varicella #2; diphtheria–tetanus–acellular pertussis (DTaP) #5 (if younger than 7 years); and inactivated poliovirus (IPV) #4

Annual influenza vaccine

Administer other immunizations if not up to date

Health Screening

Objective hearing and vision screening

Speech assessment for fluency

Hemoglobin or hematocrit

Urine for sugar and protein

Blood pressure

Fasting lipid screen if at risk

Tuberculosis (TB) screening if at risk (see Chapter 21)

Anticipatory Guidance

Provide health teaching to the child as well as to the parent

Nutrition

Follow dietary guideline–recommended servings; teach the child how to keep track of servings and to give input into meal preparation

Advise to avoid fast foods and to eat a nutritious breakfast

Watch calcium and iron intake

Vitamin D supplementation 400 international units per day if consuming less than 1 liter (33 oz) per day of milk and vitamin D–fortified foods

Elimination

Regular bowel movements according to the child's pattern; treat constipation by increasing water intake and intake of fresh fruits and vegetables

Occasional bed-wetting is within the norm; refer for more serious problems (see Chapter 20)

Dental

Provide regular dental care every 6 months

Continue regular brushing with fluoride toothpaste and flossing (may need assistance with this)

May need dental sealants as permanent molars erupt

Sleep

Facilitate an individually appropriate sleep pattern; school-age children usually go to bed by 9 PM and are up by 7 AM

If the child is not tired, advise the parent to allow a quiet reading time in bed

Safety

Review gun safety; bicycle, skating, and scooter safety; playground safety; fire safety; automobile and pedestrian safety; water safety; sun protection; good touch versus bad touch; stranger awareness

Discuss exposure to contact allergens (poison ivy, oak, sumac), tick checks, sports safety, use of reflective clothing if out at night

Play

Encourage developing collections, playing complicated board and card games, crafts, electronic and science-related games

Advise limiting television watching to no more than 2 hours a day

Self-Esteem and Competence

See Patient-Centered Teaching box, p. 134.

Realistic expectations, clearly defined rules, and logical consequences help children develop self-discipline and increased self-esteem. Some families have meetings where they discuss how responsibilities in the family will be shared. The child is made to feel more a part of the solution rather than the problem.

Responsibility can be developed in children through the use of natural and logical consequences related to actions. Children become accountable for their actions. If a child leaves a toy outside and it is damaged, the parent is empathetic but does not replace the toy. The parent does not get in a power struggle, nor does the parent verbally

? CRITICAL THINKING EXERCISE 7-1

Mrs. George states that Megan, 11 years old, has recently started to leave her belongings throughout the house and that her room is always a mess. Mrs. George states that she is frustrated and feels as if she is constantly asking Megan to pick up her things and clean her room.
1. What assumptions might a nurse make on the basis of Mrs. George's report about her daughter's behavior?
2. What other data does the nurse need to clarify to best help Mrs. George and Megan in this situation?
3. What are some possible approaches the nurse might suggest to Mrs. George?

attack the child. The child begins to understand that there are consequences to actions. This type of discipline, correctly used, will allow the parent to separate the deed from the doer; not pass moral judgment; focus on the present, not the past; and show respect and firm kindness. In addition, the child will be given choices and the consequence will relate to the logic of the situation.

Teachers' disciplinary efforts are often thwarted when parents do not support them or when they show no concern about their children's misbehavior in school. Teamwork between parents and teachers is essential for effective discipline. Regular parent-teacher conferences help make discipline effective.

Safety

Unintentional injury is the leading cause of death in children of every age-group beyond 1 year of age (National Center for Health Statistics, 2011). Although the death rate from unintentional injury is lower in children ages 5 to 9 years than it is during early childhood, the patterns of injury differ. Aside from injury from falls, the leading causes of nonfatal unintentional injury in children of this age-group include being struck by or striking an object that resulted in injury, lacerations, bites and stings, bicycle injuries, and motor vehicle passenger injuries (Centers for Disease Control and Prevention [CDC], 2011a).

Approaches to safety education vary as the child grows older. Physically, middle childhood is a period of great activity, with the child moving back and forth between the home environment and the community. The school-age child has less fear when playing and frequently imitates adults by using tools and household items. Children in this age-group enjoy helping with adult routines and chores around the home. Anticipatory guidance related to safety is very important as children develop and try new projects that require use of more dangerous or sophisticated equipment.

Safety education is best accomplished by simply stating safety rules and providing reinforcement through short projects and immediate rewards. Role-playing activities and error-detection picture games are excellent ways to reinforce safety lessons. Children in this age-group are inquisitive and will frequently ask questions. The answers to their questions should contain concrete rationales. Group projects with safety topics help foster independent thinking while promoting interactions with the child's peer group.

Car Safety

If the child has attained a height of 4 feet 9 inches and is between ages 8 and 12 years, the child may be large enough to use the vehicle's three-point restraining system (AAP, 2011). The child needs to be tall enough that the shoulder belt crosses the middle of the chest and the lap belt rides low onto the thighs (AAP, 2011). Smaller and younger children can remain in an approved booster seat, which will position the belts

properly in relation to the child (AAP, 2011). Parents should be aware of the state laws regarding child automobile safety seats for school-age children in the area where they reside as well as in other areas when they travel, as most states have specific ages or height/weight requirements for when a child must use the vehicle restraint system. Adherence often is determined by family values, with use or nonuse reflecting parental practices. Children should sit in a rear seat away from car passenger safety airbags.

Fire and Burn Safety

Parents should continue to reinforce safety procedures associated with fire safety. Routine fire drills should be practiced in the home. Repetition of family drills helps ensure that the child will respond correctly and automatically to smoke alarms. Children of this age can better comprehend cause-and-effect relationships, so they can understand why they should not play with potentially flammable substances.

⚡ SAFETY ALERT

Fire Safety Rules

Know two specific escape routes from each area in the home.
Know how to dial 911.
Know how to crawl under the smoke to leave a burning house.
Have a predetermined meeting area outside the house.
Never return to a burning house.
Practice fire drills.

School-age children are eager to help parents with daily chores such as cooking or ironing. Parents need to invest the time to teach their children how to use tools and appliances properly and must establish guidelines to avoid burn injuries as a result of the child's inexperience.

Fireworks create another burn hazard for children. Each summer, many children are seriously burned or permanently scarred by fireworks. To prevent serious burn injuries, the federal government, under the federal Hazardous Substance Act, prohibits the sale of the more dangerous fireworks to the general public. However, a degree of risk always is associated with any fireworks. There are no absolutely safe fireworks for children or adults. Fireworks are best left to the experts and viewed from a safe distance. Encourage families to enjoy the many community-sponsored fireworks displays.

Bicycle, In-line Skating, Scooter, and Skateboard Safety

Mastering the ability to ride a bicycle is a milestone in a child's life, leading to independence. The bicycle is typically considered a toy but is actually a vehicle that is capable of speedy transportation. Bicycle injuries are a leading cause of nonfatal injury in children 5 to 15 years old. Children ages 10 to 15 years sustain more bicycle injuries than those of any other age-group in the United States (CDC, 2011a). For this reason, the public health community supports the mandatory use of bicycle helmets. Research has demonstrated that the use of a helmet can reduce the incidence of head injury by as much as 88% when it is fitted properly (AAP, Committee on Injury and Poison Prevention, 2001/2008).

Bicycle safety practices actually begin when the child is a passenger in a bicycle seat on the back of a parent's bicycle. They continue as the child learns to ride a tricycle and progressively build as the child becomes more skilled and begins to ride a bicycle. A helmet and other safety accessories are essential for protection, but they are only an adjunct to the child's skill level and knowledge of the rules of the road.

A young cyclist is unpredictable and may be preoccupied with managing the bicycle itself. For this reason, parents should set limits on where, when, and how far the child may ride until the child can competently maneuver the bicycle. When parents on bicycles accompany children, it is essential that the parents wear helmets and follow the rules of the road to role model appropriate safety and emphasize the importance of the helmet and the rules. In-line skating and skateboarding are recreational activities that are popular with school-age children. Balancing, stopping, and turning are challenging and require motor skills

PATIENT-CENTERED TEACHING

Bicycle, In-line Skating, Scooter, and Skateboard Safety

- Children should always wear a helmet when bicycle riding, in-line skating, or skateboarding. This safety practice should begin when the child begins to learn these activities.
- Helmets should fit properly and snugly on the head. Helmets need to be lightweight and ventilated and have reflective trim. Write your child's name and phone number in indelible ink on the inside of the helmet.
- Children should be taught not to ride at dusk or in the dark. They should always call home for a ride if it is after dark.
- Children should not ride two on a bicycle.
- Riding barefoot, in thongs, or in slippers is dangerous.
- Children need to avoid using audio headsets while riding a bicycle because headsets can diminish hearing capabilities.
- Encourage children to stay on sidewalks, paths, or driveways until they have mastered advanced bicycling skills and know the rules of the road.
- While bicycling or in-line skating, children should avoid uneven road surfaces, gravel, potholes, and bumps.
- Bicycles should be equipped with reflectors and lights. With their parents' help, encourage children to routinely inspect their own bicycles to ensure that they are functioning properly (e.g., brakes, tires, lights).
- Proper sizing is important when purchasing a bicycle for a child. Oversized bicycles are responsible for many injuries. The child should be able to place the balls of both feet on the ground when sitting on the seat with the hands on the handlebars.
- The child should be able to straddle the center bar with both feet flat on the ground. There should be about 1 inch of clearance between the crotch and the bar.
- The handlebars should be within easy reach for the child.

Rules of the Road

- Children younger than 8 years old should ride only with adult supervision and not in the street. Limit in-line skating or skateboarding to areas where there is no car traffic.
- Children should not ride bicycles on roads with heavy traffic.
- A bicycle should be ridden on the right side of the road, with the traffic. Bicycle riders must obey all traffic laws, traffic signs, and lights.
- Children need to learn the appropriate hand signals and use them every time before turning.
- Bicycles should be walked across busy intersections, not ridden.
- Children need to learn to stop, look left, look right, and look left again before entering a street or leaving a driveway, alley, or parking lot.
- Children should stop at all intersections, marked and unmarked.
- Children riding bicycles should obey all stop signs and red lights.
- Children should look back and yield to traffic coming from behind before turning left at intersections.
- Basic bicycle safety rules apply to scooters, in-line skates, and skateboards.

similar to those required for bicycling. As the child begins to learn these skills, falls are frequent and protective gear is essential. Helmets and protective pads covering the knees and elbows help protect the most vulnerable areas of the child's body from serious injury. Key educational points and an overview of safety principles are described in the Patient-Centered Teaching box on this page.

Unpowered scooters are very lightweight, small versions of an older, more stable type of scooter used by children in the 1950s. They are propelled by one foot and have a very narrow base and small wheels. Because of their portability, both adults and children use them, many times on crowded city sidewalks. Since the introduction of unpowered scooters in the late 1990s, scooter-related injuries have markedly increased, representing a significant percentage of the children annually seen in emergency departments. Injuries related to unpowered scooter use are mainly to the upper extremities, head and neck (Griffin, Parks, Rue, & McGwin, 2008). Recommendations for safe operation of scooters are similar to those for in-line skating, with the exception of wrist pad use.

Pedestrian Safety

Children between ages 5 and 9 years are at great risk for automobile-pedestrian injuries (CDC, 2011a). The tremendous forces of impact and the lack of protection for the pedestrian can lead to severe injury. Children are commonly struck when they dart into traffic, especially where parked cars obscure the driver's view of the child (e.g., crossing the street in front of a school bus, playing near cars in driveways or yards). Several factors predispose this age-group to such injuries. Their smaller physical stature limits their visibility to drivers until too late. In addition, children in this age-group have the misconception that if they can see the car, the driver must be able to see them and will be able to stop instantly. Focused on play activities, they often impulsively dart into the street, oblivious to boundaries and potential traffic dangers.

Children learn traffic safety by watching and doing. Exposure to traffic increases as the child begins to walk to and from school and friends' houses. Parents have the responsibility of practicing pedestrian safety hundreds of times before the child is allowed to venture across streets alone.

Water Safety

School-age children learn to swim well enough to keep their heads above water for a short time at about 8 years old. The length of time they can keep their heads above water and their swimming ability increase with age and experience. The incidence of drowning decreases in this age-group; however, drowning is the third leading cause of death after motor vehicle injury in the 5- to 9-year-old age-group (CDC, 2011c). Adult supervision is still needed to prevent a water-related injury in this age-group. School-age children often overestimate their swimming capabilities and endurance. As their swimming abilities improve, anticipatory guidance can include general swimming safety. Children should be taught to stay away from canals and the fast-moving waters of creeks and rivers. Advise parents to teach children to wade into shallow water or to jump feet first into water of unknown depth to prevent neck injuries. Safety near the water includes never running, pushing, or jumping on others who are in the water.

Selected Issues Related to the School-Age Child
Adjustment to School

Most children are eager to start school, particularly if they have older siblings. They even look forward to bringing home their books and doing "real" homework. This enthusiasm usually fades quickly,

HEALTH PROMOTION
The 9- to 11-Year-Old Child

Focused Assessment

Ask the child the following:

- Can you tell me how often and what foods you like to eat? How often do you eat at fast-food restaurants? How do you feel about how much you weigh? Do you think you need to gain or lose any weight?
- What types of physical activities do you like to do? How often and for how long do you do them? Do you have any quiet hobbies that interest you? How many hours each day do you watch television or movies, use the computer, or play video games? What is your favorite television program?
- How often do you brush your teeth, floss, and see the dentist? Do you take fluoride?
- What time do you go to bed at night? What time do you get up in the morning? Do you have any trouble falling asleep or do you wake up in the middle of the night?
- How often do you have a bowel movement? Are there any problems with urination? (Use the child's familiar terminology if known.) Do you wet the bed? If so, how often?
- What grade in school are you? Are you doing well in school or having any problems? Do you feel safe at school? In what before- or after-school programs do you participate?
- What kinds of activities do you enjoy doing with friends? Do you sometimes feel pressured to do things you don't want to do or know you shouldn't? Do you or your friends smoke or take any substances (alcohol, drugs)?
- How do you get along with other members of your family? Is there a special family member you could talk to if you are having a problem? If so, who?
- Do you do any or all of the following: use a seatbelt every time you get in a car; wear a helmet every time you ride a bicycle; wear a helmet and protective pads every time you skate or use a scooter; use sunscreen; swim with a buddy and only when an adult is present; always look both ways before crossing the street; use the right equipment when you play sports; know to avoid strangers and how to call for help if needed?
- Has anyone ever physically hurt you or touched you in a way that made you uncomfortable? Have you ever thought about hurting yourself?

Ask the parent the following:

- Are there any concerns related to the child's nutrition, body image, physical activity, oral health, sleep, elimination, school, family interactions, self-esteem, and ability to practice safety precautions?
- Is there a gun in the home? If so, is it locked away and the ammunition stored locked in a separate place?
- Do you have a fire escape plan that you practice regularly?
- What types of information have you given to your child about puberty, sexual activity, and high-risk behaviors such as drug and alcohol use? Do you feel uncomfortable talking with your child about these issues?

Developmental Milestones

Personal/social: Peers' opinions become more important than parents'; clubs, with secret codes and rituals, are at a peak; hero worship; fairly responsible, dependable, and polite to adults; boys tease girls, and girls may become "boy crazy"; may become angry but is learning to control it; critical of own work; rebelliousness may begin; ready for away-from-home experiences, such as camp

Fine motor: Hand-eye coordination fully developed; fine motor control approximates adults'

Language/cognitive: Reads more and enjoys comics and newspapers; understands fractions, conservation of volume and weight; likes to talk on the telephone; interested in how things work

Gross motor: May begin to be more awkward as growth spurt begins; may drop out of team sports to avoid embarrassment

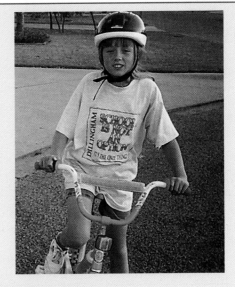

Health Maintenance
Physical Measurements

Girls are 2.54 cm (1 inch) taller and 0.9 kg (2 lb) heavier on average than boys

About 90% of facial growth has been attained

Boys have greater physical strength

Girls may have rapid growth spurt and menarche

Compute and plot BMI

Immunizations

Review immunization records

Administer immunizations if not up to date; some children may need measles-mumps-rubella (MMR) #2; varicella; hepatitis B series; tetanus and diphtheria (Td) if more than 5 years since last dose; give tetanus-diphtheria-acellular pertussis (Tdap) if child is 11 years old and has had the primary diphtheria-tetanus-pertussis series

Consider meningococcal vaccine if child is 11 years old

Consider human papillomavirus (HPV) vaccine (see Chapters 4 and 8)

Annual influenza vaccine

Health Screening

Objective hearing and vision screening (may become myopic as growth spurt begins)

Hemoglobin or hematocrit

Urine for sugar and protein

Blood pressure

Baseline fasting lipid screen

Tuberculosis (TB) screening if at risk (see Chapter 21)

Scoliosis screening

Anticipatory Guidance

Provide health teaching to the child and the parent

Nutrition

- Follow recommended servings according to the dietary guidelines; teach the child how to keep track of servings, to read labels, and to give input into meal preparation
- Advise to avoid fast foods and to eat a nutritious breakfast
- Watch calcium and iron intake
- Vitamin D supplementation 400 international units per day if consuming less than 1 liter (33 oz) per day of milk and vitamin D–fortified foods
- Assess adequacy of diet and snacks

Continued

HEALTH PROMOTION—cont'd
The 9- to 11-Year-Old Child

Elimination
Regular bowel movements according to the child's pattern

Dental
Provide regular dental care every 6 months
Continue regular brushing with fluoride toothpaste and flossing
May need dental sealants as permanent molars erupt
May need referral to orthodontist for malocclusion

Sleep
Facilitate an individually appropriate sleep pattern; school-age children usually go to bed by 9 PM and are up by 7 AM
If the child is not tired, advise the parent to allow a quiet reading time in bed

Hygiene
May resist baths and showers, may wear the same clothes every day, bedroom is usually messy
Early reluctance to keep clean may be followed by a period of overcleanliness (multiple showers daily, new outfit after each shower)

Safety
Review gun safety; bicycle, skating, and scooter safety; playground safety; fire safety; automobile and pedestrian safety; water safety; sun protection; exposure to outside allergens and ticks; sports safety; use of reflective clothing if out at night
Continue to have child belted in the back seat of the car away from airbags
Discuss not allowing others into the home if parent is not there; how to contact emergency services; not to open doors to strangers; avoiding listening to loud music through earphones

Play
Encourage reading age-appropriate fiction, developing collections, playing complicated board and card games, crafts, electronic and science-related games
Advise limiting television watching to no more than 2 hours a day

Self-Esteem and Competence
See Patient-Centered Teaching box, p. 134.

however. Most children adjust well to first grade, enjoying the opportunities it provides for peer interaction and stimulating experiences. First grade may be the child's first experience of being away from home. For these children, starting school may be a frightening experience. Even children who have attended preschool have some anxiety about beginning first grade. Adjustment to school depends on a variety of factors, including the child's physical and emotional maturity, the child's experiences, and the parents' ability to support the child and accept the separation (see Chapter 6).

Peer Influence. School is often the first experience a child has with a large number of children of the same age. From peers children learn how to cooperate, compete, bargain, and follow rules. Peer approval is of major importance as children look to their friends for recognition and support. The influence of peers becomes stronger as the child grows older.

Influence of Teachers. Teachers have a significant influence on children's social and intellectual development. An effective teacher makes learning fun and capitalizes on the child's interests and talents. Teachers guide the child's learning by rewarding success and helping the child learn from and deal with failures. The teacher plays an important role in preventing feelings of inferiority in the child. By structuring the learning environment so that the child experiences success, the teacher bolsters feelings of industry.

The student-teacher relationship is a key factor in school success. Effective teachers motivate students by being warm and understanding, showing interest, and communicating at the child's level. Children value the opinion of such teachers and will work to gain their approval. Favorite teachers serve as role models and are often objects of hero worship by their students.

Even excellent teachers cannot do an effective job alone. They need the support of parents and school administrators to maximize children's learning potential.

Parents' Role. Parents play a key role in their children's academic success. By taking an active interest in children's progress and encouraging them to do their best, parents can foster learning. Positive reinforcement is given for honest efforts, not just good grades. Parents should enforce rules that encourage self-discipline and good study

habits (e.g., no television until homework is finished). The child must create and adhere to a schedule for completing large assignments to prevent last-minute panic. If the child does not have a desk or another private place for homework, the kitchen table or another quiet, well-lighted area should be made available during study time. The television should be turned off during study time and distractions kept to a minimum. Adequate sleep is important for school performance. Parents may need to enforce bedtime rules to meet the child's needs. Rewarding children for meeting deadlines and for being organized encourages them to take responsibility for their learning and fosters skills that are important for success in jobs as adults.

Parents need to communicate with teachers and stay informed about their children's progress. Visiting the classroom and attending parent-teacher conferences and school activities are important. Showing respect and support for the teacher facilitates learning.

School Refusal. School refusal is a descriptive term for behavior that may indicate the presence of a specific anxiety disorder, truancy, or social disorder (Alday, 2009). In the past, the term was used interchangeably with the terms *school phobia* and *school avoidance*. School refusal has been defined as frequent absences from school, academic disengagement or disruption, or dropping out (Dube & Orpinas, 2009). Some school-refusing children show specific fears of school or school-related situations (e.g., tests, bullies, teacher reprimands, undressing for gym); others refuse to attend school because of feelings of boredom or disengagement, and prefer to engage in more pleasant activities at home (e.g., watching television, playing video games) (Dube & Orpinas, 2009). Because some children with school-refusal behaviors have intense emotional distress related to school attendance, they are labeled *phobic*. The confusion over the use of these terms can make assessment and treatment of these children difficult. For an additional discussion of separation anxiety, see Chapter 29.

Children may go to school unwillingly or may refuse and have temper tantrums if the parents insist on taking the child to school. Younger children may complain of stomachaches, headaches, nausea, and vomiting. Older children may complain of palpitations and feeling faint. These symptoms typically resolve when the child returns home.

Helping a child overcome school refusal. In uncomplicated cases, the parent needs to return the child to school as soon as possible. If symptoms are severe, a limited period of part-time or modified school attendance may be necessary. For example, part of the day may be spent in the counselor's or school nurse's office, with assignments obtained from the teacher. The child should be gently questioned about factors at school that cause worry or fear. Specific causes, such as a bully or an overly critical teacher, should be dealt with immediately. Parents must support each other because the child may play one parent against the other to avoid school. It is important to explain to parents that mild anxiety is not dangerous to the child (Alday, 2009). Parents should be empathetic yet firm and consistent in their insistence that the child attend school. Parents should not pick the child up at school once the child is there. Positive reinforcement for school attendance is essential. Encouraging and maintaining peer contacts and emphasizing the positive aspects of school are helpful. The principal and teacher should be told about the situation so that they can cooperate with the treatment plan. More complicated cases require more in-depth evaluation and referral for the treatment of potential underlying issues. Cognitive-behavioral therapy may be helpful (Alday, 2009).

Self-Care Children

The number of children who let themselves into their homes after school and are left alone continues to grow as the number of dual-income and single-parent families increases. These children are called self-care children or *home-alone children,* previously referred to as *latch-key children.* Eleven percent of children ages 9 to 11 years and 36% of children 12 to 14 years care for themselves regularly; 2% of self-care children are between 5 and 8 years of age (Forum on Child and Family Statistics, 2011).

Parents often feel guilty about leaving children alone and may feel concern for their children's safety. Potential positive outcomes of this experience are learning to be independent and responsible. Because of time spent unsupervised at home, the risk of children engaging in problem behaviors (smoking, alcohol use, inappropriate eating) increases. The quality of the parent-child relationship and having parents who are emotionally supportive and establish firm rules play a role in moderating adverse effects on the child in self-care.

Nurses can help families by offering support and education to parents and children to reduce the risks for self-care children. Parents need to know when and how to prepare their children for self-care, teaching them specific strategies for staying safe at home alone. When considering whether a child is ready to stay home alone, parents should think not only about age, but maturity level. Parents can consider whether the child follows instructions well, exercises good judgment, knows how to contact the parent and emergency personnel, and seems comfortable being alone (Child Welfare Information Gateway, 2007). An additional consideration includes the safety of the neighborhood and the home itself (Child Welfare Information Gateway, 2007). Nurses can serve as child advocates by working to develop expanded after-school child-care programs in the community. A number of communities have established after-school telephone help lines to provide information, support, and assistance to self-care children. Nurses should also know the laws relating to self-care in their state of practice, as some states have established a minimum age at which children may be left home alone.

Obesity

When intake of food exceeds expenditure, the excess is stored as fat. Obesity is an excessive accumulation of fat in the body and is assessed in children as a body mass index (BMI) that exceeds the 95th percentile for age.

Obesity can be a precursor of hyperlipidemia, sleep apnea, cholelithiasis (gallstones), orthopedic problems, hypertension, and diabetes. In addition, children who are obese can have psychosocial difficulties, particularly in the areas of self-esteem and body image (Cornette, 2008; United States Preventive Services Task Force [USPSTF], 2010). Because the obese child develops increased numbers of fat cells, which are carried into adulthood, preventing obesity in childhood can reduce the risk of obesity in adulthood and plays a role in preventing disease.

Cultural, genetic, behavioral, environmental, and socioeconomic factors are linked to childhood obesity (Barlow, 2007). Children with low metabolic rates and more fat cells tend to gain more weight. Of the 17% of children in the United States who are obese, prevalence is highest in Hispanic boys, non-Hispanic black girls, and those of low socioeconomic status (CDC, 2011b). Family influences in the development of childhood obesity are extremely strong, with inconsistent patterns of eating within families related to childhood obesity (Kime, 2009). Children with one or both parents overweight are at increased risk for obesity (Gahagan, 2011). Obese children also are at risk for developing metabolic (insulin resistance) syndrome (Bindler, Massey, Shultz, et al., 2007; Daniels, Greer, & the Committee on Nutrition, 2008). Features of this syndrome include obesity, elevated lipid levels, increased blood pressure, and elevated fasting blood sugar (Daniels et al., 2008). It is often difficult to isolate factors contributing to obesity in a family in which the parents are obese. When a parent lacks nutritional knowledge, it is reflected in the meals and snacks provided in the home. The child is at risk for development of the same habits. Unstructured meals, "meals on the run," and meals at fast-food restaurants can lack proper nutrition and be high in calories. Lack of exercise also contributes to obesity. Studies have shown that, as school-age children get older, they are less likely to be involved in regular physical exercise (CDC, 2007). The child who is given food for reward or punishment attaches more to eating than gaining nutrition. Some people still think that a fat baby is a healthy baby. This type of thinking leads to overfeeding.

Unfortunately, the long-term success rate for the elimination of childhood obesity is poor. Positive outcomes are increased when the child has a support system and understands the importance of diet and exercise.

Assessing the Scope of the Problem. The child who is obese looks overweight. Experts define childhood overweight as being a BMI between the 85th and 94th percentile for age and gender; BMI greater than or equal to the 95th percentile characterizes obesity (USPSTF, 2010).

Generally, obesity is caused by increased calorie intake combined with decreased physical activity. The amount of time spent watching television, at a computer, and playing video games takes away from time the child could be participating in active exercise. The possibility of disease as a contributing factor must be evaluated. Increased weight gain has been associated with central nervous system tumors, hypothyroidism, Cushing syndrome, and Turner syndrome.

Prevention. Early identification of risk factors can target the child who needs special attention and support. All children should be taught healthy eating habits and the importance of regular exercise. School- and community-based interventions can, along with regular guidance from health providers, assist with obesity prevention. The USPSTF (2010) has provided evidence that an appropriate screening and counseling program throughout childhood can prevent obesity. The AAP (Barlow, 2007) recommends regular assessment of obesity risk beginning in infancy, combined with counseling about appropriate dietary and physical activity requirements of childhood, as obesity prevention measures.

Interventions and Anticipatory Guidance. A successful program that addresses weight control in school-age children involves a combination of physical activity, nutrition education, goal setting, and improving self-esteem (USPSTF, 2010). Take a dietary history and evaluate the child's eating habits and patterns. The child or parents (or both) should keep a food diary for 1 week. The diary should include the time, place, and type and amount of food eaten and the reason for eating. The general dietary habits of the family should also be assessed.

One of the key elements of successful weight reduction in the child or adolescent is ownership by the child of whatever plan is proposed. Care should be taken to avoid a power struggle between the parent and child. Obviously the young child will need more parental involvement than the older child or adolescent. The family should be willing to support the child but should not take on the role of watchdog (see the Patient-Centered Teaching: How to Prevent and Manage Obesity box).

PATIENT-CENTERED TEACHING
How to Prevent and Manage Obesity

You can help prevent and manage obesity in your child by doing the following:
- Do not use food as a reward.
- Establish consistent times for meals and snacks and discourage in-between eating.
- Offer only healthy food options (ask the child to choose between an apple or popcorn, not an apple or a cookie).
- Avoid keeping unhealthy food in the house and minimize trips to fast-food restaurants.
- Be a role model by improving your own eating habits and levels of activity.
- Encourage the child to do fun, physical activities with the family.
- Praise the child for making appropriate food choices and for increasing physical-activity levels.

Caloric requirements vary depending on the age and gender of the child. By changing the obese child's lifestyle to include exercise and nutritious foods in smaller servings, the possibility of success is increased. Teach the family and child how to select and prepare foods that are tasty and how to restrict serving size. Reading labels assists with healthier food choices. The nurse should be mindful of considering cultural food preferences and traditions and including them in the child's daily meal plan, if possible. Teach family members how to assess culturally significant foods for nutritional value and encourage the family to provide a variety of foods from all the food groups (Sealy, 2010). The child's favorite foods should be identified and incorporated whenever possible. Because snacks are an important aspect in childhood nutrition, nutritious snacks should be identified. Involving the whole family will create family behaviors that support the child's new eating and activity behaviors.

The parent needs to limit television and computer game time. Children should be involved in regular physical exercise at school and at home. Children can be encouraged to ride their bicycles or to walk rather than ride in a car to a friend's house to play. Planned physical activities should be part of the child's after-school and weekend routine.

Some older children and adolescents may find success in a support group, such as Weight Watchers or Overeaters Anonymous. Some

EVIDENCE-BASED PRACTICE
Family Influence on Obesity

Evidence Level VI

Childhood overweight and obesity is a concerning issue in American children and, because of its increasing prevalence, addressing it is a priority in the *Healthy People 2020* goals. Statistics demonstrate that obesity is a particular problem for boys, poor children, and children from certain minority populations (National Center for Health Statistics, 2011). Although it is generally acknowledged that causes of obesity are multifactorial (e.g., genetic, environmental, cultural, and behavioral), Kelly and Patterson (2006) state that there is little research available that describes the ways parents, in particular, influence childhood obesity.

Using an evidence level VI qualitative study design, in which they conducted focus groups with 17 caretakers of young school-age children from a low-income urban community, Kelly and Patterson (2006) aimed to describe three aspects of caretakers' influences on the dietary patterns of their children—perceptions about nutrition, choices made when preparing meals, and barriers/facilitators for choosing and providing a healthy diet given the restrictions of the urban environment (e.g., no grocery stores nearby, readily available fast-food restaurants). The study design allowed the researchers to gather information gained by participants' piggybacking ideas that they might not have shared in individual interviews.

Verbatim transcripts of the audiotaped focus sessions were analyzed by qualitative research software and the researchers, and significant statements were categorized into major themes that addressed the goals of the study. Participants expressed the desire to provide healthy foods for their children and tried to balance healthy alternatives with unhealthy meals, but identified a variety of obstacles to doing so. Among other overlapping themes that can enlighten nursing practice are the following (Kelly & Patterson, 2006):
- Although caretakers appeared knowledgeable about nutrition principles and healthy eating, they were not as knowledgeable about how unhealthy eating could affect their children immediately and in the future.
- Healthy foods are more expensive, are less available in an urban setting, and take more time to prepare than less healthy foods.
- Financial constraints influenced food choices. Restaurants where large quantities of food were available for a reasonable price were preferred for families where both time to prepare food and finances were limited.
- Tradition, family rituals, and cultural food preferences are important vehicles for transmitting food preferences and eating habits. Parents are role models for their children's eating patterns.
- Government programs, such as WIC, do not offer fresh fruits and vegetables as part of their programs.
- Positive nutritional habits are integrally related to an overall lifestyle and competing needs.

If you were assisting a school nurse to develop an educational program to improve nutrition and reduce the prevalence of obesity in the children in the school, what considerations would you think to be most important, given the results of this study? What types of advocacy issues are raised by the study results? Think about what steps you might take to address these issues.

Kelly, L., & Patterson, B. (2006). Childhood nutrition: Perceptions of caretakers in a low-income urban setting. *Journal of School Nursing, 22*(6), 345-351.

centers have a special group for children. Other support groups may be associated with schools, summer camps, and children's hospitals in the community.

A team approach is often necessary for successful weight reduction. Psychological support may be essential for the child and family to be successful. A registered dietitian can provide expertise in the identification and planning of foods that are not only nutritional but also items that the child likes.

The school nurse can assist children and families both by addressing individual needs and by advocating for healthy food practices within the school setting. The CDC reports that school districts have made some progress with providing regular recess time and reducing low-nutrient foods in snack machines and school lunches (CDC, 2007). Problems that still need to be addressed, however, include the availability of soda and lack of regular daily physical education programs. Nurses can assist with developing wellness policies that address nutrition and physical exercise within the school setting.

Stress

Today's children are subjected to stress as no generation has been before. Alarming increases in drug abuse, childhood suicide, child abduction and murder, and school failure attest to the overwhelming stress that children experience. Rapid, bewildering social change and ever-increasing demands for achievement often pressure children to grow up too quickly.

Stressed children may not show serious symptoms during childhood but may develop patterns of emotional response that can lead to serious illness as adults (Box 7-2).

Sources of Stress in Children. Growing up is stressful, even for well-adjusted children with loving, supportive families. Children experience stress from societal change, family relationships, school, competitive athletics, rushed schedules, and the media.

Middle-class children in particular are pressured to grow up quickly. Achievement-oriented parents, focused on success and financial gain, often view children as extensions of themselves and unwittingly expect too much of their children. Pressure on children to succeed, to win, and to be the best and brightest is great, especially when parents value academic achievement. Children are often pressured into a frenzied schedule of music, dance, sport, and art lessons and may have little time for family meals or playing with friends. Self-esteem and peer relationships often suffer. Byrne, Thomas, Burchell et al., (2011) researched the primary daily stressors experienced by school-aged children. They found that stressors can be categorized into three main areas—family, peers, and school—and relate often to transitions in development. School-age children describe frequent stressors to include problems in relationships with friends (moodiness, arguments), impatient or upset parents, illness or injury of a family member, concerns about schoolwork or homework, being victims of inappropriate touching, and not being listened to by others (Byrne et al., 2011). Economically deprived children must cope with an even greater burden of stress. Faced with the dangers of violence, drug and alcohol addiction, and gangs, these children must fight daily for survival. Children from lower-income families travel dangerous streets to and from school and suffer from the insecurity and uncertainty of poverty. Children who are homeless—as is increasingly common—have the added stress of living on the street or in shelters and having decreased access to appropriate nutritional, health, and educational resources.

School pressures. School can be a source of stress for children. Some children are unable to cope with the competitive, test-regulated curricula of school. They find it difficult to keep up with the unrelenting academic pressure. School imposes long-term stress on these children, and they tend to dislike school and stay home whenever they can. They are often tardy and may abuse alcohol and drugs. Eventually, they may drop out of school. These children rarely return to complete their education.

Other children, particularly those who are academically gifted, find school stressful because it is tedious or uninteresting. Boredom can be stressful. Meaningless, repetitive schoolwork can cause bright, talented children to become chronically fatigued, inattentive, and careless.

Physical threats. Children also face other types of stress at school. Violence and theft in schools are national problems. School-age children commonly voice fears of being beaten up or held up. The child who leaves a bicycle unlocked or a watch or jacket unattended quickly learns the hazards of such carelessness. Students who abuse drugs or participate in gang activity create a pervasive attitude of wariness and fear and are a real source of stress for children.

Competitive sports. Participation in competitive sports is stressful for some children. Fear of failure, especially in front of a cheering crowd, can be overwhelming. Some parents contribute to competitive stress by overemphasizing the importance of winning. Because of their own needs or interests, some parents push their children to participate in organized sports at an early age (Figure 7-2).

Tight schedules and adaptation overload. As the number of single parents and working mothers increases, so does the stress on children who must adapt to parents' work schedules. Many children are rushed from home to school to carpool to daycare or a babysitter. Children must draw on their energy reserves to exercise self-control in these varying situations and may not be able to cope. Fatigue and exhaustion from such demands often result in behavioral problems and regression.

Family pressures. In today's mobile society it is not unusual for families to move and for children to have to leave other family members and friends. Attending a new school, making new friends, and losing former support systems can be very stressful for children. This happens at a time when one or both parents are also making major adjustments in their lives, and they may not have the time and energy to meet all of the child's needs.

Overhearing parents quarrel produces anxiety and fear in children and erodes a child's sense of security. Some parents, although physically present, may be emotionally unavailable to children because of their own stresses. Divorce and separation are especially painful. Changes frequently caused by divorce, such as moving to a new house, attending a new school, and, usually the most stressful of all, separation from one of the parents, can cause great stress for children.

Media influence. The media are a common source of stress for today's children. Sexual and violent material portraying loss of

---

BOX 7-2 MANIFESTATIONS OF STRESS IN CHILDREN

How children perceive stress influences its effects. It is not just the stress but how the child perceives and responds to the stress that determines whether the child has symptoms of stress.

Intervention is needed when a child shows the following signs of stress:

- Unhappiness, moodiness
- Irritability, increased aggressive behavior
- Fatigue, inability to concentrate
- Hyperactivity
- Changes in eating or sleeping habits
- Physical complaints (nausea, headaches, stomachaches)
- Bed-wetting
- Substance abuse
- Diminished school performance

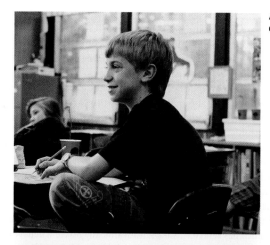

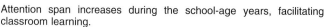

Attention span increases during the school-age years, facilitating classroom learning.

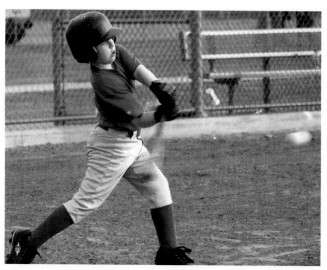

The nurse is in an excellent position to help parents and children identify factors that produce stress and to suggest ways to cope with its effects. Participation in competitive sports is stressful for some children, especially if parents push their child to play organized sports at an early age or overemphasize the importance of winning. Focusing on having fun and on the excitement of the game decreases competitive stress.

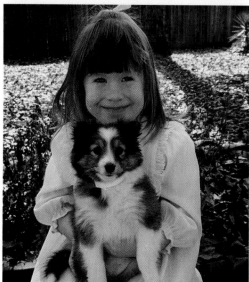

Spending time playing with and caring for pets can be fun and relaxing. Children who are given time and encouragement to play are better able to deal with the stresses of life.

FIG 7-2 Health promotion for the school-age child and family.

control may frighten children because it suggests that they may not be able to master their own sexual and aggressive impulses. Television exposes children to vivid portrayals of the problems of today's society for many hours of their day. It also tends to isolate children from their parents and peers. Hours spent watching television can limit children's participation in more creative play and contact and interaction with others.

The AAP (2009a) issued a policy statement on violent media exposure, which suggested that prolonged or frequent exposure to violence in the media can "desensitize" children to violence, and lead to violent behavior toward others and emotional difficulties (irrational fears, nightmares). Specific recommendations from the AAP include assessing media exposure at every well-child visit; encouraging parents to support the recommended daily limits for television and computer time; advising parents to be aware of potentially violent videos, programs, or computer games; and advocating for more positive media to be available for children along with an accurate rating system for various forms of media (AAP, 2009a).

Interventions and Anticipatory Guidance. The nurse is in an ideal position to help parents and children identify factors that produce stress and to suggest ways to cope with its effects. Parents can meet basic psychological needs, influence self-esteem, shape values, control exposure to stressful events, and provide support. Parents may need guidance about realistic expectations from their children. Parents should watch for behavior changes in their children that may indicate signs of stress and offer appropriate reassurance. If significant tension is in the home, parents can try to resolve conflicts by negotiating rather than continuing to build an emotionally charged atmosphere. Parents should examine the child's schedule to make sure the child is not overburdened with school and extracurricular activities.

Close communication with teachers is important to prevent and deal with school-related stress. Becoming interested in and involved with the child's schoolwork conveys support and caring. Parents need to become active in parent-teacher associations and other community organizations to find solutions to the problems of violence and crime in the schools.

! NURSING QUALITY ALERT

Sources of Stress for School-Age Children

- Societal change
- School
- Competitive sports
- Tight schedules
- Family pressures
- Influence of the media
- Being bullied
- Fear of violence
- Chaotic living conditions

Children should be allowed to decide whether to participate in competitive athletics. It is important for parents to talk to coaches to determine what is expected of their children. Corrective instruction rather than punishment should be given for errors. A parent should serve as a role model for good sportsmanship.

Limiting the number of hours that children watch television and helping them select appropriate programs can decrease its negative effects. Watching television with children and discussing the content of programs are also helpful.

Children need to have time just to play. Parents should recognize that play is the child's work. Whether it is shooting baskets in the driveway, working on a collection, or building a model, play reduces stress for children. Toys and games that provide the greatest opportunity to use imagination are the best stress relievers. Most children love animals. Spending time playing with and caring for pets can be relaxing and fun. Children who are given the time and encouragement to play are better able to deal with the stresses of life (see Chapter 4).

One of the most effective antidotes for childhood stress is a loving, attentive parent who takes the time to listen. A sympathetic adult who understands the stresses of childhood can offer valuable support. Discussion and modeling of ways to deal with the inevitable stresses of life can teach the child valuable lessons for living in today's society.

Peer Victimization

Peer victimization, often called bullying, is becoming a significant problem for school-age children and adolescents in the United States. Its prevalence has been difficult to determine because there is no standard definition, which makes measurement less accurate (Turner, Finkelhor, Hamby et al., 2011). To accurately measure the prevalence of peer victimization, Turner et al. (2011) defined it as being comprised of six different aspects: physical assault (attacking, pushing); physical intimidation; emotional victimization (berating, isolating, teasing, name calling); sexual victimization; property victimization (robbery, destruction of property); and Internet bullying (cyberbullying). Using a national sample of nearly 3000 children, Turner et al. (2011) found that primary causes of peer victimization in school-age children are emotional, physical intimidation, and property victimization. Although Internet harassment is not common in young school age children, it increases during the late school-age years and, in adolescence, 5.6% report cyberbullying (Turner et al., 2011). Victimization can occur both in school and outside of school, and the underlying mechanism that causes emotional and psychological consequences of bullying in children is feelings of powerlessness (United States Department of Health and Human Services [USDHHS], 2011).

The signs that may indicate a child is being bullied are similar to signs of other types of stress and include nonspecific ailments or complaints, withdrawal, depression, school refusal, and decreased school performance (Weston, 2010). Children may express fear of going to school or ask to be driven instead of riding the school bus. Some children spend inordinate amounts of time in the school nurse's office with vague complaints. Other children will have belongings that are missing or damaged for no known reason. Very often children will not talk about what is happening to them.

Nurses should encourage parents to be "tuned in" to their children, to identify when there are problems with children being bullied, or with possible bullying behavior in their child. Parents can be encouraged to talk with their children about bullying, empathize with the child who is being bullied, and reassure their child that it is not the child's fault (USDHHS, 2011). A strategy that helps children deal with victimization includes role-playing actions to take when being bullied (speak up, walk away, don't retaliate, tell someone). It is most important for the parent to emphasize that no one should be bullied. Notifying the child's school can ensure that the child will be monitored in the school setting (USDHHS, 2011).

If parents think their child is bullying others, intervention is also warranted. Children who victimize other children can have long-term emotional consequences. Talking with the child, setting limits, stating that bullying is unacceptable, emphasizing the child's positive characteristics, and using appropriate discipline for misbehavior are all interventions to reduce bullying behavior (USDHHS, 2011).

The AAP (2009b) discusses the role of the pediatrician in violence prevention. The AAP has sponsored a program called *Connected Kids: Safe, Strong, and Secure*, which has resources for professionals and parents to manage bullying. Many school districts have introduced a variety of anti-bullying programs; school nurses are often involved with planning and executing these programs. Additional information and resources are available through www.stopbullying.gov, a website maintained by the USDHHS.

▌ KEY CONCEPTS

- Slow, steady physical growth (steady increases in height and weight, increased muscle mass, and maturation of body systems) and rapid social, emotional, moral, and cognitive development characterize the school-age period, from 6 to 12 years. During the school-age years, children gradually move away from home and parents as a primary source of support, and they enter the wider world of peers and school.
- The age at onset of puberty varies widely, but puberty is occurring at an earlier age than in the past.
- School-age children enjoy a variety of activities. Cooperative play and team sports are typical of this age-group.

- School-age children experience an increase in appetite, and older school-age children have increased energy needs as they approach puberty. Obesity is an important public health issue for which vigorous prevention approaches are necessary.
- Safety issues are related to the child moving more from the home environment to the community, less fear when playing, and the increased use of tools and household items. Important safety issues that impact school-age children include prevention of fire and burn injuries, pedestrian and motor vehicle injuries, pedestrian injury, and drowning.

- Sources of stress for school-age children include societal change, school, competitive athletics, rushed schedules, fear of violence, chaotic living conditions if homeless, and the media. Teaching children coping strategies can reduce the effects of stress.

- Peer victimization, or bullying, is becoming an important health issue for school-age children. It can occur within or outside the school setting and, without intervention, can cause long-term emotional problems for both the child being bullied and the bullier.

REFERENCES

Alday, C. S. (2009, January 1). Anxiety-based school refusal: Helping parents cope. *Brown University Child and Adolescent Behavior Letter*, 5-7.

American Academy of Pediatrics. (2011). *Car safety seats: Information for families for 2011*. Retrieved from www.healthychildren.org.

American Academy of Pediatrics. (2009a). Policy statement—media violence. *Pediatrics, 124*(5), 1495-1503.

American Academy of Pediatrics. (2009b). Policy statement—role of the pediatrician in youth violence prevention. *Pediatrics, 124*(1), 393-402.

American Academy of Pediatrics. (2008). Preventive oral health intervention for pediatricians. *Pediatrics, 122*(6), 1387-1394.

American Academy of Pediatrics, Committee on Injury and Poison Prevention. (2001, reaffirmed 2007, 2008). Policy statement: Bicycle helmets. *Pediatrics, 108*(4), 1030-1032.

American Dental Association. (2011). *Mouthguards.* Retrieved from www.ada.org.

Barlow, S. (2007). Expert Committee recommendations regarding the prevention assessment and treatment of child and adolescent overweight and obesity: Summary report. *Pediatrics, 120*, S164-S192.

Bindler, R., Massey, L., Shultz, J., et al. (2007). Metabolic syndrome in a multiethnic sample of school children: Implications for the pediatric nurse. *Journal of Pediatric Nursing, 22*, 43-58.

Biro, F., Galvez, M., Greenspan, L., et al. (2010). Pubertal assessment method and baseline characteristics in a mixed longitudinal study of girls. *Pediatrics, 126*(3), e583-e590.

Byrne, D., Thomas, K., Burchell, J., et al. (2011). Stressor experience in primary school-aged children: Development of a scale to assess profiles of exposure and effects on psychological well-being. *International Journal of Stress Management, 18*(1), 88-111.

Centers for Disease Control and Prevention. (2007). *United States schools making progress in decreasing availability of junk food and promoting physical activity*. Retrieved from www.cdc.gov.

Centers for Disease Control and Prevention. (2011a). *National estimates of the 10 leading causes of nonfatal injuries treated in hospital emergency departments, United States—2008*. Retrieved from www.cdc.gov.

Centers for Disease Control and Prevention. (2011b). *Overweight and obesity*. Retrieved from www.cdc.gov.

Centers for Disease Control and Prevention. (2011c). *Ten leading causes of injury deaths by age group highlighting unintentional injury deaths, United States 2007.* Retrieved from www.cdc.gov.

Child Welfare Information Gateway. (2007). *Leaving your child home alone*. Retrieved from www.childwelfare.gov.

Cornette, R. (2008). The emotional impact of obesity on children. *Worldviews on Evidence-Based Nursing, 5*(3), 136-141.

Daniels, S., Greer, F., & the Committee on Nutrition. (2008). Lipid screening and cardiovascular health in childhood. *Pediatrics, 122,*(1), 198-208.

Dube, S., & Orpinas, P. (2009). Understanding excessive school absenteeism as school refusal behavior. *Children and Schools, 31*(2), 87-95.

Erikson, E. (1963). *Childhood and society* (2nd ed.). New York: Norton.

Forum for Child and Family Statistics. (2011). *America's children: Key national indicators of well-being, 2011*. Retrieved from www.childstats.gov.

Gahagan, S. (2011). Overweight and obesity. In R. Kliegman, B. Stanton, J. St. Geme, et al. (Eds.), *Nelson textbook of pediatrics* (19th ed., pp. 179-188). Philadelphia: Elsevier Saunders.

Griffin, R., Parks, C., Rue, L., & McGwin, G. (2008). Comparison of severe injuries between powered and nonpowered scooters among children aged 2 to 12 in the United States. *Ambulatory Pediatrics, 8*, 379-382.

Kelly, L., & Patterson, B. (2006). Childhood nutrition: Perceptions of caretakers in a low-income urban setting. *Journal of School Nursing, 22*(6), 345-351.

Kime, N. (2009). How children eat may contribute to rising levels of obesity. Children's eating behaviors: An intergenerational study of family influences. *International Journal of Health Promotion and Education, 47*(1), 4-11.

Kohlberg, L. (1964). Development of moral character. In M. Hoffman & L. Hoffman (Eds.), *Review of child development research*, Vol. 1. New York: Russell Sage Foundation.

National Center for Health Statistics (NCHS). (2011). *Health, United States, 2010 with special feature on death and dying.* Hyattsville, MD: Author.

Piaget, J. (1962). *Play, dreams, and imitation in childhood* (C. Gattegno & F. M. Hodgson, Trans.). New York: Norton.

Rozier, G., Adair, S., Graham, et al. (2010). Evidence-based clinical recommendations on the prescription of dietary fluoride supplements for caries prevention. A report of the American Dental Association Council on Scientific Affairs. *Journal of the American Dental Association, 141*(12), 1480-1489.

Sealy, Y. (2010). Parents' food choices: Obesity among minority parents and children. *Journal of Community Health Nursing, 27*, 1-11.

Turner, H., Finkelhor, D., Hamby, S., et al. (2011). Specifying type and location of peer victimization in a national sample of children and youth. *Journal of Youth and Adolescence, 40*, 1052-1067.

United States Department of Agriculture. (2011). *Dietary guidelines for Americans, 2010.* Retrieved from www.cnpp.usda.gov/DietaryGuidelines.html.

United States Department of Health and Human Services. (2011). *Bullying is a serious problem.* Retrieved from www.stopbullyingnow.gov.

United States Preventive Services Task Force. (2010). Screening for obesity in children and adolescents: US Preventive Services Task Force recommendation statement. *Pediatrics, 125*, 361-367.

Weston, F. (2010). Working with children who have been bullied. *British Journal of School Nursing, 5*(4), 172-176.

Health Promotion
for the Adolescent

℮volve WEBSITE

http://evolve.elsevier.com/James/ncoc

LEARNING OBJECTIVES

After studying this chapter, you should be able to:

- Describe the adolescent's normal growth and development.
- Identify the sexual maturity rating and Tanner stages and recognize deviations from normal.
- Describe the developmental tasks of adolescence.
- Describe the concept of identity formation in relation to adolescent psychosocial development.
- Describe appropriate health-promoting behaviors for adolescents and young adults.

- Provide anticipatory guidance for adolescents and their families regarding risk-taking behaviors, nutrition, and safety.
- Discuss the prevalence of adolescent violence and strategies to deal with aggressive behavior.
- Discuss adolescent sexuality and related health risks.

Adolescence spans ages 11 to 21 years, although the developmental tasks of early adolescence, as well as the beginning stages of sexual maturation, may overlap with the school-age years. Adolescence is a time of change for teenagers and their families, a transition from childhood to adulthood. During this transition period, dramatic physical, cognitive, psychosocial, and psychosexual changes take place that are exciting and, at the same time, frightening.

Healthy People 2020 (U.S. Department of Health and Human Services [USDHHS], 2010) objectives address many areas of adolescent health, some of which are contained in a new topic area specifically directed toward adolescents. These areas include access to comprehensive health care and education about, and practice of, appropriate reproductive health practices, violence reduction, and decrease in risk factors.

ADOLESCENT GROWTH AND DEVELOPMENT

The adolescent tries out many new roles during this time as part of the important developmental task of identity formation. The peer group is of the utmost importance as adolescents experiment with new roles outside the confines of the family unit. When identity formation is complete, the young adult is emancipated from the family and establishes independence.

The rapid rate of physical growth during adolescence is second only to that of infancy. Adolescents come in many shapes and sizes, and the changes that take place during the teen years are obvious and dramatic. With physical changes come the development of secondary sexual characteristics and an intense interest in romantic relationships. In general, adolescents move from the same-sex friendships of childhood to the capacity for intimate, long-lasting relationships as young adults. Sexual orientation and gender identity are often recognized during adolescence as the teenager engages in exploration and self-discovery.

Both parents and adolescents need the nurse's support and guidance in understanding and facilitating health-promoting behaviors. Nurses can assist adolescents and their families in the areas of health promotion, disease prevention, and management of common problems by using effective communication strategies, knowledge of normal growth and development, anticipatory guidance, and early identification of potential problems.

Physical Growth and Development

℮ Physical development during the adolescent years is characterized by dramatic changes in size and appearance. Girls experience budding of the breasts followed by the appearance of pubic hair. Approximately 1 year after breast development, height increases rapidly until it reaches

Video—Female Breasts, Sitting Position

149

HEALTH PROMOTION

Selected Healthy People 2020 Objectives for Adolescents

AH-1	Increase the proportion of adolescents who have had a wellness checkup in the past 12 months.
AH-3	Increase the proportion of adolescents who are connected to a parent or other positive adult caregiver.
AH-5.1	Increase the proportion of students who graduate with a regular diploma 4 years after starting 9th grade.
AH-7	Reduce the proportion of adolescents who have been offered, sold, or given an illegal drug on school property.
AH-11	Reduce adolescent and young adult perpetration of, as well as victimization by, crimes.
ECBP-2	Increase the proportion of senior high schools that provide comprehensive school health education to prevent health problems in the following areas: unintentional injury; violence; suicide; tobacco use and addiction; alcohol or other drug use; unintended pregnancy, HIV/AIDS, and STD infection; unhealthy dietary patterns; and inadequate physical activity.
FP-8	Reduce pregnancies among adolescent females.
FP-9	Increase the proportion of adolescents aged 17 years and under who have never had sexual intercourse.
FP-10 and 11	Increase the proportion of sexually active persons aged 15 to 19 years who use contraception to both effectively prevent pregnancy and provide barrier protection against disease.
FP-12 and 13	Increase the proportion of adolescents who received formal instruction or talked to a parent about reproductive health topics, including all of the following: abstinence, birth control methods, safer sex to prevent HIV, and prevention of STDs before they were 18 years old.
HIV-2, 3, and 4	Reduce the rate of HIV/AIDS transmission and infection among adolescents.
IID-11	Increase routine vaccination coverage levels of adolescents.
IVP-29	Reduce homicides.
IVP-34	Reduce physical fighting among adolescents.
IVP-35	Reduce bullying among adolescents.
IVP-36	Reduce weapon carrying by adolescents on school property.
IVP-41	Reduce nonfatal intentional self-harm injuries.
NWS-21	Reduce iron deficiency among young children and females of childbearing age.
PA-3	Increase the proportion of adolescents who meet current federal physical activity guidelines for aerobic physical activity and for muscle-strengthening activity.
SA-1	Reduce the proportion of adolescents who report that they rode, during the previous 30 days, with a driver who had been drinking alcohol.
SA-2 and 3	Increase the proportion of adolescents never using substances and who disapprove of substance use.
TU-2 and 3	Reduce tobacco use by adolescents and reduce the initiation of tobacco use.

Modified from U.S. Department of Health and Human Services. (2010). *Healthy People 2020*. Retrieved from www.healthypeople.gov.

its peak (peak height velocity [PHV]). Growth in height in girls typically ceases 2 to $2\frac{1}{2}$ years after menarche.

Boys also experience physical changes, but those changes are not as obvious as in girls. Boys first experience testicular enlargement, followed in approximately 1 year by penile enlargement. Pubic hair usually precedes the growth of the penis. The growth spurt in boys occurs later than it does in girls, beginning between ages $10\frac{1}{2}$ and 16 years and ending between $13\frac{1}{2}$ and $17\frac{1}{2}$ years. Growth continues at a much slower pace for several years after the spurt but usually ceases between 18 and 20 years of age.

Muscle mass increases in boys, and fat deposits increase in girls. Because of greater muscle mass, fully developed adolescent boys tend to be larger and stronger than adolescent girls.

Psychosexual Development, Hormonal Changes, and Sexual Maturation

The physical development, hormonal changes, and sexual maturation that occur during adolescence correspond to Freud's final stage of psychosexual development, the genital stage (Freud, 1960) (see Chapter 4). The genital stage begins with the production of sex hormones and maturation of the reproductive system. Sexual tension and energy are manifested in the development of sexual relationships with others, and sexual gratification is sought. Freud's theory suggests that personality development is closely related to psychosexual development, with an emphasis on aggressive and sexual impulses as determining factors of personality. Freud's theories about male dominance, sexual repression,

and the Oedipus and Electra complexes make the psychosexual theory of development highly controversial even today.

Girls generally reach physical maturation before boys with the onset and establishment of menstruation *(menarche)*. Menarche usually occurs between ages 9 and 15 years, however recent evidence suggests that the initiation of pubertal development (Tanner stage 2) is occurring at an earlier age than previously thought (Biro, Galvez, Greenspan et al., 2010). Biro et al. (2010), in a study of pubertal development in a sample of over 1200 girls ages 7 to 8 years, found that by 8 years of age, 18.3% of white, 42.6% of non-Hispanic black, and 30.4% of Hispanic girls had attained Tanner 2 breast development. Reasons for earlier maturity are uncertain, but may include genetic influences, elevated body mass index (BMI), exposure to environmental chemicals, diet, and racial predisposition (Biro et al., 2010). Most young women achieve reproductive maturity 2 to 5 years after the start of menstruation. During the 2 to 5 years before reproductive maturity, the female sex hormones gradually increase, ovulation occurs more frequently, and menstrual periods become more regular.

Ultimately, diet, exercise, and hereditary factors influence adolescents' height, weight, and body build. The earlier onset of puberty has implications for the timing of sex education programs and anticipatory guidance. It also has implications for health issues, such as breast cancer, that have hormonal components.

The physical growth of boys and girls is directly related to sexual maturation and occurs in a relatively predictable sequence. The secretion of sex hormones—estrogen in girls and testosterone in boys—stimulates the development of breast tissue, pubic hair, and genitalia. Hormonal secretion at the time of puberty is the result of a complex regulatory process among the environment, the central nervous system, the hypothalamus, the pituitary gland, the gonads, and the adrenal glands. Puberty is a biologic process that brings about PHV, or the "growth spurt," the changes in body composition, and the development of primary and secondary sexual characteristics in both sexes. Although variable in both sexes, the PHV occurs at approximately age 12 years in girls and age 13½ years in boys. Table 8-1 describes five distinct stages in a sexual maturity rating (SMR) based on breast and pubic hair development in girls and genital and pubic hair development in boys and includes approximate age ranges for early, middle, and late puberty (Tanner, 1962). The beginning Tanner stages frequently occur in the school-age child, and Tanner stages 3 to 5 occur in adolescence.

In boys, puberty is considered delayed if testicular enlargement or pubic hair development has not occurred by age 14 years. Absence of breast budding or pubic hair development in girls by 13 years is reason for referral. Some of the more common causes of delayed puberty are chronic illnesses, malnutrition, extreme exercise, and hypothyroidism.

Female Sexual Maturation

Sexual maturation in girls begins with the appearance of breast buds (thelarche), which is the first sign of ovarian function. Thelarche occurs at approximately age 8 to 11 years and is followed by the growth of pubic hair. The PHV is reached during thelarche, usually in Tanner stage 2 or 3. Linear growth slows, and menarche begins approximately 1 year after the PHV. As pubic hair increases in amount and becomes

---

! NURSING QUALITY ALERT

Understanding Tanner Staging

> Knowledge of Tanner staging is essential for nurses to assess normal growth and development and provide adolescents and their parents with anticipatory guidance regarding sexual development. Nurses must remember, however, that sexual maturation and physical development are highly variable and that Tanner stages may overlap one another. A description of the adolescent's SMR provides greater information about the child's physical development than does chronologic age (age in years).

dark, coarse, and curly, axillary hair develops and the apocrine sweat glands reach secretory capacity in Tanner stage 3 or 4. Frequent showers and deodorants become important to the adolescent. With increasing hormonal activity, girls develop a more adult body contour. As breasts mature, the nipples project more and the pubic hair extends to the medial thighs; the young female is estimated to be at Tanner stage 5. Ovulation may be established, and conception can occur.

Male Sexual Maturation

The first sign of pubertal changes in boys is testicular enlargement in response to testosterone secretion, which usually occurs in Tanner stage 2. Slight pubic hair is present and the smooth skin texture of the scrotum is somewhat altered. As testosterone secretion increases, the penis, testes, and scrotum enlarge. The PHV usually occurs during Tanner stages 3 and 4, and the voice deepens and "cracks" as the cartilage in the larynx enlarges. Axillary hair develops, and the eccrine and apocrine sweat glands respond to stressful or emotional stimuli. Skin

---

TABLE 8-1 · SEXUAL MATURITY RATING (SMR): TANNER STAGES OF ADOLESCENT SEXUAL DEVELOPMENT

BOYS

STAGE 1	STAGE 2	STAGE 3	STAGE 4	STAGE 5
Pubic hair: none	Pubic hair: slight, long, straight, slightly pigmented at the base of the penis	Pubic hair: darker in color, starts to curl, small amount	Pubic hair: coarse, curly, similar to adult but less quantity	Pubic hair: adult distribution spread to inner thighs
Penis: preadolescent	Penis: slight enlargement	Penis: longer	Penis: larger, glans and breadth increase in size	Penis: adult in size and shape
Testes: preadolescent	Testes: enlarged scrotum, pink, slight alteration in texture	Testes: larger	Testes: larger, scrotum darker	Testes: adult

Early puberty: Testes, 9½-13½ yr; penis, 10½-14½ yr; pubic hair, 12-12½ yr

Middle puberty: Testes, 13½-14½ yr; penis, 13½-15 yr; pubic hair, 12½-14½ yr

Late puberty: Testes, 13½-17 yr; penis, 13½-16 yr; pubic hair, 13½-16½ yr

Continued

TABLE 8-1   SEXUAL MATURITY RATING (SMR): TANNER STAGES OF ADOLESCENT SEXUAL DEVELOPMENT—cont'd

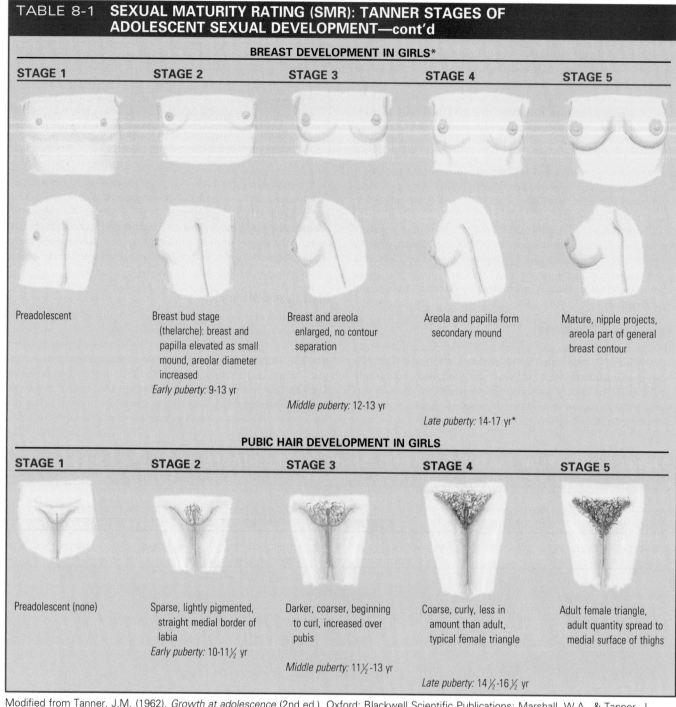

BREAST DEVELOPMENT IN GIRLS*

STAGE 1	STAGE 2	STAGE 3	STAGE 4	STAGE 5
Preadolescent	Breast bud stage (thelarche): breast and papilla elevated as small mound, areolar diameter increased *Early puberty: 9-13 yr*	Breast and areola enlarged, no contour separation *Middle puberty: 12-13 yr*	Areola and papilla form secondary mound *Late puberty: 14-17 yr* *	Mature, nipple projects, areola part of general breast contour

PUBIC HAIR DEVELOPMENT IN GIRLS

STAGE 1	STAGE 2	STAGE 3	STAGE 4	STAGE 5
Preadolescent (none)	Sparse, lightly pigmented, straight medial border of labia *Early puberty: 10-11½ yr*	Darker, coarser, beginning to curl, increased over pubis *Middle puberty: 11½-13 yr*	Coarse, curly, less in amount than adult, typical female triangle *Late puberty: 14½-16½ yr*	Adult female triangle, adult quantity spread to medial surface of thighs

Modified from Tanner, J.M. (1962). *Growth at adolescence* (2nd ed.). Oxford: Blackwell Scientific Publications; Marshall, W.A., & Tanner, J. (1969). Variations in pattern of pubertal changes in girls. *Archives of Disease in Childhood, 44*(235), 291-303. Modified with permission from Blackwell Scientific Publications and The BMJ Publishing Group.
*Breast and pubic hair development may continue into late adolescence and may increase with pregnancy.

surface bacteria metabolize secretions from the apocrine glands, and body odor develops. *Gynecomastia* (male breast enlargement) occurs in approximately two thirds of young males during early adolescence and may be unilateral or bilateral (Ali & Donohoue, 2011). This phenomenon is often disturbing to boys, and they need considerable reassurance that the breast tissue will decrease over time. During Tanner stages 4 and 5, rising levels of testosterone cause sebaceous glands to enlarge, and excessive sebum may result in acne. The voice continues to deepen, facial hair appears at the corners of the upper lip and chin, and ejaculation may occur. Nurses need to provide anticipatory guidance to adolescent boys regarding involuntary nocturnal emissions of seminal fluid ("wet dreams") and assure them that this occurrence is normal. By Tanner stage 5, genital maturation is complete, spermatogenesis is well established, facial hair is present on the sides of the face, and the male physique is adultlike in appearance. Gynecomastia significantly decreases or disappears, much to the adolescent male's relief.

Motor Development

Adolescents often engage in various forms of motor activity, from aerobic exercise to football. Motor activities such as sports and dancing provide an outlet for the adolescent's energy, as well as an opportunity for competition, teamwork, and social relationships. Large muscle mass increases in adolescents, and coordination of gross and fine muscle groups improves. With practice, adolescents become more adept at athletics and also at art, music, sewing, and other activities that require fine motor skills. The bones are not completely calcified until after puberty and are still fairly resistant to breaking in the young adolescent. Participants in sports activities should be grouped according to their size and their sexual maturity rating rather than their chronologic age. A small, thin, late-maturing boy is less capable of competing with an early-maturing, muscular classmate, and injuries are more likely to occur if they are grouped together.

⚡ SAFETY ALERT

The Adolescent Who Is Involved in Athletics

Adolescents participating in athletics need the following:
- Adequate equipment
- Appropriate training schedules
- Frequent rest periods
- Adequate fluids to prevent injury, dehydration, and exhaustion

---

Nurses, particularly school nurses, may be helpful in assessing adolescents' growth and development and counseling them about sports activities in which they can succeed rather than those in which they will meet with physical and psychological failure. Adolescents should have a yearly physical examination if participating in high school athletics (Box 8-1); the school nurse keeps documentation of this matter. Because it is generally superficial, the school sports examination should not substitute for the recommended complete adolescent physical examination with counseling.

The development of the cardiovascular pump plays an essential role in the adolescent's participation in gross motor activities. Cardiopulmonary capacity increases during adolescence and is relatively mature in the late adolescent. The cardiovascular pump is not as efficient in young adolescents, whose lungs are smaller. Adolescents generally cannot run as fast or as long as young adults. The athlete's aerobic power, body composition, joint flexibility, and strength of skeletal muscles determine physical fitness.

Cognitive Development

Cognitive development influences every aspect of adolescent psychosocial development. Cognition moves from concrete to abstract thinking during the three phases of adolescent development. According to

---

BOX 8-1 NURSING GOALS FOR PREPARTICIPATION SPORTS PHYSICAL EXAMINATION

- Assess the adolescent athlete's general health.
- Identify conditions that could limit participation or predispose to injury.
- Assess the adolescent athlete's physical and psychosocial maturity.
- Determine the athlete's fitness relative to performance requirements.
- Assess legal insurance requirements for participation.
- Provide wellness counseling and anticipatory guidance.

Piaget (1969), formal operations, or abstract thinking, characterize the last stage of cognitive development. Early abstract thinking encompasses inductive and deductive reasoning, the ability to connect separate events, and the ability to understand later consequences. Abstract thinking in late adolescence is increasingly logical, and young adults are capable of using scientific reasoning, understanding complex concepts, and using analytic methods. Because of logical reasoning, adolescents are able to differentiate between others' perceptions and their own and to view social situations from a societal perspective.

In a review of adolescent cognitive development, Herrman (2005) cites research suggesting that the brain is still maturing during adolescence, and this maturational process affects cognitive and emotional processing. Areas of the brain that control coordination and physical skills as well as emotional intensity develop during early adolescence, with increased myelinization occurring in the cerebellum and amygdala. At this age, adolescents are physically capable of many skills and emotionally more likely to take physical risks. They have a heightened sensitivity to stress, demonstrated by an exacerbated stress response. During middle adolescence maturation in the midbrain allows for increased organization and problem-solving skills and critical thinking. Finally, maturation in the frontal cortex assists the late adolescent to use rational thought to mediate intense emotion (Herrman, 2005).

The implications of this finding for nurses are especially apparent for health teaching. Adolescents think in different ways than adults. For example, sex education for ninth graders is quite different from that for college freshmen or adolescents with their first full-time jobs. The college freshman should be able to appreciate the later consequences of sexual behavior, whereas the young adolescent is focused on the here and now. For example, one should ask the ninth grader and the college freshman how an unintended baby will affect their lives, and compare their answers.

For a variety of reasons (including, for example, poor comprehension ability, lack of education, and chronic substance abuse), some older adolescents remain concrete thinkers. Nurses and educators need to know their audiences and address them appropriately. Nurses may need to help parents learn how to communicate with their teens appropriately. Counseling a group of adolescent substance abusers may be ineffective if the consequence of their behavior is tied to the future when their thinking is in the present. A professional approach to communicating with teens includes the following:

- Enjoy them.
- Be patient and flexible.
- Know adolescent development; consider how a teen will look to peers.
- Be open to their ideas and opinions and willing to negotiate choices.
- Listen nonjudgmentally, keeping criticism to a minimum.
- Encourage problem solving and mutual decision making.
- Maintain confidentiality.
- Be an advocate, but do not take sides against a parent.
- Explore feelings about health care choices, and allow for questions and analysis of health care options.

Sensory Development

Adolescents' eyes and ears are fully developed, and with the exception of refractive errors and occasional minor infections of the eyes, ears, and sinuses, the sensory system remains quite healthy. Myopia occurs in early adolescence, between ages 11 and 13 years, often requiring frequent changes in corrective lenses.

Because of increased participation in competitive sports and outdoor activities, eye injuries are common in adolescence. Boys are more prone to eye injuries than are girls. Adolescents should always be required to wear safety or protective equipment when competing in sports or participating in any activity that may compromise eye safety.

Language Development

With the acquisition of formal operational thought and adequate intellectual capacity, adolescents are able to understand abstract concepts, process complex thoughts, and express themselves verbally. Adolescents who read extensively are generally more articulate and have a larger vocabulary than those who do not. Social development and self-confidence play a significant role in how well adolescents express themselves verbally to others. Shy, introverted adolescents may have difficulty speaking to a group or members of the opposite sex but may write expressively. Conversely, extroverted, social adolescents who have no trouble with verbal expression may lack the reading and writing skills for effective written communication.

Computer technology has added to the adolescent's avenues for creative expression. Adolescents are capable of expressing ideas in symbols and abstract concepts, and many enjoy interpreting or even developing complex computer programs. Computers have a symbolic language of their own that some adolescents find fascinating. Teens may become more proficient with computer technology than their parents. In addition to teaching teens basic computer literacy, many high schools have computer clubs where students who excel in computer languages share ideas and knowledge of computer information systems. Because of safety concerns with young adolescents using the Internet, parents need to monitor computer use and investigate whether parental controls available through some Internet access companies are appropriate for their child.

Electronic or digital vehicles for communication have had an impact on language communication as well. Social media websites, e-mail, telephone text messaging, instant messaging, blogs, and Twitter all contribute to abbreviated communication techniques, which eliminate not only grammar and sentence construction, but also word construction (e.g., using "ur" for "you are").

Communicating with adolescents sometimes presents a challenge to parents and other adults. Although adolescents are capable of verbal expression, they are also intensely private and may not wish to divulge their thoughts and feelings to others. Developmentally, the verbally expressive 12-year-old may turn into a relatively uncommunicative 14-year-old. Conflict with parents increases tension in communication (see Patient-Centered Teaching: Communicating with Adolescents box).

PATIENT-CENTERED TEACHING

Communicating with Adolescents

Parents need encouragement to maintain open communication with their teenager while not appearing too intrusive. Inundating adolescents with questions or going through their belongings causes feelings of invasion and a lack of trust. Adolescents get more out of discussions in which they participate than they do out of lectures and are more likely to respond positively to adults who listen and appear interested in what they have to say.

Nurses who work with adolescents must develop communication skills that include assuring confidentiality, making no assumptions, remaining nonjudgmental, and posing open-ended questions. Questions such as "Tell me about your plans for the future" will glean more information than "Do you plan to go to college?" The question "Do you live with your parents?" makes an assumption about the living situation that could make the adolescent feel uncomfortable. "Describe where you live and who lives with you" gives the adolescent an opportunity to discuss the living situation.

Psychosocial Development

Identity formation is the major developmental task of adolescence; other tasks include the formation of a sexual and vocational identity and the ability to emancipate oneself from the family or become independent (Figure 8-1). Energy is focused within the self, and the adolescent is described as egocentric or self-absorbed. Frustrated parents often describe teenagers during this phase as self-centered, lazy, or irresponsible. In fact, they just need time to think, concentrate on themselves, and determine who they are going to be. Erikson (1968) described the conflict of this phase of psychosocial development as identity formation versus role confusion; this phase corresponds to Freud's genital stage of psychosexual development (see Chapter 4 for information on developmental theories).

In the transition period from childhood to adulthood, adolescents try new roles and experiment with the environment until they find a role that fits. The phase of experimentation has been termed the *moratorium,* meaning a period of delay granted to someone not yet ready to make more than a tentative commitment (Erikson, 1968). The adolescent's changing interests from year to year illustrate the lack of commitment. Parents may invest in expensive sports equipment or a musical instrument only to find it abandoned after a short time.

The peer group plays an essential role in adolescent identity formation. Teenagers take their cues on appearance, social behavior, and language from the peer group. The peer group serves as a safe haven as adolescents emotionally move away from the family and struggle to determine who they are. The peer group validates acceptable behavior, and teenagers feel secure in trying on new roles with peer-group approval. Teens frequently spend all day with friends in school and all evening rehashing the day's events over the phone or through postings on social media websites (Box 8-2). Changes in the adolescent's body image, psychosocial development, and peer group acceptance are closely related. Early and middle adolescents are particularly audience conscious and feel that they are the focus of everyone's attention. A bad hair day or a blemish may throw the adolescent into despair. Clothing, hairstyles, and material possessions that are accepted by the group become the most important. Nurses counsel parents to negotiate choices with teens but always consider how peers will judge the child.

! NURSING QUALITY ALERT

The Adolescent and Erikson

- Identity formation and establishment of autonomy
- Acquisition of abstract reasoning leading to the following:
  - Analytic thinking
  - Problem solving
  - Planning for the future

Early adolescence and middle adolescence are the periods when teens are prone to gang formation and activities. Peer modeling and peer acceptance, being of the utmost importance, lead some adolescents to form gangs that provide a collective identity and give them a sense of belonging. Peer pressure, companionship, and protection are the most frequently reported reasons for joining gangs, particularly those associated with violent or criminal acts.

Early and late adolescence have marked developmental differences. Each age-group has unique reactions to the developmental tasks,

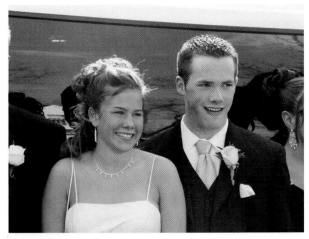

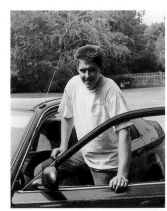

Relationships with the opposite sex are more mature by late adolescence. Individuals in late adolescence have more realistic expectations of both themselves and those who are important to them. They devote many hours and much anxious thought to making events such as prom night memorable for a lifetime. Some adolescents may be left out because they are unpopular or shy or do not have the financial resources to participate in these special events.

With the freedom driving brings to the adolescent comes responsibility. The adolescent's inexperience and risk-taking behaviors can be a lethal combination.

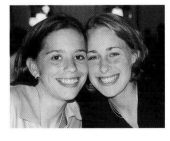

Although teens often have friends of both sexes, they are more comfortable sharing their hopes, dreams, secrets, and even embarrassing incidents with friends of the same sex.

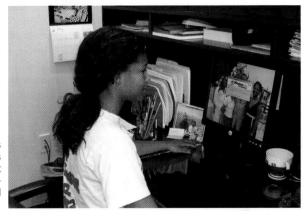

Computers in school and in many homes provide the adolescent with opportunities for learning, creative expression, communication, and entertainment. Adolescents often enjoy "surfing" the Internet, which can provide them with information not readily available locally. Parents must monitor their adolescent's computer connections, however, for these networks sometimes allow access to people and activities that conflict with family values.

FIG 8-1 Adolescent growth and development.

BOX 8-2 AGE-RELATED ACTIVITIES AND GAMES FOR ADOLESCENTS

General Activities
Games and athletics are the most common forms of play.
Strict rules are in place.
Competition is important.

Games and Special Types of Play
Sports, videos, movies, reading, parties, hobbies, listening to favorite music, experimenting with makeup and hairstyles, talking on the telephone or cell phone, playing computer games, participating in social media discourse.

---

which are influenced by the adolescent's cognitive thinking. According to Piaget (1969), adolescent cognition is characterized by the transition from concrete operational thought to formal operational thought, the ability to think logically and use deductive and abstract reasoning (see Chapters 4 through 7). The acquisition of formal operational thinking allows the adolescent to recall past experience and to apply knowledge to the future by drawing logical consequences from a set of observations. Adolescents are capable of using abstract symbols such as those derived from higher-order mathematics, making and

testing hypotheses, and considering and arguing philosophic issues. Problem-solving and decision-making skills become more highly developed, although adolescents may still be conflicted about idealism versus reality.

Early Adolescence

The early adolescent (11 to 14 years) has intense feelings about body image and the many physical changes taking place. Less confident with members of the opposite sex, early adolescents tend to group together and have best friends of the same sex. One has only to visit the local mall or a movie theater to see groups of young teens of the same sex, observing but rarely speaking to groups of the opposite sex.

The early adolescent is quite egocentric and may move from obedience to rebellion regarding parental authority. Parents are often shocked by the sudden turn of events and are hurt by the teen's rejection. Providing parents with anticipatory guidance regarding age-specific developmental changes is a primary nursing function. For example, the happy-go-lucky 11-year-old may turn into the shy, self-absorbed 12-year-old who seems comfortable only in the presence of friends. Young teens, who are developmentally egocentric, fail to differentiate between how others see them and their own mental preoccupations, thinking everyone is as obsessed with them as they are with themselves. Elkind (1993) describes this phenomenon as a reaction to the imaginary audience. The belief in the imaginary audience is probably why young teens are so self-conscious; they believe everyone is critical of them, and indeed teens are quite critical of one another, especially those who are different. Self-conscious behavior may also be the result of the physical and emotional transition to middle adolescence. The early adolescent is losing the familiar role of the child but does not yet feel comfortable with the role of the adult. Ambivalence toward independence is common, and the teen who feels too grown up for a good-night kiss from a parent still falls asleep with a favorite teddy bear.

Elkind (1993) believes that because young teens are so audience conscious, they see themselves as unique and tell themselves a "personal fable" that supports feelings of invulnerability. They believe bad things will happen to others but not to them. Adolescent suicide attempts, for example, serve as a dramatic message to others, but young teens often do not realize the final consequences of their actions.

Middle Adolescence

Middle adolescence (15 to 17 years) is often described by parents as the most frustrating period of adolescent development. The real audience gradually replaces the imaginary audience, and teens become even more introspective and narcissistic. Conformity to peer-group norms becomes even more important, and conflicts between teenagers and parents often escalate. Testing of limits, sulky withdrawal, and overt rebellion may occur over conflicts regarding curfews, friends, activities, appearance, cars, and money. The adolescent may feel more secure by associating with or becoming a member of a gang (Box 8-3). Nurses counsel parents to negotiate choices when possible and set limits that are perceived as reasonable by the adolescent. Consistent discipline and structure actually make adolescents feel more secure and assist them with decision making. With parental guidance, adolescents are able to make decisions that will result in desirable outcomes. Adults must keep in mind that middle adolescents are impulsive and impatient, however. Parental concern may be seen as interference rather than guidance and may be met with resistance and resentment.

Feelings about self-image and social relationships are intense. Middle adolescence is generally a time of transition from same-sex

---

BOX 8-3   SIGNS OF GANG INVOLVEMENT

- Associating with new friends while ignoring old friends. The adolescent usually will not talk about the new friends or what they do together.
- A change in hairstyle or clothing and associating with other youths with the same style. Usually some of the clothing, such as a hat or jacket, has the gang's colors, initials, or "street" name on it. Parents may note tattoos on the body.
- Unexplained source of money or possessions (e.g., stereos, jewelry, cars).
- Indications of drug, alcohol, or inhalant abuse (e.g., paint or correction fluid on the clothes, the smell of chemicals on the breath or clothes).
- Change in attitude toward activities such as sports, Scouting, or church. Discipline problems at school, in public, or at home. Youth no longer accepts parents' authority and challenges it frequently.
- Problems at school, such as failing classes, skipping school, and causing problems in class.
- Fear of the police.
- Unexplained signs of fighting, such as bruises, cuts, and reports of pain.
- Graffiti on or around residence or possessions.
- Threats from rival gang members. Sometimes a family member is a victim of a drive-by shooting before the family realizes the youth is involved in a gang.

---

friendships to an extreme interest in the opposite sex; it is also a time when adolescents may acknowledge homosexual feelings. The proportion of teens who are sexually experienced and sexually active has declined slightly, as has the teen birth rate (Centers for Disease Control and prevention, 2011a, 2011b). Nurses and other health care providers cannot become complacent in response to this change in trends. The United States still has one of the highest adolescent birth rates compared to other developed countries (CDC, 2011a). In a recent survey by the CDC (2010), 5.9% of adolescents reported initiating sexual intercourse before age 13 years, and 46% of the ninth through twelfth graders surveyed had had sexual intercourse at least once. Of concern is the trend for early initiation of sexual intercourse.

Sexual activity is often related to peer pressure and self-esteem issues. Adolescents with low self-esteem are more vulnerable and are more apt to engage in negative risk-taking activities associated with sexuality. Decisions about sexual activity are often impulsive and made with little regard to later consequences or prior preparation. In fact, according to the 2009 Youth Risk Behavior Surveillance (CDC, 2010), of the teenagers who reported being currently sexually active, 39.9% reported they did not use a condom at last intercourse.

Another concerning trend among adolescents is the increasing participation in oral sex. Recent reports of national statistics suggest that the prevalence of oral sex among adolescents 15 to 19 years old exceeds 50% (Lindberg, Jones, & Santelli, 2008). Questions about oral sexual activity are not currently included in the Youth Risk Behavior Surveillance. Halpern-Felsher (2008) states that adolescents tend to have oral sex for a variety of reasons, but primarily because they believe it is more socially acceptable than vaginal intercourse and does not carry the same risks. This and other evidence-based information (CDC, 2009; Lindberg et al., 2008) suggests that, although many adolescents may know that human immunodeficiency virus (HIV) and other infectious diseases can be contracted from engaging in oral sex, they nevertheless do not consider oral sex to be as risky as vaginal sex.

Nurses and other health professionals who assess adolescent health status need to be more specific when interviewing adolescents about sexual activity. The question of whether an adolescent is sexually active is no longer sufficient; questions should be directed toward assessing participation in various specific types of sexual activity as well as the method of barrier protection used. Nurses may help by providing accurate information to assist adolescents in making appropriate sexual choices. Parents need encouragement to maintain open communication and guide teenagers in sexual decision making. Providing parental guidance about sexual behavior is not easy during middle adolescence, when privacy is of extreme importance and communication with parents tends to decrease. In addition, some parents may find sexual behavior a difficult topic to discuss and often avoid talking with teens about sexual issues altogether.

Vocational Exploration. In the initial stages of establishing a vocational identity, adolescents are more likely to experience role confusion and have unrealistic expectations of themselves. Some adolescents identify a role that holds their interest, whereas others experiment with many roles, moving quickly from one role to another. Overidentification with glamorous roles takes precedence over reality and is enriched by daydreams and fantasy. A 15-year-old girl may spend time with her friends describing her future as a popular media star while failing to fold the laundry or do the dishes.

During middle adolescence, some teens acquire part-time jobs and identify various skills and interests. Part-time jobs are often a source of income for material possessions and activities not provided by parents. Such experiences help adolescents set realistic expectations

---

> **! NURSING QUALITY ALERT**
>
> ### Elements of Adolescent Care
>
> Nurses working with middle adolescents must:
> - Be approachable
> - Maintain objectivity
> - Encourage confidence
> - Support parental authority
> - Be a child advocate while not coming between adolescents and their parents
> - Encourage the family to work as a mutually respectful unit

about work, become more independent, and develop self-esteem. Those who are successful in the working world demonstrate a sense of responsibility and tend to have more positive social interactions. However, some adolescents may allow work to interfere with educational activity and have difficulty setting priorities. School nurses, in collaboration with parents and teachers, are in an excellent position to identify working students and assist them in setting realistic guidelines for work and education.

Late Adolescence (18 to 21 Years)

Late adolescence is characterized by the ability to think abstractly, conceptualize verbally, and express thoughts and feelings about various aspects of life. Late adolescents tend to be idealistic about love, social issues, ethics, and lifestyles until their experiences modify their beliefs. Conformity becomes less important as teens progress through late adolescence. With the development of a unique identity, self-esteem increases and adolescents are able to resist group pressure if it is not in their best interest. Interactions with parents are less turbulent unless values clash, and relationships with both friends and family are maintained.

Emancipation (leaving home) is a major issue; late adolescents prepare themselves to meet this task through education or vocational training. Identifying realistic career goals is important, but many adolescents are not yet ready to make lifelong commitments. Changing career goals is not uncommon, but the nurse should watch for those adolescents who have set no career goals, who demonstrate apathy about the future, and who appear committed only to the present. Boredom and apathy are often symptoms of a greater problem: depression.

Social relationships are more mature, although partner selection often continues to fluctuate. Friendships developed in late adolescence may last a lifetime, and expectations of friends and lovers become more realistic and less self-serving. The ability to consider others' needs increases, and recognition of societal needs is more apparent as the adolescent moves from adolescence to adulthood.

Failure to achieve identity formation may leave adolescents in role confusion and impede the successful mastery of the tasks of young adulthood. A positive ego identity depends on the adolescent's ability to accept the past, learn from experience, and become engaged in the future. Most adolescents move through the identity versus role confusion stage of development with minimal difficulty.

Moral and Spiritual Development

Children develop moral reasoning in a sequential manner, as described by American psychologist Lawrence Kohlberg (1964). As adolescents move from concrete to analytic thinking, they advance to Kohlberg's stage 4 conventional level or Kohlberg's stage 5 postconventional level of moral development. Adolescents who remain concrete thinkers may never advance beyond Kohlberg's stage 3 of moral reasoning: conformity to please others and avoid punishment. The teenager's sense of justice is developed through interpersonal relationships with peers, family, and other adult role models. Behaviors that are modeled and rewarded, such as helping the less fortunate and showing loyalty to friends, contribute to the development of a conscience, which operates as a moral guide for subsequent behavior. The middle to late teenager can appreciate that stealing from others is wrong regardless of whether one is caught and punished.

Adolescents and young adults develop a respect for law and order and a society-maintaining orientation (Kohlberg's stage 4). Young adults may even advance to the societal-perspective stage (Kohlberg's stage 5), which honors the moral rules of right and wrong, contractual agreements, majority opinion, and overall utility or the greatest good for the greatest number (see Chapter 4).

Older adolescents and young adults question the values of family and society and challenge existing moral codes before integrating their experiences and beliefs into a personal moral framework. Once the moral framework is developed, interpersonal relationships tend to be with those whose values and beliefs are similar.

Young adolescents in the stage of concrete operational thought are able to think logically. In this stage, children deal well with the observable but also begin to see other points of view and examine what they have learned. The young adolescent will accept religious teaching and examine how religious concepts relate to everyday life. Young adolescents are especially inclined to look to God for guidance when troubled.

Individuals in middle to late adolescence are capable of analytic thought and may begin to question the religious affiliation of the family, much as they question other family values. Older adolescents may explore different kinds of religion and share religious activities with the peer group.

Evidence suggests that spirituality has a positive effect on health-related quality of life in adolescents (Cotton, Tsevat, & Yi, 2007). Spirituality may also be protective for both physical and emotional well-being (Rubin, Dodd, Desai, et al., 2009) as part of providing holistic nursing care, nurses need to include an assessment of spiritual beliefs and values when working with adolescents and incorporate these values in nursing interventions.

HEALTH PROMOTION FOR THE ADOLESCENT AND FAMILY

Adolescence is generally a period of wellness. Young people may seek health care for school or sports physicals, skin conditions (acne, contact dermatitis), acute minor illnesses (colds, flu), conditions related to sexuality (birth control, pregnancy, sexually transmissible infections [STIs]), and the management of chronic illness (diabetes, epilepsy). Health promotion and disease prevention are achieved through adequate nutrition, rest, balanced exercise, and proper immunization against disease.

During well visits for health promotion, adolescents confer privately with the nurse and the health provider; separately, parents are asked about any concerns they might have. Confidentiality is often an issue when adolescents are seen in the health care setting. Nurses should encourage adolescents to involve their parents, but adolescents frequently ask that communication be kept confidential. The adolescent must understand that the nurse will respect this confidentiality unless the information shared suggests a potentially life-threatening danger either to the adolescent or to others.

CRITICAL THINKING EXERCISE 8-1

The nurse is caring for a 15-year-old girl, Heidi, who has been admitted to the hospital with dehydration. She is quiet and answers questions with a simple "yes" or "no." On the day Heidi is to be discharged, she says, "I'll tell you something, but you can't tell anyone else."

1. What factors must the nurse consider in this situation?
2. What would be the nurse's best response?

BOX 8-4 FACTORS INFLUENCING THE ADOLESCENT'S DIET

- Busy schedule (sports, activities, jobs)
- Body image concerns, which can lead to undereating
- Skipping breakfast
- Eating away from home
- Eating fast food frequently
- Beginning to buy and prepare own food
- Peer pressure
- Psychological and emotional problems

Adolescents need to be directly asked questions about their health. These include questions about diet and exercise, sexual risk behavior, substance use, preventive safety measures (e.g., seat belt, bicycle helmet, protective sports equipment), violence, peer and family relationships, and emotional health (AAP Committee on Adolescence, 2008). Screening tools are available that can be used to perform an adolescent assessment in an organized manner. Guidelines for Adolescent Preventive Services (GAPS) is an assessment program that looks at parenting, development, drugs, sex, learning problems, depression, abuse, safety, and diet and fitness. GAPS is a comprehensive packet of services that includes screening and preventive services (American Medical Association, 1997). There are specific screening tools that assess for emotional and mental health issues. One of these is the Diagnostic Predictive Scales-8 (DPS-8), which is a questionnaire about mental health issues including suicide (ideation, attempts), phobias, general anxiety, substance use, and depressive symptoms (Husky, Miller, McGuire, et al., 2011). Questionnaires can be administered before the adolescent comes to the provider or in the provider's office, either by paper and pencil or by computer (Husky et al., 2011).Some providers publically display their policy on confidentiality, always underlining the need to share information only if someone is in danger. Issues related to the time necessary for an adequate interview may arise in the current managed care environment. Nurses should be knowledgeable about communicating with adolescents and aware of when referral is warranted.

Access to regular quality health care for adolescents has become an increasing issue of concern because of its importance to the prevention of illness related to adolescent risk behavior (AAP Committee on Adolescence, 2008). Regular health promotion visits to a provider during adolescence facilitates comprehensive health screening, preventive intervention, counseling, and referral. Many adolescents and their parents perceive the yearly sports physical as being sufficient. However, this physical examination—often performed by a school physician—is not comprehensive enough to identify subtle problems, nor is it likely to provide time for confidential communication of adolescent concerns to the provider (AAP Committee on Adolescence, 2008). For this reason the AAP Committee on Adolescence (2008) recommends that access to comprehensive health care for adolescents be widely available in a variety of venues, including school-based health clinics, physicians' offices, community or public health clinics, and hospitals. In addition, the Committee recommends offering assurance of confidentiality, comprehensive services, care that is culturally and ethnically relevant, and health insurance coverage for all adolescents (AAP Committee on Adolescence, 2008).

Nutrition during Adolescence

The accelerated growth (in linear height, weight, and muscle mass) and sexual maturation during adolescence increase teenagers' nutritional needs, including needs for protein, calories, zinc, calcium, and iron. Periods of intense growth require increased caloric intake, and the adolescent appears constantly hungry. Snacks and regular meals need to contain adequate nutrients to meet the body's anabolic needs.

Adolescents are generally interested in nutrition and the effect food has on their bodies. Teenagers tend to be concerned about their weight, complexion, sexual development, and acceptance by their peers. These issues, together with the adolescent's growing independence, can have nutritional implications.

Age-Related Nutritional Challenges

The adolescent's food habits are influenced by many factors (Box 8-4). Unfortunately, this happens at a time when the body has greater nutritional needs. Boys tend to have fewer nutritional deficiencies than girls because they take in more food and are less likely to be dieting. Soft drinks frequently replace milk. Fast foods and low-nutrient "junk foods" sometimes become the mainstay of the adolescent's diet. The social aspect of food consumption gains importance, and adolescents may prefer to eat meals with peers at social gatherings and restaurants of their choice. Parental supervision of meals declines as the adolescent spends more time away from home and engages in extracurricular activities with peers.

Nutritional Guidance for the Adolescent

The nurse needs to understand growth and development to be successful in counseling adolescents and their parents about nutrition. Adolescents' increasing need to be independent and make their own choices should guide the nurse in teaching nutrition. The adolescent should always be involved in the planning.

The nurse should assess the adolescent's present diet and determine habits and eating patterns. The assessment should elicit how often the adolescent eats food from the different food groups and what foods the adolescent does not eat. On the basis of this information, nutritious foods for meals can be identified and a plan developed. In general, the U.S. Department of Agriculture (USDA) (2011) recommends 1600 to 1800 calories/day for adolescent girls and 1800 to 2200 calories/day for adolescent boys, with foods coming from a variety of groups—whole grains, fruits and vegetables, dairy, and protein (plant and animal). Adolescents should drink at least three cups of milk a day and limit fats to 25% to 35% of total daily calories consumed. Adolescents need calcium to prevent future osteoporosis, and adolescent girls require adequate iron and folic acid (400 mcg/day from supplements or folic acid–fortified foods) (USDA, 2011).

The nurse can also assist the adolescent by pointing out nutritious fast foods and snacks. An awareness of nutritious fast foods can also aid the adolescent in meal selection. Many fast-food chains have salads with nonfat or low-fat dressings, grilled chicken sandwiches, pasta, and nonfat yogurt. Fat and salt contents have been reduced, and vegetable fats have replaced animal fats at some restaurants. Adolescents should be guided to mix an occasional hamburger and fries with a regular selection of more nutritious foods. Permission should be given to eat foods that may be untraditional at a particular meal, such as pizza for breakfast.

Many adolescents decide to follow a vegetarian diet during their teen years. Several dietary organizations have suggested that a vegetarian diet, if correctly followed, is healthy for this population because the low-fat aspect of the diet can prevent future cardiovascular problems (Stettler, Bhatia, Parish, & Stallings, 2011). If an adolescent wishes to follow a vegetarian diet, the nurse can assist with planning food choices that will provide sufficient calories and necessary nutrients. The focus is on obtaining sufficient calories for growth and energy through a variety of fruits and vegetables, whole grains, nuts, legumes, seeds, tofu, and soy milk; some vegetarians choose to eat eggs and dairy products as well (Stettler et al., 2011). As with any adolescent, nurses need to advise adolescents who follow a vegetarian eating plan to avoid low-nutrient, high-fat foods.

Body image is of particular importance to adolescents. The media reinforce the belief that "thin is in." Adolescents hold themselves to standards set by the entertainment and advertising worlds, which emphasize fitness, glamour, and sexuality. Products that promise a quick weight loss or enhanced muscle mass with a lean physique are appealing to adolescents. Weight management techniques may include fasting, diet pills and laxatives, self-induced vomiting, and fad diets instead of low-fat, low-calorie, nutritionally sound diets and more aerobic exercise. Adolescents may not realize that unsound nutritional habits often follow them for a lifetime or that growth and development may be delayed or permanently impaired. School nurses are in an excellent position to identify adolescents who have nutritional problems or eating disorders and provide counseling or referral for adolescents and their families (see Chapter 29).

Hygiene

Adolescents in general are meticulous about personal hygiene. A major concern, however, is acne. Acne contributes to adolescent self-consciousness and, if severe, to decreased self-image. Nursing interventions to address acne are discussed in detail in Chapter 25.

Dental Care

The incidence of dental caries decreases in adolescence, but dental hygiene remains important. Most permanent teeth have erupted, with the possible exception of the third molars (wisdom teeth), which erupt by late adolescence or remain impacted and may be removed surgically. Several dental conditions are prevalent during the adolescent years: gingivitis, malocclusion, and dental trauma. Gingivitis is the inflammation and breakdown of the gingival epithelium; the gums appear pale and swollen and bleed easily. Increased hormonal activity at the time of puberty, diets high in sugar and simple carbohydrates, and the use of dental braces and appliances that make cleaning less effective are thought to contribute to the development of gingivitis.

PATIENT-CENTERED TEACHING
Caring for a Child with an Avulsed Tooth

A tooth that has been completely knocked out of the mouth (avulsed) can sometimes be reimplanted. The sooner the reimplantation occurs, the greater is the likelihood of success. If the tooth can be recovered, it should be rinsed in lukewarm tap water and placed in saline, water, milk, or a commercial tooth-preserving liquid. The tooth should not be scrubbed, and cleaning agents and disinfectants should be avoided. The child should be seen as soon as possible by a dentist or taken to the emergency department. The prognosis is best if the injury is treated within 30 minutes.

Malocclusion (improper contact) occurs in approximately 50% of adolescents because of facial and mandibular bone growth and dental crowding. Treatment varies but generally entails dental devices such as braces to correct tooth position and redirect facial growth. Adolescents may be self-conscious if their peers are no longer in braces and may need reassurance that the condition is temporary. For economic reasons, some adolescents are unable to undergo correction of malocclusions and suffer the consequences indefinitely. Nurses can help by referring adolescents with no dental care to free clinics or agencies providing dental care at low cost. People with uncorrected malocclusions are at greater risk for dental trauma.

A tooth that has been completely knocked out of the mouth (avulsed) can sometimes be reimplanted. The sooner the reimplantation occurs, the greater is the likelihood of success. The prognosis is best if the injury is treated within 30 minutes. School and clinic nurses may be the first health professionals to see a child with a complete tooth avulsion and should be aware of the proper procedure (see Chapter 10). Parents should also know how to care for their child if such an incident occurs (see Patient-Centered Teaching: Caring for a Child with an Avulsed Tooth box).

Sleep and Rest

Along with increasingly independent activities, adolescents show a propensity for staying up late (particularly if working on a school project or attending a weekend party) and having difficulty waking up in the morning. Setting one's own bedtime and sleeping late on weekends are behaviors associated with gaining independence, although it may result in adverse effects of decreased amounts of sleep. Hours of sleep may vary from 6 to 8 hours during the week to 12 hours on the weekends, but an overall average of 9 hours per night is recommended for adolescents and young adults. Babcock (2011) suggests that adolescents are more often than not in a state of sleep deprivation. Contributing factors include hectic after-school activities that postpone homework until late at night, electronic devices in the adolescent's bedroom, and the need to socialize late into the night. Effects of sleep deprivation include moodiness, fatigue (including falling asleep in classes), inattention, poor grades, psychological problems, and biologic effects, such as immune suppression (Carskadon, 2011).

Rapid physical growth and increased activities contribute to the adolescent's fatigue, and frustrated parents may complain that their teenager has energy for everything but household and family chores. Nurses can educate teens and their parents to set realistic schedules that allow time for adequate rest and relaxation. Some teens may find themselves so overscheduled that they develop sleep disturbances from excess fatigue and anxiety. Adult sleep cycles are formed during adolescence, and sleep disturbances continue into the adult years. Persistent difficulty in falling asleep, wakefulness during the night, and early waking may be signs of emotional problems associated with tension, anxiety, or depression and may warrant referral.

Several studies have suggested that adolescents' sleep patterns can interfere with their academic performance because the interaction between natural circadian sleep rhythm and social activities makes them less alert in the early morning (Carskadon, 2011). These findings have implications for schools in terms of scheduling start times and planning tests for high school students. School districts in various sections of the country are beginning to address this issue by looking at later start times.

Exercise and Activity

Although adolescents are often involved in many activities, these activities do not always promote physical fitness. One goal of *Healthy People*

HEALTH PROMOTION

Focused Assessment

Ask the adolescent the following:

- Can you tell me how often and what foods you like to eat? How often do you eat at fast-food restaurants? How do you feel about how much you weigh and the shape of your body? Do you think you need to gain or lose any weight? Do you try to control your weight by making yourself vomit, by taking diet pills or laxatives, or by exercising too much?
- Can you describe how much physical activity and what kinds of physical activity you participate in daily?
- How often do you brush your teeth, floss, and see the dentist?
- What time do you go to bed at night? What time do you get up in the morning? Do you have any trouble falling asleep, or do you wake up in the middle of the night?
- How often do you have a bowel movement? Are there any problems with urination?
- What grade in school are you? How well do you think you are doing in school? Do any circumstances at school make you feel unsafe or threatened?
- Tell me about your friends. What types of enjoyable activities do you do together? Do your friends pressure you to do things you would rather not do? Do you or your friends smoke cigarettes or take any substances (alcohol, drugs)?
- Tell me about your relationship with other members of your family. Do you have a special family member to talk to if you are having a problem? If so, whom?
- Do you do any or all of the following: use a seatbelt every time you get in a car; refuse to get into a car if the driver has been drinking or taking drugs; avoid talking on a cell phone or texting while driving; wear a helmet every time you ride a bicycle or motorcycle; wear a helmet and protective pads every time you skate; use sunscreen; swim with a buddy; protect yourself by not putting your personal information on social media websites (e.g., Twitter, Facebook, gaming sites) or reveal it to others in chat rooms or blogs?
- Has anyone ever physically harmed you or touched you in a way that made you uncomfortable? Have you ever thought about harming yourself? Do you or does anyone you know own a gun?
- Have you begun dating? Have you been or are you sexually active? (If sexually active, ask about condom use and birth control methods and any incidence of sexually transmissible infections (STIs).) Do you have any questions or concerns about your sexual development (ask girls about the pattern and frequency of menstruation)?
- What kind of job do you have, if any? How many hours per week do you work?
- What kinds of things do you do to stay healthy? Do you regularly take any medications or dietary supplements? Do you regularly perform breast or testicular self-examinations? Do you have any concerns about any aspect of your health?

Ask the parent the following:

- Do you have any concerns related to your adolescent's nutrition, body image, physical activity, oral health, sleep, elimination, school, family interactions, self-esteem, or ability to practice safety precautions?
- Do you continue to stay involved in your child's life?
- What types of family rules do you consistently enforce?

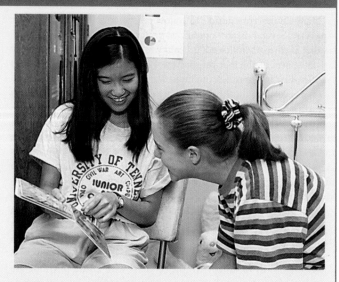

Developmental Milestones

Personal/social: Experiences emotional and social turmoil associated with rapid changes in development and altered body image; is interested in opposite-sex relationships (some lead to a level of intimacy for which the adolescent is not ready); assumes varying roles to integrate social skills with new aspirations and to gain a sense of self; clarifies values and career directions; has more stable emotional control in later adolescence; may exhibit imaginary audience ("Everyone is staring at me") or personal fable ("It will never happen to me")

Fine motor: Adult fine motor control

Language/cognitive: Becomes future oriented; views the world in broad perspective; hypothesizes several alternatives to a problem; thinks and reasons abstractly; develops moral reasoning

Gross motor: Early growth-related awkwardness develops into coordinated muscle control

Health Maintenance

Physical Measurements

Girls achieve PHV approximately 2 years before boys

Average weight gain during growth spurt is 50% of adult weight, largely from body fat in girls and muscle mass in boys

Average height gain is 20% to 25% of adult height over a 2- to 3-year period (girls, 8.3 cm/yr; boys, 9.4 cm/yr)

Achieve Tanner stage 5 (see Table 8-1)

Compute and plot BMI

Immunizations

Review immunization records; administer immunizations if not up to date

Administer tetanus-diphtheria–acellular pertussis (Tdap) at age 11 to 12 years if primary DTaP series is complete and it has been 5 years since the last dose of DTaP. If adult tetanus-diphtheria (Td) booster has already been given, consider immunizing with Tdap if it has been 5 years since the Td booster dose.

Meningococcal conjugate vaccine quadrivalent (MCV4) at age 11 to 12 years or at entrance to high school, if not administered earlier. Administer a booster dose at age 16 years.

Human papillomavirus (HPV) vaccine—recommended at 11 to 12 years old (three doses—give second dose 2 months after the first; give third dose 6 months after the first); may be considered for boys as well as girls (CDC, 2011a)

Influenza vaccine annually

HEALTH PROMOTION—cont'd

Health Screening
Objective hearing and vision screening (adolescent may become myopic as growth spurt begins)
Scoliosis screening
Hemoglobin or hematocrit
Urinalysis by dipstick
Blood pressure
Fasting lipid screen if at risk
Tuberculosis (TB) screening if at risk (see Chapter 21)
Papanicolaou (Pap) smear for sexually active girls
STI screening if applicable
Emotional and stress screening

Anticipatory Guidance
Nutrition
Follow recommended servings according to the USDA's MyPlate system (www.choosemyplate.gov); teach the adolescent how to keep track of servings and give input into meal preparation
Advise to avoid fast foods and eat a nutritious breakfast; watch calcium and iron intake; assess adequacy of diet and snacks; recommend folic acid supplementation for adolescent girls
Vitamin D supplementation 400 international units per day if consuming less than 1 L (33 oz) per day of milk and vitamin D–fortified foods
Teach principles of a vegetarian diet if applicable

Elimination
Regular bowel movements according to individual pattern

Dental
Provide regular dental care every 6 months
Continue regular flossing and brushing with fluoride toothpaste
Discuss emergency care for fractured or avulsed teeth (see Patient-Centered Care: Caring for a Child with an Avulsed Tooth box)

Sleep
Facilitate an individually appropriate sleep pattern; adolescent usually needs 8 hours

Safety
Review gun safety; automobile and motorized vehicle driver and passenger safety; water safety; sun protection; fire safety; avoiding listening to loud music through earphones
Discuss techniques to combat violence, particularly dating violence; wear protective equipment in the workplace; no drinking and driving; preventing STIs and pregnancy (if applicable); learn cardiopulmonary resuscitation (CPR)

Emotional Health
Tell another if concerned about a friend
Take every threat of suicide as real
Try to resist peer pressure
Learn stress-reduction techniques
Seek help if depressed or angry

2020 is to increase physical activity in children of all ages. Surveys reveal that only 18.4% of adolescents meet the recommended levels of participation in regular exercise (60 minutes of mostly aerobic exercise daily, with some time allocated three times a week for both muscle- and bone-strengthening exercise) (USDHHS, 2010; USDA, 2011). Regular exercise enhances physical and emotional development and promotes healthy sleep patterns. Healthy diet and exercise habits formed during adolescence can follow into adulthood and significantly reduce the risk of cardiovascular disease.

Adolescence is an ideal time to initiate an exercise program, either as a team sport or as an individual activity. Exercise need not always involve an athletic activity but should provide for a program that gradually increases exercise over a 1- to 3-week period with a goal of vigorous exercise of at least 60 minutes daily to enhance cardiovascular fitness (USDA, 2011). Nurses can assist adolescents in designing an exercise program that allows gradual fitness and provides warm-up and cool-down sessions. Exercise programs are highly personal and should be structured for enjoyment, with consideration of physical capabilities and limitations.

Safety

Injuries claim more lives during adolescence than all other causes of death combined. The predominance of injuries during adolescence results from a combination of factors: physical growth, psychomotor function, insufficient physical coordination for the task, energy, impulsivity, peer pressure, and inexperience. Impulsivity, inexperience, and peer pressure may place adolescents in unsafe situations. Feelings of invulnerability ("It can't happen to me") persist, and little thought may be given to the negative consequences of certain behaviors. Alcohol and other drugs that impair judgment are known to contribute to fatal injuries among adolescents, especially those involving firearms and motor vehicles (see Chapter 29 for a complete discussion of alcohol and substance abuse). The sad fact is that most serious or fatal injuries involving adolescents are preventable.

Nurses need to educate adolescents and their families about safety issues and injury prevention. Nurses in school and community action programs are increasingly focusing on preventing firearm and traumatic head injuries. Factual information with supportive explanations should be provided. Expressing a genuine interest in adolescents as individuals and listening in a nonjudgmental way are also important steps to gain confidence and trust. Helping the adolescent recognize choices when faced with difficult or potentially dangerous situations is an important component of safety promotion with this age-group.

The adolescent period is also a frightening time for parents because they are aware of the risks predisposing the adolescent to injury or death. Parents may request guidance from health care professionals in setting appropriate limits and establishing methods of effective enforcement. Parents should be encouraged to model the safe behaviors that they expect from the adolescent.

Car Safety

Obtaining a driver's license signifies a passage into adulthood and provides the adolescent with the means to explore and experience the world more freely. Driving is a complex activity, and proficiency in it requires skill, judgment, and experience. The adolescent's lack of judgment, opposition to authority, and need to express independence often result in a disregard for sound defensive driving practices. Risk-taking behaviors appear to play a major role in the high incidence of car-related injuries and deaths among teenagers. The young, inexperienced driver tends to drive faster and take more chances while operating a car than older drivers do. The 2009 Youth Risk Behavior Surveillance Survey of high school students found that 9.7% had rarely or never worn a seatbelt, which has not changed statistically since the previous survey (CDC, 2010). However, during the 30 days preceding the survey, 28.3% had ridden with a driver who had been drinking alcohol (CDC, 2010).

The association between alcohol use and motor vehicle crashes by adolescents is alarming. Despite legal drinking age laws, alcohol is easily accessible to adolescents. The teenager's greater social activity, combined with the availability of alcohol, increases the incidence of impaired driving.

Nurses can promote car safety by supporting driver education programs for teenagers and the use of seatbelts, and discouraging teens from using a cell phone or texting while driving. In addition, many schools and community organizations have developed prevention programs that are helpful in presenting the facts about drinking and driving to adolescents. Nurses should encourage teens and their parents to set up a ride-home agreement to discourage any driving after drinking alcohol. Adolescents need to know that they have an option available to them if they find themselves in a situation in which the driver has been drinking. Dealing with the inconveniences of finding another ride home is much better than dealing with the injuries and damages of motor vehicle crashes.

Water Safety

Drowning is a needless cause of death in teenagers, but it is the fourth leading cause of death from unintentional injury in the 10- to 14-year-old age-group and the seventh leading cause of unintentional injury death in the 15- to 24-year old age-group (National Center for Health Statistics [NCHS], 2011b). Most drowning deaths occur in lakes, rivers, and ponds, with the rest occurring in public or private swimming pools. Risk-taking behaviors contribute greatly to deaths from drowning and to the incidence of spinal cord injuries. Adolescents are able to travel to areas that are free of adult supervision. Frequently, alcohol and drugs are contributing factors. Given the combination of freedom and alcohol, adolescents may inadvertently place themselves at risk for injury by exceeding the limits for safe swimming and diving.

Safety promotion includes encouraging swimming lessons, water safety classes, and the completion of a course in cardiopulmonary resuscitation. Adolescents need to know how alcohol and drugs impair their ability to perform activities at which they are usually competent.

Suicide

Suicide is the seventh leading cause of death for children 5 to 14 years of age and the second leading cause of death in adolescents and young adults 15 to 24 years of age (NCHS, 2011b). In a survey of adolescents, 13.8% had seriously considered committing suicide during the previous 12 months (CDC, 2010). The identification of adolescents at risk for suicide is a priority. Depression is a common finding among suicidal youths; other risk factors are declining mental health, poor impulse control, poor school performance, family disorganization, conduct disorders, substance abuse, homosexuality, and recent stress. Nurses must be involved in identifying high-risk adolescents through the scientific study of these phenomena. Adolescents identified as at risk for suicide

and their families should be targeted for supportive guidance and counseling before a crisis situation. Nurses should counsel parents that all adolescent suicidal gestures should be taken very seriously. Many adolescents do not know what type of drug ingestion or action will actually harm them. The suicidal gestures may appear minor to adults, but the actions may have serious intent (see Chapter 29).

Violence toward Others

Violence continues to threaten the health and well-being of adolescents and society as a whole (see Chapter 1). Homicide is the fourth leading cause of death in children ages 10 to 14 years, and for teens and young adults ages 15 to 24 years it is the second leading cause of death, after unintentional injury (NCHS, 2011). Factors contributing to violence are multiple and complex (Box 8-5). There is a growing body of evidence that suggests that exposure to violence at a young age contributes to later violent behavior. Exposure to violence in the family, community, and through various types of media (e.g., television, movies, video games, Internet) desensitizes children to the effects of violence on others and increases the likelihood that a child will use violent means to solve problematic relationships (AAP, 2009a, 2009b). Contributing factors related to behavior provide the greatest opportunity for interventions initiated by health care professionals.

Nurses working with children, adolescents, and their families have the opportunity to include violence prevention as a component of anticipatory guidance. Ideally, prevention should begin when the child is young. Violence is a learned behavior. It is often reinforced by the actions of those closest to the child and by ever-increasing exposure to violence in the media. Assessing how a family deals with anger and resolves conflict provides insight into the way the child will likely react in similar situations. A family with violent tendencies should be referred to a counselor. Learning to react to anger or stress with nonviolent actions through conflict resolution is the goal for the youth. Unfortunately, intervention cannot be a one-time educational session. Efforts must be reinforced in multiple facets of the adolescent's life, such as in school, youth organizations, and religious organizations, and at home.

Parents need to be aware of the amount and type of violence to which their children are exposed in the media. Parents cannot isolate their children from all media violence, but they can be encouraged to monitor and limit their children's television viewing and to co-view and discuss with their children the implications of violence shown.

The availability of firearms is related to violent acts. In a survey of students in grades 9 through 12 conducted by the CDC, 17.5% reported having carried a weapon within the 30 days preceding the survey

---

BOX 8-5   FACTORS CONTRIBUTING TO ADOLESCENT VIOLENCE

- Low socioeconomic status
- Crowded urban housing
- Single-parent family or limited parental supervision
- History of family violence or child abuse
- Access to guns
- Peer pressure or gang involvement
- Limited education
- Racism
- Drug or alcohol use or abuse
- Low self-esteem and hopelessness about the future
- Aggression

(CDC, 2010). Carrying a weapon can establish a feeling of control or power, or it may be a response to fear of those with power. Regardless of the reasons, firearms in the hands of adolescents are used impulsively, before the ramifications of such actions can be logically considered.

As society urgently seeks a solution to the growing problem of violence, health care professionals must become advocates of violence prevention. Opportunities for adolescents to discover and use less violent means to express themselves or resolve day-to-day issues should be taught and promoted. Peer mediation programs in schools have been successful in preventing violent behavior among teens. Given the tragic effects of violence on the safety and health of American children, nurses should participate in efforts to resolve the complex issues of violence in society.

Selected Issues Related to the Adolescent
Body Piercing

Ear lobe piercing has been popular with teens for many years. Today the ear cartilage, tongue, lip, eyebrow, nose, navel, and nipple are also common sites. Generally, body piercing is harmless, but nurses should caution teens about performing these procedures under unsterile conditions and should educate them about complications, such as bleeding, infection, keloid formation, and allergies to metal. There is a risk for contracting bloodborne diseases or infection from improperly sterilized needles (American Academy of Dermatology [AAD], 2011). Qualified personnel using sterile needles should perform piercing procedures; piercing guns should be avoided unless all parts that touch the skin are sterile (AAD, 2011).

Depending on the site of the piercing, healing time can take anywhere from 6 weeks to up to a year. Important principles for caring for the piercing site include the following: refraining from touching the site or removing the jewelry until fully healed, appropriate hand hygiene, cleaning at least once each day (more often for a tongue piercing) with a recommended saline or antibacterial soap, protecting the site from friction stress, and teaching the adolescent to monitor for signs of infection (Association of Professional Piercers, 2010).

Tattoos

Tattoos are increasingly popular among mainstream adolescents. Like clothing and hairstyles, tattoos serve to define one's identity. Unfortunately, tattoos are often the result of an impulsive decision by the adolescent and are performed by amateurs who are not qualified to do the procedure.

Because of the invasiveness of the tattoo procedure, it should be considered a health-risk situation. Little regulation exists in the tattoo industry, and nurses should educate adolescents about the risks of bloodborne infections, skin infections, and allergic reactions to dyes used in the tattoo process. In addition, nurses need to be informed about tattoo removal to provide correct information to adolescents and their families (see Patient-Centered Teaching: Tattooing box). Impulsive decisions to have a tattoo are often regretted, and teens or their parents may want the tattoo removed. Laser therapy is available for tattoo removal but is painful, costly, and not usually covered by insurance (AAP, 2010). Amateur tattoos are removed quite easily, but studio tattoos made with red and green dyes are difficult to remove. Tattoo removal requires several visits, and adolescents have to tolerate the tattoo's appearance during the removal process (AAD, 2011). Nurses need to caution adolescents with tattoos to notify health professionals of the tattoo if magnetic resonance imaging (MRI) is to be performed because many of the tattoo inks contain metal, such as iron.

PATIENT-CENTERED TEACHING
Tattooing

- Carefully consider tattooing by talking with others about the process.
- Avoid making an impulsive decision about obtaining the tattoo, the location of the tattoo, or what the tattoo will represent.
- Understand that tattooing carries a risk for complications such as infection, allergic reaction to the dye, scarring or keloid formation, and bloodborne diseases such as hepatitis B and HIV; be sure you are immunized against hepatitis B. Tattoos are permanent and are expensive and painful to remove.
- Check the artist's technique; be sure that all equipment is sterile (e.g., ink and needles removed from the package and used just for you), the artist wears gloves and replaces them after touching anything else, and the artist displays a certificate of inspection by the health department.
- Be sure to obtain written instructions about caring for your skin after tattooing.

Data from American Academy of Dermatology. (2011). *Tattoos and body piercings.* Retrieved from www.aad.org; American Academy of Pediatrics. (2010). *I'm thinking about getting a tattoo. What will it be like?* Retrieved from www.aap.org.

Additionally, in general, individuals must wait 12 months after receiving a tattoo before donating blood.

Tanning

A "good" suntan does not exist. Persuading adolescents that tanning is harmful to their skin and is a risk factor for developing skin cancer later in life is difficult, however. The media (advertising, movies, television) promote the image of beach glamour: young, well built, and tanned. Although most companies that manufacture tanning products promote the sun protection factor (SPF) in their products, the advertised image remains a bronzed, attractive, young person. Most exposure to ultraviolet radiation occurs during childhood and adolescence, and skin cancers could be prevented with the appropriate and consistent use of sunscreens and sun blocks.

The estimated prevalence of indoor tanning salon use is approximately 17% of adolescent girls in the United States and 3% of boys (Mayer, Woodruff, Slymen et al., 2011). An area of concern is the fact that a percentage of the adolescents who use tanning salons do not use sun protection (either in the salon or when under natural sunlight) and are not aware of the dangers of exposure to this type of ultraviolet light. Adverse effects from tanning beds include eye injury, premature aging of the skin, and increased risk of skin cancer of all types (Balk & the Committee on Environmental Health and Section on Dermatology, 2011). There is also some evidence that regular use of a tanning salon is addictive for adolescents and there is proposed legislation that no one younger than 18 years be permitted to use a tanning salon (Balk et al., 2011). Nurses who are doing anticipatory guidance with teens must address these issues along with teaching about the risks of tanning in natural sunlight.

Nurses need to educate teens about the benefits and side effects of different sun protection products and to encourage their use during water sports and all activities that involve sun exposure. Teens involved in athletic activities are often exposed to the sun for long periods without protection. Teenagers may be cognizant of body exposure at a beach but may forget about the exposure of body parts during a long tennis match or a baseball game, especially on a cloudy day, when up to 80% of the sun's radiation reaches the ground. Nurses should caution teens receiving any type of medication about the side effects related to sun exposure. Some medications may potentiate the sun's ultraviolet rays, resulting in quicker burning. The side effects of sunscreen products include itching, burning, and redness immediately or up to 24 hours after application. Some people are allergic or sensitive to the sunscreen agent (e.g., para-aminobenzoic acid [PABA], PABA esters, cinnamates, anthranilates, benzophenones) or other ingredients used, such as fragrances and preservatives. Sunscreen use should be discontinued if an allergic dermatitis is noted, and the teen should try another type of sunscreen. Numerous products are on the market with various ingredients that have protective capabilities. Sun damage can be prevented, and simple measures can minimize the effects of ultraviolet radiation on the skin. Many products are available over the counter or through professional salons that have the look of a tan when applied. Nurses can encourage adolescents to use these products rather than expose themselves to ultraviolet light.

Sexual Activity

Adolescent Sexuality. *Adolescent sexuality* refers to the thoughts, feelings, and behaviors related to the adolescent's sexual identity. Middle adolescence typically marks the initial period of dating and experimentation with heterosexual and homosexual behaviors, although in some cultures sexual experimentation occurs much earlier. Initially, group dating may be popular, but this is quickly replaced by dating in couples, who might be sexual partners. Intimate relationships in middle adolescence are usually short lived as adolescents experiment with their sexual identity. Of greatest concern to parents during the adolescent's stage of sexual experimentation are unwanted pregnancies, STIs, and the teen's feelings of despair over failed relationships. Adolescents themselves are often impervious to the possibility of negative consequences of their sexual experimentation and believe that "It can't happen to me."

Although homosexual behavior in adolescence does not necessarily indicate that the adolescent will maintain a homosexual orientation, gay and lesbian adolescents face many challenges growing up in a society that is often unaccepting. Those adolescents who self-identify their sexual preference as homosexual during high school are at increased risk for a variety of health risks and problem behaviors, including suicide, victimization, risky sexual behaviors, and abuse of multiple substances (Pathela & Schillinger, 2010).

Most very young teens have not had intercourse. The likelihood that teenagers will have vaginal intercourse increases with age, however. The 2009 Youth Risk Behavior Surveillance System (YRBSS) showed that 5.9% of the group had had sexual intercourse before age 13 years and that 46% of all adolescents had been involved in sexual activity at some point during adolescence (CDC, 2010). At present, this system does not ask questions about oral sex, although it is believed that a substantial percentage of teens engage in this behavior (CDC, 2009; CDC, National Center for Chronic Disease Prevention and Health Promotion, 2007; Halpern-Felsher, 2008). Adolescence is a period of risk taking, and many adolescents choose to be sexually active and to do so unprotected. Sexual activity in adolescents is greatly correlated with other risk behaviors, especially alcohol and other substance use, so nurses must approach the issue from multiple perspectives.

Some underlying themes influence whether an adolescent delays engaging in sexual activity. Adolescents who demonstrate high levels of self-esteem, who have few other behavioral risk factors (e.g., smoking, drinking), and who are looking for romantic relationships based on desirable personal characteristics in others are more

likely to delay intercourse (Royer, Keller, & Heidrich, 2009). The AAP Council on Communications and Media (2010) suggests that exposure to sexually explicit music, videos, movies, and television programs can contribute to early initiation of sexual activity in adolescents.

A troublesome trend is that adolescents more frequently are obtaining information about sex and sexual relationships through social networking sites or through information searches on the Internet (AAP Council on Communications and Media, 2010; Brown, Keller, & Stern, 2009). One of the major effects of this trend is that adolescents are being exposed to an environment in which sexuality and sexual behavior are presented as desirable, without the presentation of the associated risks and responsibilities (Brown, Keller, & Stern, 2009). In addition, adolescents may be obtaining inaccurate information on which they base decisions about whether to engage in active sexual behavior. Social media can facilitate adolescent sharing of personal information and inappropriate photographs, and can contribute to both the objectification of sex and the risk for sexual victimization (Brown et al., 2009). The adolescent's limited cognitive abilities or lack of abstract thinking may influence contraceptive practices. Adolescents who feel invulnerable to pregnancy often cannot assimilate and apply to themselves information about sexual behavior, conception, and birth control. Lack of self-esteem and peer pressure also play a role in determining adolescents' sexual behavior. Teens may use sex to feel loved or desired, and they may fear abandonment by a partner if sex is refused. Some teens lack correct reproductive information and do not plan ahead for sexual encounters. Sexual activity is often impulsive, erratic, and unplanned because the relationships are relatively short term.

Nurses in schools and community clinics are in a position to identify teens at risk for pregnancy and provide guidance with appropriate information and referral in a confidential atmosphere. Nurses should strongly encourage adolescents to discuss sexuality, sexual behavior, and contraception with their parents whenever possible but must guarantee confidentiality of nurse-adolescent communication.

School sex education programs have had varying success. Many are either abstinence based or protection based. A comprehensive program that provides information about protection methods while emphasizing the benefits of abstinence may be more successful than either emphasis alone (Royer et al., 2009).

The nurse's professional role is to ensure that adolescents have the knowledge, skills, and opportunities that enable them to make responsible decisions about sexual behavior. Education regarding sexuality and contraception should be oriented to the developmental level of the individual or group. The nurse uses primary preventive intervention by assisting adolescents to develop coping strategies to meet their needs in ways other than through sexual behavior. The AAP Council on Communications and Media (2010) suggests that the media could be used to send positive messages about sexuality and healthy relationships, but that this can only occur through advocacy and collaboration with the broadcast and entertainment industry. In addition, the Council recommends that parents limit their adolescents' exposure to sexually explicit media through monitoring adolescents' television viewing, use of social media websites, and access to R-rated movies.

Contraception. Complete protection from pregnancy and STIs is achievable only through sexual abstinence. Because approximately half of adolescents between ages 15 and 19 years are sexually active, however, nurses need to feel comfortable with managing health concerns related to sexuality. Comprehensive health care includes providing services for sexually active adolescents. Health care providers should provide

! NURSING QUALITY ALERT

Factors to Consider in Selecting Adolescent Contraception

- Cognitive development (concrete vs. abstract thinking)
- Understanding and acceptance of attitudes and values
- Sexual maturity rating
- Communication between partners
- Opportunity to counsel both partners
- Use of more than one method
- Frequency of intercourse
- Appropriate information (three messages per visit)
- Problem-solving abilities (appeal to logic and feelings of power over body)
- Communication with parents or other adults
- Physical and mental health
- Motivation of both partners
- Concrete, graphic instruction in all methods
- Number and gender of partners
- Encouragement that abstinence is all right

screening for and management of STIs, contraceptive services, and psychosocial counseling.

In the United States in 2007, births to adolescents younger than 18 years of age accounted for 3.4% of all live births (NCHS, 2011a). This percentage has stabilized, but is considerably less than the 4.1% in 2000. Most teens do not seek contraceptive information for 1 year after first intercourse, resulting in unintended pregnancy frequently occurring within the first several months after intercourse is initiated (Klein, 2005). When the nurse is educating adolescents about birth control methods, consultation with the two partners together is ideal. Open communication between partners is essential, and decisions about contraception should be mutual. Both male and female adolescents need to assume responsibility for sexually active behavior. Regardless of the method of birth control selected, all adolescents need frequent follow-up to maintain consistent contraception behaviors. Table 8-2 presents selected contraception methods available to adolescents. Counseling teens about sexuality and contraception requires nurses who are open, forthright, and respectful of the decisions teens make about sexual activity. (See Chapter 4 for a discussion of media violence and Chapter 17 for information about STIs.)

TABLE 8-2 METHODS OF CONTRACEPTION FOR ADOLESCENTS

METHOD	ADVANTAGES	DISADVANTAGES
Chance (no protection)	No cost; requires no preparation	High failure rate No disease prevention
Abstinence (no sexual intercourse)	No cost; requires no preparation	May be difficult for sexually active teens
Withdrawal (withdrawal of penis from vagina before ejaculation)	No cost; requires no preparation	High failure rate Requires control and motivation by male No disease prevention
Periodic abstinence (rhythm method; no sexual intercourse during fertile/ovulation period)	No cost; natural family planning	High failure rate Requires awareness of fertility times, motivation, and predictable menstrual cycle No disease prevention
Condom (male: latex, or non-latex, penile sheath to trap sperm; female: sheath inserted into the vagina)	Male condoms are inexpensive; allows for planning; effective with spermicide Disease prevention in general; not for some, such as human papillomavirus (HPV) and herpes simplex (HSV) Male condoms readily available over the counter	Moderate failure rate; should be used in conjunction with other contraceptive method Requires planning Non-latex condoms may be used if allergic to latex Best used with spermicide Requires new condom with each successive intercourse Female condom more difficult to insert, not widely available
Spermicides (creams, jelly, foam, suppositories placed in vagina to kill sperm before it enters cervix)	Available over the counter Effective if used with barrier method Relatively inexpensive Allows for planning Prescription not required	Requires planning High failure rate it used alone Messy Must reapply with each successive intercourse No disease prevention
Vaginal ring (medicated device inserted in the vagina by the user that releases continuous low doses of hormone, which is absorbed by vaginal mucosa)	Not tied to sexual activity Three week on, 1 week off schedule Nearly immediate contraceptive protection Effectiveness similar to oral contraception	Must be prescribed by a physician Backup contraception required if removed and not replaced immediately Vaginal discomfort, inflammation, or infection may occur Other side effects similar to oral contraceptives Medical intervention and prescription needed No disease prevention

Data from Hatcher, J., Trussell, J., & Stewart, F. (1994). The essentials of contraception: effectiveness, safety, and personal considerations. In *Contraceptive technology* (p. 113). New York: Irvington Publishers, Inc.; Fuller, J. (2007/2008). Adolescents and contraception: The nurse's role as counselor. *Nursing for Women's Health, 11*(6), 547-556.

Continued

TABLE 8-2   METHODS OF CONTRACEPTION FOR ADOLESCENTS—cont'd

METHOD	ADVANTAGES	DISADVANTAGES
Combined oral contraceptives (combination products suppress ovulation, increase thickness of cervical mucus, decrease thickness of uterine lining)	Not tied to sexual activity Highly effective; failure rate is <1% Allows for planning Some available in various extended-cycle regimens that decrease breakthrough bleeding	Requires knowledge and motivation for use Adherence to pill schedule is imperative for adequate contraception Expensive for teens Side effects include breakthrough bleeding during cycles (varies with pill and patient); mood changes; needs to be avoided if at risk for thrombolytic or embolic disorders Usually requires pelvic examination and regular follow-up No disease prevention
Contraceptive patch (thickens the cervical mucus and suppresses ovulation; applied to skin in upper torso [not breasts], upper outer arm, buttocks or abdominal area)	Not tied to sexual activity Patch is worn continuously, changed weekly for 3 weeks, then 1 week off; no need to remember to take medication daily Highly effective	Prescription required and periodic medical evaluation Side effects include skin irritation, nausea, vomiting, headache, breast tenderness; usually disappear after continued use Usually covered by Medicaid Requires back-up contraceptive method if schedule of patching is not closely followed or the patch comes off inadvertently Risk for thromboembolic event is higher than that for oral contraceptives, related to increased estrogen exposure
Injectable contraceptive (Depo-Provera [DMPA], injectable progestin given every 3 months; suppresses ovulation for up to 15 weeks)	Highly effective Not tied to sexual activity No planning once medication has been injected Stops menses in 50% of users Can be used by lactating females, those with selected cardiac disease, or chronic illnesses, and drug addicts	Requires medical intervention and intramuscular injection every 3 months May have delay in fertility after discontinuation Side effects of progestin: irregular, heavy, or no bleeding; headaches; weight gain; depression Expensive Should not be used longer than 2 years because of increased risk for osteoporosis; regular long bone activity should be encouraged
Emergency contraceptive pills (combined estrogen and progestin taken within 72 hours and again 12 hours later; Plan B-progestin only)	Approximately 70% to 85% effective in preventing pregnancy, depending on the medication used and the elapsed time since intercourse	Should not be used as routine contraception Requires medical intervention for adolescents; sold over the counter in some states for women over 18 years of age Contraindicated in teens who cannot use oral contraceptives or if longer than 72 hours after intercourse Nausea is the main side effect Pregnancy test required if no menses after 3 weeks of taking the medication Most physicians will require counseling for STI prevention and routine contraception

KEY CONCEPTS

- Adolescence is a period of transition from childhood to adulthood that is marked by important biologic, psychological, emotional, and social changes.
- The hallmark of physical development during adolescence is the development of primary and secondary sexual characteristics, which are acquired through the influence of reproductive hormones in males and females and assessed through a sexual maturity rating (SMR, or Tanner stage).
- Social development during adolescence is concerned with identity and self-perception, and cognitive thinking moves from concrete to abstract reasoning.

- Poor eating habits and lack of aerobic exercise contribute to obesity and decreased overall physical fitness; it is imperative that adolescents consume a well-rounded diet, combined with at least 60 minutes of aerobic exercise daily to prevent obesity.
- Health and safety issues pertinent to adolescents that require nursing intervention, include tanning, body piercing, tattooing, and other high-risk behaviors, such as substance abuse, sexual activity (e.g., teen pregnancy and STIs), violence, and reckless operation of motor vehicles.

REFERENCES

Ali, O. & Donohoue, P. (2011). Gynecomastia. In R. Kliegman, B. Stanton, J. St Geme, et al. (Eds.). *Nelson textbook of pediatrics* (19th ed., pp. 1950-1951). Philadelphia, PA: Elsevier Saunders.

American Academy of Dermatology. (2011). *Tattoos and body piercings*. Retrieved from www.aad.org.

American Academy of Pediatrics. (2009a). Policy statement: Media violence. *Pediatrics, 124*(5), 1495-1503.

American Academy of Pediatrics. (2009b). Policy statement: Role of the pediatrician in youth violence prevention. *Pediatrics, 124*(1), 393-402.

American Academy of Pediatrics. (2010). *I'm thinking about getting a tattoo. What will it be like?* Retrieved from www.aap.org

American Academy of Pediatrics Committee on Adolescence. (2008). Achieving quality health services for adolescents. *Pediatrics, 121*(6), 1263-1270.

American Academy of Pediatrics Council on Communications and Media. (2010). Sexuality, contraception and the media. *Pediatrics, 126*, 576-582.

American Heart Association. (2011). *Dietary recommendations for healthy children*. Retrieved from www.heart.org.

American Medical Association. (1997). *Guideline for adolescent preventive services (GAPS) recommendations monograph*. Retrieved from www.ama.assn.org.

Association of Professional Piercers. (2010). *Suggested aftercare guidelines for body piercings*. Retrieved from www.safepiercing.org.

Babcock, D. (2011). Evaluating sleep and sleep disorders in the pediatric primary care setting. *Pediatric Clinics of North America, 58*, 543-554.

Balk, S. and the Council on Environmental Health and Section on Dermatology. (2011). Technical report: Ultraviolet radiation: A hazard to children and adolescents. *Pediatrics, 127*(3), e791-e817.

Biro, F., Galvez, M., Greenspan, L., et al. (2010). Pubertal assessment and baseline characteristics in a mixed longitudinal study of girls. *Pediatrics, 126*, e583-e590.

Brown, J., Keller, S., & Stern, S. (2009). Sex, sexuality, sexting, and sex ed: Adolescents and the media. *The Prevention Researcher, 16*(4), 12-16.

Carskadon, M. (2011). Sleep in adolescents: The perfect storm. *Pediatric Clinics of North America, 58*, 637-647.

Centers for Disease Control and Prevention. (2009). *Oral sex and HIV risk*. Retrieved from www.cdc.gov.

Centers for Disease Control and Prevention. (2010). Youth Risk Behavior Surveillance—United States, 2009. *MMWR, 59*(SS-5), 1-148.

Centers for Disease Control and Prevention. (2011a). *Recommended immunization schedule for persons aged 7 through 18 years—United States 2011*. Retrieved from www.cdc.gov.

Centers for Disease Control and Prevention. (2011b). *Teen birth rates decline again in 2009*. Retrieved from www.cdc.gov.

Centers for Disease Control and Prevention. (2011c). Teen pregnancy, the importance of prevention. Retrieved from www.cdc.gov.

Centers for Disease Control and Prevention, National Center for Chronic Disease Prevention and Health Promotion. (2007). *Healthy youth health topics, sexual risk behaviors*. Retrieved from www.cdc.gov.

Cotton, S., Tsevat, J., & Yi, M. (2007). Existential well-being, depressive symptoms, and health-related quality of life in adolescents. *Journal of Adolescent Health, 40*(2), S43-S44.

Elkind, D. (1993). *Parenting your teenager*. New York: Ballantine Books.

Erikson, E. (1968). *Identity: Youth and crisis*. New York: Norton.

Freud, S. (1960). *The ego and the id* (J. Riviere, Trans.). New York: Norton.

Halpern-Felsher, B. (2008). Oral sex behavior: Harm reduction or gateway behavior? *Journal of Adolescent Health, 43*(3), 207-208.

Herrman, J. (2005). The teen brain as a work in progress: Implications for pediatric nurses. *Pediatric Nursing, 31*(2), 144-147.

Husky, M., Miller, K., McGuire, L., & et al. (2011). Mental health screening of adolescents in pediatric practice. *Journal of Behavioral Health Services and Research, 38*(2), 159-169.

Klein, J. & Committee on Adolescence. (2005). Adolescent pregnancy: Current trends and issues. *Pediatrics, 116*(1), 281-286.

Kohlberg, L. (1964). Development of moral character. In M. Hoffman & L. Hoffman (Eds.), *Review of child development research*, Vol. 1. New York: Russell Sage Foundation.

Lindberg, L., Jones, R., & Santelli, J. (2008). Non-coital sexual activities among adolescents. *Journal of Adolescent Health, 43*(3), 231-238.

Mayer, J., Woodruff, S., Slymen, D., et al. (2011). Adolescents' use of tanning: A large-scale evaluation of psychosocial, environmental, and policy level correlates. *American Journal of Public Health, 101*(5), 930-938.

National Center for Health Statistics (NCHS). (2011a). *Health, United States, 2010 with special feature on death and dying*. Hyattsville, MD: Author.

National Center for Health Statistics. (2011b). *Ten leading causes of injury deaths by age group highlighting unintentional injury, United States—2007*. Retrieved from www.cdc.gov/nchs.

Pathela, P., & Schillinger, J. (2010). Sexual behaviors and sexual violence: Adolescents with opposite-, same-, or both-sex partners. *Pediatrics, 126*, 879-886.

Piaget, J. (1969). *The theory of stages in cognitive development*. New York: McGraw-Hill.

Royer, H., Keller, M., & Heidrich, S. (2009). Young adolescents' perceptions of romantic relationships and sexual activiey. *Sex Education, 9*(4), 395-408.

Rubin, D., Dodd, M., Desai, N., et al. (2009). Spirituality in well and ill adolescents and their parents: The use of two assessment scales. *Pediatric Nursing, 35*(1), 37-42.

Stettler, N., Bhatia, J., Parish, A., & Stallings, B. (2011). Feeding healthy infants, children, and adolescents. In R. Kliegman, B. Stanton, St. J. Geme, et al. (Eds.). *Nelson textbook of pediatrics* (19th ed., pp. 168-169). Philadelphia: Elsevier Saunders.

Tanner, J. (1962). *Growth at adolescence* (2nd ed.). Oxford: Blackwell Scientific Publications.

United States Department of Agriculture. (2011). *Dietary guidelines for Americans, 2010*. Retrieved from www.cnpp.usda.gov/DietaryGuidelines.html.

U.S. Department of Health and Human Services. (2010). *Healthy People 2020*. Retrieved from www.healthypeople.gov.

Physical Assessment
of Children

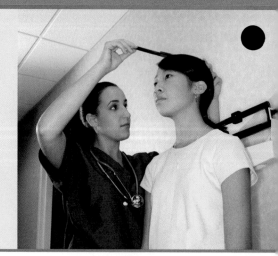

evolve WEBSITE

http://evolve.elsevier.com/James/ncoc

LEARNING OBJECTIVES

After studying this chapter, you should be able to:

- Apply principles of anatomy and physiology to the systematic physical assessment of the child.
- Describe the major components of a pediatric health history.
- Identify the principal techniques for performing a physical examination.
- Use a systematic and developmentally appropriate approach for examining a child.

- Describe the general sequence of the physical examination of the infant, the young child, the school-age child, and the adolescent.
- Describe normal physical examination findings.
- List common terms used to describe the findings on physical examination.
- Record physical examination findings in a systematic way.

Nurses perform physical assessments of infants and children in various settings—the clinic, the hospital, the school, and the home. The physical examination may be part of a well-child assessment, it may be the admission examination when a child enters the hospital, or it may be part of an initial assessment for home health care. The physical examination provides objective and subjective information about the child. The ability to perform a physical examination is fundamental to nursing care of the child. Findings from a thorough physical examination help to determine a child's health status, which is the basis of all nursing interventions.

GENERAL APPROACHES TO PHYSICAL ASSESSMENT

As when providing any nursing care for infants and children, the nurse applies knowledge of growth and development when preparing the child and parents for performance of the physical examination. Involving parents as much as possible in the examination and allowing the child to handle safe, clean instruments, such as the stethoscope, reduce anxiety and increase the likelihood of examining a cooperative child.

The physical examination is often the first direct contact between the nurse and the child. Establishing a trusting relationship between the child and the examiner is important. Throughout the examination the nurse should be sensitive to the cultural needs of and differences among children. Providing a quiet, private environment for the history and physical examination is important. The classic systematic approach to the physical examination is to begin at the head and proceed through the entire body to the toes. When examining a child, however, the examiner tailors the physical assessment to the child's age and developmental level.

Infants from Birth to 6 Months

Infants ages birth to 6 months are responsive to human faces, are increasingly interested in their environment, and do not mind being undressed (see Chapter 5). Their examination should therefore be relatively easy. If the infant is nursing or asleep in the parent's arms, auscultate the heart, lungs, and abdomen without waking the baby. Even if the infant is awake, effective examination can still be accomplished with the infant laying or sitting in the parent's arms or on the lap. As body parts are examined, incorporate evaluation of the primitive reflexes—palmar grasp, plantar grasp, placing, stepping, and tonic neck reflexes. Leave all uncomfortable procedures, such as abduction of the hips, speculum examination of the tympanic membranes, and elicitation of the Moro reflex, until last. Before beginning the examination, undress the infant, leaving the diaper on a male child. Refocus an unhappy infant by calmly talking in a soft voice, distracting with a rattle, or offering a pacifier.

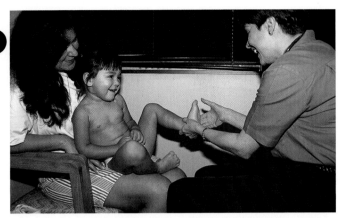

FIG 9-1 During the assessment, the nurse allows the child to remain on her mother's lap, enlisting the child's trust and increasing the likelihood of a successful physical examination. (Photo courtesy Parkland Health and Hospital System, Community Oriented Primary Care Clinics, Dallas, TX.)

Infants from 6 to 12 Months

For an older infant, follow the same procedures used for the infant from birth to 6 months, but keep in mind that infants 6 months and older feel stranger anxiety and so are more difficult to examine. Distracting a child of this age with a toy or object may be useful. It is easier to do as much of the examination as possible with the child held on the parent's lap. Leave ear, oral, and other uncomfortable procedures until last.

Toddlers

Toddlers are the most challenging to examine because they are least likely to cooperate (see Chapter 6). To form a supportive relationship with the parent and toddler, the examiner begins by sitting or standing next to the parent (Figure 9-1). To facilitate relaxation, the examiner can provide a few toys and books and encourage the child to explore. Allowing the child to handle objects used during the examination can decrease fears. Communicating with the child, using age-appropriate words to describe what is about to be done, can also help decrease fear.

! NURSING QUALITY ALERT

Adapting the Physical Examination to the Child

The classic systematic approach to the physical examination is to begin at the head and proceed to the toes. For children, painful or frightening procedures should be left until last. Involving parents by asking them to hold or stand by the child can decrease children's anxiety and assist them in relaxing.

Portions of the examination can be done before the child is totally undressed. The order of the examination is flexible, proceeding from least to most invasive procedures. Resistance and crying are common with toddlers. The nurse assures the parent that the child's response to the examination is normal. The parent is the best resource for gaining the child's cooperation during the examination. Parents' use of approaches to soothing and comforting that are familiar to a child can do much to facilitate examination.

Preschoolers

Preschool children are usually more cooperative than toddlers but still like to have their parents nearby (see Chapter 6). Preschool children are happy to show nurses that they can undress themselves. They can

also be expected to cooperate. The nurse may proceed with the examination from the head to the toe but should still save the more invasive procedures, such as the speculum ear examination and the oral examination, until last. The examiner can reinforce the child's interest by allowing the child to participate in the examination and by praising the child for cooperating.

School-Age Children

To establish trust with the school-age child, the examiner asks the child questions the child can answer. Children in elementary school will talk about school, favorite friends, and activities (see Chapter 7). Older school-age children may have to be encouraged to talk about their school performance and activities. The examiner encourages the parent to support and reinforce the child's participation in the examination.

The examination proceeds from head to toe. Children of this age prefer a simple drape over their underpants or a colorful examination gown, and the examiner should be sensitive to the child's modesty. The examination is a wonderful opportunity to teach the child about the body and personal care. The nurse answers questions openly and in simple terms.

Adolescents

Adolescents are most comfortable with a straightforward, noncondescending approach (see Chapter 8). Decisions about who should be present during the examination should be openly discussed with the adolescent. In most cases adolescents should be examined without the parent present. However, the parent should be given the opportunity to talk to the nurse about any concerns. The order of the examination is the same as for the school-age child.

It is best to incorporate the genital examination into the middle of the examination. If possible, proceed from the abdominal examination to the genital examination, to allow ample time for questions and discussions about this part of the examination. The physical examination provides the opportunity to assure the pubertal child about normal developmental stages and to answer concerns children this age frequently have about what is happening to their bodies. The adolescent is expected to undress and wear a gown. The adolescent is draped appropriately during the examination.

TECHNIQUES FOR PHYSICAL EXAMINATION

When performing the physical assessment, the nurse uses the four basic techniques of inspection, palpation, percussion, and auscultation, generally in that order. During the abdominal examination, the sequence is altered: inspection is performed first, and then auscultation, percussion, and palpation. The sequence of the abdominal examination is changed so as not to alter bowel sounds before determining their presence and characteristics. Percussion is performed to determine the size of abdominal organs before palpation.

Inspection

Most information is gathered during the physical examination by systematic and deliberate visual observations. The nurse first surveys an entire area of the body and then focuses on specifics, such as color, shape, size, and movement. Inspection can be both direct and indirect. Direct inspection relies on the examiner's senses of sight and hearing. Indirect inspection is accomplished with the use of special equipment, such as an otoscope, to examine a specific body area.

Palpation

During palpation, the nurse uses the sense of touch to make judgments about pulsations and vibrations and to locate structures and masses. Palpation allows the nurse to determine characteristics such as size, texture, warmth, mobility, and tenderness of various areas of the body.

Different parts of the hands are used to detect different characteristics. The finger pads are used to palpate the breast, while fingertips are used to palpate the lymph nodes and pulses. The back of the hand is used to assess temperature. The palm of the hand is used to detect vibrations.

The type of palpation used is governed by the structure to be examined and the need to avoid any unnecessary discomfort to the child. Light palpation is accomplished by gently applying fingertip pressure to depress the skin surface approximately $\frac{1}{2}$ to $\frac{3}{4}$ inch and then moving the fingertips in a circular motion.

⚠ NURSING QUALITY ALERT

Using the Hands for Palpation

- Finger pads are used to palpate the breast.
- Fingertips are used to palpate lymph nodes, and pulses.
- The back of the hand is used to assess temperature.
- The palm of the hand is used to identify vibrations.

Deep palpation identifies abdominal structures such as the liver, spleen, and kidneys and detects abdominal masses. Deep palpation follows light palpation. The surface is depressed approximately $1\frac{1}{2}$ to 2 inches to identify underlying masses and abdominal structures. Bimanual palpation is performed with both hands. The examiner superimposes one hand over the other to increase pressure or places one hand near the other to capture and trap a mass or structure between them, such as a kidney or the spleen.

Percussion

To percuss, the nurse uses quick, sharp tapping of the fingers or hands to produce sounds. Percussion is performed to locate the position, size, and density of underlying structures. The three basic methods are as follows:

- *Mediate,* or *indirect percussion,* in which the finger of one hand is placed against the body surface and the finger of the other hand acts as the hammer
- *Immediate percussion,* performed by striking the finger of one hand directly against the body
- *Fist percussion,* in which the ulnar aspect of the fist is used to deliver a firm blow directly to the area

The method used depends on the area to be percussed. The nurse uses quick, light blows to create vibrations that penetrate approximately 2 inches below the surface. Sounds identified by percussion are classified as *flat, dull, resonant, hyperresonant,* or *tympanic* (Box 9-1).

Auscultation

Auscultation entails eliciting and listening to body sounds created in the lungs, heart, blood vessels, and abdominal viscera. The most common way to auscultate is to use a stethoscope. Most auscultated sounds result from air or fluid movement within the body. The diaphragm of the stethoscope is most effective in assessing high-pitched sounds, such as heart and breath sounds. The bell of the stethoscope is most effective in hearing low-pitched sounds, such as blood pressure and vascular sounds. Auscultation requires a quiet environment. The

---

BOX 9-1   SOUNDS IDENTIFIED DURING PERCUSSION

Flat: High-pitched, soft-intensity sound elicited by percussing over solid masses, such as bone or muscle

Dull: Medium-pitched, medium-intensity sound elicited when percussing over high-density structures, such as the liver

Resonance: Low-pitched, loud-intensity sound elicited over a hollow organ, such as the lungs

Hyperresonance: Very low, very loud, with a booming quality heard over the lungs in young children

Tympany: High-pitched, loud-intensity sound heard over air-filled body parts, such as the bowel or stomach

---

BOX 9-2   POTENTIAL INDICATORS OF CHILD ABUSE

Dress: Inappropriate for the weather; ragged or excessively dirty

Grooming and personal hygiene: Dirty teeth; broken and dirty fingernails; matted and dirty hair

Posture and movements: Crouching in a corner; slow, concentrated movements

Body image distortion: Being thin but describing self as fat

Speech and communication: Answering questions in words of one syllable; looking to others to respond first; seeking approval for answers

Facial characteristics and expressions: Fearful, anxious, tearful, sad, or angry expressions

Psychological state: Labile, demanding, bizarre, overly dramatic, or condescending

---

nurse places the stethoscope on the skin in the appropriate area. Sounds heard are described according to pitch, intensity, duration, and quality.

Smell

While examining the child, the nurse uses the sense of smell to detect general body odors, common in children who are neglected or dirty. Odor may also indicate infection. Odors from the mouth, urine, or feces can be important. In particular, some diseases are characterized by odors coming from the mouth (Seidel, Ball, Dains et al., 2010).

SEQUENCE OF PHYSICAL EXAMINATION

General Appearance

During the first contact with the child and parent, the examiner forms an initial impression by making a general survey. The nurse determines the child's age, sex, and race, and identifies clues concerning the child's behavior and health status. Because each child is a unique human, individual differences in behavior and health status related to growth and development will be evident. During the general survey, the examiner continually notes the parent-child interaction and the way the parent responds to the child's needs and behavior. Physical and emotional neglect, as well as inadequate parental supervision for the child's age, may be subtle or overt. These observations, together with other indicators of the child's health status, may provide clues to distress or abuse (Box 9-2).

BOX 9-3 THE COMPLETE HISTORY

The complete or initial history includes the following:

1. *Statistical information:* Name, age, address, telephone number, birth date, names of parents or guardians, and source of support.
2. *Client profile:* Times the child eats and sleeps, educational level, developmental level, race, ethnicity, nationality, religion, economic status, and health status perception. If an interpreter is used to gather the health history, the person's name is included in the record, usually in this section of the history. Also included is a statement about the reliability of an informant, such as an older sibling who answers questions concerning a younger sibling or an aunt or uncle who answers questions regarding a child.
3. *Health history:* Birth history, growth and development, common childhood illnesses, immunizations, previous hospitalizations, accidents or injuries, and allergies or allergic reactions and exact symptoms the allergy produced. The person taking the history should ask about medications taken daily or for an acute episode of an illness and should list all medications being taken, including dose and frequency. The parent should name both prescription and over-the-counter medications as well as herbal remedies and supplements. The examiner also asks whether the child has ever had a blood transfusion or has received any blood products. For any hospitalizations, serious illnesses, and injuries, the nurse should obtain the following information:
   a. Reason for admission
   b. Place of admission
   c. Length of stay
   d. Surgical procedures
   e. Other treatments
   f. Outcomes
   g. Follow-up
4. *Family history:* Information concerning the health status of the child's mother, father, siblings, and specific blood relatives such as aunts, uncles, and grandparents. If any are deceased, the history includes the age and cause of death. The purpose is to determine constitutional and hereditary factors that are likely to affect the child's health.
5. *Lifestyle and life patterns:* The child's interaction with the social, psychological, physical, and cultural environment. Growth and development; use of street drugs, alcohol, and tobacco; roles and relationships; and family life information are all important.
6. *Review of systems:* A systematic review of the major anatomic and physiologic parts. A head-to-toe review focusing on the health function and maintenance of each body part should occur in this order:
   a. General appearance
   b. Head
   c. Hair
   d. Face
   e. Eyes
   f. Ears
   g. Nose and sinuses
   h. Mouth
   i. Throat
   j. Neck
   k. Lungs
   l. Heart
   m. Breasts
   n. Abdomen
   o. Kidneys and bladder
   p. Bowels, rectum, and anus
   q. Genitals
   r. Extremities

Animation: Organ Systems 3-D Tour

BOX 9-4 PROBLEM-ORIENTED HISTORY

Chief complaint: Use the child's own words.
Body location: Place the problem somewhere on the body.
Quality: Define what the problem is like for the child.
Quantity: Describe the intensity of the problem for the child.
Chronology: Determine when the problem began, the periodicity and frequency, and the course of symptoms.
Setting: Identify where the problem occurs.
Aggravating and alleviating factors: Find out what makes the problem better or worse.
Associated manifestations: Document other related information.
Treatment: Document what has been used to treat the problem. Be sure to ask about complementary therapies as well as traditional approaches.

History Taking

Taking an accurate history is the single most important component of the physical examination. Practitioners obtain three different types of health histories: the complete or initial history; the well, interim history; and the episodic or problem-oriented, history.

In the *complete* or *initial history* (Box 9-3), data are gathered about the child from the time of conception to the child's current status. The *well, interim history* includes data gathered about the child from the last well visit to the current visit. When doing a well, interim history, the examiner assumes that a database is in place. In a *problem-oriented,* or *episodic history* (Box 9-4), information is gathered about a current problem. Information about the specific problem is then added to the existing database.

CRITICAL THINKING EXERCISE 9-1

Ann Maloney, a 17-year-old single mother, brings her 6-month-old daughter, Kerrie, to the clinic. This is Kerrie's first visit. Ms. Maloney made several earlier appointments for Kerrie but was always unable to keep them. She states, "I am very busy trying to work and care for Kerrie. I had to miss work because Kerrie has lots of colds. I hate to take time off when she is well. My supervisor at work said that it is important for her to have her immunizations and a physical examination. I guess I messed up."

1. What assumptions could the nurse make about Ms. Maloney?
2. How should the nurse respond to Ms. Maloney's comment?
3. How can the nurse best act as an advocate for both Kerrie and her mother?

Recording Data

The information gathered during the history is documented concisely to provide all necessary information from pregnancy to the child's current status. Milestones in growth and development, immunizations, and family status are always included in the child's history.

Vital Signs

Vital signs are taken for every child during every visit in ambulatory care settings and are monitored throughout the day in a hospitalized child. Assessment of vital signs (temperature, pulse, respirations, and

TABLE 9-1   NORMAL VITAL SIGNS BY AGE

AGE	TEMPERATURE* DEGREES FAHRENHEIT	DEGREES CELSIUS	PULSE RATE (BEATS/MIN)	RESPIRATORY RATE (BREATHS/MIN)	BLOOD PRESSURE RANGE (mm Hg)†
Newborn	97.7-99.1 (axillary)	36.5-37.3 (axillary)	120-160	30-60	Systolic: 65-95‡ Diastolic: 30-60‡
4 yr	97.5-98.6 (axillary)	36.4-37 (axillary)	80-125	20-30	Girls Systolic: 91-104 Diastolic: 52-66 Boys Systolic: 93-107 Diastolic: 50-65
10 yr	97.5-98.6 (oral)	36.4-37 (oral)	70-110§	16-22	Girls Systolic: 102-115 Diastolic: 60-74 Boys Systolic: 102-115 Diastolic: 61-75
16 yr	97.5-98.6 (oral)	36.4-37 (oral)	55-90	15-20	Girls Systolic: 111-124 Diastolic: 66-80 Boys Systolic: 116-130 Diastolic: 65-80

*The normal range of the child's temperature depends on the method used. Temperatures exhibit circadian rhythms at all ages.
†Blood pressures represent values for the 50th and 90th percentiles at age and average height.
‡Taken by Doppler measurement.
§After age 12 yr, a boy's pulse is 5 beats/min slower than a girl's.

blood pressure) is an important way to measure and monitor vital body functions. Measuring vital signs provides the basis for decisions concerning the child's overall health and illness. In children, changes in vital signs are important signs of changes in health status. Table 9-1 describes normal vital signs by age, and Chapter 13 details the procedure for taking vital signs in children.

Temperature

The method for measuring children's temperature may vary from one setting to another. Some parents are comfortable taking a rectal or axillary temperature. Health care providers may use a tympanic membrane or temporal artery sensor or an electronic, digital thermometer. Currently, parents are encouraged to take axillary rather than rectal temperatures. Reasons for the recommendation are the invasive nature of rectal temperature measurements, the risk of injury, and their questionable accuracy with febrile children because feces retain body heat for hours after a fever has diminished. Axillary temperatures, when taken correctly, provide accurate information concerning changes in the child's health status.

Tympanic temperature measurements are frequently used in health care agencies because they can be performed quickly and involve less cross contamination; however, studies have shown mixed results as to their accuracy in determining fever (Devrim et al., 2007; Holzhauer, Reith, Sawin, & Yen, 2009). When recording a tympanic temperature, the nurse notes the side on which the temperature was elicited. Variation can occur from one ear to the other in the same child.

An oral thermometer may be used with older children, usually starting at 5 or 6 years old. For oral temperature measurements, an electronic thermometer is unbreakable and registers quickly.

A temporal artery thermometer (TemporalScanner, Exergen Corp., Watertown, MA) is a noninvasive system with advanced infrared technology. It measures temperatures with a gentle stroke across the forehead and then down to the ear. This thermometer can be used with infants, children, or adolescents. As the probe crosses over the temporal artery, the sensor inside the probe measures ambient temperatures, mathematically replaces the small temperature loss from cooling at the skin, and displays an accurate arterial temperature (Exergen Corporation, 2005). (See Chapter 13 for a discussion of various methods of assessing temperature.)

Pulse

Apical pulse rates are measured in children younger than 2 years and in any child who has an irregular heart rate or known congenital heart disease. Radial pulse rates may be taken in children older than 2 years. To compensate for normal irregularities, the nurse counts the pulse for 1 full minute. Chapter 13 details the procedure for measuring the pulse rate.

Arterial pulses are palpated to determine pulse rate and rhythm and to evaluate blood flow, arterial wall elasticity, and vessel patency. To determine the position of the heart in the anterior precordium, the nurse palpates the apical impulse in infants and children younger than 6 years. In the acute care setting, an apical impulse is always palpated in every child and the location of the apical impulse is noted. Simultaneously, the examiner palpates and compares femoral, radial, and carotid pulses in children of any age. The nurse may also compare a carotid pulse with a femoral or radial pulse for equality of pulses. In infants, the nurse notes the pulsating anterior fontanel. The pulse may be increased significantly above normal in infants and children with anxiety, fever, exercise, inflammatory illnesses, shock, or heart disease. The resting heart rate changes with increasing age.

The rhythm of the heartbeat is assessed for equal spacing between consecutive beats. Irregular cardiac rhythms are not uncommon in children and are often related to changes in rhythm that occur in response to respiratory inspiration and expiration.

Respirations

The nurse observes the rate, depth, and ease of respiration in the child. Respirations vary with age. The respiratory rate, like the heart rate, is significantly influenced by emotion and exercise. In infants, the rate may be determined by observing abdominal excursion. In toddlers and older children, the nurse observes thoracic excursion. Because the movements are irregular, the rate should be assessed for 1 minute in infants and young children. Respirations are best counted when the child is not paying attention to the examiner. Respirations should be counted while the examiner continues to keep fingers on a pulse or the stethoscope on the chest, as though checking the pulses. This effort will ensure that the child is unaware that the examiner is counting respirations.

The depth and rhythm of respirations are determined subjectively and compared with norms for a particular age group. The ease or difficulty of respirations is a somewhat subjective observation. Respirations should be quiet and appear effortless. *Stridor,* a crowing noise heard on inspiration and heard louder over the neck, is worrisome in a child and may be a sign of croup or a late sign in epiglottitis (Roosevelt, 2011) (see Chapter 21). Inspiratory stridor indicates a partial obstruction of the airway. Continuous inspiratory and expiratory stridor may be related to delayed development of the cartilage in the tracheal rings or to a relatively small larynx.

Blood Pressure

Blood pressure measurements are taken for all children at every ambulatory visit; in an acute-care setting, blood pressure is measured at least daily, and often more frequently, depending on the child's condition. The appropriate-size cuff must be used in order to obtain an accurate blood pressure. Blood pressure measurements in healthy ambulatory children are compared with standard norms (see Table 9-1 for the effects of age on vital signs). An auscultated blood pressure measurement that is equal to or exceeds the 90th percentile for the child's sex, height, and age (see Evolve Website) must be confirmed before the child is described as being hypertensive. An average of at least three abnormal blood pressure measurements taken on separate occasions requires further evaluation. If an adolescent's blood pressure is greater than 120/80 mm Hg, the adolescent is considered to be prehypertensive even if this value is below the 90th percentile (American Academy of Pediatrics [AAP], National High Blood Pressure Education Program Working Group on High Blood Pressure in Children and Adolescents, 2004).

The size of the cuff is important. Cuffs that are too small will cause falsely elevated values; those that are too large will cause inaccurate low values (see Chapter 13 for determining appropriate cuff size). Several determinations may be needed to obtain values unaffected by anxiety (Feld & Corey, 2007). Instructing the child that the "balloon" will gently squeeze the arm or give the arm a "hug" will usually decrease anxiety. To alleviate anxiety, the child can also assist with taking a blood pressure on a doll, a stuffed animal, or the parent.

Pain Assessment

For children in acute and ambulatory care settings, the initial and ongoing assessment of pain is essential (see Chapter 15). The American Pain Society introduced the phrase "pain as the 5th vital sign" to emphasize the importance of assessing pain along with the standard four vital signs (American Pain Society, n.d.). The Joint Commission standards include requirements that all health care providers identify patients in pain using methods that are consistent with the patient's age, condition and ability to understand (2010). Use of a pain assessment tool that is developmentally appropriate for the pediatric patient is recommended (Jarvis, 2008). See Table 15-2 for a list of Pain Assessment Tools.

Anthropometric Measurement

Anthropometrics entails measuring the human body and assessing nutritional status, as well as growth and development. Weight, height, and head circumference are always measured in children and are compared with averages for age-group and sex. The amount of body fat should be measured on the basis of the body mass index (BMI), which is calculated according to a simple formula:

$$BMI = \frac{Weight\ (kg)}{Height\ (m)^2} \quad or \quad BMI = \frac{Weight\ (lb) \times 703}{Height\ (in)^2}$$

See Evolve website for BMI charts for children. Midarm muscle circumference, skinfold thickness, and weight provide information about three body tissues (subcutaneous tissue, muscle, and fat) altered by nutrition. Because children's body fat varies with age and sex, anthropometric measurements are most valuable when they are plotted on a growth curve and evaluated serially so that trends can be monitored.

Measuring height and weight are routine procedures that provide valuable information about a child's health. Children grow and develop rapidly, and this growth and development must be constantly evaluated. A child's serial physical measurements reflect the rate of growth. A failure in growth, an acceleration in growth, or any change in growth pattern may be the first clue to serious health problems. When a child's weight or height stops following the child's own growth curve, this is the most significant indicator of a change in health status. Measurements must be correct and accurate and are taken at every visit from birth to adulthood.

The methods of measuring a child vary with the child's age. Infant and toddler length is best measured with the child lying down on a flat measuring board. This method is used until the child is able to stand independently. The child's head is held securely to the headboard, and the movable footboard is stretched to touch the child's heel. If a measuring board is not available for the infant and young child, it is possible to position the child's body on a flat surface, mark the point where the heel touches the surface, and then mark the point where the top of the head is lying on the surface, taking care to ensure that the child's legs and body are straight on the surface. The examiner then removes the child and measures the distance between the two points with a measuring tape. Measuring the length of the child in this manner is not as accurate as using a measuring board.

! NURSING QUALITY ALERT

Importance of Anthropometric Measurements

Anthropometric measurements reflect any change in the growth pattern and may be the first clue to a serious problem. Measurements must be taken at every health care visit from birth to adulthood. If a child's weight or height stops following the child's own growth curve, this is a significant indicator of a change in health status.

When a child is able to cooperate and stand without support, around age 2 years, the examiner stands the child in stocking feet next to a standard measuring tape that begins at the child's heel and is not displaced by room molding. A flat, hard surface is used to reach from the top of the child's head to the tape so that the examiner does not guess or add height because of the hair. If this is the first standing measurement, there may be a slight discrepancy from the lying measurement.

Once the measurement is taken, it must be plotted on a standardized growth chart appropriate for length or height measurement (see Evolve website). Height and weight are evaluated by determining whether the child is following a predictable percentile curve on a growth chart. Height and weight are related to hereditary factors and will vary from child to child.

Weight

The method and equipment for weighing vary with the child's age. All scales must be balanced or zeroed first before weight is measured. Infants are placed in a lying position on a regular baby scale with all their clothing removed. Older children who are able to stand or walk without support may be weighed on the adult standing scale. On the older child, remove all clothing except underwear. Like height, weight is plotted on a standardized growth chart (see Evolve website).

Head Circumference

Head circumference is measured in all children from birth to age 36 months and is plotted on a standard growth chart on all visits. In the child older than 3 years with any questionable head size—macrocephaly or microcephaly—the head circumference should be measured at every visit. To measure the head circumference, a nonstretching measuring tape is wrapped above the supraorbital ridges and over the most prominent part of the occiput (Figure 9-2).

The head circumference is plotted on a standardized growth chart. During the first year of life, the head circumference normally increases

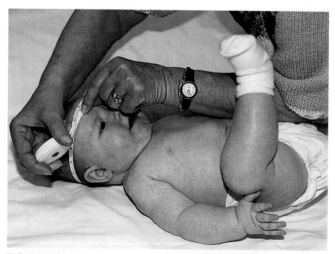

FIG 9-2 Measuring head circumference. The head circumference is measured from birth through age 36 months. The nurse uses a nonstretching tape and measures in a "hat band" position, just above the eyebrows and around the occipital prominence in the back. Chest circumference is also routinely measured in the newborn; it is usually smaller than the newborn's head circumference. (Courtesy The University of Texas at Arlington College of Nursing, Arlington, TX.)

by 1.2 cm (0.5 inch) each month. Head circumference can reflect an abnormal rate of development, give some indication of nutritional status, and possibly indicate tumor growth or an abnormal accumulation of cerebrospinal fluid (CSF) known as hydrocephalus.

Chest Circumference

Chest circumference is routinely measured only in the newborn infant. The newborn's head circumference is larger than the chest circumference. Chest circumference is almost equal to head circumference after age 1 year. To measure chest circumference, the measuring tape is wrapped around the chest at the nipple line. The measurement is taken between inspiration and expiration.

Midarm Circumference

Midarm circumference reflects muscle mass and fat. To measure midarm circumference, the midpoint on the arm between the acromial process and the olecranon process is determined. Then, with the arm hanging loosely at the side, the child's arm is measured at the midpoint with a tape measure. The measurement is recorded in centimeters. With a decrease in fat or muscle atrophy, the midarm circumference decreases. It will increase with weight gain.

Triceps Skinfold

Triceps skinfold thickness indicates total body fat because at least half of body fat is directly below the skin. Metal calipers are used to obtain this measurement. On the nondominant arm, the midpoint of the arm is determined with the same method that is used for measuring midarm circumference. With the arm hanging loosely at the side, a fold of skin at the midpoint on the posterior aspect of the arm is grasped. To avoid error, the child is asked to flex the arm muscle after the examiner grasps the skin. If contraction is felt, muscle as well as fat has been grasped. The examiner applies the caliper and takes a reading after waiting 3 seconds. Fat stores decrease with long-term undernutrition and malnutrition.

Use of Growth Charts

An accurate record of a child's overall pattern of growth is best determined by measurements over months or years. The Centers for Disease Control and Prevention (CDC) provides growth charts—a series of percentile curves for selected measurements—that are used to assess body size and monitor growth in infants, children, and adolescents in the United States (CDC, 2010).

The CDC recommends that health care providers use the World Health Organization (WHO) growth standards to monitor growth for infants and children ages 0 to 2 years and the CDC growth charts for children age 2 years and older (CDC, 2010). The reason is that the data collected for the WHO growth charts represent infants and children who were breastfed during their first year of life; this is considered optimal nutrition and the standard to which all infants and children should be compared (Grummer-Strawn, Reinold, & Krebs, 2010).

There are separate sets of growth charts for girls and boys. WHO growth charts for ages birth to age 2 years, plot length, weight, and head circumference measurements for age. They also plot the weight-to-length relationship, which can be used as an indicator of overweight or obesity in children. The CDC charts for ages 2 through 20 years, plot measurements of stature (height), weight, and BMI for age (see Evolve website). BMI is used primarily to screen for children who are overweight, though it may also be used to describe children who are underweight (CDC, 2010). Special growth charts for premature, very low birth weight infants (<1500 g) and children with specific conditions that may affect size and growth (such as Down syndrome) are available, although most of these were developed from limited data (see Evolve website). Plotting on a growth chart proceeds as follows: The exact age of the child is located on the chart's horizontal axis. The corresponding measurement is noted on the chart's vertical axis. The chart is marked where the two lines intersect. The percentile lines on these charts indicate the number of children whose measurements are expected to fall above and below the child's measurement.

Weight and height measurements above the 97th percentile or below the 3rd percentile on a standard growth chart may indicate a growth disturbance and need further investigation. Brain growth can be assessed by serial head circumference measurements (see Chapter 28). BMIs from the 85th to below the 95th percentile indicate a risk for being overweight; BMIs at or above the 95th percentile in children older than 2 years indicate overweight (CDC, 2010).

Skin, Hair, and Nails

Skin

Skin assessment includes inspection and palpation. The entire skin surface is examined for color, texture, turgor, and presence of lesions. This examination may be combined with assessment of other areas of the body.

Inspection. The nurse observes the color and pigmentation of the skin. Skin color reflects the amount of melanin and can range from pink to black (Box 9-5). In dark-skinned infants and children, erythema appears dusky red or violet, cyanosis appears black, and jaundice appears diffusely darker. In dark-skinned infants and children, it is best to determine the normal skin color and then compare any color change with the normal color. Increased pigmentation and thickening of the skin on the posterior neck, the armpits, and behind the knees and elbows (acanthosis nigricans) can be an indication of non–insulin-dependent diabetes mellitus in children (Morelli, 2011). Skin color changes may be related to sun exposure or tattooing.

! NURSING QUALITY ALERT

Skin Inspection in Dark-Skinned Children

Erythema: Dusky red or violet
Cyanosis: Black or dusky
Jaundice: Diffusely darker than the child's normal color

BOX 9-5   SKIN COLOR TERMINOLOGY

Vitiligo: Areas of depigmentation
Nevi: Areas of increased pigmentation
Jaundice: A yellow discoloration of the skin, best seen in the sclera of the eyes
Cyanosis: A blue discoloration of the skin, best seen in all races in the mucous membranes of the mouth, particularly under the tongue
Carotenemia: An orange color of the skin, best seen on the soles of the feet and palms of the hands
Pallor: Loss of skin color
Erythema: Diffusely red
Mottling: Discolored areas of the skin

Palpation. The examiner palpates the skin to assess moisture, temperature, texture, turgor, edema, and lesions, as follows:

Moisture is assessed by lightly stroking the skin surface and body creases. The external skin on exposed areas is normally drier than unexposed areas of the skin.

Temperature is assessed by using the back of the hand because it is more sensitive to skin changes. The two sides of the child's body are compared.

Normal *texture* of the skin is described as being smooth and soft. Scars or excessive scar tissue should be noted.

Turgor is assessed by grasping the skin between the thumb and index finger and quickly releasing it (see Figure 16-1). The skin normally returns to place without excessive skin markings. Skin that "tents" when released indicates dehydration. The abdomen and upper arm are the best places to test for tissue turgor on a child.

Edema is the accumulation of excessive salt and water in the interstitial spaces. It is identified by pressing the thumb into an area of the body that may appear swollen and noting if an indentation persists after the release of pressure. The extremities and buttocks are classic areas to palpate for edema in the child. Periorbital edema is observed on the eyelids.

Lesions are identified, noting configuration, distribution, color, and size. Skin lesions are identified as primary lesions, arising from normal skin (e.g., freckle), or secondary lesions, resulting from an alteration of a primary lesion (e.g., scab). Configuration of a skin lesion is the arrangement or position of several lesions in relation to one another or to the arrangement of a single lesion. Distribution is the body location and the symmetry or asymmetry of lesions.

Hair

Hair normally covers the entire body except for the palms, soles, and parts of the genitalia. Hair is examined for texture, changes in color, unusual distribution, and cleanliness.

Scalp hair has a wide range of normal textures, including straight, curly, and kinky. The hair is usually shiny, silky, and strong. The examiner should keep in mind the child's age and development. Fine, downy hair is normal for a newborn infant, whereas in an older child it would lead the examiner to consider nutritional and endocrine abnormalities. Brittle hair, identified when the hairs break off easily when bent between the fingers, also might indicate endocrine and nutritional abnormalities.

The color of the hair is genetically determined and may be anything from pale blond to black. Changes in color may be caused by depigmentation, hereditary factors, or chemicals applied to the hair. Hair texture varies widely with race.

The distribution of the hair over the head is identified. In most children, the hair begins in a whorl and then is distributed over the head. Some children may have more than one whorl. Scalp hair does not grow beyond the nape of the neck or down to the eyebrows. *Hirsutism* is defined as excessive hair growth; *alopecia* is unusual hair loss.

The hair is separated and examined for cleanliness, signs of trauma, lesions, and scaling. The scalp should be clean and free of any infestations. Most cases of head lice (*Pediculosis capitis*) are first detected when one or more children are seen scratching the head. Closer observation may reveal nits adhering to the hairs. Depending on their distance from the scalp, these usually are the whitish to sand-colored empty shells of eggs that have hatched (see Chapter 25 for further discussion of the integumentary system).

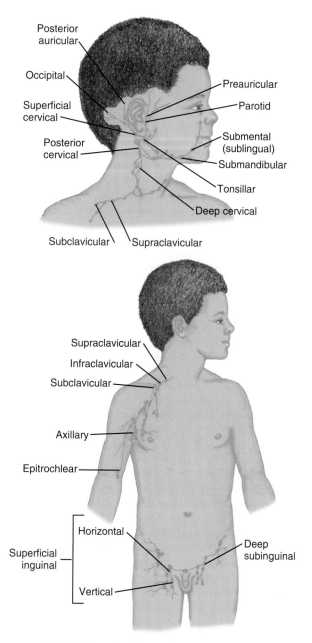

FIG 9-3 Location of superficial lymph nodes.

Nails

Nails are inspected and palpated for shape and contour. The nail surface is normally flat or slightly convex. The edges of the nails should be smooth, rounded, and clean. Clubbing of fingernails can be identified by looking at the index finger to see if the nail bulges upward. If the angle between the nail base and the fingertip is greater than 160 degrees, clubbing is present. On palpation, the base of the fingernail should be firm. On touching the index fingernails back to back, a diamond of light below the knuckle and above where the fingernails touch will be present. In early clubbing, the diamond shape is decreased or not apparent (see Chapter 22).

Pressing and releasing on the nail edge assess capillary refill; the nail will blanch, and then color will normally return to the nail within 1 to 2 seconds. A capillary refill time of more than 2 seconds may be caused by anemia, peripheral edema, vasoconstriction, or decreased cardiac output as a result of hypovolemia, shock, or congestive heart failure (Jarvis, 2008).

Lymph Nodes

Lymph nodes are inspected and palpated. Lymph tissue is found all over the body and must be evaluated as the examiner assesses body systems. The examiner should always assess for enlarged lymph nodes in the head and neck, the supraclavicular area, the axillary region, the arms, and the inguinal region (Figure 9-3). At the time these areas are examined, the lymph nodes are assessed as well. When an enlarged lymph node or a mass is found during examination, its characteristics should be described (Box 9-6).

To palpate for most lymph nodes, the examiner uses the distal portion of the fingers and gently but firmly moves the fingers in a circular motion to determine the node's characteristics and mobility.

Lymph nodes that are enlarged, warm, firm, and fluctuant indicate infection. Lymph nodes that are small, firm, and shotty (freely palpable and very small) are often palpable in healthy infants and children, in the cervical, axillary, and inguinal areas (Tower & Camitta, 2011). An enlarged supraclavicular lymph node on the left in young children is called the *sentinel node* because it may suggest the presence of Wilms tumor or other neoplastic disease.

Head, Neck, and Face
Head

The head is inspected and palpated. To examine the head, the examiner must see and feel. The head is evaluated from the front, the back, and the sides. The head is examined for symmetry, paralysis, weakness, and movement (Box 9-7).

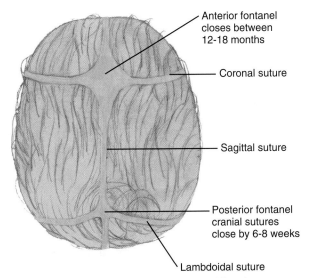

Anterior fontanel closes between 12-18 months

Coronal suture

Sagittal suture

Posterior fontanel cranial sutures close by 6-8 weeks

Lambdoidal suture

FIG 9-4 Fontanels are inspected and palpated for size, tenseness, and pulsation.

BOX 9-7 HEAD SHAPE TERMINOLOGY

Normocephalic: Normal-size head
Microcephalic: Head small for body size and age
Macrocephalic: Abnormally large head
Bossing: Frontal enlargement

Symmetry is assessed by looking at and feeling the entire head. If any lumps or bumps are seen or felt, the examiner notes their exact location, size, and density. The suture lines in infants should be palpated. Sutures are felt as prominent ridges in the neonate but usually flatten by 6 months of age.

Paralysis and weakness of the head are directly related to the condition of the neck muscles. That is, paralysis and weakness of the head occur with paralysis or weakness of the neck muscles.

Head movement is evaluated by observing the child's spontaneous head movement. Head control is observed with the infant in a supine position and while the examiner grasps the infants hands and pulls the infant into a sitting position. An infant younger than 4 months may show some head lag, but the infant in an upright position should be able to maintain the head upright for several seconds. Head lag after age 6 months may indicate poor muscle development. However, increased neck extensor and axial tone in the young infant may make head control appear better than it actually is and may be suggestive of neuromuscular problems such as cerebral palsy, a form of static encephalopathy (Lee & Johnston, 2010). The head should be put through a full range of motion by asking the older child to look up, down, and sideways. After age 4 months, inability to move the head or to hold the head in an upright position may be related to paralysis or weakness of the neck muscles.

The fontanels are inspected and palpated for size, tenseness, and pulsation (Figure 9-4). The posterior fontanel is closed by age 2 to 3 months. The anterior fontanel should be soft and flat when the child is sitting. Measure the width and length of an open anterior fontanel. The anterior fontanel should be less than 5 cm in length and width after age 12 months and should be completely closed by age 12 to 24 months (Jarvis, 2008). A sunken fontanel is associated with dehydration, and a bulging fontanel can be associated with increased intracranial pressure. A bulging fontanel is normally seen when an infant cries, coughs, or vomits. Inability to palpate the anterior fontanel may be an indicator of premature closure known as craniosynostosis (see Chapter 28).

Neck

In the child, the neck is inspected and palpated for symmetry, size, and shape, which is directly related to use or disuse of the neck muscles. The infant's neck is relatively short and lengthens as the child grows. The neck is viewed from the front, back, and both sides. Webbing of the neck—the presence of an extra fold of skin posteriorly—is associated with some chromosomal abnormalities such as trisomy 21, or Down syndrome.

The neck is mobile and supple. While palpating the child's neck, the examiner palpates the thyroid gland by identifying the isthmus of the thyroid across the trachea. To identify an enlarged thyroid in a child, the examiner gently displaces the thyroid gland laterally and palpates thyroid tissue with the opposite thumb and fingers. The lobe may be more palpable when the child swallows.

Face

The child's face is inspected and palpated for dysmorphic features. Spacing and symmetry of facial features are noted. The face is observed for any changes in color or the presence of edema, such as cellulitis. The eyes are examined for size, position, and configuration. *Hypertelorism* is a condition in which the eyes are unusually widely spaced; in *hypotelorism,* the eyes are unusually close together. The child's nostrils should be oval in shape and equal in size, with no evidence of a hypoplastic philtrum (shallow crease or absence of a crease below the nose). The lips should be equal on either side of the midline. The child's ears are inspected for alignment. Low-set ears are identified when the auricle of the ear does not cross or touch the eye-occiput line. The position of the auricle should be almost vertical, with no more than a 10-degree lateral posterior angle (Figure 9-5).

The functions of cranial nerve V (trigeminal nerve) and cranial nerve VII (facial nerve) are evaluated during assessment of the face. Cranial nerve V is evaluated by observing chewing or sucking, which demonstrates the strength of the temporomandibular joint, and by touching the child's forehead and cheeks with a piece of cotton. The child should move the head or bat the object away. Cranial nerve VII is evaluated by asking a child to frown, smile, or make a face while the examiner observes for symmetry of movement. Having the child puff out the cheeks or whistle also allows the examiner to evaluate cranial nerve VII (Jarvis, 2008).

Nose, Mouth, and Throat
Nose

The examiner should wear gloves when doing the nasal examination, noting any drainage coming from the nose and describing the amount, color, and consistency.

The external nose is inspected and palpated. Patency can be determined by occluding one nostril and having the child sniff, and then repeating on the other side. The external nose is observed for symmetry, deformity, inflammation, or skin lesions. The "allergic salute," frequent wiping of the nose because of drainage, produces a transverse crease on the child's nose and is suggestive that the child has allergies. The entire external nose is palpated for septal deviation or other deformities. The sense of smell is mediated by cranial nerve I. This function can be evaluated by having the child close the eyes, occlude one nostril, and identify familiar odors, such as cinnamon, peppermint, orange, and cherry.

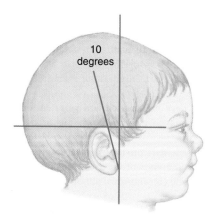

10 degrees

Normal alignment

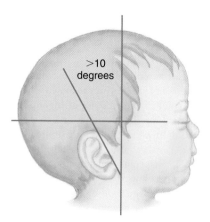

>10 degrees

Low-set ears and deviation in alignment

FIG 9-5 The child's ears are inspected for alignment. Low-set ears could indicate a cognitive disability or renal anomalies.

The nasal cavity can be examined by inserting the short, wide-tipped speculum on the otoscope into the nasal vestibule, with precautions taken to not put pressure on the nasal septum. The nasal mucosa is inspected for color and moisture. The nasal mucosa is normally smooth and moist, with a bright pink color. In children with allergies, the mucosa is pale and appears boggy. With infectious diseases (viral or bacterial), the mucosa is erythematous and swollen; the nasal drainage may be yellow or green. The nasal septum is examined for intactness and for any deviation.

The *frontal* and *maxillary sinuses* are inspected and palpated (Figure 9-6). The areas over the sinuses are examined for color and swelling. Puffiness and redness over the sinuses and dark circles under the eyes may indicate an inflammatory process in children. The frontal sinuses are palpated by pressing over the sinuses below the eyebrow. The maxillary sinuses are palpated by pressing upward with the thumbs under the maxillary bones.

Mouth and Throat

Assessment of the mouth in a young child should be performed at the end of the physical examination because it may create anxiety. The examination should proceed from the anterior structures to the internal structures of the mouth.

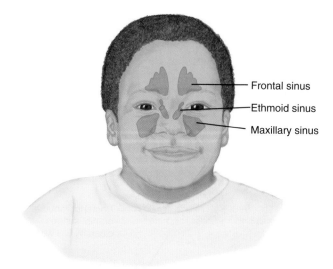

Frontal sinus
Ethmoid sinus
Maxillary sinus

FIG 9-6 The frontal, ethmoid, and maxillary sinuses.

The *philtrum,* the little notch between the nose and upper lip, should be intact. In children with dysmorphic features, the philtrum is absent or shallow.

The examiner should wear gloves when doing the oral examination. A tongue blade and a penlight assist with visualization of the oral cavity. When the child opens his or her mouth, the examiner evaluates mouth odors. The mouth and internal structures are examined by inspection, palpation, and the sense of smell.

Lips are inspected for symmetry, color, moisture, cracking, and the presence of any lesions. The alveolar frenulum, which attaches the lips to the gums, should be intact. The lips are palpated to identify any masses.

The *buccal mucosa* is examined by holding the cheeks open with a tongue blade and observing for color, nodules, and lesions. Significant mouth odors should be noted. For many children, this part of the examination can be unpleasant. To facilitate the child's cooperation, the examiner may want to demonstrate on a doll or on the parent or allow the child to place the tongue blade in the parent's mouth. The buccal mucosa should be pink, smooth, and moist. Dark-skinned children may have patchy areas of hyperpigmentation. The opening of the *parotid gland* is found as a small dimple on the buccal mucosa opposite the upper second molar. The entire surface of the buccal mucosa is palpated for changes in consistency or masses.

Teeth are inspected for number, cavities, tooth formation, and occlusion. The number and characteristics of the teeth will change with growth and development (Figure 9-7). The eruption of deciduous teeth begins around the sixth month of extrauterine life; all 20 deciduous teeth are present by age 30 months. After having the child bite down, the examiner gently parts the lips and notes the position of the teeth. The upper teeth slightly override the lower teeth. The color and shape of each tooth should be noted. The crown is white, with some variation from person to person. Permanent teeth are larger and have a darker color than deciduous teeth. Brown or black discoloration of the teeth is usually caused by dental caries. Long-term use of certain medications (e.g., tetracycline, iron) may stain teeth. With excessive fluoride ingestion, the enamel of the permanent teeth may appear mottled. The shape of a tooth is determined by age, development, and the amount of wear.

The gums (*gingivae*) are inspected and palpated for color and swelling. The gum surface has a pink, stippled appearance and feels firm.

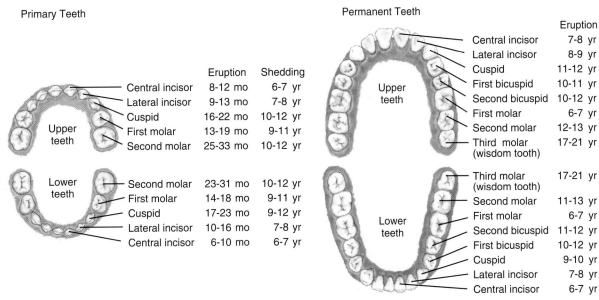

FIG 9-7 Sequence of eruption of primary and secondary teeth. (Data from American Dental Association, retrieved from www.ada.org.)

Dark-skinned children may have a dark-pigmented line along the gingival margin.

The floor of the mouth can be inspected by asking the child to lift the tongue to the roof of the mouth. The examiner observes the frenulum, the sublingual ridge, and Wharton's ducts, which lie on either side of the frenulum. The color of the floor of the mouth is pink.

The tongue is inspected and palpated. The dorsum of the tongue should appear dull red, moist, and glistening, with a white coat. The anterior portion of the tongue should have a slightly roughened appearance with papillae and small fissures. The tongue is palpated for indurations or ulcerations. While palpating the mouth of a young child, the examiner can prevent being bitten by holding the child's cheeks.

Cranial nerve XII *(hypoglossal nerve)* is examined by asking the child to stick out the tongue as though licking a lollipop and observe for any deviation of the tongue to one side. The examiner can determine the strength of the tongue by placing a finger to the side of the child's cheek and asking the child to press the tongue against the examiner's finger. The tongue should feel equally strong on the two sides.

To evaluate the hard palate, soft palate, and uvula, the examiner asks the child to tilt the head back. The examiner inspects the hard palate for shape and color. The hard palate is whitish and convex, with transverse rugae. The examiner palpates the hard palate for the height of the arch and for intactness. The examiner can allow the infant to suck on a gloved finger while palpating the hard palate to determine the strength of the sucking reflex. The soft palate is continuous with the hard palate and is concave and pinker. The uvula varies in length and thickness and is located in midline as a continuation of the soft palate. Cranial nerves IX *(glossopharyngeal nerve)* and X *(vagus nerve)* are evaluated at this time. The child is asked to say "ah"; normally, the soft palate and the uvula rise symmetrically and phonation of "ah" is understood.

A tongue blade is used to depress the tongue and observe the oropharynx. This action can be unpleasant for the child. To minimize discomfort, the examiner slides the tongue blade along the side of the tongue until it reaches the soft palate and then compresses the tongue to elicit the gag reflex (cranial nerve X) and observe the back of the throat. The tonsillar pillars are inspected with particular notation of size and color of tonsils. The tonsils are pink.

The size of tonsils varies; large tonsils are common in young children. Tonsils may have crypts where food particles collect. With inflammatory processes, the crypts may contain exudate. A child whose parents comment on the child's snoring or being awakened by snoring may have grossly enlarged tonsils. The posterior wall of the pharynx should be smooth and glistening pink; the wall may have small, irregular spots of lymphatic tissue and small blood vessels (Seidel et al., 2010).

Eyes

The eyes are inspected, palpated, and evaluated for visual acuity and extraocular muscle function.

Visual Acuity

Visual acuity can be difficult to evaluate in a young child. Acuity develops over time, and evaluation requires the child's cooperation. Items needed for evaluating visual acuity in a child are an eye cover and vision charts (Box 9-8). The chart chosen is determined by the child's age and development. The infant from birth to age 1 or 2 months gazes at black-and-white contrasting figures and faces. At age 4 weeks or older, an infant fixates on a brightly colored object and follows it.

Visual acuity testing for all children beginning no later than age 3 years is recommended (American Academy of Ophthalmology, 2007). Several groups have been researching the reliability and validity of vision screening methods for preschool-age children (National Eye Institute, Ocular Epidemiology Strategic Planning Panel, 2007). Visual acuity tests that have evidence to support reliability and validity for preschool children include the Lea chart, tumbling E, and the HOTV matching test (U.S. Preventive Services Task Force, 2004b).

Preschool children can be tested using the HOTV chart at 10 feet. A card printed with *H, O, T,* and *V* is given to the child to hold. One eye is covered, and the child is instructed to match the letters on the

BOX 9-8   TYPES OF EYE CHARTS

Snellen chart: A standardized chart with graduated letters for testing far vision of children at 20 feet. Used with children older than 6 years.
Tumbling E (Snellen E): A standardized chart using the letter *E* in various directions that is used with preschoolers ages 3 to 6 years to test far vision at 20 feet. Also available for a distance of 10 feet.
Lea chart: A chart with four different symbols. Used for preschool-age children. Designed for use at 10 feet.

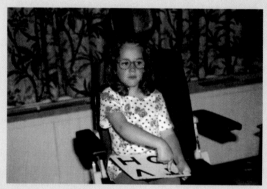

HOTV chart: A standardized chart with the letters *H, O, T,* and *V* in graduated sizes. Designed for use at 10 feet with children ages 3 to 6 years.

HOTV chart for children ages 3 to 6 years. The letters *H, O, T,* and *V* are presented at a distance, and the child points to the corresponding letter on the card resting on her lap.*

Jaeger chart: Standardized chart with graduated letters for testing near vision at 12 to 14 inches from the eyes. Used with children older than 6 years.
Ishihara chart: A series of polychromatic cards with a pattern of dots printed against a background of many colored dots. Designed to test for color vision between ages 4 and 6 years.

*From Goldbloom, R.B. (2011). *Pediatric clinical skills* (4th ed.). Philadelphia: Saunders Elsevier.

held card with the chart at 10 feet using the uncovered eye. The child holds the card, or it is placed on a table directly in front of the child. Screening is begun at the 20/40 line for children younger than 4 years and at the 20/30 line for older children. The child passes the screening if the child correctly identifies four of the five symbols.

Older children's visual acuity can be tested by use of the Snellen chart, placed on a wall 20 feet away from the child. The chart should have no glare and should be well illuminated. No other materials should be around or near the chart. Both eyes are tested together first, and then each eye is tested separately. If the child has corrective lenses, the procedure should be repeated with the corrective lenses on. Unless the child is known to have very poor vision, testing is begun at the line on the chart for 40 feet. To determine at what level the child cannot see, the examiner finds the distance at which the child misses half plus one of the symbols on a line of the chart. The visual acuity is then designated as the smallest line at which the child is able to identify more than half the symbols on the line. For corrective lenses, the examiner notes the last date the child was examined for a prescription. Findings are recorded by noting the distance of the line correctly read

for both eyes (i.e., right eye 20/20, left eye 20/20). This annotation means that the child has correctly interpreted the letters on the chart for 20 feet at a distance of 20 feet, which matches what the average child can see at that distance. If the child correctly identifies the letters on the line labeled *40 feet,* that child can see at 20 feet what the average child can see at 40 feet (20/40). Visual acuity changes with age and varies according to the test used. Normal ranges are as follows:

- *Birth:* Fixates on objects (8 to 12 inches), 20/100 to 20/150
- *4 months:* 20/50 to 20/80
- *1 year:* 20/40 to 20/70
- *4 years:* 20/30 to 20/40
- *5 years:* 20/20 to 20/30

Color Vision

Color vision deficit, less correctly termed *color blindness,* is an inherited recessive X-linked trait that, in varying degrees, may affect the child's ability to discern traffic lights, brake lights, and color-coordinated clothing. Color discrimination occurs through integration of information from the cone pigments in the retinal layers of the eye. The genes for some colors are located on the X chromosome, and because boys have only one X chromosome, they are more likely to have color vision deficit. Color vision deficit may affect learning if the learning is color related. The condition is very rare in females but affects 8% to 10% of males.

Color vision is evaluated by Ishihara charts—a series of polychromatic cards. These cards have a pattern of colored pictures embedded in the charts. Children between ages 4 and 8 years are tested once and are asked to touch or identify the embedded patterns. A child with this deficit cannot see the patterns against the field of color.

Peripheral Vision

Visual fields are evaluated in older children to identify peripheral vision. The examiner's face is positioned directly in front and on the level of the child, about 2 feet away. The child's visual fields should roughly mirror those of the examiner. The examiner covers one eye and has the child mimic by covering the opposite eye. Slowly a puppet or some other test object is brought from the periphery into the child's field of vision. The object should come from a position slightly behind the child's head, and the child is asked to say "now" when the object is in view (Figure 9-8). Testing for visual acuity and visual fields evaluates cranial nerve II, the optic nerve, which mediates vision.

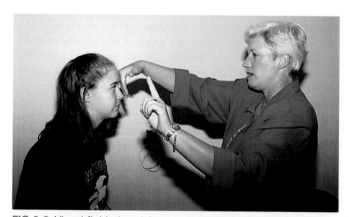

FIG 9-8 Visual fields (cranial nerve II) are tested in each eye separately. One eye is covered as the child stares straight ahead. An object is slowly moved from the side of the head into the field of vision. The child says "now" upon first seeing the object.

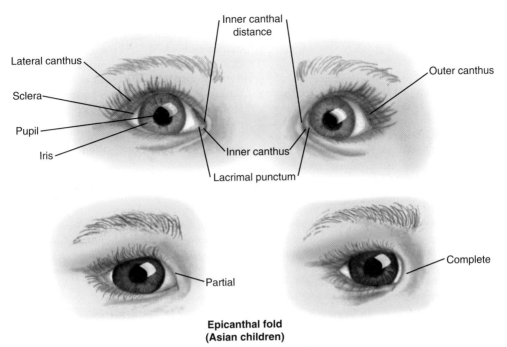

FIG 9-9 External structures of the eye.

Binocular Vision and Strabismus

Extraocular muscle function is evaluated to test binocular vision and the presence of strabismus. Strabismus, or "crossed eyes," is the abnormal or incomplete development of binocular visual alignment. Three tests are performed: the corneal light reflex (Hirschberg) test, field-of-vision test, and cover/uncover (alternate cover) test.

Corneal Light Reflex Test. The corneal light reflex is assessed by shining a light directly onto the irises from a distance of about 40.5 cm (16 in). The reflection of the light should appear in exactly the same spot on both eyes. If the light falls off center in one eye, the eyes are malaligned. Children with *epicanthal folds*—vertical folds that partially or completely cover the inner canthi (Figure 9-9) may give a false impression of malalignment (pseudostrabismus).

Field-of-Vision Test. The six cardinal fields of vision are tested by holding the child's chin so that the head does not move and asking the child to follow a puppet or a familiar object held approximately 12 inches away from the face as the object is moved to each of the six cardinal positions. As the object is moved to the margins of each cardinal position, the examiner holds it momentarily in that position before proceeding back to the center. The eyes will track in a parallel fashion to each position. As the eyes are in the margins of each position, the examiner can note *end-stage nystagmus,* a gentle oscillation of the eye, which is considered normal. Children younger than 2 to 3 years may not be able to cooperate with this test.

Tests for Eye Muscle Function. Testing for extraocular muscle function in children younger than 5 years is critical to identifying any muscle imbalance so that it can be corrected at an early age to preserve vision. Extraocular muscle function evaluates three cranial nerves: cranial nerve VI, the *abducent* nerve, which innervates the lateral rectus muscle (responsible for abducting the eye); cranial nerve IV, the *trochlear* nerve, which innervates the superior oblique muscle (responsible for downward and inward movement of the eye); and cranial nerve III, the *oculomotor* nerve, which innervates the superior, inferior, and medial rectus and the inferior oblique muscles (Seidel et al., 2010).

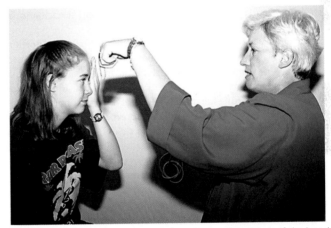

FIG 9-10 The cover/uncover test detects small degrees of deviated eye alignment. With one eye covered, the child gazes straight ahead with the uncovered eye. The cover is then removed, and the eye should continue to stare straight ahead. Movement in either eye suggests muscle weakness. Extraocular muscle function is controlled by cranial nerves III, IV, and VI.

The cover/uncover test is used to detect deficits in binocular vision by interrupting fusion of the eyes as they gaze at a fixed object. One eye is covered with an opaque card while the child stares straight ahead, at which time the examiner observes the uncovered eye. A steady, fixed gaze is maintained by the uncovered eye. Next the covered eye is uncovered and observed for any movement; it should continue to stare straight ahead (Figure 9-10). The procedure is repeated with the opposite eye. Any movement in either eye in the process of covering or uncovering may indicate muscle weakness.

The random dot E stereo test, in which the child looks through special glasses to identify an E on a card, is now recommended as part of comprehensive vision testing for preschoolers and young school-age children and helps to identify conditions such as amblyopia or strabismus (Hartmann et al., 2006).

External Eye

The external eye is evaluated for position and placement (see Figure 9-9). The examiner notes whether the eyes are set wide apart or close together. Epicanthal folds are seen in Asian children and in some non-Asian children as well. The slant of the eyes is determined by drawing an imaginary line across the inner canthi (see Figure 9-9).

The eyebrows are inspected for symmetry and hair growth and eyelashes for even distribution. The *lacrimal apparatus* is assessed by asking the child to look down. The outer part of the upper lid is palpated along the bony orbit for any discomfort, swelling, or redness. The *punctum* (tear duct) on the inner canthus is palpated for obstruction in the infant.

The eye globe is palpated for firmness and can be gently pushed into the orbit without causing discomfort. Palpation of the eye may cause anxiety in small children and should not be done unless there is a serious concern about the size of the eye.

Eyelids are inspected for color, swelling, discharge, and lesions. The position of the eyelids on the globe should be noted. With the eyelids open, the upper lid normally falls below the superior limbus but does not cover any of the pupil. The lower lids normally fall just at the inferior limbus. The limbus is the point where the sclera of the eye meets the color portion of the iris. When closed, the eyelids approximate each other completely, without tremor, fasciculations, or tics.

The *conjunctiva* has two portions to evaluate. The palpebral portion of the conjunctiva lines the lids. The palpebral conjunctiva is examined by pulling down as the child looks up. It is normally clear, with a pink color, and several small blood vessels may be visible. The upper lid can be inspected by everting the upper eyelid over a cotton-tipped applicator. Eversion of the upper eyelid is not normally done because eye manipulation may cause apprehension in a child. The bulbar portion of the conjunctiva is transparent and lies over the sclera, allowing the white of the sclera to be clearly visible.

The following anterior structures of the eye are inspected: sclerae, cornea and lens, anterior chamber, and irises. The sclerae are white. The sclerae of dark-skinned children may have gray-blue or "muddy" color variations. Dark-skinned children may have small brown macules around the limbus (where the iris meets the sclera). These variations are normal. The corneas are clear, transparent, and very sensitive. Shining a light obliquely across the cornea highlights any abnormal irregularities on the corneal surface. The examiner illuminates the anterior chamber by shining a light across the eye from the temporal side to illuminate the entire iris without producing a shadow. The irises are round and contain muscle fibers that contract or expand in response to light. The pigmentation of the irises is unique for each individual. The two irises are similar in color but may exhibit some variation.

Pupils appear round, regular, and of equal size in the two eyes. The *pupillary light reflex* is tested by darkening the room and asking the child to gaze into the distance. A light is brought from the side (temporally), and the examiner notes the change in the size of the pupil. Shining a light directly into a pupil causes the pupil to constrict (direct light reflex). The procedure is repeated while the opposite eye is observed. The opposite eye constricts (consensual light reflex) in response to the light shone in the first eye. Pupils should constrict at equal speeds and to the same degree.

Pupil size should be the same in both eyes. In some children, pupils of unequal size are normal, but in general, unequal pupils call for a consideration of central nervous system injury. Asking the child to focus on a distant object can test accommodation. The pupils normally dilate. An object such as a puppet or a finger brought into the line of vision about 7 to 8 cm from the nose should cause pupillary constriction and convergence of the axes of the eyes (Seidel et al., 2010).

Ophthalmoscopic Examination

The ophthalmoscopic examination requires a cooperative child, practice, and patience. Lights in the room should be dim. Most children enjoy playing with the light of the "flashlight" and having them watch the light as the examiner moves it around the room facilitates cooperation. Minimally, all practitioners view the red reflex, but the procedure requires demonstration and practice. When the ophthalmoscope is placed in front of the pupil and the light hits the lens, a red color is reflected from the retina to the examiner. The retina, choroid, optic disc, macula, fovea centralis, and retinal vessels are also visible with the ophthalmoscope.

Ears

Assessment of the ears includes testing for hearing acuity, inspection and palpation of the external ear, and examination of the internal ear with the otoscope.

Hearing Acuity

Infant Assessment. Newborn infants born in a hospital are tested for response of the acoustic nerve at the time of birth and before discharge. In an older infant, hearing is assessed by asking the parent to speak to the infant from behind and observing the infant's response to the parent's voice. The examiner can stand behind the infant and ring a bell or make a sound the infant is familiar with and observe the infant turning to locate the sound. A very young infant, younger than 4 months, may demonstrate a startle reflex to loud sounds.

Preschool and School-Age Assessment by Audiometry. In preschool and school-age children, the audiometer gives a precise (quantitative) assessment of the ability to hear. The child is placed in a soundproof room and is asked to identify tones played at a level the child can hear. With the audiometer, two tests are used to evaluate hearing: the sweep test and the pure tone hearing test. The *sweep test* is used to screen for hearing losses. The *pure tone test* is used to determine the exact extent of the hearing loss.

Preschool, School-Age, and Adolescent Assessment: The Whisper Test. The examiner stands approximately 0.6 m (2 feet) behind the child (to prevent lip reading); then exhales and whispers a series of three numbers and letters (i.e., 4-K-2). If the child correctly repeats the letter/number series, hearing is considered normal. Adaptations for preschool children may be necessary; the examiner whispers a command such as "Please put the toy on the floor" and then observes to see if the child follows the command, indicating normal hearing.

Conduction Tests (Tuning Fork Hearing Tests). Tuning fork tests are qualitative tests that determine the ability to hear by air conduction and by bone conduction. In the normal child, air conduction of sound is greater than bone conduction. The *Rinne hearing test* is used to determine whether air conduction is greater than bone conduction. The *Weber hearing test* determines the child's ability to hear by bone conduction. Testing the child's hearing evaluates cranial nerve VIII (*acoustic nerve*).

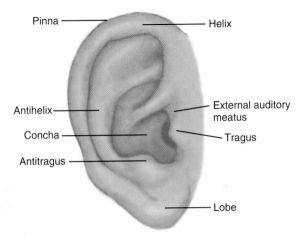

FIG 9-11 Landmarks of the external ear.

External Ear

The external ear is inspected and palpated. Ear placement and position are evaluated during assessment of the face (see Figure 9-5), but the external ear is also examined for any malformations or unusual markings (Figure 9-11). Any discharge coming from the auditory meatus is noted, and its amount and characteristics are described. Soft, yellow-brown cerumen (ear wax) is normally seen in the external auditory meatus.

The bony prominence of the mastoid process behind the ear is palpated for tenderness. The auricles are gently pulled to determine whether this action causes discomfort.

Otoscopic Examination

The *tympanic membrane* is examined with the otoscope (Figure 9-12). Many children may be apprehensive about this examination. If necessary, a small child is positioned on the parent's lap and the parent secures the child's arms. The examiner uses the largest speculum that will fit comfortably into the ear canal. In a child younger than 3 years, the ear canal is straightened by pulling the pinna of the ear down and back. If a child is 3 years or older, the pinna is pulled up and back. As much of the canal as possible should be visible before the speculum is inserted into the auditory meatus.

The canal is inspected for any lesions and for cerumen. The tympanic membrane is inspected for landmarks, color, and mobility. A puff of air is injected into the canal with an insufflation bulb, and the tympanic membrane is observed for movement. Normally, the tympanic membrane moves inward with a slight puff and outward with a slight release.

Thorax and Lungs

Assessment of the thorax and lungs consists of inspection, palpation, percussion, and auscultation, although not necessarily in that order, to optimize the accuracy of findings. For example, in a sleeping infant, the nurse is wise to seize the opportunity to inspect and auscultate breath sounds. To assist with localizing findings on the thorax, anatomic landmarks such as the ribs and intercostal spaces are identified and imaginary lines are drawn on the surface (Figure 9-13, p. 185).

Location of lung tissue depends on the age and development of the child. In an infant, lung tissue on the anterior chest can be located from the apex, above the clavicle, to the level of the fifth rib in the midclavicular line. By age 6 years, lung tissue is assessed from the apex to the level of the sixth rib in the midclavicular line. Laterally, lung tissue is assessed from the axilla to the level of the eighth rib. Posteriorly, lungs are assessed from the level of the first thoracic vertebra to the tenth thoracic vertebra.

Inspection

The child's shirt or clothing covering the chest is removed. In adolescent females, the breasts should be kept covered and exposed only when necessary. Inspection of the chest includes observing the child for any cough, stridor, grunting, hoarseness, snoring, wheezing, and type and amount of any sputum, if present. Respiratory rate and pattern are observed. In young children and infants, breathing is more diaphragmatic or abdominal (see Table 9-1 for the effect of age on vital signs). The chest wall should expand symmetrically during respiration. Respirations should be easy, regular, and without apparent distress. Rapid respirations, retractions, nasal flaring, and head bobbing may indicate respiratory difficulty.

Thoracic configuration is evaluated by determining the shape and symmetry of the chest from the front, sides, and back (Figure 9-14, p. 186). In infants and young children the thorax is more rounded. Some children may have "Harrison groove," a horizontal line in the rib cage extending from the sternum to the midaxillary line. Two common alterations in structure in the anterior chest are *pectus carinatum* (pigeon chest) and *pectus excavatum* (funnel chest). *Scoliosis*, a lateral S-shaped curvature of the thoracic and lumbar vertebrae, is a common alteration of the posterior chest that may cause impaired pulmonary function.

Palpation

Palpation of the chest begins with the posterior chest. To alleviate fear in a young child, the examiner should stand in a position that allows the child to see the examiner at all times. The posterior chest is palpated for areas of tenderness, tactile fremitus, and chest excursion.

To palpate for tenderness, the examiner touches the entire thorax with the palmar aspects of the fingers. This process elicits any points of discomfort or pain. The examiner notes any masses or edema (Figure 9-15, p. 186). The presence or absence of tactile fremitus, vibration felt on the chest wall when the child is crying or speaking, may indicate airway alterations and thus must be assessed.

Percussion of the chest is performed by advanced practitioners to determine changes in sound produced by the density of the underlying tissues. Hyperresonance is normal in the infant and young child because of the thin chest wall.

Auscultation

Auscultating the chest with a stethoscope determines the characteristics of breath sounds. Breath sounds heard with the stethoscope are made by the flow of air through the respiratory tree and are characterized by intensity, pitch, quality, and duration.

It is best to listen to breath sounds with the child sitting upright if possible. Infants and toddlers can be held in the parent's lap; have the parent assist with removal of clothing and positioning of the child. The examiner's position is on the side of the child, allowing the child to observe the examiner's movements. Before touching the chest, the examiner allows the young child to hold or play with the stethoscope and warms the stethoscope before placing it on the child's chest. The head of the stethoscope is cleaned with alcohol between patients.

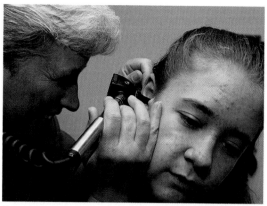

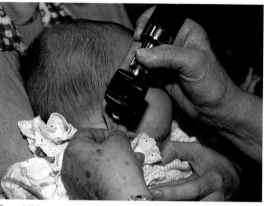

To straighten the ear canal of a child older than 3 years, the nurse pulls the child's pinna up and back.

For children younger than 3 years, the pinna is pulled down and back.

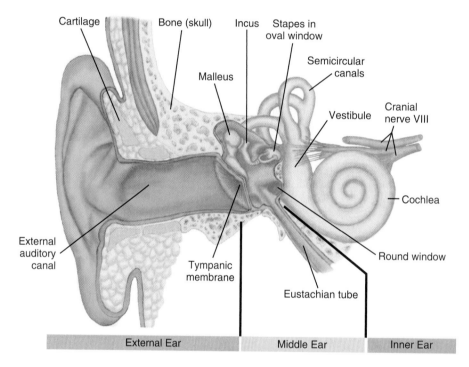

Cartilage   Bone (skull)   Incus   Stapes in oval window

Malleus

Semicircular canals

Vestibule   Cranial nerve VIII

External auditory canal

Tympanic membrane

Cochlea

Round window

Eustachian tube

| External Ear | Middle Ear | Inner Ear |

Landmarks of Tympanic Membrane

Malleolar folds

Pars flaccida

Long crus of incus

Umbo

Short process of malleus

Long process of malleus (manubrium)

Annulus

Light reflex

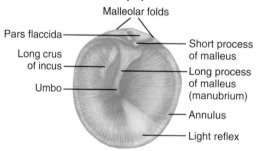

FIG 9-12 Inspection of the tympanic membrane with the otoscope. The auditory canal is inspected before the otoscope is inserted to see the child's tympanic membrane.

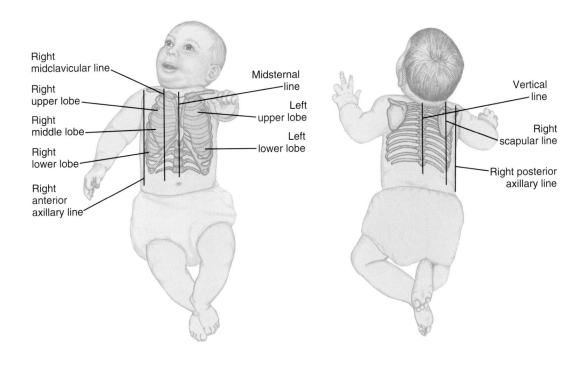

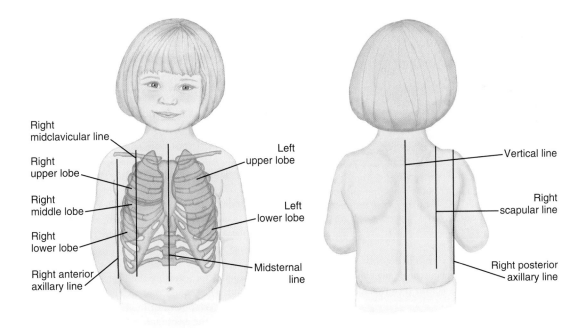

FIG 9-13 Anatomic landmarks of the thorax in infants and children.

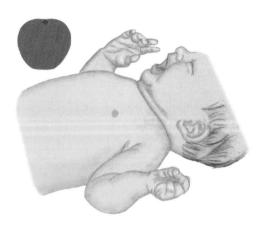

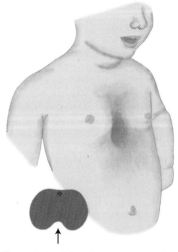

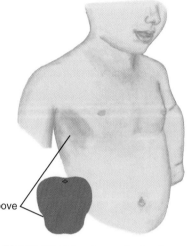

Normal infant: The chest of the normal infant is approximately round or barrel-shaped in cross section. A barrel chest in a child older than 6 years suggests a chronic pulmonary disease, such as asthma or cystic fibrosis.

Funnel chest (pectus excavatum): A funnel chest has a depression in the lower portion of the sternum. Compression of the heart and great vessels may cause murmurs.

Groove

Pigeon chest (pectus carinatum): In pigeon chest, the sternum is displaced anteriorly, increasing the anteroposterior diameter. Grooves in the chest wall accentuate the deformity.

FIG 9-14 Common alterations in chest configuration.

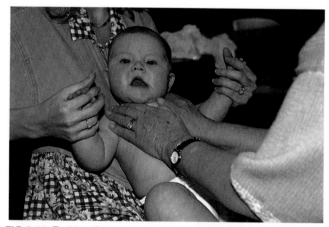

FIG 9-15 To identify areas of fremitus, tenderness, symmetry, and depth and equality of expansion, the nurse palpates the child's posterior and anterior chest. When palpating any area, warm hands increase the child's comfort. (Courtesy The University of Texas at Arlington College of Nursing, Arlington, TX.)

An anxious or frightened child may cry during this part of the examination. Distracting the child or having the young child focus on another activity may facilitate listening. For the inconsolable child, the examiner listens to breath sounds between cries. If the young child is sleeping or comfortable in the parent's arms, the examiner listens to the chest first before proceeding to the rest of the examination.

For listening to the posterior thorax, the child is positioned with the head bent forward and hands folded in front. Having the child raise the arms overhead while sitting erect allows the examiner to listen laterally. To auscultate the anterior chest, have the child sit erect with the shoulders back (Figure 9-16).

The examiner begins on the posterior thorax and has the child open the mouth and breathe in and out while the examiner listens with the diaphragm of the stethoscope. Having the young child blow bubbles, pretend to blow out birthday candles, or blow a tissue increases breath sounds. Compressing the hand holding the stethoscope on the chest

wall while placing the other hand on the opposite side of the chest accentuates expiration and makes end-expiratory sounds (e.g., wheezes) easier to hear. Having the child inhale deeply and then blow the breath out forcibly may assist with identification of adventitious breath sounds. Lung auscultation follows a zigzag pattern, comparing sounds from right to left. The usual sequence for listening to breath sounds is posterior chest, right and left lateral chest, and anterior chest (Figure 9-17); however, adjustments may be made in order to encourage the child's cooperation.

Adventitious Breath Sounds

In addition to normal breath sounds, *adventitious sounds* may be audible with the stethoscope. Table 9-2 on p. 188 describes the origin and characteristics of adventitious sounds. Adventitious sounds are additional sounds heard in an abnormal clinical state. They are described by their quality. The examiner notes whether they are continuous or discontinuous and where they occur in the respiratory phase. The effects of coughing are also noted. When adventitious sounds are heard, they are described as to location, timing, and intensity.

Heart

The techniques for assessing the heart are inspection, palpation, and auscultation. The sequence of this examination depends on the age, growth, and development of the child being examined. For an infant or young child, the examiner may want to listen to the child's heart while the parent is holding the child, before doing other parts of the examination. Infants and children have varying degrees of dependence on parents and may be fearful of the examination. Percussion of the heart indicates primarily the size and shape of the heart and is not routinely done. The heart is assessed with the child in a supine position, in a left lateral recumbent position, and in a sitting position while leaning forward slightly.

Inspection

The anterior chest is systematically inspected, with special attention paid to the following five areas: second right intercostal space (aortic

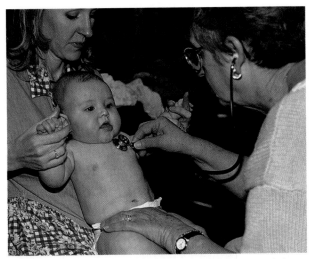
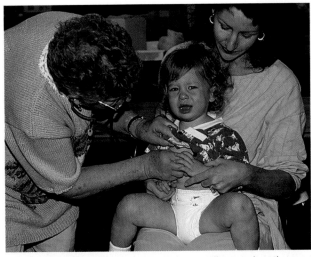

Infants and toddlers can be held sitting upright in the parent's lap while the nurse listens to breath sounds.

If the child is upset, the examiner may have to listen to breath sounds between cries. Keeping this child in the comfort of her mother's arms lessens distress.

FIG 9-16 Auscultation is most easily done when the child is quiet, so this part of the examination is best performed first if the child is quiet or asleep. To allay fears, the child can play with the stethoscope first and can be distracted with a toy while the nurse is listening. Warming the stethoscope bell increases comfort. (Courtesy The University of Texas at Arlington College of Nursing, Arlington, TX.)

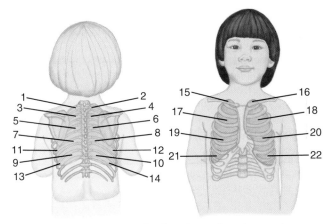

FIG 9-17 Sequence for listening to breath sounds.

area), second left intercostal space (pulmonic area), left sternal border (right ventricular area), fifth left intercostal space in the midclavicular line (apex), and just below the xiphoid process (epigastric area). The location of these areas will differ with a child's age (Figure 9-18, p. 189). During infancy, the heart is more horizontal in the thorax, and the apex is one or two intercostal spaces above the fifth intercostal space and lateral to the midclavicular line. The examiner locates the second intercostal space by identifying the sternal angle. The second rib is attached to the sternum just below or at the sternal angle. The second intercostal space is below the second rib. Other ribs and intercostal spaces are identified by their relationship to the second rib.

The precordium (anterior chest overlying the heart and great vessels) is inspected for *bulges, lifts, heaves,* and *apical impulse.* The apical impulse is seen as a pulsation of the anterior chest wall every time the heart beats. The location of the apical impulse will change gradually as the child matures and by age 7 years it can be seen at the fifth intercostal space in the midclavicular line.

Palpation

The examiner palpates the precordium with the fingertips for the presence of any pulsations at each individual area (see Figure 9-18). The examiner locates the apical pulse, sometimes identified as the *point of maximal impulse (PMI),* or the point where the light tapping of the heart is felt the best. The location of the PMI varies with age. In a child younger than 7 years, the PMI is located in the fourth intercostal space, lateral to the midclavicular line. The PMI in a child older than 7 years is located in the fifth intercostal space in the midclavicular line. Using the palmar aspect of the hand to feel for *thrills,* palpable vibrations of the heart, the examiner then palpates each area of the precordium.

Auscultation

Auscultation of the heart is done by listening both with the bell and with the diaphragm of the stethoscope as the child is lying supine, in a left lateral recumbent position, and sitting up. To auscultate heart sounds, the examiner uses a systematic approach. Sounds heard with the stethoscope are predominantly produced with the closing of the heart valves. The four traditional areas for listening to heart sounds are the aortic valve area in the second right intercostal space, the pulmonic valve area in the second left intercostal space, the tricuspid valve area in the left lower sternal border, and the mitral valve area in the fifth intercostal space at the left midclavicular line (see Figure 9-18). The position for listening to these areas depends on the age of the child. It is best to listen to heart sounds by inching the stethoscope across the precordium in a Z-shaped pattern, from the base of the heart across and down, or from the apex upward. All areas are auscultated with both the bell and the diaphragm of the stethoscope.

Sounds produced by the closing of the valves can be heard all over the precordium, so it is necessary to concentrate on one heart sound at a time. The heart sounds are divided into two components, the first heart sound (S_1) and the second heart sound (S_2), and are auscultated using the diaphragm of the stethoscope. S_1 is heard best at the apex of

TABLE 9-2 ORIGIN AND CHARACTERISTICS OF ADVENTITIOUS BREATH SOUNDS

SOUND	DESCRIPTION	MECHANISM	CLINICAL EXAMPLE
Discontinuous Sounds			
Crackles—fine (rales, crepitations); heard when fluid is in airways	Discontinuous, high-pitched, short, crackling, popping sounds heard during inspiration and not cleared by coughing. You can simulate this sound by rolling a strand of hair between your fingers near your ear or by moistening your thumb and index finger and separating them near your ear. Described as discrete (short), discontinuous.	Inhaled air collides with previously deflated airways; airways suddenly pop open, creating crackling sound as gas pressures between the two compartments equalize.	*Late inspiratory* crackles occur with restrictive disease: pneumonia, congestive heart failure, and interstitial fibrosis. *Early inspiratory* crackles occur with obstructive disease: chronic bronchitis and asthma.
Pleural friction rub	A very superficial sound that is coarse and low-pitched; it has a grating quality, as if two pieces of leather were being rubbed together. A pleural friction rub may sound just like crackles but close to the ear. It sounds louder if you push the stethoscope harder into the chest wall.	Caused when pleurae become inflamed and lose their normal lubricating fluid. Their opposing roughened pleural surfaces rub together during respiration. This sound is heard best in the anterolateral wall, where lung mobility is greatest.	Pleuritis, accompanied by pain with breathing. (Rub disappears after a few days if pleural fluid accumulates and separates pleurae.)
Continuous Sounds			
High-pitched wheeze heard with narrowing of the air passages from fluid, swelling, spasm, and tumors	High-pitched, musical squeaking sounds that predominate in expiration but may occur in both expiration and inspiration. Coughing frequently will change the character of the sound.	Air squeezed or compressed through passageways narrowed almost to closure by collapsing, swelling, secretions, or tumors. The passageway walls oscillate in apposition between the closed and barely open positions. The resulting sound is similar to that produced by a vibrating reed.	Obstructive lung disease, such as asthma.
Low-pitched wheeze (sonorous rhonchi)	Low-pitched, musical snoring, moaning sounds. They are heard throughout the cycle, although they are more prominent on expiration and may clear somewhat with coughing.	Airflow obstruction as described by the vibrating reed mechanism. The pitch of the wheeze does not correlate with the size of the passageway that generates it.	Bronchitis.

NOTE: Although nothing in clinical practice seems to differ more than the nomenclature of adventitious sounds, most authorities concur on two categories: (1) discontinuous, discrete crackling sounds and (2) continuous, coarse, or wheezing sounds.

the heart in the tricuspid and mitral area, and S_2 is heard best at the base in the aortic and pulmonic area (see Figure 9-18). S_1, phonetically described as *lub*, is produced by the closing of the mitral and tricuspid valves. S_2, phonetically described as *dub*, is produced by the closing of the aortic and pulmonic valves.

The physiologic splitting of S_2, an audible pause between the closing of the aortic and pulmonic valves, frequently heard in children of all ages, is considered normal. Splitting of S_2 can be heard best at the pulmonic area because ejection times on the right side of the heart are slightly longer than on the left side. Splitting of S_2 is greatest at the peak of inspiration and decreases or goes away during expiration.

The routine for assessing heart sounds follows this sequence:
1. Identify the rate and rhythm.
2. Identify S_1 and S_2.
3. Assess S_1 and S_2 separately to determine where they are best heard.
4. Listen for extra heart sounds.
5. Identify murmurs.

Normal Rate and Rhythm. The normal rate of a child's heart is different at various ages (see Table 9-1). Children's heart rates often increase with inspiration and slow down during expiration. To decrease the irregular rhythm associated with respirations, the examiner has the child hold the breath as the examiner continues to listen to the heart.

! NURSING QUALITY ALERT
Normal Findings in Children

- Small, firm, nontender, and shotty (freely palpable and very small) lymph nodes may be palpable.
- Tonsils of varying sizes; often larger in young children.
- Pupils of equal size, round, and reactive to light and accommodation (PERRLA).
- Pulses in upper and lower extremities; bilaterally symmetrical.

Extra Heart Sounds, Including Murmurs. Extra sounds (sounds heard over and above the normal heart sounds) may be described as opening snaps, ejection clicks, midsystolic to late systolic clicks, and murmurs. Snaps and clicks are short, high-pitched sounds heard with valve disorders and do not vary with respirations. *Murmurs* are blowing, swooshing sounds that occur because of turbulence of the

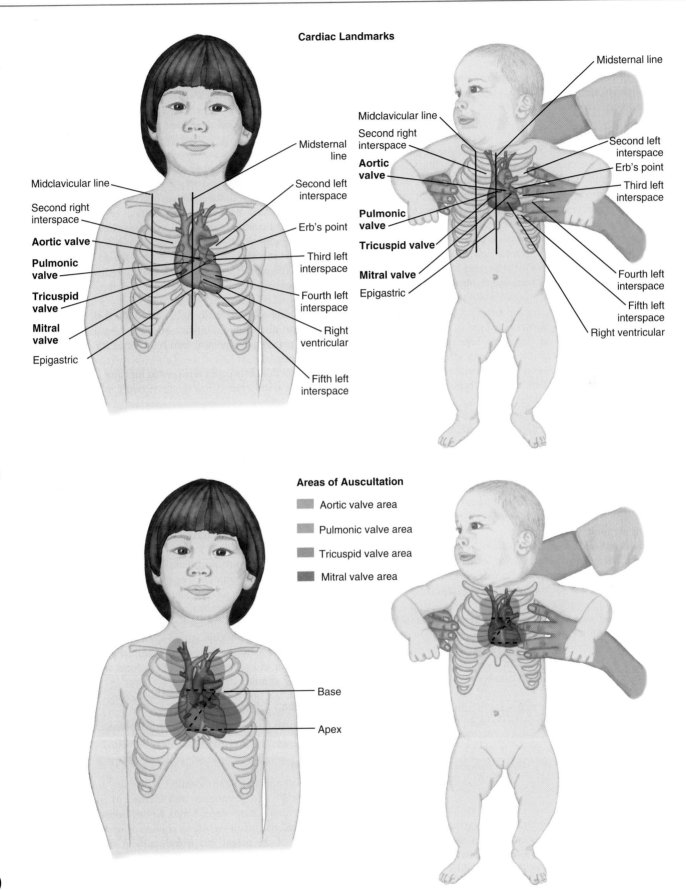

FIG 9-18 Location of the heart within the thorax in the infant and the older child, showing landmarks and areas of auscultation.

blood flow into, through, or out of the heart and are best heard with the bell of the stethoscope. Innocent or functional heart murmurs are frequently heard in children. Innocent murmurs occur during systole, are heard best along the left sternal border, do not radiate, and change with position change. To describe and classify extra heart sounds, the nurse needs advanced training and practice.

Peripheral Vascular System

Arterial pulses are examined for decrease or absence of pulses. Pulses are palpated, with the examiner noting the rate, rhythm, elasticity of the vessel wall, and equal force of bilateral pulses. The pulse force should be symmetrical and should be the same for upper and lower extremities. Comparing opposite pulses is necessary in children. The examiner compares one femoral pulse with the opposite radial pulse for equality and compares one lower extremity pulse with an upper extremity pulse for equality. A femoral pulse that is diminished (or absent), in comparison to the radial pulse, may be the sole indication of coarctation of the aorta in infants and children (see Chapter 22).

Breast

The examiner inspects and palpates breast tissue. Developmental differences occur in response to circulating hormones and affect the appearance of breast tissue. In infants of both sexes, the breasts may appear engorged because of maternal estrogen crossing the placenta. *Thelarche,* or breast development, marks the beginning of puberty in preadolescent girls and can occur as early as age 7 years.

The examiner inspects the nipples for position and appearance. In infants, the nipple is flat and symmetrical with darker areolar pigmentation. In preadolescent and adolescent girls, the Tanner sexual maturity rating is used to evaluate developmental levels (see Table 8-1). The nipples should be symmetrical on the chest and should point in the same direction. Nipples may appear to be inverted or everted. An inverted nipple is significant if the inversion has recently occurred. The breast skin should be smooth and free of any dimpling. It is common to see some asymmetry during growth.

All adolescent girls should be taught how to do breast self-examination once they have reached menarche. Teaching self-examination to the adolescent and reinforcing its importance at every visit are important roles for the nurse. Many adolescents do not do breast self-examinations because of lack of knowledge or fear of finding something wrong. Once the adolescent is familiar with how her breasts look and feel, the natural and normal changes that occur in the breast as a result of hormonal fluctuations can be easily identified. The adolescent girl is taught to do breast self-examination 3 to 4 days after menses because the breasts usually are least tender and sensitive at that time.

The examiner uses the same technique to palpate the breast tissue and the axilla of the adolescent boy. In the male, the examiner expects to feel a thin layer of fatty tissue overlying the muscle. During puberty, some boys experience *gynecomastia,* an enlargement of breast tissue, felt as a smooth, firm, movable disk. It frequently affects only one breast and can be temporary.

Abdomen

The child's comfort should be considered during the abdominal examination. Abdominal relaxation is enhanced if the child's bladder is empty, the examiner's hands are warm, and the child is positioned supine on the examining table with a pillow under the head and the knees flexed. For an infant or young child, most of the abdominal examination can be done while the child is lying in the parent's lap.

For an older child, the genitalia and breasts are draped. The child and parent should be questioned about urinary and bowel patterns.

The abdomen is divided into four quadrants that correlate with underlying anatomic structures (Figure 9-19). Because bowel sounds are disturbed by percussion and palpation, the sequence of techniques differs in abdominal assessment. The abdomen is first inspected, then auscultated, then percussed, and last palpated.

Inspection

Abdominal inspection assesses contour, symmetry, characteristics of the umbilicus and skin, pulsations or movement, and hair distribution. *Contour* is the profile of the abdomen from the rib margin to the pubic bone and is best determined by looking tangentially across the abdomen. The contour is described as flat, scaphoid, rounded, or protuberant (Figure 9-20). The abdominal contour provides an overall indicator of nutritional state. The abdomen should be bilaterally symmetrical. The examiner looks for distention, bulging, a visible mass, and asymmetrical shape. A protuberant abdomen is typical for the toddler.

The umbilicus is normally midline and inverted. There should be no signs of discoloration, inflammation, or hernia. Throughout the neonatal period, the umbilical cord is inspected for signs of infection and bleeding.

The skin of the abdomen is inspected for color and the presence of scars, lesions, and striae. A fine venous network may be seen in infants and small children.

The abdomen is inspected for pulsations and movement. In thin children, the examiner may see the pulsations from the aorta beneath the skin in the epigastric area. Most children have abdominal movement with respirations. Peristalsis of the abdomen should not be visible.

Auscultation

Auscultation of the abdomen follows inspection. The diaphragm of the stethoscope is held lightly against the skin to note the character and frequency of bowel sounds. Bowel sounds are high-pitched, gurgling sounds heard in all four quadrants. They are irregular and can occur from 5 to 34 times per minute. The examiner begins in the lower right quadrant and listens in all four quadrants. To determine that there are no bowel sounds, the examiner must listen for up to 5 minutes in an area where no bowel sounds are heard.

The bell of the stethoscope is used to listen for bruits over the aortic, renal, iliac, and femoral arteries. The examiner also listens in the epigastric region and around the umbilicus for a venous hum—a soft, low-pitched, continuous sound.

Percussion

Advanced practitioners perform abdominal percussion. The technique reveals tympany, liver span, and splenic dullness.

Palpation

Abdominal palpation can identify any mass or tenderness and determine the size, consistency, and location of certain organs. The examiner should have warm hands before palpating the abdomen. Palpation of the infant or young child can be done with the child in the lap of the parent and examiner, who sit facing each other. The child lays with the head and thorax across the parent's legs and the child's abdomen and legs extending across the examiner's legs. The child's knees are flexed to prepare the child for palpation of the abdomen.

Animation—Abdominal Anatomy

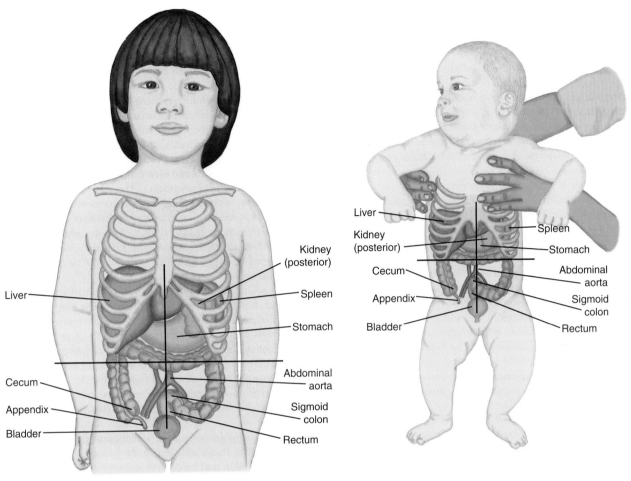

FIG 9-19 Abdominal quadrants and structures.

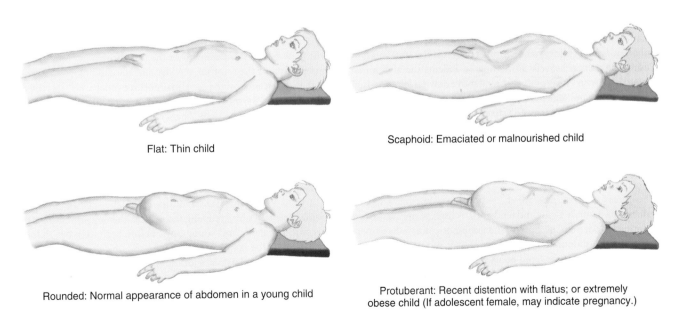

Flat: Thin child

Scaphoid: Emaciated or malnourished child

Rounded: Normal appearance of abdomen in a young child

Protuberant: Recent distention with flatus; or extremely obese child (If adolescent female, may indicate pregnancy.)

FIG 9-20 Abdominal contours. The contour of the abdomen provides an indication of the child's overall nutritional state.

Fear and anxiety may cause the child to resist when the examiner touches the abdomen. Distracting the young child with a toy or by talking is helpful. Beginning with light palpation shows the child that palpation will not hurt.

The examiner asks an older child who is anxious or ticklish, to assist with this part of the examination. The child places a hand on the abdomen, and the examiner places a hand, with fingers touching the abdomen, on top of the child's hand and asks the child to push as the examiner pushes. This technique allows the child some control as the examination begins, and it reduces the sensation of tickling. To assist with relaxation of the abdominal muscles, the examiner can ask the child to take deep breaths.

The examiner begins with light palpation of all four quadrants using light, even pressure and pressing the palmar surface of the fingers no more than 1 cm into the abdomen. The hand is lifted while moving from area to area. Sudden jabs should be avoided. As the examiner circles around the abdomen, the abdomen should feel soft and smooth. Light palpation is useful in identifying areas of tenderness and muscular resistance. Guarding, resistance, or tenderness should alert the examiner to move cautiously with deeper palpation.

Tenseness can be either voluntary or involuntary. In a child, tenseness and rigidity may be caused by fear and anxiety. Distracting the child or waiting for the child to breathe helps determine whether the tenseness is voluntary or involuntary. The examiner gently indents the fingers into the abdominal wall during inspiration. With even pressure, the abdomen should feel soft. Rigidity, a constant, boardlike hardness, of the abdomen is usually associated with an acute inflammation of the peritoneum.

Using the same techniques, the examiner performs deep palpation of the abdomen. The examiner pushes down about 5 to 8 cm into the abdominal wall, beginning in the right lower quadrant. The entire abdomen is examined to identify palpable organs and masses.

To palpate the liver's edge, the examiner begins at the level of the umbilicus in the midclavicular line, using the side of the hand to indent the abdomen about 5 to 8 cm. With deep penetration of the abdominal wall, the hand is gently inverted toward the costal margin. Then the examiner progresses upward with the same maneuver until palpating the border of the liver. The edge of the liver is felt as soft and smooth. The firm border moves downward when the child takes a deep breath. In infants and young children, the examiner begins at the costal margin and, using the palmar aspects of the fingers, indents the abdominal wall about 5 to 8 cm. The examiner should move down from the costal margin until the hand falls off the edge of the liver border. In infants and toddlers, the liver edge may be palpated 1 to 3 cm below the costal margin.

While palpating the abdomen, the examiner checks skin turgor and palpates the femoral pulses and inguinal lymph nodes. Advanced practitioners palpate the spleen and kidneys to determine the presence and size of masses and enlargement.

When areas of tenderness are elicited during palpation, a special procedure for identifying rebound tenderness is used. A site away from the identified tenderness is chosen. The examiner places a hand perpendicular to the abdomen, pushes down slowly and deeply into the abdomen, and then lifts the hand quickly. With peritoneal inflammation, the sudden release of the pressure will cause severe pain and muscle rigidity.

The child is turned over, and the buttocks are inspected. The buttocks in children are full, with symmetrical folds. No evidence of scars or ecchymosis should appear on the buttocks. The sacrococcygeal area is examined for dimples and tufts of hair.

Male Genitalia

The approach to examining the male genitals depends on the child's growth and development. For an infant, toddler, or young child, the nurse tells the child what will occur and then the parent or guardian concurs that the nurse should proceed to examine the child's genitalia.

Objective signs of pubertal changes and the adolescent's perception of these changes have an impact on understanding physical signs experienced by this age-group. Adolescent boys are normally apprehensive about the genital examination. Concerns arise from modesty, fear of pain, negative judgment, or a previous uncomfortable experience. A matter-of-fact approach and direct communication will facilitate this part of the physical examination. The genital examination is performed during or immediately after the abdominal examination. In the adolescent, the physical examination should not conclude with the genital examination, so as to allow further opportunities for communication. A good practice is to conclude the physical examination with the musculoskeletal and neurologic examination after the genital examination has been completed.

Gloves should be worn during every genital examination. The examiner begins by inspecting the penis. The size of the penis is directly related to age and to growth and development. In infants and young boys, the penis is approximately 2 to 3 cm. Genital hair distribution is noted. The adolescent shows a wide variation in normal development of the genitals. Tanner stages are used for determining the level of development in the adolescent (see Chapter 8).

The skin on the penis normally appears wrinkled, hairless, and without lesions. In the adolescent, a dorsal vein may be prominent. Any indurations on the penile shaft should be noted. In the circumcised male, the glans looks smooth and without lesions. In an uncircumcised infant, the glans may not be visible. By the time the male is age 5 to 6 years, the foreskin may be easily retractable behind the corona of the glans. The adolescent is asked to retract the foreskin himself.

The meatus is evaluated by compressing the glans between the thumb and forefinger anteroposteriorly. The adolescent may be requested to compress the glans so that the examiner can see the meatus. The meatus in the male has a slitlike or tear-shaped configuration and is located on the ventral surface, just millimeters from the tip of the glans. The meatus opening is pink, smooth, and without discharge.

The scrotum is inspected for size and configuration, which changes with growth and development. In the infant or young boy, the proximal portion of the scrotum is wider and the distal portion narrower. In the adolescent boy, the proximal portion is narrower and the distal portion wider. Asymmetry of the scrotum is normal, with the left half slightly lower than the right. The scrotum is movable and, to maintain optimal temperature of the testes, moves closer to or away from the body in response to environmental temperature.

The contents of the scrotum are palpated. The *cremasteric* reflex in young boys may cause the testes to withdraw into the inguinal canal, making palpation more difficult. If the boy is old enough, have him sit in a cross-legged, or "tailor" position, which will help prevent the cremasteric reflex by stretching the muscle, thereby preventing its contraction. In infants and young boys, before beginning the abdominal examination, the examiner warms the hands, blocks the inguinal canal with one hand, and palpates for the scrotal contents (Figure 9-21). The examiner uses the thumb and first two fingers to palpate each testis and epididymis. The testes should be smooth, rubbery, and free of nodules. The size of the testes changes with growth and development. Tanner growth and development stages are used for appropriate interpretation. Because of the high incidence of testicular tumors in young men, adolescents should be taught to do testicular self-examination.

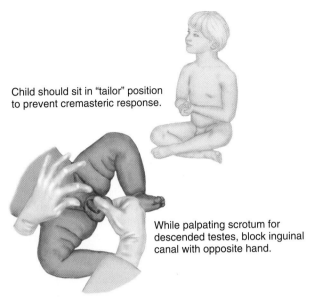

Child should sit in "tailor" position to prevent cremasteric response.

While palpating scrotum for descended testes, block inguinal canal with opposite hand.

FIG 9-21 When a boy's scrotum is examined, the cremasteric reflex may cause the testes to withdraw into the inguinal canal. To prevent this reflex, the examiner can have the boy sit in a tailor position. The examiner uses one hand to block the inguinal canal and the other to palpate.

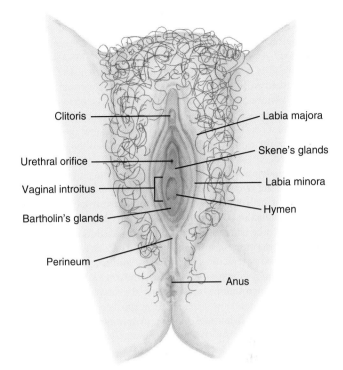

Clitoris — Labia majora
Urethral orifice — Skene's glands
— Labia minora
Vaginal introitus — Hymen
Bartholin's glands —
Perineum —
— Anus

FIG 9-22 Postpubertal female genitalia.

Female Genitalia

In general, the anogenital examination in prepubescent girls is limited to visual inspection and gentle palpation of the external area. Internal speculum examinations are not routine in prepubescent children. The appearance of the external genitalia in females varies from child to child and with growth and development. A relaxed, caring attitude on the part of the examiner will reassure both the child and parent.

To safeguard privacy, reinforce modesty, and decrease anxiety, the child is draped appropriately. The examiner communicates to the child what will be done, and the parent or guardian concurs that it is appropriate to examine the genitalia. With the child in different positions, the genitals differ in tone, relaxation, and appearance. Generally, the genitalia in a young girl are examined with the child supine; the legs are gently drawn up onto the abdomen to expose the genitalia.

The examiner dons gloves and begins by inspecting the *mons pubis* and *labia majora*. The skin should be smooth and clean. The examiner notes the distribution of pubic hair. Tanner stages are used to determine appropriate growth and development (see Chapter 8).

In the newborn infant, the labia majora and minora may be edematous, with the *labia minora* often more prominent. In the infant, the *hymen* may protrude and may appear thick and vascular. The clitoris may appear relatively large. The hymen is centrally located and is about 0.5 cm in diameter. The examiner determines whether the hymen has an opening.

In the young girl or adolescent, the labia majora may be gaping or closed, shriveled or full, dry or moist, depending on the age and development of the child. The labia majora are usually symmetrical (Figure 9-22).

The examiner uses the fingers to gently spread the labia majora and then inspects and palpates the labia minora, the *clitoris*, the urethral orifice, and the *vaginal introitus*. The labia minora should appear symmetrical, dark pink, and moist. On palpation, the tissue should be soft and homogeneous with no tenderness.

With the labia majora spread, the examiner inspects the clitoris for size and length. The clitoris varies with growth and development.

Moving toward the anus, the examiner locates the urethral meatus, which may be close to or inside the vaginal introitus. The urethral meatus is usually in the midline and appears as a dimple posterior to the clitoris.

The vaginal introitus may be a thin, vertical slit or a large orifice with irregular edges, depending on the characteristics of the hymen. The hymen may or may not be stretched across the vaginal opening. By menarche, the opening should be at least 1 cm wide. The tissue is usually moist. The amount and characteristics of any vaginal discharge depend on the circulating hormones in the child. A normal vaginal discharge is odorless and may be cloudy or clear, thick or thin, and there may be a slippery sensation around the time of ovulation.

Normally, *Skene's glands*, located just inferior to the urethral meatus, are not seen or felt and have no discharge. Any discharge from Skene's glands indicates an infection. The examiner inspects and palpates *Bartholin's glands*, located in the posterolateral portion of the labia majora. Bartholin's glands should not be swollen or tender.

A speculum examination of the internal reproductive organs is not indicated for young girls. The adolescent girl has special needs during the genital examination, which is performed by advanced practitioners.

Musculoskeletal System

The musculoskeletal system is composed of the bones, joints, cartilage, ligaments, and muscles. Joint motions are defined as flexion, extension, abduction, adduction, internal rotation, external rotation, and circumduction. The musculoskeletal examination focuses principally on the upper and lower extremities and the spinal column. Musculoskeletal evaluation begins with observing the child during play or history taking. Observation of the child climbing, jumping, hopping, rising from a sitting position, and manipulating toys and other objects provides evidence of joint function, range of motion, bone stability, and muscle strength. Assessment of fine motor and gross motor ability is accomplished during the Denver II test for the child younger than 5 years old (see Chapter 4 and Evolve website).

General inspection begins with visual scanning of the body with use of a *cephalocaudal* (head-to-toe) organization. The child can be dressed in shorts or underwear during the examination. The examiner compares the two sides of the body for symmetry, contour, size, and involuntary movement. The examiner then inspects the two sides for areas of swelling or edema and for ecchymoses or other discolorations. The structural relationship of the feet with the legs and the hips to the pelvis, the upper extremities, the shoulder girdle, and the upper trunk are evaluated.

Common deformities of the extremities are *varus* and *valgus* deformities. With the reference point of the midline of the body, a varus deformity is a medial adduction, or turning inward. A valgus deformity is a medial abduction, or turning outward (see Chapter 26).

Injuries to the extremities caused by overexertion and strenuous movements are common in children. Sprains are the most common injury, followed by fractures, dislocations, and lacerations. Overuse injuries, common in school-age children and adolescents, are caused by repetitive microtrauma that exceeds the body's rate of repair. Overuse injuries occur most frequently in sports emphasizing repetitive motion such as swimming, running, gymnastics and skating. Children's participation in sports should be evaluated for the specifics of conditioning and training.

Deformities of the spine are *scoliosis, kyphosis,* and *lordosis,* which are discussed in Chapter 26.

Palpation of the skull, extremities, and ribs for tenderness, swelling, deformity, and crepitus is performed on any child if injuries are suspected or if there are circumstances that point to possible abuse.

Infants

During infancy, symmetrical flexion of the arms and legs is noted. Limbs should be freely movable, with symmetry of the axillary, gluteal, femoral, and popliteal creases. The examiner inspects the hands, noting the shape, number, and position of the fingers and palmar creases. The clavicle should feel smooth, regular, and without crepitus. By age 2 months, the infant can lift the head while prone.

The examiner observes range of motion as the infant spontaneously moves the extremities. The infant with normal muscle strength wedges securely between the examiner's hands when lifted under the axilla. The examiner checks the hips for congenital dislocation by comparing leg lengths. The baby's feet are placed flat on the table, and the knees flexed up. The examiner looks for the top of the knees to be the same height (Allis test). Posterior gluteal folds should be equal on both sides. The *Ortolani* and *Barlow maneuvers* are performed by a trained examiner on every visit until the infant is 1 year old (see Figure 26-9).

Toddlers, Preschoolers, and School-Age Children

The examiner may want to start with the child's hands and arms by checking for range of motion and the presence of pain while the child is sitting. Children are willing to show their hands, so this is an excellent way to make contact with the child.

The child should stand so that the examiner can observe the posture from behind. The shoulders should be level and the scapulae symmetrical. Lordosis is common in young children. Anteriorly, the examiner begins with the feet and observes for adduction and pronation of the foot. Pronation is common between ages 12 and 30 months because of the young child's broad-based stance. Adduction, or toeing in, is demonstrated when the child walks on the lateral side of the foot. Adduction tends to correct itself by age 3 years as long as the foot is flexible. *Genu varum* (bowleg) is present when a space of more than 2.5 cm is measured between the knees as the medial malleoli are held

together. Genu varum is normal after the child has begun to walk and may persist until the child is 3 years old. With *genu valgum*, more than 2.5 cm remains between the medial malleoli when the knees are held together. Genu valgum is present between ages 2 and 3½ years (see Chapter 26).

The child is instructed to stand on one leg and then the other while the examiner watches from behind. The iliac crest should stay level when the weight is shifted.

Adolescents

For adolescents, the examiner follows the sequence described for school-age children but with special attention to the spine. Adolescents frequently have kyphosis (see Chapter 26, Figure 26-5) caused by poor posture. Although the U.S. Preventive Services Task Force (2004a) found no good evidence that routine community screening for scoliosis in asymptomatic children or adolescents alters the eventual progression of scoliosis, children ages 9 through 15 years are often screened for scoliosis, and the nurse needs to know the correct screening procedure. While standing, the child is told to bend forward, allowing the shoulders to droop with the arms hanging freely. The nurse looks for unilateral elevation of the lower thoracic ribs and flank (Box 9-9).

Range of Motion

The examiner notes the child's ability to perform active range-of-motion movements when the child is sitting, standing, and moving about the examination room. The quality of movement for each joint and equality of movement for contralateral joints should be noted. There should be no pain, limitation of movement, spastic movement, joint instability, deformity, or crepitation during movement. Passive range-of-motion movements are performed on joints in which limitations are noted. Passive range-of-motion movement is accomplished by the examiner, who anchors the joint with one hand while using the other hand to slowly move the joint to its limit. Active and passive ranges of motion should be the same.

Muscle Strength and Mass

The examiner assesses the strength of each muscle group. The child is asked to flex the muscle and then resist as opposing force is applied against flexion. Muscle tone should be firm on palpation. When appropriate, the evaluation of muscle strength is integrated with examination of the associated joint for range of motion. The motor segment of cranial nerve V *(trigeminal nerve)* is evaluated by the application of opposing force to the temporalis muscle while the child clenches the teeth. Cranial nerve XI *(accessory nerve)* is tested by assessing the strength of the sternocleidomastoid and trapezius muscles with rotation of the head from side to side and chin to shoulder.

When atrophy or hypertrophy is suspected, the examiner measures muscle mass. Muscles are best measured at their greatest circumference. With the joint used as a landmark, the distance from the joint to a point on the extremity is measured and compared with the opposite muscle. One measurement is not as significant as a series of measurements to determine changes in size of muscles.

Joints

The examiner palpates each joint for temperature, tenderness, swelling, crepitation, and masses. In children, fatigue, stiffness, or weakness, along with heat and redness, are frequently associated with disorders of the joints. Children usually do not move a joint if it is painful.

Gait

Assessment of the child's gait and the ability to ambulate is an essential part of both the musculoskeletal and the neurologic assessments. The

BOX 9-9 SCREENING PROCEDURE FOR SCOLIOSIS

To ensure early detection and treatment, children ages 9 through 15 years may be screened for scoliosis. At greatest risk are girls from 10 years old through adolescence.

The child should be unclothed or wearing only underpants so that the chest, back, and hips can be clearly seen. Have the child stand with his or her weight distributed equally on the feet, with legs straight and arms hanging loosely at the sides. Observe for the following signs of scoliosis:

- Nonpainful lateral curvature of the spine.
- A curve with one turn (C curve) or two compensating curves (S curve).
- Lateral deviation and rotation of each vertebra, observed better by looking at the ribs, as well as the spinal column itself.
- Unequal shoulder heights.
- Unequal scapular prominences and heights. (Note that the muscle masses may be somewhat unequal, especially if the child uses one shoulder more than the other, as in carrying books. Look for bony, not muscular, prominence.)
- Unequal waist angles.
- Unequal rib prominences and chest asymmetry.
- Unequal rib heights when the child stands in Adam's position (see photograph).

The physical examination should also include the following:

- Observation for equal leg lengths
- Examination of the skin for hairy patches, nevi, café au lait spots, lipomas, and dimples
- Neurologic examination
- Cardiac examination for Marfan syndrome
- Congenital scoliosis is visible in the infant lying prone; the condition is sometimes more prominent if the infant is suspended prone.

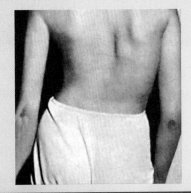
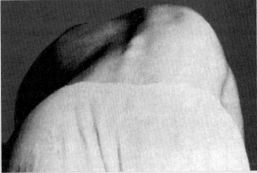

Adam's position demonstrates the rib hump of structural scoliosis. Lateral curvature of thoracic and lumbar segments of the spine, usually with some rotation of involved vertebral bodies. Functional scoliosis is flexible; it is apparent with standing and disappears with forward bending. It may be compensatory for other abnormalities such as leg-length discrepancy.

Structural scoliosis is fixed; the curvature is evident both when the individual stands and when the individual bends forward. Note the rib hump with forward flexion. When the child is standing, unequal shoulder elevation, unequal scapulae, obvious curvature, unequal elbow level, and unequal hip level is seen.

Data from Burns, C. (2008). Musculoskeletal disorders. In C. Burns, A. Dunn, M. Brady, N. Starr, & C. Blosser (Eds.), *Pediatric primary care* (4th ed.). Philadelphia: Saunders Elsevier. Photographs from Delp, M.H., & Manning, R.T. (1981). *Major's physical diagnosis: An introduction to the clinical process* (9th ed., p. 450). Philadelphia: Elsevier.

developmental acquisition of the ability to walk follows a prescribed sequence in infants and toddlers (Table 9-3) (see Chapter 5).

Gait is assessed in two phases—stance and swing. The stance phase begins when the heel strikes the floor; then the weight is transferred to the ball of the foot, and the toes push off the floor. The swing phase occurs when the foot is off the floor and consists of acceleration, swing through, and deceleration.

Neurologic System

The purpose of the neurologic examination in the child and adolescent is to identify any nervous system malfunction and to ascertain the extent of nervous system development and functioning. In cases of neurologic deficit, the examiner needs to determine the degree, type, and location of nervous system lesions. In the child, the examiner determines the degree to which the nervous system is functioning so that the healthy portion of the nervous system can be used for habilitation or rehabilitation. For the child younger than 5 years, neurologic functioning is best evaluated with the Denver II test or other reliable and valid developmental screening test (see Chapter 4 and Evolve website). For the child older than 5 years, the sequence of the

neurologic examination is adapted to the child's ability to understand and cooperate.

Brain dysfunction in infants and young children may be manifested by apnea, loss of consciousness, and seizures. Very young children may have milder nonspecific clinical signs, such as irritability, recurrent vomiting, fever, and loss of appetite.

Testing cerebral function, cranial nerves, and cerebellar function gives a picture of nervous system functioning above the spinal cord. The child's age and development determine the sequence of the neurologic examination. Infants and younger children are not able to cooperate with neurologic testing. A review of developmental milestones attained helps establish the rate and consistency of development in the infant and younger child. The 3- or 4-year-old cooperates with testing when it is approached as a game.

Cerebral Function

The evaluation of cognitive function focuses on appearance, behavior, orientation, speech patterns, memory, logic, and affect. The examiner needs to obtain information from the primary caregiver about changes in the child's behavior, personality, appearance, and age-appropriate

TABLE 9-3 GROSS MOTOR DEVELOPMENT IN THE INFANT: PROGRESSION TO WALKING

ACTIVITY	AGE
Raises head and holds position	2 wk-2 mo
Moves all extremities, kicking arms and legs when prone	2 mo
Draws up knees and raises abdomen off table; rocks back and forth while up on hands and knees; rolls over	3-6 mo
Sits alone, using hands for support (tripod fashion)	By 7 mo
Lurches forward and pulls legs to chest in "inchworm" fashion, may move backward in same fashion; creeps and rolls	By 9 mo
Crawls in one-sided manner (moves arm and leg on same side of body, then other side)	6-9 mo
Crawls in regular fashion, alternating arm and opposite leg	6-9 mo
Begins to pull up	By 11 mo
Cruises: attempts to walk with support or holding on to something stable	By 12 mo
Momentarily lets go and maintains balance for a few seconds	Once comfortable standing and holding on
Takes first steps (a broad stance with arms flexed for balance)	Once standing balance accomplished
Sits from a standing posture	By 12 mo
Walks alone	By 15 mo

BOX 9-10 SPECIFIC CEREBRAL FUNCTION TESTS

Sound recognition: Can the child identify familiar sounds with the eyes closed?

Auditory and verbal comprehension: Does the child answer questions and carry out instructions appropriate for age?

Recognition of body parts and sidedness: Does the child recognize the parts of the body? Does the child know right from left?

Performance of skilled motor acts: Can the child drink from a cup, button clothes, use a common tool?

Visual object recognition: Can the child identify a familiar toy or object (e.g., ball)?

Visual and verbal comprehension: Can the child read appropriately and explain the meaning?

Motor speech: Does the child imitate different sounds and phrases?

Automatic speech: Can the child repeat a series of learned words (e.g., nursery rhymes, days of the week)?

Volitional speech: Does the child answer questions relevantly?

Writing: Can the child write his or her name or the name of an object?

school performance. Evaluation of cognitive function in the older child and adolescent is based on observation of level of consciousness, awareness, thought processes, and communication.

The degree of response to sensory stimuli provides information about the older child's or adolescent's level of consciousness. The child is described as alert, lethargic, obtunded, stuporous, or comatose.

The older child and the adolescent have the ability to understand, think, feel emotions, and appreciate sensory information about self and surroundings. Awareness is evaluated by observing the older child's or adolescent's level of orientation in relation to person, place, and time. The normally functioning child is oriented to person, place, and time.

Thought processes include abstract thinking, problem solving (simple calculations and concentration), insight, memory (recent and remote), and judgment. The child's school performance may or may not be an accurate indicator of thought processes. Factors that may influence thought processes are attention span, communication, perceptual problems, and emotional withdrawal and depression.

Language ability is evaluated through speech patterns and comprehension. The child is questioned about reading and writing ability. Is the child's speech intelligible? Does the child answer questions appropriately for age and developmental level? Typically, older children and adolescents are able to speak fluently, name objects correctly, and write both name and address (Box 9-10).

Cranial Nerves

Assessment of the cranial nerves (Table 9-4, p. 198) should be incorporated into the examination of the system each nerve affects. Games, such as making faces and performing tests on a parent or the examiner, will enhance cooperation.

Cerebellar Function

Proprioception, balance, and coordination are tested by having the child perform specific movements. The cerebellum controls balance and coordination. Proprioception evaluates laterality and orientation in space. The techniques used vary with the child's age and development. The child should attempt the technique and show continued improvement with maturation (Box 9-11).

Motor System

Muscle size, muscle tone, involuntary movements, and muscle strength are assessed during the musculoskeletal examination.

While the child is at rest, the muscles are inspected and palpated for size, consistency, and possible atrophy. The examiner notes symmetry of posture and of muscle contours and outlines.

Muscle tone is evaluated by palpating the muscles at rest and noting resistance to passive movement. The examiner inspects the muscles for involuntary movements. Muscle strength is tested first without resistance and then against resistance. Corresponding muscles on the two sides are compared. The examiner then tests the major joints for flexion, extension, and other movements.

Sensory System

Sensory testing depends on the child's perception and interpretation of the stimuli and on the child's age and development. Sensory tests should first be done in an educational practice session before being done in a testing situation. Sensory testing compares the two sides of the body, corresponding extremities, and the sensitivity of the distal and proximal parts of each extremity for each form of sensation. Sensory testing is performed to determine whether sensory changes involve one entire side of the body, are *dermatomal* (along nerve pathways in the skin) in distribution, or are confined to the peripheral nerves (Box 9-12). In an older child, primary forms of sensation, such as superficial tactile, superficial pain, sensitivity to temperature, sensitivity to vibration, deep pressure pain, and motion and position, can be tested. Cortical and discriminatory forms of sensation require interpretation by the cerebral cortex. They are evaluated by two-point discrimination, point localization, texture discrimination, *stereognostic* (touch recognition of objects) function, *graphesthesia* (identification of figures traced on the skin), and extinction phenomenon.

BOX 9-11 CEREBELLAR FUNCTION: TESTS OF BALANCE AND COORDINATION

Balance and coordination are tested by having the child perform the following movements:

Finger-to-nose test. Child performs first with one hand, then with the other; first with the eyes open, then with the eyes closed. Ask child first to touch her finger to her nose and then to your finger as you change the position of your finger. Repeat this action with increasing rapidity. The tests are performed with each hand.

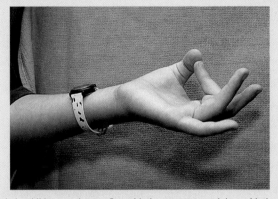

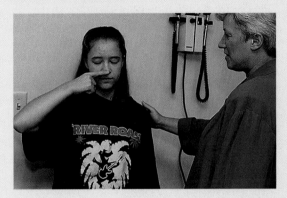

Ask the child to stand erect, first with the eyes open and then with the eyes closed. Stand near the child to prevent injury if the child begins to fall.

Rapid alternating movements. Ask the child to rapidly pat his knee with the palms and backs of his hands by pronating and supinating the hands *(demonstrate first)*. Ask the child to touch his thumb to each of his fingers in rapid succession *(demonstrate first)*.

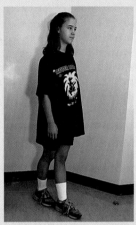

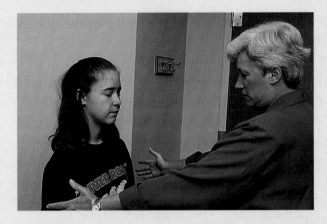

Ask the sitting child to run each heel down the opposite shin. With the child lying down, ask the child to point to your hand with each big toe.

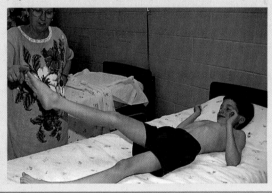

Ask the child to walk in tandem fashion, placing her heel immediately in front of her opposite foot's toe and alternating while walking a straight line.

Reflex Status

Most brain growth occurs in the first year of life. Primitive reflexes in the neonate are inhibited when more advanced cortical functions and voluntary control take over as the child matures and grows. Commonly elicited reflexes are illustrated in Table 9-5 on p. 199.

Motor maturation proceeds in a cephalocaudal direction. The ability to elicit a reflex requires an intact afferent nerve fiber, functional synapses in the spinal cord, intact motor nerve fibers, functional neuromuscular junctions, and competent muscle fibers. The examiner compares the responses on the right and left sides, which should be equal. Diminished or hyperreflexic responses are reported for further evaluation.

Neurologic "Soft" Signs

Neurologic "soft" signs are findings that indicate the child's inability to perform certain activities related to the child's age. They may provide subtle clues to an underlying central nervous system deficit or neurologic maturation delay.

Although these findings may fall in a gray area, they should be recorded and reported when they are observed. Children with multiple "soft" signs are often found to have learning problems (Seidel et al., 2010).

Children with neurologic "soft" signs need evaluation and monitoring because some children with medical, mental, or emotional problems may also demonstrate such signs (Box 9-13).

TABLE 9-4 ASSESSING CRANIAL NERVES*

CRANIAL NERVE	PROCEDURE
I (olfactory nerve)	The child is asked to identify familiar odors with the eyes closed. Each side of the nose is tested separately.
II (optic nerve)	Visual acuity is tested using the Snellen chart, the HOTV chart for young children, or the tumbling E chart for very young children. Each eye is tested separately and then both eyes together. If corrective lenses are worn, the eyes are tested both with and without correction.
III, IV, VI (oculomotor, trochlear, abducent nerve)	The child is asked to follow a toy or the examiner's finger as the object moves in all directions of gaze (six cardinal fields of gaze).
V (trigeminal nerve)	The child is asked to identify a wisp of cotton on the face. Corneal reflex is tested by observing for blinking when the examiner approaches the face closely. The masseter and temporal muscles' strength can be evaluated by having the child bite down on a tongue blade as the examiner tries to remove it.
VII (facial nerve)	The child is asked to imitate the examiner's frown, wrinkled forehead, smile, and raised eyebrow. The child tries to keep the eyes closed while the examiner attempts to open them, to test the strength of the eyelid muscles. The sensory portion of the facial nerve can be evaluated by having the child identify the taste of sugar and salt placed on the anterior part of the tongue on each side.
VIII (acoustic nerve)	Cochlear nerve tests assess hearing. Audiometric testing is a quantitative evaluation of hearing. The Weber (lateralization) and Rinne (air and bone conduction) tests are qualitative evaluations of hearing.
IX, X (glossopharyngeal nerve, vagus nerve)	The glossopharyngeal and vagus nerves are tested together. With a tongue depressor, the gag reflex is tested by touching the posterior pharyngeal wall. The palatal reflex is tested by stroking each side of the mucous membrane of the uvula. The side touched should rise. Normal function of the vagus nerve is revealed by the child's ability to swallow and to speak clearly.
XI (accessory nerve)	The examiner palpates and notes the strength of the trapezius and sternocleidomastoid muscles against resistance, or the child shrugs the shoulders against resistance.
XII (hypoglossal nerve)	The child is asked to stick out the tongue, and the examiner notes any lateral deviation when it is protruded. The strength of the tongue is assessed by having the child push the tongue against the examiner's finger pressed against the cheek.

*Cranial nerves are tested when the system in which they occur is assessed.

BOX 9-12 TESTS FOR EVALUATING SENSORY FUNCTION

Primary Forms of Sensation
Check in sequence the hands, forearms, upper arms, trunk, thighs, lower legs, and feet for the following:

Superficial tactile sensation: Touch the child with a wisp of cotton.

Superficial pain: Touch the child with a pin or other sharp object. Be careful not to injure or frighten the child.

Sensitivity to temperature: Touch the various parts of the child's body with test tubes containing warm and cold water. This test is infrequently done with children because of the difficulty of keeping water warm or cold enough for the child to distinguish the difference.

Sensitivity to vibration: Hold a vibrating tuning fork to the bony prominences, noting the child's ability to perceive the vibration and tell you when the vibration stops.

Deep pressure pain: Press the tip of your fingernail against the child's fingernail. The child will feel discomfort. You may also squeeze the Achilles tendon, calf, and forearm muscles, noting sensitivity.

Motion and position: Hold the sides of the toes, thumbs, and fingers by grasping them between your index finger and thumb. Move the fingers and toes passively and ask the child to tell you the final position of the digit.

Cortical and Discriminatory Forms of Sensation
These forms of sensation are complex somatic sensory impressions that require interpretation by the cerebral cortex.

The following sensations can be evaluated, depending on the age and development of the child being tested:

Two-point discrimination: Can the child differentiate between one and two points? With the child's eyes closed, various parts of the body are touched simultaneously with two sharp objects. Then alternate touching the child with one point or two points is done. Different areas of the body vary in the distance by which the child can differentiate one from two points. This test is more appropriate for older children.

Point localization: With the eyes closed, can the child locate the spot where the child was touched?

Texture discrimination: Can the child recognize with the hands the difference in the feel of materials such as cotton, wool, and silk?

Stereognostic function: Can the child identify familiar objects placed in each hand? Place several objects in a paper bag, and have the child identify them with each hand and show you the object.

Graphesthesia: Can the child identify letters or numbers traced on the palm or back of the hand with a blunt point? Numbers are easier than letters for a young child to recognize.

Extinction phenomenon: With the eyes closed, can the child identify touch on both sides? Touch opposite sides of the body in identical areas simultaneously. This test is used for older children only.

BOX 9-13 EXAMPLES OF NEUROLOGIC "SOFT" SIGNS

- Short attention span
- Poor motor coordination
- Clumsiness
- Frequent falling
- Hyperkinesis, voluntary or involuntary
- Uneven perceptual development

- Incomplete laterality, with no side clearly dominant
- Language disturbances: articulation disorders, dyslexia
- Motor outflow (movements involving more muscles than intended)
- Mirroring movements of the extremities (e.g., both hands in motion when only one is performing a function)

TABLE 9-5   EVALUATING COMMON REFLEXES

REFLEX	EVALUATION
Deep tendon reflexes	Evaluation elicited by tapping briskly on a tendon or a bony prominence, evoking a sudden stretching of certain muscles and their resulting contraction. For an adequate response, the limb should be relaxed and the muscle partially stretched. The reflex is stimulated by directing a sharp blow of the reflex hammer onto the muscle's insertion tendon.
Biceps reflex 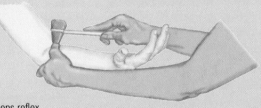	The child's arm should be flexed up to 45 degrees at the elbow. The biceps tendon in the antecubital fossa is palpated. The thumb is then placed on the biceps tendon, and a blow is struck on the thumb. The response is a visible or palpable flexion of the forearm.
Triceps reflex 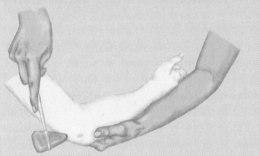	The arm is suspended by holding the upper arm and instructing the child to just let the arm "go limp." Alternatively, the forearm can be supported on the examiner's arm. The triceps tendon is struck directly just above the elbow. The response is extension of the forearm.
Brachioradialis reflex 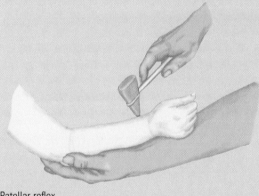	The child's arm is supported on the examiner's arm, and the elbow is flexed up to 45 degrees. The brachioradial tendon is struck with the reflex hammer 2.5 to 5 cm (1 to 2 in) above the radial styloid process. The response is pronation and flexion of the elbow.
Patellar reflex 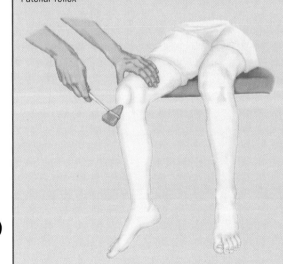	The lower leg is allowed to dangle freely by flexing the child's knee up to 90 degrees. The examiner supports the upper leg with the hand and strikes the patellar tendon just below the patella. The response is extension of the lower leg.

Continued

TABLE 9-5   EVALUATING COMMON REFLEXES—cont'd

REFLEX	EVALUATION
Achilles reflex 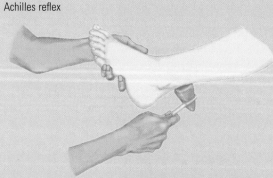	The hip is externally rotated, and the foot is held in dorsiflexion. The Achilles tendon is struck directly. The response is plantar flexion of the foot. An alternative way to elicit this reflex is to have the child kneel on a chair with the toes pointing toward the floor; the examiner then strikes the Achilles tendon directly.
Clonus reflex	Eliciting a *clonus*—a continued, rapid flexion and extension of the foot and hand—is attempted in children. Clonus is elicited by suddenly and briskly dorsiflexing the foot or hand and applying sustained and moderate pressure. No rhythmic oscillating movements should be palpated.
Superficial reflexes	Tested by stroking the skin with an object that is moderately sharp but not sharp enough to break the skin. The receptors are in the skin rather than the muscles.
Upper and lower abdominal reflexes and cremasteric reflex 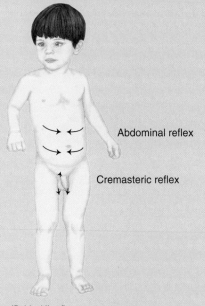 Abdominal reflex Cremasteric reflex	*Upper and lower abdominal reflexes:* While the child is in a supine position and with the abdomen exposed and knees slightly bent, the skin of the abdomen is stroked. Movement of stroking is from the side of the abdomen toward the midline at both the upper and lower abdominal levels. The response is ipsilateral contraction of the abdominal muscle with an observable movement of the umbilicus toward the side being stroked. *Cremasteric reflex:* In the male, light stroking of the inner aspect of the thigh causes the ipsilateral testicle to elevate. This reflex may cause withdrawal of the testicles into the inguinal canal when the abdomen is touched with very cold hands.
Plantar (Babinski) reflex 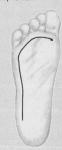	The lateral aspect of the sole of the foot, from the heel to the ball of the foot, is stroked in a movement curving medially across the ball. A fingernail or the wooden end of an applicator stick may be used. The response in an infant is dorsiflexion, fanning of the toes, and hyperextension of the great toe. Once a child is walking, the response is plantar flexion of the toes. Some children withdraw from this stimulus by flexing the hip and the knee.
Gluteal reflex	When the buttocks are separated, the skin tenses at the gluteal area.

CONCLUSION AND DOCUMENTATION

When the physical examination has been completed, the examiner should ask the parents and child, if age appropriate, whether they have any questions concerning the examination. Findings are documented in a complete and concise manner. Deviations from normal and risk factors should be identified and documented. Depending on the setting, referrals may be made.

KEY CONCEPTS

- Systematic physical examination is tailored to the child's developmental level, includes all body systems, and generally proceeds from head to toe.
- Developmentally appropriate assessment of children requires flexibility and creativity in the examiner.
- Collection of accurate subjective and objective data is foundational to identifying nursing needs of children.
- Vital signs should be assessed during each visit in ambulatory care settings and monitored on a regular basis in the hospitalized child.
- Assessment of vital signs is an important way to measure and monitor vital body functions.
- Examination findings are recorded completely and concisely. Deviations from normal and risk factors are identified, documented and, when appropriate, reported for further evaluation.
- Serial recordings of growth, development, anthropometrics, and nutritional status provide important clues to a child's health status.
- The skin is inspected and palpated to determine color, moisture, temperature, turgor, edema, and lesions.
- A child's general appearance is observed for signs of abuse, both physical and psychological.
- Lymph nodes are palpated as part of the examination of different anatomical areas of the body.
- The head is inspected for symmetry, movement, control, and shape.
- The fontanels are inspected and palpated for size, tenseness, and pulsation.

- The eyelids, eyebrows, palpebral fissures, nasolabial folds, mouth, and nose are inspected for spacing and symmetry.
- The nasal mucosa is inspected for color and moisture.
- Assessment of the mouth in a young child is performed at the end of the examination as it may cause anxiety.
- Selection of an eye chart to assess visual acuity is based on the child's age and developmental level; it must be reliable and valid.
- Assessment of the thorax and lungs entails inspection, palpation, percussion, and auscultation.
- The heart is auscultated with use of both the bell and diaphragm of the stethoscope, with the child in the supine, left lateral recumbent, and sitting upright positions.
- An empty bladder, a warm room, and a supine position with a pillow under the head and knees flexed will enhance abdominal relaxation.
- Examination of the genitalia may evoke concerns for some children. A matter-of-fact approach and clear communication of what will occur will help create a positive experience.
- The musculoskeletal examination is directed predominantly toward the upper and lower extremities and the spinal column.
- The neurologic examination is done to identify any nervous system malfunction and to evaluate current nervous system development and functioning.
- When the physical examination has been completed, the examiner should ask the child and parents whether they have any questions concerning the examination.

REFERENCES

American Academy of Ophthalmology. (2007, March). Policy statement: Eye examination in infants, children, and young adults by pediatricians. *One Network: The Ophthalmic News and Education Network.* Retrieved from www.one.aao.org/CE/PracticeGuidelines/Clinical Statements_Content.aspx?cid=e57de45b-2c03-4fbd-9c83-02374a6c09e0.

American Academy of Pediatrics (AAP), National High Blood Pressure Education Program Working Group on High Blood Pressure in Children and Adolescents. (2004). The fourth report on the diagnosis, evaluation, and treatment of high blood pressure in children and adolescents. *Pediatrics, 114*(2), 555-576.

American Pain Society. (n.d.). *Pain: Current understanding of assessment, management, and treatments.* Retrieved from www.ampainsoc.org/ce/enduring/downloads/npc/npc.pdf.

Centers for Disease Control and Prevention (CDC). (2010). *Growth charts.* Retrieved from www.cdc.gov/growth charts.

Devrim, I., Kara, A., Ceyhan, M., et al. (2007). Measurement accuracy of fever by tympanic and axillary thermometry. *Pediatric Emergency Care, 23*(1), 16-19.

Exergen Corporation. (2005). Exergen *Temporal artery: Instructions for use.* Retrieved from www.exergen.com/medical/PDFs/tat2000instrev6.pdf.

Feld, L. G. & Corey, H. (2007). Hypertension in childhood. *Pediatrics in Review,* (28), 283-298.

Grummer-Strawn, L., Reinold, C., & Krebs, N. (2010). Use of world health organization and CDC growth charts for children aged 0-59 months in the United States. *MMWR Morbidity and Mortality Weekly Report, 59*(RR-9), 1-15.

Hartmann, E. E., Bradford, G., Nottingham Chaplin, P. K., et al. (2006). Project Universal Preschool vision screening: A demonstration project [electronic version]. *Pediatrics, 117*(2), e226-e237.

Holzhauer, J., Reith, V., Sawin, K. J. & Yen, K. (2009). Evaluation of temporal artery thermometry in children 3-36 months old. *Journal for Specialists in Pediatric Nursing, 14*(4), 239-244.

Jarvis, C. (2008). *Physical examination and health assessment* (4th ed.). St. Louis: Elsevier.

Lee, R. & Johnston, M. (2010). Clinical summary: Cerebral palsy. *Neurology MedLink.* Retrieved from www.medlink.com/medlinkcontent.asp.

Morelli, J. (2011). Acanthosis nigricans. In R. Kliegman, B. Stanton, J. St. Geme, et al. (Eds.). *Nelson textbook of pediatrics* (19th ed., pp. 2266-2267). Philadelphia: Elsevier.

National Eye Institute, Ocular Epidemiology Strategic Planning Panel. (2007). *Epidemiological research: From populations through interventions to translation.* Retrieved from www.nei.nih.gov/strategicplanning/finalreport.asp#pediatric.

Roosevelt, G. (2011). Infectious upper airway obstruction. In R. Kliegman, B. Stanton, J. St. Geme, et al. (Eds.). *Nelson textbook of pediatrics* (19th ed., pp. 1445-1449). Philadelphia: Elsevier Saunders.

Seidel, H. B., Ball, J., Dains, J., et al. (2010). *Mosby's guide to physical examination* (7th ed.). St. Louis: Elsevier Mosby.

The Joint Commission. (2010). *Approaches to pain management: An essential guide for clinical leaders* (2nd ed.). Oakbrook Terrace, IL: Joint Commission Resources, Inc.

Tower, R., & Camitta, B. (2011). Lymphadenopathy. In R. Kliegman, B. Stanton, J. St. Geme, N. Schor, & R. Behrman (Eds.). *Nelson textbook of pediatrics* (19th ed., p. 1724). Philadelphia: Elsevier Saunders.

U.S. Preventive Services Task Force. (2004a). *Screening for idiopathic scoliosis in adolescents.* Retrieved from www.uspreventiveservicestaskforce.org/uspstf/uspsaisc.htm.

U.S. Preventive Services Task Force. (2004b). *Screening for visual impairment in children younger than age 5 years: Recommendation statement.* Retrieved from www.uspreventiveservicestaskforce.org/3rduspstf/visionscr/vischrs.htm.

Emergency Care of the Child

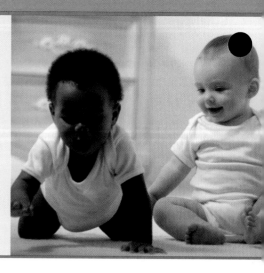

evolve WEBSITE

http://evolve.elsevier.com/James/ncoc

LEARNING OBJECTIVES

After studying this chapter, you should be able to:

- Describe general principles that encourage cooperation and help make examination and treatment of children in emergency settings more comfortable for the child and family.
- List significant developmental issues when caring for infants, toddlers, preschool and school-age children, and adolescents in emergency care settings.
- Compare the child's airway anatomy with that of an adult and explain the significance of the differences in managing the pediatric airway.
- Assess the early signs of shock in infants and children, recognizing that changes in heart rate and skin signs are more accurate signs of early shock than is decreased blood pressure.

- Define *triage* and list the most important factors to assess when obtaining an overall ("across the room") impression of an infant's or a child's condition.
- Describe the general guidelines for cardiopulmonary resuscitation in infants and children and discuss what additional precautions and procedures are required for infants and children with traumatic injuries.
- List indications that suggest a child brought into the emergency care setting has been neglected or abused, and discuss the nurse's responsibility for reporting possible neglect or abuse.
- Identify several possible roles for nurses in preventing traumatic injuries, poison ingestion, and environmental injuries.

CLINICAL REFERENCE

GENERAL GUIDELINES FOR EMERGENCY NURSING CARE

Many factors affect the psychological impact of an emergency on both the child and family. In addition to the expected fears children have at various developmental stages (e.g., separation, pain, altered body image); an overriding concern expressed by both children and parents in emergency care settings is fear of the unknown. The suddenness with which the child and family come in contact with emergency personnel, the necessity for rapid assessment and intervention, and the relative seriousness of the child's condition can intensify a fearful response and overwhelm normal coping mechanisms. In addition, children and families are unfamiliar with the setting, the staff of the health care facility, the equipment, and the procedures. Emergency nurses can use some simple interventions to make examination and

treatment of children in the emergency setting more comfortable for the child and for the family and to decrease the adverse psychological effects of the experience.

Communicate an attitude of calm confidence. This attitude can be difficult to maintain when the situation is critical, but families in crisis look to nurses for reassurance and expect to see competent, professional behavior. Speak quietly and calmly to the child and parents, and remain firmly in charge. Remember to talk to the family often throughout the visit; silence is a form of communication that is easily misinterpreted. Create a communication plan with the parent or family that specifies when they should be called if they are away from the department and that lists numbers where they can be reached (Mullen & Pate, 2006). Acknowledge and address the child's and family's fears. Poor communication is the cause of 35% to 70% of medicolegal actions, including failure to update the family on the plan of care and failure to understand and incorporate patient and family perspectives in the plan of care (Levetown, 2008).

Establish a trusting relationship with the child and family. Make eye contact with the child and family when you speak to them. Call the child by name to personalize care. Treat the child and family kindly and gently. To establish a trusting relationship, check back with the family and provide periodic updates if the child and family are separated. When parents are confident that they are being kept informed, they are less likely to make demands for additional attention and information. When speaking to the child and family, use simple, nonmedical terms and remember that children (and sometimes adults) can have inaccurate ideas of how their bodies function and the location of body parts. Providing comfort measures to the family members also builds a trusting relationship. It is important to protect their privacy, direct them to a public telephone or cafeteria, and provide space where they can talk quietly.

Encourage caregivers to stay with the child. Family-centered care recognizes the partnership between health care workers and family in ensuring the well being of the child. Nursing care is driven by the needs of the family and child rather than controlled by health care providers. According to comfort levels and ability, include the parents as partners in their child's treatment. Unless the child does not want a parent in the room (e.g., some adolescents), a parent can help calm the child, and many examinations and procedures can be performed with the child on a parent's lap. Although having the family remain with the child can be calming and supportive, respect the family's right to leave if the child's condition or the painful nature of a procedure provokes more anxiety than the family member is able to handle.

For parents who do not know exactly how to be of assistance in these situations, it can help to explain how a parent might help, such as "I think he might stay calmer if you hold his hand and tell him a story while I clean this burn" or "Try counting to 10 with her while I start this intravenous line."

Whenever possible, designate one staff member as the child's caretaker and liaison to the parents. In the unfamiliar emergency setting, the child and family find that having one contact person is less confusing. Consistency is helpful in a crisis because the child and family may feel overwhelmed in the busy and sometimes confusing emergency department environment.

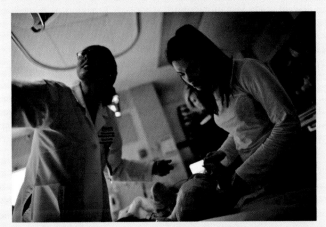

Encouraging parents to remain with their child in the emergency setting can bolster the family's coping. (Courtesy Children's Medical Center, Dallas, TX.)

Tell the truth. To establish a trusting relationship, be as honest as possible. If a procedure will be painful, tell the child (usually briefly beforehand). Only then can the child believe health care providers when they say that a procedure will *not* be painful. When a painful procedure is completed, tell the child you are finished and there will be no more pain. Keeping a child informed of what will occur by describing sensations (e.g., "This will feel cold and wet as I clean your arm.") is more helpful than describing the actual procedure.

Provide incentives and rewards. Provide positive feedback when either the child or the parents are being helpful. Children from 3 to 12 years of age especially appreciate verbal praise and concrete rewards for good behavior, such as stickers, fancy bandages, or inexpensive toys (Hawkins, 2004). Adults also appreciate being thanked for their patience and for their assistance in their child's care. All these techniques help create as positive an experience as possible.

Assess the child's unspoken thoughts and feelings. Try to determine what the child is thinking or feeling but not verbalizing. Encourage the child to express thoughts and feelings; sometimes the child might be misinterpreting a situation or need to express emotions.

PEDIATRIC EMERGENCY EQUIPMENT

Airways
  Oropharyngeal airway: sizes 4-10 cm
  Nasopharyngeal: sizes 12-36 Fr
  Laryngeal mask airway
Endotracheal tubes: ID in mm
  Cuffed: infant = 3; 1-2 yr = 3.5; over 2 yr = 3.5+(age/4)
  Uncuffed ID: infant = 3.5; 1-2 yr = 4; over 2 yr = 4+(age/4)
Laryngoscope with blades
  Straight: sizes #0-3
  Curved: sizes #2-3
Magill forceps
Oxygen equipment: infant, pediatric, and adult masks and cannulas
Bag-mask ventilation device: infant, pediatric, and adult sizes
Chest tubes: sizes 8-30 Fr
Flexible suction catheters: sizes 5-14 Fr (tracheal)
Yankauer suction tip (oropharyngeal)
Pediatric peripheral IV equipment and solutions (cannulas: 18-24 gauge)
Intraosseous device: 15-18 gauge
Nasogastric tubes: sizes 5-18 Fr
Urinary catheters: sizes 5-12 Fr
Length-based resuscitation tape (Broselow)
Defibrillator with adult and pediatric paddles
ECG monitors with pediatric-size electrodes and sensors
Pulse oximeter
Capnometer to measure exhaled CO_2
Heating source
  Fluid warmer
  Infrared lamp
  Overhead warmer

Data from Kleinman, M.E., Chameides, L., Schexnayder, S.M., et al. (2010). Part 14: Pediatric advanced life support: 2010 American Heart Association guidelines for cardiopulmonary resuscitation and emergency cardiovascular care. *Circulation, 122*(suppl 3), S876-S908; and Susil, G. (2009). Emergency management. In J. Custer & R. Rau (Eds.), *The Harriet Lane handbook* (18th ed., pp. 3-17). St. Louis: Elsevier Mosby.

CLINICAL REFERENCE

PEDIATRIC EMERGENCY MEDICATIONS

MEDICATION	USE
Adenosine	Treats supraventricular tachycardia
Amiodarone	Treats pulseless arrest, supraventricular and ventricular tachycardia
Atropine sulfate	Treats symptomatic bradycardia and toxins/overdose (i.e., organophosphates)
Calcium chloride 10%	Treats hypocalcemia, hypermagnesemia, hyperkalemia, and calcium channel blocker overdose
Dextrose (25%, 50%)	Treats hypoglycemia, a common complication of dehydration, sepsis, and resuscitation
Inotropic agents	Treat hypotension or hypoperfusion, severe congestive heart failure, or cardiovascular shock
Epinephrine (1:1000 [endotracheal], 1:10,000 [intravenous/intraosseous])	Treats bradycardia or pulseless arrest, hypotensive shock, anaphylaxis, toxins/overdose (i.e., beta blockers, calcium channel blockers)
Lidocaine	Treats pulseless ventricular tachycardia, ventricular fibrillation, or wide complex tachycardia (with pulses)
Magnesium sulfate	Treats torsades de pointes arrhythmia, hypomagnesemia, or severe asthma
Naloxone hydrochloride	Reverses effects of opiate narcotics
Sodium bicarbonate (4.2%)	Treats severe metabolic acidosis, hyperkalemia, and sodium channel blocker overdose

Data from Kleinman, M.E., Chameides, L., Schexnayder, S.M., et al. (2010). Part 14: Pediatric advanced life support: 2010 American Heart Association guidelines for cardiopulmonary resuscitation and emergency cardiovascular care. *Circulation, 122*(suppl 3), S876-S908.

In some cases, however, the child's and family's coping mechanisms break down, causing inappropriate behavior. If violence or abusive behavior is an issue, you might need to obtain assistance from law enforcement or hospital security officers. For an emotional crisis that does not involve abusive or aggressive behavior, the following simple rules apply:

- Encourage the person in crisis to move to a quiet place. Observers and stimuli from other sources tend to aggravate a crisis.
- Encourage the child or parent to talk about feelings, as well as the "facts" of the situation. Use reflective statements.
- Avoid defensiveness, explanation, or justification of your own or others' behavior.
- Speak in simple sentences. Use sentences of no more than five words, with words no longer than five letters (e.g., "Let's sit down over here," "Let me help," "Please let go of that").

- Set limits. Avoid "yes" or "no" responses. Rather than saying, "Will you take this medicine?" (the small child will probably say "NO!"), ask "Would you rather take the pink or the yellow medicine first?"

When interacting with families in distress, a good general rule is to try to listen rather than talk. Simply being present for children and families and empathizing with them are useful interventions. Help families identify specific problems and their effective coping mechanisms and assist them to explore reasonable solutions.

When coping mechanisms break down entirely, however, some direction is necessary. Consulting social services, spiritual counselors (e.g., chaplain), or crisis intervention professionals can be helpful. Early intervention and support for appropriate coping mechanisms are far easier and less time consuming than intervening after a child's or parent's emotional decompensation.

Very few experiences are as frightening to a family as a child's sudden illness or injury. Caring for children and families in the emergency setting therefore presents special challenges to the health care team. Nurses play an important role in emergency settings because they are most often responsible for the initial contact, *triage,* and continuing care throughout an emergency visit. The goals of emergency nursing care include addressing the child's physical problems, supporting the child's and family's coping mechanisms, and creating an atmosphere in which the family is valued and kept as intact as possible.

GROWTH AND DEVELOPMENT ISSUES IN EMERGENCY CARE

Emergency nursing care of children needs to address both the physiologic and psychological differences in children in terms of age and development. Paying close attention to developmental issues assists in obtaining a more accurate assessment and can affect the course of care (see Chapters 5 through 8 for approaches to children of different ages). The nurse treats each child as an individual and avoids becoming judgmental when a child regresses to a "safer" developmental level.

Although children of the same age-group are similar, past experiences, cultural differences, and maturity levels may result in a range of behaviors. One toddler might be much more mature than another, and one adolescent might lean more toward school-age behaviors than another (Box 10-1).

The Infant

An infant experiences the world through the senses; hunger, satiation, cold, warmth, quiet, and noise affect the infant's comfort or discomfort. An infant has not learned patience and has little tolerance for physical or emotional discomfort, including pain (see Chapter 15 for management of pain in infants and children). Crying can be stressful for caregivers; pacifiers are an adequate self-comforting measure when analgesia is not indicated. Stress can cause increased metabolic demands in the infant so offer rest periods during procedures to maintain normothermia.

Although infants are able to discriminate their parents from others, older infants (9 to 18 months of age, or earlier in some infants) can exhibit signs of both separation and stranger anxiety. The nurse should allow the parent to hold the infant as much as possible for examination and treatment. This may not be possible in a critical

BOX 10-1   WORKING WITH CHILDREN IN EMERGENCIES: DEVELOPMENTAL GUIDELINES

Infants
- Allow the use of a pacifier.
- Use a quiet, soothing voice.
- Touch, rock, or cuddle the infant. Holding the infant securely or swaddling a young infant can also be comforting.
- Keep the infant warm; if the infant must be left undressed, use warming lights to ensure a comfortable temperature.
- As much as possible, allay parents' fears so they will not be communicated to the infant.
- Remember that infants feel pain (see Chapter 15 for pain interventions).

Toddlers
- Give treatments and perform procedures with the toddler sitting up on the stretcher or examining table or on the parent's lap.
- Perform the most distressing or intrusive parts of the examination last.
- Reassure family members as much as possible; the child will benefit from their confidence.
- Allow the child to have familiar objects (transitional objects) such as a blanket, doll, or toy to help feel safe.
- Keep frightening objects out of the child's line of vision. Also try to keep machines that make loud noises away.
- Praise (e.g., "You are being so brave") and distraction (e.g., bubbles, puzzles) will decrease anxiety and increase cooperation.

Preschoolers
- Explain a procedure or treatment a few seconds rather than minutes beforehand, because allowing the young child time to think about it may result in frightening fantasies or exaggerations.
- Talk to preschool children throughout procedures, describing the sensations they are feeling or will feel and telling them how they can help.
- Distract the child with noises or bright objects. Counting with some preschool children might help calm them during procedures.
- Avoid criticizing the preschool child for crying, struggling, or fighting during a procedure.
- Reassuring a child that the child did try his or her best to cooperate will help to build a positive self-image.
- Encourage the preschool child to talk about how the illness or injury occurred. If the child is inappropriately taking responsibility for the illness or injury, try to reassure that the child is not to blame for the situation.

- Remember that preschool children can seem to understand more than they actually do. Health care providers often overestimate understanding in a child of this age, so be sure to explain things in words the child understands.
- Use positive terms, such as "make better" and "help," and avoid more frightening terms, such as "shot" and "cut."
- Use adhesive bandages over small wounds and injection sites. Preschool children might imagine their blood leaking out through puncture wounds.

School-Age Children
- Offer simple choices whenever possible to help the child feel more in control. The school-age child is capable of deciding in which arm to have an injection or in which hand to hold a nebulizer. Talk directly to the child, explaining procedures in simple terms. When explaining treatments or care options to the parent, include the child.
- Ask the child about the level of understanding and allow time for questions.
- Address the child's fears or concerns directly rather than treating them as foolish or inconsequential.
- Give rewards, such as a sticker or an inexpensive toy, after a procedure regardless of the child's behavior. Think of this gesture as a reward for undergoing the procedure, not as a judgment of "good" or "bad" behavior.

Adolescents
- Preserve the adolescent's modesty; offer adolescents a choice regarding whether they want their parents present when obtaining history and during the examination.
- Consider the legal issues regarding the right to privacy for pregnant adolescents and adolescents with sexually transmissible diseases.
- Provide an opportunity for questions.
- Listen to the adolescent's concerns nonjudgmentally and without belittling the young person.
- Developing a teasing relationship with an adolescent is often a temptation, but this has potential for harm; the adolescent is easily embarrassed.
- Explain procedures or treatments carefully and allow choices. Adolescents are capable of complex abstract thinking and can make intelligent and reasoned decisions about their own care.

---

situation, but nurses need to remember to reunite parent and child whenever feasible.

The Toddler

Toddlers are just beginning to explore the world and seem to have limitless energy and curiosity. They are also beginning to have a clearer image of themselves as autonomous and distinct beings. For this reason, they do not respond well to restrictions and tend to push any limits imposed. This tendency can be a problem in the emergency setting because some nursing care might involve securing and restraining the toddler, which makes the toddler feel vulnerable. The nurse should be sure to remove any restriction or restraint as soon as safety permits. Toddlers have little understanding of time, so procedures should be introduced just before they are initiated.

The Preschooler

The preschool child is talking and beginning to be more independent. This outward appearance of organization is somewhat misleading, however, because the preschool period is also the stage of fear and

fantasy. Because of their imaginative nature, preschoolers need little time lag between the explanation of a procedure and its completion. Additionally, avoid using terms such as "stick" or "cut" to prevent literal misinterpretations of meanings. Preschoolers are strong believers in cause-and-effect relations and tend to blame themselves for illnesses and injuries.

The preschool child may be more willing than the toddler to be separated from parents, but the nurse should keep this separation as brief as possible. The nurse can include the parents in treatments and provide them with instructions on calming the child if they seem unsure. The nurse should not ask a parent to restrain the child because this role may be confusing to the child and difficult for the parent.

The School-Age Child

School-age children are interested in learning and gradually acquire reasoning skills, including some abstract thinking. They are able to understand the cause of illness and injury and are much less likely to fantasize and exaggerate. School-age children have extensive vocabularies, and they can understand simple explanations of procedures.

They are also able to make decisions about their own care. By this time, they have developed personal techniques to help them through painful times. The nurse helps them use coping techniques that work for them. Because risk-taking behaviors may begin during this age, caregivers must stress the importance of injury prevention behaviors.

The Adolescent

Although adolescents are at varying stages of puberty, they begin to resemble adults in appearance. They are also beginning to explore the adult world and develop their own unique identities. The nurse needs to remember, however, that even though adolescents may appear physically mature, they might not be emotionally mature and they continue to require support. Coping with extraordinary changes in their physical appearance, they are often concerned with whether they are "normal" and whether others have similar thoughts and feelings.

Although this is an age of risk taking, which can make them prone to serious injury, adolescents can be quite fearful of death. Although they are aware of the possibility of their own death, they avoid thinking about its reality. Adolescents consider themselves invincible and many experience overwhelming emotions when a friend dies unexpectedly.

Adolescence is an age of extremes—teenagers might either exaggerate or underplay the seriousness of a condition. Sometimes assessing the full extent of an adolescent's illness or injury is difficult. Expert care of the adolescent requires sensitivity to both verbal and nonverbal cues. Adolescents' privacy should be respected; nurses should approach them as one would an adult, giving them full attention and respect for their thoughts and feelings.

THE FAMILY OF A CHILD IN EMERGENCY CARE

Stress on the family results directly and indirectly from the child's illness or injury. The way a child perceives an illness or injury often is related to the parents' attitude, so caring for the child requires assessment of and intervention with the family.

The most common emotions experienced by parents of children cared for in emergencies are fear and anxiety. Past experiences may lessen or increase these emotions. Parents are afraid of the following possibilities.

- *Their child might die.* This fear is the greatest source of anxiety and can be present even when death is highly unlikely, such as in the case of minor illnesses or injuries. This anxiety is often the underlying cause of parents' anger toward health care providers.
- *Their child might experience pain.* As a rule, parents try very hard to protect children from pain. Even when pain is necessary, it is difficult for parents to understand and accept.
- *The child's body may be permanently altered.* Parents often fear that their children will have permanent scars or body changes.

Parental guilt is another frequently seen emotion. Parents can feel guilty for the following reasons:

- They feel responsible for their child's illness or injury.
- They are submitting their child to a painful experience.
- They do not have enough knowledge to make educated decisions about their child's care.

In addition, parents may have had negative experiences with health care providers in the past or have other concerns about siblings, financial arrangements, and work schedules.

The particular causes of stress for families in emergencies are unique to the circumstances and to the family involved. The nurse needs to define the family (e.g., single parent, two parents, grandparent, other caregiver) and who are the decision makers (e.g., family members, religious leaders) and communicate accordingly. All the

stressors combined could stretch parents' coping mechanisms to the limit and result in anger, withdrawal, or tearfulness. Stress also can manifest itself in hyperactivity—making numerous phone calls, repeating questions, and involving a large number of people.

Including family members in their child's care can reduce feelings of helplessness and promote positive coping mechanisms. Nurses should facilitate family presence during procedures and encourage them to support their child. Although it is not appropriate to solicit family members to help hold or restrain a child for a procedure, they can offer emotional support. Early assessment and appropriate support before problems occur are advantageous for both health care workers and the family.

EMERGENCY ASSESSMENT OF INFANTS AND CHILDREN

In the emergency setting, assessment of the ill or injured child must be rapid and accurate to identify abnormal findings quickly. In children, initial evidence of life-threatening conditions can be subtle, with few signs of impending respiratory or cardiopulmonary arrest. Making as many initial observations as possible without touching the child is extremely important so that assessments can reflect the child's baseline, or resting condition. For an apparently stable infant or young child, most of the examination required for general triage can be performed with the child on the parent's lap. The nurse also observes the relationship between the parents and child during the examination process.

The triage nurse usually performs the initial observation in the emergency setting and decides the level of care needed for the child. Triaging is an important skill that improves with experience. The nurse bases much of the initial assessment on an overall sense of how the child looks—sick or well (an "across the room" assessment). Because children do not try to cover up either how they feel or how they look, the nurse immediately receives a fairly accurate impression of illness or wellness.

Three essential factors combine to form a first impression: respiratory rate and effort, skin color, and response to the environment. Abnormalities are compared with the parent's or caregiver's perception ("Is this his normal color?"). If results of this assessment appear to be normal, the nurse completes a more thorough and in-depth evaluation. If the general impression is that the child is seriously ill, the nurse must intervene immediately and combine any additional evaluation with interventions.

Primary Assessment

Primary assessment, which is part of the initial triage assessment, consists of assessing the ABCDEs—*a*irway, *b*reathing, *c*irculation, level of consciousness (*d*isability), and *e*xposure. Because the two most common pathways to death in children are respiratory failure and shock, interventions include providing respiratory and circulatory support. When head, neck, or back trauma is suspected, cervical spine protection should be initiated by maintaining the spine in a neutral position. Cervical and spinal cord injury can be difficult to detect without radiologic intervention in children who cannot effectively verbalize their pain or symptoms.

Airway Assessment

Although determining the cause of respiratory distress or failure in an ill child ultimately will be important, more important is recognizing symptoms and signs of respiratory distress. In the emergency setting, initial treatment is the same regardless of the cause. Remember that apparent respiratory distress can originate from causes such as rib fractures and metabolic acidosis.

Initial Observations for Triage

Respiratory rate and effort: Is the child's breathing rapid or shallow, or is the child using accessory muscles? What is the child's position of comfort? When children are having difficulty breathing, they use accessory muscles to help. Substernal, intercostal, or subclavicular retractions are all signs of serious breathing difficulties. Nasal flaring, head bobbing, grunting, stridor, upright position, and prolonged expirations signal increased work of breathing. A slow respiratory rate is of great concern; a child who seems to be breathing at a rate normal for an adult is almost certainly hypoventilating. This respiratory rate can signal imminent respiratory arrest. Observe for abnormal breath sounds, and assess oxygen saturation by pulse oximeter.

Skin color: Is the child's skin pale, mottled, or cyanotic? Abnormal skin color could result from the two greatest threats to a child's life: respiratory distress or failure, and inadequate tissue perfusion (shock).

Response to the environment: Is the child alert, interactive, crying, sleepy, or limp? Is the child smiling and able to play? Does the child make eye contact and interact appropriately? Although response to the environment is more difficult to evaluate in the preverbal child, responsiveness is an important component of the assessment. A well child should look around, fixate on objects, and appear to recognize caretakers. An anxious-appearing child may be in respiratory distress; a flaccid, disinterested child may be in respiratory failure or frank shock.

Because of some differences in airway anatomy and physiology, children are at greater risk of airway problems than are adults (Table 10-1). When assessing children's airways, the nurse pays particular attention to breath sounds (often audible to the naked ear) as well as snoring, stridor, wheezing, and grunting. Snoring is caused by obstruction in the upper airway (often the tongue relaxing against the posterior pharynx) and can be heard in a child with decreased mental status. Stridor is a high-pitched sound heard on inspiration (laryngeal obstruction) or on both inspiration and expiration (midtracheal obstruction). Wheezing, a high-pitched, musical sound heard primarily on expiration, signals obstruction of the lower airway. Crackles or rales are fine, popping noises heard on inspiration; they usually indicate fluid in the lungs, such as in pneumonia.

Breathing Assessment

Level of consciousness, rate and depth of breathing, breath sounds, and the child's respiratory effort are indicative of relative oxygenation. Anxiety or decreased responsiveness may denote hypoxia. A rapid respiratory rate with shallow breathing indicates respiratory distress. Very slow breathing in an ill child is an ominous sign, indicating respiratory failure. A slowly breathing child might no longer have the energy for adequate ventilation. Increased work of breathing with quiet breath sounds may indicate an absence of air entry into lung fields. Abdominal breathing is normal in the infant or young child, so the nurse observes the rise and fall of the abdomen instead of the chest.

The use of accessory muscles for breathing invariably indicates respiratory distress. The child's chest wall is relatively weak and unstable, so retractions occur with increased work of breathing. Assessment of breathing includes observing the child for intercostal, substernal, suprasternal, supraclavicular, and infraclavicular retractions. As a child becomes exhausted, retractions may diminish, usually indicating respiratory failure. Nasal flaring with inspiration is another form of accessory muscle use. Grunting, a sound made by the expiration of air

against partially closed vocal cords, is a sign of hypoxemia and represents the body's effort to improve oxygenation by generating positive end-expiratory pressure.

The nurse observes the child's preferred body posture. A child in respiratory distress is upright with the jaw thrust forward, leaning forward on outstretched arms—the tripod position. This position, often referred to as "tripoding," helps maximize airway opening and the use of accessory muscles of respiration.

Once the work of breathing has been carefully observed, listening to the chest provides some useful information. Children have small chests, and breath sounds can be transmitted throughout the chest. The nurse therefore auscultates a child's chest at both sides of the body at the midaxillary line and over the trachea to confirm equality of breath sounds and distinguish upper from lower airway noises.

Normal respiratory rates for children vary by age and are faster than for adults (see Table 9-1). A respiratory rate greater than 60 breaths/min, however, is abnormal for any age. Another important adjunct for respiratory assessment is the pulse oximetry reading (see Chapter 13). Measuring exhaled CO_2 using capnography (even in nonintubated patients) may provide a more sensitive detection of hypoventilation, impaired gas exchange and perfusion, metabolic acidosis, and carbon monoxide poisoning (Anderson, 2006).

Cardiovascular Assessment

Cardiovascular assessment includes observing the child's skin color and temperature, checking capillary refill, and assessing central and peripheral pulse rate and quality. A child can compensate more effectively for fluid loss, through increased heart rate and peripheral vasoconstriction, than an adult can. Tachycardia and decreased peripheral perfusion are early signs of cardiovascular compromise in a child and require immediate intervention to prevent decompensation. Hypotension is a late finding in a child with shock. Hypotension manifests only after significant fluid loss because of the compensatory mechanisms that result in vasoconstriction (Kleinman, Chameides, Schexnayder et al., 2010). Hypotension in children suggests that compensatory mechanisms are no longer adequate to maintain cardiac output.

Disability: Neurologic Assessment

The infant's or child's level of consciousness is an essential component of the primary assessment. Alteration in level of consciousness (irritability or agitation, lethargy, or inability to recognize parents or caregivers) can be the first sign of respiratory compromise or worsening condition.

A rapid neurologic assessment consists of two components: (1) pupillary reactivity and size; and (2) a brief mental status assessment (*AVPU: a*lert, responds to *v*oice, responds to *p*ain, *u*nresponsive). More thorough and sophisticated means of assessment are used later if needed (see Chapter 28). Serial assessment is imperative. Progressive loss of consciousness may be a result of hypoxemia, hypoglycemia, increased intracranial pressure, or another life-threatening condition.

Exposure

Primary assessment ends with exposure, or removing the child's clothing to identify additional injuries or indicators of illness. The nurse needs to preserve the child's clothing appropriately if it will be needed for evidence in any potential civil or criminal proceeding. Infants and children have a larger body surface area/weight ratio, making them at higher risk for hypothermia. Maintaining body temperature by shivering increases metabolic needs, such as oxygen and glucose, and the child has limited reserves. The risk of hypoxia and hypoglycemia is

TABLE 10-1   PRIMARY ASSESSMENT IN PEDIATRIC EMERGENCIES

ASSESSMENT	PEDIATRIC DIFFERENCES	NURSING IMPLICATIONS
A: Airway Patency, positioning for air entry, audible sounds, airway obstruction (blood, mucus, edema)	The child's airway is narrower than an adult's and more easily obstructed by foreign bodies, small amounts of mucus, or tissue edema. Infants are preferential nasal breathers for the first several months of life; therefore nasal secretions can cause respiratory compromise. Children are more susceptible to infectious respiratory diseases that contribute to risk of airway obstruction. Edema and mucus in a narrow airway cause incrementally more obstruction than in a wider one. The tongue is relatively large in relation to the oral cavity and can more easily fall into the airway in the unconscious child. Cartilage of the larynx is relatively soft, and the trachea is thinner and more flexible than an adult's. The larynx is higher and more anterior, increasing the risk of obstruction and aspiration. The submandibular area is softer and can be more easily compressed to occlude the airway. Deciduous teeth are poorly anchored and easily dislodged. Altered mental status is an early sign of hypoxia.	Allow the child to maintain a position of comfort or manually position the airway (jaw thrust or head-tilt/chin-lift); encourage the child to avoid flexing or hyperextending the neck; use spinal immobilization and airway adjuncts as required.
B: Breathing Decreased level of consciousness, increased or decreased work of breathing, nasal flaring, use of accessory muscles of respiration (retractions), rate, pattern, quality, oxygen saturation	The chest wall is thin, softer, and more compliant. Rib alignment is more horizontal. The younger child is more susceptible to respiratory distress and failure. Retractions commonly occur with respiratory distress and can compromise the ability to increase tidal volume. The diaphragm is the predominant muscle of respiration. Pressure above or below the diaphragm can impede respiratory effort. Infants and children have a higher metabolic rate and increased oxygen demand. Hypoxia occurs more rapidly.	Provide supplemental oxygen; initiate assisted ventilation with bag-valve-mask ventilation device, and prepare for intubation as indicated; provide gastric decompression with orogastric or nasogastric tube; provide comfort measures; encourage family presence to decrease anxiety.
C: Circulation Skin color, temperature, and capillary refill (<2 sec); rate and strength of peripheral and central pulses	The child's circulating blood volume per body weight is much larger than an adult's, even though actual blood volume is much smaller. Therefore small volume losses have more severe circulatory consequences. A higher percentage of fluid is located in the extracellular compartment, causing more rapid fluid shifts. A higher metabolic rate and oxygen demand require an increased heart rate; tachycardia is the first compensatory mechanism for decreased oxygenation—not hypotension.	Control bleeding through application of direct pressure; obtain vascular access; initiate volume replacement; perform chest compressions; defibrillate or provide synchronized cardioversion; initiate drug therapy.
D: Disability Level of consciousness or activity level; response to the environment (especially caregivers); pupillary response	A larger head/body ratio and weak neck muscles contribute to more serious head injury from shaking or impact. The anterior fontanel remains open until approximately age 18 mo. An open fontanel allows for expanded cranial volume, so signs of increased intracranial pressure, which indicate underlying traumatic brain injury, may be delayed. A thinner skull predisposes the child to more severe injury. Nerve myelinization is incomplete during infancy; unmyelinated tissue is more vulnerable to shearing injury.	Treat the underlying cause (e.g., signs of increased intracranial pressure; fluid or blood volume deficit; hypoglycemia; hypothermia; hypoxia); compare assessment with parent's perception (a deeply sleeping child may be difficult to arouse, which is "normal" to caregivers).
E: Exposure To identify underlying injuries or additional signs of illness	Bulging fontanel, periorbital edema, unusual rashes, and edema or exudate in the pharynx can indicate a variety of severe childhood communicable diseases. Bruising, unusual burns, vaginal tearing, rectal bleeding, and discharge suggest child abuse. Swelling, deformities can indicate underlying trauma to vital organs.	Remove all clothing, including diapers; save any clothing needed for evidence; maintain an appropriately warm environment.

Data from Emergency Nurses Association. (2007). *Trauma nursing core course provider manual* (6th ed.). Des Plaines, IL: Author.

Animation—Bag Ventilation

TABLE 10-2	**SECONDARY ASSESSMENT IN PEDIATRIC EMERGENCIES**
ASSESSMENT	**NURSING IMPLICATIONS**
F: Full Set of Vital Signs; Family Presence Evaluate the child's vital signs, including temperature, for abnormal findings; obtain weight in kilograms. Family presence: assess the needs of the family for support and inclusion in care.	Continuously monitor the child's vital signs, including temperature; weigh child or obtain estimated weight if child's condition prohibits measured weight. Facilitate family presence and support in a culturally appropriate way.
G: Give Comfort Measures Discomfort is usually related to the underlying problem; use pain assessment scales for children.	Frequently monitor pain level and response to pain-relief measures; include nonpharmacologic techniques for reducing pain.
H: Head-to-Toe Assessment; Obtain History Perform a complete head-to-toe assessment and obtain a history; during triage assessment, a focused assessment related to the chief complaint may be used.	Continuously monitor the child for changes in condition; assess for any unusual odors.
I: Inspect the Back Observe the back for obvious or hidden injuries; assess for communicable illness or susceptibility to illness (immunocompromised patients).	Reinspect the back as indicated.

Data from Emergency Nurses Association. (2007). *Trauma nursing core course provider manual* (6th ed.). Des Plaines, IL: Author.

higher in neonates from utilization of brown fat for nonshivering thermogenesis and an increased metabolic demand secondary to an infectious or physiologic process. Methods to help the child maintain a normothermic state or help with warming include overhead warmers and heat lamps, warmed intravenous (IV) fluids and humidified oxygen, removal of wet clothes, and providing warmed blankets.

Secondary Assessment

After the primary assessment is complete and interventions (if necessary) have stabilized the child, the nurse begins the secondary assessment. Components of the secondary assessment include vital signs, assessing for pain, history and head-to-toe assessment, and inspection (Table 10-2).

Vital Signs

Vital signs are useful in the triage assessment of the child, but because age variations make their significance more difficult to interpret, they are not as reliable an indicator as in adult assessment. This variation is especially applicable to temperature. For example, an infant has an immature thermoregulatory system and may not have a fever or may even be hypothermic in the presence of infection, so the nurse needs to be alert for supporting signs. The nurse remembers that an alteration in one part of the vital signs may result in abnormal values in other parts. For example, an abnormally high heart rate and respiratory rate may be a result of hyperthermia, crying, pain, hypoxemia, or hypovolemia (see Chapter 13 for methods of obtaining a temperature).

When taking a child's vital signs, the nurse observes the respiratory rate first and then obtains the pulse; the nurse obtains the temperature and blood pressure last because these procedures can be more upsetting for children. The nurse should be certain to use the correct size blood pressure cuff and take both the respiratory and heart rates for 1 full minute because subtle differences are important in the child. Normal pediatric respiratory and heart rates are faster than adult rates, whereas the blood pressure is lower on average (see Table 9-1 and Evolve website for normal vital signs by age). An accurate weight should be obtained at this time, and monitors such as a cardiac or a pulse oximeter should be applied as indicated.

History and Head-to-Toe Assessment

A brief history provides information about prior illness or injury that might affect the emergency care of the child. One format often used for pediatric clients is the mnemonic *SAMPLE*:

S   signs and symptoms
A   allergies
M   medications taken (prescription, over the counter, and herbal or home remedies) and immunization history
P   prior illness or injury
L   last meal and eating habits
E   events surrounding this injury or illness (e.g., length of illness, mechanism of injury)

This mnemonic gives sufficient information to determine whether the child's medical history will play an important role in assessment and treatment of the current illness or injury. In emergency departments that care for children, a list of immunizations and the appropriate ages should be posted in a convenient location (see www2.aap.org/immunization/IZschedule.html).

After obtaining an appropriate history, the nurse begins to perform a head-to-toe assessment, documenting any findings that might affect the child's condition. Assessment findings are compared with the history to aid in diagnosis and look for inconsistencies. The nurse inspects all body surfaces, looking for fractures, lacerations, contusions, and penetrating injuries. The nurse also observes the skin for petechiae or rashes. The presence and pattern of any pain are described. The nurse pays particular attention to signs of pneumothorax or hemothorax (e.g., decreased breath sounds on the affected side, signs of hypoxemia, and signs of shock). The nurse then palpates the child's abdomen and auscultates for the presence of bowel sounds. Any sign of hematuria suggests genitourinary injury or infection. Blood found at the urinary meatus suggests disruptive injury of the lower urinary tract, and a urinary catheter should not be inserted.

Diagnostic Tests

Once the child has arrived in the emergency setting and has undergone initial assessment and interventions, diagnostic tests are performed that assist in the evaluation process. Standard protocols for laboratory tests usually include a complete blood count (CBC) with differential count, serum electrolytes, bedside glucose, and urinalysis. Additional studies may be necessary for the child who has multiple trauma. These include coagulation profiles, blood urea nitrogen (BUN), creatinine, glucose, amylase, lipase, SGOT (serum glutamic-oxaloacetic transaminase, also known as AST [aspartate aminotransferase]), SGPT (serum glutamic-pyruvate transaminase, also known as ALT [alanine aminotransferase]), and blood type and crossmatch.

Radiologic films may be obtained depending on the presenting problem and assessment data. Placement of a gastric tube, urinary catheter, or other device may be required. Orogastric tubes should be placed in children with suspected head trauma because of the risk of misplacement and injury with a nasogastric tube in children with basilar skull and facial fractures. Gastric tubes are placed to reduce gastric inflation that can place pressure on the diaphragm and decrease ventilation effectiveness because children are diaphragmatic breathers (Kleinman et al., 2010).

Weight

Determining the child's weight is essential in emergency care because all medication dosages and fluid amounts are calculated according to the child's weight in kilograms. The nurse weighs the child on an appropriately calibrated scale if possible, following agency procedure for measuring and recording weight (e.g., with or without clothing, diaper on vs. diaper off).

Another way to determine the child's weight and medication dosages is through the use of a length-based resuscitation tape, such as the Broselow tape. Tapes with precalculated medication doses calculated at various lengths have been proven more accurate in the prediction of body weight than provider or parent estimate-based methods (Kleinman et al., 2010). A length-based resuscitation tape is placed on a gurney or stretcher next to the child, and the child's length is measured. The length is keyed to emergency medication dosages, usually listed on the tape. The tape also indicates fluid bolus volumes, defibrillation energy levels, and sizes of the pediatric airway, bag-valve-mask ventilation device, laryngoscope, endotracheal tube, gastric tube, urinary catheter, chest tube, and intravenous (IV) catheter. The validity of length-based resuscitation tapes is questioned with the growing trends in childhood obesity, and these tapes should be used with caution in overweight children.

Parent-Child Relationship

Rapid triage assessment of the child also includes observation of the child in relation to the parents. If the relationship does not appear to be close, comfortable, and trusting, the nurse may want to explore this further.

EVIDENCE-BASED PRACTICE

Obtaining an Accurate Allergy History

Level IV

The triage area in an emergency department is extremely busy, and nurses working in that area are subject to many distractions from patients, families, and the environment itself. The purpose of triage is to make a rapid and accurate assessment of patients and a decision about the needed level of care. Because data collected at the point of care in triage are used subsequently by professionals treating the child, it is essential that important information be accurately assessed and documented. One critical piece of information is whether or not a child is allergic to medication.

Porter, Manzi, Volpe, and Stack (2006) questioned whether errors in assessment, documentation, or communication (via both documentation and placement of an allergy alert wristband) of a child's medication allergy continued systematically through the child's treatment phase in the emergency setting. The specific purposes of their observational research were to identify how specific information provided by parents determines whether or not the child is allergic to medication and also whether errors in assessing or communicating medication allergy persist throughout the child's emergency department encounter.

Using observations of triage nurse assessments, a convenience sample of 211 parent-child dyads, who used emergency department services in a busy urban emergency department was identified. The researchers collected data on ways nurses questioned parents about medication allergy, whether parents' responses were clarified, whether a potential allergy was appropriately documented in the child's record, and whether the child was given an allergy alert band (Porter et al., 2006). Additionally, through parent interview and chart review, researchers were able to identify whether treating professionals clarified or re-inquired about medication allergy and whether the reported allergy met the standard criteria for allergy diagnosis.

Results from this study have important implications for nurses in any setting. This research demonstrated "significant gaps" in the assessment and communication of children's medication allergy in an emergent care setting. The researchers described errors (both positive and negative) they identified during triage and that were carried throughout the treatment phase. The results from the Porter et al. (2006) study suggest several communication issues that apply specifically to nurses:

- Many parents identify their child as being allergic without describing data that support a hypersensitivity reaction, or are not able to identify specific

medications to which the child may be allergic. Listing the patient's reaction to an allergen can differentiate between allergies, adverse drug reactions, and normal medication side effects, such as nausea, that are interpreted as allergies (Paparella, 2009).

- If nurses are not precise with terminology when asking about medication allergy, or if nurses do not clarify specific allergic manifestations, they risk identifying an allergy incorrectly or not identifying an allergy that actually exists.
- Reviewing an allergy history at all phases of an encounter to validate initial reports can assist with identification of incorrect allergy information.

Porter et al. (2006) recommend that nurses more precisely inquire about medication allergy when taking a nursing history. Asking "Has your child ever had a problem or reaction to any medicine that was given?" rather than "Does your child have any allergies?" decreases the risk of error related to parents' incomplete understanding of what constitutes an allergy. It also provides an opportunity for the nurse to clarify the child's specific history of reactions to medications. Additional barriers to effective allergy identification include the use of social cause bands that can distract providers and cause confusion, and the lack of a standardized system or color for allergy alert bands (Dean, 2010).

A more recent study by Porter and colleagues compared the quality of data obtained from parent use of a health information technology *(ParentLink)* to that obtained by nurses and physicians (Porter, Forbes, Manzi, & Kalish, 2010). In the emergency department, parents entered information about their child's medication allergies and history of present illness related to head trauma, into a computer located on a mobile kiosk. The *ParentLink* child allergy data were more accurate and the history of present illness data more comprehensive than the information documented in the medical record by nurses and physicians (Porter et al., 2010).

Think about how you have obtained a child's allergy history on admission to the hospital. Could you have been more precise in identifying or clarifying information provided by the parents? What methods do you think are essential for conveying medication allergy information to other nurses and health care providers? What is the potential influence of cultural or language differences? How might electronic health information technologies streamline the process of gathering key information as well as improve the accuracy of documentation?

CARDIOPULMONARY RESUSCITATION OF THE CHILD

Airway and Breathing

Initial Assessment and Intervention

Whereas lethal arrhythmias related to heart disease are the most common causes of cardiopulmonary arrest in adults, factors leading to shock and respiratory failure are the most common causes of cardiopulmonary arrest in children. Early recognition of and intervention for respiratory distress and compensated shock can be lifesaving for the child. Assistance with ventilation and administration of fluids may prevent further deterioration in the child's condition. Once the child progresses to respiratory failure and shock, **cardiopulmonary resuscitation** (CPR) is necessary. Resuscitation of children requires attention to the differences between adults and children (see Table 10-1).

If a child is unresponsive and not breathing, basic life-support measures will be initiated. However, the child with spontaneous respiratory effort or a pulse will require more evaluation to determine the need for CPR. Cardiac arrests in infants and children are more commonly caused by asphyxiation, and though research has shown that resuscitation outcomes are better with a combination of ventilations and chest compressions, it is unknown whether the sequence makes a difference (Berg, Schexnayder, Chameides et al., 2010). To avoid delays in initiating CPR, the American Heart Association (AHA) recommends the CAB sequence (circulation, airway, breathing) beginning with 30 chest compressions followed by opening the airway and two rescue breaths (Berg et al., 2010). The early initiation of high-quality chest compressions improves blood flow to vital organs and will improve chances of survival (Kleinman et al., 2010).

Because of the proportionately larger size of the child's head with a weaker supporting muscle structure, repositioning the head and placing a rolled-up towel under the child's shoulders can often facilitate improved air exchange. Additionally, the tongue of the young child is larger in relation to the oropharynx and is often the cause of airway obstruction. When administering assisted ventilations, the nurse should stop inflating the lungs when the chest just begins to rise and allow enough time for exhalation (longer than inhalation). Endotracheal intubation by a provider skilled in the technique is necessary if the child cannot be ventilated adequately with these measures or if prolonged ventilation is anticipated. Ventilations should be given at a rate of 12 to 20 per minute or approximately one breath every 3 to 5 seconds; each breath should be given over 1 second (Berg et al., 2010).

A pressure gauge attached to the bag-valve-mask ventilation device helps deliver breaths at the correct pressure, especially for infants and young children. Choosing the appropriate-size mask and the correct volume bag is important. The mask should cover the child's mouth and nose but not place pressure on the eyes. A good fit ensures a seal around the face and under the chin. Gastric decompression by use of an orogastric or nasogastric tube is indicated during assisted ventilation.

Obstructed Airway Management

Inability to inflate the lungs suggests airway obstruction, a life-threatening emergency. When ventilation is not possible, the infant or child will die in a very short time.

Management of airway obstruction depends on the cause and on the child's age. Definitive treatment depends on diagnosis. Whereas adults more commonly choke while eating, children can choke while eating or playing. Foreign body aspiration, for example, is a problem frequently seen in young children, with a large number of aspirations attributed to coins, small toy parts, and certain foods, particularly candy, nuts, and grapes. More than 90% of pediatric deaths related to choking occur in children younger than 5 years of age (Berg et al., 2010). When a child is unable to ventilate adequately and aspiration of a foreign body is suspected as the cause, the nurse initiates maneuvers to remove the obstruction.

Although controversy remains about how to clear a foreign body from the airway, for conscious children older than 1 year the American Heart Association recommends using the Heimlich maneuver. CPR should be initiated for all unresponsive infants and children with a foreign body aspiration. The rescuer tries to visualize the foreign body for removal before each ventilation sequence (Berg et al., 2010). Removal of a foreign body from an infant involves placing the infant in a downward slant position and giving five back blows alternating with five chest compressions. Abdominal thrusts are not used in infants because of the risk of liver injury. Blind finger sweeps used in an attempt to remove a possible foreign object are not recommended because of the risk of forcing the object farther down the airway or causing injury to the supraglottic area. If an object is seen, it should be removed.

If obstruction continues after these maneuvers, subsequent actions may include direct laryngoscopy and use of a Magill forceps to remove the foreign body. Tracheostomy is used as a last resort. When the lower airway is obstructed because of a disease process, such as asthma, medication to open the airway may be necessary.

⚡ SAFETY ALERT

Airway Obstruction in Children

When a child is in significant respiratory distress and the child is coughing or able to breathe adequately despite partial obstruction, the child should be allowed to maintain *whatever position is comfortable* until specialized care is available. In the smaller child, this position may be in the parent's or caregiver's arms. The nurse remains with the child and encourages the child to remain calm by reassuring in a soothing manner.

Circulation

The nurse feels for the pulse in the child older than 1 year by palpating the carotid or femoral artery and looking for signs of circulation such as movement. For an infant younger than 1 year, the nurse uses the brachial artery because the infant's relatively short, thick neck makes palpation of the carotid artery difficult. The nurse begins chest compressions if no pulse is palpated after approximately 10 seconds, or if the infant's or child's heart rate is less than 60 beats/min and perfusion is poor. Compressions should be administered at a rate of at least 100 compressions per minute with enough pressure to depress at least one third of the chest and allowing complete recoil after each compression (Berg et al., 2010) (Table 10-3).

Automatic external defibrillators (AEDs) are becoming increasingly more available in community settings. They are effective for correcting serious rhythm disturbances in adults, and it is recommended that AEDs be used for infants and children as well. AEDs with high specificity in recognizing pediatric shockable rhythms and a system to decrease or attenuate the delivery of energy (shock) are best for use in children under 8 years (Berg et al., 2010). In a witnessed arrest, the AED should be used as soon as it is available. If the arrest is not witnessed, CPR should be performed for at least five cycles (2 minutes) with minimal interruptions in chest compressions before the AED is used (Berg et al., 2010).

TABLE 10-3 HEALTH CARE PROFESSIONAL BASIC LIFE SUPPORT ELEMENTS FOR INFANTS AND CHILDREN

ELEMENT	INFANT (<1 YEAR)	CHILD (1 YEAR-ONSET OF PUBERTY)	ADULTS (ADOLESCENTS)
Discovery	Unresponsive No breathing or only gasping No brachial pulse palpated in 10 sec	No carotid or femoral pulse palpated in 10 sec	No carotid pulse palpated in 10 sec
Sequence for CPR = C-A-B (Circulation-Airway-Breathing)			
Circulation Compressions		At least 100 compressions/min "Push fast" "Push hard"	
Location	Compress just below nipple line	Compress lower half of sternum	
Technique	Two fingers or two thumbs encircling hands around chest; two rescuers	Heel of one or two hands	Heel of two hands
Depth	About 1.5 in (4 cm)	About 2 in (5 cm)	At least 2 in (5 cm)
Ratio	30:2 one rescuer; 15:2 two rescuers	30:2 one rescuer; 15:2 two rescuers	30:2 one rescuer or two rescuers
Compressions/Ventilations		Allow chest to fully recoil after each compression Limit interruptions in compressions to under 10 sec	
Airway		Head-tilt/chin-lift (if trauma is present, use jaw thrust)	
Breathing		8 to 10 breaths/min; not correlated with chest compressions	
Advanced airway in place		1 breath every 6 to 8 sec 1 second for each breath; look for chest to rise	
Defibrillation	Defibrillate as soon as possible; use manual defibrillator or AED with pediatric dose attenuator	Defibrillate soon as possible; use automatic external defibrillator (AED)	
Foreign body airway obstruction	Back blows, chest compressions	Heimlich maneuver (abdominal thrusts)	

Data from Berg, M.D., Schexnayder, S.M., Chameides, L., et al. (2010). Part 13: Pediatric basic life support: 2010 American Heart Association guidelines for cardiopulmonary resuscitation and emergency cardiovascular care. *Circulation, 122*(suppl 3), S862-S875.

Rapid venous access for fluid resuscitation and medication administration is essential in the child with compromised circulation. Because peripheral venous access can be challenging in critically ill children, attempts should be limited and intraosseous access should be established during CPR or treatment of severe shock (Kleinman et al., 2010). An intraosseous (IO) line, placed in the anteromedial tibia or distal femur serves as a rapidly accessible and safe form of vascular access in children. Immediate availability of a fluid access site is more important than the route of administration. Children should be given IV fluid (usually lactated Ringer's or normal saline solution), 20 mL/kg, as a rapid bolus for symptoms of shock. The nurse administers additional boluses as needed after reassessing cardiovascular status and warms the solution before any rapid infusion. If more than three boluses are required for hemodynamic stability, administration of blood products may be required.

Epinephrine is the drug of choice for management of cardiac arrest, arrhythmias, and hemodynamic instability. It can be given through the endotracheal tube when necessary. Atropine diminishes vagally mediated bradycardia. Sodium bicarbonate is given on the basis of arterial blood gas results, and dextrose can be used on the basis of blood glucose results, for children unresponsive to other resuscitative efforts.

Although cardiac rhythm disturbances in children are rare, rapid heart rates can occur, including sinus tachycardia, supraventricular tachycardia, and ventricular tachycardia. Cardiac output is a function of stroke volume and heart rate. Because children are unable to increase stroke volume, they can increase cardiac output only by increasing their heart rate. As heart rates increase, cardiac filling time decreases and cardiac output falls.

Sinus tachycardia usually requires observation and determination of the cause (e.g., fever, shock, toxic ingestion). Vagal maneuvers (e.g., applying ice water to the face), synchronized cardioversion at 0.5 to 1.0 joules/kg, or adenosine may be necessary for symptomatic supraventricular tachycardia (heart rate greater than 200 beats/min) (Kleinman et al., 2010). Ventricular tachycardia in a child is usually the result of congenital abnormalities, toxic ingestion, or chronic cardiac disease and requires complex interventions.

Resuscitation of the child requires a team effort. Training and rehearsal, such as mock codes, are needed. National courses such as the AHA's Pediatric Advanced Life Support (PALS) program and the Emergency Nursing Pediatric Course (ENPC) provided by the Emergency Nurses Association, are available.

THE CHILD IN SHOCK

Shock is an acute, complex, unstable physiologic state of inadequate oxygen delivery to tissues. Decreased tissue perfusion (circulation of blood through the vascular bed of tissue) leads to a cascade of physiologic consequences and, if prolonged, irreversible tissue and organ damage (Turner & Cheifetz, 2011). The causes of shock can be classified into three major categories: hypovolemic, cardiogenic, and distributive, with some overlaps (Kleinman et al., 2010). Regardless of the cause, the body will respond similarly to compensate for the alterations in perfusion and transport of oxygen and metabolic substrates that have occurred.

Etiology
Hypovolemic Shock
Hypovolemic shock is the most common cause of shock in children and is characterized by an overall decrease in circulating blood or fluid volume. Hemorrhage, burns, and dehydration are the most common causes of hypovolemic shock. Blood loss can be caused by trauma or surgery; fluid and plasma losses can occur with vomiting and diarrhea, burns, and diabetic ketoacidosis.

Distributive Shock
Distributive shock is the result of an abnormality in the distribution of blood flow or inability of the body to maintain vascular tone through vasoconstriction.

Septic shock is the most common form of distributive shock and occurs when microbial toxins (from bacteria, viruses, fungi, or rickettsiae) are present in the blood. These toxins cause a cascade of metabolic, hemodynamic, and clinical changes, resulting in impaired organ perfusion and hypotension. Despite major advances in vaccines in the past two decades, septic shock continues to be a frequent reason for admission to pediatric intensive care units. Organisms responsible for septic shock vary with age and immunocompetence, but include group B beta-hemolytic streptococci, enteric gram-negative rods (*Escherichia coli*, *Klebsiella*, Enterobacteriaceae), *Listeria monocytogenes*, and *Staphylococcus aureus* in neonates; and *Streptococcus pneumoniae*, *S. aureus*, *Neisseria meningitides*, and group A *Streptococcus* in infants and children (Kleinman et al., 2010). Infants and children with debilitating illnesses, and prolonged hospitalizations in the intensive care unit with many invasive lines, as well as those who are immunosuppressed, are at greatest risk for development of septic shock. Anaphylaxis, central nervous system or spinal injury, and drug intoxication are other forms of distributive shock.

Cardiogenic Shock
Cardiogenic shock occurs when myocardial function is impaired and cardiac output is not sufficient to meet the body's metabolic demands. It is characterized by low cardiac output, cyanosis, respiratory distress, differentiated extremity blood pressures, poor tissue perfusion, and poor response to fluid resuscitation (Kleinman et al., 2010). The causes of cardiogenic shock include structural abnormalities related to congenital heart disease, infectious and noninfectious cardiomyopathies, intractable arrhythmias, trauma, ischemia, metabolic abnormalities, drug intoxication, and impaired cardiac function after intracardiac surgical repair.

Manifestations
Recognition of the clinical manifestations, with early intervention, is imperative for optimal treatment of shock (Box 10-2). In the early stages, the child is able to compensate with tachycardia, tachypnea, and vasoconstriction to maintain cardiac output. If the condition cannot be reversed, a decompensated state arises with altered perfusion (delayed capillary refill, weak pulses, cool extremities, and hypotension) and profoundly altered mental status. Progression results in cardiovascular collapse and death. Table 10-4 presents the general appearance of a child in shock.

PATHOPHYSIOLOGY
Shock

Hypovolemic Shock
Hypovolemic shock results from an abnormal decrease in circulating volume. Water constitutes a much greater portion of an infant's or a child's body weight than it does an adult's, and because the bulk of fluid volume in young children is located in the extracellular tissue spaces, infants and young children are more susceptible to hypovolemic shock. Infants, with their large body surface area and increased metabolic rate, also experience increased insensible fluid loss, thus compounding hypovolemia. Because of their small body size, even relatively small blood losses can result in hypovolemia.

When intravascular volume is reduced, the body initially compensates by increasing the peripheral vascular resistance, stroke volume, and heart rate and redistributing the blood flow to the vital organs (brain, heart). If a fluid resuscitation is not initiated within an appropriate time frame, altered sensorium and oliguria will be noted and hypovolemic shock will eventually result in irreversible tissue and organ damage (Turner & Cheifetz, 2011).

Distributive Shock
Septic shock, the most common form of distributive shock, occurs when an invading organism infects a susceptible host, overwhelms the host's first and second lines of defense, and enters the bloodstream. The body's response to toxins or organisms in the blood, including endocrine, metabolic, and immunologic reactions, can result in inflammatory and coagulation abnormalities. Endotoxins, produced by lysis of bacteria, cause maldistributed blood flow, cardiac dysfunction, oxygen supply-and-demand imbalance, and metabolic alterations. The end result can be organ ischemia, multiple organ dysfunction syndrome, and death (Kleinman et al., 2010).

Cardiogenic Shock
Cardiogenic shock is characterized by low cardiac output and hypotension, which result in inadequate oxygen delivery to the tissues. Unlike hypovolemic shock, the compensatory mechanisms that occur in a child with cardiogenic shock can cause further myocardial dysfunction. These compensatory mechanisms redistribute blood away from the peripheral, splenic, and mesenteric circulation to help maintain the circulation to the vital organs: the heart and brain. Initially, compensatory mechanisms increase the heart rate, myocardial contractility, and vasoconstriction. Subsequent events result in sodium and fluid retention, producing a greater workload on the left ventricle (afterload). The increased workload causes increased oxygen demands on the myocardium in response to a depleted oxygen supply. This process leads to myocardial ischemia, which further depresses cardiac function, thereby establishing a vicious cycle.

An alteration in contractility, as seen in an injury to the myocardium and myocarditis, results in a decreased stroke volume and the ventricle being unable to eject blood.

⚡ SAFETY ALERT
Hypotension in Children with Shock
Children can compensate for a 25% blood loss with an increase in heart rate and peripheral vascular resistance, so hypotension is a late sign of shock (Emergency Nurses Association, 2007). The lower limits for systolic blood pressure (BP) in children are as follows:
- Infants younger than 1 month: 60 mm Hg
- Infants ages 1 to 12 months: 70 mm Hg
- Children older than 1 year: 70 mm Hg plus the number that is double the child's age in years (e.g., 10-year-old child: 70 + 20 = 90 mm Hg, the lower limit for systolic BP)

BOX 10-2 MANIFESTATIONS OF SHOCK IN CHILDREN

Hypovolemic Shock
- Dry mucous membranes
- Depressed fontanel
- Cold, clammy skin
- Oliguria
- Poor skin turgor
- Delayed capillary refill

Distributive (Septic) Shock: Early
- Vasodilation
- Extremities that are warm to the touch
- Tachycardia, tachypnea

Septic Shock: Late
- Rapid, thready pulse
- Cyanosis
- Cold, clammy skin
- Purpuric skin lesions
- Narrow pulse pressure
- Oliguria or anuria

Cardiogenic Shock
- Hepatomegaly
- Cardiomegaly
- Increased central venous pressure
- Periorbital edema
- Crackles
- Diaphoresis
- Oliguria
- Reduced capillary refill
- Differences in proximal and distal pulses

TABLE 10-4 ASSESSING A CHILD'S GENERAL APPEARANCE: "LOOKS GOOD" VERSUS "LOOKS BAD"

	"LOOKS GOOD"	"LOOKS BAD"
Color	Pink mucous membranes Consistent color over the trunk and extremities	Mottled color, "gray" or pale
Skin perfusion	Warm Brisk capillary refill (<2 sec)	Cold (peripheral to proximal cooling) Sluggish capillary refill (>2 sec)
Activity	Age-appropriate (may be frightened, unhappy, unwilling to be separated from parents) Will engage in play	Fretful, then lethargic
Responsiveness	Age-appropriate	Irritable (early), then lethargic Decreased response to painful stimulus is worrisome
Infant feeding	Eats well	Weak suck Tires during feeding May have respiratory distress during feedings

Data from Kleinman, M.E., Chameides, L., Schexnayder, S.M., et al. (2010). Part 14: Pediatric advanced life support: 2010 American Heart Association guidelines for cardiopulmonary resuscitation and emergency cardiovascular care. *Circulation, 122*(suppl 3), S876-S908.

Diagnostic Evaluation

The diagnosis of shock in infants and children is established chiefly on the basis of clinical manifestations and medical history. A chest radiograph may help differentiate cardiogenic shock from hypovolemic and distributive shock. In cardiogenic shock, the heart is usually enlarged and the chest x-ray film may show signs of pulmonary edema. In hypovolemic or distributive shock, the chest radiograph is usually normal or shows signs of infiltrates (indicative of pneumonia) and the heart is smaller than normal (indicative of a decrease in circulating volume). An echocardiogram can identify underlying structural cardiac disease.

Laboratory studies used in a differential diagnosis include blood cultures and cultures of other sites that may be the source of infection (e.g., spinal fluid, urine, sputum, wound drainage, indwelling lines), arterial blood gas values, glucose levels, electrolytes, BUN, creatinine levels, CBC, and coagulation studies.

Therapeutic Management

The therapeutic management of the child in shock includes basic life support (maintaining airway, breathing, and circulation) and treating signs and symptoms.

Monitoring with pulse oximetry and increasing ambient oxygen are indicated in most cases. If vascular access cannot be obtained, an IO line can be used until the child is resuscitated, at which time the temporary IO line can be replaced with an IV line.

Hypovolemic Shock

Once the airway, breathing, and circulation are established, the next priority is adequate vascular access. An intravenous crystalloid infusion of warm normal saline or lactated Ringer's solution should be promptly initiated. If hypovolemic shock is caused by hemorrhage and symptoms persist after administration of crystalloid boluses, blood transfusions may be considered (Hartman & Cheifetz, 2011).

Colloids (albumin) are protein-containing fluids that may be used in volume resuscitation after the initial treatment with crystalloids. Colloids are used primarily for dehydration or body fluid losses other than blood.

Distributive Shock

The therapeutic management of distributive shock involves restoring hemodynamic status with fluid resuscitation and promptly treating the underlying cause. For septic shock, parenteral antibiotics are administered promptly. Inotropic medications and vasodilators are used to manage the cardiovascular instability. Vasoconstrictors may be used to increase vascular tone and counteract the effects of toxins. Steroids, medications to treat hypoglycemia and electrolyte imbalances, and administration of blood products may be required to combat complications of distributive shock (Kleinman et al., 2010). Maintaining a secure, patent airway may be necessary if significant respiratory distress occurs. Surgery also might be indicated to eliminate the source of infection (e.g., an abscess) or stabilize a central nervous system/spinal injury.

Cardiogenic Shock

Supplemental oxygen, vascular access, hemodynamic monitoring, and frequent assessments are imperative in shock management. The nurse uses assessment skills to recognize early signs of deterioration and response to therapeutic interventions. Invasive monitoring of central venous pressure, arterial blood pressure, and pulmonary artery pressure help identify hemodynamic changes and the subtle clinical signs and symptoms of decreased cardiac output (e.g., cyanosis, decreased skin temperature, and delayed capillary refill).

With an excess of intravascular fluid volume, diuretics may be prescribed. Usually furosemide (Lasix), 1 mg/kg IV, provides effective diuresis.

The heart rate must be in the normal range or higher than normal to improve the cardiac output. Children, especially infants younger than 6 months, have a decreased ability to increase stroke volume and thus depend much more on an increased heart rate as a compensatory mechanism to improve cardiac output. Pharmacologic therapy is the mainstay of medical treatment in children with cardiogenic shock. Frequently a combination of pharmacologic agents is necessary to stabilize the child. Dopamine, dobutamine, and milrinone are the initial drugs of choice for treating cardiogenic shock (Kleinman et al., 2010).

Extracorporeal life support (ECLS) is a means of providing short-term circulatory and respiratory support for infants and children with underlying cardiac disease and/or when other methods of treatment are not effective. It has been successfully used in distributive and cardiogenic shock. Vital organ perfusion is maintained by ECLS to allow for prolonged delivery of oxygen to tissues (Kleinman et al., 2010).

NURSING CARE OF THE CHILD IN SHOCK

Assessment

Nursing assessment of a child in shock should be thorough, with attention focused on the child's cardiopulmonary system and neurologic status. A changing level of consciousness is one of the first indicators of a worsening condition, and early identification and treatment of shock in infants and children are crucial to decreasing morbidity and mortality rates. Initial concerns are ensuring a patent airway and monitoring the child's respiratory effort to confirm adequate air exchange with good chest expansion. Central circulation is assessed by checking a brachial, carotid, or femoral pulse. Assessment of level of consciousness is performed serially to detect early changes.

Hypovolemic Shock. A child in hypovolemic shock may have a history of trauma, vomiting and diarrhea, or anorexia. The parent may report a decrease in wet diapers or explain that the child has not voided recently. With trauma, the child may demonstrate obvious signs of injury or bleeding or covert symptoms suggestive of blunt trauma.

The child in hypovolemic shock requires frequent assessment of vital signs, including blood pressure (every 15 to 60 minutes). Skin color, turgor, and temperature should be closely monitored. The anterior fontanel (if present) should be assessed to determine whether it is depressed or full. A depressed fontanel may be a manifestation of dehydration, whereas a full or level fontanel usually suggests that fluid volume is adequate.

In addition, the nurse assesses and monitors the child's neurologic status closely. A decreased or deteriorating level of consciousness should be reported promptly. The nurse auscultates heart and lungs and palpates peripheral pulses. Capillary refill time, moistness of mucous membranes, and general muscle tone and strength should be assessed and urine output closely monitored. In very young children, weighing the diapers quantifies urine output. If the child has diarrhea, a urine bag or Foley catheter should be placed to monitor urinary output. The abdomen should be palpated and auscultated for the presence of bowel sounds. Abdominal injury must be ruled out, especially if the abdominal girth appears to be increasing, with evidence of abdominal distention. Any abnormal bruising or obvious trauma must be recognized quickly, because blunt abdominal trauma is a major cause of shock in children.

Distributive Shock. Early signs of distributive shock include hyperthermia or hypothermia. The temperature should be closely monitored. In early shock (the hyperdynamic phase), the skin is typically warm and flushed. In late shock (the hypodynamic phase), skin is ashen and cold. An exception is in the case of spinal injury, in which the body cannot maintain a normal temperature. Shock of any etiology may cause microcirculatory dysfunction leading to abnormal function of coagulation factors and platelets. Therefore the nurse observes the skin closely for signs of petechiae, oozing of blood from invasive lines, or purpuric lesions. The presence of petechiae that are spread diffusely over the body may indicate severe sepsis. In children, hypotension is a late sign of all types of shock.

Cardiogenic Shock. A child with cardiogenic shock requires close monitoring of the heart and lungs for adventitious sounds. The liver should be palpated and its size measured. The child's respiratory effort must also be assessed. Retractions, grunting, and nasal flaring may be apparent. Periorbital and peripheral edema or other signs of cardiac failure may be present. Close monitoring of the peripheral pulses and capillary refill is extremely important.

Nursing Diagnosis and Planning

The following nursing diagnoses and expected outcomes may be appropriate after assessment of the child with shock:

- Ineffective Tissue Perfusion (cardiopulmonary, cerebral, peripheral) related to decreased fluid volume (in hypovolemic shock); abnormal distribution of blood flow, metabolic acidosis, or both (in distributive shock); or decreased cardiac contractility (in cardiogenic shock).

Expected Outcome. The child will maintain adequate tissue perfusion, as evidenced by strong peripheral pulses, appropriate skin turgor, normal capillary refill time, pink and warm mucous membranes and nail beds, vital signs within normal limits for age, and no evidence of dyspnea or altered mental status.

- Impaired Gas Exchange related to possible decreased pulmonary blood flow, increased interstitial fluid in alveoli, and inflammatory response of alveoli.

Expected Outcome. The child will have adequate gas exchange, as evidenced by oxygen saturation level between 95% and 100% and normal arterial blood gas measurements.

- Risk for Infection related to invasive venous and arterial lines, indwelling catheters, presence of endotracheal tube, possible incisional wounds, and compromised state.

Expected Outcome. The child will remain free from signs of infection, as evidenced by normal temperature, white blood cell (WBC) count within normal limits, no signs of redness or purulence from access sites, and negative blood cultures.

- Anxiety related to threat of a possible grave prognosis in a critically ill child.

Expected Outcomes. The child, if verbal, and parents will verbalize symptoms of anxiety, seek information to ensure understanding of the condition, and demonstrate adequate coping skills.

Interventions

Interventions for the child in shock are directed toward maintaining tissue perfusion by improving cardiac output, ensuring adequate oxygenation, preventing infection, and enhancing child and family coping.

Maintaining Tissue Perfusion. The nurse performs careful and frequent observation of the child's cardiovascular status. Take vital signs and assess circulation every 1 to 2 hours. After establishing an adequate IV access, administer appropriate fluid replacement. Maintain strict intake and output records, and report urine output that is abnormal for age (see Chapter 16) or any major discrepancy between intake and output. Weigh the child daily on the same scale. Report any rapid weight gain to the physician.

Because infants have high glucose requirements and low glycogen stores, alterations in glucose metabolism are frequently seen in response to stress. Monitor blood glucose levels every 2 to 4 hours.

Administer ordered medications by IV pump to ensure appropriate delivery of medication. Because vasoactive drugs can cause tissue necrosis if infiltration occurs in peripheral tissues, these agents are administered preferably through a central line.

Ensuring Oxygenation. The nurse observes and records respiratory rate and effort, skin color, chest expansion, and aeration. Note signs of respiratory distress and report them to the physician promptly. Oxygen is administered as ordered, ensuring that the delivery mode is appropriate for the child's age. Monitor oxygen saturation, arterial blood gases, and hemoglobin levels. Maintain a patent airway, and have emergency endotracheal intubation and ventilation equipment available. Ensure normothermia and control pain and anxiety to decrease oxygen demands. Place a gastric tube to decompress the stomach and allow full expansion of the thoracic cavity.

Preventing Infection. Because children in a compromised state are prone to infection, the nurse must maintain strict aseptic technique when handling IV lines, invasive tubes, and incisional or puncture sites. Closely monitor the child's temperature and report any rectal temperature greater than 38° C (100.4° F) or less than 36° C (96.8° F). Observe secretions and body fluids, incisions, and puncture sites for erythema, edema, or purulent drainage. Positive culture results and elevated WBCs are reported promptly to the physician. Administer ordered antipyretics as indicated and ensure adequate caloric intake. If the child is unable to tolerate oral or nasogastric feedings, discuss alternative methods of feeding with the physician.

Enhancing Coping. The nurse provides concise, accurate information to parents at frequent intervals. Further, the nurse determines the child's developmental level and level of comprehension and provides simple explanations to the child and parents of procedures before initiating them. Information is given in a calm, relaxed, and empathetic manner, answering all questions honestly. Allow the child and parents to express their feelings, concerns, and anxieties. Encourage the parents to participate in the child's care as appropriate (e.g., bathing, combing hair, feeding). This assistance provides them with some degree of control. Be nonjudgmental in response to parents' actions. Use available resources (e.g., social worker, chaplain, other family members) to help calm parents who are exhibiting uncontrolled feelings.

Elicit the parents' perceptions of the events and provide reassurance or clarify any misconceptions. Determine the availability of support systems and encourage their use. Help the parents identify coping mechanisms that have been effective in the past, and encourage parents to use these mechanisms during the current crisis.

■ Evaluation

- Does the child demonstrate pink mucous membranes, brisk capillary refill, alertness, responsiveness, and normal vital signs for age?
- Is the oxygen saturation at least 95% on room air, and are blood gas values within normal limits?

- Does the child demonstrate a normal breathing rate, pattern, and work of breathing?
- Is the child afebrile with negative culture results?
- Can the parents and child express their feelings to staff and significant others?
- Is the family demonstrating decreased anxiety by using available resources and effective coping mechanisms?

PEDIATRIC TRAUMA

Despite a marked decline in injury deaths among children since 1980, unintentional injuries are still the leading cause of morbidity and mortality among children in the United States (Borse, Gilchrist, Dellinger et al., 2008). The Centers for Disease Control and Prevention (CDC) has consistently found that motor vehicle injuries have the highest death rate in all children younger than 19 years of age (Borse et al., 2008). For infants under 1 year of age, two thirds of deaths are caused by suffocation, and drowning is the leading cause of injury deaths in those 1 to 4 years of age. Burns, poisoning, and falls are other unintentional injuries that are leading causes of fatal as well as nonfatal injuries requiring emergency department treatment (Borse et al., 2008). The term *injury* is used in preference to *accident* when describing trauma because some trauma is not accidental and much of it is preventable. Serious and fatal motor vehicle injuries can be reduced by over half with the use of age- and size-appropriate car and booster seats (National Highway Traffic Safety Administration [NHTSA], 2010b).

Injury prevention and education have been credited with a decrease in unintentional deaths among children. Despite this, much more needs to be done. Successful prevention and educational steps include motor vehicle safety restraints, firearm education, bicycle helmet programs, safety caps and locked medications, and eliminating potential hazards, such as old refrigerators and unfenced pools. Up-to-date educational resources can be obtained through organizations and websites such as those offered by the national Safe Kids USA campaign, the CDC, and the U.S. Consumer Product Safety Commission. When child victims of trauma are discharged from the emergency department, the nurse provides injury prevention information to the families. Injury prevention is also discussed at every well-child visit through adolescence (see Chapters 5 through 8).

Mechanism of Injury

Injuries can be categorized as *blunt, penetrating,* and *multiple trauma.* The most common areas of bodily injury (in order of frequency) are head, musculoskeletal system, abdomen, and thorax (Emergency Nurses Association [ENA], 2007). Knowing the mechanism of injury and recognizing anatomic and physiologic differences in the pediatric population help identify common injury patterns and predict the child's needs and outcomes.

Blunt Trauma

Blunt or penetrating force causes tissue trauma. Blunt trauma occurs more frequently than all other injuries combined (Roskind, Dayan, & Klein, 2011). Blunt trauma accounts for 80% of pediatric injuries (ENA, 2007). Injuries sustained from blunt trauma are often less apparent but, nevertheless, can be extremely serious.

Motor Vehicle Trauma. A common cause of blunt trauma is acceleration-deceleration force, often from motor vehicle collisions or falls. Just before a motor vehicle collision, both the occupant and the vehicle are traveling at the same speed. When the vehicle meets an opposing force, the speed of both the occupant and the vehicle rapidly decelerate. When this change occurs, four collisions take place: (1) the

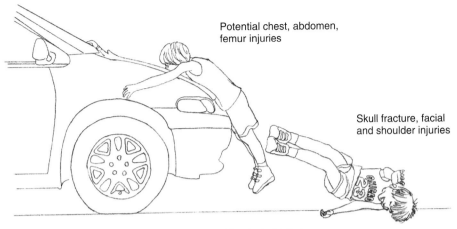

Potential chest, abdomen, femur injuries

Skull fracture, facial and shoulder injuries

FIG 10-1 Waddell's triad of injuries.

moving vehicle collides with the opposing object; (2) the occupant's body collides with the interior portion of the vehicle; (3) the occupant's internal organs and tissues collide with rigid internal structures; and (4) loose objects in the vehicle become projectile forces (Hawkins, 2004). Factors that affect the severity of motor vehicle collision injuries are the individual's location in the vehicle, impact speed, stopping distance, vehicle type, and restraint use (ENA, 2007).

Unrestrained occupants in a motor vehicle collision have a higher incidence of injury than restrained occupants have because they are tossed around the interior of the vehicle or are ejected at the point of collision. This principle applies also to children riding unrestrained in the back of open pickup trucks; they become missiles ejected out of the vehicle into oncoming traffic or onto the road. Children who are held on an adult's lap during a motor vehicle collision can be instantly crushed between the rigid part of the automobile and the moving adult.

Child safety seats and safety belts, *when appropriately sized and correctly installed,* can prevent injury and save lives. Since 1990, there have been approximately 260 child fatalities as a result of frontal airbag deployment (NHTSA, 2009). These injuries have been almost completely eradicated over the past 5 years thanks in part to a national safety campaign educating parents about placing children in the backseat, strict child passenger laws, and mandated car safety standards and airbag advancements (NHTSA, 2009). In 2011, the American Academy of Pediatrics issued recommendations for best safety practices related to child restraint systems and passenger vehicle safety: (1) rear-facing car safety seats for most infants up to 2 years of age; (2) forward-facing car safety seats for most children through 4 years of age; (3) belt-positioning booster seats for most children through 8 years of age; (4) lap-and-shoulder seatbelts for all who have outgrown booster seats; and (5) all children younger than 13 years ride in the rear seats of vehicles (Durbin, 2011).

Pedestrian Injury. Pedestrian injuries in children are also a significant problem, with the largest number of incidences occurring in children 5 to 14 years of age (Safe Kids USA, 2009b). In 2008, one in every five children between the ages of 5 and 9 years killed in traffic crashes were pedestrians (NHTSA, 2010a). Many of these injuries occur as the child darts out into the middle of the street between parked cars or stands unnoticed behind a vehicle backing out of a driveway. In general, pedestrian injuries occur in urban areas, at non-intersections, in normal weather conditions, and at night (NHTSA, 2010a).

When a child is hit by a motor vehicle, a triad of injuries, referred to as Waddell's triad, occurs (Figure 10-1). This one traumatic event results in three different types of injuries:

1. After being struck by the bumper and hood of the car, the child sustains abdominal or thoracic injuries.
2. The child is then propelled into the air, lands on the ground, and sustains femur or other leg injury, as well as surface trauma.
3. As the child is propelled like a missile to the ground, the large size and weight of the child's head result in skull fracture or closed head injury to the contralateral side of the head.

Penetrating Trauma

Penetrating trauma includes stabbing, firearms, blasting, and impaling injuries. Damage to the body tissue can result from the penetrating object itself and secondarily from radiating energy forces along the pathway of the penetrating object. The severity of an injury depends on the location of impact and the type of object. For example, with gunshot wounds, what might seem like a fairly innocuous wound can actually be severe, depending on factors such as projectile, fragmentation, type of tissue struck, and striking velocity. Injuries from a stab wound depend on length of the instrument, applied velocity, and angle of entry. Penetrating injuries account for 20% of pediatric injuries, and the incidence of gunshot wounds and nonfatal stabbing injuries is on the rise as a result of increased violence in younger children (ENA, 2007).

Multiple Trauma

A child with multiple trauma incurs injuries to more than one body system. A positive outcome for a child who has sustained multiple trauma depends on rapid assessment and intervention, which begin at the scene of the accident and continue through the trauma center emergency department, the critical care and acute care units, and the rehabilitation phase. Ideally, a critically injured child should be rapidly transported to a trauma facility with the personnel, equipment, and commitment to provide specialized care to children.

At the trauma center, and even in the emergency department of the community hospital, the presence of qualified trauma team members to assess and treat the trauma patient is crucial. A trauma team consists of skilled surgeons, other physicians, nurses, social workers, and other health care professionals, each with a specific role and duties during trauma resuscitation. The team assembles after notification of a patient's pending arrival and readies the trauma room with appropriate personnel and equipment.

All children with multiple trauma require a rapid, complete, and thorough assessment to determine the extent of injuries. The assessment of a child with multiple trauma includes primary and secondary surveys, with concurrent suitable interventions.

Primary Survey

The goal of the primary survey is to assess and manage life-threatening injuries. The primary assessment (see "Primary Assessment" section) proceeds with the following additions.

Airway Assessment and Management. Airway management is the priority. The airway is opened and maintained using the jaw-thrust maneuver to prevent movement of the cervical spine. The nurse inspects for loose teeth or other potential airway obstructions. Because the child's lower airway is narrow and easily obstructed by edema and mucus, oral suctioning may be required to keep the airway clear. All unresponsive and/or nonverbal trauma patients should have cervical spine protection until definitive diagnosis can be made (ENA, 2007). Cervical spine injury is uncommon, but the long-term results can be devastating. A pediatric cervical collar and immobilization board secure a child when spinal cord injury is a concern (Figure 10-2). To determine a correct fit, the cervical collar is measured for maximal stability: the chin must rest securely in the chin holder, with the collar below the ears and the lower end not extending below the upper part of the sternum. Any movement can worsen spinal cord injury and compromise the airway. The cervical immobilization device and spinal immobilization device (long backboard) must remain in place until spinal injury has been ruled out. Because of children's proportionately large occiput (head), it may be necessary to place padding under the shoulders for neutral alignment of the cervical spine to prevent flexion and airway compromise.

When an alert child is brought to the emergency setting in the car seat, the nurse places rolled towels on either side of the child's head and secures these with tape to maintain cervical immobilization without removing the child from the seat. The child can then remain in the car seat until radiographs have shown no injury to the cervical spine or until a change in status is noted.

Breathing Assessment and Management. Pulse oximetry readings are an adjunct to evaluating ventilation and adequate oxygenation. Oxygen use in the child with multiple trauma is not contraindicated; therefore the nurse starts supplemental oxygen at a rate of 10 to 15 L/min by mask. If the child is alert and does not tolerate the mask, using blow-by oxygen with the tubing only or using a plastic cup attached to the end of the tubing might be less threatening to a child.

If ventilation is inadequate or absent, the nurse begins to ventilate the child (see Table 10-1) using a bag-valve-mask ventilation device with a reservoir and high-flow oxygen. An oropharyngeal or nasopharyngeal airway maintains patency in a child with altered consciousness.

Endotracheal intubation may be needed for airway control and oxygenation in children with altered levels of consciousness, lack of spontaneous respirations, or severe head injuries. The nurse assists in evaluation of endotracheal tube placement after the procedure.

While observing the child for respiratory difficulty, the nurse checks the neck for obvious injuries. Jugular vein distention or tracheal deviation is difficult to assess in a child because of a shorter neck. If visualized, both findings are late signs of a tension pneumothorax. Because respiratory difficulty can be caused by chest injury, the nurse observes the chest for contusions, penetrations, abrasions, and paradoxic movement. Chest tube insertion or interventions for cardiac tamponade may be indicated for a penetrating chest injury, or an occlusive dressing may be taped on three sides for an open pneumothorax.

Severe facial trauma, although rare in children younger than 5 years, can be life threatening, primarily because of the potential to obstruct ventilation. Both fractures and soft tissue injury can cause narrowing of the airway. Facial trauma in children is treated as it is in adults. Nursing interventions include ensuring an adequate airway and breathing, observing for possible progressive obstruction, and keeping the injured areas clean to prevent infection.

Circulation Assessment and Management. Cardiovascular assessment of the child focuses on early recognition and treatment of hypovolemia. Blood loss in children is usually caused by internal abdominal or chest injury, severe injuries to the extremities, or surface head trauma. As previously discussed, early indicators of shock in children are tachycardia, increased capillary refill time (longer than 2 seconds), mottled skin, agitation or apprehension, pallor, and cool extremities. Decreased level of consciousness, dusky skin color, clammy extremities, bradycardia, and hypotension are late signs, indicating that cardiac arrest is imminent.

> **! NURSING QUALITY ALERT**
> ### *Artificial Airways*
>
> *Oropharyngeal airway:* Used in the unconscious child only. Determine the length of the airway by measuring the distance from the corner of the mouth to the tip of the earlobe. Use a tongue blade to depress and displace the tongue while inserting the airway curve down (in the anatomic position) and over the tongue.
>
> *Nasopharyngeal airway:* Select an airway with a diameter slightly less than the diameter of the child's nares, and determine the length of the airway by measuring the distance from the nares to the tragus of the ear. Make sure the bevel faces the septum regardless of which naris is used. Nasopharyngeal airways should be avoided in children with suspected or actual facial or head trauma.

Cardiac monitoring and frequent cardiovascular assessments are necessary during the acute stage. During this stage, any external hemorrhage is noted and controlled and IV or other access to the circulatory system is obtained.

The nurse assesses extremities for fractures and decreased peripheral circulation and splints any suspected fracture, assessing peripheral

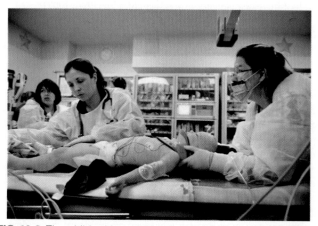

FIG 10-2 The child with multiple trauma injuries must remain on an immobilization board (long backboard) with a cervical immobilization device in place until the child has been evaluated for spinal injuries. (Courtesy Children's Medical Center, Dallas, TX.)

circulation after applying a splint. Assessment includes motor (Can the child move the extremity? Does the child feel pain?), circulatory (Does the child have good color, a strong pulse, and good capillary refill?), and neural function (Is sensation to the area intact? Does the child have any numbness or tingling in the extremity?). If neurovascular or circulatory compromise is present, immediate intervention is necessary.

Disability. During the primary survey phase, a brief neurologic examination is performed to establish level of consciousness, pupil size and reactivity, and muscle movement. AVPU can assess mental status. Sudden changes, such as agitation or somnolence, may indicate hypoxia or decreased cerebral perfusion.

Secondary Survey

After exposing the child by removing all of the child's clothing and providing warming measures, the trauma staff assesses for pain, carefully inspects and documents all signs of injury by performing the head-to-toe assessment (including log rolling the child to inspect the back), and obtains a history of the injury.

Obtaining a History of the Injury. Determining the degree and severity of injuries is both an art and a science. Diagnosis depends on knowing the mechanism of injury, as well as the presenting signs and symptoms. Nurses can obtain a comprehensive history by asking specific questions (Box 10-3). Thorough assessment depends on a systematic trauma evaluation, which takes place along with lifesaving intervention.

Trauma Scoring. On-site emergency medical personnel and nursing staff perform and document various kinds of scoring as part of the assessment process. A trauma score is used as an objective measure of the severity of the injury caused by a traumatic event and may be used to decide the facility most appropriate for treating the child. Most scoring systems are for the assessment of injury to adults and do not take into account the anatomical differences of children (Box 10-4).

Assessing for Child Abuse. Child maltreatment can be a cause of injury (see Chapter 29 for an in-depth discussion of child abuse).

Nurses working in emergency settings play an important role in both the assessment and reporting of child maltreatment. However, it is rare to have adequate time to assess parent-child interactions or observe at length the child's behavioral indicators, although these actions may provide important information. The following important indicators raise the suspicion of child maltreatment in the emergency setting:

- A history inconsistent with physical findings
- Activity reportedly leading to the trauma that seems inconsistent with the age and condition of the child
- Delay in seeking treatment for the trauma
- A history of other emergency-department visits

The following physical findings should also raise the level of suspicion for child maltreatment:

- Fractures in various stages of healing noted on radiography
- Injuries rarely found in children (e.g., long bone or rib fractures) when the history is not appropriate for the injury
- Patterns of injury indicating that a specific object caused injury (e.g., belt marks, cigarette burns)

The nurse carefully assesses these indicators in the context of the injury and in relation to the affect of the child and family. Bruises can be an indicator of abuse, but must be carefully evaluated in the appropriate developmental context. Children less than 9 months old rarely have bruising, but toddlers who are beginning to crawl and walk may have bruising on bony prominences. Caution should be used when evaluating the stages of bruising, as increasing evidence suggests this may not be an objective science (Harris, 2010). Bleeding conditions, Mongolian spots, and brittle bone disease can mimic the signs of abuse and should also be considered. The nurse observes the family's reaction to the child and staff, keeping in mind that people behave differently depending on culture, ethnicity, experience, and psychological makeup. Above all, health care providers do not assume an investigative role—that is law enforcement's responsibility. Nurses are required to report the suspicion of child maltreatment, however, and must carefully document all observations in detail. When child maltreatment is suspected, the intervention of child protective services is essential to ensure the safety of the child (and that of other children in the home) and to prevent additional injury.

Nursing Considerations
The Child and Family

The most critical aspect of nursing care of the child with traumatic injury is continuous assessment of respiratory, circulatory, and neurologic status. The nurse observes injured children for the early signs of shock and intervenes immediately to prevent rapid and irreversible

---

BOX 10-3   HISTORY OF INJURY QUESTIONS

For a Victim of a Motor Vehicle Collision
- Was the child wearing a seatbelt or in a child's car seat?
- What was the type of seatbelt (lap or lap-and-shoulder or car seat)?
- What was the speed of the motor vehicle?
- With what did the motor vehicle collide?
- At what location on the motor vehicle was the point of impact?
- Where was the victim seated in the motor vehicle?
- How much damage was done to the motor vehicle?

For a Victim of a Fall
- How far did the child fall?
- How did the child land (on what part of the body)?
- On what type of surface did the child land?
- Was the child's fall broken by any objects?

For a Victim of a Penetrating Injury
- How long and how wide was the blade of the knife?
- How far away was the gun when it was fired?
- What type of gun was used, and what was the caliber of the gun?

BOX 10-4   TRAUMA SCORING SYSTEMS

Trauma Score (TS)
- Adult scoring tool sometimes used with children
- Assesses respiratory rate and effort, blood pressure, and capillary refill
- Includes the Glasgow Coma Scale (GCS)

Revised Trauma Score (RTS)
- Composed of the GCS, blood pressure, and respiratory rate

Pediatric Trauma Score (PTS)
- Adapted for the pediatric client
- Assesses size, airway, central nervous system response, systolic blood pressure, open wounds, and skeletal fractures

deterioration. Preparing for the many procedures and examinations required and observing the equipment used for monitoring should not interfere with close and continuous observation of the child's signs and symptoms.

Nursing care of the child also requires care of the family. When the family arrives at the hospital, one staff member should become the contact person and provide regular updates. The hospital staff supports family members when they visit their critically ill child. Information concerning their child's condition should be provided simply but completely, incorporating the family's educational and emotional status and readiness to learn. Family members are encouraged to touch and talk to their child if they so desire. Family presence during resuscitation and invasive procedures has been shown to facilitate healthy grieving and support the belief that everything possible was done in the event that their child dies as a result of injury or illness (ENA, 2007). Additionally, health care providers report there is no interruption in care delivery when someone (e.g., chaplain, social worker) is designated to stay with the family and provide updates. Remember that informed consent must be obtained from the families of children for all procedures unless the intervention is required to save the child's life.

The Child during Recovery

Regardless of the cause of the injury, most children with traumatic injury do well unless the injuries are extremely severe. Their cardiovascular systems are strong and their bodies are growing, allowing them to compensate for even the most serious injuries. Even children with severe traumatic brain injuries (TBIs) have far more favorable chances of recovery than do adults. Children 0 to 4 years old sustain TBIs 30% more often than any age-group, but comprise the lowest number of TBI-related hospitalizations and deaths (Faul, Xu, Wald, & Coronado, 2010). Children and their families require nursing support to recover from both the physical and psychological effects of trauma; the need for rehabilitation must be considered from the moment the child arrives in the emergency setting.

? CRITICAL THINKING EXERCISE 10-1

You are working in a small emergency department when a father brings in his 6-year-old daughter, who has been struck by a car while riding a bicycle. She is in her father's arms, her eyes are closed, and she is pale with mottled lower extremities. Blood is on the father's clothes.

1. What are the key elements of your primary assessment? What are you looking for?
2. What questions would you ask the father to obtain the history?
3. What do you think is wrong with her? Is this an emergency? Why or why not?
4. What interventions would you do? Which would you do first? Why?
5. What responses to your interventions would be expected? Why?

INGESTIONS AND POISONINGS

The term *poison exposure* is defined as the ingestion of or contact with a substance that can produce toxic effects (National Center for Injury Prevention and Control [NCIPC] Division of Unintentional Injury Prevention, 2008). The combination of small weight and size, curiosity, lack of fear, and evolving mobility places all children at risk of injury or death from toxic exposure and ingestion. Differences exist, however, in types of incident by age-group. Younger children (1 through 5 years of age) are indiscriminately curious and can innocently ingest a toxic

substance in a matter of seconds. As children grow, they gradually learn from parents to avoid dangerous substances, but accidental ingestions and exposures still can occur. In adolescence, the risk is higher for deliberate ingestion.

Incidence

More than half of all poison exposures occur among children younger than 6 years. The mortality rate from poisonings is higher in the adolescent population as a result of adolescents using poisons to cause self-harm (NCIPC, 2008). More than 90% of all poison exposures occur in homes. Most poisonings occur as a result of oral ingestion. Ocular or dermal exposure, inhalation, parenteral exposure, and envenomation (e.g., an animal or insect bite) account for the remainder of poisoning incidents. Children are poisoned by plants; household and personal care products such as cosmetics, cleaning substances, and medicines; lead; and carbon monoxide. Adolescent poisoning tends to occur as a result of alcohol, and prescription and nonprescription drug ingestions.

Manifestations

Assessment and treatment of toxic exposure and ingestion go hand in hand. Although identification of the type and amount of the exposure is important, the child must initially be treated on the basis of physical signs and symptoms.

An accurate history of the ingestion is useful in planning for the child's care. History given by the child, parent, friend, or caretaker may not always be accurate or complete—areas of confusion are often present, especially in cases of unwitnessed ingestions. The information obtained in the history of the ingestion is combined with the child's presenting physical assessment to provide a complete picture of the event and plan treatment. Laboratory analysis in some cases may provide definitive diagnosis.

Most ingestions seen in emergency settings occur acutely, and the child is brought in immediately or when parents realize the event has occurred. An exception to this is lead poisoning. Although lead poisoning is relatively common, with an estimated 1 million children having elevated levels, it is rarely identified in the emergency setting. A child who has unusual neurologic signs or symptoms, neuropathy, or anemia that cannot be attributed to other causes may have lead poisoning. Elevated blood lead levels result primarily from exposure to lead-based paint or lead-contaminated dust and soil. Older miniblinds, improperly glazed pottery, folk remedies, toys, and cosmetics are also reported sources of lead poisoning (National Center for Environmental Health [NCEH], 2009b). A careful history can assist in the diagnosis of lead poisoning, but testing serum lead levels provides the only accurate diagnosis. The child with a markedly elevated lead level usually is admitted to the hospital. Chelation therapy, if needed, is administered on an inpatient basis to remove lead from the blood and tissue. When a child is found to have elevated lead levels, other children in the home should be tested as well because of the environmental nature of the ingestion.

Diagnostic Evaluation

In cases of known or suspected ingestion, laboratory tests can be performed to assess serum levels of the substance and the effects of the toxin on body systems. Regional poison control centers and clinical pharmacists should be included as members of the treatment team. Measurements of serum glucose level and toxicology analysis of urine, serum, and stomach contents are the most common laboratory tests ordered for possible toxic exposure or ingestion. Blood gases and chest radiographs are required if the child is hypoventilating, has other respiratory difficulties, or has been exposed to a hydrocarbon (e.g., gasoline) or bleach. Baseline liver enzymes and kidney function tests may be checked if the suspected substance is known to be toxic to these organs.

Therapeutic Management

The first step in treatment of a toxic exposure or ingestion is to assess ABCDEs and stabilize the child. Oxygen can be given and breathing supported with a bag-valve-mask ventilation device if necessary. If the child's level of consciousness is altered, endotracheal intubation may be necessary to protect the airway. When the child has ingested a sufficient amount of a substance to cause rapid deterioration in mental status, an intubation tray should be at the bedside even when the child is awake and alert. If the child is in shock or shows signs of compensated shock, IV fluid resuscitation is initiated. Cardiac rhythm disturbances can result from many ingested substances, so placement of a cardiac monitor and pulse oximeter is also indicated. Seizure precautions should be instituted in exposures to toxins with neurologic or metabolic side effects.

Care of the child who has been exposed to or ingested a toxic substance depends on the amount ingested and the toxicity of the ingested substance (Table 10-5). After initial stabilization, removing the poison, preventing its absorption, and limiting complications are primary goals. Several methods frequently used to treat toxic exposures and ingestions include removal of dermal and ocular toxins, dilution of the toxin, administration of activated charcoal, and administration of an antidote. For most pediatric poison ingestion cases, gastric lavage is no longer recommended because of the risk of aspiration and further injury (O'Donnell & Ewald, 2011).

Removal of Dermal and Ocular Toxins

Removing the child from a toxic environment, including removing contaminated clothes, brushing chemical powders from skin, and liberal washing, is mandatory with skin exposure. Copious irrigation of the eyes with water or normal saline is imperative with an ocular exposure. In cases of exposure to an alkaline substance, irrigation proceeds until the eyes return to a normal pH (see Chapter 31).

Diluting the Ingested Toxin

Acid or alkali substances, when ingested, can cause burning of tissue along the gastrointestinal tract. Because these caustic substances continue to cause damage until neutralized, inducing emesis is contraindicated.

Administration of syrup of ipecac in the home setting is no longer recommended. Parents are advised to call the poison control center immediately if they suspect their child has ingested a poisonous substance.

Activated Charcoal

Activated charcoal is a charcoal substance with a porous surface that binds to the toxin and passes it through the gastrointestinal system. Activated charcoal has become the recommended treatment for acute poisonings in the pediatric population and is most effective when

TABLE 10-5   COMMON POISONOUS SUBSTANCES

SUBSTANCE	PATHOPHYSIOLOGY	CLINICAL MANIFESTATIONS	TREATMENT
Acetaminophen (Tylenol, in many over-the-counter products)			
Toxic dose: uncertain, do not exceed recommended levels Seriousness of ingestion determined by amount ingested and length of time before intervention and if toxicity is acute or cumulative Other factors, such as decreased oral intake, have been linked with hepatotoxicity	Metabolic byproducts deplete liver glutathione and cause damage to hepatic cells. Children younger than 6 yr seem to be more resistant to development of hepatotoxicity than older children and adults.	*First stage* (first 24 hr): malaise, nausea, vomiting, sweating, pallor, weakness. *Second stage* (24-48 hr): latent period with a rise in liver enzymes (aspartate and alanine aminotransferase) and bilirubin; right upper quadrant pain; prolonged prothrombin time. *Third stage* (3-7 days): jaundice, liver necrosis, signs of hepatic failure. *Fourth stage* (5-7 days): recovery or progression to death.	Administer antidote: *N*-acetylcysteine (Mucomyst) as ordered. IV fluids. Within 1-2 hr post-ingestion, administer activated charcoal. Sodium-restricted, high-calorie, high-protein diet.
Salicylates (aspirin, in many over-the-counter products, oil of wintergreen)			
Toxic dose: single dose exceeding 200-280 mg/kg Peak gastric absorption occurs within 2 hr of ingestion	*First stage:* stimulation of respiratory center, leading to respiratory alkalosis. *Second stage:* loss of potassium; increase in metabolic rate; accumulation of ketones leading to metabolic acidosis, hypokalemia, and dehydration. Inhibition of prothrombin formation, decreased platelet levels and adhesiveness, capillary fragility (chronic poisoning).	Gastrointestinal effects: nausea, vomiting, thirst. Central nervous system effects: hyperventilation, tinnitus, confusion, seizures, coma, respiratory failure, circulatory collapse. Renal effect: oliguria. Hematopoietic effects: bleeding tendencies. Metabolic effects: sweating, dehydration, fever, hyponatremia, hypokalemia, dehydration, hypoglycemia.	Administer activated charcoal to decrease absorption. IV fluids, sodium bicarbonate (enhances excretion), potassium replacement; volume expanders as needed to support circulation. Vitamin K for bleeding tendencies (chronic poisoning). Glucose for hypoglycemia. Hemodialysis in severe cases if child unresponsive to therapy.

Continued

TABLE 10-5 COMMON POISONOUS SUBSTANCES—cont'd

SUBSTANCE	PATHOPHYSIOLOGY	CLINICAL MANIFESTATIONS	TREATMENT
Corrosives (toilet and drain cleaners, bleach, ammonia)			
Extent of damage depends on causticity of substance and amount ingested	Severe chemical burns of mouth, throat, esophagus. "Splash" burns of eyes and skin. Alkali substances can continue to cause damage after initial contact. If damage is severe, long-term care is needed, including gastric button or tube, repeated esophageal dilations, and surgical repair of esophagus, sometimes with colon tissue transplant (done when child is older).	Whitish burns of mouth and pharynx, color darkens (red, swollen, oozing as ulcerations form and tissue erodes). Edema, difficulty swallowing, drooling. Respiratory distress, pain. Residual difficulty swallowing; subsequent healing of burns can produce esophageal strictures. Severe burns causing perforation can lead to vascular collapse and shock.	IV fluids while NPO (nothing by mouth). Analgesics, steroids, antibiotics, nasogastric tube feedings.
Hydrocarbons (gasoline, paint thinner, lighter fluid, turpentine, furniture polish)			
	Chemical pneumonitis from aspiration of hydrocarbon. Pneumonia and acute hemorrhagic necrotizing disease, usually in 24 hr.	Burning sensation in mouth and pharynx. Characteristic petroleum breath odor. Nausea, vomiting, anorexia, central nervous system depression, fever. Respiratory distress, wheezing.	Prevent vomiting. Support ventilation; administer oxygen. IV fluids.
Lead (paint chips from older homes, soil contaminated with lead, lead solder used in plumbing, vinyl miniblinds, improperly glazed pottery, toys)			
Diet high in fat and low in iron and calcium increases lead absorption Serum lead level >10 mcg/dL: considered harmful; 10-15 mcg/dL: more frequent screening indicated; 15-20 mcg/dL: nutritional and educational interventions and environmental investigation; 20 mcg/dL: possible removal and treatment	Gastrointestinal tract is major route of absorption. Lead is deposited in blood, bone, and soft tissue. Major toxic effects occur in bone marrow, nervous system, and kidney. Amount of lead ingested, size of the particle, and repeated ingestion over time contribute to severity of lead poisoning.	Symptoms may be vague with insidious onset. Central nervous system effects: irritability, lethargy, hyperactivity, cognitive and perceptual motor difficulties, clumsiness, seizures, coma, and death (associated with blood level of 100 mg/dL). Hematopoietic effect: anemia. Gastrointestinal effects: anorexia, nausea, vomiting, constipation, lead line along gums. Skeletal effects: increased density of long bones, lead line in long bones. Renal effects: glycosuria, proteinuria, possible acute or chronic renal failure. Kidney damage is reversible early in the disease, but with continued lead exposure, permanent kidney damage may occur.	Level >25 mcg/dL: remove child from lead source, hospitalize if level is significantly higher. Administer chelating agents: Succimer (Chemet) orally for lead level of 35-45 mcg/dL; EDTA for level >70 mcg/dL given IV over several hours for 5 days (causes lead to be deposited in bone and excreted by kidneys); bronchoalveolar lavage every 4 hr for six doses for level >70 mcg/dL. Monitor kidney function because EDTA is nephrotoxic; monitor calcium levels because EDTA enhances excretion of calcium. Provide adequate hydration. Calcium, phosphorus, and vitamins C and D. Anticonvulsants. Oral or intramuscular iron for anemia. Follow-up lead levels to monitor progress (lead is excreted more slowly than it accumulates in the body).
Carbon Monoxide			
Most often from improperly ventilated heaters; also from poorly ventilated vehicles. Cause of the exposure should be determined and eliminated.	An odorless, colorless gas that binds to receptors on hemoglobin more effectively than does oxygen, thereby causing hypoxia.	Headache, visual disturbances. Altered level of consciousness, cherry-red lips and cheeks, nausea, and vomiting.	100% oxygen by rebreathing mask. Serum carboxyhemoglobin levels, hyperbaric chamber treatment may be necessary for clients with high carboxyhemoglobin levels. Other interventions based on signs and symptoms. Prevention—carbon monoxide detectors in every home

administered within 60 minutes of ingestion. Activated charcoal can bind to the toxin at any point along the gastrointestinal tract.

Activated charcoal may be administered with sorbitol to facilitate elimination of bound substances and prevent constipation. Administering activated charcoal is a nursing challenge because the substance is unpalatable in both taste and appearance to young children. In the toddler, having the child sit on a parent's lap and administering charcoal by oral syringe may be successful. Mixing the activated charcoal with chocolate milk or other flavoring sometimes makes it easier to drink. Placing the charcoal in a covered opaque or decorated container prevents the child from seeing the substance while drinking. Activated charcoal administration can be repeated, especially in delayed release suspensions, to prevent reabsorption of the toxin from fluid secreted in the biliary tract. The dosage is usually 1 g/kg in children.

Antidotes

Specific antidotes can be used to inhibit the absorption of the toxin at the receptor site or reduce the concentration. Examples of commonly used antidotes are *N*-acetylcysteine (Mucomyst) for significant acetaminophen ingestion and naloxone (Narcan) for narcotics (see Table 10-5).

NURSING CARE OF THE CHILD WHO HAS INGESTED A TOXIC SUBSTANCE

■ Assessment

Accurate and rapid assessment of the poisoned child can mean the difference between life and death. The nurse starts by assessing ABCDEs and taking frequent vital signs. Initiate respiratory or circulatory support as needed. Because shock is a result of ingestion of many toxic substances, blood pressure, tissue perfusion, and urine output are carefully monitored. Observe and document the child's mental status frequently to determine any changes in level of consciousness. Assess changes in pupil size or reactivity, as well as the occurrence of seizures.

The nurse needs to take the responsibility for assessing the cause of poisoning. A poison exposure is extremely distressing to parents. If the ingestion was purposeful, psychological consultation and referral should be provided. In some cases, child abuse must be ruled out.

■ Nursing Diagnosis and Planning

The following diagnoses apply to the child and family:

- Risk for Injury related to insufficient parental knowledge about first aid for toxic ingestion and accidental poisonings.

Expected Outcome. The parent will describe how to assess the child and access appropriate treatment if accidental poisoning occurs.

- Ineffective Breathing Pattern related to effects of toxic substances.

Expected Outcome. The child will breathe in a way that maintains adequate oxygenation and ventilation, as evidenced by normal arterial blood gases and serum pH or pulse oximetry readings.

- Risk for Deficient Fluid Volume related to effects of ingested substances, treatment modalities, or decreased fluid intake.

Expected Outcome. The child will maintain an hourly urine output appropriate for weight and age, with age-appropriate specific gravity.

- Compromised Family Coping related to sudden hospitalization and emergency aspects of illness.

Expected Outcomes. The family will appropriately discuss the child's condition and treatment, verbalize feelings and concerns, and remain with the child as much as possible.

- Risk for Poisoning related to insufficient parental knowledge about poisoning prevention.

Expected Outcome. The parent makes the necessary changes in the home environment to prevent future poisoning.

■ Interventions

Stabilizing the child is the nurse's priority in caring for the child who has ingested a poisonous substance. Nursing care also includes reducing the child's and the family's fear and anxiety, providing preventive teaching concerning the storage of poisons and supervision of children, and removal of the poison from the child's skin and mucous membranes to reduce further injury.

> **! NURSING QUALITY ALERT**
>
> *Assessment of Poison Ingestion*
>
> Obtain information about the following:
> - Substance ingested, if known
> - Amount ingested (how many pills are missing?)
> - Approximate time of ingestion
> - Change in the child's condition
> - Treatment administered at home

Parents usually are overwhelmed by feelings of guilt, fear, and anger when their child has ingested a poisonous substance. Providing an opportunity for them to express their feelings in a nonjudgmental atmosphere helps parents cope with this experience. Some aspects of treatment, such as placement of a gastric tube or support of ventilation, are disturbing and frightening to parents. Offer support by explaining treatment, including the parents in care (as appropriate), and informing them about their child's status.

Ideally, nurses intervene with parents (and other caregivers such as grandparents, older siblings, and childcare providers) before a poison exposure occurs. Knowledge of safety and "safe proofing" the child's environment is important. Discussion of safe storage of medications and other potentially toxic substances and age-appropriate supervision of children are essential aspects of poison prevention. Advise the parent to post the poison control phone number clearly and to call the poison center before treating the child. This and other injury prevention information should be readily available in daycare, primary care, and emergency care settings and should be given to families proactively. Education through community programs to prevent poisoning and reduce drug abuse should be directed to the parents and caretakers of young children, as well as to adolescents. Simple ideas such as storing medication in the original containers and placing in locked cabinets, labeling all cleaning product containers and placing these out of the reach of children, and never calling medication "candy" should be promoted.

■ Evaluation

- Do parents describe the appropriate actions to take in the event of a future poisoning?
- Are the child's oxygen saturation, blood gas measurements, and level of consciousness within normal limits?
- Is the child's hourly urine output appropriate for age and weight?
- Are family members remaining with the child and able to provide adequate support?
- Can parents and other caregivers describe poison prevention (e.g., keeping common poisonous household hazards out of the child's reach)? Do they have easy access to the poison control telephone number?

ENVIRONMENTAL EMERGENCIES

Active children are exposed to a variety of environmental hazards. Injuries from animal and snake bites, submersion injuries, and sun- and heat-related illnesses account for the majority of environmental injuries. This section focuses on animal, human, and snake and spider bites; submersion injuries; and heat-related illnesses. Sunburn is discussed in Chapter 25.

Animal, Human, Snake, and Spider Bites

Etiology

Animal and Human Bites. Both animal and human bites involve soft tissue damage from crushing, lacerations, and puncture wounds. All animal bites have potential for infection. Although human bites are relatively rare, they carry the greatest risk of infection if they break the skin, particularly if they are on the scalp, face, hands, wrists, or feet. Serious injury can result from any type of bite, but most bites are not life threatening.

Snake and Spider Bites. Envenomation of children on land is usually from snakes, scorpions, and spiders. Envenomation can also result from marine animals, such as jellyfish, sea urchins, and stingrays. Fatalities from envenomation are rare; most fatalities occur from snake bites.

Incidence

Animal bites in children are most often from dogs and have the highest incidence in boys ages 5 to 9 years old (CDC, 2008). Breed-specific data is difficult to obtain because of the large number of mixed-breed dogs and reporting challenges, but anecdotal data regarding aggressive breeds have prompted breed-specific legislation (CDC, 2008). There are relatively few fatalities as a result of dog bites, and most injuries in children are in the head and neck region (CDC, 2008).

Bites from pet birds, rats, ferrets, pigs, hamsters, turtles, fish, alligators, snakes, horses, and many other animals have been seen in emergency settings, as have bites from a variety of wild animals, such as raccoons, skunks, and coyotes.

In the United States, there are two groups of poisonous snakes: Crotalids or pit vipers such as rattlesnakes, water moccasins, and copperheads; and Elapids such as coral snakes. Children should be taught to avoid snakes, and health care providers should be familiar with snakes indigenous to their area. Bites from only two types of spiders in the United States can cause significant illness: the black widow spider and the brown recluse spider.

Manifestations

Animal and Human Bites. Because of the risk of infection, human bites are more serious and can be differentiated from dog bites by the distance between the canine teeth; in human bites the distance is generally greater than 3 cm. A human bite is horseshoe shaped and rarely breaks the skin. Localized tissue damage and multibacterial infections are serious manifestations of animal and human bites. Dog bites run an additional risk because of the crush injuries that ensue.

Snake Bites. To determine the cause of envenomation, medical staff in emergency settings should have some knowledge of the venomous snakes likely to be encountered in the surrounding geographic area.

Smaller children are usually bitten on the hand or foot, whereas older children are more commonly bitten on lower extremities.

Regardless of whether the snake can be positively identified, treatment should be based on physical assessment and symptoms. The following local signs and symptoms most commonly suggest envenomation from a snake:

- Bite marks that look like fang marks
- Burning at the site
- Ecchymosis and erythema
- Pain or numbness
- Progressing edema

The following systemic signs and symptoms suggest severe envenomation:

- Nausea, vomiting
- Sweating, chills
- Numbness, paresthesia of the tongue and perioral region
- Hypotension
- Coagulopathies

When a substantial amount of venom has been injected and when treatment is delayed, envenomation can progress to coagulopathies, respiratory failure, renal failure, seizures, shock, and (rarely) death. Because of advancements in antivenin preparation and availability, significant injury can be prevented with early treatment. However, any child with a suspected or actual venomous snake bite should be monitored closely in the hospital for at least 24 hours even if antivenin has been administered (Schroeder & Norris, 2011).

Spider Bites. Bites from neurotoxic spiders such as the black widow are very painful and possible systemic effects include hypertension, tachycardia, bradycardia, diaphoresis, increased salivation, and muscle spasms. A bite from a brown recluse spider can cause significant local tissue necrosis and, in rare cases, systemic toxicity with presenting signs of fever, chills, nausea, malaise, rash, and petechiae progressing to hemolysis, coagulopathy, and renal failure (Schroeder & Norris, 2011).

Therapeutic Management

Animal Bites. Emergency care for animal bites depends on the type of bite but usually includes thorough irrigation and débridement. The affected extremity should be kept in a dependent position to prevent changes in toxicity related to gravity or circulatory impairment. Tetanus prophylaxis is given if the child's immunization is not up to date or if documentation is unavailable. Antibiotics are prescribed when a high probability of infection exists. Smaller bite wounds are often left open rather than sutured because puncture wounds and wounds closed with sutures have more potential for infection. A specialist should be consulted if tendon, bone, or compartment injury is suspected. Treatment of the child for rabies may be necessary, especially in cases of wild-animal (e.g., raccoon, rat, and skunk) bites.

Snake Bites. The following three factors influence the severity of bite from a venomous snake:

- The child's age, size, and general health
- Size of the snake (larger snakes produce more venom)
- Location of the injury (peripheral injuries account for 90% of the bites and are less severe)

When assessing the child with a snake bite, identification of the type of snake is helpful, but this is not always possible. In most cases, an expert in the treatment of snake bites should be consulted. Emergency treatments (e.g., use of a tourniquet, incision, and extraction of the venom; electric shock therapy; cryotherapy) are not recommended and can result in complications. First aid (after assessment and maintenance of the ABCs) includes washing with soap and water; immobilization of the extremity in a dependent position; removal of clothes, rings, and other constricting items; and rapid transport to an emergency facility.

In the hospital setting, emergency management continues assessment and maintenance of the ABCs, insertion of an IV line if envenomation is suspected, and laboratory studies, including CBC, coagulation studies, electrolytes, creatinine phosphokinase, and urinalysis, to assist in determination of need for antivenin therapy. Children with symptoms should be admitted to the hospital. In cases of moderate to severe envenomation, the negative side effects of antivenin must be weighed against the positive effects. Antivenin therapy is the mainstay of treatment for snake bites. Indications for administration include worsening injury, coagulation abnormalities, or systemic effects.

Spider Bites. Supportive care is the focus for management of spider bites. In severe cases, antivenin may be administered to reduce pain and reverse systemic effects from a black widow spider bite. The wound from a brown recluse spider bite requires daily cleansing and intermittent ice therapy for the first 3 days; antibiotics are given to prevent a secondary bacterial infection. Systemic disease is managed with medications and IV fluids because recluse spider antivenin is not available in the United States.

Nursing Considerations

With severe bites, significant envenomation, or anaphylaxis, nursing interventions for bites and envenomation begin with attention to the ABCDEs and support of vital body functions. With envenomation, nursing care includes keeping the child as calm as possible to help prevent spread of the toxin or venom. Hospitals may not have sufficient antivenin for severe envenomations, so nurses should make sure that available protocols include the location of centers to contact for additional antivenin.

The injury site of all bites is carefully cleaned and tetanus prophylaxis is administered if immunizations are not up to date. When the bite or envenomation is located on an extremity, the nurse immobilizes the extremity. Measuring the circumference of the affected extremity every 20 to 30 minutes will track progression of the injury, as well as results of treatment.

If antivenin is to be administered, a thorough history of allergies is obtained because the most common antivenins are made from horse serum. Antivenin is most effective if given within 4 to 6 hours after injury, but it may be repeated if coagulopathies or bleeding is present. The nurse documents the type and location of the injury, the length of time since the injury, and the signs and symptoms resulting from the injury. All children who require antivenin should be monitored in an intensive care setting. To assess hypersensitivity, a small test dose of antivenin is given intradermally before the full dose.

Education concerning avoiding snake habitats, wearing protective clothing, and avoiding provocative behavior around snakes should be emphasized.

In most states, notification of the local animal control agency is required for animal bites. The rabies immunization status of the animal, if available, should be documented in nursing notes. Quarantine of the animal responsible for the attack may be necessary if the animal can be found. Nurses should advise parents to observe the child closely for changes in behavior and refer for counseling, if needed.

Discharge instructions should include observation for signs and symptoms of infection and wound care. The nurse provides injury prevention education to all families. This includes giving parents information about how to teach their children to avoid animal bites by avoiding strange animals and provocative behavior in dealing with enraged animals.

Submersion Injuries (Near Drowning)

Known as the "silent event," submersion injury is the second and third leading cause of unintentional death in children 1 to 4 years old and 10 to 14 years, respectively (Borse et al., 2008). *Drowning* is submersion that results in asphyxia and death within 24 hours. If the child survives longer than 24 hours after submersion, the event is referred to as *near drowning.*

One of the most important nursing responsibilities related to drowning is prevention of injury, including water safety education and training, support of legislative efforts to pass drowning prevention measures, and teaching CPR to families. Nurses must emphasize the importance of adequate adult supervision when children are in or around bodies of water.

Etiology

Most drownings happen in residential swimming pools, although drownings can occur in any body of water, including hot tubs, spas, bathtubs, toilets, and even buckets. Open water sites, such as lakes, rivers, and oceans, are more likely to be the site of accidents among teenagers. Alcohol is often a factor in teenage drownings because it alters judgment and increases risk-taking behaviors.

Incidence

Although death by drowning in the child younger than 14 years of age has decreased over the past 15 years, more than 800 children in this age-group die annually and in excess of 4000 children require emergency department treatment (Safe Kids USA, 2009a). Nearly 40% of these children are in the toddler age-group. Boys are two to four times more likely than girls to die from drowning. Swimming pools, lakes, ponds, and bathtubs are common locations of drownings.

PATHOPHYSIOLOGY

Submersion Injury

Hypoxia causes the injury to organ systems when drowning occurs. Drowning progresses in a predictable sequence of events. Drowning victims panic, struggle, and attempt to hold their breath. In doing so, they begin to swallow water, which is then vomited and aspirated. This process can cause laryngospasm, which leads to hypoxia, seizures, and death (called *dry drowning* because laryngospasm prevents large amounts of water from entering the respiratory system). If the child becomes unconscious before laryngospasm, hypoxia causes loss of airway reflexes and subsequent aspiration of large amounts of water (leading to *wet drowning*). As hypoxia and acidosis progress, cardiopulmonary arrest occurs. Swallowing large amounts of fresh water also causes electrolyte shifts into the intracellular spaces, resulting in hyponatremia and cerebral edema.

Submerged children lose body heat quickly in cold water because of their relatively large body surface area. Severe hypothermia offers some protection to the brain through the diving reflex, which is stimulated when the face is submerged in cold water. This neurologic reflex shunts blood away from the periphery, increasing blood flow to the brain and heart. The diving reflex is stronger in young children. Irreversible brain damage usually occurs after 4 to 6 minutes of submersion, but some children have had a complete recovery after lengthy submersion (10 to 40 minutes) in very cold water.

Manifestations

The child's condition after near drowning varies with the extent of injury. Factors that may contribute to the child's eventual prognosis are: (1) age, (2) submersion time, (3) water temperature, (4) elapsed time before resuscitation efforts are instituted, and (5) neurologic status. A child with the poorest prognosis is one who was submerged longer than 10 minutes, received CPR for longer than 25 minutes, arrived at the emergency department in deep coma (Glasgow Coma Scale score of 5 or lower), and did not regain consciousness within the first 48 to 72 hours of hospitalization (Shephard & Quan, 2011).

The child who is conscious with adequate respirations might have mild hypothermia, show slight pulmonary changes on radiography, and demonstrate minor blood gas alterations. Children who are unconscious (stuporous or comatose) demonstrate consequences related to whether respirations are present or absent. If respirations are adequate, the child may have mild to moderate hypothermia and mild to moderate respiratory distress with abnormal chest radiography and arterial blood gas results. The child who has required resuscitative efforts is in markedly poorer condition, with altered mental status, metabolic acidosis and other arterial blood gas abnormalities, electrolyte disturbances, possible seizures, or shock, and may develop disseminated intravascular coagulation. Death is the result of complete cardiopulmonary arrest or cerebral anoxic-ischemic injury. Most long-term sequelae of near drowning are neurologic in origin (Shephard & Quan, 2011).

Therapeutic Management

Prehospital Emergency Management. Treatment begins at the scene of the submersion with rescue and removal from the water. The prehospital care the child receives can significantly affect the chances for a normal recovery. Prompt initiation of CPR and activation of the emergency medical system are imperative. The goal of prehospital care is to maintain adequate oxygenation and circulation, minimize secondary organ damage, and take proper precautions to stabilize possible cervical spine injuries.

Every child with submersion injury is considered hypoxic. When the brain is deprived of oxygen for even a short period, irreversible brain damage can occur. After the child's airway is opened, the nurse suctions the child's oropharynx to remove mucus and fluid and delivers 100% oxygen by mask or by bag-valve-mask ventilation device in the child with inadequate respiratory rate or effort. Overinflation of the lungs must be avoided to prevent a pneumothorax. Pulse oximetry may not be available in prehospital management or may be inaccurate in the child with hypothermia. Assessment of breath sounds, chest symmetry and rise and fall, and central color are more reliable indicators of adequate respirations.

Elevating the head of the bed to 30 degrees may help lower intracranial pressure but should be done only if no spinal injury or shock is present. Intubation should be performed for unconscious and non-breathing children.

A cardiac monitor is used for ongoing assessment of heart rate and rhythm. Ventricular fibrillation or asystole that is unresponsive to resuscitative efforts can occur in the severely hypothermic (92.4° F [28° C]) child. Resuscitative efforts continue while aggressive warming measures are instituted. Children have been successfully resuscitated up to 40 minutes after a cold-water immersion. Because the presence of a cardiac rhythm does not ensure perfusion of the tissues, the prehospital team assesses the child's cardiovascular status at regular intervals in addition to observing the rhythm on the cardiac monitor.

The wet clothes are removed, and the child is covered with warm blankets. Increasing the ambient temperature of the transport vehicle may be indicated. Rapid transport to the local emergency department or tertiary care center is critical for the severely hypothermic child.

Two IV lines should be started immediately in critically ill children with submersion injuries. Because of the electrolyte and fluid shifts into the intracellular space, children can become hypovolemic and fluid resuscitation is required. Adequate circulation is necessary to maintain organ perfusion. The rescuer may obtain blood for laboratory analysis while inserting the IV lines. Standard blood studies for the submerged child include CBC, serum electrolytes, BUN, creatinine level, and serum amylase. If the child is in shock or has experienced significant trauma, typing and crossmatching of two to four units of blood should be included.

Both air and water can be swallowed during a submersion incident. Air may also be forced into the stomach with resuscitative efforts. Because gastric distention resulting from air and water in the stomach can prevent full expansion of the lungs, a gastric tube should be inserted to decompress the stomach, ensure full respiratory excursion, and prevent aspiration of stomach contents from vomiting.

Hospital Management. Emergency care, on reaching the emergency department, continues the prehospital goals of maintaining adequate oxygenation and circulation. Additional treatments are initiated on the basis of laboratory and radiologic findings. Arterial blood gases may indicate the need to correct acidosis with sodium bicarbonate administration. Continued hypothermia is addressed providing warmed IV fluids and oxygen, overhead lights, and warmed blankets. Fluid and electrolyte corrections can be instituted.

The child is admitted to the hospital for observation, even if in stable condition after initial rescue and emergency treatment.

NURSING CARE OF THE CHILD WITH A SUBMERSION INJURY

Nursing care of the child with a submersion injury requires obtaining an accurate history, ensuring adequate oxygenation and tissue perfusion, and maintaining body temperature.

■ Assessment

Assessment of the child with a submersion injury focuses on the respiratory system. Airway and breathing are the priorities. The nurse observes the child for rate and depth of respiration, work of breathing, and any change in mental status. Cardiovascular assessment includes assessment of capillary refill and heart rate. The child's temperature is taken as soon as possible to determine any hypothermia.

Obtaining an accurate history of the injury is important although often difficult. Whether the submersion incident occurred in salt or fresh water is irrelevant for early treatment, but subsequent intensive care may vary somewhat depending on the immersion fluid.

■ Nursing Diagnosis and Planning

The following diagnoses are applicable to the child with a submersion injury:

- Impaired Gas Exchange (actual or potential) related to bronchospasm, aspiration of fluid, surfactant elimination, or pulmonary edema.

Expected Outcome. The child will demonstrate normal oxygen saturation, blood gas measurements, and clear breath sounds.

- Risk for Imbalanced Fluid Volume related to electrolyte imbalances that cause volume shifts from interstitial to intravascular space.

Expected Outcomes. The child will maintain hourly urine output appropriate for weight and age and vital signs within normal limits; electrolytes will return to normal.

- Hypothermia related to prolonged exposure to cold water.

Expected Outcome. The child will maintain body temperature between 97.7° to 99.3° F (36.5° to 37.4° C).

- Compromised Family Coping related to the child's critical status.

Expected Outcomes. The family will verbalize feelings (including feelings of guilt and anger) and concerns appropriately, exhibit an attitude of confidence in the care being provided, and provide support to the child.

Interventions

After the initial assessment and emergency management have been completed, the nurse monitors for changes from the baseline, anticipates the development of complications, and implements therapeutic management.

Providing Respiratory Support.
Because hypoxia is the primary problem, with potential for damage to all major organ systems, attention to the pulmonary system is a priority. The nurse assesses the child's level of consciousness and listens for adventitious breath sounds, which can signal the development of complications such as pulmonary edema, atelectasis, or pneumonia. Persistent hypoxemia, dyspnea, tachycardia, and respiratory alkalosis can also signal these pulmonary complications. If the child is intubated, airway maintenance is a priority with frequent observations for signs of tube displacement or pneumothorax.

Restoring Appropriate Circulatory Status.
Cardiovascular monitoring includes measuring vital signs, pulses, level of consciousness, skin temperature, color, and urine output. The well-perfused child is alert with age-appropriate behavior and has a capillary refill time of less than 2 seconds and urine output according to age (see Chapter 16). The nurse maintains IV lines and administers fluid volume replacement as ordered.

Identifying and Preventing Neurologic Consequences.
The neurologic system is monitored frequently. Common parameters include level of consciousness, pupillary response, movement of extremities, reflexes, and vital signs. The nurse anticipates signs and symptoms of increased intracranial pressure up to 24 hours after the submersion event. Conventional measures to prevent increased intracranial pressure, such as positioning the head in the midline, elevating the head of the bed 20 to 30 degrees, preventing or managing elevated body temperature, and controlling pain and agitation, are instituted as ordered.

Restoring Fluid Balance.
As a result of ingestion of large amounts of water during the near-drowning event, the child is at risk for development of alterations in fluid and electrolyte balance. The nurse carefully monitors urine output, laboratory data, and physical signs and symptoms. Hyponatremia and water intoxication should be anticipated, particularly with a fresh-water submersion. Observe for changes in central nervous system functioning, especially seizures, as the serum sodium level drops.

Controlling Infection.
The acutely ill child is at risk for local or systemic infection. Complications from organ damage, intubation and ventilation tubes, invasive monitoring lines, and urinary catheters are possible sources for infection. If infection is present, antibiotic therapy is started. The nurse must monitor the child's response to this therapy.

Maintaining Nutritional Status.
In the gastrointestinal system, hypoxia leads to decreased blood supply to the bowel. Stress ulcers and gastrointestinal bleeding are not uncommon. Gastrointestinal function in all areas must be monitored. This includes intake (nothing by mouth [NPO], oral or enteral feedings), internal systems (bowel sounds, residual feedings), and output (presence or absence of blood; amount, color, and consistency of stool).

The child's increased metabolic demands, along with disruption of gastrointestinal functioning, can result in a nutritional deficit. Nutritional therapy is implemented as ordered in the form of enteral feedings or total parenteral nutrition. If enteral feedings are ordered, monitor weight gain, residuals, amount and consistency of stools, and vomiting to ascertain tolerance of the feedings. If total parenteral nutrition is ordered, the nurse checks the product label with the order, administers the solution as ordered, monitors laboratory values, and assesses for any side effects.

Providing Emotional Care for the Family.
Because seriously ill children brought to the emergency department may not have a positive outcome, an important element of nursing care is psychological intervention and support for the child's family. The most important nursing interventions with the family of any critically ill or injured child initially include attention to the family's physical needs and provision of information and hope.

Families should be encouraged to participate in the decision regarding their presence in the treatment area, especially if the child is likely to die and the family may not have an opportunity to see the child alive again. If the parents choose to be brought into the resuscitation room, one person should be their liaison, bringing them in, answering questions, and escorting them out at appropriate times. The American Heart Association guidelines for CPR and emergency care state that often families do not ask to be present during resuscitative efforts; nurses should be sensitive to this and offer the opportunity for family members to be present (Berg et al., 2010).

Be honest with the family. If the child is in full arrest, make a simple statement such as, "Your child (use the child's name if possible) is not breathing and has no heartbeat. We are supporting his breathing and helping his heart to beat right now." This statement is far better than "We're doing everything we can," which leaves much more room for doubt.

Parents react in many different ways, according to their cultures, religious beliefs, individual personalities, and past experiences. Remember that denial can initially be protective and allow the family to accept information gradually. Ask family members if they want other family members or clergy contacted. Religious rites, including baptism, may be extremely important to families. A list of clergy from a variety of religions should be readily available for use by the nursing staff in emergency care settings.

Providing hope for the family is always important. At times, the only hope may be that the child is not suffering, or did not suffer, and that the child is, or was, not alone. If the child survives the incident, the parents will have ample time to adjust to any adverse consequences, so insisting on their acceptance is not necessary at this point. Many miraculous recoveries have occurred after lengthy submersions, usually in very cold water. In the emergency setting, however, predicting the ultimate outcome for a child is impossible. The nurse needs to convey to the family a realistic, positive attitude, while acknowledging the strong possibility of long-term effects for the child.

Evaluation

- Does the child demonstrate adequate oxygenation and independent breathing? Are lung sounds clear?
- Is the child's urine output appropriate for weight and age? Have electrolyte levels returned to normal?
- Is the child's body temperature between 97.7° to 99.3° F (36.5° to 37.4° C)?
- Do the parents verbalize their feelings and concerns appropriately, and do they provide appropriate support for the child?

! NURSING QUALITY ALERT

Needs Expressed by Families of Critically Ill Children

The highest ranked need identified for families in most research studies is the need for hope. Needs for privacy and comfort are also consistently identified as extremely important by the families of critically ill and injured children; these needs are usually ranked higher than the need for psychological support from nursing staff. Another commonly cited need is to have a contact person to provide updates and answer questions.

Heat-Related Illnesses

Heat-related illnesses include sunburn, heat cramps, heat rash, heat exhaustion, and heat stroke. The most serious types are heat exhaustion and heat stroke, both of which can ultimately result in death. Two important factors in evaluating the possibility of heat-related illnesses are environmental temperature and humidity. If the body is unable to maintain normal temperature through evaporation of sweat, as in the case of high humidity and exertion, thermoregulation systems can be overwhelmed, creating a cascade of potentially life-threatening events (NCEH, 2009a).

Incidence

Children's anatomic and physiologic differences make them more susceptible to sun- and heat-related illnesses. On average, there are approximately 650 deaths from exposure to extreme heat each year; 7% of these are children under age 15 years (CDC, 2006). The majority of pediatric deaths are a result of small children being left alone in closed vehicles. Infants and young children are sensitive to the effects of high temperatures related to rapid fluid loss and impaired compensatory mechanisms. They rely on others to regulate their environments and provide adequate liquids (NCEH, 2009a). Prophylactic measures such as use of sunscreen and adequate fluid and electrolyte intake should be carried out. Both parents and children, early in life, should be taught to use these prophylactic measures. This section focuses on heat-related illnesses; sunburn is discussed in Chapter 25.

Children involved in physical activity sweat less, create more heat in proportion to their body size and weight, and take longer to adapt to warm environments than do adults (Landry, 2011). In addition, younger children have a greater body surface area–to-mass ratio, which causes their bodies to gain heat from the environment on a hot day. Obese children are vulnerable because of increased insulation. Active children may continue playing without feeling the need to drink adequate amounts of fluids even in extremely hot environments.

Manifestations and Therapeutic Management

Symptoms of heat-related illness are wide ranging and, if left unrecognized or untreated, can quickly progress to heat exhaustion and the life-threatening state of heat stroke. Management of heat-related illness is dictated by the severity of symptoms. The first priority in all cases is to move the child to a cool place and start cooling measures such as loosening and removing wet clothes and applying cool cloths. Rehydration is instituted, either by oral rehydration solution in cases of overexertion or by IV fluid and electrolyte administration if the child is unable to tolerate the oral route. In cases of heat stroke, this is not sufficient. The child's temperature-controlling mechanisms are not working, the child is unable to sweat, and brain damage and death could result if the body is not cooled rapidly. Concurrent assessment and prompt stabilization of cardiopulmonary circulation are critical (Table 10-6).

Nursing Considerations

The nurse caring for a child with a heat-related emergency will initially assess and possibly intervene in stabilizing the ABCDEs, provide cooling measures aimed at progressively decreasing core body temperature without causing shivering or increased metabolic demands, giving the child fluids with electrolytes as indicated, and provide emotional support for the child and family.

Depending on the severity of symptoms, the nurse will assess for respiratory compromise and intervene with the appropriate method of oxygen delivery. In the hospital setting, the child with heat exhaustion may benefit from cool oxygen blow-by or nasal cannula, whereas the child with heat stroke will require oxygen by nonrebreathing mask or even intubation in the case of an insufficient respiratory effort. The nurse performs serial assessments of circulation and disability to determine the effectiveness of oral and/or IV fluid resuscitation.

As in other pediatric emergencies, the family should be involved early and to the extent they are comfortable. Family presence is encouraged, with the nurse or other member of the health care team available to provide clear explanations of procedures, answer questions, and give support.

Following stabilization of the child's condition, the nurse provides education to the family and child regarding prevention of heat-related illnesses. Even in cool temperatures, young children should *never* be left alone in a car or other type of vehicle. Even with the windows partially opened, the interior temperature can increase by 20 degrees (F) in the first 10 minutes, putting children at great risk for heat stroke and death (CDC, 2009). Parents, children, and members of the

TABLE 10-6	**HEAT-RELATED ILLNESS**		
TYPE	**PATHOPHYSIOLOGY**	**CLINICAL MANIFESTATIONS**	**TREATMENT**
Overexertion	Muscles generate heat during strenuous exercise; body fluids are being lost through sweating; rapid breathing; increased metabolic demands	Dizziness; flushed skin; diffuse muscle cramps	Move to cool environment; offer oral fluids; loosen clothing
Heat exhaustion	Increased loss of body fluids; increased blood flow to the skin with resulting decreased oxygen and blood flow to vital organs	Heavy sweating; nausea; vomiting; dizziness or fainting; exhaustion; headache; cramps; cool, moist, or flushed skin; core body temperature may be slightly elevated	Move to cool environment; apply cool, moist cloths to skin; remove clothing or change to dry clothing; elevate legs; offer oral rehydration fluids if no altered mental status or vomiting
Heat stroke	Thermoregulation is ineffective; sweating has stopped; vascular collapse and severe central nervous system abnormalities are noted because of hyperthermia and insufficient circulating volume	Hot, dry, red skin; change in level of consciousness or coma; rapid, weak pulse; rapid, shallow breathing; elevated core body temperatures ≥105° F (40.6°C)	Emergency transport if not in an emergency setting; rapid cooling with moist, cool cloths and fans; administer oxygen by nonrebreather, or intubate for respiratory insufficiency; aggressive IV rehydration; intervene as needed to maintain vital functions

community need to gain an understanding about the dangers of sun and heat exposure and the importance of adequate fluid and electrolyte intake, wearing light-colored, loose-fitting clothing, and adjusting activity levels according to temperature and humidity of the environment.

> **❓ CRITICAL THINKING EXERCISE 10-2**
>
> You are at a seventh-grade baseball game when you are asked by a parent to look at her previously healthy child who is reporting nausea, leg and arm cramps, and dizziness. His baseball uniform is wet, and the child is sweating profusely. It is 33.3° C (92° F) outside and it had rained earlier in the day.
> 1. What do you think is wrong with the child? Why?
> 2. What are your interventions while on the baseball field?
> 3. If he starts vomiting, what interventions may be anticipated?

DENTAL EMERGENCIES

Incidence and Etiology

Injury to the teeth, particularly the anterior teeth, is common in children. Toddlers, because of their lack of coordination, receive dental injuries from falling from or onto furniture. School-age children are more likely to have their teeth injured on playgrounds and during sports activities. The first teeth begin to erupt at approximately 6 months of age. By approximately 2 years of age, a child has all 20 primary teeth. Permanent teeth come in at approximately 5 or 6 years of age. By adolescence, a child usually has the full complement of 32 permanent teeth, although the eruption of wisdom teeth may be delayed. Injury to primary and permanent teeth is considered equally serious. Teeth are embedded in the bones of the maxilla and mandible. Injuries to teeth are usually divided into the following categories:

Concussion: The tooth is not displaced, but pressure may cause pain.
Subluxation: The tooth is moveable within the socket but is displaced less than 2 mm. The socket is not damaged.
Intrusion: The tooth is pushed into its socket with injury to the underlying structures.
Extrusion: An upper tooth is dislodged downward from the socket, or a lower tooth is dislodged upward.
Luxation: The tooth is moved laterally with tearing of the periodontal ligament.

Avulsion: The tooth is no longer in the socket, and the socket itself may be damaged.

Therapeutic Management

Dental emergencies require specialized care, which is often difficult to obtain immediately. Survival of the tooth depends on the periodontal ligament attachment, so concussion, subluxation, lateral luxation, and extrusion, in which the periodontal ligament is still attached, have a better prognosis than complete avulsion of a tooth. Intrusion of a tooth may damage underlying structures to a greater extent and diminish chances for tooth survival.

Time is of the essence in caring for dental injuries. With injury to a child's mouth, the nurse observes for missing teeth. If a missing tooth cannot be found in the oral cavity, possible aspiration should be considered in the presence of dyspnea. To determine whether other teeth are loose or malpositioned, the nurse gently palpates (using Standard Precautions) the teeth for movement and asks the child to check. A tooth that is loose in the socket should not be removed. If the position is not correct, repositioning may be necessary by a specialist.

In general, primary teeth are not replanted because damage to the developing tooth bud can occur. Complete avulsion of a permanent tooth requires care of the socket and the tooth itself. Survival of an avulsed tooth depends on prompt evaluation and replacement. Irreversible damage to the periodontal ligament because of dehydration of the open socket may occur after 60 minutes.

Emergency care by the dentist includes cleaning the tooth and socket, placing the tooth in the socket, and splinting the tooth. Tetanus immunization is given if needed, and an antibiotic may be prescribed.

Nursing Considerations

Parents should be instructed to keep the tooth moist. The tooth may be immersed in saline, water, milk, or a commercial tooth-preserving liquid. The tooth should not be cleaned or scrubbed. These actions increase the chances of tooth survival. The child should see a dentist, if possible, or should go to an emergency facility for care without delay.

Parents should be given careful discharge instructions and appropriate referrals for continuing dental care. When appropriate, reassure the family that with proper care, a good cosmetic outcome is possible with injury to or loss of a child's primary as well as secondary teeth.

KEY CONCEPTS

- Nursing care of ill and injured children may seem more complicated than care of adults because of their size, medication dosing, equipment, and age-related psychological differences.
- Familiarity with the issues related to the child's growth and development and careful organization of pediatric equipment can improve the care of children in emergency settings.
- Airway management is the most critical element in pediatric emergency care.
- Shock must be recognized early and must be taken into account when children begin to decompensate.

- Care of the family and the child's developmental stage should always be considered when providing nursing interventions in the emergency setting.
- Trauma assessment of the child includes the standard primary and secondary survey and intervention but must also include skin assessment, level of consciousness, and prevention of hypothermia.
- Injury prevention plays an important role in the nursing care of children. Motor vehicle injuries, ingestions, poisonings, and environmental injuries are largely preventable.

REFERENCES

Anderson, M. (2006). Capnography: Considerations for its use in the emergency department. *JEN: Journal of Emergency Nursing, 32*(2), 149-153.

Berg, M. D., Schexnayder, S. M., Chameides, L., et al. (2010). Part 13: Pediatric basic life support: 2010 American Heart Association guidelines for cardiopulmonary resuscitation and emergency cardiovascular care. *Circulation, 122*(suppl 3), S862-S875.

Borse, N., Gilchrist, J., Dellinger, A., et al. (2008). *CDC childhood injury report: Patterns of unintentional injuries among 0-19 year olds in the United States, 2000-2006.* Atlanta: Centers for Disease Control and Prevention National Center for Injury Prevention and Control Division of Unintentional Injury Prevention.

Centers for Disease Control and Prevention. (2006). Heat-related deaths: 1999-2003. *MMWR Morbidity and Mortality Weekly Report, 55*(29), 796-798. Retrieved from www.cdc.gov/mmwr/preview/mmwrhtml/mm5529a2.htm.

Centers for Disease Control and Prevention. (2008). *Dog bites: Fact sheet.* Retrieved from www.cdc.gov/HomeandRecreationalSafety/Dog-Bites/dogbite-factsheet.html.

Centers for Disease Control and Prevention (2009). *Extreme heat: A prevention guide to promote your personal health and safety.* Retrieved from www.bt.cdc.gov/disasters/extremeheat/heat_guide.asp.

Dean, C. (2010). Triage nurses influence safety by cutting the color: Removal of non–health care colored wristbands reduces risk for error. *JEN: Journal of Emergency Nursing, 36*(6), 599-600.

Durbin, D. (2011). Policy statement from the American Academy of Pediatrics, Committee on Injury, Violence, and Poison Prevention: Child passenger safety. *Pediatrics, 127*(4), 788-793.

Emergency Nurses Association. (2007). *Trauma nursing core course provider manual* (6th ed.). Des Plaines, IL: Author.

Faul, M., Xu, L., Wald, M., & Coronado, V. (2010). *Traumatic brain injury in the United States: Emergency department visits, hospitalizations and deaths 2002-2006.* Atlanta: Centers for Disease Control and Prevention, National Center for Injury Prevention and Control.

Harris, T. S. (2010). Bruises in children: Normal or child abuse? Journal of Pediatric Healthcare, 24(4), 216-221.

Hartman, M., & Cheifetz, I. (2011). Pediatric emergencies and resuscitation. In R. Kliegman, B. Stanton, J. St. Geme, et al. (Eds.), *Nelson textbook of pediatrics* (19th ed., pp. 279-296). Philadelphia: Elsevier Saunders.

Hawkins, H. (Ed.). (2004). *Emergency nursing pediatric course provider manual* (3rd ed.). Park Ridge, IL: Emergency Nurses Association.

Kleinman, M. E., Chameides, L., Schexnayder, S. M., et al. (2010). *Part 14: Pediatric advanced life support:* 2010 American Heart Association guidelines for cardiopulmonary resuscitation and emergency cardiovascular care. *Circulation, 122*(suppl 3), S876-S908.

Landry, G. (2011). Heat injuries. In R. Kliegman, B. Stanton, J. St. Geme, et al. (Eds.), *Nelson textbook of pediatrics* (19th ed., pp. 2420-2421). Philadelphia: Elsevier Saunders.

Levetown, M. (2008). Communicating with children and families: From everyday interactions to skill in conveying distressing information. *Pediatrics, 121*(5), e1441-e1460.

Mullen, J., & Pate, M. F. (2006). Caring for critically ill children and their families. In M. Slota (Ed.), *Core curriculum for pediatric critical care nursing* (2nd ed., pp. 20-31). St. Louis: Elsevier Mosby.

National Center for Environmental Health. (2009a). *Extreme heat: A prevention guide to promote your personal health and safety.* Retrieved from http://emergency.cdc.gov/disasters/extremeheat/heat_guide.asp.

National Center for Environmental Health. (2009b). *Lead poisoning: Prevention tips.* Retrieved from www.cdc.gov/nceh/lead/tips.htm.

National Center for Injury Prevention and Control, Division of Unintentional Injury Prevention. (2008). *Poisoning in the United States: Fact sheet.* Retrieved from www.cdc.gov/ncipc/factsheets/poisoning.htm.

National Highway Traffic Safety Administration. (2009). *Special crash investigations—Counts of frontal air bag related fatalities and seriously injured persons.* Retrieved from www.nhtsa.gov/people/ncsa/scireps.html#abfatal.

National Highway Traffic Safety Administration. (2010a). *Traffic safety facts 2008: Pedestrians.* Retrieved from www.nrd.nhtsa.dot.gov/Pubs/811163.pdf.

National Highway Traffic Safety Administration. (2010b). *Traffic safety facts 2009: Children.* Retrieved from www-nrd.nhtsa.dot.gov/Pubs/811387.pdf.

O'Donnell, K., & Ewald, M. (2011). Poisonings. In R. Kliegman, B. Stanton, J. St. Geme, et al. (Eds.), *Nelson textbook of pediatrics* (19th ed., pp. 250-270). Philadelphia: Elsevier Saunders.

Paparella, S. (2009). Allergies: Essential patient information for safe practice. *JEN: Journal of Emergency Nursing, 35*(3), 239-241.

Porter, S., Forbes, P., Manzi, S., & Kalish, L. (2010). Patients providing the answers: Narrowing the gap in data quality for emergency care. *Quality and Safety in Health Care, 19*(5), 1-5.

Porter, S., Manzi, S., Volpe, D., & Stack, A. (2006). Getting the data right: Information accuracy in pediatric emergency medicine. *Quality and Safety in Health Care, 15*, 296-301.

Roskind, C., Dayan, P. & Klein, B. (2011). Acute care of the victim of multiple trauma. In R. Kliegman, B. Stanton, J. St. Geme, et al. (Eds.), *Nelson textbook of pediatrics* (19th ed., pp. 333-340). Philadelphia: Elsevier Saunders.

Safe Kids USA. (2009a). *Drowning prevention fact sheet.* Retrieved from www.safekids.org/our-work/research/fact-sheets/drowning-prevention-fact-sheet.html.

Safe Kids USA. (2009b). *Pedestrian safety fact sheet.* Retrieved from www.safekids.org/our-work/research/fact-sheets/pedestrian-safety-fact-sheet.html.

Schroder, B., & Norris, R. (2011). Envenomations. In R. Kliegman, B. Stanton, J. St. Geme, et al. (Eds.), *Nelson textbook of pediatrics* (19th ed., pp. 2460-2465). Philadelphia: Elsevier Saunders.

Shephard, E., & Quan, L. (2011). Drowning and submersion injury. In R. Kliegman, B. Stanton, J. St. Geme, et al. (Eds.), *Nelson textbook of pediatrics* (19th ed., pp. 341-348). Philadelphia: Elsevier Saunders.

Turner, D., & Cheifetz, I. (2011). Shock. In R. Kliegman, B. Stanton, J. St. Geme, et al. (Eds.), *Nelson textbook of pediatrics* (19th ed., pp. 305-314). Philadelphia: Elsevier Saunders.

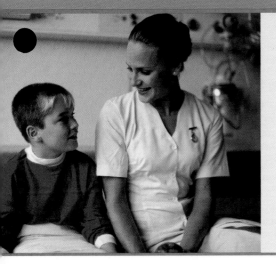

The Ill Child in the Hospital and Other Care Settings

evolve WEBSITE

http://evolve.elsevier.com/James/ncoc

After studying this chapter, you should be able to:

- Discuss the nurse's role in various settings where care is given to ill children.
- List common stressors affecting hospitalized children.
- Describe the child's response to illness.
- Discuss the stages of separation anxiety.

- Describe the factors that affect children's responses to hospitalization and treatment.
- Discuss the psychological responses of families to the illness of a child in the family.

Because of current trends in health care management, the care of ill children continues to move from the traditional acute-care hospital setting to community-based settings and the home. Hospitalized children are more acutely ill than in the past, and their stays are shorter. In addition, the hospitalized child is more likely to have a chronic or terminal disease or to have special needs that require specialized care. These changes do not mean that the need for pediatric nurses has diminished; their role is ever changing and expanding. Pediatric nurses will continue to care for children in hospitals, schools, clinics, and homes.

All children experience some form of illness at some time. The ways in which stressors and developmental needs are addressed are important factors in resolving the immediate crisis and in dealing with future illnesses. The nurse is often the first person the child sees when the child enters the health care system, and the nurse spends more time with an ill child than does any other health care provider. The nurse therefore has a unique opportunity to influence that child's physical and emotional health.

SETTINGS OF CARE

The Hospital

Entering the hospital is somewhat like visiting a foreign country. The language, culture, activities, and expectations may be unfamiliar to the child and the family. The nurse acts as a coordinator and provides a safe environment, both physically and emotionally. Being the

coordinator includes activities as diverse as explaining the jargon (e.g., NPO, IV, "vitals"), explaining procedures that are often painful, and facilitating the parents' access to hospital resources, such as social services, case managers, spiritual counselors, and ethics specialists. Above all, the nurse must educate the child and family about the disease process, its treatment, hospital procedures, and discharge issues.

Hospitalizations can be categorized according to length of stay, planned or unplanned admission, surgical or medical intervention, and outpatient (day) or inpatient status. Although they overlap, these categories provide a framework for examining the child's experience.

Another variable is the type of facility. Children may be hospitalized in a pediatric hospital, on a pediatric unit within a general hospital, or in a general hospital that occasionally admits children. Pediatric units within a general hospital or hospitals that do not have a specific pediatric unit may not have as many child-oriented services as a pediatric hospital has. Special play areas and child-size equipment and fixtures are often not available in general hospitals. Staff members who routinely do not care for children may be less comfortable in those roles.

The nurse in this situation is aware of these challenges and can provide support for the child and the family, for example, by taking extra time when the child is admitted to explain routines and procedures or by placing the child close to the nurses' station. This support might include moving a cot into the room for the parent and ordering special foods for the child. Sometimes it means removing part of the food from a tray that is about to be served so that the child is not overwhelmed by large servings intended for an adult. Ultimately, it means being sensitive to the needs of the child and the family.

24-Hour Observation

Many children with acute illnesses become ill quickly and recover quickly. For this reason, they may need acute care for a short time, such as when they are dehydrated or are having an acute asthma episode. At the end of 24 hours, the child is evaluated to determine whether further hospitalization is needed or whether discharge with home care instructions is appropriate.

The nurse must prepare the child and family for discharge and assess the parents' ability to care for the child at home. Instructions should be written in the language the parent can read, and the parent should be encouraged to ask questions. The nurse informs the parent about when to notify the primary health care provider in the event the child's condition worsens. An awareness of cultural and language differences enhances the nurse's ability to assess the child's and family's educational needs and develop an individualized teaching plan. For example, is the parent smiling because of contentment, or is the parent embarrassed to ask a question? Are parents nodding because they understand or are they too embarrassed to say they cannot understand English or cannot read? Many children's hospital units have a policy of contacting caregivers 1 to 2 days after the child is discharged, especially if the child left the facility at the end of 24 hours. Arrangements are made with the parent for a convenient time to be contacted. This policy allows the nurse to check on the child's condition and reinforce discharge teaching.

Emergency Hospitalization

An emergency admission can be distressing since there is little time for the child and family to prepare. The admission can be the result of traumatic injury or acute illness. The family may arrive at the hospital with little money, clothing, or other resources. Siblings may also be present, competing with the sick child for the parent's attention. In addition to caring for the sick child, the staff may be called on to help meet the family's basic needs for food, clothing, and a place to stay. A social service referral is appropriate in such situations.

Because of the intense level of activity in emergency departments, care of the family is often overlooked. The family may fear that the child will die or be permanently disabled. Although nurses may see many similar situations each day in which children do well, they must be sensitive to the family's fears, keep the family informed of the child's condition and care, and encourage a family member to stay with the child.

The time for preparing a child is usually limited in emergencies. Nurses must seize every opportunity to prepare children for the care they will receive. Holding and touching the child, talking softly, distracting the child, and involving the child in the procedure are methods of support used in emergencies. After the child is stable, the nurse returns and uses therapeutic communication to talk about the event. A child life specialist may also help the child express feelings. The use of dolls, puppets, and hospital equipment can aid children in communicating their feelings. (Chapter 10 provides more detailed information about caring for children and their families in an emergency setting.)

A 7-year-old boy was admitted to the general pediatrics unit after spending several hours in the emergency department because of acute asthma. Although his mother brought him to the hospital, she had his younger brother and sister with her and could not stay with him in the room. The boy remained quiet, but the nurse noticed that he watched every move she made. In such a case, the nurse might say, "Some kids

say it's scary to come to the hospital and especially to be in the emergency room, with the bright lights and everyone rushing around. If you'd like, I can spend a little time with you and we can talk about being in the hospital."

Outpatient and Day Facilities

Outpatient facilities have evolved in an effort to keep children out of the hospital unless absolutely necessary. The outpatient facility may be part of a hospital, or it may be free standing. The child arrives in the morning; undergoes a procedure, test, or surgical procedure; and goes home by the evening. Common procedures performed during such admissions include tympanostomy tube placement, hernia repair, tonsillectomy, cystoscopy, and bronchoscopy.

This mode of care has three main advantages: (1) it minimizes separation of the child from the family, (2) it decreases the risk of infection, and (3) it reduces cost. A disadvantage is that outpatient facilities that are not connected to a hospital may not be equipped for overnight stays. If complications develop that require continued observation and treatment, the child may have to be transferred to a hospital. This situation can be upsetting to the child and the family.

Although the procedure may be short, teaching the child and the parent is as important as in the acute-care setting. When possible, a tour of the facility before the procedure can decrease fear of the unknown. Parents have indicated that, although they like the idea of outpatient care, taking a child home afterward can be frightening.

Assessing the parent can assist the nurse in deciding whether the parent is capable of managing the child's care at home or whether home health care is needed. Written instructions specific to the child and procedure are helpful and reassuring. At the very least, a follow-up phone call to the home should be required. Parents must also be encouraged to call the facility if they have any concerns, and they should be given other resources to contact after the facility closes. Families who live far from the health care facility may want to spend the night at a nearby hotel or consider an overnight admission.

Rehabilitative Care

After a serious illness or trauma, the child's ability to function may change. After the acute situation has resolved, the child may be admitted to a rehabilitation hospital. Staff members from nursing, medicine, physical therapy, occupational therapy, and other areas collaborate to develop a treatment plan by which the child, family, and health professionals work to help the child regain previous abilities. Children with neurologic injuries, such as head injuries, or children with serious burns may thrive in this environment, which usually resembles a home environment with facilities available for the child to relearn activities of daily living.

Nurses in rehabilitative settings must balance nurturing and firm discipline as they help children reclaim independence. Parents often need encouragement and support because they are torn between "doing for" their child and watching the child struggle to function independently. Overprotection is a common reaction, and parents can be assisted in identifying the child's developmental need to master the environment. The focus should be on what the child can do rather than on the child's limitations.

The Medical-Surgical Unit

Children admitted to the hospital are usually acutely ill or have a chronic disease or disability that requires frequent, often long-term hospitalizations. (Care of the child with a chronic disease is discussed in Chapter 12.) The average length of hospital stay for the acutely ill child has shortened significantly, and the need for teaching has increased in proportion.

Preparation for a planned hospitalization is essential. Some hospitals provide an opportunity for the child to visit the hospital before admission, and many pediatric hospitals host preoperative parties or classes to introduce children to the strange sights and sounds they will experience during surgery. Literature is available from public libraries and hospital sources. These types of literature may be presented in pamphlet, video, and book formats. Parents should make sure that these present a realistic picture of the hospital experience (Ono, Hirabayashi, Oikawa, & Manabe, 2008). Parents should encourage the child to talk about the hospitalization and answer questions honestly. Videos may also be available for family members to view together and then discuss.

The Intensive Care Unit

When a child is admitted to the intensive care unit, both the child and the family may experience increased stress related to factors such as the seriousness of the admitting diagnosis, the rapid onset of the illness, and the high-technology, unfamiliar environment (Aldridge, 2005). In addition, the child often is experiencing pain, uncomfortable procedures, noise, and constant lighting. In many instances, the child cannot eat or talk. Meanwhile, the parents are experiencing a parent's worst fear—the possible loss of a child.

The child and family need intense emotional support. All the normal responses to hospitalization are magnified and need to be assessed. When possible, planned admissions to the intensive care unit (e.g., for cardiac surgery) should be preceded by visits to the unit or special classes that provide information about procedures and operations at a level the child can understand.

The parent should be encouraged to remain with the child and be kept informed of the child's condition (Figure 11-1). Procedures, equipment, and treatments should be explained, in appropriate language, to both the child and the parent. If the parent leaves and the child's condition changes or a new tube or piece of equipment has been added, the nurse should prepare the parent for the change before the parent sees the child. Nurses need to encourage parents to provide care and to touch their child as much as possible. The nurse's active listening is essential.

Siblings of the seriously ill, hospitalized child can easily be overlooked. Siblings may need to talk, to be comforted, or to have the hospital experience explained to them. Parents may feel pulled between the ill child and the rest of the family. Often family members want to help but do not know what to do. Suggesting that a grandparent or other relative relieve a parent so that the parent has time with the ill child's sibling can help both the parent and the child. Supporting parents by discussing options can relieve stress and may lead to solutions. Inclusion of family members in the provision of care, such as bathing and feeding, is important to both the family members and the child.

School-Based Clinics

The traditional areas of school health nursing that are still prevalent in many school systems include the following:

- *Health screening:* Vision, hearing, and growth checks can provide information about problems that may affect a child's ability to learn. When problems are identified, referral and follow-up services are provided.
- *Emergency care:* School nurses are the first to provide care for children experiencing an unintentional injury, both on the playground and in the school building. Excellent assessment skills

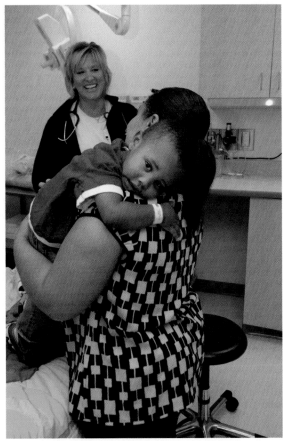

FIG 11-1 Parents are encouraged to stay with their child whenever possible. This mother is holding her child in the post-anesthesia recovery room, a setting that in the past was off limits to parents. (Courtesy St. Louis Children's Hospital, St. Louis, MO.)

are necessary to determine the need for health care provider visits or emergency care.

- *Communicable disease management:* The nurse must assess children for illnesses that may be transmitted to other children, provide care and isolation until the parent can pick up the child from school, and give advice concerning the safe time for re-entry into the school setting.
- *Health care advice:* The school nurse can be a source of referral for families in need of services.
- *Provision of specialized care for children with chronic health needs:* School attendance by children with many health care needs, including catheterization, gastric tube feedings, and suctioning, requires variation in the school nurse role to provide or supervise these specialized services.

School-based clinics have been part of health care for more than 25 years, but with the recent changes in health care delivery, this setting is now a site for expanding primary care. School-based clinics play an important role in providing care for children in remote rural communities and in underserved inner-city areas. School nurses, nurse practitioners, physicians, social workers, and other health care providers typically staff these clinics. This area of practice will continue to grow, and many believe that school-based clinics are the perfect setting for providing primary care for selected groups of children and adolescents because they are well situated to influence the health and well-being of underserved or disadvantaged students (Richardson, 2007).

Prevention remains the focus of school-based care as children learn healthy habits to prevent development of acute problems. Nurses identify children who need immunizations and provide immunizations when necessary. Screening that once required referral can often be handled on-site. Through school-based clinics, children can receive medical services in a timely manner and avoid expensive emergency visits. For example, a child with an earache at school can be seen on-site, treated, and sent home, if warranted. The child's adherence to treatment can be monitored and a follow-up visit scheduled to determine whether treatment has been effective. Funding for school-based clinics is increasing, and they will continue to be a focus of health care delivery in the community.

Nurses in school-based clinics must be sensitive to parental concerns about certain topics in health care, especially areas related to sexuality (e.g., birth control, sexually transmissible diseases, abortion). Community involvement and support can dispel concerns and assist in setting guidelines for such clinics. School-based clinic nurses must also be team members who act in collaboration with other health care providers and have a strong background in preventive health care and the ability to think critically.

The school-based clinic provides a setting for parental education in preventive health care, growth and development, anticipatory guidance, parenting skills, and care of acutely and chronically ill children. The nurse respects the rights and wishes of the parents, but respecting parents' wishes can be a challenge when the value systems of the health care provider and the parent differ. The pediatric nurse is a child advocate but must exercise caution unless the child is being harmed. (Child abuse is discussed in Chapter 29.)

The school nurse is an integral part of the health education program addressing both health and educational goals for school children (American Academy of Pediatrics [AAP], 2008). A comprehensive health education program is an important part of the curriculum in most school systems, for children in kindergarten through high school (AAP Healthy Children, 2010). The goals for this program are to increase students' health knowledge, generate positive attitudes towards health maintenance, and encourage healthy behaviors. To achieve these goals, active participation by students and involvement of parents are essential. Topics addressed include nutrition, disease prevention, physical growth and development, reproduction, mental health, drug and alcohol abuse prevention, consumer health, and safety (crossing streets, riding bikes, first aid, the Heimlich maneuver) (AAP Healthy Children, 2010).

Community Clinics

Community health clinics provide primary care for children and their families. In these settings, nurses, nurse practitioners, and physicians provide both case management of illness and health promotion. Because most children enter these settings during illness, preventive health care is integrated into the child's acute care. Support services and groups (e.g., social services, a dental clinic, daycare) may be available in the same center, and referrals to medical specialists and other health care providers are also available.

Although many children seen at community health clinics are ill, nurses must use the opportunity to obtain a health history, determine if immunizations are up to date, and assess nutritional status and growth and development. Needs for anticipatory guidance and education are evaluated as well. If the child is ill at the time of the visit, the nurse can set an appointment for the child to return for immunizations or other care that cannot be given when the child is ill (see www2.aap.org/immunization/IZschedule.html).

In some urban areas, nurses are involved in primary prevention and offer information and education about childhood immunization, the

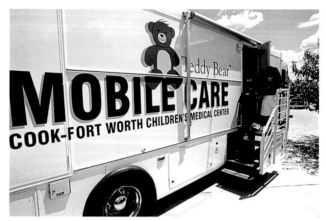

FIG 11-2 Nurses today help take health care on the road to provide services to those who otherwise might not obtain them. This mobile van is stationed at a public school, where it offers health screenings and prevention services to children. (Courtesy Cook Children's Medical Center, Fort Worth, TX.)

signs and symptoms of childhood illnesses, injury prevention, and parenting skills (Figure 11-2).

Home Care

Pediatric home care is the provision of skilled care within the child's home. Nurses in this setting are part of a multidisciplinary team that often is comprised of physicians, respiratory therapists, physical therapists, speech therapists, occupational therapists, and social workers. Children cared for at home include those receiving respiratory therapy, having dressing changes, receiving total parenteral nutrition, or needing skilled care because of a chronic illness or an injury.

Nurses who work in home care should have previous hospital experience in their practice area. The nurse must be able to make independent decisions and think critically and should have good clinical, documentation, communication, and teaching skills. To meet the needs of each child and family, the nurse must understand various cultures and socioeconomic backgrounds.

Although the separation of the child from the family is not a problem in home health care, the child may display many other effects of illness, such as fear of the unknown, loss of control, anger, guilt, and regression. In addition, care is taking place in the family's domain and the nurse is a guest in the home. Family members may have to adjust to unfamiliar noises and equipment, such as special beds, ventilators, and intravenous (IV) pumps, in their home. They may feel that they have lost their privacy and cannot "be themselves" because someone outside the family is frequently present. Awareness of siblings' needs is also a nursing goal in this setting.

The nurse's role as a teacher is especially important because many tasks that the nurse might perform in the hospital are delegated to the family, with the nurse monitoring the care. In this case, the nurse acts as a case manager and coordinator of care.

STRESSORS ASSOCIATED WITH ILLNESS AND HOSPITALIZATION

Age, cognitive development, preparation, coping skills, and culture influence a child's reaction to illness. Previous experience with the health care system and the parent's reaction to the illness also affect the child.

Each child is unique, so predicting reactions to an illness is often difficult. In general, hospitalization can create a number of threats or fears for children that have been grouped into the following five main categories: (1) bodily injury and pain, (2) separation from parents, (3) unknown or strange, (4) uncertainty about limits and expected behaviors, and (5) loss of control and autonomy (Visintainer & Wolfer, 1975). Educating parents about what to expect when their child is hospitalized and supporting their participation in their child's care decreases parental stress and enables them to better facilitate their child's adjustment (Melnyk, Carno, & Small, 2004; Melnyk, Feinstein, & Fairbanks, 2006).

! NURSING QUALITY ALERT

Children's Responses to Illness

- Fear of the unknown
- Separation anxiety
- Fear of pain or mutilation
- Loss of control
- Anger
- Guilt
- Regression

Although preschoolers and young school-age children experience separation anxiety, it is most significant in infants and toddlers, especially those ages 6 to 30 months. In times of stress, anxiety related to separation increases.

Each age-group has its own fears related to pain and injury. The past decade has seen an expansion of knowledge about pain and its treatment, negating many erroneous beliefs about children and pain. Children quickly learn to associate health care activities and professionals with pain and injury. The fear is usually focused on injections ("shots"). (Chapter 15 discusses issues related to pain.)

A child's feeling of having control over a situation has been shown to affect the child's management of stressors (Board, 2005). If children believe that they have personal control over a situation, they are more likely to feel confident and master a task, whether it is holding still while a needle is inserted or lying still while radiography is performed.

Although specific fears are related to the child's age, hospitalization puts all children at high risk for fears related to their unfamiliarity with the people, surroundings, and events. The child has not developed trust in the health care provider and therefore does not know what to expect. The child may have real or imagined fears: Will the nurse know when I am hungry or hurting? Will the nurse hurt me?

The Infant and Toddler
Separation Anxiety

Infants and toddlers, especially those between 6 and 30 months of age, often experience separation anxiety. Separation is this age-group's major stressor, and it is traumatic to both the child and the parent. The child passes through several stages in reaction to the separation: protest, despair, and detachment (Box 11-1).

In the initial phase, known as protest, the child demonstrates distress by crying and rejecting anyone other than the parents (Figure 11-3). The child appears angry and upset. During the despair phase, the child feels hopeless and becomes quiet and withdrawn. Crying decreases and the child becomes apathetic. If separation from the parent continues, the child enters the detachment phase. During this phase, the child again becomes interested in the environment and begins to play. Nurses may misinterpret this phase as a positive sign that the child has adjusted to the hospitalization. In reality, the child

---

BOX 11-1   STAGES OF SEPARATION

- *Protest:* Child is agitated, resists caregivers, cries, and is inconsolable.
- *Despair:* Child feels hopeless and becomes quiet, withdrawn, and apathetic.
- *Detachment:* Child becomes interested in the environment, plays, and seems to form relationships with caregivers and other children. If parents reappear, the child may ignore them.

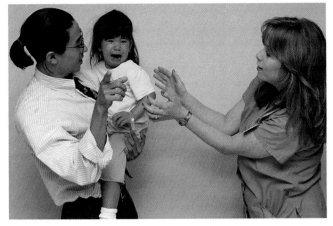

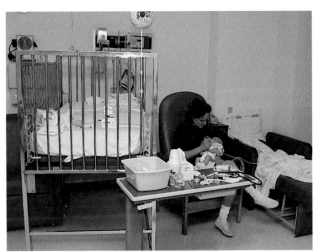

A toddler exhibits separation anxiety by reacting with protest to leaving her parent's arms.

Rooming-in reduces the stress of hospitalization and provides opportunities for parent teaching.

FIG 11-3 Separation is one of the stressors of hospitalization that affects both child and parent. (Courtesy T.C. Thompson Children's Hospital, Chattanooga, TN.)

has "given up." If the parents return during this stage, the child may ignore them and the parents may think that the child does not want to see them. This reaction, however, is a coping mechanism to protect the child from further emotional pain related to the separation.

Nurses in acute-care settings see the first two stages of separation—protest and despair—much more frequently than the final stage, detachment, which is more common in long-term separations. Parents may misunderstand their child's behavior. They may even perceive the child's reaction as a behavior problem. Nurses need to reassure parents that this reaction is a normal response to separation and that most children will not have any permanent effects from the event. As understanding of separation anxiety has evolved, visiting times for hospitalized pediatric patients have changed from structured hours to more flexible rooming-in situations (see Figure 11-3).

Most practitioners believe that, if separation can be avoided, the child will be much more resilient during a hospitalization. Infants and toddlers go through the stages of separation. For this age-group, the older the child's age, the more elaborate the child's protests. The child not only cries but also may cling to the parent, kick, and generally create a scene. Parents need to understand that this behavior is a sign of healthy parent-child attachment. The toddler may resist bedtime and eating and may have temper tantrums more frequently than normal for this age. Regression may occur in toileting and eating. Nurses need to explain to parents that regression is normal and to encourage parents to reinforce appropriate behavior while allowing the regressive behavior to occur.

A parent might ask whether someone from the family needs to be with a hospitalized toddler all the time and may be especially concerned because the parents work and have other children. The nurse responds, "We encourage parents to stay with their children when they are in the hospital. If you have to leave, however, we will spend time with your child and check on your child frequently. You may call us at any time, day or night. When you return, perhaps you could bring a favorite toy or stuffed animal and something that reminds the child of you. A picture or a piece of clothing [transition object] will make your child feel more secure because it is familiar."

Fear of Injury and Pain

Previous experiences, separation from parents, restraint, and preparation affect the reaction of infants and toddlers to pain and bodily injury. The young child views injury and pain concretely. Nurses who have worked with toddlers know that most toddlers react to any intrusive procedure, whether it is painful or not. (See Chapter 15 for a more extensive discussion of pain in infants and toddlers.)

Loss of Control

According to Erikson (1963), the major task of the toddler period is developing autonomy. Control is a major issue with this age-group. The toddler experiences the environment through all the senses and loves to explore the environment. At the same time, toddlers need sameness (rituals, routines). Because of the changes in growth and development taking place in the toddler, familiar rituals and routines (e.g., those for eating, sleeping, playing) provide reassurance and stability.

Hospitalization, which has its own set of rituals and routines, can severely disrupt the toddler's life. The child may be confined to a crib, and the crib may have a cover over it. Because of safety issues, the child is not allowed to run in the halls. If the parents are unable to be with the child, the way the child is put to bed or bathed may be unfamiliar. Information obtained from parents about routines for feeding, going to bed, and playing can assist the nurse in maintaining usual and comforting routines. When children are unable to do things themselves, their sense of control and autonomy is weakened. They are frustrated and may have temper tantrums. Choices, even simple ones, can return some control to the child.

This lack of control is often exhibited in behaviors related to feeding, toileting, playing, and bedtime. The nurse should remember that each of these activities may have associated rituals and routines and that the child may also show some regression in these areas.

The Preschooler
Separation Anxiety

Separation anxiety occurs among preschoolers but it is generally less obvious and less serious than in the toddler. Although the preschooler may already be spending some time away from parents at a daycare center or preschool, illness adds a stressor that makes separation more difficult.

The preschooler expresses the same protest as the toddler but tends to be less direct. The nurse may find a preschooler quietly crying because the parents have told the child to "act like a big boy (girl)." Children of this age may refuse to eat or take medications, and they may be generally uncooperative. They may repeatedly ask when their parents will be coming for a visit; with access to a phone, the child may constantly call the parents. All these behaviors are signs that the child is having difficulty coping with the situation.

Fear of Injury and Pain

The preschooler fears mutilation. The child who must have surgery affecting a limb or other body part feels greater fear. The preschooler generally does not understand body integrity. Children of this age report a predominant fear of pain and procedures that may cause pain such as injections (shots) and blood sample–taking/tests (Salmela, Salantera, & Aronen, 2009). Procedures that may be painful should be performed in the treatment room so children see their hospital rooms as safe places. Because of their literal interpretation of words, they often imagine treatments to be much worse than they are. A child's imagination can become extremely active during illness. The preschooler may believe that the illness occurred because of some personal deed or thought or perhaps just because the child touched something or someone. (The preschooler's specific reactions to pain are discussed further in Chapter 15.)

> **! NURSING QUALITY ALERT**
> ### Maintaining a Safe Place
>
> A designated safe area can enhance the child's security. For example, intrusive procedures may cause discomfort or anxiety and might better be done in the treatment room rather than the child's room. The playroom should also be a place for playing, not treatments and administration of medications. Nurses should consider the child's age, developmental level, coping skills, and parent/child preference when deciding where to perform procedures that may be painful or distressing.

Adapted from Fanurick, D., Schmitz, M., Martin, G., et al. (2000). Hospital room or treatment room: Where should inpatient pediatric procedures be performed? *Children's Health Care, 29*, 103-111.

Loss of Control

The preschooler has attained a good deal of independence in self-care and has been given more independence at home, preschool, or daycare. Some children expect to maintain their independence in the hospital. For example, the preschooler may like to wander about the unit and may not be happy when restricted to the bed or room. Like the toddler, a preschooler likes familiar routines and rituals and may show some regression if not allowed to maintain some areas of control.

One 5-year-old boy refused to have his dressing changed by the nurse who had cared for him the previous day. She reported that he cried, pulled up the covers, and said that she was "mean." This behavior was unusual for him, and the nurse suspected that he had been told to do too many things and had not been given choices. In response, the nurse might say, "I know there have been many changes for you since you came to the hospital. Today, we are going to decide together what is going to happen. I see you have chosen a video to watch. Would you like me to change your dressing before you watch the video or after?" This approach gives the preschooler a choice and some control while maintaining boundaries.

Guilt and Shame

Because their thinking is egocentric and magical, preschoolers may believe that their illness is somehow related to a thought or deed. This belief can lead to feelings of guilt, shame, and increased stress at a time when the child has to cope with several other stressors. Because the child typically does not share these feelings with adults, parents and caregivers must be aware of the possibility of guilt and shame in this age-group.

The nurse's role is to assess the child for this type of thinking and, through therapeutic communication, assist the child in identifying unfounded fears and beliefs. The child may be able to relate perceptions of what is happening. The use of puppets, dolls, and drawings can help children deal with their feelings. A tremendous decrease in anxiety can result when the nurse helps the child identify a perceived punishment and then reassures the child that nothing the child did could cause the illness.

The School-Age Child
Separation

The school-age child is accustomed to periods of separation from parents, but, as in the preschooler, as stressors are added the separation becomes more difficult. The younger school-age child may already have been feeling separation anxiety related to starting school.

Older children may be more concerned with missing school and the fear that their friends will forget them. The need to adjust to an unfamiliar environment and the regression seen in ill children, however, increase the likelihood that some separation anxiety will take place.

Fear of Injury and Pain

The school-age child is concerned with body disability and death. The child is more relaxed about having a physical examination or having the eyes or an ear examined but is uncomfortable with any type of genital examination. School-age children want to know the reasons for procedures and tests, and they ask relevant questions about their illness. Because they can understand cause and effect, they can relate actions to becoming ill. Their parents may tell them that if they do not get enough rest, wear warm clothes, or eat nutritious meals, they will get a cold. If they become ill, they associate their actions with the disease. (For further discussion of pain in the school-age child, see Chapter 15.)

Loss of Control

School-age children are "movers and shakers." They control their self-care and typically are highly social. They like being involved, and most fill their days with activities. Illness can change all these patterns. If children of this age have physical limitations, they can feel helpless and dependent (Figure 11-4). Anxiety in response to loss of control, environmental changes, and the hospitalization experience can alter the way school-age children appraise both the experience and the amount

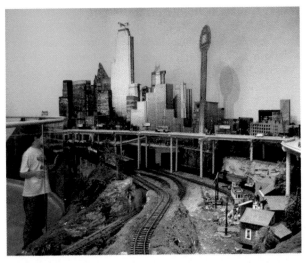

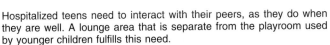

Hospitalized teens need to interact with their peers, as they do when they are well. A lounge area that is separate from the playroom used by younger children fulfills this need.

This model railroad "trainscape" in a pediatric hospital provides children and adults with a welcome respite from real-life stresses. (Courtesy Frolin Marek, Marek Mountain RR, www.Frolin.com.)

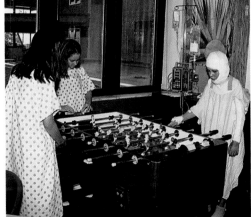

FIG 11-4 Activities for the hospitalized child are important for growth and development, stress relief, socialization, and a sense of control.

of resulting stress. School-age children can view the hospital experience as a threat. Children use coping strategies that include sleeping, talking with others, distraction (e.g., television, music, video games), and play. Ineffective coping can occur if the child sees the strategies as unsuccessful for regaining control (Board, 2005).

Friends are important to children of this age-group, and school-age children may think that their friends will forget them while they are ill. They are also accustomed to making choices about meals and activities. By capitalizing on their abilities and needs, the nurse can encourage children of this age to become involved in their own care. School-age children can select their own menus, assist with some treatments, keep their rooms neat, and visit with other children when it is appropriate for both. With these opportunities for independence, children retain a sense of control, enhance their self-esteem, and continue to work toward achieving a sense of industry.

The Adolescent
Separation
Adolescents often are unsure whether they want their parents with them when they are hospitalized. Some enjoy the freedom and the period of independence. Others, in response to the stress of illness, become more dependent and want their parents nearby. A third group cannot decide what they want, and this situation can be frustrating to parents. All of these responses are consistent with normal adolescent growth and development.

Because of the importance of the peer group, separation from friends is a source of anxiety to the adolescent. Ideally, the peer group will support the ill friend. Some adolescents are reluctant to visit friends in the hospital, either because of their own health fears or because the reality of illness in someone their age is difficult for them to handle. Hospitalized adolescents may be upset if their friends simply go on with their lives, excluding them. It is important to provide special activity areas and other opportunities for the adolescent to meet and interact with other hospitalized adolescents (see Figure 11-4).

Fear of Injury and Pain
To the adolescent, appearance is crucial. Therefore an illness or injury that changes an adolescent's self-perception can have a major impact. Even children who have seemingly adjusted to a chronic disease in their earlier years may have difficulty during adolescence simply because they do not want to be different. The adolescent who has diabetes may not want to eat different foods or take time out from an activity for injections. Adolescents do not want attention drawn to them, so they may eat the wrong foods and skip their medication.

Adolescents may also give the impression that they are not afraid, although they are terrified. Adolescents may think that being "cool" means being in control. They may question everything, or they may appear overly confident. Because of their concern with their bodies, they are guarded when any areas connected with sexual development are examined. Nurses need to be sensitive to adolescents' concerns and reassure them that they are normal, if in fact they are. Some adolescents also believe that they are invincible and that nothing can hurt them or cause death. This belief can cause them to take risks and to be nonadherent to treatment because they may not see the consequences of their behavior. (Pain management is discussed in Chapter 15.)

Loss of Control
Control is important to the adolescent. Thus, nurses must understand that many of the challenges they face caring for an ill adolescent stem from control issues. Giving the adolescent some control avoids endless power struggles. Behaviors exhibited in response to loss of control include anger, withdrawal, and general uncooperativeness.

Control issues can cause a major conflict between adolescents and parents. Parents often feel like "ping-pong balls" as they are bounced back and forth by a child who wants help one minute and rejects it the next. Parents who do not understand growth and development can become frustrated and angry over such behavior. Providing information about developmental issues, as well as information about the child's illness and care, facilitates communication (Sarajärvi, Haapamäki, & Paavilainen, 2006).

Adolescents may also feel that they are losing control of their social lives as they sit on the sidelines of activities. Time to plan for the separation (e.g., scheduled surgery) allows a greater sense of control than an unplanned hospitalization (e.g., trauma).

Fear of the Unknown
The sights and sounds of the hospital can be frightening and confusing to children. The child may have many questions: Why are the nurses wearing masks? Why does that alarm keep ringing? Am I dying? Why are they putting tubes in me?

The child's routines and rituals may have been disrupted, and the child may wonder what will happen next. Understanding these fears can assist the nurse in structuring care and teaching in a way that avoids unnecessary anxiety.

Regression
Children may regress in toileting or may cry for a bottle although they have been weaned for several months. They may want more attention at bedtime or have temper tantrums. The older child may react to separation by clinging or crying or may have fears about shadows on the walls or noises in the halls.

Parents may be overly concerned about regression. They should be told that the child might continue some regressive behaviors at home for a period of time following hospital discharge. The child may need more emotional support while the parent slowly returns the child to normal routines. If the child has regressed in toileting, the parent should wait until the child has returned to a daily routine and then begin the toilet training again. Behavior that is appropriate for the child's age should be reinforced.

The nurse might explain, "I know that you are concerned because your son has been soiling his pants since he has been in the hospital. This is an expected reaction to the stress of being ill and in the hospital. When he returns home and things return to normal for him, he will likely resume his previous schedule for using the toilet."

FACTORS AFFECTING A CHILD'S RESPONSE TO ILLNESS AND HOSPITALIZATION

Each child responds to illness or hospitalization differently. The expression "perception is everything" certainly applies to the ill child. How children perceive the incident will affect their responses before, during, and after the illness or hospitalization. How a child reacts is often related to the parents' response to the illness and the child's age, level of cognitive development, preparation, previous experiences, and coping skills. Research suggests that the stress some children experience when injured and during the subsequent hospitalization can result in symptoms of posttraumatic stress. As a part of trauma care, all children need to be screened for acute stress and provided appropriate care for emotional trauma (Rzucidio & Campbell, 2009).

For children who have had a previous illness or hospitalization, how that event unfolded and the child's response to it will greatly affect the child's view of future experiences. Children with chronic diseases who undergo multiple hospitalizations have a different perception of illness from those who have an occasional cold (see Chapter 12). A visit to a pediatrician's office will show the wide range of responses children exhibit. Some older children have more negative responses as they begin to associate certain people, colors, and surroundings with what was for them an unpleasant experience.

The Expert Panel on Child/Adolescent/Family of the American Academy of Nursing (AAN) has developed the *Indicators of Nursing Excellence* that consists of 18 guidelines for nurses and other health professionals to follow when working with children and their families in hospital and community settings. Some guidelines that pertain to the care of a hospitalized child and family are as follows: (1) The families of children and youth are partners in decisions, planning, and delivery of care; (2) family values, beliefs, and preferences are a part of care; (3) children, youth, and families' privacy and rights are protected; and (4) children, youth, and families receive comfort care (Craft-Rosenberg & Krajicek, 2006). Also included are questions that the child and family can ask to determine whether care providers are following each guideline. Some questions that families can ask are: Does your provider give you enough information about your child's care? Do you have a chance to share your cultural values and beliefs? Does your provider make you feel sure that your families' health information is kept private? Does the provider give you useful information about your child's pain? (Craft-Rosenberg & Krajicek, 2006.)

Age and Cognitive Development

Children's developmental levels affect their reactions to illness. These differences should be considered during the planning of nursing care. Preparing a toddler for hospitalization or a procedure differs from preparing a school-age child. The content, the time frame, the setting, and the method of preparation are all based on the child's growth and development. Pediatric nurses must have a clear understanding of the cognitive abilities of children in each age-group (Box 11-2).

Parental Response

Children have sharp observation skills and know when their parents are anxious and upset. This anxiety is transferred to the child, and the child's anxiety then increases. If the parents talk outside their child's room or within hearing range but in whispers, the child begins to imagine what the parents are saying. All children, but especially pre-schoolers, who have such active imaginations, can invent elaborate stories to explain what is happening.

The parent who does not answer the child's questions or who does not tell the truth for fear it will frighten the child only confuses the child and weakens the child's trust in the parent. The child wants to believe that someone is in control and that he or she can trust that person. Some parents cannot be honest with their children because of their own fears and insecurities. The nurse needs to assess for all of these issues.

EVIDENCE-BASED PRACTICE

Evaluation of Nursing Care by Hospitalized Children

Level V

An integral part of the nursing process is evaluation. Following implementation of a patient's nursing care plan, the nurse carefully evaluates whether the expected outcomes for the patient have been met. This process then allows the nurse to revise the plan of care as indicated to optimize nursing care. Findings from qualitative research studies (Schmidt, Bernaix, Koski et al., 2007; Lindeke, Nakai & Johnson, 2006; Pelander & Leino-Kilpi, 2004) provide pediatric nurses with the unique opportunity to evaluate their behaviors and actions from the perspective of their patients: hospitalized children whose voices are not often directly and clearly heard.

Schmidt et al. (2007) conducted semi-structured interviews of 65 children ages 5 to 18 years of age who were in the hospital for a minimum of two nights and medically stable. Boys and girls were equally represented; 64% of participants had a chronic illness and 34% had at least one previous hospital admission. Younger children provided verbal responses to the interviewer and older children gave written responses for eight interview questions with no input from parents. Questions were designed to elicit both positive and negative descriptions of the children's experiences (i.e., children were asked to recall nurse behaviors that helped them feel "less scared" and that they "liked" or "disliked").

The analysis of the children's responses revealed seven nurse behavior themes: positive affect/attitude, physical comfort, entertainment/humor, advocacy, meeting basic needs, acknowledgment, and reassurance. The most predominant theme was positive affect/attitude; the majority of children appreciated nurses who smiled, were "nice," used "kind words," and were "happy and helpful" (Schmidt et al., 2007). Nearly 50% of participants in all age-groups indicated that nursing actions to decrease pain or limit the infliction of pain were highly important to them. When asked what nurses did that the children did not like, the most frequent responses were "starting IVs" and "shots." Other important nurse behaviors included making children laugh; providing toys, craft supplies, and books, and playing with children; explaining what is going on; coming to the room when called; talking to the child directly even when parents were present; and offering reassurance through words and nonverbal actions (letting a child squeeze a nurse's hand). Children acknowledged being most frightened at the time of hospital admission and during intrusive procedures, and that they did not appreciate nurses who failed to make eye contact and interact with them when in their rooms (Schmidt et al., 2007).

Findings from this study by Schmidt et al. (2007) were consistent with those from earlier studies (Lindeke et al., 2006; Pelander & Leino-Kilpi, 2004). In conclusion, Schmidt et al. (2007) offer the following guidance for pediatric nursing practice:

- Remember to enter a child's room with a smile and establish eye contact.
- Ask children directly how they feel and what they need. Assume that children, even as young as 5 years, can provide such information.
- Do not assume that because a child's parent or caregiver is present, the need for individualized, sensitive nursing care and presence is diminished.
- Acknowledge children with each interaction by using each child's name and engaging them in conversation about their concerns related to hospitalization and their life outside of the hospital.
- Provide age-appropriate diversion and friendly interaction.
- Provide basic needs in a gentle, organized manner.
- Step into a child's room frequently, even if only for a brief moment, to ensure the child's safety and well-being.
- Remember that older children continue to need physical comfort, reassurance, and conversation, and they appreciate the advocacy roles that nurses assume.
- Children/teens respect professionalism in their nurse and want to be respected as individuals.
- Make special efforts at the time of hospital admission to explain the role of the nurse to children inexperienced with hospitalization.
- Provide children with age-appropriate explanations of treatments, timely care, truthful responses, and privacy.

BOX 11-2   DEVELOPMENTAL APPROACHES TO THE HOSPITALIZED CHILD

Neonate

- Anticipate needs and fulfill them in a timely manner.
- Provide opportunities for nonnutritive (comfort) sucking and oral stimulation with a pacifier.
- Provide swaddling, with the infant's hands drawn to the midline and close to the face. Use soft talking to soothe.
- If the infant is very ill, provide a quiet, soothing environment. Pay close attention to light and sound stimulation.
- When stimulation is appropriate, provide stimulation for each sense (e.g., mobiles, music, smell, soft stuffed animals). Use contrasting colors and textures.
- Watch for cues of overstimulation, such as eye avoidance, extension of arms, splaying of fingers, and "zoning-out" behavior.
- Before painful procedures, provide comforting touch and nonnutritive sucking. Follow painful procedures with tucking, holding, and cuddling.
- Model and share appropriate behaviors with family members regarding stimulation, touch, verbalization, and feeding.
- Provide consistent caregivers when parents are not available.
- Collaborate with parents on ways to provide care to the neonate.
- Involve the parents in the care of their neonate as much as possible.
- Encourage parents to room-in if possible.

Infant

- For the younger infant, provide the same care given for a neonate.
- The older infant will begin to anticipate painful procedures and fight. Use sheets and blankets to provide swaddling if necessary. Allow nonnutritive sucking for comfort.
- Expect regression and inform parents to expect it and why.
- Limit the number of caregivers to whom the infant must adjust.
- Request that parents bring the infant's security object (e.g., blanket, stuffed animal).
- Encourage parents to be present during procedures.

Toddler

- Expect regression and inform parents about behaviors.
- Follow home routines and rituals.
- Involve parents in the care of the toddler.
- Provide for rooming-in if possible.
- Allow opportunities for mobility when it can be done safely.
- Use all possible methods of pain control when the child must have a painful procedure.
- Anticipate temper tantrums when the child's frustration level is high.
- Maintain a safe environment for the toddler's physical acting out and temper tantrums.
- Encourage the child to be independent (e.g., feed self, use potty chair, put on socks).
- Provide support when the toddler needs to be dependent (e.g., hold after a procedure, comfort if parents leave).
- Approach with a positive attitude ("I am going to give you your medicine.").

Preschooler

- Provide safe ways to act out aggression (e.g., with punching bags, painting, clay).
- Take time for communication. Answer questions with simple, concrete explanations. Explain all procedures honestly. Allow for choices whenever possible.
- Expect egocentric behavior.
- Provide for a safe and secure environment (e.g., with a night light, view of others, objects from home).
- Be consistent.
- Ask the parents how the child usually copes in new situations.
- Tell the child that he or she did not cause the illness.
- Involve parents in care and follow home routines.
- Place the child with other children of the same age if possible.
- Provide for play activities in the playroom and in the room.
- Accept regression if it occurs and explain it to parents.
- Encourage the child to be independent (e.g., feeding, dressing, toileting).

School-Age Child

- Inform the child of limits, and enforce them (e.g., no water fights, no wheelchair races, no leaving the unit).
- Involve the child in planning and implementing care (e.g., allow child to choose from menu and assist with some procedures).
- Explain all procedures and allow the child time for questions and answers. Use medical and scientific terminology and diagrams, body outlines, or anatomically correct dolls to explain the procedure.
- Accept regression but encourage independence.
- Provide privacy.
- Encourage the child to assist in keeping the room and belongings in order.
- Assist the child in contacting friends. Encourage parents to contact the teacher and have school friends send mail.
- If the child's condition supports visits and calls from friends, encourage this contact.
- Provide for the child's educational needs by encouraging parents to bring in the child's homework and by scheduling study times. If the child will have a prolonged period of hospital or home care, arrange for a teacher to work with the child. Some hospitals have a hospital-based teacher.

Adolescent

- Provide privacy for care and visiting.
- Encourage the adolescent to wear street clothes and perform normal grooming.
- Encourage questions about appearance and the effects of illness on the adolescent's future.
- Use scientific and medical terminology to prepare the adolescent for procedures.
- Use body outlines and diagrams and give the rationale for the procedure.
- When possible, provide for a special activity area that is limited to adolescent use. Introduce the child to other adolescents on the unit.
- Encourage peers to call and visit if the adolescent's condition can tolerate this action.
- Assist parents in communicating, supporting, and guiding adolescents by providing them with information about growth and development.
- Allow favorite foods to be brought in if the adolescent does not need a special diet.
- Approach the adolescent with caring, understanding, and acceptance.
- Provide for educational needs, as for a school-age child.

Preparing the Child and Family

Stress has been defined as a nonspecific response of the body to any demand made on it. Perceived stressors, the conditioning factors brought to the situation, and the coping mechanisms used to adapt all affect each person's adaptation to a stress-producing situation. Preparing for an event (in this case, hospitalization) can decrease stress in several ways. During preparation, the child's and the parents' perceptions of the event can be explored. In addition, previous experiences that might affect the impending hospitalization and the use of previous coping strategies can be identified and discussed.

The depth and method of preparation vary among children and are based on an understanding of the child's individual needs. Variables that the nurse should consider are the child's age and developmental level, involvement of the family, timing, child's physiologic status and psychological status, setting, sociocultural factors, and the child's past experiences with illness and hospitalization.

Preparation sessions should be planned. Teaching is more effective if the nurse and family develop trust. Honesty and use of language appropriate for the child's age are imperative. When possible, all of the child's senses should be involved. The child should be allowed to see the intensive care area or surgery area before being admitted, to take the blood pressure of a stuffed animal, or to handle the mask that will be used in surgery. Preparing children through the use of therapeutic play interventions have been shown to lower the anxiety levels of children and to increase parent satisfaction (Li & Lopez, 2008). The nurse should avoid using medical terms that children and their parents may not understand. Literal interpretation of some words may be confusing and scary to some children, especially preschoolers (see Chapter 3). Some children assume that certain procedures involve pain. Explanation and the opportunity to handle equipment, when possible, can help children master the fear of hospitalization and treatment.

Special attention should be given to prepare the family as well. Assuming that parents will understand complicated aspects of a child's care is a mistake. In fact, to thoroughly include families in the child's care, nurses must give information to family members that, like information given to the child, includes what the family will see, hear, and need to do (Melnyk et al., 2006).

Coping Skills of the Child and Family

Coping is the process of contending with difficulties in an effort to overcome or work through them. How the child copes with illness or hospitalization is related to age, perception of the event, previous hospitalizations and encounters with the health care profession, support from significant others, and the child's and parents' coping skills.

Depending on age, children use words, behaviors, and physical actions to help them through stressful situations. The child may also cope by ignoring or negating the event. The younger child is more likely to use emotional expression, whereas the older child and adolescent are more likely to withdraw or practice more self-control behaviors. For example, although the younger child might scream and kick during a procedure, the older child might remain stoic and say that it did not hurt, even though it did. Some children try to appear brave and meet self-imposed or parental expectations.

Breathing (e.g., blowing bubbles, pinwheels, party blowers) or singing helps with relaxation and offers a focus for the child. Teaching coping mechanisms and practicing them before a procedure can help a child feel more in control and successful. Distraction (e.g., water wheels, games, books, music) and imagery (e.g., tapes, scenarios) for older children are effective tools for coping. Parents, nurses, and child life specialists may all serve as facilitators for these techniques.

Psychological Benefits of Hospitalization

Some think that hospitalization causes only negative psychological effects. The stress of illness and hospitalization can actually enhance growth and development by promoting a child's use of coping skills and bolstering self-esteem. Children can increase their self-confidence as they overcome anxiety related to hospitalization and perhaps master some self-care skills. They feel positive about their recovery or increased ability to cope with any disability they have. In addition, hospitalization offers an opportunity for children to ask questions and obtain new information. Some even become interested in a career in health care while observing professionals caring for them. Hospitalization can also be an opportunity to teach parents about children's growth and development, improve parenting skills, and assess the child's well care and immunizations.

PLAY FOR THE ILL CHILD

Play for the ill child is believed to decrease the potential negative effects of hospitalization by promoting expression of feelings and enabling control over stressful experiences (Bolig, Ferne, & Klein, 1986). Because play is familiar and comfortable for children, child life programs provide opportunities for play in a variety of health care settings, including inpatient units, ICUs, outpatient clinics, emergency departments, and presurgical waiting areas (AAP Child Life Council and Committee on Hospital Care, 2006). Preferred play activities vary according to the stage of development. For example, a young child engages in make-believe play, a school-age child joins others in a structured game, and an adolescent uses a computer to electronically communicate with peers outside the hospital (AAP Child Life Council and Committee on Hospital Care, 2006). Nurses should ensure that children with complex and continuing health needs are allowed the same rights as their peers and are given opportunities to communicate, play, and enjoy leisure activities (Hewitt-Taylor, 2010).

Playrooms

Hospitals and clinics often provide playrooms where children may go to play with toys, participate in age-appropriate arts and crafts, and socialize with other children. Children should always see this area as a safe place where procedures and treatments do not take place. Children, when their condition is stable, may be taken to the playroom in their beds and wheelchairs (Figure 11-5). A separate activity area

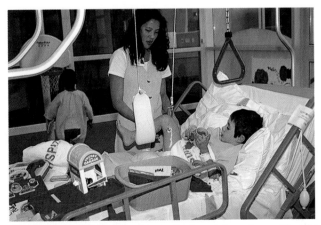

FIG 11-5 To provide diversion and allow interaction with other children, the play therapist wheels the child, while still in bed with traction in place, to the playroom. (Courtesy Parkland Health and Hospital System, Dallas, TX.)

should be provided, when possible, for adolescents to listen to music, play video games, use computers to access e-mail and Internet sites, and visit with their peers. If playrooms are not available, a supply of developmentally appropriate toys, games, and books should be maintained so nurses can give them to pediatric patients.

Therapeutic Play

When a child is hospitalized, one component of the child's plan of care is the use of therapeutic play. Therapeutic play differs from normal play in its design and intent. Members of the health care team guide it, and activities are planned to meet the physical and psychological needs of the child. Interpretations of the child's play behavior and some types of play therapy require guidance by a trained play therapist. Therapeutic play can provide an emotional outlet, instruct, and improve physiologic abilities (AAP Child Life, 2006). Supervised play with medical equipment helps reduce fear and separate reality from fantasy.

Child life specialists are available in many hospitals to share their expertise in child growth and development and the use of play. Child life program goals include maintaining normal living patterns, minimizing psychological trauma, and promoting optimal development of the child. Using a collaborative approach with the nurse, child life therapists systematically prepare children for surgery, and this may lead to increased positive outcomes for these patients and their families (Sorensen, Card, Malley, & Strzelecki, 2009).

Emotional Outlet Play

Emotional outlet play is often called dramatic play. During this type of play, the child acts out or dramatizes real-life stressors. These might include emotional stressors, such as abuse or neglect, or a painful physical stressor, such as a bone marrow aspiration. The hospitalized child who is separated from family and friends might use a wooden hammer and pegs to express anger over the separation. A child who has been sexually abused might not be able to communicate the experience verbally but may be able to use an anatomically correct doll to show what happened. Terminally ill children have been reported to use play to tell their stories and to express thoughts and feelings, an important part of the emotional healing process for children and parents (van Breeman, 2009).

Many commercially crafted toys are available for dramatic play. Anatomically correct dolls and puppets are available. Some dolls have removable parts that enable the child to see the various organs of the body.

Children can express their inner beliefs and perceptions through drawing (Wikstrom, 2005) (Figure 11-6). For example, a child may draw a very big bed with a tiny child on it surrounded by large, hovering adults or a huge syringe with a long needle. Driessnack (2005), in a meta-analysis of research into facilitative drawing, suggests that allowing a child to draw while being interviewed and then attending to the child's story about the drawing facilitates communication. Skybo, Ryan-Wenger, and Su (2006) suggest that encouraging children to draw a human figure can reveal important information about their developmental and emotional status. Human figure drawing can be most valuable when the child is either developmentally or physically unable to communicate verbally (Skybo et al., 2006).

Injection play is an appropriate intervention with the child who has to undergo frequent blood work, injections, IV therapy, or any other therapy involving syringes and needles. If a needle is used for this type of activity, safety is of the utmost importance, and the nurse should assess the child's growth and development level before using this type of directed play. An adult is always present if a needle is used. The child

can give a doll an injection and can thereby work through anger and anxiety. Wooden hammers and pegboards, foam (Nerf) balls, and boxing gloves are all avenues for release of stress or anger.

Teaching through Play

Play can also be used to educate. It can be used in preoperative teaching and teaching before a new, painful, or extensive procedure (see Figure 11-6). The nurse assesses the child's cognitive level before this type of teaching, and the play should be appropriate to the child's level.

Hospital equipment is often used in this type of play. The nurse might demonstrate taking a blood pressure on the child's stuffed animal before putting the cuff on the child. A breathing treatment might be "given" to the child's doll before the child is given the treatment. The nurse might use drawings and diagrams to explain procedures or surgery. Use of play for children experiencing invasive, painful procedures such as IV line insertion has been shown to be effective in teaching what to expect before the procedure and to improve coping skills (Breiner, 2009).

Some hospitals have preoperative visits during which children come to meet the people who will be taking care of them and see the physical surroundings. They may see the scrub gowns and masks worn by the surgical staff and visit a typical room. Children and parents can ask questions and meet other children and parents who are going through a similar experience as they tour the area.

Enhancing Cooperation through Play

Children with illnesses that require unpleasant or painful therapies often are uncooperative. Developing a plan that will stimulate and engage such a child in the activity is a challenge. The nurse should include age-appropriate growth and development activities when planning care. The school-age child who loves competition and games is more likely to increase range of motion of an arm if points can be made each time a foam ball is thrown through a hoop.

Allowing the child to blow bubbles, a whistle, or a pinwheel or to simulate blowing out the nurse's penlight can enhance deep-breathing exercises. Range of motion can be accomplished by throwing foam balls, beanbags, and paper balls. The child who needs to increase intake can sometimes be motivated to drink more fluids if a graph shows the amount taken in and the child receives a reward when a selected goal is reached. Including the child in planning and identifying rewards and goals enhances motivation. Colorful stickers, baseball cards, small toys, and special pencils can be used as rewards.

Unstructured Play

In addition to therapeutic play, the nurse encourages unstructured play in the hospital setting. Through unstructured play, children can control events, ideas, and relationships. Music therapy can give children choices to play instruments such as drums and bells or to join in while a music therapist leads songs and plays a guitar. A study by Hendon and Bohon (2007) showed that music therapy was more likely to improve the mood of an ill child than play therapy.

Evaluation of Play

Therapeutic play should be reflected in the child's nursing care plan. During the evaluation step of the nursing process, the nurse looks at the outcome criteria to determine whether play has facilitated the achievement of goals. Is the child coughing and deep breathing every 2 hours? Is the child expressing feelings over the separation from parents? Is the child eating or sleeping? If the pediatric patient's goals have been achieved, the interventions have been effective.

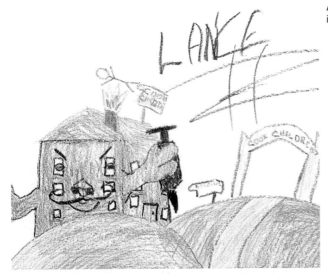

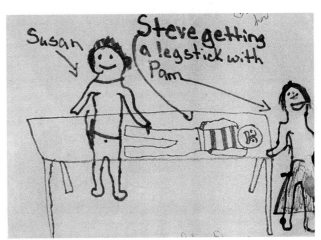

Art materials allow children to express their thoughts and feelings about illness and hospitalization.

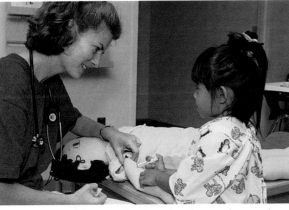

Giving a doll an injection can help a child work through anxiety and anger about injections she may be receiving.

FIG 11-6 Therapeutic play can be used to teach children about medical procedures or help them work through their feelings about what has happened to them in the health care setting. Child life specialists are often members of the team in children's hospitals to provide expert guidance for therapeutic play.

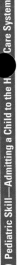

Pediatric Skill—Admitting a Child to the Health Care System

ADMITTING THE CHILD TO A HOSPITAL SETTING

Taking the History

The admission procedure sets the tone for the hospitalization. It should not just consist of a series of questions but rather serve as a time of collaboration between the nurse and the family. The amount of time the family has spent in the emergency department, the seriousness of the illness, and other family needs (e.g., other children staying with grandparents or left with neighbors) may affect the interview process.

The nurse should acknowledge a parent's concerns. For example, the nurse might say to a parent, "I know you're concerned about your other children. Would you like to call your neighbor to check on them before I ask you some questions about your daughter and her illness?"

Most hospitals provide an admission interview form. Some of the information is essential for providing immediate care, and some can be collected later. By recognizing the family's needs, the nurse can structure each admission to fit that child and family. If the parent has entered the system through the emergency department, some of the questions may have previously been answered. Looking at the information already obtained by other departments can avoid repetition. Critical data about allergies, medications taken at home, and recent illness history, however, must be obtained again.

Although hospitals have policies and procedures for admission, the routine may need to be altered because of the child's condition. For example, an IV infusion should be started for a severely dehydrated child, and a child in pain should be medicated immediately. The primary needs of the child and family may be emotional. A parent who has just been told that her child may have a terminal disease may have difficulty remembering the dates of the child's immunizations. In this situation, the nurse should provide the parent with support and assistance in mobilizing coping mechanisms and support systems rather than focusing on data gathering.

After the child and family are made comfortable (Figure 11-7), the nurse obtains a thorough physical, health, and psychosocial history. This is followed by a detailed physical examination. For all types of admissions, the history is recorded on an admission data sheet, which, depending on the facility, may be in electronic format. The format of the admission data sheet varies from hospital to hospital, but most admission forms ask for much of the same information:

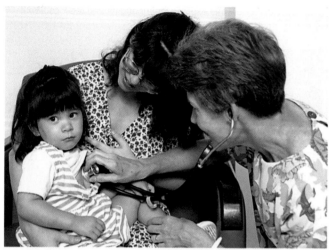

FIG 11-7 To reduce the stress of unfamiliar surroundings and people, the nurse assesses the child who remains in the security of her mother's arms. (Courtesy T.C. Thompson Children's Hospital, Chattanooga, TN.)

history, allergies, and nutritional, sleep, elimination, and psychosocial information.

Physical Examination
Initial Inspection

The initial inspection determines the need for any immediate or emergency care that must be provided before other information can be obtained.

Baseline Data

The physical examination should be thorough, and special attention should be given to the body system or systems involved in the child's chief complaint. Many admission forms have an outline of the child's body on which the nurse should indicate any bruises, scratches, or other skin markings that provide specific objective data. (The process of interviewing, taking a history, and physical assessment is explained in Chapter 9.)

Data collected at admission are used to formulate nursing diagnoses and the child's plan of care and should be accessible to all health care providers. Placing the information in a location that is difficult to access diminishes its importance for care planning.

◎ NURSING CARE PLAN

The Child and Family in a Hospital Setting

Focused Assessment

- Provide a comprehensive hospital admission assessment of the child and family
  - Review the child's past medical history and records of previous hospital experiences
  - Analyze physical examination data
- Assess factors that impact the hospitalized child
  - *Nutrition:* Calorie intake compared to requirements for age and weight; height and weight percentiles; favorite foods; mealtime rituals; cultural or religious customs
  - *Elimination:* Bowel and bladder control norms; terms child uses for elimination; signs of regression and whether regression is distressing to the child or family
  - *Sleep:* Usual sleep patterns, bedtime, hygiene practices, and rituals (rocking, prayers, snacks, stories); compare to norms for age; changes in hours of sleep per day
  - *Self-Care:* Typical level of function (e.g., eating, bathing, dressing, brushing teeth); note any alterations due to stress
  - *Emotional/Social Status:* Signs of anxiety or fear of hospital setting (crying, tantrums, withdrawal, not communicating); participation in activities/play; maintaining contact with peers
- Assess factors that affect the family's adjustment to their child's illness and hospitalization
  - Stress levels of parents
  - Stress levels of siblings and other family members
  - Quality of past hospital experiences
  - Concerns about severity of child's illness and prognosis
  - Need for sleep, food/fluid intake, health care, psychosocial/spiritual support, financial assistance, information, and education

Planning
Nursing Diagnosis

Imbalanced Nutrition: Less Than Body Requirements related to unfamiliar foods, separation from caregiver, strange environment, or disease process.

Expected Outcomes

The child will eat the appropriate number of calories and variety of nutrients according to age.
The child will maintain prehospital weight.

Intervention/*Rationale*

1. Identify the cause of the child's decreased intake.
   Identification can facilitate problem solving.
2. Encourage parents to bring foods from home and to be with the child during meals
   The parents' presence simulates the home environment and increases the likelihood that the child will eat.
3. Allow the child to select food from the menu. Communicate to other staff the foods the child likes to eat.
   Choice gives the child control and may prompt the child to eat.
4. Offer frequent, nutritious snacks and encourage parents to do the same.
   Children need to eat foods with high nutritious value during meals and snacks.
5. Offer small portions. Use colorful, small dishes, cups, and utensils.
   Children may be overwhelmed by large portions and refuse to eat. Child-size tableware, that is decorated, is more appealing to children.
6. Request a consultation with the dietitian.
   A dietitian can assist in planning age-appropriate nutritious meals.

Evaluation

Is the child's nutritional intake appropriate for age?
Did the child maintain baseline body weight during hospitalization?

Planning
Nursing Diagnosis

Delayed Growth and Development, regression in toilet training or self-care skills, related to separation and hospitalization.

Expected Outcomes

The child will maintain usual self-care activities of feeding, toileting, dressing, and bathing. Any regression reverses quickly after discharge.

NURSING CARE PLAN

The Child and Family in a Hospital Setting—cont'd

Intervention/Rationale

1. Follow home routines of elimination, when possible.
   Cooperation will increase and anxiety will decrease if the child's normal routines are maintained.
2. Support the child if regression in toileting skills occurs. Provide diapers and incontinence pads as needed.
   Incontinence (day and/or night) may occur because of the stress of hospitalization and illness.
3. Explain to parents that some temporary regression in self-care activities is expected for ill and hospitalized children.
   Parents may be concerned about the child's regression and may increase their child's anxiety.
4. Encourage the child to participate in self-care activities according to developmental abilities. Provide assistance when factors related to illness impair performance.
   Self-care increases the child's self-esteem and feeling of control. Fatigue, pain, and other symptoms may limit the child's ability to perform self-care independently.
5. Provide the necessary equipment for self-care and place it within reach of the child.
   These actions make it easier for the child to engage in self-care activities and facilitates independence.
6. Offer choices and allow the child to make decisions when appropriate.
   Making choices increases the child's sense of control and may decrease anxiety.

Evaluation

Is the child able to feed, toilet, dress, and bathe at the same level as before the illness?

Does the child readily participate in self-care activities?

Planning
Nursing Diagnosis

Disturbed Sleep Pattern related to unfamiliar environment, anxiety, or discomfort.

Expected Outcome

The child will sleep the appropriate number of hours for age.

Intervention/Rationale

1. Plan for periods throughout the day for sleep. Group nursing care activities.
   Planning to perform multiple tasks while in the child's room (i.e., measure vital signs, conduct shift assessment, and give medications) provides time for uninterrupted sleep.
2. Post a sign on the door when the child is asleep to prevent staff and visitors from waking the child. Eliminate other distractions.
   Minimizing staff and environmental distractions (blinds closed; TV, phone, and lights turned off; door closed, if safe) will facilitate uninterrupted sleep for the child and parents.
3. Reassure the child and family that the nurses will closely monitor the child during periods of sleep, day and night. Provide a night light if indicated.
   Feelings of security are increased if the child and family understand that the nurses are watching and available. Some children fear darkness and need a light on to be comfortable.

Evaluation

Does the child take naps and sleep an appropriate amount of time according to age requirements?

Planning
Nursing Diagnosis

Anxiety related to fear of the unknown and separation from significant others and familiar surroundings.

Expected Outcomes

The child will display decreased indicators of distress (e.g., crying, withdrawal, irritability).

The child will verbalize feelings of anxiety.

The child will play appropriately and maintain contact with peers.

Intervention/Rationale

1. Orient the child and family to the hospital's layout and unit routines.
   Familiarity with the environment and routines will decrease anxiety caused by fear of the unknown.
2. Prepare the child for all procedures and events in an age-appropriate way. Educate parents in advance to decrease anxiety and fear.
   Parents can better support their child if they are knowledgeable.
3. Encourage parents to stay with the child when possible and to be involved in the child's care.
   Presence of parents supports the parental role and decreases the child's separation anxiety.
4. Hold, rock, and cuddle the infant or young child.
   Physical contact increases feelings of security.
5. If the parents cannot stay with the child, provide for a consistent caregiver.
   Continuity of care provides the child the opportunity to develop a trusting relationship.
6. Follow home routines and rituals when possible.
   Familiar routines help the child predict events, resulting in decreased anxiety caused by the unfamiliar setting.
7. Encourage parents to honestly tell their child when they must leave and when they will return. Obtain contact information from parents. Encourage parents to call their child and the nurses while away.
   Trust is increased and anxiety and fear are decreased when parents are honest with their child. Open communication between the parents and nurses can decrease stress.
8. Encourage parents to provide their child with transition objects (e.g., blanket, teddy bear) and reminders of family (e.g., pictures, scarf, handkerchief).
   Transitional objects and family reminders give the child a feeling of security and comfort, which can decrease anxiety particularly during times of separation.
9. Plan play activities for the child throughout the day. Take children to the playroom; promote interaction with other children. Provide toys and other items (books, coloring books, crayons, video games) as well as time for play in the hospital room if the child cannot leave.
   The playroom provides a safe place for the child to engage in activities that facilitate expression and distraction. Interaction with other children can support adaptation to the environment. All children need to be encouraged and given time for play.
10. For the older child, arrange for peer contact through visits, phone calls/texts, e-mails, and cards/letters.
    The older child may fear losing contact with peers. Maintaining contact supports positive self-esteem and security.
11. Offer choices and allow the child to make some decisions.
    These actions increase the child's sense of control.

Continued

⊚ **NURSING CARE PLAN**

The Child and Family in a Hospital Setting—cont'd

Intervention/*Rationale*—cont'd

12. Encourage the children to wear their own clothes and to decorate their hospital room.

    Giving children an opportunity for self-expression helps them feel more comfortable in the hospital environment.

13. Provide opportunities for the older child to verbalize feelings about the illness and hospitalization; inform the child life specialist about the child's concerns and needs.

    Fear and anxiety may decrease if the child has an opportunity to communicate feelings, have them validated, and participate in problem-solving techniques.

Evaluation

Is the child playing and communicating with other children and staff and showing decreased signs of distress?

Is the child able to express feelings of anxiety either verbally or through play?

Planning

Nursing Diagnosis

Interrupted Family Processes related to the child's hospitalization and illness.

Expected Outcomes

The parents and family members will participate in the child's care.

The parents and family members will maintain a baseline level of physical health.

The parents and family members will use appropriate support systems.

The parents and family members will identify ways to cope.

The parents and family members will assist the child to move from a sick role to a well role.

Intervention/*Rationale*

1. Orient the parents and family to the hospital and provide information related to their physical needs (e.g., fluids/food, sleep, bathing, medications).

The parents and family's physical needs must be met for them to meet the child's needs and their own emotional needs. Meeting their needs indicates support by the caregiver.

2. Encourage family members (parents, siblings) to express their feelings and to ask questions about the child's illness.

   Open communication decreases anxiety and clarifies misconceptions.

3. Provide the family with information about the child's condition, treatment, and support systems. Begin to prepare them for the child's discharge (see Patient-Centered Teaching Information for Discharge box).

   Information gives parents a sense of control and decreases their anxiety.

4. Identify with the family the ways in which they are coping; support their parenting skills.

   Individuals are not always aware of their coping mechanisms, and the nurse should help the family evaluate the effectiveness of theirs.

5. Refer the family to other professionals (e.g., social worker, clinical psychologist, clinical specialist, psychiatrist, clergy) when their problems are not within the scope of nursing.

   Early identification of family problems can decrease the possibility of escalation of the problems. Collaboration with other health professionals can bring a holistic approach to the care of child and family.

6. Provide information to the parents about diagnosis, treatment, and prognosis. Attend to their needs for sleep and nutrition.

   The child is affected by parents' anxiety. Helping the parents cope will help decrease their anxiety, which will in turn decrease the child's anxiety.

Evaluation

Are the parents and family members able to participate in the child's care while meeting their own basic physical needs?

Do family members support each other and seek other resources when necessary?

Are family members able to describe and use positive coping skills?

Are the parents able to assist the child to move from a sick role to a well role?

THE ILL CHILD'S FAMILY

Through family-centered care, the nursing care is provided to the child in the context of the family. The nurse's patient is the entire family. Further, the nurse acknowledges that the parents and family are the primary and continuing providers of care for the child.

Parents

A child's illness may create a situational crisis for the family. If the illness leads to hospitalization, either planned or unplanned, the family's anxiety increases. Ill children become the parents' central focus; parents can become very vigilant and committed to protecting the child and ensuring optimal care (Hopia, Tomlinson, Paavilainen, & Astedt-Kurki, 2005). The parental role often changes when the child is admitted to the hospital. The parent who had been in control before the admission is now in an unfamiliar environment. Parents have identified significant stress regarding their ability to fulfill their parental role and care for their ill child (Salisbury, LaMontagne, Hepworth, & Cohen, 2007). Parents may be confused as to what they can and cannot do. Can they bathe their child? Can they hold their child, or will they dislodge the tubes? When nurses, through education and support, assist parents to provide care to their ill child, anxiety levels are reduced for the family as a whole (Salisbury et al., 2007; Keefe, Karlsen, Lobo et al., 2006).

Effective parent/family/child/nurse collaborations are essential to achieving positive outcomes from the hospital experience. Communication between the health care team and the child and family is vital to promoting trust, which promotes high quality, effective care (Precht & Schlucter, 2007). Nurses are responsible for ensuring that children and parents are prepared for hospital experiences, allowed to participate in care activities, and kept informed regarding the child's response to treatment (Ygge, 2007). Research related to critically ill children has shown parents to have significantly reduced stress when they can stay in the pediatric ICU (room-in) with their child (Smith, Hefley, & Anand, 2007). Language barriers and cultural differences can impair effective communication with families. In the United States, children in households where English is not the primary language have been shown to receive lower quality health care services than children in English-speaking households (Flores & Tomany-Korman, 2008). Use of medical interpreters may be effective in improving care for these children (Figure 11-8).

Parents have varied responses to a child's illness. They may have guilt feelings related to the belief that if they had sought treatment

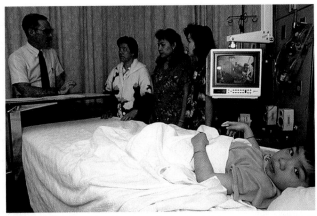

FIG 11-8 The family of a hospitalized child may not speak the prevailing language. Interpreters are available (on-site or on-call) at many hospitals to help parents and children communicate with health care team members. This arrangement provides a familiar link to the parents' and child's culture and language. (Courtesy Cook Children's Medical Center, Fort Worth, TX.)

❓ CRITICAL THINKING EXERCISE 11-1

Tommy, 4 years old, was admitted to the hospital with pneumonia. Tommy has cystic fibrosis. His family has recently moved to the area, and this is his first admission to your hospital. Tommy loves to play with his dinosaur collection and spends much of his day playing and watching his favorite DVDs. His mother visits for short periods during the lunch hour, and his father visits in the evening. Tommy cries when his parents leave. You mention to a colleague that you think Tommy's parents should spend more time with him. She responds, "We don't know what their other responsibilities are."

1. What other responsibilities might the family have?
2. What are some of the nursing interventions that would support a family with a child in the hospital?

PATIENT-CENTERED TEACHING

Information for Discharge

After assessing the family's knowledge, the nurse provides the information families need to know to help the child's transition from hospital to home:

- Information about the illness or trauma and expected outcomes. Tell the parents when they should consult the primary care physician or nurse.
- Medications or treatments to be given at home and information about times, route, side effects, and any special care to be taken when giving the medication. Providing written information is valuable.
- Information about any special nutritional needs.
- Specific activities the child may or may not participate in.
- The date when the child may return to school.
- The date to bring the child back to the hospital, clinic, or office for follow-up care.
- Information about any referral agency needed for the child or family.
- The unit phone number and primary nurse's name.

The nurse explains, demonstrates, and then requests a return demonstration by the parents (and child if age-appropriate) of any treatments or procedures that will be done at home. This teaching should be a continuing process and not left until the time of discharge because learning takes place at different rates.

---

earlier, the child would not be so ill, or they may initially deny that their child is ill. A period of **denial** may be followed by anger. This anger may be directed at the nurse, at another family member, or sometimes at a deity. When the immediate crisis is over, a period of depression can occur. Many times parents become exhausted, both physically and psychologically, because of spending long hours at the hospital in addition to working and caring for their other children. It is essential that nurses address the health needs of family members (Hopia et al., 2005) and provide support for identified psychosocial needs (Aldridge, 2005). This may include encouraging parents to express their feelings, active listening, assistance with processing feelings, and referral for counseling and social work services.

The needs of fathers are sometimes forgotten. The father may come to the hospital only after he has spent a day at work and then, after a short visit, may need to go home to be with other children. He may not be there when the primary care physician makes rounds and therefore receives most of his medical information from someone else. The father may think that he needs to be the strong one in the family and not show his fear and anxiety. In some families, the mother works outside the home while the father stays with the child. In either case, an awareness of each parent's role will assist the nurse in identifying the individual needs of the parents.

Because of dual roles, long separations, increased stress, and numerous other factors, the parents' marriage may be strained. This situation is especially likely in marriages that are already at risk. Even when both partners are at the hospital, they may not have any time alone.

Many children have stepmothers and stepfathers or may be cared for by grandparents. In such cases, all caregivers need recognition, support, and education. How the family copes with the child's illness depends on use of its coping strategies. A family that is already in crisis or one without support systems (e.g., family, friends, church) will have more difficulty adjusting to the change than a family that is organized and adjusted. A family that deals successfully with the crisis is strengthened by the experience. (For further discussion of the effects of illness on the family, see Chapter 2. For a discussion of the family with a child with a chronic illness, see Chapter 12.)

Siblings

The illness or hospitalization of a brother or sister can be difficult for children. The ill child's siblings may experience jealousy, insecurity, resentment, confusion, and anxiety. Children often have difficulty understanding why their ill sibling is getting all the attention and why their parents have so little time for them. They may worry that if their sibling could get sick, so could they. Preschool children, who engage in magical thinking, may worry that they somehow caused the illness. All of these thoughts and feelings are compounded by children's difficulty expressing their feelings (Box 11-3). A review of several studies looking at the psychological adjustment of siblings whose brother or sister has cancer reveals that the siblings experience stress symptoms, negative emotional reactions (fear, sadness, anger, helplessness, guilt), and school difficulties along with positive outcomes of increased maturity and empathy (Alderfer, Long, Lown et al., 2010). The ability of siblings to cope with stress can vary with age and developmental level, relationship with the ill child, and frequency of visits to see the ill child. In addition, parents significantly influence how siblings cope. Research findings for siblings of children with cystic fibrosis have shown that increased parental stress and less family social support result in poorer adaptation to stress by the well sibling (O'Haver, Moore, Insel et al., 2010). Siblings are a part of the family unit and their needs must be assessed so that appropriate interventions by nurses and other health care team members can be provided.

BOX 11-3 CARING FOR THE SIBLINGS OF AN ILL OR HOSPITALIZED CHILD

Factors that Add to the Stress of Siblings

- Age younger than 10 years
- Emotional closeness to the hospitalized child
- Receiving only a limited explanation of the experience
- Fear of getting the illness themselves
- Being cared for outside their own home
- Perceiving that their parents are acting differently toward them
- Having a sibling who is progressively ill

Nursing Care Guidelines for Meeting the Needs of Siblings

- Encourage caregivers to have the ill child retell what happened. This experience may be uncomfortable for the adult, but it helps the sibling put the illness or accident in perspective.
- If the sibling has feelings of guilt, address the child's concerns directly. If the feelings of guilt continue, suggest a consultation with a counselor.
- Give parents educational materials, and show them how to use them with the sibling.
- Schedule a time for the sibling to visit. Prepare the sibling for the medical equipment and any changes in the ill child's appearance that may cause concern.
- If the sibling cannot visit, send photographs.
- Encourage the sibling to talk with the child on the telephone.

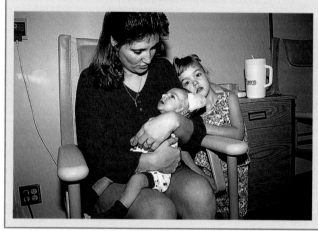

Siblings of ill children may experience jealousy, insecurity, resentment, confusion, and anxiety. The nurse can help them cope by assessing and implementing care to meet their needs. (Courtesy Children's Medical Center, Dallas, TX.)

Modified from Craft, M., Wyatt, N., & Sandell, B. (1985). Behavior and feeling changes in siblings of hospitalized children. *Clinical Pediatrics, 24,* 374-378.

■ KEY CONCEPTS

- Pediatric nurses provide specialized care for children in different settings—hospital, school, community, and home.
- Common stressors that affect hospitalized children are separation anxiety, fear of pain or mutilation, fear of the unknown, and loss of control.
- Children may respond to illness with anger, guilt, and regression.
- The stages of separation anxiety are protest, despair, and detachment.
- With increased stress, it is more difficult for children to separate from their parents.
- A child's reactions to pain and fear of injury are related to developmental stage, previous experiences, separation from parents, restraint, and preparation.
- When ill children feel they have control, they are more likely to be cooperative.

- Children commonly return to an earlier stage of behavior (regression) when stressed due to illness.
- Children's responses to illness and hospitalization are affected by their perception of events, age, developmental level, cognitive ability, preparation, previous experiences, coping skills, and parent and family responses.
- Nursing care of the ill child focuses on promoting self-care, minimizing separation anxiety, understanding growth and development, providing diversion/play, involving family, allowing control, and managing pain.
- Parents may feel guilt, denial, anger, and depression when their child is hospitalized.
- Therapeutic play allows for emotional expression and enhances development. It is used by nurses to educate children and prepare them for procedures.

REFERENCES

Alderfer, M., Long, K., Lown, E., et al. (2010). Psychosocial adjustment of siblings of children with cancer: A systematic review. *Psycho-Oncology, 19*(8), 789-805.

Aldridge, M. (2005). Decreasing parental stress in the pediatric intensive care unit: One unit's experience. *Critical Care Nurse, 25*(6), 40-50.

American Academy of Pediatrics. (2008). Policy statement: Role of the school nurse in providing school health services. *Pediatrics, 121*(5), 1052-1056.

American Academy of Pediatrics Child Life Council and Committee on Hospital Care (2006). Child life services. *Pediatrics, 118*(4), 1757-1763.

American Academy of Pediatrics Healthy Children. (2010). *Ages and stages: Teaching health education in schools.*

Retrieved from www.healthychildren.org/English/ages-stages/gradeschool/school/pages/Teaching-Health-Education-in-School.aspx.

Board, R. (2005). School-age children's perceptions of their PICU hospitalization. *Pediatric Nursing, 31,* 166-175.

Bolig, R., Ferne, D., & Klein, E. (1986). Unstructured play in hospital settings: An internal locus of control rationale. *Children's Health Care, 15*(2), 101-107.

Breiner, S. (2009). Preparation of the pediatric patient for invasive procedures. *Journal of Infusion Nursing, 32*(5), 252-256.

Craft-Rosenberg, M., & Krajicek, M. J. (Eds.), (2006). *Nursing excellence for children and families.* New York: Springer.

Driessnack, M. (2005). Children's drawings as facilitators of communication: A meta-analysis. *Journal of Pediatric Nursing, 20,* 415-423.

Erikson, E. (1963). *Childhood and society* (2nd ed.). New York: Norton.

Flores, G., & Tomany-Korman, S. (2008). The language spoken at home and disparities in medical and dental health, access to care, and use of services in U.S. children. *Pediatrics, 121*(6), e1703-e1714.

Hendon, C., & Bohon, L. (2007). Hospitalized children's mood differences during play and music therapy. *Child: Care, Health and Development, 34*(2), 141-144.

Hewitt-Taylor, J. (2010). Supporting children with complex health needs. *Nursing Standard, 24*(19), 50-56.

Hopia, H., Tomlinson, P., Paavilainen, E., & Astedt-Kurki, P. (2005). Child in hospital: Family experiences and expectations of how nurses can promote family health. *Journal of Clinical Nursing, 14*, 212-222.

Keefe, M., Karlsen, K., Lobo, M., et al. (2006). Reducing parenting stress in families with irritable infants. *Nursing Research, 55*(3), 198-205.

Li, H. C. W., & Lopez, V. (2008). Effectiveness and appropriateness of therapeutic play intervention in preparing children for surgery: A randomized controlled trial study. *Journal of Specialists in Pediatric Nursing, 13*(2), 63-73.

Lindeke, L., Nakai, M., & Johnson, L. (2006). Capturing children's voices for quality improvement. *MCN The American Journal of Maternal-Child Nursing, 31*(5), 290-295.

Melnyk, B. M., Carno, M-A., & Small, L. (2004). The effectiveness of parent-focused interventions in improving coping/mental health outcomes of critically ill children and their parents: An evidence base to guide clinical practice. *Pediatric Nursing, 30*(2), 143-148.

Melnyk, B. M., Feinstein, N., & Fairbanks, E. (2006). Two decades of evidence to support implementation of the COPE program as standard practice with parents of young unexpectedly hospitalized/critically ill children and premature infants. *Pediatric Nursing, 32*(5), 474-481.

O'Haver, J., Moore, I., Insel, K., et al. (2010). Parental perceptions of risk and protective factors associated with the adaptation of siblings of children with cystic fibrosis. *Pediatric Nursing, 36*(6), 284-291.

Ono, S., Hirabayashi, Y., Oikawa, I., & Manabe, Y. (2008). Preparation of a picture book to support parents and autonomy in preschool children facing day surgery. *Pediatric Nursing, 34*(1), 82-83, 88.

Pelander, T., & Leino-Kilpi, H. (2004). Quality in pediatric nursing care: Children's expectations. *Issues in Comprehensive Pediatric Nursing, 27*(3), 139-151.

Precht, B., & Schlucter, J. (2007). Family partnerships key to family-centered care model. *Patient Education Management, 14*(1), 3-4.

Richardson, J. (2007). Building bridges between school-based health clinics and schools. *Journal of School Health, 77*(7), 337-343.

Rzucidio, S., & Campbell, M. (2009). Beyond the physical injuries: Child and parent coping with medical traumatic stress after pediatric trauma. *Journal of Trauma Nursing, 16*(3), 130-135.

Salisbury, M., LaMontagne, L., Hepworth, J., & Cohen, F. (2007). Parents' self-identified stressors and coping strategies during adolescents' spinal surgery experiences. *Clinical Nursing Research, 16*(3), 212-230.

Salmela, M., Salantera, S., & Aronen, E. (2009). Child-reported hospital fears in 4 to 6-year-old children. *Pediatric Nursing 35*(5), 269-303.

Sarajärvi, A., Haapamäki, M., & Paavilainen, E. (2006). Emotional and informational support for families during their child's illness. *International Nursing Review, 53*, 205-210.

Schmidt, C., Bernaix, L., Koski, A., et al. (2007). Hospitalized children's perceptions of nurses and nurse behaviors.

MCN The American Journal of Maternal Child Nursing, 32(6), 336-342.

Skybo, T., Ryan-Wenger, N., & Su, Y. (2006). Human figure drawings as a measure of children's emotional status: Critical review for practice. *Journal of Pediatric Nursing, 22*, 15-28.

Smith, A., Hefley, G., & Anand, K. (2007). Parent bed spaces in the PICU: Effect on parental stress. *Pediatric Nursing, 33*(3), 215-221.

Sorensen, H., Card, C., Malley, M., & Strzelecki, J. (2009). Using a collaborative child life approach for continuous surgical preparation. *AORN, 90*(4), 557-566.

van Breeman, C. (2009). Using play therapy in paediatric palliative care: Listening to the story and caring for the body. *International Journal of Palliative Nursing, 15*(10), 510-514.

Visintainer, M., & Wolfer, J. (1975). Psychological preparation for surgical pediatric patient: The effect on children's and parents' stress response and adjustment. *Pediatrics, 56*(2), 187-202.

Wikstrom, B. (2005). Communicating via expressive arts: The natural medium of self-expression for hospitalized children. *Pediatric Nursing, 31*, 480-485.

Ygge, B. M. (2007). Nurses' perceptions of parental involvement in hospital care. *Paediatric Nursing, 19*(5), 38-40.

The Child with a Chronic Condition or Terminal Illness

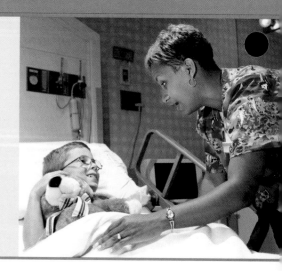

evolve WEBSITE

http://evolve.elsevier.com/James/ncoc

LEARNING OBJECTIVES

After studying this chapter, you should be able to:

- Define chronic illness.
- Analyze the effects of a chronic illness on the child and family.
- Discuss the concerns and needs of the child and family dealing with a chronic illness.
- Compare the stages of death and dying.
- Apply the concepts of death and dying as they relate to the pediatric patient.

- Explain the concerns and needs of the child and family facing an impending death.
- Analyze the nurse's response to death and dying in the pediatric population.
- Use the nursing process to describe nursing care of the chronically ill and dying child.

Rapid advances in health care have changed the experience of chronic illness in childhood. Increasing numbers of children who previously would have died from their illnesses early in their lives are living longer (Chamberlain & Wise, 2011). Improvements in early diagnostic testing and treatment have enhanced quality of life, as well as longevity.

CHRONIC ILLNESS DEFINED

A chronic illness or condition is long term, persisting more than 3 months. It does not spontaneously resolve, is usually without complete cure, frequently has residual characteristics that limit activities of daily living (ADLs), and requires adaptation or special assistance. Box 12-1 lists some of the common chronic conditions of childhood. Severity varies among chronic conditions. Many, such as epilepsy, diabetes, or sickle cell disease, although not physically apparent, may have a tremendous impact on the child and family. A chronic condition that is terminal but lasts only a short time may also have serious long-term effects on the surviving family. Although the first section of this chapter refers only to chronic conditions, this information also applies to terminal conditions. The U.S. Department of Health and Human Services, Health Resources and Services Administration, Maternal and Child Health Bureau (2008) developed the following definition regarding the special needs of chronically and terminally ill children for planning and advocacy purposes.

Children with special health care needs are those who have or are at increased risk for a chronic physical, developmental, behavioral, or emotional condition and who also require health and related services of a type and amount beyond that required for children generally.

THE FAMILY OF THE CHILD WITH SPECIAL HEALTH CARE NEEDS

Family Dynamics and Impact on the Family

Improvements in technology, reimbursement provisions (e.g., insurance, state and federal funding), and allocation of health care resources have all affected the family's role in caring for the child with a chronic illness. Children with special needs can now be safely cared for in the home setting, with minimal periods of hospitalization. Such care, which includes psychosocial support, is the most desirable and cost-effective care for both child and family.

Although improved quality of life and longevity are positive developments, they do present certain difficulties. Despite health care advances, the child and family must live with a constant physical problem and uncertainty that require consistent, ongoing attention and adaptation. This is referred to as the illness trajectory: the course of a chronic illness and the impact on the lives of all those involved. For children, it is difficult to predict accurately the progression of

BOX 12-1 COMMON CHRONIC CONDITIONS OF CHILDHOOD

- Attention deficit hyperactivity disorder (ADHD)
- Attention deficit disorder (ADD)
- Asthma (reactive airway disease)
- Autism
- Bleeding disorders (e.g., hemophilia)
- Bronchopulmonary dysplasia
- Cancer
- Cardiac disorders
- Cerebral palsy
- Chronic renal failure
- Congenital heart disease and other heart conditions
- Cystic fibrosis
- Developmental delay
- Diabetes mellitus

- Down syndrome
- Hepatitis
- Human immunodeficiency virus (HIV) infection
- Acquired immunodeficiency syndrome (AIDS)
- Hydrocephalus
- Inborn errors of metabolism
- Intellectual impairment (formerly, mental retardation)
- Juvenile arthritis
- Lupus erythematosus
- Muscular dystrophy
- Neural tube defects
- Phenylketonuria
- Seizure disorders
- Sickle cell disease

many serious, long-term illnesses (Ullrich, Duncan, Joselow, & Wolfe, 2011).

Chronic illness is stressful and can create situational crises for families. A situational crisis is an unexpected crisis for which the family's usual problem-solving abilities are not adequate. However, various studies show that some families reorganize and actually become stronger in response to a situational crisis. These families are considered resilient; that is, they are able to recover from adversities associated with chronic illness. They do this through normalization, making necessary changes in their lives and adjusting to the presence of the chronic illness. They actively work on responses that will help counteract the illness and resulting abnormal behaviors to maintain social roles that are appropriate and valued.

Family resiliency implies present and future success at managing complex aspects of a crisis, such as having a child with a chronic condition. Resilient families are able to focus on their strengths to assist them with problem solving (Frain, Berven, Tschopp et al., 2007). Resilient families exhibit many important traits, but a predominant trait is family cohesiveness. This cohesion is achieved through active efforts to keep the family intact by sharing the new responsibilities related to the chronic condition, as well as the routine, enjoyable activities of family life. Although family life may be altered by the crisis, resilient families become skilled at successfully managing day-to-day tasks, even though roles within the family structure might need to be altered (Frain et al., 2007). Families accomplish this by developing protective factors to counteract the stress inherent in caring for a child with a chronic illness and by accessing resources to assist them. Processes that enhance family resilience include the following (Frain et al., 2007; Patterson, 2002):

- Establishing and accessing both internal and external sources of physical, social, and financial support
- Reframing the situation to identify positive rather than negative aspects
- Successful coping that increases family self-efficacy, or the belief that the family can problem solve in new ways to meet the new challenges
- Maintaining high-quality and open communication patterns
- Being flexible
- Maintaining social integration
- Preserving family boundaries

Maintaining social integration involves balancing the needs of the family with the needs imposed by the child's condition, as well as reciprocal interactions with the community relative to the child's needs. Resilient families are careful in allocating resources, including money, time, and energy, as they balance various needs. This balance ensures that no child in the family, ill or well, is neglected or overindulged. Additionally, it ensures that the condition-related needs of the ill child are balanced with normal growth and development needs and that needs are met without overprotection. In resilient families, the child's condition-related needs are incorporated into the family's daily life; they do not become the focus around which the activities of the entire family revolve. This integration helps achieve and maintain the family's new normality imposed by the illness. In such a family setting, baseball practices, school activities, ballet recitals, and other activities do not stop for either the ill child or the well siblings. Rather, care of the child, medical appointments, and treatments for the ill child are arranged around these activities to the degree possible. When conflicts do arise, parents (or other family members or friends) alternate responsibility for maintaining the activities of both the ill child and well siblings.

Equitable allocation of caregiving and encouragement of parental involvement with each other and well siblings help maintain appropriate family boundaries. When either of the two parents becomes primarily involved in meeting the needs of the ill child, the parental relationship suffers. To keep these boundaries intact, resilient families pay specific attention to maintaining a positive parental relationship. They also work to avoid showing favoritism toward the ill child.

Single-parent families may encounter additional difficulties that heighten the risks that the chronic condition will negatively affect resilience and impede normalization. Social support may not be inherent in the family structure, so these families are at increased risk for social isolation. Health care providers can refer single parents to support groups, put them in contact with other parents who have a child with a similar chronic condition, or organize group-sharing experiences between parents experienced in the care of the child with a particular chronic condition and parents of newly diagnosed children.

Boundary problems of a different sort can arise when the need for outside care and assistance increases, such as the presence of home health or hospice personnel. Whether they are in the home around the clock or for various shifts throughout the week, external family boundaries can be negatively affected. However, difficulties can be minimized if family members adopt an assertive role in managing the child's care and, along with the health care personnel, work to maintain professional relationships and boundaries with caregivers.

Resilient families consistently work to ensure appropriate communication, which may be more difficult because of new, condition-related language (medical or otherwise); an increased need for problem-solving based communication; and, most important, the need to express emotions. Accepting the validity of all emotions and learning suitable means of expressing them may be difficult. However, many families report that the experience of living with a chronic illness brings about positive life changes, such as increased empathy, increased family unity, and new meanings to life.

Even when positive meaning is attached to a child's chronic condition, much flexibility is required of family members regarding family roles and expectations. This flexibility is also required of the health care team, both for the benefit of the family and as a means of achieving a positive, collaborative relationship between the team and the family. The team becomes an integral part of family life. The quality of this relationship may affect how the entire family adapts to and copes with the child's condition.

For resilient families, coping is an active process that entails learning about their child's illness and available resources. These families do not sit idly by, letting others meet their child's needs. They are also the strongest advocates for their child. Subsequently, they have a tremendous need for any information concerning their child's condition. The nurse has an important role in helping families educate themselves and learn to meet their child's special health care needs.

At times of extreme stress, such as periods of unexpected physical setbacks, exacerbations, worsening or relapse of the condition, as well as at the time of death, families may slip into less effective patterns of behavior and coping. Gentle reminders, support, and encouragement may be all the assistance that a resilient family needs to help members resume the behaviors that foster resiliency despite the many ongoing stressors and uncertainties of a chronic condition.

Coping and the Grieving Process

The most important aspect of a chronic illness is that it affects the entire family, not just the ill child. This scope of concern necessitates consistent family-centered nursing care (see Chapter 2). All family members respond to the child's chronic condition. However, responses of individual family members vary according to their age and developmental level, their relationship and involvement with the ill child, and any previous experiences they have had with a health care problem.

Chronic and terminal conditions involve the loss of health and result in grief. Grief is a normal psychophysiologic process that occurs in response to a specific loss. A normal and frequent response to such conditions includes the five stages of grief as defined by Elisabeth Kübler-Ross (1969). Her work identified the stages in relation to the anticipated death of an adult. However, they apply to children as well as adults and to the grief associated with a chronic condition as well as a terminal illness. The ill child, siblings, parents, and other family members may experience these stages.

The stages include denial, anger, bargaining, sadness or depression, and acceptance. During the first stage, *denial*, individuals react with disbelief and shock. Feelings of "no, not me" and "no, not my loved one" occur whether the person is explicitly told of the diagnosis or, in the case of some children, they figure it out on their own. *Anger* usually follows denial. This may include feelings of rage and resentment directed at themselves or at others. At this point, the questions of "why me?" and "why my loved one?" may also occur. Anger may recur at any time during the process of the illness. *Bargaining* then happens, whereby the individual attempts to postpone the inevitable. Although most bargaining is with a spiritual deity, bargaining with oneself or others may also take place.

Depression is the next stage. Such sadness may be for either past losses or those impending losses. Past losses may include physical losses, such as a change in appearance (e.g., hair loss), lifestyle changes, or changes in physical ability. Impending losses may include imminent

loss of loved ones. It may also include preparing loved ones for the absence created by death. The last stage is *acceptance*, whereby the individual is no longer depressed or angry. Although acceptance is not necessarily a happy stage, it is generally a time of comfort and peace.

Individuals need different periods of time to work through and resolve the feelings of one stage before proceeding to the next stage. The stages are not always experienced sequentially. Some fluctuation may recur across stages before acceptance and comfort are reached. Acceptance of a chronic illness can take place even in the presence of noticeable denial. Such denial might appear to be maintained throughout the course of the illness. Because children have less predictable and more variable protective mechanisms, they may use denial more frequently than adults. An individual who has a positive, optimistic outlook and who focuses on concerns and tasks of the day rather than on fears about the condition may appear to be adjusting well; however, he or she also may be using denial as a protective coping mechanism.

The period for the presence of denial is important. Short-term, true denial, although often considered maladaptive, may truly be adaptive. Denial that persists may be maladaptive and part of a prolonged grief response (Maciejewski, Zhang, Block, & Prigerson, 2007). Persistent denial can be contributory to dysfunctional coping patterns and can interfere with problem solving. Attempting to establish whether true, ongoing denial is present is important. Many times what appears to be denial is simply the individual's expression of lost hopes for the ill child. This might be seen as a mother's talk of how beautiful her daughter will look as a bride. It might be a sibling's discussion as to how much fun he or she will have with the ill child next summer at camp. Families need to recognize and express the most difficult aspects of their impending loss in order to grieve fully and appropriately. Another aspect of what appears to be denial is the expression of the faith that a miracle will occur and that the child will not die after all.

As adjustment to the condition progresses, many parents experience chronic sorrow related to the unending nature of the child's condition and the ongoing feelings of loss (George, Vickers, Wilkes, & Barton, 2006-2007). Contributing to this are feelings of helplessness, emotional and psychological stress, and uncertainty related to the unpredictable course of the child's illness or condition (George et al., 2006-2007). Chronic sorrow is a normal process and may never resolve. However, adaptation to the presence of the illness occurs. The family establishes a "new normal," and their life continues. Chronic sorrow, however, is not the same as prolonged or chronic grief. Chronic grief refers to mourning that is of excessive duration and interferes with the individual's ability to return to normal living after the death of a significant person (Maciejewski et al., 2007).

The first step in supporting families and helping them deal with chronic sorrow is to listen, and then recognize and acknowledge their emotions. The family can be assisted to recognize the normality of such feelings and emotions themselves. Family members should be gently encouraged to acknowledge and express feelings of chronic sorrow, to the degree with which they are comfortable. However, at the same time, they should be encouraged and assisted to verbalize and demonstrate realistic hopes and dreams.

George and colleagues (2006-2007) found that thoughtlessness on the part of caring professionals can trigger or exacerbate feelings of chronic sorrow in parents of children with chronic illness. Not recognizing parents as experts in their child's care, making hurtful or insensitive comments about the child, repeatedly asking for the child's history, or not providing appropriate support or understanding of the parents' emotional needs were seen as triggers for feelings of grief. Nurses need to be particularly aware of how they communicate with parents. Showing concern and an attitude of support, while facilitating the expression of feelings by the parents, is optimal nursing care for parents coping with chronic sorrow (Thurgate, 2006).

Many support organizations, both general and disease specific, offer a wealth of information, support, and assistance to families of a child with a chronic or terminal illness. They offer much beyond the information related to the child's condition. The nurse should introduce the family to such services and, as necessary, assist them to use these services fully. Conversely, a family's decision not to use support services should be respected.

Supportive services may be particularly important when observation and assessment of family behaviors indicate problems that may necessitate referral to a mental health professional. In caring for children with a chronic or terminal illness and their families, one issue that is frequently overlooked is that death may occur unexpectedly or earlier than anticipated. This is an important but difficult issue to address with families. It should be done in the early stage of the condition to prepare them if the death does happen in an unexpected manner. The nurse should support children and their families through all stages of the grief process. Supporting the family requires understanding the family's current knowledge base, coping skills, and personal beliefs, as well as recognizing and attending to the grief-related problems that arise.

THE CHILD WITH SPECIAL HEALTH CARE NEEDS

Coping and Growth and Development Concerns

Children with chronic disorders have many different concerns and needs related to their conditions, not the least of which is successful navigation of the stages of growth and development. Children's responses to illness are influenced by their age at the onset of the disorder, as well as growth and development considerations throughout the course of the illness. Nursing care is planned accordingly.

Chronic and terminal conditions often span a number of years and developmental stages. Regardless of the stage, concerns related to self-esteem, self-reliance, and autonomy are prevalent among children with chronic conditions. Many will experience altered body awareness and body image as a result of physical changes related to the illness or treatment. These changes frequently have a negative impact on children's self-esteem. Control and autonomy may be decreased because of hospitalizations and treatment regimens that offer few decision-making opportunities for the child. Socialization activities and adjustment may be limited as a result of hospitalization and the side effects of the illness or treatment. Side effects, including altered appearance, decreased physical ability, or increased susceptibility to infection, may interfere with age-appropriate socialization. There can be times when a medical condition (e.g., infection risk, bleeding risk) may not keep the child from participating; rather, the child declines to do so because of fears regarding his or her appearance or physical abilities.

Such factors may profoundly affect a child's acquisition of age-appropriate growth and developmental skills, especially during adolescence. An important goal is to minimize the effects of illness and hospitalization and to maximize the child's developmental potential. This is true regardless of the age or developmental stage, and the nurse should understand issues concerning self-esteem and autonomy in relation to each stage of growth and development (Box 12-2).

Despite the understanding and interventions of family and staff, a variety of consequences may frequently occur among children with a chronic condition or illness. Most are minimal, short lived, and expected as a part of the course of a chronic condition. For example, stranger anxiety may be heightened or may reappear months after previous resolution among infants and toddlers.

Temporary regression may be seen with children of all ages, including adolescents. However, it is more prevalent among older infants through the young school-age years. Toddlers use regression frequently as they attempt to cope with the stress of a serious illness. Despite the normalcy of regression, it may be unsettling to the child and family because it involves the loss of recently acquired skills or the reappearance of behaviors seen when the child was younger. Common regressive behaviors include reverting back to a bottle, pacifier, or thumb-sucking; a change in toileting skills; an increased incidence of bed-wetting; and an increased use of "baby talk" or communication techniques more appropriate for younger children.

Another possible difficulty is a fluctuation in the child's age-appropriate communication patterns between family and members of the health care team. Lack of communication or altered communication patterns with health care providers may occur in the clinic or hospital setting, with regular patterns of communication resuming at home. Among older preschoolers, a lack of communication may be a form of withdrawal or an expression of stubbornness and a refusal to cooperate. This problem may also be seen in school-age children and adolescents, usually related to issues involving independence and self-esteem.

Coping and Parental Responses to Developmental Issues

Regardless of the developmental stage or the number of years that a chronic illness has existed, the basic guidelines for child rearing still apply to all children in the family. Boundaries, discipline, and consistency are equally important to both the ill child and the well siblings. A good example is the mother of a 3-year-old with cancer who would frequently remind both the ill child and her older sibling that cancer is no excuse for bad manners!

Experiencing a chronic illness is confusing, especially for children whose cognitive abilities are not sufficiently developed to allow understanding that could help them cope with the stress. When changes in a child's world begin to affect the only constant he or she knows, the family, this is often reflected in the child's behavior. Negative behavior may result from the stress of the illness and changes in the family and environment. Previously existing negative behaviors may worsen, making treatment and a positive, cooperative relationship with health care team members difficult. Future behavior and long-term development may be affected as well. At the time their child is diagnosed, parents should be reminded about the importance of maintaining previous rules and expectations. Chronically ill children are more likely to experience behavioral and psychological issues. Despite this, most children with chronic health problems will experience the same level of behavioral and psychological issues as other children in the same age-group (Chamberlain & Wise, 2011).

! **NURSING QUALITY ALERT**

Goals for Chronic Care

Goals for the Child
- Achieve and maintain normalization
- Obtain the highest level of health and function possible—physically, emotionally, and psychosocially

Goals for the Family
- Remain intact
- Achieve and maintain normalization
- Maximize function throughout the course of the illness

BOX 12-2 THE ILLNESS EXPERIENCE: THE CHILD AND ADOLESCENT

Infant

Developmental task: Achievement of awareness of being separate from significant other.

Impact of illness: Potential distortion of differentiation of self from parents or significant others.

Cognitive age/stage: Sensorimotor (birth to 2 years).

Major fears: Separation, strangers.

Interventions: Provide consistent caregivers. Minimize separation from parents and significant others. Decrease parental anxiety, which is projected to infant. Maintain crib and nursery as "safe place" where no invasive procedures are performed.

Toddler

Developmental task: Initiation of autonomy.

Impact of illness: Interference with or loss of developing sense of control, independence.

Cognitive age/stage: Preoperational (2 to 7 years): egocentric, magical, little concept of body integrity.

Major fears: Separation, loss of control.

Concept of illness: Phenomenism (2 to 7 years)—perceives external, unrelated, concrete phenomena as cause of illness (e.g., "being sick because you don't feel well"). Contagion—perceives cause of illness as proximity between two events that occurs by "magic" (e.g., "getting a cold because you are near someone who has a cold").

Interventions: Minimize separation from parents or significant others. Keep security objects at hand. Provide simple, brief explanations. Explain and maintain consistent limits. Encourage participation in daily care. Provide opportunities for play.

Preschooler

Developmental task: Creation of a sense of initiative.

Impact of illness: Interference with or loss of accomplishments, such as walking, talking, controlling basic body functions.

Cognitive age/stage: Preoperational thought—egocentric, magical, tendency to use and repeat words child does not understand, providing own explanations and definitions. Literal translation of words. Inability to abstract.

Major fears: Body injury and mutilation, loss of control, the unknown, the dark, being left alone.

Concept of illness: Phenomenism, contagion.

Interventions: Provide simple, concrete explanations. Advance preparation is important: days for major events, hours for minor events. Verbal explanations are usually insufficient, so use pictures, models, actual equipment, and medical play.

School-Age Child

Developmental task: Sense of industry.

Impact of illness: Potential feelings of inadequacy or inferiority if autonomy and independence are compromised.

Cognitive age/stage: Concrete operational thought (7 to 10 years).

Major fears: Loss of control, body injury and mutilation, failure to live up to expectations of important others, death.

Concept of illness: Contamination—perceives cause as a person, an object, or an action external to the child that is "bad" or "harmful" to the body (e.g., "getting a cold because you didn't wear a hat"). Internalization—perceives illness as having an external cause but being located inside the body (e.g., "getting a cold by breathing in air and bacteria").

Interventions: Provide choices whenever possible to increase the child's sense of control. Emphasize contact with peer group. Use diagrams, pictures, and models for explanations because thinking is concrete. Emphasize the "normal" things the child can do because the child does not want to be seen as different. Reassure children that they have done nothing wrong; hospitalization, for example, is not punishment.

Adolescent

Developmental task: Achieving a sense of identity.

Impact of illness: Potential alteration in or relinquishment of newly acquired roles and responsibilities.

Cognitive age/stage: Formal operational thought (11+ years): beginning of ability to think abstractly. Existence of some magical thinking (e.g., feeling guilty for illness) and egocentrism.

Major fears: Loss of control, altered body image, separation from peer group.

Concept of illness: Physiologic—perceives cause as malfunctioning or nonfunctioning organ or process; can explain illness in sequence of events. Psychophysiologic—realizes that psychological actions and attitudes affect health and illness.

Interventions: Allow adolescent to be an integral part of decision making regarding care. Give information sensitively because adolescents react both to the content of information and to the manner in which it is delivered. Allow as many choices and as much control as possible. Be honest about treatment and its consequences. Stress the importance of cooperation and adherence. Additionally, emphasize decision making in which the adolescent can participate, as well as the areas in life over which control can be maintained. Assist in maintaining contact with peer group.

Data from Gibbons, M. B. (1993). Psychosocial aspects of serious illness in childhood and adolescence. In A. Armstrong-Dailey & S. Goltzer (Eds.), *Hospice care for children.* New York: Oxford University Press; Bibace, R., & Walsh, M. E. (1980). Development of children's concepts of illness. *Pediatrics, 66*(6), 912-918.

THE CHILD WITH A CHRONIC ILLNESS

The goals for any child with a chronic illness are to achieve and maintain the highest level of health and function possible—cognitively, emotionally, physically, and psychosocially. The aim is similar for the family system, including parents or guardians, siblings, and extended family members. Goals for the entire family are to remain intact, achieve and maintain normalization, and maximize function throughout the illness. This necessitates a family-centered approach to nursing care.

The nursing process for the child with a chronic illness is ongoing for the duration of the illness. It may be more complex because of goals that are both physical and psychosocial. The psychosocial environment is significant in that it greatly influences the manner in which the child relates to others and copes with stress. In addition, the entire family is involved, as well as the ill child. Care is provided over a span of years and must often incorporate rapid changes in the child's growth and development. The nurse is prepared for a changing assessment, both physical and psychosocial, related to duration of care and fluctuations of the illness.

Planning and implementation of nursing care are based on several factors. The child's physical condition is the first consideration. Generalization across broad categories of illnesses, such as cancer, respiratory conditions, or cardiac problems, is not possible. Each illness has specific implications, including subsequent disabilities that impact the child's growth and development across the span of the illness. Additionally, the needs, coping mechanisms, and available resources of child and family are influencing factors. Nursing care includes assisting the child and family to accept, understand, and incorporate the illness appropriately into each stage of growth and development, regardless of the child's age at diagnosis.

Ongoing Care

Evaluations, as well as subsequent modifications in the planning and implementation of nursing care, often take place on a daily basis because of the child's frequent physical changes. Unexpected setbacks, such as an exacerbation, a relapse, a critical infection, an undesirable response to medication, a lack of physical progress, or the need to undergo a medical or surgical procedure unexpectedly or sooner than anticipated, may be a standard part of the chronic illness. Goals may have to be repeatedly altered. All changes may be stressful and difficult for the child and family to handle even though they have been coping with an illness for a long period. Continuous support and reassurance are necessary throughout the course of the illness.

Education

With an illness that continues for several years, numerous changes may occur because of the child's physical condition or the child's increasing age. Education involves the child and family, addressing both physical and psychosocial needs. It is imperative that the family has an accurate knowledge base in order to provide care to the child at home

One important consideration in relation to education and support for the ill child and siblings is use of a child life specialist (Figure 12-1). The child life specialist uses methods that are educational, supportive, and therapeutic. These may include medical play and art, and therapeutic play and art. All are similar in that they present the child with opportunities for learning, for increased expression of feelings, and for development of additional coping methods. The nurse may also use some of these techniques in daily care or when a child life specialist cannot be present. Child life services are available for siblings.

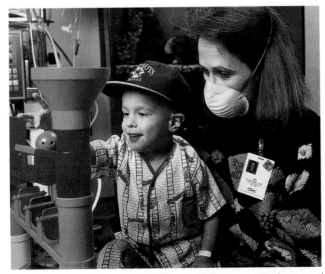

FIG 12-1 The nurse or a child life specialist can use therapeutic play, medical play, and therapeutic art to enhance self-expression, education, and growth and development. (Courtesy Norm Tindell for Cook Children's Medical Center, Fort Worth, TX.)

Communication

Communication with the ill child may be more difficult than physical care (see Chapter 3). Communication is the most important factor in establishing a good relationship with the child and family. *Appropriate communication involves both honesty and compassion. It is always based on the child's age and development.* Following these principles can help decrease the child's fears and misunderstandings. This may also help increase the child's confidence in nurses and other members of the health care team. Increased cooperation with the therapeutic regimen is an additional benefit. If fears and misunderstandings are not alleviated at the beginning and caregivers do not gain the child's trust, establishing trust at a later date can be more difficult. This is particularly true when the nursing care involves unpleasant or painful medications and treatments.

To prevent misinterpretations and misunderstandings, the nurse can ask children to explain what they know and understand. The nurse should also strive to understand what the child is really asking. The classic example of miscommunication is the child who asks where she comes from and hears the entire story of reproduction, when all she really wanted to know was whether her family was from Texas or Oklahoma. Clarifying questions can help the nurse avoid providing more information than the child wants or can handle emotionally. Providing too much information may be overwhelming and frightening to the child. It may also inhibit future questions and interaction with the nurses.

Honesty and trust must be maintained at all times when caring for the child. These principles should be encouraged among the family and other members of the health care team. Complete honesty may cause problems for some family and staff members, especially when they face the difficult questions that often arise when caring for a chronically or terminally ill child. The most difficult and feared questions are usually centered on whether the child is going to die and why he or she became sick and is dying. These are followed closely by questions concerning the deaths of other children whom the child has known or with whom the child has developed a close relationship.

Children are often reluctant to ask questions of adults and to ask questions when they fear the answers. Many times the child already knows the answer, so the question is really a test concerning honesty and a point of reference in the child's relationship with the adult (parent or health care provider). As with adults, children need honesty to establish trust. They may not understand the use of dishonesty as a means of protecting them against emotional pain or unpleasantness. Once children have experienced dishonesty from an adult, they may feel that they cannot and will not trust any of the adults around them, parents or health care providers. Dishonesty may have damaging effects, particularly when trying to reassure a child and gain cooperation. If a chronic condition becomes terminal, the child's trust can be paramount to achieving comfort and peace.

For children with a chronic condition, honesty may increase their emotional pain to some degree and, conversely, help comfort them at the same time. Honest answers to a child's difficult questions are not always handled well by family members. The nurse strives to help family members understand the importance of maintaining the child's trust, to explore their feelings about providing honest answers to the child's questions, and to establish communication guidelines. The family may give instructions about communication that brings about conflict for the nurse, both professionally and personally. The family may ask that the nurse answer deceitfully concerning the serious nature of the illness or the fact that the child is expected to die. In many situations, a compromise is reached in that the nurse will not initiate conversations that may lead to questions about whether the child is expected to die. However, if the child initiates the conversation and asks questions directly, the nurse will reply honestly, in terms approved by the family. This may not work with some families. In such instances, other members of the health care team (physicians, child life therapists, social workers, pastoral care providers) can become involved to make communication decisions that best suit the needs of all involved.

Caring for Parents

Health care professionals can support parents in the following ways (Lindblad, Rasmussen, & Sandman, 2005):

- Increase parents' confidence
- Acknowledge the parent as a person
- Acknowledge the parent as the child's caregiver and the expert on the child
- Ease the parents' daily worries by providing information and easy access to the health care provider when questions and problems arise
- Acknowledge the child as valuable and unique
- Help the parents see the child's potential and abilities
- Help the parents understand the child's normal growth and development needs

Grief Education and Support

Nursing care should include education about the child's condition and treatment, as well as education concerning any grief issues. The nurse helps all family members, including the child, to understand and express their grief in the manner most comfortable for them. Taking time to provide care and support in this area is as important as physical care. Many adults have not experienced illness or death before the child's diagnosis and are not accustomed to the idea of grief, much less grief as a normal, healthy process. In addition, some family members may have had a previous experience with dying, death, and grief that they perceived as negative and distressing. Both situations may increase support needs among the family.

The nurse educates the family about the importance of the grief process and provides opportunities for grieving. Nursing care may include conversations and time "being present" with family. Being present for all family members as the need arises entails the important aspect of listening and sitting in silence. Many times family members do not need or want conversation; they just want to be with someone who knows their child and is familiar with what they might be experiencing. This may be true even for siblings. Children who just want to be with an adult may require only that the person sit with them while they play. The expression of emotions is recognized to be more beneficial for most individuals than holding the emotions inside. However, for some, emotional expressions are not a normal or comfortable part of their lives before their child's illness. The nurse accepts each family member's choice to express or not express emotions while letting them know that a caring individual is available at any time should the need for talking and sharing arise.

Cultural and Religious Beliefs

Groves (2010) notes that culture is a unique and dynamic force that includes learned values, beliefs, and practices that can be affected by the social environment. Culture and religion influence the meaning of illness and death, as well as customs observed by the family. Assessing the perceptions of the child and family regarding chronic illness, hospitalization, and disability in light of the family's culture facilitates culturally sensitive nursing care. When faced with an unfamiliar culture or religion, the nurse becomes familiar with beliefs and practices honored and used by the family. The nurse and the entire health care team should communicate acceptance of the family's beliefs. Team members must not assume that a family belongs to a particular religion or denomination based solely on their cultural background. In addition, they should not assume that a family adheres to all beliefs and practices of its religion or denomination. If in doubt, the nurse should ask questions of the family, stressing the need for information to provide the most comprehensive and appropriate care possible.

Referrals

To the degree possible, the nurse should endeavor to make sure that the physical, emotional, psychosocial, and cognitive needs of the child and family are met. Additionally, nursing care includes assisting family members to provide for the child's physical and psychosocial needs. The nurse works as a member of an extensive health care team and determines when referrals need to be made to professionals with expertise needed by the child and family. For example, the child with a chronic illness and the family may need services from clergy members, psychologists, and social workers. Hospital chaplains generally have access to information on various religious beliefs, as well as to clergy members from different religious groups. Psychologists can provide ongoing counseling to the child and family on an individual or group basis. Social workers are able to provide information concerning available resources for the family related to finances, insurance, government assistance, housing, transportation, and medical care and supplies.

Schooling

The face of public education and the child with special health care needs has changed dramatically. The Education for All Handicapped Children Act (PL 94-142), now codified as Individuals with Disabilities Education Act (IDEA), and subsequent amendments (most notably the Individuals with Disabilities Education Act, 1997) ensure a free, public education for each child with a disability or other chronic condition. The act also mandates that special education and support services be provided in the least restrictive environment for children ages 3 years and older. Consequently, children with a wide variety of physical needs are able to receive appropriate educational services and attend public school. These needs range from relatively simple needs (e.g., medication administration, respiratory treatments) to more extensive needs (e.g., gastrostomy tube feedings, tracheostomy tubes, ventilators). Facilitating the start of school or return to school for the child with special needs requires preparation and assistance from a health care team that includes the child, family, hospital or clinic nurse, school nurse, teacher, counselor, and director of special education for the school district.

A specific, structured plan of care is developed before the child's return to school. This is accomplished by the school system through a legally mandated process referred to as an *individualized educational program* (IEP) or *admission, review, and dismissal* (ARD) meeting. This plan is developed with input from the health care team, who are encouraged to attend the actual meeting, if possible. The plan addresses cognitive and physical needs in relation to the child's school attendance. This plan includes learning goals that might require some modifications as a result of the child's special needs and chronic condition, as well as the specific tasks for achieving such goals. The plan also addresses any special health care that needs to be provided while the child is in school, such as medications, feedings, or breathing treatments. Planning conferences are held before the child is scheduled to start school for the first time after his or her condition has been diagnosed. After the initial plan, an IEP or ARD meeting must take place at least once a year and when changes in the child's condition occur that will necessitate changes in the schooling plan. Most schools offer children the opportunity to attend school full or part time as their conditions allow and receive homebound instruction when necessary. Regardless of the type of school services the child is receiving, the hospital or clinic nurse may need to provide ongoing education and support to the school nurse and other school personnel.

Special considerations are given in the school setting for a child who is immunosuppressed, whether related to a disease or to treatment. Preventing the infection that can occur with immunosuppression is a challenge in the school setting regardless of the age of the child. Reasons include the crowded conditions in school classrooms and the often inadequate infection control practices of children (e.g., good hand hygiene). The school nurse should alert teachers to be particularly vigilant and notify the nurse if any children with an infectious disease are present in the classroom. Families of all schoolchildren are asked to notify the school if their children contract a serious communicable illness such as strep throat and to keep their children out of school until their disease is no longer contagious. The school nurse may also visit classrooms and present health-teaching modules on general infection-prevention practices. The school nurse must obtain information about the specific signs to look for when monitoring the condition of the chronically ill child and how to contact the child's health care team directly and quickly if concerns arise.

Ongoing psychosocial support may also be necessary for the child and family in relation to school. Parents may experience mixed emotions regarding their child's return to school. They are likely to be pleased and excited that the child is well enough to attend school. At the same time, they may be concerned about the child's well-being during school hours, particularly whether the child's special health care needs will be met appropriately. For children with a terminal condition, parents may also experience a degree of sorrow about being apart during what limited time they have with their child. The child's siblings may also experience similar feelings. The nurse can best provide support by maintaining ongoing communication with the family and recognizing that problems and concerns with school may vary over time. Referral to a spiritual counselor, social worker, or mental health professional may also be helpful for the psychosocial support of the child and family.

Regardless of whether the child is transitioning into or re-entering school, the child, parents, other family members, school nurse, teacher, school personnel, and health care providers need to understand the child's chronic condition and should partner in facilitating needed accommodations within the school setting (Erickson, Splett, Mullett, & Heiman, 2006). The goal of this partnership is to enhance the child's independence and create a positive climate for learning.

The Nurse as Liaison

The nurse is a liaison for the family in many different situations. The most important liaison work, however, is to link the family with other members of the health care team, particularly the physician. In this capacity, the nurse can help guarantee that family members receive accurate information and have an appropriate understanding of their child's condition, as well as resulting psychosocial and physical needs. These efforts can facilitate the family's health care planning, working relationship with the health care team, communication with care providers, and compliance with the treatment plan.

Caring for Siblings

The concerns and needs of siblings in relation to their brother or sister's chronic illness vary according to age and developmental stage. Thus, fluctuations are common when the child's chronic condition exists for several years. Siblings may have many of the same anxieties and fears as their parents.

Siblings often have feelings of guilt regarding their perceived role in the ill child's condition. Many children have had thoughts of what life would be like without having to share material possessions and parental love with their sibling(s). When a sibling then becomes ill, the guilt and associated emotions may be overwhelming. The well siblings should be reassured about the normalcy of such feelings and that the illness is not the result of anything that they said, thought, or did.

Nursing care of siblings involves education regarding the ill child's condition, treatment, physical changes, disabilities, and expected disease progression. The siblings should ideally be kept up to date regarding changes in the ill child's condition, both positive and negative. The same principles of honest communication apply both to siblings and to the child with the illness. However, what information is ultimately shared with siblings is at the parents' discretion. The hospital setting's rules, equipment, and personnel must also be explained to siblings in terms appropriate for their developmental level. If possible and suitable, siblings may be allowed to participate in physically caring for the ill child.

Siblings may regress in developmental stage and activities. Parents frequently do not expect such behavioral changes from a well sibling. They may need to be reminded that in the presence of a stressful event, regression is a normal coping mechanism for all children, both ill and well.

The nurse can help siblings understand that illness creates stress, which may result in difficult or painful emotions, such as anger and jealousy. Children need to know that these emotions are a normal part of life, although they are often perceived as negative and harmful. Siblings must be allowed to have and express these feelings (Figure 12-2). Health care professionals and the family must provide care and support to meet the psychosocial and emotional needs of the siblings in order to prevent added stress for the family that may negatively affect the ill child.

The nurse and family should include siblings as much as possible in the life and activities of the ill child, whether the child is hospitalized or receives outpatient care. The family will require education and input from the health care team regarding the pros and cons of sibling involvement. Spiritual or cultural beliefs may affect this type of

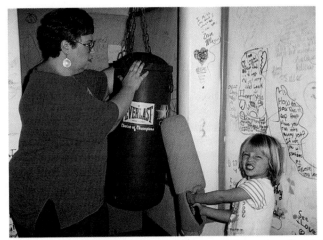

FIG 12-2 Chronic illness is stressful for the siblings of an ill child. Siblings' emotional needs may be overlooked. Siblings should be given the opportunity to express negative feelings, such as anger and jealousy, through therapeutic art and play, as well as through physical outlets such as striking a punching bag, as this little girl is doing. (Courtesy Gwen T. Martin, R.N., Fort Worth, TX.)

decision. Many families choose to minimize siblings' time and involvement in the health care setting as a means of keeping the siblings' lives as normal and uninterrupted as possible. Other families try to maintain the existing degree of closeness between the siblings and the ill child and choose to have the siblings closely involved in the ill child's care at the hospital, including siblings being present during the day and for overnight visits, if permitted. The family's decisions related to sibling involvement should be supported by the health care team.

The nurse ensures that siblings receive appropriate education to decrease misunderstandings and fears related to the ill child's condition and treatments as well as the emotions and behaviors of their parents and other adults. Medical play, therapeutic play, and therapeutic art are excellent means of educating and providing support to the siblings. These interventions may also assist siblings to gain understanding of their intense and confusing emotional responses, as well as how to express them in a healthy, appropriate manner. Nurses striving to teach, support, and include siblings in the care of the ill child should collaborate with the child life specialist.

Extensive sibling involvement may bring with it additional risks. Siblings may be exposed to the ill child's severe physical and emotional experiences, which can have emotional consequences for the siblings. Close attention from health care team and family members can help determine if siblings have needs for interventions by nurses, physicians, child life specialists, clergy, social workers, or professional counselors.

The relationship between the ill child and siblings may be altered because of normal feelings of resentment, jealousy, and competition as the siblings see the ill child receiving additional attention. Siblings may experience guilt and shame about such feelings. The nursing staff, child life specialist, social worker, and chaplain can give individual attention to the siblings separately from the ill child. Siblings may also be referred to support groups. These interventions provide siblings the opportunity to gain understanding and accept the normality of their feelings by verbalizing emotions, interacting with caring, nonjudgmental adults, and talking with peers who share similar experiences.

Because the ill child often receives extra attention, including gifts, from family and friends, siblings may associate illness with extra attention and gifts, and subsequently experience real or imagined illnesses as a bid for similar attention. The nurse should encourage family and friends to give attention and gifts to the siblings as well as to the ill child. It is also helpful to acknowledge siblings' accomplishments and special times, such as birthdays. Encouraging the parent to spend some time every day with each sibling is essential for the family to maintain positive relationships.

! NURSING QUALITY ALERT

Nursing Care for Children with Chronic Conditions and Their Families

- Care for a child with a chronic condition means attending to the needs of the family system. Both parents and siblings may need additional support.
- The age and developmental level of the chronically ill child affect both the child's understanding and the family's needs. Goals may need to be frequently revised to meet the child's changing developmental needs.
- The nurse should listen carefully to the child's perception of the condition. A child's illness experience does not always match an adult's view of the physical limitations and emotional stress.

? CRITICAL THINKING EXERCISE 12-1

How can the nurse apply the principles of family-centered nursing to the family with a chronically ill child?

◎ NURSING CARE PLAN

The Child with a Chronic Condition in the Community Setting

Focused Assessment

- Provide a comprehensive and collaborative assessment of the chronically ill child
  - Involve child, family, school personnel, and multidisciplinary health care team members
  - Assess the child's development level and cognitive, physical, and psychosocial abilities
  - Use as a baseline for developing a hospitalization plan or school IEP
  - Determine expectations and the level of assistance the child will require
- Assess the child's perception of physical changes related to the chronic illness and treatments
  - Address impact on self-esteem, self-reliance, and autonomy
  - Determine if altered body awareness or image negatively affects self-esteem
  - Assess over time the perception changes that occur at different developmental stages and school (grade) levels
- Assess the child and the entire family system for:
  - Communication and behavior patterns and emotional concerns
  - Existing coping and adaptive mechanisms; when child is at home, school, or hospital
  - Inappropriate coping behaviors, considering interventions to support change to beneficial/healthy coping mechanisms

- Explore family's response to the child's illness
  - Verify the family's recognition that the illness affects the entire family system
  - Determine each family member's understandings about the disease process and treatment regimen, correcting misinformation or misinterpretations
- Assess coping over the course of the chronic disease
  - Consider the physiologic progression of the disease
  - Note that as the child's condition changes, the impact on the family will change and different coping mechanisms will be needed
- Evaluate and document the family's community support system
  - Address the influence on family's beliefs, responses, and coping methods

Planning
Nursing Diagnosis
Risk for Delayed Development related to the effects of chronic illness or disability.

Expected Outcomes
The child will experience minimal disturbance of normal growth and development (physical, cognitive, emotional, and psychological), as evidenced by minimal delays and documented by an age-appropriate and reliable developmental screening tool.

NURSING CARE PLAN

The Child with a Chronic Condition in the Community Setting—cont'd

The child will experience minimal disturbance of normal growth and development, as evidenced by ability to interact in an age-appropriate manner cognitively, emotionally, physically, and socially to the degree allowed by the existing disability.

The child will experience minimal disturbance of normal growth and development, as evidenced by the ability to perform usual, age-appropriate ADLs as allowed by the existing disability.

Intervention/*Rationale*

1. Educate the child and family about the physical conditions, expected physical changes or disabilities, and prescribed treatment. Education should be in a manner appropriate for the child's cognitive abilities.

   This encourages a sense of control and acceptance of the physical changes as well as increased cooperation with treatment. Some children with chronic conditions have cognitive abilities beyond their chronologic age and may be able to discuss medical matters knowledgeably.

2. Involve the child, family, school personnel, and interdisciplinary health care team in setting reasonable goals for improving and maximizing abilities in relation to the existing disability.

   Goal setting assists children and families to increase their abilities and self-esteem through successful accomplishment of tasks. It may also increase a sense of situational control.

3. Assist the child to develop a sense of pride in existing physical abilities and to set goals expanding the range of activities.

   Focusing on regaining skills and participating in preferred activities can provide incentive for achieving new goals (i.e., obtain a driver's license).

4. Collaborate with the child and school personnel to modify school routines to better fit the child's educational and social schedule and needs.

   Involving the child in setting meaningful goals will support achievement.

5. Offer child as many choices and opportunities to make age-appropriate treatment decisions as possible.

   Offering choices and opportunities to the child promotes autonomy and situational control that are often lost as a result of limitations imposed by the condition or treatment. May improve self-esteem.

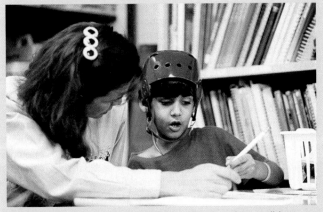

FIG 12-3 Because more children with chronic conditions are living longer, more attend public school. However, these children are likely to be frequently hospitalized, so hospitals often provide an area where teachers can help them with their studies. (Courtesy Cook Children's Medical Center, Fort Worth, TX.)

6. Encourage the child to engage in age-appropriate ADLs and self-care. Provide and teach the child to use assistive devices, at home and school.

   Self-care encourages independence and gives the child an opportunity to practice and improve abilities.

7. During hospital stays, provide child's own clothes and items from home for grooming, eating, and recreation. Encourage completion of schoolwork and peer visits (e.g., invite peers to special events).

   Use of personal items, maintaining school involvement, and engaging with peers promote normalization, minimize disturbances in usual routines, and maximize the child's sense of control. School nurses or child life therapists can educate and support peers if fears exist.

8. Provide social activities both in and out of the hospital and encourage peer interactions to the degree allowed by the child's physical condition or treatments. Advise family to schedule clinic visits and treatments to avoid conflicts with social events.

   Ongoing social activities (e.g., sports, school clubs or activities, church, social groups) and peer connections encourage maintenance and acquisition of developmental skills as well as contribute to the child's positive self-esteem and autonomy.

9. Encourage the child to join general or disease-specific peer support groups and attend special camp programs for children with chronic illness. Respect the decision if child decides to not participate.

   Support, acceptance, understanding, and learning can be derived from regular interactions with peers who have similar chronic conditions. Support groups may be most beneficial after initial diagnosis, when fears and concerns are increased. Considering the individual support needs for each child is essential.

Evaluation

Does the child exhibit minimal developmental delays?

Does the child exhibit age-appropriate cognitive, emotional, physical, and social interactions?

Does the child perform age-appropriate ADLs as allowed by the existing disability?

Planning
Nursing Diagnosis

Interrupted Family Processes related to intermittent situational crisis of chronic illness.

Expected Outcomes

The child and family will experience normal family functioning, as evidenced by maintaining usual family routines, meeting developmental needs of all family members, and maintaining usual expectations for the ill child.

The child and family will experience appropriate psychosocial adjustment, as evidenced by expressing feelings, identifying ways to cope effectively, and using appropriate support systems.

Intervention/*Rationale*

1. Provide information to the family that facilitates a positive, realistic view of their child in relation to the chronic condition. Discuss appropriate behavioral expectations for the chronically ill child.

   Education decreases fears and misconceptions, encourages appropriate interactions between family members and with the health care team, and prompts adherence to treatment.

Continued

◎ NURSING CARE PLAN

The Child with a Chronic Condition in the Community Setting—cont'd

2. Assist the family to identify and express fears and emotions pertaining to the child's illness. Convey acceptance of feelings and explain that expression is a healthy part of coping.
   Verbalization of feelings, with positive feedback, can help decrease stress and facilitate resolution of negative emotions.

3. Act as a role model for appropriate, accepting, positive attitudes and behaviors concerning the child.
   A positive role model may facilitate acceptance and adjustment by the family of a chronically ill child.

4. Discuss with the family approaches to maintaining usual routines for the chronically ill child and the entire family.
   By including some adaptations, families can maintain usual routines and meet the needs of all family members.

5. Refer the family and child to resources (e.g., social worker, clergy, counselor) for additional psychosocial interventions, as indicated.
   Psychosocial assistance beyond the nurse's scope of practice, or as requested by the family, may be needed for certain families and children.

Evaluation

Is the family able to maintain its usual routine and meet the needs of all family members?

Does the family treat the ill child as normally as possible to avoid overdependence?

Do family members express their feelings? Has the family identified and utilized appropriate coping mechanisms, and are they using appropriate support systems?

Maintaining close contact with each sibling's school personnel and keeping them up to date regarding the current circumstances of the ill child are important. This can help personnel understand and support the siblings if behavioral issues are noted in school or if increased absences occur due to circumstances with the ill child. Siblings may also turn more frequently to their teacher and other school personnel for support. School personnel working with the siblings may need similar educational support as those working with the ill child. The hospital or clinic nurse and child life therapist can make school visits and provide education to personnel, as well as to the siblings' peers and classmates. The family and members of the health care team determine the extent of information given to the children.

THE TERMINALLY ILL OR DYING CHILD

Coping and the Child's Concept of Death

An understanding of death and dying in relation to childhood is necessary when caring for the child approaching death. The established and accepted guidelines concerning children's concepts of death are based on the stages of growth and development. As Wass (1985) explains, these concepts correlate with age and cognition (Table 12-1). In addition, a child's response to death is affected by culture, environment, social setting, spirituality, and personal experiences with death (Bluebond-Langner, 1978).

Infants and Toddlers

Infants and toddlers view death in relation to the loss of a caregiver and the subsequent emptiness in their lives. They are also affected by the loss of comfort measures, such as when they experience pain or cold. Consequently, time with primary caregivers is quite important. As they approach death, they often sense the severity of their condition through their parents' nonverbal communication. Children of this age may react to the dying process based on the sadness, anger, and anxiety conveyed by their parents. Reactions will be expressed through crying, attachment to the primary caregiver, and separation anxiety.

Preschoolers

Preschoolers view death as a separation or departure and believe it to be only temporary. Death is also seen as reversible. Magical thinking and egocentricity at this age often lead to guilt and shame because children may believe that their thoughts or actions caused the death.

TABLE 12-1	**THE CHILD'S CONCEPT OF DEATH**	
AGE	**COGNITIVE STAGE**	**CONCEPT**
Infancy and toddlerhood (0-2 yr)	Sensorimotor	Death as loss of the caregiver
Early childhood (2-7 yr)	Preoperational	Death as a reversible and temporary separation
Middle childhood (school-age; 7-12 yr)	Concrete operations	Death as sad and irreversible but not necessarily inevitable
Adolescence (12+ yr)	Formal operations	Death as inevitable and irreversible but often a distant event

The child's first exposure to death frequently involves a dead animal, such as an insect, bird, or pet.

Preschoolers facing impending death frequently view their condition as punishment for behaviors or thoughts. They respond with guilt, anger, sadness, and fear. Their self-imposed guilt may cause them to believe that others, including parents, see them as "bad" and are angry with them. Feelings are kept inside, and children this age may withdraw from everyone, including those whom they love and on whom they depend. Their anger at those they care about and the intensity of that anger frightens them. Great patience and understanding are required of their parents and nurses, particularly when emotions are labile and subject to frequent, sudden changes. Indeed, all children feel greater security when adults maintain discipline and suitable, customary limits; this is especially true for dying children who are experiencing multiple changes and discrepancies in their daily lives.

School-Age Children

By the school-age years, death begins to be understood as a sad and irreversible event, yet it still may be considered inevitable only for adults. Children at age 10 years begin to understand that they too can die. Some associated feelings of guilt often persist for school-age children. They may continue to believe that thoughts or actions can cause death or that death serves as a punishment for wrongdoing.

The school-age child has increased cognition and other resources necessary to cope with the dying process. However, these same abilities may lead to additional questions and fears. School-age children may wonder why they are ill and must die so young. Fear about the process of dying and what follows may also arise. Even in children who have a foundation of spiritual beliefs, this fear may persist because they do not have a concrete knowledge of what it is like after a person dies. The school-age child may fear being without the love and support of parents and other close family members. Moreover, school-age children may feel vulnerable and doubt their ability to cope with the knowledge of their impending death, as well as the experience itself.

Adolescents

Most adolescents have a fully developed understanding of death as inevitable and irreversible. However, many adolescents view death as a distant event and may consider themselves invulnerable to death, related to their increasingly independent frame of reference. Although adolescents may understand death and dying, they do not necessarily have an emotional acceptance of their impending death. Adolescents who are attempting to separate from their parents often test and break rules as they strive for independence. This process may cause guilt for the dying child, especially when contemplating the spiritual aspects of life and death.

As the result of their illness, adolescents may become isolated from their peers. The terminal illness or disability of a peer forces healthy adolescents to abruptly and unwillingly face and question their own mortality. Discomfort may prompt the healthy adolescent to decrease or stop contacting and visiting even a close friend who is seriously ill. Adolescents who are dying may become isolated from caring adults, family, and health care providers because they feel adults do not understand them. Consequently, many feel lonely and fear that they will die without the love and support they need and desire. Realizing that they are facing death when their lives are just beginning, adolescents can respond with anger and sadness, particularly when considering what they will never be able to experience as an adult. This may contribute to the onset of depression.

Coping and Responses to Death and Dying

The process of dying, as well as the actual death of a child, is a unique and complex situation. The responses of all persons involved; the child, family, and health care providers, are affected by various factors including personal and spiritual beliefs, previous experiences with illness and death, the quality of the relationship with the dying child, and experiences with this child during the current illness and dying process. Another very important factor is the individual's progression through the stages of grief. At any given time, the child, parents, and siblings may all be experiencing a different stage of grief and expressing that grief in different ways.

The Child's Response

A child who is dying wants to feel safe and does not want to be alone or in pain. These concerns are frequently more intense for school-age children and adolescents. The child's responses to death and dying will be multiple and varied, not always fully correlating with the child's chronologic age and expected stage of development and cognition. The traumatizing experiences associated with a chronic condition and treatments tend to make children more mature and "wise beyond their years." As dying children work through the five stages of grief, they may reach a point where they consider their illness and treatment to be worse than dying, and then experience relief and acceptance of death. The responses and actions of the dying child are also affected by the

behaviors and feelings of those around them, particularly family, friends, and health care providers.

The child's response to dying and the resulting actions are often more precocious than would be expected, particularly among preschool children. Family or hospital staff members may consider precocious actions to be inappropriate and some statements of a spiritual nature to be unbelievable. They possibly attribute these responses to physical changes, such as a low hemoglobin level, altered neurologic status, or medications such as analgesics or sedatives.

Spiritual beliefs may influence the child and be reflected in conversations and actions. Children may speak of seeing or even interacting with angels or the Higher Being recognized by their specific faith. They may also speak of going to heaven to be with the angels or other spiritual beings. In addition, children may speak of going to play or be with another child or relative who has already died. This type of conversation may take place anywhere from several weeks to days or hours before death, with children actually giving specifics as to when they will see or be with deceased individuals. Such behaviors are commonly referred to as *nearing death awareness.*

Dying children often experience a heightened sense of understanding and awareness, particularly as death nears. Many know specifically when they will die. As seen with adults, death often occurs after children have successfully achieved closure of some type. Closure may be a special event in their life or that of a loved one, such as a graduation, holiday, or birthday. Frequently, closure also involves resolution of unfinished business, such as interacting with a loved one who has been absent or apologizing for things they have said or done.

One concept of pediatric death that families may have difficulty understanding and accepting is "allowing" their child to die. As noted by Kübler-Ross (1983), children are afraid not of death but of abandonment. Children who are enveloped by hope, joy, and love may sustain their grasp on life. For most children, allowing them to die means giving the child permission to die. A predominant issue of childhood is that children should obey their parents. This assumption is based on the knowledge that parents know best and provide guidance for their child to do what is safe and correct. A child's dying process may not occur until parents tell the child it is "all right" to die.

Accordingly, some children, particularly those who are younger, need verbal "permission" to die, reassurance that it is safe to do so, and a description of what to expect as they die and in the time afterward. Children may also need to know that the family, friends, and loved ones who are left behind will grieve and yet will be all right and will take care of each other. Equally important to children of all ages is the knowledge that loved ones will remember them always.

The Parents' Response

When a child is initially diagnosed with any condition that is life threatening, every parent faces and begins to cope with the *possibility* of their child's death. When they are informed that nothing more can be done medically to treat their child's illness, parents face the *reality* of their child's death. They begin to experience anticipatory grief, the processes of mourning, coping, interacting, planning, and psychosocial reorganizing that occurs as part of the response to the impending death of a loved one.

The stages of grief associated with the child's illness must now be experienced in relation to the child's death. Acceptance does not always occur. Some parents may find it difficult or unacceptable to discontinue treatment. They may choose to continue treatment of a curative rather than a palliative nature. Such a choice, however, does not always indicate denial. It may simply represent a belief system based on spiritual or personal convictions. Legally, emotionally, and psychosocially, the family's decision must be upheld and supported by members of the health care team. However, such treatment may prolong and worsen the child's dying experience by causing pain or other uncomfortable symptoms. The health care team should strive as diligently as possible to remain the child's advocate; looking carefully at whether treatment is *doing for* the child as opposed to *doing to* the child.

At such times, the team's experience with other children in similar situations may be useful in gently guiding the parents towards palliative care services. The provision of palliative care optimizes quality of life, communication, and symptom control (Ullrich et al., 2011). The aim of palliative care treatments and procedures is to promote comfort and improve the quality of the child's life. Palliative care can occur while a child with a life-threatening illness is still receiving treatment focused on sustaining life. The interdisciplinary palliative care team provides comprehensive physical, psychological, social, and spiritual care to the entire family including the child, with consideration of cultural, religious, and family values (Ullrich et al., 2011).

Parents will exhibit the need to talk about their child and the experience of their child's illness and death. They talk to assimilate the experience, but more important, they talk to remember their child.

When a chronic condition has extended over time, the parents' initial reaction to their child's death is often relief that the child is no longer suffering, physically or emotionally, and that the uncertainty of the illness has ended. Many times, this relief and feeling of peace may begin when death is known to be inevitable and imminent. Such relief may evoke feelings of guilt. Support and explanations regarding the normalcy of these feelings may be necessary for parents. Relief at the death is followed by numbness, intense sadness, and a sense of profound loss and emptiness. The grief of the child's grandparents can be greater than that of the parents, because they grieve the loss of their grandchild and also grieve for *their own child,* the parent, who has experienced the death of a child.

The Siblings' Response

The responses of siblings to death and dying, as well as their progression through the stages of grief, vary according to age and developmental level. Although children usually experience all five stages of grief, this may not necessarily occur in the given sequence. Frequently, children move between the stages in a seemingly random fashion, often experiencing one stage several times. This process is an appropriate coping mechanism for some children. Issues dealt with successfully earlier in the course of the illness, such as concerns about causing the illness or death of the brother or sister, may resurface. Siblings may experience emotions similar to those experienced by their parents, however, they may not yet have the cognitive and developmental abilities to understand and work through the grieving process. The result is unresolved grief which may contribute to emotional problems in adult life.

Because children work through the grieving process differently than adults, siblings often need guidance and support from parents and others to resolve issues and complete the grieving process. Grief support centers are available to provide assistance to children who have experienced the death of a loved one, including a sibling. Health care providers and professional counselors can also intervene as indicated.

The most important aspect of providing support to a grieving sibling is acknowledging that the loss experience of the sibling is *just as significant* as the loss experience of the parents. Although it is common practice for the health care team members to send sympathy cards and other correspondence to parents after their child's death, it is important to also communicate sympathy and concern to the siblings individually through cards and phones calls. Such validation of

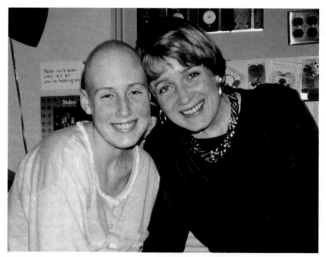

FIG 12-4 The family of the child with a terminal condition needs compassion and support from the nurse. Nursing care includes physical care and support of the family's caregiving efforts, and assistance with the grieving process. (Courtesy Gwen T. Martin, R.N., Fort Worth, TX.)

the sibling's grief can support their successful navigation of the grieving process.

Caring for the Dying Child

Despite medical advances and current technology, many chronic disorders ultimately end in death. Providing nursing care to the child with a terminal illness who is nearing death, as well as to family members, requires a heightened level of understanding, compassion, and support. A family's coping abilities are often tested beyond measure. Nursing care includes assisting the child and family to withstand the intense pressures and emotional demands of the situation (Figure 12-4).

Nursing Professionalism and Boundaries

Caring for dying children involves certain stressors for all involved, including the nurse. An important aspect of self-care is for nurses to recognize and acknowledge the impact of these stressors. Caring for the child who is approaching death can be rewarding, but it may also severely test the nurse's coping skills. Compassion is necessary, but also essential are awareness and maintenance of professional boundaries. These boundaries are necessary for the nurses to provide clinically sound, compassionate care while maintaining their own emotional, physical, and spiritual health.

To maintain professionalism and boundaries, nurses must understand and accept their own feelings and beliefs about death. Unresolved emotions may interfere with providing appropriate nursing care. Hospital resources for nurses seeking support and assistance include the pastoral care team, social workers, and nursing support groups. Attending patient care conferences or ethics committee meetings may help the nurse better understand and participate in patient care decisions. The nurse also learns more about the education and services the family is receiving and how these are supporting their decision-making process. In some situations, nurses may choose to obtain personal counseling services privately or through a hospital employee support program.

Communication

Nursing staff and family members must be aware of, understand, and accept the dying child's communication needs and patterns. The dying child should consistently be reassured that the illness and approaching death are not the result of any action or omission committed by the child. Parents and nurses must make certain that dying children know they will never be left alone; a family member or health care professional must always be with these children.

Children who are dying need to experience complete love and acceptance; they must receive assurances that their feelings and thoughts are not wrong. Children, parents, and siblings may need assistance to understand their intense emotions, especially anger and guilt. Parents, other adult family members, and siblings need opportunities away from the dying child to express their feelings. This can help to minimize or prevent the dying child from feeling responsible for the emotions of others, particularly the parents. The goal is to have the child and family together in an environment that is as soothing, comfortable, and as stress free as possible.

Most dying children will follow the family's rules and patterns for communication. As death approaches, communication between child and family can decline in both extent and effectiveness. The nurse should consider communication strategies the family has used effectively during previously stressful times (e.g., at diagnosis, with relapses), and encourage the family to use those same approaches again. The nurse carefully evaluates each child and family on an individual basis and assists them to experience effective, comfortable communication.

The most common issue that arises when a family is facing the impending death of their child is whether to inform the child of the grave prognosis. Though the needs of the parents, siblings, other family members, and health care providers are considered, the needs of the dying child must take precedence. One suggested approach is to allow the child to maintain open communication with trusted individuals who are comfortable talking with the child about death. This supports the child's need for someone to acknowledge that the child is dying and be willing to talk with the child at the child's request. Simultaneously, it allows mutual pretense and decreased communication with those who prefer to not talk about the child's death. This flexible approach has been found to be effective and is prevalent.

Nurses may be caught between children who wish to talk about their death and parents who forbid any such conversation. As the caregiver and primary advocate, the nurse should first meet the child's needs. Any skirting of the issues or dishonesty with the child may damage the nurse-patient relationship, possibly denying the child a much-needed source of comfort and support. It is critically important that the nurse maintain the trust of the dying child in order to provide the child with optimal nursing care including administering medications to manage pain and other symptoms. Nurses should inform parents that they will not initiate any discussion of the child's death but need and intend to respond openly and honestly if the child asks questions or wants to talk. This practice allows nurses both to respect the wishes of the parents and provide support to the child when needed.

Words are not always necessary to provide assistance and care to the dying child. Presence—simply sitting with the child—or a light touch, such as holding a hand, may be exactly what the child needs. The silence itself may be a therapeutic intervention, or it may help open the door for desired verbal communication.

Family Dynamics, Beliefs, and Practices

To fully support parents during the time surrounding the death of their child, nursing care must impart consistent respect and acceptance; regardless of any differences between the spiritual or cultural beliefs and practices of the family and those of the nurse (Box 12-3).

| BOX 12-3 | **RESOURCES ON DEATH AND DYING FOR FAMILIES AND HEALTH CARE PROFESSIONALS** |

Internet Resources

Children's Hospice International (U.S.): www.chionline.org
  Information regarding children's hospice, palliative, and end-of-life care.
Compassionate Friends (U.S.): www.compassionatefriends.org/home.aspx
  Brochures for parents and siblings in both English and Spanish. Discussion support groups and chat rooms are available for siblings.
Baby Steps (Canada): www.babysteps.com
  Extensive book list, sharing rooms, and grieving rooms.

Book Selections for Children

Alley, R. W. (1998). *Sad isn't bad*. St. Meinrad, IN: Abbey Press.
Buscaglia, L. (2002). *The fall of Freddie the leaf: 20th anniversary edition*. Thorofare, NJ: Slack Inc. (all ages)
Fitzgerald, H. (2000). *A guide for teenagers and their friends*. New York: Simon & Schuster. (teens)
Peterkin, A., & Middendorf, F. (1992). *What about me? When brothers and sisters get sick*. Washington, DC: Magination Press.
Raschka, C. (2007). *The purple balloon*. New York: Schwartz & Wade.
Simon, J. (2001). *This book is for all kids, but especially my sister Libby. Libby died*. Kansas City, MO.: Andrews McMeel. (preschool)

Book Selections for Adults—Parents and Nurses

Bluebond-Langner, M. (2000). *In the shadow of illness*. Princeton, NJ: Princeton University Press.
Coloroso, B. (2000). *Parenting through crisis: Helping kids in times of loss, grief, and change*. New York: Harper Collins.
Grollman, E. A. (1990). *Talking about death*. Boston: Beacon Press.
Hilden, J. M., Tobin, D. R., & Lindsey, K. (2002). *Shelter from the storm: Caring for a child with a life-threatening condition*. Cambridge, MA: Perseus Press Group.
Ilse, S., & Leininger, L. (1985). *Grieving grandparents*. Maple Plain, MN: Wintergreen Press.
Power, P. W., & Dell Orto, A. E. (2003). *The resilient family: Living with your child's illness or disability*. Notre Dame, IN: Sorin Books.
Rothman, J. C. (1997). *The bereaved parent's survival guide*. New York: Continuum.
Schive, K., & Klein, S. D. (Eds.). (2001). *You will dream new dreams: Inspiring personal stories by parents of children with disabilities*. New York: Kensington.
Seibeti, D., Drolet, J. C., & Fetro, J. V. (2003). *Helping children live with death and loss*. Carbondale, IL: Southern Illinois University Press.
Sourkes, B. M. (1996). *Armfuls of time: The psychological experience of the child with a life-threatening illness*. Philadelphia: University of Pittsburgh Press.

Book Selections for Nurses

D'Avanzo, C. (2007). *Pocket guide to cultural assessment* (4th ed.). St. Louis: Mosby.
Field, M. J., & Behrman, R. (Eds.). (2003). *When children die: Improving palliative and end-of-life care for children and their families*. Washington, DC: National Academies Press.
Giger, J. N., & Davidhizar, R. E. (2007). *Transcultural nursing: Assessment and intervention* (5th ed.). St. Louis: Elsevier Mosby.

The nurse will encounter different beliefs and practices surrounding death and the grieving process. These practices may include wearing prayer cloths; the laying on of hands; use of holy water or oil; viewing religious pictures, icons, or other objects; extemporaneous prayer gatherings; or the preparation and serving of certain foods. Some practices may be of concern to the nurse and the health care team related to safety and the child's emotional state. Each practice by each family must be evaluated individually, addressing the potential emotional or spiritual benefits to the child and family and potential safety issues.

Many parents have difficulty moving from active treatment that is aimed at curing the disease to palliative care with an emphasis on comfort and quality of life for the dying child. Parents' final attempts to find a cure for their child's illness may include the use of unproven medications or treatments, some of which are in other countries. Although these treatments may not be approved by the U.S. Food and Drug Administration (FDA), many are not physically harmful to the child. Indeed, they may be emotionally beneficial to both parent and child providing affirmation that everything possible was tried to cure the child's terminal disease. These efforts may instill hope, which is vitally important to the child and family. If any of these unapproved medications or treatments is potentially harmful to the child, the health care team may not allow their use. The decision and the rationale are explained compassionately yet firmly to the family, noting the decision was made in the best interest of the child.

Family beliefs and practices, as well as strong emotions, influence their decision making regarding do-not-resuscitate (DNR) orders. A DNR order means that cardiopulmonary resuscitation (CPR) or other interventions designed to initiate heartbeat and respirations after a cardiopulmonary arrest, are not performed. Families, who acknowledge their child's impending death, may have great difficulty and uncertainty about the decision to not resuscitate their child. They may also change their decision several times regarding the DNR order. The health care team members need to educate family members regarding the possible choices, and encourage them to discuss their feelings and explore their wishes for their child. A DNR order does not mean withholding treatment *while the child is alive*. Rather, it involves not initiating treatment *after the child has died*. Parents are reminded that if a DNR order is chosen, they may revoke the order at any time. Most important, the health care providers assure the family that their child will be cared for and comfort will be maintained regardless of the presence or absence of a DNR order.

Parents may make treatment decisions that do not seem to be in the best interest of the child. For instance, parents may not allow their child to receive pain medication because they want the child to be more alert. They might request continued treatment that is traumatic and is not likely to provide long-term survival for the child. These situations can cause emotional, spiritual, and professional distress for the nurse, particularly when there is conflict with the nurse's beliefs. To provide appropriate care, the nurse must use coping strategies or seek assistance to resolve these distressing feelings. If resolution is not possible, the nurse should be given the option of not participating in the child's care.

Pain Control

The interventions that are seen as most important by the child with a terminal illness and the family involve pain management. The nurse educates the child and family regarding pain control methods and then provides consistent reassurance that all appropriate interventions will be done to provide for the child's continued comfort. Families and older children may express concerns about inadequate pain relief as well as fears about addiction when opioids are prescribed. The nurse reassures the child and family members that treating the child's pain symptoms is the top priority and that addiction is unlikely to occur when medications are given to the child for pain caused by the illness.

The child and family must be informed that the pain associated with terminal conditions may escalate acutely and often, with a corresponding decrease in pain relief from opioids and other medications. For this reason, it is necessary at times to increase the medication dosages or change the medication regimen in order to control escalating pain. The nurse ensures that the child and family understand that the child's pain will be assessed frequently and pain control methods evaluated regularly in order to make changes as needed so the child is kept comfortable. (For further information and discussion of pain control for children, see Chapter 15.) Education regarding appropriate pain management, including myths and realities, should begin whenever pain medications are first used during the course of the child's illness. This allows the nurse to simply reinforce information already learned during the terminal phase of the child's illness.

Hospice Care

For many terminally ill children and their families, being outside the hospital environment, either in a home hospice program or at a hospice facility, may be the preferred choice for meeting their complex needs during the dying process. Hospice care is a specialized, comprehensive system of care that provides support and assistance to patients and their families during the last phase of a terminal illness. Hospice care generally starts during the last 6 months of a patient's life. The use of hospice care for children is increasing. Specialized nursing and physician care is the cornerstone; however, other care providers and services are available. Hospice team members include social workers, chaplains, home health aides, physical and occupational therapists, child life specialists, bereavement counselors, and volunteers. Families may receive pharmacy prescriptions, health care supplies, and medical equipment that are delivered to their home.

The nurse can help families choose an appropriate hospice program by referring them to Children's Hospice International (CHI). CHI is a nonprofit organization whose mission is to promote pediatric hospice through pediatric care facilities (Children's Hospice International, 2010a). It provides resources and referrals to children with life-threatening conditions and their families. CHI also provides education and training for health care providers and has developed standards of care and practice guidelines. These standards address access to hospice care, the child and family as a unit, continuity of care, pain and symptom management, bereavement programs, policies and procedures for pediatric hospice services, and utilization review/quality improvement (Children's Hospice International, 2010b). CHI has a list of pediatric hospice care programs, as well as a variety of other resources regarding end-of-life care for children.

A child's home or a hospice care facility may provide a more comfortable and relaxed environment than the acute-care hospital unit. At home, children can have family, pets, friends, and the comfort of their own bedrooms and possessions nearby. Hospice care may be provided in a free-standing facility or in a separate unit of an acute-care hospital. Families may choose a hospice care facility for the following reasons:

- The child's physical care requirements and the emotional burdens are too great for family caregivers to manage.
- The child's physical symptoms may require aggressive management, or the child may have pain requiring intensive and complex medication control.
- The home may not be conducive to adaptations needed for the child's care (e.g., hospital bed, oxygen equipment, a private room).

Brief periods of inpatient hospice care may also be used to meet a family's needs for respite, providing an environment for the dying child that is less threatening and more home-like than an acute-care hospital setting. Family members must take care of their physical and emotional needs so they are able to care for and support their children.

Hospice care should always be offered to families along with the information necessary for making an educated choice. Some families may choose home-based hospice care but later admit the child to a hospital during the final hours or days of life. This choice, which always remains available to families, may be related to concerns about pain control, the adequacy of physical care for the child, and the emotional aspect of a death occurring in the home. Parents may be particularly anxious regarding how they or the siblings will cope with living in their home once their child's death has occurred there. This may lead parents to choose hospitalization, even when their child prefers to die at home. Health care team members need to discuss these concerns with the family early in the child's dying process to allow them time to explore their fears and emotions; ideally leading to a choice that is acceptable and comfortable for the child, siblings, and parents. If a family elects to hospitalize the child when death is imminent, health care providers must accept and support the decision.

The Dying Process and the Time of Death

The care needs of the dying child are much like those of the chronically or seriously ill child. Much of the care is directed by the physical, emotional, and spiritual needs of the child and family. The goal of nursing care is to provide a comfortable, peaceful time for the child and family with minimal disruptions. Whether the death is occurring at home, in the hospital, or at a hospice care facility, the child's room should be secluded, comfortable, and quiet. This type of surrounding contributes significantly toward creating a meaningful time for the child and family.

Privacy for the Child and Family. Privacy without interruptions is important for the dying child and the family so their physical, emotional, and spiritual needs can be met. The child's endurance will be greatly diminished, with increased needs for daytime napping and extended nighttime sleep, when possible. The child may experience sleep deprivation, frequent wakefulness, or nightmares. Privacy and careful control of the number and frequency of visitors will preserve the child's strength and promote rest and sleep. The child must be reassured that family members and care providers are close by, and always accessible and available.

Disruptions by staff and possibly even by friends or extended family should be minimized to the extent desired by the child and family. Often, members of the immediate family will request private time with the dying child. Occasionally this request may cause others to become distraught or to insist on spending time with the child. The nurse as an advocate for the child and family takes responsibility for enforcing the request for privacy. Nurses also strive to facilitate communication among family members and friends in order to convey the family's wishes and explain the need for privacy.

Changes in Family Routines. The availability of loved ones becomes more important to the child with a terminal illness, who will experience more frequent periods of prolonged sleep. Regardless of the duration—moments, minutes, or hours—intervals spent with the child can become treasured memories. The nurse should facilitate as much as possible times for the parents, siblings, and dying child to be together. Special care must be taken to explain to siblings the reasons for rearranging life around the ill child's wakeful hours.

Family Concerns about Oral Intake. Lack of interest in eating and drinking is a normal part of the dying process, yet diminishing nutritional intake can be very difficult for family members to handle. They may hold misconceptions that the child will "starve to death" and that hunger or thirst will add to the child's discomfort. Fluid intake may actually cause discomfort for the child by increasing lung secretions necessitating suctioning. The nurse must prepare the family that often days before death the child will lose the ability to swallow and oral intake will cease. The family members will need enhanced emotional support when this occurs. If kidney function declines during the dying process, the child will retain fluids and feel uncomfortable, thus fluid intake will need to be restricted.

Fluids and Oral Care. There are important nursing implications regarding fluid intake and oral care for the dying child. If the child has a dry mouth or feels thirsty, small amounts of ice chips or fluids given at the request of the child, can alleviate these symptoms.

Physical and emotional comfort can be enhanced by allowing the child who is terminally ill to drink favorite fluids, despite the risk of aspiration that exists if the ability to swallow is compromised. Promoting the child's independence and choices can give a sense of control which the child often loses during the dying process. If a lack of strength or coordination makes drinking from a glass or straw difficult, fluids can be provided using a "sippy" cup, spoon, medicine dropper, or syringe (oral or catheter-tip). Care must be taken not to deliver too much fluid at one time and cause choking. The nurse, with the help from the family, provides appropriate oral care to the dying child to promote comfort and prevent complications. Sponge swabs can be used to clean the lips and mouth and to provide moisture with the use of artificial saliva preparations. Solutions that reduce pain and inflammation can also be applied with sponge swabs. Lip balms or medicated products can be applied to dry, chapped lips. Products that contain alcohol or fragrances should not be used in the mouth or on the lips; they can have a drying effect and cause irritation and pain to inflamed or cracked areas. Appropriate and frequent oral care will minimize mouth odor and improve the child's appearance. Providing oral care may give the family a feeling of usefulness and an opportunity for regular contact with the child. The nurse encourages the family members to decide the types of amount of physical care they wish to provide to their child.

Responsiveness and Communication. A child's level of awareness or wakefulness shortly before the time of death can be an overwhelming concern for family members. The child may become unresponsive in the days or hours before death or may be intermittently responsive until the actual moment of death. The nurse explains the possible variations to family members. Many children have been noted to experience a period of time (either a few hours or an entire day) immediately before they die when they are stronger, more alert, and show increased interest in their family members. This occurrence may cause family members to have unrealistic expectations for recovery; therefore nurses must prepare and educate families about this possible event.

Though a dying child may appear unresponsive, hearing is the last sense to stop functioning before death. The nurse encourages the family members to talk to the child and maintain physical contact such as touching or holding the child's hand, until death occurs, and even after as desired by the family. Some family members may find this difficult due to personal fears or beliefs. Family members have different comfort levels in relation to the dying process, different needs for personal space, or different emotional expressions. The nurse assesses the needs of the family during the final moments of their child's death and offers assistance as indicated to facilitate contact and communication with the child.

⚠ NURSING QUALITY ALERT

Nursing Care for the Dying Child and the Child's Family

- The nurse should be available to assist both the dying child and the child's family but must not impose personal beliefs and expectations on either the child or the family members.
- The siblings of a dying child need time and attention. They, too, will experience grief and will need to resolve their feelings.
- Most family members need to talk about the experience of illness and death. Open communication helps support family resilience and helps family members remember the child after death.
- Care for the dying child includes providing adequate pain control, oral care, privacy, and information. The family needs to be aware of the signs of imminent death and what to expect in the immediate postmortem period.
- After death occurs, family members should have as much time as they desire with the child.

Indicators of Imminent Death. Family members may find security and comfort in the knowledge of the physical indicators that usually signal that the time of death is imminent. The heart rate increases, with a concomitant decrease in the strength and quality of peripheral pulses. Blood pressure also decreases. Pulses and blood pressure may become difficult or impossible to palpate, a state that can last for hours. Cardiac changes generally occur before respiratory changes. Family members more readily notice respiratory changes, which are visible and audible. The force of the respiratory effort may decline. An increased work of breathing, along with apnea, may be noted. Respirations may fluctuate between the two states—rapid, increasingly shallow breaths followed by cessation or Cheyne-Stokes respiration leading to respiratory arrest. Cheyne-Stokes respiration is a cyclic period of slowing respirations with apnea, followed by an increased respiratory rate to a peak, and then slowing and becoming apneic again. These respirations are often referred to as *agonal;* a description that may inaccurately imply they are painful, and thus the term should not be used when family members are present.

As death nears, respirations may become more audible and may be accompanied by an expiratory sigh. This sigh often resembles moaning and may alarm family members because they interpret the sound to indicate pain. If the child is otherwise without verbal or physical indications of pain, the family should be reassured that the child's pain level is well controlled. The nurse educates the family as to the cause of the sounds and noting their correlation with each breath. All these variations in respiratory patterns will result in either hypoxia or hypercapnia. If hypoxic agitation occurs, it is treated with oxygen and morphine, IV or sublingual. Both measures provide physical comfort for the child and emotional comfort for the family. A rising carbon dioxide level may actually contribute to increased comfort due to sedative and analgesic effects. Continuing respiratory and cardiac changes may lead to cool extremities and cyanosis. These effects most often begin in the lower extremities and progress upward to the face. The nurse must prepare the family for the changes they are going to see.

Noisy breathing caused by the rattling secretions in the upper airway can be very distressing to family members. This rattling—often called the *death rattle*—occurs when the child has lost the strength and ability to clear airway secretions. The nurse educates the family about the causes of noisy breathing and that they may see secretions coming from the mouth. Even with education, hearing these sounds can be extremely difficult for the family to handle. Pharyngeal suctioning can help remove secretions but may need to be done very frequently. Medications such as atropine or diphenhydramine may be given to decrease the amount of secretions. The nurse can position the child in the side-lying position to facilitate the drainage of secretions. A cloth should be placed under the mouth to collect the secretions. The child is rarely aware of these respiratory changes; the focus of nursing care is symptom management and providing support to the family. When respirations stop, there may be a brief period of seconds or minutes until the heart stops beating. A final gasping noise may occur after respiratory and cardiac function have ceased. Reassure the family that this sound is normal and not painful.

◎ NURSING CARE PLAN

The Terminally Ill or Dying Child

Focused Assessment
- Provide a comprehensive assessment of the terminally ill child and family (parents and siblings)
  - Address family relationships and involvement with the child
  - Assess the child's development level and cognitive, physical, and psychosocial abilities
  - Determine the child and family's previous experiences with illness and death
  - Examine recent experiences of the child and family related to the current illness
- Explore the child and each family member's individual progression through the stages of grief in relation to the child's impending death
- Assess the child and family for symptoms of anxiety and other negative psychosocial effects
  - Examine child for indications that anxiety is exacerbating pain or triggering other physical symptoms (e.g., dyspnea)
  - Reassess level of anxiety or other concerns during times of increased stress (e.g., time of diagnosis, disease exacerbations, relapses)
- Assess the child's and family's coping strategies and adaptive mechanisms

Planning
Nursing Diagnosis
Grieving related to the impending death of a child.

Expected Outcomes
The child and family will experience appropriate progression through the five stages of grief, as evidenced by verbalization of an understanding of the five stages of grief, expression of all emotions in an appropriate manner, and expression of feelings by each family member.
The child and family will exhibit behaviors indicating acceptance of the child's impending death and the family will provide care and support—emotional, physical, and psychosocial—in the manner desired by the child.

Intervention/Rationale
1. Explain the five stages of grief and the necessary grieving process, including resolution to acceptance.
   Explanations of the normal grieving process should facilitate grief progression and guide behaviors in each stage.

◎ NURSING CARE PLAN

The Terminally Ill or Dying Child—cont'd

2. Identify the stage of grief being experienced and provide each family member the opportunity to verbalize feelings and receive positive feedback.
   Verbalization of feelings and receiving positive feedback guide behaviors and facilitate progression through the grief stages.

3. Explain to the family the stages of grief progression characteristic for children (the dying child and any siblings). Encourage patience with the extended period of grief for children.
   Understanding the ways in which children's coping mechanisms differ from those of adults facilitates acceptance and understanding by parents.

4. Offer the child and all family members the opportunity to verbalize and convey all emotions, in an appropriate manner. Exhibit a nonjudgmental attitude toward and acceptance of verbalization and behaviors.
   Venting of emotions helps decrease stress and facilitate resolution of anger. An attitude of acceptance conveys care and support and encourages appropriate, needed expression of all emotions.

5. Encourage open, honest communication with the child (to the degree requested). Demonstrate appropriate communication techniques.
   Appropriate communication with the child will provide comfort and support as well as facilitate expression of needs and problem resolution.

6. Offer family members the opportunity to participate in the child's physical care, as desired by both parties. Demonstrate providing gentle, supportive care.
   Family members may fear the provision of physical care to a dying child. Observing the nurse may lessen fears and enhance care giving.

Evaluation

Do the child (if cognitively able) and family verbalize an understanding of the five stages of grief and express all emotions in an appropriate manner and in a communication style most comfortable for each individual?

Do the child and family exhibit behaviors that indicate acceptance of the impending death?

Does the family provide physical, emotional, and psychosocial care and support in the manner and environment desired by the child?

Planning
Nursing Diagnosis

Anxiety related to the threat of impending death.

Expected Outcomes

The child and family will achieve anxiety control, as evidenced by open verbalization of all feelings and emotions and questions concerning the diagnosis and prognosis.

The child and family will verbalize physical, emotional, and spiritual comfort.

Intervention/*Rationale*

1. Educate the child and family about the terminal phase of illness (e.g., what to expect in physical, emotional, and spiritual areas). Explain how needs will be met.
   Misconceptions may lead to increased fear and family expressions of anxiety, which can cause increased distress for the dying child.

2. Assure the child and family that the child will be kept safe and comfortable (with minimal pain), and will not be left alone. Provide frequent reassurance.
   Fears about the child's comfort (pain level) and security are the most common. Frequent reassurances are often necessary as the disease and symptoms worsen.

3. Provide as much privacy as possible for the family and the child dying in the hospital setting. Encourage parents and siblings to stay with the child if desired. Regulate visitations by those outside the immediate family, as necessary.
   Immediate family members may need extended time for processing grief and to reach closure. Increased visitations may interfere with the time and privacy needed by the family when death is imminent. The nurse needs to manage the number of visitors because this often is too difficult for the family.

4. Provide opportunities for family members to care for the child or to decline providing all or some aspects of care. As indicated, teach family members how to provide care in a suitable manner.
   Children are usually most comfortable when cared for by family members. However, at times, the child and family may be more comfortable if the nurse provides certain aspects of care.

5. Offer the family and child alternatives for care, such as hospice care in the home or an in-patient facility, if indicated.
   Hospice care programs can be individualized to meet the needs of a dying child and the family.

Evaluation

Do the child and family openly and appropriately verbalize all feelings, emotions, and questions concerning the diagnosis and prognosis?

Do the child and family exhibit physical, emotional, and spiritual comfort?

The Family after Death. After death has occurred, family members should have the opportunity to spend time with their child, even before the body is cleaned. It may be preferred to clean and prepare the body first because of the drainage, bleeding, and spontaneous elimination of body wastes that often occur at the time of death. Some families ask to make hand and foot prints or cut a lock of hair as a remembrance of the child. The nurse explains to the family what will be involved in the care of the body. Family members including siblings can be invited to assist in bathing the child's body. This final act of physical care may serve as a special means of closure. Some family members do not wish to assist with the bathing and parents may not allow siblings to participate. The nurse respects whatever decisions are made by the family. Rare occasions may occur when the family's time with the deceased child or ability to participate in after-death care may be limited, due to required procedures such as an autopsy. Families should be provided information before the child's death if an autopsy will be required and how this will affect their time and involvement with their child after death occurs.

As family members prepare to hold the deceased child, the nurse discusses the physical changes that occur very quickly after death; cooling of the body, cyanosis or paleness, and stiffening. The nurse attempts to prevent further drainage of body fluids. The nurse prepares the family emotionally and provides towels and blankets to facilitate the family's comfort.

The nurse provides privacy for the family, but remains close by and returns as needed or requested. The nurse always offers the services of pastoral care or other appropriate hospital staff members. If a funeral home has not been chosen by the family, clergy and social services personnel can provide assistance.

The nurse informs the family that the child can go to the funeral home either in a hospital gown or in personal clothes. The family including the siblings may choose the clothes and a personal item such as a blanket or toy that will go with the child to the funeral home. The clothes and item will be returned to the family after the child is dressed for burial. Some hospitals and hospices hold periodic memorials for children who have died. Attending these services and/or the funerals of children who have died supports the family through the bereavement period. It may also assist nursing staff as they deal with the death of a patient. Parents appreciate the efforts by staff both at the time of death and the period after (Barrera, O'Connor, D'Agostino et al., 2009; Meert, Briller, Schim, et al., 2009).

The Nurse's Response to the Dying Child

Not all health care providers cope well with the reality of death. This limitation may hold serious implications for the nurse who chooses to work in an area where deaths occur frequently such as the emergency department, oncology floors, and critical care units. Caring for dying children and their families can be stressful and emotionally demanding. Nurses working with terminally ill children need increased emotional and psychosocial strength, as well as clinical expertise.

The nurse's response to the dying process and death of a pediatric patient correlates to a certain degree with the stages of grief. The nurse who has become more accustomed to the reality and frequency of death may not experience each stage. Length of treatment and personal affinity may cause a nurse to become more involved with a certain child and this can lead to a more intense response or a delay in the resolution of grief. Some nurses may have difficulty maintaining appropriate boundaries between personal involvement and professional care. The nurse who is compassionate yet can maintain professionalism may be better able to provide care on a continuing basis to children with terminal illnesses and their families.

Every nurse who cares for dying children will experience loss and grief and needs support. Nurses can provide mutual support through organized support programs as well as simple acts of respect, concern, and care among colleagues. When a nurse begins working with dying children for the first time, having a more experienced nurse mentor may be helpful. In order for nurses to provide high quality care to children with chronic or terminal illnesses and their families, nurses must also take care of their physical and emotional health.

KEY CONCEPTS

- Children with chronic conditions are living longer, often with conditions once considered fatal. Despite improvements in the quality and length of life, chronic illness remains a situational crisis for families.
- Chronic illness affects the entire family, not just the child.
- With a chronically ill child, all family members must work together to meet the physical and emotional needs of the child, provide care for the rest of the family, and manage financial burdens.
- The stages of grief are applicable to children, with special considerations. A child's concepts of death and dying are based on the development level as well as age, cognition, and life experiences. Both ill children and their well siblings fluctuate in their understanding of and responses to death and dying.
- The dying child, like the dying adult, desires the comfort, safety, and presence of loved ones.

- Parents must move from *fear* to *acknowledgment* of the child's impending death.
- For parents caring for a dying child, pain is the greatest concern.
- The grief of a sibling can be more difficult for the nurse to address, related to the developmental level, cognitive abilities, and changing needs, than the grief of parents.
- Each family member (adults and children) must process grief by understanding that the person who has died is gone and experience the resulting emotions. Then, family members must reinvest in life and go forward.
- Caring for a terminally ill or dying child can be a stressful and demanding experience for the nurse. It is imperative that nurses attend to their own physical, emotional, and spiritual health so they can provide physical and psychosocial care to the child and family during this difficult time.

REFERENCES

Barrera, M., O'Connor, K., D'Agostino, N. M., et al. (2009). Early parental adjustment and bereavement after childhood cancer death. *Death Studies, 33*(6), 497-520.

Bluebond-Langner, M. (1978). *The private worlds of dying children.* Princeton, NJ: Princeton University Press.

Chamberlain, L., & Wise, P. (2011). Chronic illness in childhood. In R. Kliegman, B. Stanton, J. St. Geme, et al. (Eds.), *Nelson textbook of pediatrics* (19th ed., pp. 149). Philadelphia: Elsevier Saunders.

Children's Hospice International. (2010a). *Who we are.* Retrieved from www.chionline.org/whoweare.

Children's Hospice International. (2010b). *About children's hospice, palliative care, & end of life care; CHI standards of hospice care for children.* Retrieved from www.chionline.org/pressreleases/standards%20guidelines%20092305-1.pdf.

Erickson, C., Splett, P., Mullett, S., & Heiman, M. (2006). The healthy learner model for student chronic condition management: Part 1. *Journal of School Nursing, 22*(6), 310-318.

Frain, M., Berven, N., Tschopp, M., et al. (2007). Use of the resiliency model of family stress, adjustment and adaptation by rehabilitation counselors. *Journal of Rehabilitation, 73*(3), 18-25.

George, A., Vickers, M., Wilkes, L., & Barton, B. (2006–2007). Chronic grief: Experiences of working parents of children with chronic illness. *Contemporary Nurse, 23*(2), 228-242.

Groves, A. (2010). Cultural competency at the bedside. *Med-Surg Matters, 19*(4), 4-7.

Kübler-Ross, E. (1969). *On death and dying.* New York: Macmillan.

Kübler-Ross, E. (1983). *On children and death.* New York: Macmillan.

Lindblad, B., Rasmussen, B. H., & Sandman, P. (2005). Being invigorated in parenthood: Parents' experiences of being supported by professionals when having a disabled child. *Journal of Pediatric Nursing, 20*(4), 288-297.

Maciejewski, P., Zhang, B., Block, S., & Prigerson, H. (2007). An empirical examination of the stages of grief theory. *Journal of the American Medical Association, 297*(7), 716-723.

Meert, K. L., Briller, S., Schim, S. M., et al. (2009). Examining the needs of bereaved parents in the pediatric intensive care unit: A qualitative study. *Death Studies, 33*(8), 712-740.

Patterson, J. M. (2002). Integrating family resilience and family stress theory. *Journal of Marriage and Family, 64*(2), 349-360.

Thurgate, C. (2006). Living with disability: Part 3. Communication and care. *Paediatric Nursing, 18*(5), 38-44.

Ullrich, C., Duncan, J., Joselow, M., & Wolfe, J. (2011). Pediatric palliative care. In R. Kliegman, B. Stanton, J. St. Geme, et al. (Eds.), *Nelson textbook of pediatrics* (19th ed., pp. 149-159). Philadelphia: Elsevier Saunders.

U.S. Department of Health and Human Services, Health Resources and Services Administration, Maternal and Child Health Bureau. (2008). *The national survey of children with special health care needs chartbook 2005–2006.* Rockville, MD: U.S. Department of Health and Human Services.

Wass, H. (1985). Concepts of death: A developmental perspective. *Issues in Comprehensive Pediatric Nursing, 8*(1-6), 3-25.

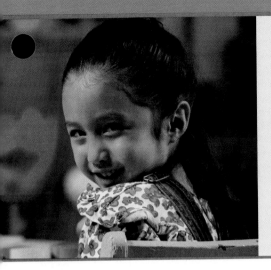

Principles and Procedures for Nursing Care of Children

⊖volve WEBSITE

http://evolve.elsevier.com/James/ncoc

LEARNING OBJECTIVES

After studying this chapter, you should be able to:
- Describe how to prepare children and families for selected procedures frequently seen in an acute-care setting and a home care setting.
- Compare anatomic and physiologic differences in children and adults as they apply to selected procedures.
- Identify psychosocial considerations unique to children undergoing selected procedures.
- Describe techniques useful for eliciting cooperation from the child undergoing selected procedures.
- Describe step-by-step nursing actions and the rationales for performing selected procedures.

Children need preparation before and accurate information about any procedure that is performed. This information is essential to promote a sense of security, decrease fear, elicit cooperation, and improve coping skills. Parents also need preparation because their anxiety about a procedure may be transferred to the child. Teaching before performing procedures increases the knowledge base of the child and family.

After assessing the child and family, the nurse needs to plan how to carry out the procedure in the most effective manner. The nurse can implement strategies to help the child and parents through all phases of a procedure: the anticipation and preparation phase, the actual procedure, and the recovery period after completion.

PREPARING CHILDREN FOR PROCEDURES

⊖ Preparing children and families for procedures, especially those that are painful, threatening, or invasive, starts with a thorough, individualized assessment. This process should include an assessment of the child's developmental stage, personality, existing level of knowledge, present level of understanding, past experiences, coping skills, and family situation. The nurse can then match explanations and teaching to the specific needs of the child and family. It is also important for the nurse to determine the communication approaches that will be most effective for the child and family based on the child's age and developmental level as well as the family's cultural preferences (see Chapter 3 for more information about communication).

Explaining Procedures

Before starting the process of preparing the child and family for a procedure, it is important for the nurse to review all the elements and hospital policies, if applicable. This is especially important if the procedure is new or performed infrequently. The nurse requests any needed medication for the child, gathers all supplies, and obtains assistance as necessary. Equipment is obtained and tested to ensure that it functions properly before beginning any procedure.

Explaining procedures includes demonstrating equipment and describing anything the child will feel, see, hear, and smell. The nurse uses a developmentally appropriate approach and words the child will understand. Relating the experience to an object or situation familiar or of interest to the child is an effective communication strategy.

Appropriately timing the explanation is critical. Many children respond better to procedures if the explanation is given either just before the procedure or step by step as the procedure unfolds. Some older children and adolescents like to be prepared well in advance in case they have questions and need more information. Advance preparation allows the child to express feelings about the procedure verbally or through role playing. Parents know their child best, so the nurse asks parents about the best timing and approach to use. Time should be allowed for the child to become familiar with the equipment and for the child and family to ask questions (Box 13-1).

Pediatric Skills—Preparing the Child for Procedures

TIPS FOR PREPARING AND SUPPORTING CHILDREN UNDERGOING PROCEDURES

Before the Procedure

- Offer the child ways to cope with pain or discomfort. For example, some children can use coping strategies such as guided imagery. Others may listen to music, increasing the volume as the discomfort level increases. Give the child permission to cry or yell if necessary.
- Use developmentally appropriate words when discussing the procedure and expectations.
- Give the child as much choice as possible over what will happen. For example, when possible, the child could be allowed to choose an injection site or a site for intravenous catheter placement.
- Be sure the consent form has been signed, if applicable.
- Always use appropriate hand hygiene before beginning any procedure and follow Standard Precautions.

During the Procedure

- Talk to the child during the procedure if the child desires. If the child is using a coping strategy such as guided imagery, however, talking will be a distraction and will decrease the child's ability to cope with what is happening.
- Keep the child informed of the procedure's progress.
- Tell the child when the procedure is nearly completed and the "worst is over."

After the Procedure

- Praise the child for attempts at cooperation even if the child did not do anything you asked. Trying counts! Specifically praise the child for accomplishing an expected task.
- Provide an opportunity for the child to vent feelings about the procedure. Remember that expressing feelings of anger is appropriate. Tell the child that you understand if the child does not want to talk with you right now and that you will return later.
- If parents were not present during the procedure, reunite the child with the parents and allow them to provide comfort and support.
- Reward the child by using age-appropriate methods such as giving stickers.
- Document the preparation process and procedure performance, who performed the procedure, the child's tolerance of the procedure, and its outcomes.

⚡ **SAFETY ALERT**

Standard Precautions

Always use appropriate hand hygiene before a procedure and when the procedure is finished. Follow Standard Precautions.

Also important for a child's successful coping with an invasive or painful procedure is the presence of someone the child trusts. Time spent establishing a trusting relationship with a child is time well spent. Trust in health care providers can enhance the child's unique coping strategies.

Before procedures, ensure the child's privacy by closing the door to the room and drawing a curtain around the bed or, optimally, by taking the child to a treatment room if appropriate and comfortable for the child and parent. The treatment room contains suitable equipment for

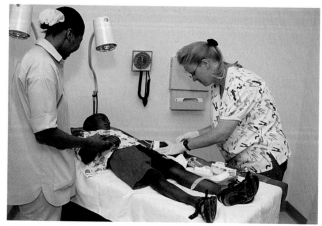

FIG 13-1 Because a child should feel that the hospital room is a safe place, a treatment room is used for invasive or painful procedures. The parent is present, not to restrain the child, but to provide emotional support.

invasive procedures and is a private area away from the safe haven of a child's room or the playroom (Figure 13-1). Visitors should be asked to leave, and parents might also choose to leave, although parental participation is supported and encouraged.

Telling children and parents in advance what they can and should do during the procedure provides a sense of control and decreases potential feelings of powerlessness. For example, a child who is having an intravenous (IV) catheter placed or a blood specimen drawn is told that to "help," he or she must hold an extremity still and not move. Parents are asked to "help" the child remember to not move.

💬 You might say to the child, "We have talked about why you need to have blood taken from your arm, but you need to know how important it is for you to hold your arm very still while we are doing this. I will tell you everything that is going to happen so you can be prepared and know when to help. Do you think you can help us, or do we need to ask someone to help you remember not to move your arm?"

The nurse offers children choices when feasible. For example, a child chooses the type of colorful bandage that will cover an injection site or whether to have a procedure done before or after the next television show. Children are never threatened with punishment if they fail to cooperate. Nurses need to have realistic expectations that are based on the child's developmental level and capacity for cooperation.

Parents are encouraged to be involved as much as they want according to what is possible during procedures. For example, a child might be much more cooperative in taking oral medications if the mother administers them. Often, by explaining what the parents will be seeing and what they can do, the nurse helps them feel comfortable staying with and supporting their child. The nurse should recognize, however, that parents might be uncomfortable remaining with their child during a painful or invasive procedure. The nurse gives parents permission to leave if they desire and assures them that they will be called if they are needed or as soon as the procedure is completed.

Consent for Procedures

All surgical or diagnostic invasive procedures, particularly those that involve risk to the child, require informed consent. Some examples are lumbar puncture, chest tube insertion, and bone marrow aspiration. Both legal and ethical requirements exist to inform the child, if appropriate, and the child's parents of the benefits and risks of the proposed procedure or treatment. Informed consent must be obtained from the parent or legal guardian before the procedure is performed.

> **! NURSING QUALITY ALERT**
>
> ### Preparation for Procedures
>
> - A treatment room is the preferred location for performing painful procedures. It is a private area away from the safe haven of a child's hospital room, and it usually contains the necessary equipment for a variety of procedures (see Figure 13-1).
> - Ensure that a person the child trusts is there for support.
> - Use terminology appropriate for the child's developmental level. Avoid using words or phrases that the child might misinterpret (e.g., dye, put to sleep, stick).
> - Offer the child choices, if appropriate.
> - Tell the child and parents how they can help with the procedure.
> - Do not threaten punishment for lack of cooperation.
> - Encourage parental participation in the procedure, but do not force an unwilling parent to stay.

Other procedures, such as IV line insertions, specimen collection, and medication and oxygen administration, are covered under the general consent to treat that is signed at admission. It is now also customary to obtain assent from children 7 years old and older. Assent means that the child has been fully informed about the procedure and concurs with those giving the informed consent. Laws on informed consent vary from state to state, so nurses should become familiar with the laws and the policies of their institution. (See Chapter 1 for information related to consent and other legal issues.)

The person performing the procedure should obtain the consent. Nurses need to check that the consent form is signed and witnessed, and they need to answer questions relating to the procedure. Occasionally an emergency or life-threatening situation arises in which contacting the parents or legal guardian for consent is not possible. In such cases administrative consent may be obtained to allow physicians to perform the indicated procedures. (See Chapter 1 for legal issues related to emergency consent provisions.)

HOLDING AND TRANSPORTING INFANTS AND CHILDREN

Infants can be held in several positions (Figure 13-2). Before the infant is discharged from the hospital, the nurse teaches new parents how to hold the infant, and nurses working on pediatric units should hold infants in similar ways. Nurses hold infants securely, anticipating sudden movement. Because infants younger than 4 months old do not have well-established head control, supporting the head and neck is essential. Infants up to 2 to 3 months of age are cradled by holding them in a horizontal position, supporting the back, and grasping the thigh (see Figure 13-2, *A*). When using the football hold, the infant is tucked between the nurse's body and elbow, with the arm carrying the infant's body and the hand supporting the head (see Figure 13-2, *B*). When carrying the infant upright, the infant erect against the nurse's chest (see Figure 13-2, *C*). The infant's buttocks rests on the forearm, and the other arms supports the infant's head and shoulders. Even for infants with well-developed neck muscles and head control, this extra support prevents infants from falling backward should they make a sudden move. Parents who use backpacks or front-facing baby carriers

are advised to be sure that the infant's head is supported at all times when in the backpack or carrier.

Hospitalized infants and children sometimes must be transported to other areas within a hospital unit or even outside the unit. A change in location might be a response to changes in the child's condition or might be done to increase parental involvement in the child's care (e.g., rooming-in). Children might be transported to different areas on the same unit (e.g., treatment room, playroom) or other hospital departments for specialized care (e.g., rehabilitation) or for diagnostic testing.

The method of transportation will depend on the child's age, developmental level, and physical condition; the destination; safety factors; and whether equipment such as oxygen, an IV pump, or a cardiac monitor is needed to accompany the child. Any special accommodations should be arranged before the time of the planned transport.

Infants and toddlers can also be transported in a bassinet or crib. The rails should always be up in the highest position, and for older infants and toddlers the protective top should be in place. Strollers and wagons can be used to transfer older infants and toddlers to other areas on the unit (see Figure 13-2, *D*). Safety belts should be used and the sides of the wagon should be in the raised position. An infant or a toddler is *never* left unattended in a wagon. With all transport methods, equipment is securely attached to a rolling cart or stand and then pushed or pulled along with the transporting vehicle. Equipment is *not* placed inside the transporting vehicle that infants or young children occupy.

Older children and adolescents are transported in wheelchairs or on stretchers with the side rails raised. In some cases, such as for a child in traction, transporting the child in the bed is preferable. Safety belts *must* be used and side rails must be in the raised and locked position. All children of all ages are supervised when in a transport vehicle.

SAFETY ISSUES IN THE HOSPITAL SETTING

Safety is of paramount concern for all children; infants and toddlers are at the greatest risk for injury. When an infant or toddler is in a crib, nurses and parents need to be especially vigilant about keeping crib sides rails locked in the raised position to prevent the child from falling out of the crib. A hand is *always* placed on the back or abdomen of an infant or young child when the crib rails are down or when the small child is on an elevated surface such as a scale or treatment table. The nurse follows this practice consistently and teaches it to parents as well. As with adult patients, when children and adolescents are in hospital beds, they are maintained in the lowest position with the rails up on each side. Small objects, such as alcohol swabs and IV line caps, must be kept out of cribs and off of bedside tables, the floor, or any area within the young child's reach. Older infants and toddlers may put these small items in their mouths, causing a significant risk for choking.

When performing a procedure on a child, techniques such as distraction by a parent or child life specialist can facilitate the child remaining calm and unmoving (Sparks, Setlik, & Luhman, 2007). Occasionally, to prevent trauma during a procedure, holding a child is necessary to restrict movement. If holding is required, it is important to enlist the cooperation of the child (if appropriate age) and parent (Brenner, 2007). Some parents may be willing to hold their child on their lap for a procedure, or provide distraction while a second nurse holds the child. Parents should not be required to hold their child during a procedure, because this has been found to cause significant distress for the family (Brenner, 2007).

Restraints should be used only as a last resort for the protection of the child and others. Some infants and young children may require protection from pulling out a tube, removing a dressing, or disrupting

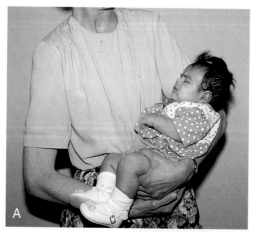

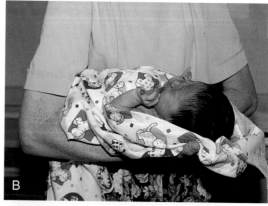

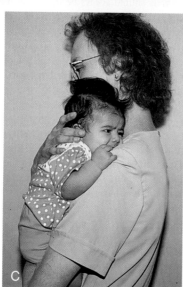

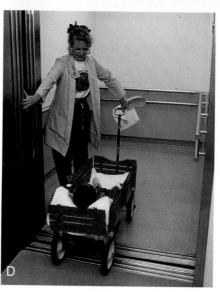

FIG 13-2 Methods of transporting infants and children. The nurse carries the infant securely, anticipating sudden movement. **A,** Cradle carry. **B,** Football hold. **C,** Over-the-shoulder carry, which can be used until the infant is 6 to 7 months old. **D,** Transport can be fun for young children, especially when it is on wheels. (**A, B,** and **C,** Courtesy Parkland Health and Hospital System District Community Oriented Primary Care Clinic, Dallas, TX; **D,** Courtesy Cook Children's Medical Center, Fort Worth, TX.)

⚡ SAFETY ALERT

Using Restraints

- Use the least restrictive restraint.
- Choose the proper device for the child's condition.
- Ensure proper fit of the device.
- Tie knots, if used, that can be easily untied for quick access.
- Secure ties to bed frames (not mattresses or side rails), to the frames of wheelchairs, or to another stable device.
- Check the extremity distal to the restraint for circulation, sensation, and motion every 15 minutes for the first hour, and subsequently as agency policy dictates.
- Remove restraints every 1 to 2 hours for range-of-motion movement and repositioning and to offer the child food or the opportunity to use the bathroom.
- Document findings from neurovascular checks; restraint removal, repositioning, and range of motion; and skin condition assessment.

a suture line by using a restraint. Thus, covering the hands with mitts, or using elbow restraints, which keep the elbows from bending so the child's hands cannot reach a vulnerable site, may be used. If a restraint is needed for the child's protection, most facilities require a physician's order stating why any restraint is needed and how long it will be in place. The restraint chosen should be the least restrictive device that will prevent injury.

Before applying any form of restraint, the nurse informs the parents and child, if appropriate, the reason for the restraint, where it will be applied, what movement it will prevent, how long it will be in place, and how often a nurse will check on the child. The call button is made readily available so the child or parent can easily reach the nurse. The child's developmental needs (e.g., thumb-sucking) are assessed and provisions are made to meet these needs when possible (e.g., restrain a toddler's arm so the thumb can still be placed in the mouth). Regardless of the type of restraint used, the nurse must remove the restraint and assess the patient on a regular and frequent basis (e.g., every 1 to 2 hours).

Many hospitalized children are physically active and may be at risk for injury from falls. There is considerable variability in how hospitals define, classify, and measure fall injury rates for children (Child Health Corporation of America, 2009). Factors that can contribute to children's falls within the hospital setting include altered mental status (e.g., sedation, conditions that cause dizziness or confusion), age (younger than 3 years), need for mobility assistance, and inattentiveness by parents due to unfamiliarity with surroundings or anxiety (Razmus, Wilson, Smith, & Newman, 2006). It is recommended that all children undergo a complete fall risk screen when admitted to the hospital and again if physiologic, motor, or sensory changes occur (Child Health Corporation of America, 2009). Children at risk for falls are then identified with ID bands, signs, and stickers.

Nurses must ensure that children, parents, and other health care team members keep side and crib rails up. Infants or small toddlers can be placed in a crib with a plastic bubble top or higher extensions to the crib sides. Older children and adolescents at risk for falls are informed to not attempt to get out of bed without assistance and how to use the call system when they need help. Other preventive actions include keeping the floors free of objects and fluids, providing adequate lighting, using assistive equipment properly, wearing nonslip footwear, and frequent patient monitoring (Child Health Corporation of America, 2009). For active children, prevention strategies might include using a sitter to stay with the child, behavior modification techniques such as a time-out, and diversional activities appropriate for the child's developmental level and condition.

INFECTION CONTROL

Hand Hygiene

Hand hygiene is the mainstay of infection control in health care settings and in the home. In 2002, the Centers for Disease Control and Prevention (CDC) published data regarding transmission of organisms by health care workers in hospital settings. Using evidence based on research that demonstrates organisms are present both in hospitalized patients and on environmental surfaces, and that alcohol-based hand rubs are more effective for eliminating organisms, the CDC (2002) issued recommendations for hand hygiene, and these have been updated in a clinical guideline for preventing transmission of infection in the hospital (Siegel, Rhinehart, Jackson, Chiarello, & the Healthcare Infection Control Practices Advisory Committee, 2007):

1. If hands are contaminated with blood or body fluids, or visibly soiled, clean hands with soap and water.
2. If hands are clean, use an alcohol-based hand rub before and after touching potentially contaminated surfaces near the patient, before and after patient contact, before putting on gloves for a procedure, and after removing gloves.
3. Put alcohol-based hand rub on the hands, rub over all surfaces of hands and fingers, and allow to thoroughly dry (total time, approximately 20 seconds).

Procedures described in this chapter assume that the nurse will use appropriate hand hygiene both before and after each procedure.

Standard Precautions

Standard Precautions, which are used in institutions and the workplace for infection prevention, apply to the following:
- Blood
- All body fluids, secretions, and excretions except sweat, regardless of whether they contain visible blood
- Nonintact skin
- Mucous membranes

Two tiers of precautions are under this system. Standard Precautions, precautions in the first tier, apply in the care of all hospitalized patients without regard for diagnosis or presumed infectious state. Second-tier precautions apply in the care of specific patients and are referred to as Transmission-Based Precautions. They are for patients known or suspected to be infected by pathogens that are transmitted through air or droplets or through contact with dry skin or contaminated surfaces.

The complete guidelines for applying Standard Precautions and Transmission-Based Precautions are highly detailed and extensive (Siegel et al., 2007). Each facility is responsible for making these guidelines available and implementing the precautions. Procedures described subsequently in this chapter assume that the nurse will use appropriate Standard Precautions.

Implementing Precautions

When Transmission-Based Precautions are in effect, the items with which the infected child comes in contact are also contaminated. These items include the bed, linens, IV pump, sink, and toys. Therefore, the nurse who is going into the room to reset an IV pump, pick up soiled linens, and so forth must use whatever protective equipment is mandated by the type of precaution (e.g., gown, mask, gloves, goggles, face shield) (Siegel et al., 2007).

Children placed on Transmission-Based Precautions often need extra attention to avert boredom. They need more diversional activities, such as games or movies, and more psychosocial support. Young children, for example, may think that they are being punished. Visitors might hesitate to enter the child's room and may need additional support or reassurance from the nurse.

Family Teaching

Family education is crucial for effective infection control or prevention. The nurse emphasizes to parents, visitors, and other health care providers that infection control precautions are important and must be closely followed. Parents often state that they are there to visit only their child and do not understand the need to wear special clothing or equipment. The nurse needs to emphasize that the organisms that cause some diseases, such as respiratory syncytial virus, can live on inanimate objects such as clothing or crib rails for many hours. Thus the disease can spread throughout the hospital or to the home if infection control or prevention measures are not followed. Family members are encouraged to visit the child frequently because visits will decrease the child's sense of isolation. Family are taught that meticulous hand hygiene, both in the hospital setting and at home, is the best way to prevent infection.

BATHING INFANTS AND CHILDREN

The nurse can use bath time to facilitate parent interaction with their infant. During the bath, the nurse demonstrates for the parents how to hold the infant securely and how to bathe the infant so that bath time is a positive experience for parents and children.

Strict observance of safety principles when bathing an infant or child can prevent falls, burns, or water aspiration. When bathing an infant or a child in the hospital setting, the nurse takes the opportunity to note any problems, such as altered skin integrity, surgical incisions, loss of sensation, abnormal skin color, bruising, paralysis, or any other condition that might warrant special consideration. Newborn infants can be immersed in water after the umbilical stump and circumcision sites (if applicable) have healed. The temperature of the child's bath water should not exceed 100° F (37.7° C)—that is, warm but not hot

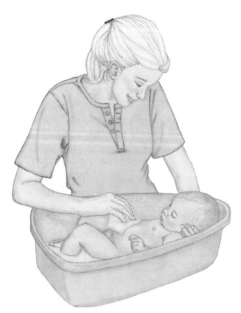 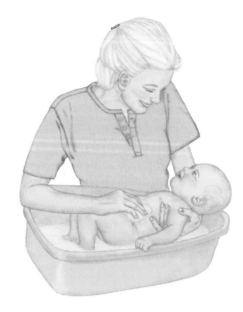

Using hand to support infant's neck and head   Using arm to support infant's neck and head

FIG 13-3 When giving an infant a tub bath, the nurse supports the infant's body at all times.

to the touch. If a bath thermometer is available, it should be used to check the temperature of the water. Otherwise, a temperature that is comfortable when tested on the inside of your wrist or elbow is appropriate.

Before bathing any child, assess the family's preferences and home practices. Factors to consider include the time of day usually set aside for the bath, bathing rituals, special equipment, any product allergies, and the type of bath preferred. This time is also used to determine the amount of assistance needed by the child and the family and to address any learning needs related to hygiene. Because bathing is one of the areas over which the parents might be allowed to retain control when their child is hospitalized, it is important to allow them to make as many decisions as possible. Decision making also allows parents to maintain a part of the home routine with their hospitalized child.

An infant who cannot sit unaided can be given either a sponge bath or a bath in an infant tub. The infant's body and head are supported at all times during the bath (Figure 13-3). Older infants and toddlers can be bathed in either an infant tub or a regular bathtub. Infants and small children are *never* left unattended in the bath. Older children can take showers if facilities are available. The nurse should use judgment in deciding how much supervision an older child needs while bathing. Privacy for the school-age child and adolescent is extremely important.

Special Considerations

Bed baths are frequently used for hospitalized infants and children. When bathing a newborn or young infant, soap is not necessary. In fact, soap can be too drying to the skin if used frequently. If soap is necessary or desired by the parent, a gentle, non-alkaline soap should be used.

To prevent chilling when giving a sponge bath, be sure to keep the child covered with a cotton blanket. The entire body except for the body part being washed or rinsed is covered. The bath begins with the face, and the diaper area is cleaned last. If eye discharge is present, the

nurse uses a clean, wet cotton ball for each eye, and cleans from the inner canthus outward. Use a clean cotton ball for each eye. The outer ears can be cleaned with a wet face cloth.

If bathing an infant, line a plastic infant tub with a towel to provide comfort, as well as traction to prevent slipping. To prevent accidental drowning should the infant slide down into the tub, fill the tub with no more than 3 inches of water.

When finished with the infant bath, the infant is wrapped in a dry towel or cotton blanket. Using the football hold and holding the infant over the tub, the nurse shampoos the infant's scalp and hair (including the area over the fontanel) with baby shampoo. Talcum powder, baby powder, and cornstarch are *not* used in the diaper area. When these substances get moist, they provide a medium for organism growth. Talcum powder and cornstarch, if accidentally inhaled, can result in respiratory complications.

Older children may choose to take a bath or shower, if their condition allows. The nurse ensures that the child has adequate towels, soap, and toiletries. Either the parent, nurse, or other staff member should remain nearby to provide assistance upon request.

Should an older child or adolescent require a bed bath, adjust the room temperature to a comfortable setting, and draw the curtain around the bed. As with any bed bath, the nurse begins with the face and proceeds in a head-to-toe progression. Obtain fresh water when it is time to rinse the child. Drape the child adequately for privacy and warmth. To prevent chilling, dry each body section as it is rinsed. The bath can be followed with application of lotion or deodorant if desired. The nurse performs the same assessment as with any child and provides assistance as necessary.

Some bathing restrictions might apply to children with surgical incisions, skin traction, IV catheters, casts, urinary catheters, artificial airways, or feeding tubes. Children may be restricted or unable to tolerate certain position changes because of their underlying conditions or treatments. It is imperative to assess for these special needs before beginning the bath.

Documentation

Documentation includes the type of bath, child or parent participation, procedure tolerance, and any abnormal findings noted, such as bruising, rashes, or excoriation. Any lotions or other skin preparations used also should be recorded.

Parent Teaching

General principles of hygiene and safety might need to be reinforced with some parents. Instruction in the use of special bathing equipment, such as infant bathtubs, safety bars, or tub grips, should be included as part of discharge teaching and preparation. To prevent injury or accidental drowning, appropriate supervision of the child should be maintained at all times. Parents are taught to *never* to leave an infant or a young child alone in the bath; the risk of drowning, even in small amounts of water, is high. Infant bath seats, which adhere to the floor of a regular bathtub by suction cups, are unsafe and should not be used because infants can slip out the sides or the seats can tip over.

ORAL HYGIENE

To remove excess food and bacteria, the nurse wipes an infant's gums gently with a wet cloth after each feeding. After teeth erupt, a soft, damp cloth, a piece of gauze, or a child's soft toothbrush can be used to clean the mouth and teeth after each feeding and before bed. Until the parent is certain that the child can perform oral care correctly and independently, young children are supervised and assisted if needed. Even then, reminders to brush might be necessary.

Children frequently need reminders to brush their teeth. Toothbrushing should be done at least twice daily with a child's soft toothbrush and a small (pea-size) amount of toothpaste. Children may ingest excessive amounts of fluoride if they are allowed to use large amounts of toothpaste or if they eat the toothpaste (CDC, 2011). Using the recommended amount of toothpaste and encouraging the child not to swallow the toothpaste will prevent fluorosis (brown spots on the teeth caused by too much fluoride).

Flossing is useful for cleaning between teeth and maintaining healthy gums. The child should begin to floss when all the primary teeth are in or when the child's molars begin to touch.

Immunosuppressed children, in particular, need excellent oral hygiene. Soft toothbrushes, sponge-covered Toothettes, or moistened gauze sponges can be used for dental care in the child who is at risk for gingival bleeding (see Chapter 24).

Discharge teaching in the area of oral hygiene is important and yet often forgotten. Many parents do not realize that an infant's gums and teeth need to be cleaned. Children should have their first visit to a dentist by the time the first teeth erupt and no later than age 2½ years. Thereafter they should be seen on a regular basis (every 6 months) for services that include checkups, professional cleaning, and fluoride application.

The risk of dental caries increases if formula, milk, or other liquids remain in a child's mouth overnight. Allowing an infant to fall asleep with a bottle containing one of these liquids can cause a condition known as bottle-mouth syndrome, which results in severely decayed primary teeth. Parents are instructed not to put a child to bed with a bottle of formula, juice, or sweetened liquid. If the child will not fall asleep without a bottle, advise the parent to use water only.

Good nutrition influences dental health. Teaching about oral hygiene often provides an opportunity to educate the child and family about proper nutrition and general health maintenance.

FEEDING

Mealtimes can be difficult for the hospitalized child. Changes in routine, diet, and surroundings, as well as dietary restrictions and illness, affect the child's ability and desire to eat. Refusing to eat might also be the way a child attempts to have some control.

The nurse assesses the child's preferences and dislikes on admission and before ordering meals. Mealtime rituals and routines, as well as cultural food variations are noted. Serving favorite and preferred foods and offering nutritious snacks can ensure appropriate caloric and nutrient intake.

The type and form of food chosen should be appropriate to the child's age and developmental level. (See Chapters 5 through 8 for a discussion of food types appropriate for each age-group.) When planning meals, the nurse must consider whether the child has any special needs or required restrictions. For example, an infant with gastric reflux may need formula that is thickened with rice cereal to prevent emesis, and an edematous child will likely be placed on a "no added salt" diet.

Feeding a hospitalized infant seldom differs from feeding an infant at home. Types of foods, feeding schedules, and routines should mimic home schedules and routines when possible. If the infant's bottle or nipple brand is not available in the hospital, ask the parents to bring what the infant uses at home. Encourage parents to be present at mealtimes and feed their children if indicated. Feeding reinforces the special bond that develops between child and parent.

Nurses facilitate breastfeeding for infants by providing a private, quiet, and relaxed location so mother and infant feel comfortable and not rushed. If the mother is pumping breast milk for use when she is absent, the nurse meticulously follows hospital policy for labeling, storing, and administering pumped breast milk to the infant.

Unless medically contraindicated, infants should be held during feedings. Because of the risk of aspiration, bottles should be **never** be propped; a pillow or rolled blanket must not be positioned next to an infant's mouth). Frequent burping during and after feedings can reduce the incidence of regurgitation. To burp the infant, the nurse can use the upright hold and gently pats or rubs the infant's back, or seat the infant on the nurse's knees with a hand supporting the infant's chin. After feeding, the infant can be positioned on the right side to facilitate the flow of the feeding toward the lower end of the stomach and allow any swallowed air to rise into the esophagus. However, if the nurse is placing an infant in the crib for sleep, the infant must be positioned supine, lying on his or her back. The supine position for sleeping infants has been shown to decrease the risk of Sudden Infant Death Syndrome (American Academy of Pediatrics, Task Force on Sudden Infant Death Syndrome, 2008).

Toddlers and preschoolers often use food as a source of control. They might exhibit "food jags," during which they will eat only one or two items for a period of several days. They enjoy finger foods but are learning to use spoons or forks fairly competently. Colorful plates and cups may encourage a reluctant child to eat. Parents are encouraged to bring the child's own cups or utensils from home to simulate usual mealtime routines as closely as possible.

For young children the nurse cuts foods into pieces appropriate in size and texture to decrease the risk of aspiration. Foods to avoid foods include hot dogs, popcorn, peanuts, and grapes, because if aspirated, these can occlude the airway. Young children *must* be supervised when eating. They are also secured at a table, in a highchair, or in bed using an overbed table during meals. "Roaming" while eating increases the risk of food aspiration and should be avoided. Children are prompted to feed themselves independently as much as possible. Mealtime is limited to 15 to 20 minutes and discontinued if the child is playing with and not eating the food.

Older children and adolescents seldom have difficulty expressing their dietary preferences. Difficulty may arise, however, when children this age are placed on a restricted or special diet. For example, the diabetic child often has difficulty staying on a restricted diet in the face of peer pressure. The nurse needs to provide support and clear limits to ensure cooperation. Referral to a dietitian may be necessary to help the child make appropriate food choices.

Special Considerations

Keeping accurate intake and output (I&O) measurements may be necessary for many hospitalized children. The nurse measures and records all intake; oral, enteral, and parenteral. All output, including output from urine and stool; drainage from tubes, stomas, or fistulas; and emesis, is also measured and recorded. When measuring urinary output for a child in diapers, weigh each wet diaper and subtract the weight of a dry diaper of the same size. One gram of weight equals approximately 1 mL of urine output.

Documentation

Documenting the child's nutritional intake assists in determining the child's overall health. The nurse records food intake and preferences, as well as observations about the child's appetite and eating patterns. Older children and adolescents are assessed for any abnormal eating patterns, because eating disorders are more prevalent in these age-groups.

Parent Teaching

Educating parents regarding feeding, special diets, and the nutritional needs of children is extremely important. The nurse should carefully instruct parents about how to manage any food or fluid restrictions, or special diets. A child with type 1 diabetes mellitus (see Chapter 27) or celiac disease (see Chapter 19) is at risk for injury if the prescribed diet is not closely followed.

VITAL SIGNS

An underlying principle for obtaining vital signs in a child is to obtain the vital signs when the child is quiet, if at all possible. Sometimes this involves measuring the pulse and respirations when the child is asleep. If this timing is not possible, note any activity that affects accurate measurement (e.g., crying, playing).

Measuring Temperature

Temperature is an objective indicator of illness, and measuring temperature is an integral part of assessing children. Oral, rectal, axillary, temporal artery (infrared), and tympanic temperature readings are often obtained using different types of electronic, digital thermometers. Beginning in 2001 and reaffirmed in 2007, the American Academy of Pediatrics recommends that thermometers containing mercury not be used for children in hospital or home settings because of toxicity risks (American Academy of Pediatrics, 2007; Goldman, Shannon, & Committee on Environmental Health, 2001). Whatever temperature measurement method is chosen, the child's temperature should be measured at the same site and with the same device to maintain consistency and allow reliable comparison and tracking of temperatures over time. (See Chapter 9, Table 9-1 for normal temperatures in children.)

Digital thermometers, which are most often run on batteries, measure the temperature quickly (usually in less than 30 seconds). To prevent cross contamination, a child may have a single thermometer kept in the hospital room. If an electronic thermometer is used for multiple patients, either use a new, disposable probe cover for each patient or cleanse the probe between patients in accordance with manufacturer guidelines.

There is considerable variation in the types of thermometers used to measure the temperature of a hospitalized child. Factors to consider when selecting the route to use for obtaining a temperature reading include the child's age and ability to cooperate with the procedure, acuity of the illness, environmental factors (room conditions, food/fluid consumption), and equipment availability. For all devices used to measure temperature by any route, the accuracy of the temperature reading is dependent on correct use of the equipment; the probe must be in the correct position and held steadily in place for the required period of time (Davie & Amoore, 2010). For infants and children who are unable to properly hold an oral thermometer in their mouth, axillary, temporal artery, or tympanic thermometers are used (Figure 13-4). Rectal temperatures are more accurate in

Axillary temperature

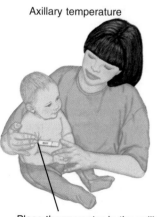

Place thermometer in the axilla and press child's arm close to body until reading is obtained.

Tympanic temperature

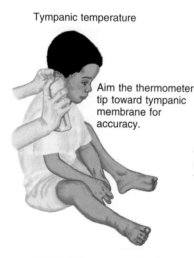

Aim the thermometer tip toward tympanic membrane for accuracy.

Temporal artery temperature

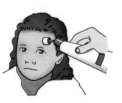

Place the thermometer probe flat on center of forehead and lightly slide horizontally across forehead to hairline.

Rectal temperature

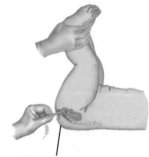

Insert lubricated thermometer no more than 1.25 cm in an infant and 2.5 cm in an older child.

FIG 13-4 Four methods of temperature measurement.

measuring core body temperature, particularly in infants (Paes, Vermeulen, Brohet, et al., 2010). However, inserting a thermometer into a child's rectum is an invasive procedure and may be contraindicated for children at risk for anal or rectal injury, infection, or bleeding (El-Radhi & Patel, 2007). For this reason, many hospital units have policies that specify when a pediatric patient should have a rectal temperature measurement.

The advantage to temporal artery and tympanic temperature measurements is that they are obtained quickly, usually within a few seconds, and cause minimal discomfort to the child. Research has shown inconsistencies when comparing tympanic temperature measurement with axillary measurement (Carbone, Flanagan, Gibbons et al., 2010; Devrim, Kara, Ceyhan et al., 2007). A temporal artery temperature reading is considered to be nearly the same as the rectal (core) temperature and approximately 0.8° F (0.4° C) higher than an oral temperature (Exergen Corporation, 2005). However, the accuracy of temporal artery temperatures is still being evaluated; studies have indicated mixed results when comparing temporal artery measurements to temperature measurements via rectal and other routes (Bahr, Senica, Gingras, & Ryan, 2010; Holzhauer, Reith, Sawin, & Yen, 2009).

Axillary temperatures are appropriate for infants and children younger than 4 to 6 years or any child who cannot safely have or hold an oral thermometer in the mouth. Axillary temperatures are approximately 1° F (0.6° C) lower than the body's core temperature. For an accurate reading, the thermometer is held in the child's axilla for a few minutes. To help the child remain still, consider holding him or her on your lap and reading a story.

Temperatures are measured orally in most children ages 6 years and older, including adolescents. Keeping a thermometer in the correct location in the mouth can be a challenge for any child. The child is instructed to keep the mouth closed, with lips in a "kiss" position, and to not bite the thermometer. Intake of foods and liquids should be avoided for 30 minutes before the oral temperature measurement. Inaccurate oral temperatures may occur because of oral intake, oxygen administration, nebulized treatments, or crying. Oral temperature measurement should not be used in any child who has had oral or tonsillar surgery or in whom **epiglottitis** is suspected (see Chapter 21).

> **! NURSING QUALITY ALERT**
>
> ### Measuring Temperature
>
> - If an elevated or low oral, axillary, temporal artery, or tympanic temperature reading is obtained, consider measuring the temperature via another route (including the rectal route), if possible.
> - Report a temperature measurement of less than 96.8° F (36° C) or more than 100.4° F (38° C). This is critical for an infant under 3 months of age.

Measuring Pulse

Apical pulse rate measurements (Figure 13-5) are recommended for infants and children younger than 2 years and in any child who has an irregular heart rate or known congenital heart disease. It is best to auscultate the apical pulse when the child is quiet, counting for one full minute. The apical heart rate must be determined before administering certain medications, such as digoxin.

Radial pulse measurements are appropriate for children older than 2 years (see Table 9-1 for normal pulse measurements).

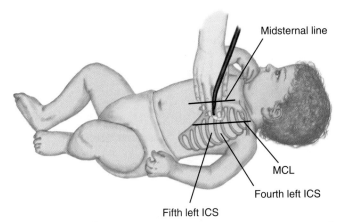

FIG 13-5 Locating the apical pulse. Apical pulse is lateral to the left midclavicular line (MCL) and fourth intercostal space (ICS) in children younger than 7 years, and to the left MCL and fifth ICS in children older than 7 years.

Evaluating Respirations

Infants often have irregular respiratory rates that change with stimulation, crying, and feeding. First, observe the pattern of inspiration and expiration to determine any irregular rhythm. Next, with an infant or young child who is quiet and at rest, measure the respiratory rate by auscultating for 1 full minute. For older children, either observe chest movement or auscultate respirations to obtain the rate (see Table 9-1 for normal respiratory rate measurements).

Measuring Blood Pressure

The blood pressure (BP) of a well child is generally assessed just once per year during routine physical examination. For the hospitalized child, blood pressure readings are obtained on admission and then every 8 to 12 hours. If abnormalities are detected or the child's condition is unstable, blood pressure checks are done more frequently. When interpreting BP results, a child's age, gender, and height must be considered (see Table 9-1 and the Evolve website for normal values). The right arm is the standard site for routine blood pressure measurement (Schell, 2006).

Choosing the appropriate cuff size is required if accurate blood pressure readings are to be obtained. A cuff that is too small may cause a BP reading to be falsely high and a cuff that is too large may result in a falsely low reading. Recommendations for how to choose an appropriate cuff size vary, but the following is a suggested procedure (Pickering, Hall, Appel et al., 2005):

- Find the midpoint of the right upper arm between the shoulder (acromion) and the elbow (olecranon).
- Holding the bladder of the cuff lengthwise, the bladder width should cover approximately 40% of the upper arm circumference at this point.
- When you wrap the cuff around the arm to take the blood pressure, the bladder should encircle 80% to 100% of the arm without overlap.
- Palpate the brachial artery, and place the stethoscope bell on the brachial artery below the cuff (medial aspect of the antecubital fossa).
- Measure the blood pressure with the arm at heart level after the child has been at rest for 3 to 5 minutes.

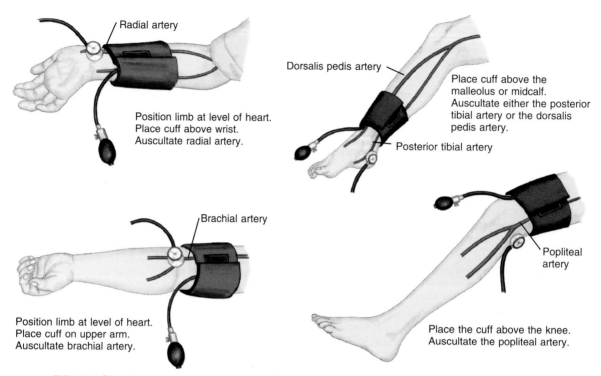

FIG 13-6 Blood pressures can be measured in the upper arm, lower arm, thigh, calf, or ankle. An appropriate-size cuff must be used to obtain accurate results.

TABLE 13-1			RECOMMENDED DIMENSIONS FOR BLOOD PRESSURE CUFF BLADDERS
AGE RANGE	WIDTH (cm)	LENGTH (cm)	MAXIMUM ARM CIRCUMFERENCE (cm)*
Newborn	4	8	10
Infant	6	12	15
Child	9	18	22
Small adult	10	24	26
Adult	13	30	34
Large adult	16	38	44
Thigh	20	42	52

Reprinted with permission from National High Blood Pressure Education Program Working Group on High Blood Pressure in Children and Adolescents. (2004). The fourth report on the diagnosis, evaluation, and treatment of high blood pressure in children and adolescents. *Pediatrics, 114*(2), 557.
*Calculated so that the largest arm would still allow the bladder to encircle arm by at least 80%.

For children, blood pressure can be measured in the upper arm, lower arm, thigh, calf, or ankle (Figure 13-6). If using a different site than the arm for blood pressure measurement, use 40% of the circumference of the site used. Commercially designated BP cuffs are standardized widths, so select the closest standard width to the 40% circumference measurement. Table 13-1 illustrates average bladder widths of commercial blood pressure cuffs.

To ensure consistency, take measurements in the same limb, in the same place, and with the child in the same position. Blood pressure measurements can differ depending on the site used, so the site must be documented.

The National High Blood Pressure Education Program Working Group on High Blood Pressure in Children and Adolescents (2004) recommends auscultated blood pressure measurements as the standard for children, and tables listing normal values are based on this method. For children, the systolic BP is determined by the onset of the first Korotkoff "tapping" sound, and the diastolic reading is the number at which the Korotkoff sound disappears. The systolic BP sometimes can be heard down to a measurement of zero. In this case, the BP measurement should be repeated with less pressure on the stethoscope. If a reading near zero is still obtained, the number when the Korotkoff sound muffles can be recorded as the diastolic BP (National High Blood Pressure Education Program, 2004).

Mercury sphygmomanometers are considered the "gold standard" but are rarely used because of mercury toxicity concerns. Aneroid sphygmomanometers are the substitute, though calibration is needed and accuracy is a concern (Schell, 2006). Automated, electronic devices are now frequently used because they make obtaining BP readings in children easier (Pickering et al., 2005). These oscillometric devices detect the mean arterial pressure, and then an algorithm is used to indirectly determine the systolic and diastolic BP values (Schell, 2006). Each type of device functions differently, so it is critical that the manufacturer's guidelines be closely followed to ensure accuracy. If the blood pressure result is low or elevated when taken electronically, retake the blood pressure using auscultation.

Documentation of Vital Sign Measurement

The nurse documents all vital signs in the child's paper or electronic medical record; the measurement result, the method used to measure each vital sign, the site where each measurement was obtained, and any action taken is included. It is essential that that the nurse reports as well as documents any abnormal findings or findings that are significantly different from the individual child's baseline.

Preparing the Child and Family

The child and family are informed about the purpose of obtaining vital sign measurements. Children should be allowed to examine or handle the equipment while the nurse explains how it is used. Many children have toy medical instruments at home and may be familiar with the concept of taking vital signs.

Tell young children that the blood pressure cuff feels like a "hug" or a "squeeze" on their arm or leg.

! NURSING QUALITY ALERT

Measuring Vital Signs

- Temperatures should not be measured rectally in the immunosuppressed child or in any child who has had rectal surgery, diarrhea, or a bleeding disorder.
- Count respirations and measure the apical heart rate before taking other vital signs. Both signs are best measured on a sleeping or quiet child.
- Measure the apical heart rate for 1 full minute on any child younger than 2 years, on a child being assessed for the first time, on any child whose heartbeat is irregular, or on a child for whom treatment decisions are made on the basis of the heart rate.
- Observe the child's respiratory rate and effort for 1 full minute while the child is quiet. Abdominal movement with breathing is normally observed in infants and young children, whereas thoracic movement can be noted in older children and adolescents.
- Evaluate the quality of respirations, symmetry of chest movement with each breath, and any noisy respirations (e.g., crackles, wheezes, friction rubs). Observe the child for any signs of respiratory distress, such as nasal flaring, grunting, stridor, retractions, increased work of breathing, cyanosis, or apneic periods.
- Always use a manual cuff and auscultation to verify electronically measured blood pressures that indicate hypertension or hypotension.

Parent Teaching

Some parents may need to learn how to take the child's temperature at home. The nurse demonstrates how to take the child's temperature, and then observes the parent perform the procedure. It is important to ensure that the parent is comfortable with the procedure and is able to read the thermometer accurately.

Some parents may need to be taught how to correctly determine their child's heart rate and respiratory rate, as well as the acceptable range for their child. Special instructions relating to when parents should notify the physician may need to be provided for children who are taking certain medications, such as digoxin.

If the child's condition requires home blood pressure monitoring, parents are taught to perform the procedure. The nurse provides information about the size of the BP cuff needed and ensures that the parents can read the dial accurately. Methods to involve the child in the procedure are discussed. For instance, parents might make a smaller BP cuff for the child's favorite doll or stuffed animal.

Special Considerations: Cardiorespiratory Monitors

Some children need cardiorespiratory monitoring so that heart rate, respiratory rate, blood pressure, and temperature can be continuously measured. Children who are acutely ill or who are undergoing procedures might be placed on a monitor to help health care providers detect subtle changes in the child's condition.

The procedure and indications for attaching a child to a cardiorespiratory monitor are no different from those for an adult. Monitors sound an alarm to warn of changes in the child's cardiorespiratory status. In accordance with the child's age, alarm parameters for each measurement are often preset based on hospital policies and physician orders. It is important that the nurse verify settings and test that the monitor is functioning correctly. False alarms can occur. Whenever a monitor alarm sounds, the nurse must first look at the child and perform an assessment, and then intervene if indicated. A flat line on the electrocardiogram (ECG) does not always signal a cardiac arrest. It may be nothing but a loose monitor lead. Check the manufacturer's recommendations for attaching leads and monitoring selected vital signs.

FEVER-REDUCING MEASURES

The body's internal thermostat, the hypothalamus, attempts to keep the body's temperature between 96.8° and 100.4° F (36° and 38° C). This regulation is done through a complex series of interactions that result in heat gain or loss. The body's mechanisms for conserving or producing heat are vasoconstriction and shivering. Heat is lost through radiation, conduction, convection, and evaporation.

Description of Fever

Fever is defined as a body temperature greater than 100.4° F (38° C) rectally or 99.5° F (37.5° C) orally that results from an insult or disease during which the body's set point temperature rises to a higher-than-normal level. After the cause of the fever is removed, the body resets its set point at the normal level.

The body's attempt to defend itself against illness is manifested by fever, which is triggered by endogenous pyrogens produced during the inflammatory response. Because research studies have not conclusively demonstrated whether fever is beneficial or detrimental, practitioners vary in their approach to managing fevers caused by infections. Mild degrees of fever may or may not require intervention, depending on the underlying cause and the child's response. Most fevers are brief and benign and resolve when the underlying infection resolves. Children with chronic cardiac or respiratory disease, those with neurologic disease, and those prone to febrile seizures should be treated for fever. Children with fevers of 104° F (40° C) or higher also should be treated.

Fever is uncomfortable, and children may become irritable. For every 1° C of temperature elevation, the body's metabolic rate increases 10% to 12%, resulting in increased insensible fluid loss, increased oxygen consumption, and increased stress on the cardiovascular system (Ward & Lentzsch-Parcells, 2009). Regardless of the fever's cause, the child's comfort is the primary reason for treating a fever in a normally healthy child.

Medications and Environmental Management

Treatment can consist of environmental measures, antipyretics, or a combination of interventions. Dressing the child appropriately (neither overdressed nor underdressed), providing adequate fluids, monitoring for signs of dehydration, and administering an appropriate antipyretic all are approaches to fever management. Studies have shown that the use of tepid sponging to reduce a fever can actually cause shivering and increase temperature as well as increase discomfort for the child (Axelrod, 2000; National Institute of Health and Clinical Excellence, 2007).

Fevers in children are treated effectively with antipyretics such as acetaminophen or ibuprofen (Perrott, Piira, Goodenough, & Champion, 2004). Aspirin is not used to treat fever in children because of its association with Reye syndrome and viral illnesses (influenza and varicella).

Children with elevated temperatures often have a loss of appetite. Dehydration can occur from decreased oral intake and increased insensible water loss through the lungs and skin. To provide for adequate hydration, offer the child oral fluids frequently. For those who refuse to ingest oral fluids or are unable to take in an adequate volume, evaluate the need for intravenous fluids.

To maintain body temperature and reduce heat loss, some infants are placed in radiant warmers or incubators (Isolettes). These microprocessor-based, servo-controlled temperature systems set the correct heating level by constantly monitoring the infant's temperature using a skin probe and the air temperature. Infants who are being cared for in these heating units must be carefully monitored, because accidental dislodgment of the skin probe can occur and excessive heating may result. Also, insensible water loss is greatly increased for infants in these units, and this must be considered when calculating fluid replacement.

SPECIMEN COLLECTION

Specimens are collected from children for the same reasons they are collected from adults, but children often need a more careful explanation of the procedures and reasons for specimen collection. All explanations should be given in age-appropriate language, and children should be prepared for any sensations that they may experience.

Regardless of the type of specimen to be obtained, use Standard Precautions. The use of personal protective equipment (PPE) including gloves, gowns, masks, goggles/face shields along with hand hygiene is required when there is the potential for the nurse to come in contact with blood and other body fluids that can contain infectious materials. The PPE used will vary according to the risk of contact with body fluids. For example, if there is potential that a "splash" could occur when collecting a specimen, a face shield and mask may need to be worn in addition to gloves and a gown. The nurse should follow health care facility policies and procedures, based on Standard Precautions, when handling body fluids.

Urine Specimens
Voided Specimens

Infants and young toddlers are not yet toilet trained and thus unable to void on request, making urine specimen collection a challenge. A commonly used, noninvasive collection device is the urine collection bag. It consists of a plastic bag with an opening lined with adhesive so that it can be attached to the perineum. It is available in two sizes, infant and pediatric. Collection bags for a 24-hour urine specimen have a tube that extends from the end of the bag, allowing each void to be removed and placed in a designated, large container.

When using a urine collection bag to obtain a nonsterile specimen, the nurse first cleans the perineal area and then applies the bag (Procedure 13-1). If obtaining a specimen for urine culture, sterile gloves and cleansing solution plus a sterile urine collection bags should be used. However, studies have indicated that urine in collection bags can become contaminated with organisms from the perineal area, causing unreliable urine culture results (Etoubleau, Reveret, Brouet, et al., 2009; McGillivray, Mok, Mulrooney, & Kramer, 2005). Many physicians choose to use urinary "in and out" catheterization or suprapubic aspiration (inserting a needle through the skin and directly into

the bladder) to obtain a "sterile" urine specimen for culture from an incontinent child.

Older children and adolescents often cooperate in the collection of urine specimens. Most can use a bedpan, urinal, or specimen cup with minimal assistance. Younger children and preschoolers who are toilet trained still have difficulty voiding on request. Parents can be helpful in obtaining urine specimens from their children. The nurse should use familiar terms, such as "pee pee," "tinkle," or "potty," when telling the preschool or young school-age child what is needed and have available a potty chair or a collection "hat" set in the toilet.

If the specimen must be collected using special techniques (e.g., a clean midstream urine sample), the nurse first carefully explains to the child and parent what preparation is needed and verifies understanding. A parent or nurse may need to assist the child during the collection. A young child may be able to sit on the toilet with the nurse or parent cleansing the perineal area and holding the specimen

---

DRUG GUIDE

Acetaminophen (Tylenol, Tempra, Panadol)

Classification
Nonnarcotic analgesic and antipyretic.

Action
Unknown; may act on hypothalamic heat-regulating center.

Indications
Mild fever and pain relief.

Dosage and Route
Dosage is age and/or weight related; administered four or five times daily. Oral, rectal. Comes in a variety of oral preparations: infant drops (80 mg/0.8 mL), liquid or suspension (160 mg/5 mL), chewable tablets (80 mg/tab), caplets and chewables for older children (160 mg/tab), adult strength (325 mg/tab). Rectal suppositories in 80, 120, 125, 300, 325, and 650 mg.

Absorption
From the gastrointestinal tract; peak action in 1 to 3 hours.

Excretion
Duration approximately 4 to 5 hours.

Contraindications
Any previous sensitivity to the medication.

Precautions
Long-term use can cause liver damage. Other over-the-counter cold preparations can contain acetaminophen; if given concurrently they can increase the amount of acetaminophen above safe levels.

Adverse Reactions
Blood dyscrasias, hypoglycemia, rashes or urticaria, liver damage with prolonged use.

Nursing Considerations
Advise parents to be extremely careful not to confuse the liquid preparations; check the label carefully before giving the medication. Never refer to this or any other medication as "candy." Acetaminophen overdose must be treated immediately to prevent hepatic toxicity. Parents need to be aware that acetaminophen can affect home glucose readings. Parents should not continue to give their children this medication for fever that lasts longer than 2 days without checking with the child's primary care provider.

PROCEDURE 13-1 URINE SPECIMEN COLLECTION FROM THE INCONTINENT CHILD

PURPOSE: To Obtain a Voided Urine Specimen for Testing

1. Before beginning the procedure, provide adequate privacy. The child may be more relaxed if a parent is present. If both blood and urine specimens need to be obtained from the incontinent child, position the collection bag before drawing the blood. Infants and toddlers often void during a painful procedure.

2. Obtain the following equipment: Nonsterile gloves, urine collection bag, sterile specimen cup, mild soap, warm water, washcloth, diaper and towel, and label and requisition form.

3. Perform hand hygiene. Put on gloves and clean the perineal area. Cleaning the perineum will remove any lotions or ointments and help the bag adhere. (If obtaining a specimen for urine culture, wear sterile gloves, use a sterile cleansing solution and apply a sterile bag.)
   - For girls: Clean from front to back and from the urinary meatus to the labia majora (in to out).
   - For boys: Clean from the tip of the penis in a circular motion. Do not retract the foreskin of an infant or young child.

4. After the perineum has been cleansed, dry it thoroughly. The skin must be completely dry for the bag to adhere properly.

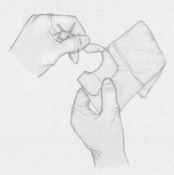

5. Remove the backing from the adhesive surface of the bottom half of the collection device.

6. Place the child in a frog-leg position to eliminate skin folds that may interfere with bag adherence. Apply the bottom half of the bag first and then remove the backing and apply the top half.

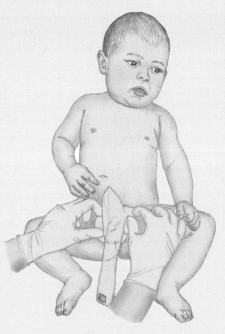

- For girls: Hold the perineum taut and apply the adhesive portion of the bag, working outward. To keep feces from contaminating the specimen, the narrow "bridge" on the adhesive patch must be placed on the tiny area of skin between the anus and the genitalia.
- For boys: Place the penis and scrotum (if small enough) inside the bag.

7. After the bag is attached, reapply a diaper. Cut a slit in the diaper and pull the end of the empty bag through the slit so that the bag protrudes from the diaper. This step reduces the chance of leaking and allows for observation of urine.

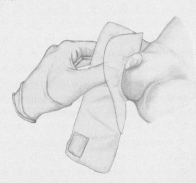

8. Check the bag every 30 minutes. Applying slight pressure over the suprapubic area or stroking along the older infant's spine will often induce voiding. As soon as urine is noticed in the bag, don gloves and gently remove the bag from the perineum.

9. Transfer the urine into a sterile specimen cup. Most bags have a small tab that can be removed to allow the urine to be poured. If the bag does not have a tab, clean the outside of the bag with an alcohol swab and withdraw the urine with a needle and syringe for placement in the appropriate container. Remove gloves and perform hand hygiene.

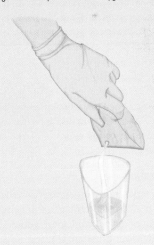

10. Label the urine specimen cup with the child's name, date, and time of collection. Place in a biohazard bag and deliver it promptly, together with a requisition form, to the laboratory. Urine for culture that cannot be tested within 30 minutes should be refrigerated.

11. Record the collection of the specimen in the child's chart. Include the date and time of collection and the amount, color, and appearance of the urine.

Home Adaptations

If a urine specimen is to be obtained at home, give instructions to the parent and provide the appropriate equipment. Parents can keep the urine collected at home in the refrigerator until they are asked to bring it to the laboratory. The specimen should be kept chilled during transport (i.e., placed in a cooler or plastic bag packed with ice).

PROCEDURE 13-2 URINARY CATHETERIZATION

PURPOSE: To Monitor Urine Output Accurately or Obtain a Sterile Urine Sample

1. Prepare the child for the procedure by using age-appropriate methods. Explain what the child will feel and what the child can do to "help." Demonstrating the procedure on a teaching doll may be helpful. Teach the child to take slow, deep breaths during the procedure, and have the child practice breathing before the procedure. Encouraging the child to sing also helps relax the appropriate muscles. The child might feel a need to urinate during the catheter insertion. Reassure the child that the feeling is normal. The assistance of another adult is often necessary with younger children.

2. Make sure the area has good lighting, and gather all necessary equipment. If equipment is not contained in the catheterization kit, obtain the appropriate-size catheter, sterile gloves (extra pairs in case of contamination), sterile cleansing solution with applicators, drapes, specimen cup, sterile topical lubricant, label, and requisition form. If the child is to have an indwelling catheter placed, use of a closed system with the catheter already attached to the drainage tube and bag is preferred. Begin by performing hand hygiene.

3. The procedure is the same as for catheterizing an adult, with the following additions:

   • When preparing to insert an indwelling catheter, the nurse considers if the balloon integrity should be tested by injecting fluid from a prefilled syringe into the balloon port and then removing this fluid by aspirating with the syringe. This is a controversial step since this may stretch the balloon and cause ridges to form which can result in injury to the urethra upon catheter insertion. It is recommended that the nurse follow the manufacturer's recommendations as well as hospital policy.

   • Take extra care to be gentle when cleansing the meatus or glans penis.

   • Choose the appropriate-size catheter. Apply the lubricant according to manufacturer's directions.

   • In girls, direct the catheter slightly upward and insert it gently through the meatus 1 to 2 inches (2.5 to 5 cm) or until urine appears. In boys, hold the penis at a 90-degree angle from the boy's body and gently insert the catheter 2 to 4 inches (5 to 10 cm) (longer in older boys) or until urine appears. Never force the catheter. The older child can assist in relaxing the external sphincter by bearing down.

4. Once urine is observed, advance the catheter approximately another $\frac{1}{2}$ inch and hold until the urine stops flowing. If obtaining a specimen, be sure urine is collected in a sterile specimen cup. For an indwelling catheter, advance to the bifurcation of drainage and balloon inflation ports before inflation of the balloon. This will be approximately 2 inches (5 cm) for girls, 3 to 4 inches (7.5 to 10 cm) for boys, newborn to preschool, and 5 inches (12.5 cm) for older boys. These distances reduce the risk of inflating the balloon in the urethra. Inflate the balloon slowly using the amount of fluid in the prefilled syringe that is recommended by the manufacturer. After inflating the balloon, remove gloves and perform hand hygiene.

5. Comfort the child if needed, offer praise for cooperation, and a reward, such as a sticker.

6. Label the specimen cup, place in a biohazard bag, and deliver promptly, together with the requisition form, to the laboratory. Refrigerate the specimen if transport to the laboratory is not immediate.

7. Document the date and time the procedure was performed, as well as the size of catheter used and the amount, color, and appearance of the urine. Note how the infant or child tolerated the procedure.

Home Adaptations

Catheterizing at home is usually a clean rather than sterile procedure used for children who have spina bifida, neurogenic bladder, or incomplete bladder emptying. Some families choose to use a new, packaged catheter each time; however, this can be extremely expensive when a child has to be catheterized several times per day. The alternative is to thoroughly rinse, clean, and dry the catheters and keep them in a clean, covered container or a plastic bag. The parent needs to follow physician protocols for cleaning the perineum; mild soap and water is often used. The infant or young child can be catheterized on a changing table, with the urine allowed to empty into a diaper or small container; the older child can be catheterized on the toilet.

---

cup while the child voids. For a boy who wishes to stand while voiding, the cup can be held in the stream as he voids. If the specimen is to be carried to another area, place the cup in a plastic biohazard bag for transport.

Urinary Catheterization

Reasons that a child needs a urinary catheter inserted include obtaining a sterile urine specimen for testing, accurately measuring urine output, and drainage of urine from the bladder (Procedure 13-2). Urinary catheterization can cause anxiety and discomfort in infants and children. Nurses need to take steps to ease the child's fears and discomfort through preparation of the child and family before the procedure, support during the procedure, selection of an appropriate-size catheter, and use of correct technique.

Children, based on their developmental level, and their parents need a complete explanation regarding the steps of procedure and what they need to do. This includes instruction on how the child can relax pelvic muscles by blowing out, pressing the buttocks against the bed, or squeezing the abdomen as if having a bowel movement. Parents can provide distraction and comfort during the procedure by reading, singing, or holding the child's hand. A second nurse may be needed to

BOX 13-2 GUIDELINES FOR URINARY CATHETER SELECTION BY AGE

- Infants up to 1 year old: 5 to 8 Fr
- Children 1 to 5 years old: 8 Fr
- School-age children: 8 to 12 Fr
- Adolescents: 10 to 14 Fr

gently hold the infant or child's legs to maintain them in the correct position.

Pediatric catheterization kits often contain a completely closed drainage system (with the catheter already attached to the drainage tube and bag). It is important that the nurse choose a urinary catheter that is the proper size for the child based on age. It should be small enough to be easily inserted into the meatus but large enough to prevent leakage of urine around the catheter (Box 13-2).

The catheter tip must be sufficiently lubricated to facilitate passage through the urethra and lessen discomfort. Some facilities recommend topical and intraurethral application of an anesthetic lubricant, such

PROCEDURE 13-3   VENIPUNCTURE

PURPOSE: To Obtain a Blood Sample for Laboratory Testing with Minimal Trauma to the Child

1. As with any procedure, prepare the child using age-appropriate language. Be sure to include what the child will see and feel. Ask the parents whether it is better to prepare their young child in advance or to describe what you are doing as you are performing the procedure. Assistance to hold the child is often necessary during the procedure. Parents are given the choice to stay with their child during the procedure or leave the room. If EMLA is to be used, it must be applied at least 45 to 60 minutes in advance of the procedure; follow the timing directions for other topical anesthetics if used.

2. Take the child to the treatment room. Have the following equipment available: 23- or 25-gauge butterfly catheter (or needle), gloves, antiseptic swabs, syringe or Vacutainer, sterile gauze, labels, appropriate collection tubes, requisition form, and tourniquet. (NOTE: Most tourniquets are composed of rubber tubing that is ½ to 1 inch wide—rubber bands should not be used for infants because they can abrade the skin.)

3. Hold the child by having one nurse place one gloved hand under the child's arm (usually at the shoulder) and the other gloved hand on the child's hand. The sampling nurse is then able to draw the blood with less likelihood of missing the vein. The vein of the antecubital area or hand is commonly used for venipuncture in children.

4. Perform hand hygiene, put on gloves, and apply a tourniquet that is tight enough to restrict venous blood flow toward the heart and distend the veins, but not so tight as to cause pain or restrict arterial blood flow. To facilitate easy removal, the tourniquet should be looped when applied. To prevent hemoconcentration, a tourniquet should be left in place no longer than 2 minutes.

5. Lightly pat or rub the sample site to help the veins become more visible.

6. With a circular motion, clean the site with an antiseptic swab and allow to dry.

7. Insert the needle of the butterfly catheter into the vein, bevel side up.

8. When blood begins to flow into the catheter, wait until the blood reaches the end of the catheter, attach the syringe, and slowly draw the appropriate amount of blood into the syringe. The tourniquet can be released when blood begins to flow into the syringe.

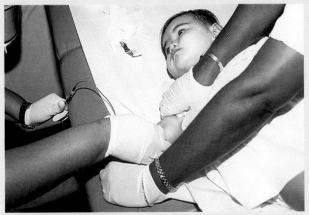

Courtesy Parkland Health and Hospital System Community Oriented Primary Care Clinic, Dallas, TX.

9. After obtaining the required amount of blood, withdraw the needle and apply pressure to the puncture site using a sterile gauze pad until the bleeding has stopped. Fill the appropriate specimen tubes or containers. Be sure to dispose of needles in the sharps container and contaminated gauze in the biohazard receptacle. Remove gloves and perform hand hygiene.

10. Comfort the child and offer praise for cooperation. Encourage the parent to provide comfort. Adhesive bandages are important because they help prevent bleeding from the puncture site. Specially colored or cartoon character bandages are available commercially and are appropriate for children's "boo-boos." The nurse can also give the child a reward, such as a sticker.

11. Label the specimen with the child's name, place in a biohazard bag, and send to the laboratory with the requisition form for the test(s) to be performed.

12. Document the date and time of collection, the amount of blood collected, the site used for puncture, and the reason blood was drawn (e.g., diagnostic test). Note the child's reaction to the procedure and the number of attempts made before a specimen was obtained.

---

as 2% lidocaine hydrochloride gel, to diminish pain during catheterization; however, research results are inconclusive regarding effectiveness (Boots & Edmundson, 2010; Mularoni, Cohen, DeGuzman, et al., 2009; Vaughan, Paton, Bush, & Pershad, 2005).

A number of children, particularly those who undergo multiple urinary tract catheterizations, are at high risk for developing latex sensitivity. At-risk children and others with known or suspected latex allergy should be identified early so that only latex-free catheters are used.

Stool Specimens

Stool specimens are obtained to test for the presence of fat, blood, viruses, bacteria, parasites, or reducing substances in the stool. If a stool specimen from an incontinent child is needed, it often can be scraped from a diaper and placed in an appropriate container. If the stool is watery, a specimen may be collected by placing a piece of gauze in the diaper to absorb some of the stool or by applying a urine specimen collection bag over the anus.

A bedpan or a specimen collector "hat" set in the toilet can be used to obtain a specimen from an older child. Because older children may be embarrassed about providing a stool sample, the nurse should use a calm, matter-of-fact manner when explaining why the specimen is needed and the procedure for handling the specimen.

Blood Specimens

Nurses use a variety of techniques to collect blood samples from children. Because blood collection is an invasive procedure, it should be performed in a treatment room if available.

Regardless of the sampling procedure used, most children find blood collection distressing. Some are concerned about the pain involved, and others fear the perceived loss of body fluid. The use of a topical anesthetic cream such as eutectic mixture of local anesthetics (EMLA) or ELA-Max (4% liposomal lidocaine) can reduce the child's discomfort. To be effective, anesthetic creams generally must remain on the site for at 30 to 60 minutes before the needle is inserted. Other anesthetic systems, such as iontophoresis, deliver lidocaine via

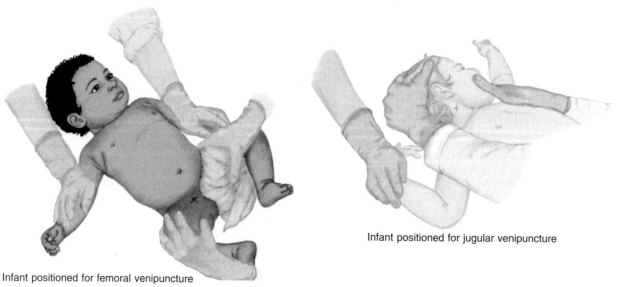

Infant positioned for femoral venipuncture

Infant positioned for jugular venipuncture

FIG 13-7 Two additional sites for obtaining blood specimens from infants and young children are the large superficial external jugular veins and the femoral veins.

PROCEDURE 13-4   CAPILLARY BLOOD SAMPLING

PURPOSE: To Obtain a Small Sample of Capillary Blood

1. Prepare the child appropriately for the procedure by using developmentally appropriate explanations (finger poke). You can warm the site before proceeding or have the older child wash the hands in warm water.

2. Bring the child or infant to the treatment room, where the following equipment should be available: Disposable lancing device, antiseptic swabs, sterile gauze, clean gloves, warm washcloth, Band-Aid, specimen containers/tubes, biohazard bag, and label and requisition form.

3. After performing hand hygiene and putting on gloves, cleanse the site, dry with sterile gauze or allow time to dry, and locate the puncture site. For the child, use the third (ring) finger of the nondominant hand and puncture halfway between the center of the ball of the finger and its side. For the infant, choose a puncture site on the lateral aspect of the heel. Hold the heel in one hand; palpate the heel bone and place the thumb over the walking surface of the heel to avoid puncturing both of these areas. Do not use fingers or areas of the heel that are bruised, edematous, or abraded, and avoid old puncture sites.

4. Puncture the child's finger or infant's heel with a lancing device that penetrates to a controlled depth and will not pierce the bone (approximately 2 mm). If possible, place the used lancing device in a sharps container before proceeding with the procedure.

5. To collect the blood sample, follow agency policy regarding whether to wipe away the first drop of blood with sterile gauze, how to collect the sample, the appropriate containers/tubes to use, amount of blood to be collected, and proper handling of the containers/tubes. To ensure adequate blood flow, it may be necessary to gently massage the heel or the finger from its base to the tip. Excessive squeezing of the foot or finger must be avoided.

6. Once collection is complete, apply pressure with sterile gauze until the bleeding stops.

7. Provide for the infant's or child's comfort. Apply a decorative Band-Aid on the finger, if the child desires; do not apply an adhesive bandage on the heel. Offer the child praise for cooperation and a reward such as a sticker.

8. Discard the lancing device in the sharps container and contaminated gauze and gloves in the biohazard receptacle. Perform hand hygiene.

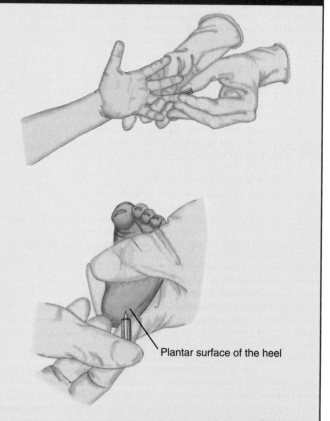

Plantar surface of the heel

9. Label the specimen with the infant/child's name, birth date, medical record number, and the time and date of collection. Place in a biohazard bag and send to the laboratory with the requisition form for the test(s) to be performed.

10. Document the date and time, amount of blood collected, site used for the puncture, if more than one puncture was done, reason for the blood draw, and the infant/child's reaction to the procedure.

an electric current and act more rapidly to produce a numbing effect at the insertion site (see Chapters 14 and 15 for more detailed information).

Children who need long-term venous access for nutrition or medications will often have a central venous catheter or port in place; the nurse can obtain blood for laboratory studies from this type of catheter or port. This procedure, however, may be performed only by specially trained nurses.

Venipuncture in children for blood specimen collection is often performed with a butterfly catheter (Procedure 13-3). The most commonly used sites are the veins of the hand and the antecubital area. Always follow Standard Precautions when performing or assisting others with blood specimen collection.

Jugular and Femoral Venipuncture

Jugular and femoral venipuncture are performed by a physician, with the nurse assisting and monitoring the child. If obtaining blood from one of the large superficial external jugular veins, assistance from a second nurse is necessary. The child's head is hyperextended to the side opposite the site, over the edge of a table or a small pillow (Figure 13-7). After the venipuncture, pressure must be applied to the site for 3 to 5 minutes or longer until bleeding stops. Care is taken to not overextend the head, because this can cause airway problems.

For a femoral venipuncture, the child is placed supine in the frog-leg position to expose the groin area (see Figure 13-7). The nurse stands above the infant's head, holding the infant's arms with the elbows and the infant's legs with the hands. To protect the venipuncture site if the infant urinates, a cloth diaper is placed over the perineal area and tucked under the buttocks, with one groin site exposed. Once the procedure is finished, the nurse applies pressure to the site for 5 minutes using a sterile gauze pad.

Capillary Blood Sampling

When a small blood sample is needed, a commercial lancing device (Microlet lancet) designed to puncture at the proper depth can be used for a child's finger or an infant's heel (Procedure 13-4). The child's hand or the infant's heel is warmed first to increase blood flow. For finger punctures, the third (ring) finger of the nondominant hand should be used. The puncture is done just to the side of the finger pad rather than at the tip. Fewer nerve endings are in this location, and the area is highly vascular. When using the lateral aspect of an infant's heel, the puncture site chosen must avoid major nerves, blood vessels, and bone. The heel is not used once the infant is walking because calluses make it more difficult to puncture.

Sputum Specimens

Sputum specimens are most frequently obtained to identify or rule out a respiratory infection. When obtaining any specimen, follow Standard Precautions. If splashing is anticipated, wear a mask and goggles or face shield in addition to gloves.

Obtaining sputum in the older child is relatively easy because older children and adolescents can cough deeply and produce a sputum sample, which can then be placed in the appropriate container. Specimens are easily obtained from children with artificial airways by attaching a mucus or suction trap to a suction catheter and suctioning the airway to obtain the specimen. A cough can be elicited by placing a suction catheter into the back of the throat in an infant or a young child.

Because younger children and infants can seldom produce a deep cough on demand and often swallow those secretions, obtaining

---

⚡ SAFETY ALERT

Throat Cultures

- Before obtaining a specimen for throat culture, assess for the presence of high fever of sudden onset, drooling, muffled voice, and erythema or exudate (signs of epiglottitis).
- Never attempt to obtain a throat specimen for culture in a child for whom a diagnosis of epiglottitis is suspected because the procedure could precipitate sudden airway obstruction.

---

sputum samples often requires a nasal washing, or lavage (Procedure 13-5). Nasal washing is particularly used to obtain a sample for identifying respiratory syncytial virus (RSV), influenza, and pertussis.

Throat and Nasopharyngeal Specimens

Throat cultures can identify the causative agent of sore throats or tonsillitis in children. Nasopharyngeal cultures are mainly used to identify pertussis (Procedure 13-6).

Cerebrospinal Fluid Specimens

Physicians and qualified advanced practice nurses perform lumbar punctures to examine the cerebrospinal fluid (CSF) for bacteria or abnormal cells, measure pressure within the cerebrospinal cavities, or inject certain medications (e.g., for pain control, to prevent or eradicate specific diseases, or as contrast agents for scans). A hollow spinal needle, inserted into the subarachnoid space between the third and fourth lumbar vertebrae, provides fluid exit and collection. An attached stopcock and manometer are used to measure spinal fluid pressure.

To minimize pain and trauma to the child, a topical anesthetic cream or spray should be used at the site of needle insertion. It is important that the topical agent be left in place the correct amount of time so the skin is numbed (see Chapter 15). Young children may require sedation because it is critical that the child not move during this procedure.

Because a lumbar puncture is frequently performed when a child is acutely ill, such as with meningitis or leukemia, the child and family may experience a high level of stress. The physician or nurse practitioner explains the procedure and obtains an informed consent from the parents or guardians. The nurse provides support and additional information to the child and family as well as assists by positioning, holding/restraining, and monitoring the child (see Chapter 28).

Bone Marrow Aspiration

Bone marrow aspiration is performed to obtain specimens of marrow for diagnostic testing, for evaluation of response to treatment, or for transplantation (see Chapter 24). The most common site of bone marrow aspiration in the child is the posterior iliac crest. Other sites include the anterior iliac crest and the tibia.

In order to tolerate this procedure, children receive a wide range of sedative, analgesic, and/or topical anesthetic agents based on age, developmental level, severity of illness, and hospital protocols. Because the reasons for a bone marrow aspiration include ruling out serious diseases, such as leukemia, or assessing the progress of cancer treatment, the nurse needs to provide the child and family thorough preparation before and a great deal of support during and after the procedure.

PROCEDURE 13-5 NASAL WASHING

PURPOSE: To Obtain a Nasopharyngeal Secretion Sample from an Infant or a Young Child

1. Prepare the child for the procedure by using developmentally appropriate language and describing any expected sensations (the procedure will make the child sneeze).
2. Gather the following equipment: Sterile syringe, sterile saline, gloves, mask, goggles or face shield, gown, small, sterile bulb syringe, sterile specimen container or pertussis kit, and labels and requisition form.
3. Ask for assistance to hold the child, or mummy wrap an infant to restrain the arms and legs.
4. Fill the syringe (without needle) with 1 to 3 mL of sterile saline.
5. Perform hand hygiene and don gloves, gown, mask, and goggles or face shield. Place the child in a supine position; gently place the tip of the syringe into one nostril.
6. Instill the saline into the nostril and immediately aspirate secretions with a small, sterile bulb syringe.
7. Place the saline and secretions into a sterile container. Remove gloves and perform hand hygiene.
8. Comfort the child and offer praise and a reward, such as a sticker, for cooperation.
9. Label the specimen with the infant/child's name, birth date, medical record number and the time and date of collection. Place in a biohazard bag and send to the laboratory with the requisition form for the test(s) to be performed.
10. Document the amount of saline instilled and the method of collection used. Note the date, time, amount, color, and consistency of secretions.

PROCEDURE 13-6 THROAT OR NASOPHARYNGEAL CULTURE

PURPOSE: To Obtain a Specimen for Culture

1. Explain the procedure to the child in appropriate language. For a throat culture, explain that the child will need to look up toward the ceiling, will need to open the mouth very wide, and may feel like coughing or gagging. Emphasize that the procedure is not painful. For a nasopharyngeal swab, tell the child to look up and explain that you will be inserting the swab into the nose. The child will feel like sneezing. Do not do these procedures immediately after the child has taken medication, eaten, or had something to drink. Assistance may be needed to hold a younger child. Encourage the parent to support and comfort the child during and after the procedure.
2. Gather the following equipment: Tongue depressor, throat or nasopharyngeal swab (cotton-tipped swab with a flexible wire extension), collection containers and labels (if not included with the swab), gloves, mask, goggles or face shield, and sterile saline.
3. An older child can sit in a chair or sit upright in bed for the culture. A younger child should be placed supine on a bed or examining table.
4. **Throat Culture**
   • Put on gloves, mask, and goggles or face shield, and have the child open the mouth and say "ahhh." Eliciting a cry from an infant will give optimal access to the pharyngeal area. Insert a tongue depressor into the mouth with the nondominant hand so that it covers the anterior half of the tongue, and depress the tongue to allow observation of the pharyngeal area. Swab the area quickly, avoiding the tongue, buccal mucosa, and palate. If the child opens the mouth wide enough for adequate visibility, a tongue depressor may not be needed. Only one swab should be used for each culture.
5. **Nasopharyngeal Culture**
   • Ask the child to look up. Bend the wire so that when the swab is inserted, the tip will go beyond the back of the nares and into the pharyngeal area. Dip the swab tip into saline and gently insert it into one nostril, down to the posterior nasopharynx. Leave it in place for several seconds and then remove.
6. After the specimen is obtained, place the swab in the appropriate culture medium. Remove gloves and perform hand hygiene.
7. Comfort the child as needed and offer praise for cooperation and a reward, such as a sticker. If possible, offer the child cool fluids to drink after the procedure.
8. Label the specimen with the infant/child's name, birth date, medical record number, and the time and date of collection. Place in a biohazard bag and send to the laboratory with the requisition form for the test(s) to be performed.
9. Document the date and time, the appearance of the specimen, and the child's response to the procedure.

GASTROINTESTINAL TUBES AND ENTERAL FEEDINGS

Because of prematurity, illness, or injury, some infants and children are unable to tolerate adequate quantities of oral nutrition, and an alternative method of feeding may be indicated. Enteral feedings are an option for infants and children with a variety of conditions, including congenital anomalies, gastrointestinal disorders, swallowing impairments, neurologic diseases, and postoperative status. Feedings are given through an orogastric, a nasogastric, or a transpyloric (nasointestinal) tube, or through a gastrostomy tube or a skin-level button (MIC-KEY) (see Chapter 19).

Tube Route and Placement

Placement of a gastrostomy tube or gastrostomy button is a surgical procedure performed by a physician. A nurse usually inserts an orogastric (OG), a nasogastric (NG), or a nasointestinal tube (Procedure 13-7). Nasogastric tubes are commonly used because with nasal placement it is easier to secure the tube and keep it in place. However, nasal placement can potentially interfere with respiratory function. Children with head or nasal anomalies or injuries and infants who are still preferential nose breathers (usually those 4 months old or younger) may require an orogastric tube. A nasointestinal tube is more difficult to insert because it must pass through the stomach's pyloric sphincter in order to enter the small intestine.

Controversy exists regarding measurement of the length of the nasogastric tube to be inserted. Two most common methods of measurement are: (1) from the nose tip to the earlobe and then to the end of the xiphoid process, or (2) from the nose tip to the earlobe and then to a point midway between the xiphoid process and umbilicus, which some consider as a more accurate method of determining correct insertion length (Beckstrand, Ellett, & McDaniel, 2007). Based on a child's age and height, mathematical predictors have been developed for nurses to use when determining the correct nasogastric tube insertion length (Beckstrand et al., 2007).

Tube Selection

Many types and sizes of tubes are commercially available. Factors influencing the selection of a feeding tube include the child's age and size, the viscosity of the formula to be administered, the reason for the enteral feeding, and whether an infusion device will be used. A feeding tube of size 5 Fr to 10 Fr is used in infants, and the size increases proportionately for older children. Selecting the smallest-diameter tube

PROCEDURE 13-7   FEEDING TUBE INSERTIONS

PURPOSE: To Provide Enteral Nutrition

1. Using developmentally appropriate language, explain the procedure to the child and parents and assess their needs and concerns (e.g., previous experience with tube insertion, ability to assist with the procedure, need for holding). Therapeutic play can be used to allay the fears of the child and parents related to the procedure.

2. Gather the following equipment before starting the procedure: Feeding tube of appropriate size and type, ¼- or ½-inch hypoallergenic tape, 30-mL syringe, sterile water for oral use, stethoscope, water-soluble lubricating jelly (for nasal insertion only), pH reagent strips, gloves, gown, mask, and goggles or face shield, feeding pump and setup (enteral feeding bag or burette), and the enteral fluid to be administered.

3. Position the child on the back or right side with the head of the bed elevated in the high Fowler position, if tolerated. To facilitate cooperation and decrease fear, a small child can be held in a parent's arms, with the child's head on the parent's shoulder. An older child may sit up in the bed. Have another staff member or parent hold the child, if necessary.

4. Measure the length of the catheter to be inserted. Mark the total insertion distance with an indelible, waterproof marker or tape:
   - To place a nasogastric tube in a child or an orogastric tube in an infant, measure the distance from the tip of the nose to the earlobe and to a point midway between the end of the xiphoid process and the umbilicus.

5. Put on gloves and other PPE. To facilitate passage through the nasopharynx, lubricate the tube with water or water-soluble lubricant. In neonates and for orogastric placement, use water only.

6. Insert the tube gently but firmly through the mouth or nose and down the throat. If you encounter obstruction or if the tube curls in the mouth, remove the tube and repeat this step. If the child gasps, coughs, gags, or turns cyanotic, withdraw the tube and wait for the response to subside before proceeding.

7. Direct the tube toward the back of the throat. Continue to advance the tube gently to the predetermined mark. While advancing the tube, ask the cooperative child to swallow repeatedly when the tube reaches the pharynx, or give small sips of water through a straw if not contraindicated. Swallowing will ease insertion into the esophagus. Giving an infant a pacifier will encourage swallowing. Advance the tube 5 to 10 cm with each swallow. Temporarily secure the tube with tape to stabilize it while checking the tube position.

8. Attach the syringe to the end of the tube and insufflate 1 to 5 mL (more for an older child or adolescent) of air. Then, after withdrawing the air, aspirate the gastric contents for observation and pH testing. Monitor the child for signs of respiratory distress, choking, or soundless coughing that may indicate placement in the trachea.

9. Check the pH of the aspirate to confirm gastric or intestinal placement. (Administration of antacid and gastric acid inhibitors will alter the pH of the aspirate, thus affecting the reliability of the pH test.) Obtain radiographic confirmation of correct placement according to hospital policy and physician orders.

10. If a nasointestinal tube with a guide wire has been used, remove the guide wire by holding the tube at the child's nostril or the corner of the mouth and slowly removing it. To allow gravity to assist in the advancement of the tube into the duodenum, keep the child on the right side. An abdominal x-ray film will be ordered by the physician to confirm tube placement in the duodenum.

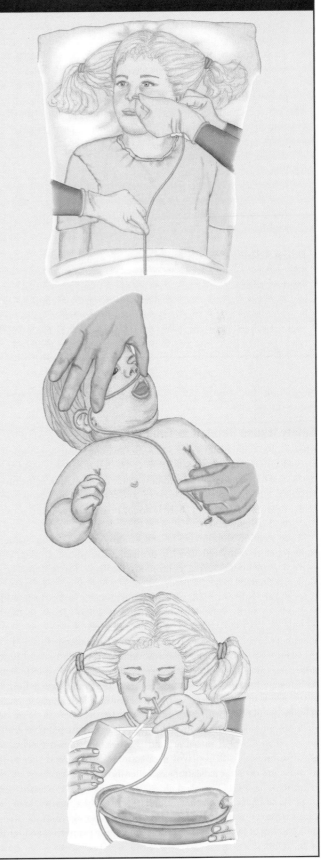

Continued

PROCEDURE 13-7   FEEDING TUBE INSERTIONS—cont'd

11. Once tube placement is confirmed, tape the tube securely in place and label the tube with the date and time of insertion. Refer to your facility's policy and procedure manual for recommended frequency of tube changes. With indelible marker or tape, mark the tube just below the insertion site. This will assist with future assessments of tube placement. Remove gloves and perform hand hygiene.

12. Comfort the child and offer praise for cooperation after initial tube placement and following radiographic confirmation of position. Encourage the parent to provide comfort during and after the procedure. The nurse can also give the child a reward, such as a sticker.

13. Document the size and type of tube used, route, and placement, air insufflation results, pH testing results, observations of gastric aspirate, assessment of respiratory status, measurement of visible tube length, date and time of insertion, child and family teaching, and the child's tolerance of the procedure.

Home Adaptations

If the child is to receive enteral nutrition at home, teach the parent how to insert and check placement of the tube. Tube placement should be confirmed before each feeding or medication administration. Describe comfort measures that may be helpful. Be sure to have the parents give a return demonstration of tube placement including use of pH strips before taking the child home. Explain to parents how to contact a health care provider with questions about tube placement.

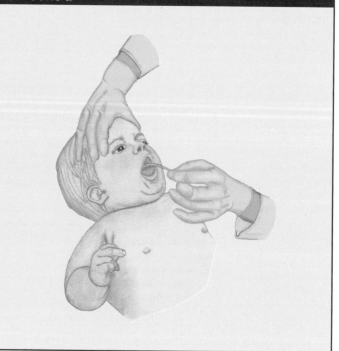

possible for the infusion and a tube of soft material will decrease the child's discomfort.

Safety Issues Related to Tube Placement

After a tube is initially inserted and *before* an enteral infusion is started or medication given, it is essential to verify that the tube is located in the stomach or small intestine. Radiographic confirmation is the most reliable method to assess tube location and is recommended following initial tube insertion and if there is doubt that a tube is in the correct position (Metheny, 2009).

Tube location should also be checked anytime a feeding is interrupted, before each bolus feeding or medication administration, and every 4 to 8 hours during continuous feedings (Farrington, Lang, Cullen, & Stewart, 2009; Metheny, 2009). The American Association of Critical Care Nurses recommends that nurses use a variety of bedside methods to verify tube location (Metheny, 2009). These methods include assessing the patient for signs of respiratory distress (indicating the tube is in the respiratory tract); checking for a change in length of the external portion of the tube (movement from the marked position); observing the volume, appearance, and color of the aspirate from the tube; and testing the pH of the aspirate. Generally, gastric fluid is grassy-green or clear/colorless, with a pH of 5 or less; however, occasionally the pH can be higher.

Respiratory secretions also can appear clear, but the pH is typically greater than 6. Small intestine fluid is often bile stained (yellow or greenish-brown) with a pH of 6 or more. Keep in mind that both formula and certain medications can alter the pH of enteral secretions (Huffman, Jarczyk, O'Brien et al., 2004). Though used in many settings, studies have shown that auscultating over the epigastric area for air insufflated through the tube is not reliable in distinguishing between tube placement in the respiratory tract and in the stomach (Farrington et al., 2009).

Nasogastric tube placement is more of a risk in children who have decreased level of consciousness; who are uncooperative or restless; who have recently been intubated or extubated; or who demonstrate decreased swallowing, cough, or gag reflexes. Measuring, marking, and documenting the external length of the tube immediately after insertion will assist in determining whether the tube has lost its original position. However, nurses cannot assume that a feeding tube has remained in proper position just because the external position has not changed. Tubes can become dislodged with suctioning, retching, or vomiting.

Contraindications to Tube Placement

It is crucial that the nurse determine if the child has any pre-existing contraindications to tube placement such as prior surgeries, trauma, or congenital anomalies (e.g., choanal atresia, tracheoesophageal fistula, esophageal strictures) that could interfere with passage of the tube. If any of these findings are present, a physician may elect to use fluoroscopy to guide the insertion. If a tube that was placed during or through a surgical repair becomes dislodged, the nurse does not attempt reinsertion and notifies the surgeon immediately.

Enteral Feedings

Following tube placement and verification, the nurse administers the enteral feeding either as a bolus (intermittent) or as a continuous feeding (Procedure 13-8). Key steps start with preparing the child and family, and then aspirating stomach contents to check the residual volume from the last feeding. During the feeding, the nurse or parent/caregiver should hold the infant or young child, when possible, to associate the feeding with pleasant sensations and facilitate bonding. A pacifier is given to infants to promote nonnutritive sucking. The nurse encourages older children to sit at a table during meals to promote normal development and socialization.

Gastrostomy Tubes and Buttons

The procedure for gastrostomy feedings is similar to that for orogastric, nasogastric, or nasointestinal feedings. Because the gastrostomy tube or button is surgically placed percutaneously into the stomach,

PROCEDURE 13-8 ADMINISTERING ENTERAL FEEDINGS (VIA THE OROGASTRIC, NASOGASTRIC, OR NASOINTESTINAL ROUTE)

PURPOSE: To Provide Adequate Nutrition in a Child Who Cannot Tolerate Oral Feedings

1. Using developmentally appropriate language, explain the procedure to the child and parent. Assess their needs and concerns related to the procedure, including previous experience with enteral feedings and the ability of the child to cooperate with the procedure. Use therapeutic play to prepare the child and family for the procedure.
2. The following equipment is needed: Stethoscope, irrigation syringe, room-temperature formula, sterile water, pacifier for neonates and infants, electronic feeding pump (for continuous tube feedings), pH testing strips, and gloves.

Intermittent Feedings (Bolus)

3. Technique:
   a. Position the child on the back or right side with the head of bed elevated and remove the syringe or cap from the tube. Perform hand hygiene and put on gloves.
   b. Check for proper tube placement using multiple bedside methods in accordance with hospital policy. Be sure the mark indicating insertion length is in its original place relative to the exit site. Aspirate residual volume from the previous feeding; note quantity and characteristics, and document. Follow hospital policy or physician's orders regarding whether the next feeding should be given based on the quantity of the residual and if the residual fluid should be discarded or re-infused.
   c. Remove the plunger from the syringe and attach the syringe to the tube.
   d. Pour room-temperature formula into the syringe and allow the feeding to flow slowly into the tube (usually over a period of 15 to 30 minutes) via gravity. Raising or lowering the level of the syringe increases or decreases the flow of formula. Encourage the infant to suck on a pacifier during the feeding. Discontinue the feeding if signs of respiratory distress, cyanosis, abdominal distention, or vomiting occur, and notify the physician.
   e. After the prescribed volume has been infused, flush the tube with sterile water and clear the tube by injecting 1 to 5 mL of air.
   f. Discard the used syringe and close or clamp the tube unless otherwise indicated. Remove gloves and perform hand hygiene.
   g. Place the child lying on the right side with the head of the bed elevated for 30 to 60 minutes after the feeding. Monitor the child closely for nausea, emesis, or respiratory difficulties during this time.

Continuous Feedings

4. Technique:
   a. Position the child on the back or right side with the head of bed elevated. Perform hand hygiene and put on gloves. Check for proper tube placement using multiple bedside methods in accordance with hospital policy. The pH is a less reliable indicator of placement when a child is on continuous feedings. Be sure the mark indicating insertion length is in its original place relative to the exit site. Aspirate the residual volume and note quantity and characteristics; it may appear like curdled milk if the tube is in the stomach or appear bile stained if the tube is in the intestine. It is likely that a small quantity of residual will be present. Follow hospital policy or physician's orders regarding whether the next feeding should be given based on the quantity of the residual and if the residual fluid should be discarded or re-infused.
   b. Fill the feeding bag, volume-control set, or syringe with the prescribed formula. Attach to infusion pump if applicable. Prime the infusion tubing with formula.
   c. Connect infusion tubing to the feeding tube and begin the infusion at the prescribed rate. Remove gloves and perform hand hygiene.
   d. Check tube placement and residual volumes every 4 to 8 hours. Flush with sterile water according to hospital policy or physician orders.
   e. To reduce the incidence of reflux and aspiration, keep the child positioned on the right side with the head of bed elevated. Encourage the infant to suck on a pacifier periodically while receiving the feeding. Monitor the child periodically for nausea, emesis, or respiratory difficulty.
5. Praise the child for cooperation during the feeding process.
6. Document the amount, color, and consistency of any residual fluids and note whether it was re-infused (returned) or discarded. Document the type and amount of formula given, the amount of sterile water given, the position the child was in after or during the feeding, and the child's tolerance of the procedure.

Home Adaptations

Assess the parent's ability to perform enteral feedings. Parents should be encouraged to make this as normal a procedure as possible (e.g., by holding the infant during feedings). Ask the parent to demonstrate the procedure before discharge. Assistance with home care can be provided by a home health agency. Advise the parent to follow manufacturer's recommendations about refrigerating and discarding opened unused formula.

! NURSING QUALITY ALERT

Enteral Feedings

- Begin the feeding only after tube placement in the stomach has been properly verified.
- Discontinue feedings and notify the physician if signs of respiratory distress, cyanosis, abdominal distention, or vomiting occur.
- Provide a pacifier to infants so that they can associate sucking with feeding. Encourage older children to sit at a table during meals to promote the normal socialization associated with eating.
- To avoid accidental overfeeding should the infusion pump malfunction, use only an amount of formula appropriate for a 4-hour feeding. Discard any formula that has been opened for more than 4 hours.
- Follow the facility's policies or procedures or physician's orders regarding discarding residual volumes and the prescribed frequency for changing feeding equipment.

verifying the location of the tube is a simpler process. Most gastrostomy tubes and buttons are sutured to the skin and have an internal inflated balloon; however, dislodgment can occur. The nurse should check external tube length and observe for indications of change from the correct position. The nurse must also assess the aspirate for volume, appearance, and color.

Special considerations for children with gastrostomy tubes or buttons include skin care around the insertion site. The nurse assesses the site for abnormal findings such as leakage of formula, skin redness, drainage, bleeding, and skin breakdown. The skin around the insertion site is cleaned with soap and water at least once daily and when soiled.

Capped gastrostomy tubes extend several inches from the insertion site. Check to ensure that no tension is on the external tube. If necessary, coil the tube and tape near the exit site. Gastrostomy buttons are placed close to the skin surface. They have a one-way valve that eliminates the need for clamping and provides a secure connection for extension tubing between the button and the feeding pump. Once the feeding is complete, the extension tube is removed and the button is capped. Gastrostomy buttons are easy for parents to use and allow children to participate in many activities.

It is important to watch for signs that the tube or button may need to be replaced and to report these to the physician if noted. The signs include leaking, tube occlusion, malfunction of the anti-reflux valve, or abnormal tube position. Many children are discharged home with gastrostomy tubes or buttons (see Chapter 19). Parents must be educated so they can provide all required care, including how to check for correct position and monitor the insertion site, what symptoms should be reported, and what to do if dislodgment occurs. Information booklets are available to assist families. Parent teaching is a major part of nursing care for a child with a feeding tube.

> ### ? CRITICAL THINKING EXERCISE 13-1
>
> The assessment of feeding tube placement has historically been a nursing responsibility, even though the only totally accurate assessment measure is radiographic confirmation.
> 1. What is the nurse's legal and ethical responsibility regarding feeding tube placement confirmation?
> 2. How does the nurse make the "best judgment" about what action to take if placement is questionable?

ENEMAS

Enemas are given when stool needs to be removed from the bowel because of severe constipation or in preparation for a diagnostic procedure or surgery. The differences between giving an enema to a child and giving an enema to an adult are the type and amount of fluid administered and the distance that the enema tip is inserted into the rectum.

Enema Administration

Rectal damage and perforation can occur with improper insertion of the enema tip. The tip is lubricated and then gently inserted 2.5 cm (1 in) to 10 cm (4 in), depending on the age and size of the child (Table 13-2). Commercially prepared, single-use enemas come with prelubricated tips of appropriate lengths.

Solutions and Volumes

The amount of the enema solution will vary with the age and size of the child. Unless the physician's orders specify a different amount, the recommended volume of enema solution based on the child's age is listed in Table 13-2. Only isotonic solutions should be used with children. Plain tap water, a hypotonic solution, should never be used because it can cause rapid fluid shifts and fluid overload.

After completing enema administration, a diaper is placed on the infant. Toddlers can use the bedpan, "potty" chair, or toilet. Older children and adolescents can use the bedpan, bedside commode, or

TABLE 13-2	**RECOMMENDED VOLUME AND DEPTH FOR ENEMA TIP INSERTION, BY AGE**	
	VOLUME (mL)	DEPTH OF INSERTION
Infants	120-240	1 in (2.5 cm)
2-4 yr	240-360	2 in (5 cm)
4-10 yr	360-480	3 in (7.5 cm)
11 yr +	480-720	4 in (10 cm)

bathroom toilet. The nurse documents the date and time the enema was given, the type and amount of solution, the amount and characteristics of the "returned" stool, other findings (e.g., presence of blood, mucus, foreign bodies, worms in the stool), and how the child tolerated the procedure.

OSTOMIES

Urinary and fecal diversion may be needed when normal methods of elimination are temporarily or permanently interrupted. Some conditions requiring the creation of a fecal stoma (ileostomy or colostomy) include imperforate anus, Hirschsprung disease, necrotizing enterocolitis, some cases of intestinal atresia, intussusception, Crohn disease, and ulcerative colitis (see Chapter 19). The anatomic location of the stoma will dictate the consistency of the stool. The higher the stoma is located in the intestinal tract, the more liquid the stool.

Urinary diversion is usually the result of obstructive uropathy, congenital anomalies, or neurogenic bladder (see Chapter 20). The ureters can be brought out through the abdominal wall (ureterostomy) or connected to a segment of small bowel (ileal conduit).

Nursing care of the child with an ostomy focuses on teaching the child and family to perform the procedures involved in the care of an ostomy. The nurse uses developmentally appropriate terminology to explain the procedures to the child and parents. A teaching model, such as a doll with a stoma, can facilitate education.

Ostomy care includes the selection and effective use of the right type and size of appliance. Maintaining the integrity of the skin around the stoma is of great importance. Parents and the child need encouragement and support as they become active participants in the treatment regimen. The nurse should make referrals to an enterostomal therapist or other support services, as indicated.

OXYGEN THERAPY

Hypoxemia, resulting from apnea or inadequate ventilation, occurs rapidly in children because of their high metabolic rate and increased oxygen consumption. Often cardiopulmonary arrest follows progressive respiratory dysfunction in a child; thus, it is vital nurses recognize the early, subtle signs and symptoms of respiratory distress.

For infants and children who are unable to maintain a normal arterial oxygen pressure (PaO_2), supplemental oxygen may be needed. A physician's order is generally required for the administration of oxygen. Some facilities may have policies that permit nurses to start oxygen therapy in certain emergency situations.

Oxygen Administration

Oxygen is commonly administered to children by nasal cannula, facemask (simple, nonrebreather, "blow-by" tube, partial rebreather, Venturi, or aerosol), an oxygen hood, or an oxygen tent (Figure 13-8). Oxygen can also be given to a child with an artificial airway such as an endotracheal tube or tracheostomy using a specialty device (e.g., a tracheostomy collar) or a ventilator (see Chapter 21). The method of delivery depends on the concentration of oxygen needed and the child's ability to cooperate with the chosen method. The nurse must always check the physician's orders for the percentage of oxygen to be delivered and the method of delivery to be used, if specified.

In most facilities, a respiratory care therapist is responsible for the setup, maintenance, and management of oxygen equipment. However, the nurse needs to have a working knowledge of the oxygen administration systems used.

Oxygen administration equipment comes in a variety of sizes designed to provide a correct fit for children in different age-groups.

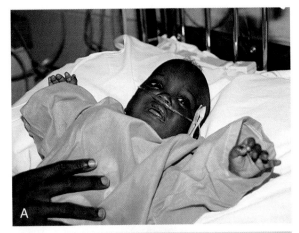

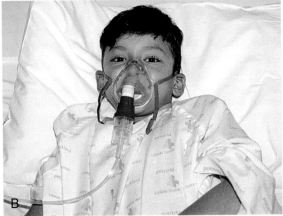

FIG 13-8 When administering oxygen to children, special consideration is given to the size and type of equipment selected, and the needs of the child and family for education and support. **A,** Nasal cannula. **B,** Simple facemask. (Courtesy Parkland Health and Hospital System, Dallas, TX.)

When delivering oxygen by mask, the correct size of mask that ensures a tight fit is selected. Masks are available in preemie, newborn, infant, child, small adult, and adult sizes. To determine the proper size for a child, the nurse determines that the mask extends from the bridge of the child's nose to the cleft of the chin. Nasal cannulas are also available in a variety of pediatric and adult sizes.

Different types of devices are used to meet the child's individual needs. Often an oxygen hood is used to provide maximal oxygenation for neonates and infants. Older infants, toddlers, and preschoolers tend to tolerate oxygen via a nasal cannula, blow-by oxygen, or facemask. School-age children and adolescents may prefer a nonrebreather mask to achieve maximal oxygenation.

A child experiencing difficulty breathing may be reluctant to have a mask or cannula placed on the face. The nurse must first explain to the child and parents, in developmentally appropriate language, what will happen, why the mask is needed, and how it will feel. The nurse encourages the child and parents to handle the equipment and to assist the nurse with placement. If needed, supports are provided to keep the oxygen delivery system in place, such as putting elbow restraints on an infant or taping nasal cannula tubing to the side of the child's face.

A nasal cannula is a low-flow delivery system indicated for infants and children who need modest amounts of supplemental oxygen (up to 40%, or a flow rate of 1 to 6 L/min). The loop of the cannula can be enlarged and then slipped easily over the child's ears. Prongs are placed in the nares and the loop tightened slightly. Flow rates should not exceed 6 L/min; higher flow rates can irritate the nasopharynx and cause gastric distention and regurgitation.

The simple facemask and the Venturi mask are indicated for infants and children who need modest amounts of supplemental oxygen (35% to 60%, or a flow rate of 6 to 10 L/min). The Venturi mask can be adjusted to deliver specific concentrations of oxygen (e.g., 24%, 28%, 35%, 50%, or 60%). The nurse attaches the mask to the humidified oxygen source and adjusts the flow rate to the prescribed level. The mask is placed on the child's face and then the nose clip and head strap are adjusted. A minimum flow rate of 4 to 6 L/min must be maintained to prevent rebreathing of exhaled carbon dioxide.

A partial or full nonrebreather mask is a facemask with an attached reservoir that allows a portion of exhaled gas to remain in the bag and mix with oxygen. Partial nonrebreather masks supply oxygen concentrations of 50% to 60% at a rate of 10 to 12 L/min. A full nonrebreather system can deliver close to 100% oxygen at a flow rate of 10 to 15 L/min if a tight seal can be maintained.

In rare circumstances when a child needs a high-humidity environment with oxygen, a cool mist tent may be indicated. In this instance, the nurse must ensure that the sides of the tent are completely tucked in to prevent escape of oxygen. To keep the child as dry as possible, cotton clothing is used and clothing and bed linens are changed when needed.

With the use of any oxygen administration system, safety is of great concern. Signs stating "oxygen in use/no smoking" are posted outside the child's door and over the bed. Although most health care facilities are nonsmoking facilities, parents and visitors are reminded that smoking is not allowed in the room. Toys that have the potential for producing a spark, including those that are battery powered, should not be permitted near the oxygen.

Documentation

Documentation in the nurse's notes includes the date and time oxygen was started; the type of oxygen administration system used; the percentage of oxygen delivered and the flow rate; the child's vital signs, skin color, respiratory effort, and lung sounds; the child's response to the procedure; and any teaching done with the child or family.

Parent Teaching

Infants and children often receive home oxygen therapy. The nurse and other health care providers such as respiratory care therapists educate the parents or caregivers about the operation of equipment to be used at home, equipment cleaning, safety factors, cardiopulmonary resuscitation, and available support services.

ASSESSING OXYGENATION

Pulse oximetry is a sensitive, reliable, noninvasive means of measuring oxygen saturation (SaO_2) in the blood. Oxygen saturation is the percentage of hemoglobin that is carrying the full complement of oxygen molecules (completely saturated = 100%). The pulse oximeter measures the absorption of light waves as they pass through highly perfused areas of the body. It provides the nurse with valuable information regarding a child's oxygenation status and may serve as an early warning sign of hypoxemia (Figure 13-9; Procedure 13-9).

A pulse oximeter can be used to measure oxygen saturation at intervals or on a continuous basis. The relationship between oxygen saturation and actual oxygenation (as measured by PaO_2) is not 1:1. In general, a small decrease in oxygen saturation can represent a much larger decrease in PaO_2. Nurses must immediately report significant decreases in oxygen saturation and intervene according to the physician's orders and hospital policies (see Chapter 21).

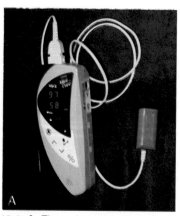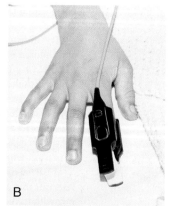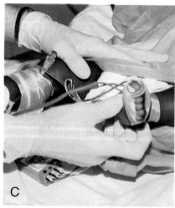

FIG 13-9 A, The pulse oximeter is a reliable, noninvasive method that allows periodic or continuous measurement of blood oxygen saturation. The sensor is applied to a child's finger **(B)** or an infant's toe **(C).** (**A,** Courtesy Randall W. Nelson, N. Richland Hills, TX.; **B** and **C,** Courtesy of Parkland Health and Hospital System, Dallas, TX.)

PROCEDURE 13-9 PULSE OXIMETRY

PURPOSE: To Assess the Child's Oxygen Saturation

1. Explain to the child and parents the indication for the procedure.
2. Bring the oximeter and sensor (finger probe, adhesive probe, or ear clip) to the child's room and allow the child to gently handle the equipment. The sensor will differ depending on whether the oximetry is intermittent or continuous.
3. Set the parameters for the alarm on a continuous measuring oximeter.
4. Place the probe on the finger, toe, or earlobe. Avoid placing the probe on an extremity with an arterial line, blood pressure cuff, or intravenous (IV) line in place. Fingernail polish or artificial nails will need to be removed before placing the sensor. Do not wrap the sensor so tightly as to prevent venous flow and cause inaccurate readings.
5. Observe and document the pulse rate and oxygen saturation. The pulse rate on the oximeter should coincide with an apical pulse or pulse rate on a cardiac monitor. If no pulse is detected, reposition the sensor.
6. To check the skin condition, remove the sensor from the site at least every 2 hours. If using a portable oximeter, be sure to clean the sensor with the manufacturer's recommended cleaning solution.
7. Document the child's response to the procedure and the pulse oximetry reading obtained, the percentage and flow rate of oxygen (if being administered), and the activity level of the child. Report any abnormal findings to the physician based on the individual child's condition. In general, a pulse oximeter reading of less than 95% is considered abnormal.
8. Inform the child and family that an alarm will sound if the child's oxygen saturation falls below the set parameter. The alarm may also sound if the child is particularly active or the sensor becomes dislodged.
9. Praise the child for cooperation with the procedure.

Pulse oximeter measurements reflect the child's oxygen saturation as well as perfusion status. Potential sources of error in measurements include an abnormal hemoglobin value (e.g., in hyperbilirubinemia or carbon monoxide poisoning), decreased peripheral perfusion (e.g., in hypotension or hypothermia), ambient light interference, motion artifact, and skin breakdown from the adhesive used to secure the sensor. To eliminate the effects of ambient light, an opaque shield can be placed over the sensor site. Sites should be rotated to prevent skin breakdown.

Under certain circumstances, arterial or capillary blood gases and pH may need to be measured to establish correlation of oxygenation with pulse oximetry readings and to monitor the child's acid-base balance. Both arterial and capillary blood sampling are invasive procedures; obtaining a capillary blood specimen is an easier procedure and less painful.

A sample of arterial blood can be obtained from an indwelling arterial catheter or an arterial puncture. The preferred site in children is the radial artery, although alternative sites (e.g., brachial artery) can be used. Based on the child's age and size, an appropriate needle length and gauge should be selected for use.

Specially trained respiratory care therapists, nurses, or other personnel must draw arterial blood samples. Nurses are often responsible for supporting and holding/restraining the child as well as assisting with the procedure. Once the specimen has been obtained, the nurse must hold pressure on the arterial puncture site for at least 5 minutes. The arterial blood gas specimen must be placed on ice immediately and then transported to the laboratory.

! NURSING QUALITY ALERT

Assisting with Arterial Blood Gas Sampling

- Position the child's wrist with the palm up but not hyperextended. Stabilize the extremity, allowing neither twisting of the wrist nor jerking of the shoulder.
- Do not hold the child's arm too tightly because a tight grip occludes arterial blood flow.
- The skin is punctured at an angle of 15 to 45 degrees. When the needle is withdrawn, it is withdrawn slowly to decrease the incidence of arterial spasm.
- After the needle is withdrawn, apply direct pressure to the site using a sterile 2- × 2-inch sterile gauze for at least 5 minutes.
- Place the sample on ice until the laboratory analysis is performed.
- Record the puncture site and the child's activity level at the time of the sampling.

CHEST PHYSIOTHERAPY

Chest physiotherapy (CPT) includes postural drainage, chest percussion and vibration, and coughing and deep-breathing exercises. These techniques can mobilize and remove secretions, reexpand the lungs, and promote efficient use of the respiratory muscles, particularly in children with chronic pulmonary diseases such as cystic fibrosis. CPT also may be used prophylactically in postoperative patients to prevent atelectasis and pneumonia. Contraindications to CPT include head injury, acute asthma, chest trauma, osteogenesis imperfecta, thrombocytopenia, and lung tumor.

Initiation of CPT requires a physician's order. In most health care settings, CPT is the responsibility of the respiratory care or physical therapist; however, nurses may perform this procedure. Nurses may also participate in educating the family to perform CPT at home for certain children with chronic lung disease. See the Evolve website for detailed procedure information and illustration.

TRACHEOSTOMY CARE

A tracheostomy is a surgically created opening (stoma) in the trachea. It is performed in children to bypass an upper airway obstruction, facilitate pulmonary secretion removal, or optimize mechanical ventilation. A tracheostomy can be either temporary or permanent. Tracheostomies continue to be used for long-term management of problem airways, with parents performing tracheostomy care in the home setting (Parrilla, Scarano, Guidi, et al., 2007; Wilson, 2005). Pacifiers should be given to infants with tracheostomies to encourage nonnutritive sucking.

Pediatric tracheostomy tubes vary in size and type. The tube most commonly used is made of Silastic (plastic), which is soft and flexible. It consists of two pieces: the outer cannula, which stays in the trachea to keep the stoma open, and an obturator, which guides the tube into place during tube changes. Some tubes have an inner cannula that can be removed for cleaning. Tracheostomy tubes with inner cannulas are often used for older children and for those who have increased mucus production.

Shiley or Bivona single-lumen tracheostomy tubes are often used for children. Tube size is categorized by the internal diameter (ID) of the tube measured in millimeters (mm). Pediatric sizes range from 2.5 mm for newborns to 5.5 mm for children. Adult-size tubes, with a 6- to 8-mm ID are often used for adolescents.

Suctioning

When a child has a tracheostomy, suctioning is often required to remove secretions and keep the airway patent. Suctioning should not be done on a routine basis; the frequency of suctioning is determined by the needs of the individual child (Wilson, 2005). The nurse should frequently assess the child's breath sounds, respiratory rate, and character of respirations as well as the quantity and quality of secretions (sputum) to determine if a child needs suctioning.

Use of appropriate techniques and equipment for suctioning can prevent complications such as hypoxia, tissue damage, and infection (Procedure 13-10). Suctioning infants and children requires the use of smaller suction catheters and lower suction pressures than for adults. Catheter sizes range from 5 Fr to 14 Fr, with smaller sizes used for smaller tubes. To avoid total airway occlusion, catheter size should be approximately half the inner diameter of the tracheostomy tube.

PROCEDURE 13-10 SUCTIONING A TRACHEOSTOMY TUBE

PURPOSE: To Maintain Patency of the Tracheostomy Tube

1. After using developmentally appropriate language to explain the procedure, its purpose, and other pertinent information to the child and parent, gather the following equipment: A sterile suction catheter of appropriate size, sterile gloves, mask, goggles or face shield, sterile normal saline, and sterile cup. Have equipment available to administer oxygen and a bag-valve-mask device, if applicable. Perform hand hygiene.
2. Auscultate the child's breath sounds. Assess respiratory rate and effort, and the presence of secretions.
3. Administer oxygen to the child, if indicated, using a tracheostomy collar. Adjust the suction vacuum pressure to the prescribed level and put on the mask and goggles or face shield. Pour normal saline into the sterile cup. Put on sterile gloves.
4. Remove the tracheostomy collar with the nondominant hand. Hold the catheter in the other hand covered in a sterile glove. Lubricate the catheter with normal saline, and then insert the catheter the length of the tracheostomy tube (pre-measured using another tracheostomy tube of the same size) with suction off.
5. Withdraw the catheter using a twisting or twirling motion and apply intermittent suction. Limit insertion and suctioning time to 5 seconds to prevent hypoxia.
6. Reapply the tracheostomy collar and reoxygenate, as indicated. Allow time for the child to rest and take a few breaths. If needed, give oxygen using a bag-valve-mask device by "bagging" the child. If the child is on a ventilator, "bagging" is imperative.
7. Auscultate the child's breath sounds and assess respiratory rate and effort to determine effectiveness of suctioning and if secretions are still present. A pulse oximeter may be used to assess oxygenation status, if indicated. Repeat the procedure again to clear the airway, rinsing the suction catheter with sterile normal saline before the second insertion.
8. Often the oral cavity requires suctioning as well. This is performed at the end of the procedure *after* suctioning of the tracheostomy is completed. The catheter is inserted into the mouth, and then suction is applied while the catheter is withdrawn.

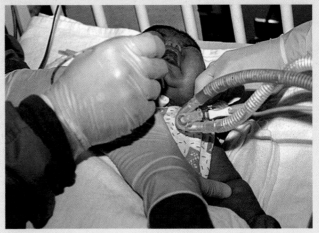

(Courtesy of Parkland Health and Hospital System, Dallas, TX.)

9. Discard the suction catheter, other equipment, and PPE in an appropriate receptacle. Perform hand hygiene.
10. Comfort the child and offer praise for cooperation. Encourage the parent to provide comfort to the infant or child.
11. Document in the child's medical record, the date and time the procedure was performed, the amount and characteristics of the secretions obtained, the character of the breath sounds before and after suctioning, the child's response to the procedure, and any teaching done with the child and parents, as well as their level of understanding and their response to the teaching.

Home Adaptations

Tracheostomy suctioning at home is a clean rather than sterile procedure, though a new, sterile suction catheter is used each time. The family will need a powered suction apparatus, suction catheters of appropriate size, normal saline, and gloves. The procedure for suctioning is as previously discussed, including presuctioning and postsuctioning assessments.

Procedure—Chest Phys ... apy

PROCEDURE 13-11   CARE OF A TRACHEOSTOMY

PURPOSE: To Maintain a Patent Airway and Prevent Infection

1. Using developmentally appropriate language, explain the procedure, its purpose, and other pertinent information to the child and parents. Some hospital facilities use videos (DVDs) and stoma dolls to demonstrate the procedure.

2. Obtain a tracheostomy care kit with the following: Cotton-tipped applicators, pipe cleaners or a brush for cleaning the inner cannula, tracheostomy ties, sterile precut drain sponge, sterile gauze, gloves (sterile and nonsterile), towel or blanket roll, hydrogen peroxide, sterile normal saline, mask, and goggles or face shield.

3. To hyperextend the head and neck to expose the site, position the child with a towel or blanket under the shoulders.

4. Use appropriate hand hygiene and open the tray, creating a sterile field.

5. Pour equal parts of normal saline and hydrogen peroxide in one small tray and normal saline in the other small tray. Use the large tray for holding cotton-tipped applicators, clean tracheostomy ties, and sterile gauze.

6. Don nonsterile gloves, mask, and goggles or face shield, and remove the dressing around the tracheostomy, if present. Discard the dressing and gloves according to hospital policy. Assess the stoma for redness, drainage or discharge, and skin breakdown. Perform hand hygiene.

7. Don sterile gloves and, using cotton-tipped applicators moistened in half-strength hydrogen peroxide solution, clean the child's neck under the tracheostomy tube flanges and tracheostomy ties and dry with sterile gauze. If the child has a tracheostomy without an inner cannula, skip to steps 8 and 9.

8. Unlock the inner cannula (if using a three-piece tracheostomy system) by rotating it counterclockwise. Remove the inner cannula and, using pipe cleaners or a brush, quickly clean it in half-strength hydrogen peroxide solution. (Alternatively, it may be replaced with a new inner cannula.) Rinse the cannula thoroughly in sterile normal saline and inspect it for cleanliness. Repeat the cleaning procedure if necessary.

9. To remove excess moisture, tap the cleaned inner cannula on the edge of the sterile container. Do not dry the outside of the inner cannula because moisture will act as a lubricant during reinsertion. Reinsert the inner cannula into the tracheostomy tube and lock it in place by rotating it clockwise.

10. It is recommended for two people to change ties. While the assistant (wearing sterile gloves, mask, and goggles or face shield) gently holds the tracheostomy tube in place, remove the existing ties from the flanges by untying or cutting with clean safety scissors. Clean and dry the skin under the ties, and inspect the skin for breakdown caused by the ties.

11. Loop the new tracheostomy ties through the flange on one side of the tracheostomy. Bring the ties around the back of the child's neck and tie them securely to the opposite flange, on the side of the neck. Ties must be tight enough to keep the tracheostomy tube in the correct position; only one finger should be able to be inserted between the ties and neck. Use a

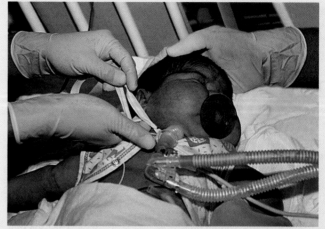

(Courtesy of Parkland Health and Hospital System, Dallas, TX.)

double square knot to prevent accidental untying and dislodging of the tracheostomy.

12. If an assistant is not available, the soiled tracheostomy ties are removed *after* the new ties are securely tied and are maintaining the tracheostomy tube in the correct position.

13. Discard used supplies and PPE in appropriate receptacles. Perform hand hygiene.

14. Comfort the child and offer praise for cooperation. Encourage the parent to provide comfort and support. The nurse can also give the child a reward, such as a sticker.

15. Document in the child's medical record the date, time, and type of procedure; the condition of the stoma and skin; any abnormal findings or complications and the nursing action taken; and the child's tolerance of the procedure. Document child and family teaching as well as their understanding of and involvement in the tracheostomy care.

Home Adaptations

Assess the parents' ability to perform the procedure. It may be necessary to engage the assistance of a home health agency. Begin to teach tracheostomy care early in the child's hospitalization, and teach more than one family member. Provide clear, written instructions. It is imperative to observe all caregivers during return demonstrations of the procedure before discharge from the hospital. All those caring for the child must have cardiopulmonary resuscitation (CPR) training.

The family may need a great deal of support and encouragement to feel comfortable with suctioning and tracheostomy care. The child can take baths, but care should be taken to prevent water from entering the trachea. Showers are not recommended. To avoid tracheal spasm, the tracheostomy can be covered loosely during cold or windy days.

Recommended pressures for tracheostomy suctioning vary by age (Ireton, 2007):

- Neonates and infants: 60 to 80 mm Hg
- Children: 80 to 100 mm Hg
- Adolescents: 80 to 120 mm Hg

The suction catheter should not be inserted beyond the end of the tracheostomy tube. Standard Precautions are used; PPE includes mask, goggles or face shield, and sterile gloves on both hands. The sterile suction catheter must be held in a sterile-gloved hand that remains sterile throughout the procedure. Instillation of saline into the tracheostomy to thin secretions has been linked to decreased oxygen saturation and should not be done on a routine basis (Ireton, 2007). Providing a humidified environment keeps secretions thin and easier to remove with suctioning.

Stoma Care

Tracheostomy site care (Procedure 13-11) includes assessing the stoma area for signs of infection and skin breakdown, changing tracheostomy ties, cleaning the tracheostomy site and inner cannula, changing the tracheostomy tube, and suctioning. The areas around the tube and the inner cannula are cleaned, the ties changed, and a new, precut drain sponge applied as often as necessary to keep the site clean and dry. To prevent the tube from being accidentally dislodged while the ties are being changed, an assistant should be present to hold the child and keep the tube in place. The tracheostomy tube is usually changed weekly, often by the physician or respiratory care therapist. Because tracheostomy care is often tiring, the child is allowed to rest after the procedure.

An extra tracheostomy tube that is the same size or slightly smaller than the child's current tube is kept at the bedside (or taped to the head of the bed) for easy access if an emergency reinsertion is required. Because of the risk of aspiration and possible obstruction of the trachea, the child with a tracheostomy should not play with small toys or toys with small parts and should not use plastic bibs or bedding. In addition, powders and aerosol products should not be used near children with tracheostomies because of the risk of inhalation injury from breathing the particles.

SURGICAL PROCEDURES

Although each child is unique and each surgical procedure is different, there is a general body of knowledge that is relevant to all children experiencing surgery. Surgery can be a traumatic event for children of all ages and their families. Stressors associated with surgery include separation from family members, care by strangers, unfamiliar surroundings, fear of the unknown, disruption in routine, lack of privacy, preoperative testing and medications, pain, and fear of mutilation, disfigurement, or disability. The nurse must identify the individual needs that the child and the family have for nursing care associated with the disorder and surgical treatment of the disorder.

Surgery can be scheduled weeks or months in advance or be performed on an emergency basis. Often surgery for a child is done in the operating room of an acute-care facility with at least one overnight stay in the hospital. However, surgery performed on an outpatient basis is increasing. Ambulatory, or same-day surgery adheres to the same standards of care as inpatient surgery but has the added benefits of the child spending less time away from home and family, lower infection rates, and reduced costs.

Preparation for Surgery

Family-centered preparation involves educating and preparing all children and their families in advance of the surgical procedure. Overall goals are to increase knowledge and decrease anxiety for the child and the parents (Chorney & Kain, 2010). A multidisciplinary approach is used that involves parents and other family members, nurses, child life specialists, physicians, anesthesiologists, and other specialists. In determining how to best prepare the child and family, the nurse considers the type of procedure to be performed, the setting (inpatient or outpatient), intensity of the child's illness or injury, the child's age and developmental level, and family coping skills (see Chapter 11).

Preparing the child and parents for surgery establishes a foundation of trust between the nurse, the child, and the family. Education sessions generally start 1 week before a scheduled surgery, although younger children may need preparation closer to the operative day. The evidence indicates that children benefit from receiving information about what will be done during the surgical procedure as well as what sensory experiences they should expect (e.g., what they will feel, hear, see, smell and taste), including pain (Chorney & Kain, 2010).

All education sessions are carefully planned, employ a developmental approach, and provide information that is simple, accurate, and presented in a non-emotional manner (Chorney & Kain, 2010). Often, a tour of the perioperative area is included. Children are allowed to see and touch some of the equipment that will be used. Therapeutic play is an essential tool and can be facilitated by nurses, child life therapists, and parents (see Chapter 11). Adequate time must be provided so questions posed by the child and family can be answered and they feel ready to undergo the procedure.

With the increase in same-day surgery, parents are often the primary educators for their child's surgical experience. Parents need to explain to the child as clearly as possible why the child is going to the hospital or surgery center and what will happen during the stay. Nurses need to first educate the parents and then offer them additional support and assistance. Books and videos written for children that explain hospitalization and surgery can be used by parents in preparing their child.

On the day of surgery, the nurse reviews key points with the child and family. The nurse verifies that the parents or guardians have been fully informed and have signed the surgical consent form. According to the child's age and hospital policy, the nurse ensures that the child has assented to the procedure as well. Involving nurses and child life therapists who participated in the child's preparation will promote continuity of care and trust. If a waiting period is required before the scheduled surgery time, it is important to keep the child busy (distracted) in order to reduce anxiety. Age-appropriate toys and activities should be provided in the holding area or in the child's room.

Children often require physical preparation before surgical procedures. Routine preoperative activities include laboratory testing (complete blood cell count, chemistry profile/electrolytes, urinalysis, and chest radiograph); withholding food and/or drink for a specified number of hours before surgery; and administering preoperative medications ordered by the physician. Nurses are also responsible for checking the child's identification, confirming the consent form is completed and signed, obtaining laboratory results, and gathering other documentation. Most hospitals and surgical centers have preoperative checklists that assist the nurse in documenting the child's preparation for surgery.

Because infants and children are at greater risk for dehydration, the period during which they can have nothing by mouth (NPO) may be shorter than for adolescents and adults (see Chapter 16). This period varies according to the protocols of the facility and the anesthesiologist (Box 13-3). It is critical that the nurse frequently monitors the hydration status of the infant or child who is NPO and waiting to go to surgery.

Preoperative Medication and Anesthesia Induction

Two interventions are primarily used to manage anxiety in children just prior to the start of surgery: preoperative sedative medication and parental presence during anesthesia induction. When providing family-centered care, the decision about which intervention to use should be jointly made by the parents and the anesthesiologist (Chorney & Kain, 2010). Though premedication is generally effective in reducing anxiety, inconsistencies have been found (Finley, Stewart, Buffett-Jerrott, et al., 2006). Other concerns about giving the child sedative medications include uncomfortable side effects (dizziness, nausea), the child's fear of injection pain, fall risk, and possible airway obstruction. After the preanesthetic medication has been administered, the child must be constantly monitored by the nurse and parents with the side rails raised on the bed or stretcher.

Premedication may not be given if parents are present when anesthesia is induced. Research results vary as to whether parental presence

BOX 13-3   GUIDELINES FOR PREOPERATIVE FASTING

1. Fast from solid food and full liquids from the night before as directed. Some physicians allow a light breakfast early in the morning if surgery will be late in the afternoon (at least 6 hours after ingestion).
2. Stop breastfeeding at least 2 hours before the hospital arrival time. Unless otherwise instructed, stop formula feeding from the night before surgery.
3. Clear liquids, such as water, broth, ice pops, gelatin, and clear juices, can be taken up to 2 hours before time of arrival at the hospital.

during anesthesia induction is more effective in lowering a child's anxiety than other nonpharmacologic, distraction interventions such as playing video games or interacting with a clown (Mainer, 2010; Rieker & Krowchuk, 2007). When a parent is with the child during the start of anesthesia, it is important that the parent stays calm. Parents must have preparation in advance regarding what they will see happen to their child as anesthesia begins to take effect (e.g., sudden muscle relaxation, intubation) and what their role is in supporting their child (MacLaren & Kain, 2008; Romino, Keatley, Secrest, & Good, 2005). Once the child is "asleep," the parent is escorted from the operating room to the surgical waiting area. Parents should be informed of the anticipated length of the surgery and receive periodic status reports throughout the course of the procedure.

Postanesthesia Care

After surgery, the child is taken to the postanesthesia care unit (PACU) or recovery room. As the child gradually regains consciousness, the nurse performs frequent assessments of the child's neurologic, cardiorespiratory, and circulatory systems. Once the child is "awake," the parents should be present to comfort and calm the child. The child may also want a favorite toy or object. Providing warm blankets and a rocking chair as comfort measures can assist both the child and the parent. Pain medication should be given as indicated (see Chapter 15). Depending on the procedure performed, the child may be discharged to home from the PACU or admitted to an inpatient unit.

Postoperative Care

Most inpatient units have a specific protocol for postoperative care that is followed after a child has been transferred from the recovery room. At regular intervals, the child's vital signs are monitored, the surgical site is checked for drainage, fluid and electrolyte status is evaluated, and pain level is assessed. The use of patient-controlled analgesia (PCA)

and the routine administration of analgesics can provide acceptable pain control. It is imperative for the nurse to assess and document the child's pain level within a designated time period following medication administration to evaluate effectiveness. (See Chapter 15 for a more detailed discussion of pain management in children.)

Atelectasis, a common complication of surgery, can result from the effects of anesthesia combined with other factors such as inadequate lung expansion because of pain. Frequent lung auscultation is done to determine if adventitious breath sounds are present or if there are areas of diminished or absent breath sounds. A pulse oximeter may be used to check oxygen saturation. Children are prompted to perform deep breathing and coughing. The use of an incentive spirometer and games where the child blows cotton, a pinwheel, or bubbles can facilitate air exchange and lung expansion. Sitting the child up on the side of the bed or in a chair as well as early ambulation can also prevent atelectasis.

To facilitate their recuperation, children are discharged from the hospital as soon as safely possible after surgery. It is essential to thoroughly educate the child and family regarding how to monitor the child's condition and provide appropriate care at home. The parents must receive clear information on what signs and symptoms, if present, indicate a possible complication and require that the physician or another health care team member be contacted. The nurse should review with the parents written schedules and instructions for medications, incision care, bathing, diet, and activity, allowing time for questions. Regarding procedures such as dressing changes, the nurse should instruct and demonstrate first and then allow the parents to perform a return demonstration before leaving the hospital.

When a child undergoes an outpatient surgery, the parents manage the postoperative recovery of their child at home, including pain management. Studies have shown that parents and children may have misconceptions about pain medications and some children do not receive the recommended doses of pain medication at home (Chorney & Kain, 2010). Children may refuse to swallow a pill or liquid suspension, and parents can be reluctant to administer pain medications because of concern over side effects. More complete education on pain medications, provided at a time when the child and parents are able to focus and comprehend, is needed (Chorney & Kain, 2010).

With decreased lengths of stay, discharge planning has to begin at the time of admission. The nurse identifies the child and family's specific needs and determines the resources that are required to support home care for the child. Some children need specialized services after discharge. Home health care agencies can provide supplies and equipment, additional family education, and nursing care in the home. The overall goal of discharge planning is a smooth transition from hospital to home for the child and family.

▌ KEY CONCEPTS

- Whenever possible, procedures are performed in the treatment room, not in the child's room.
- Certain procedures require informed consent. Children ages 7 years and older may need to assent to some procedures. Nurses must be familiar with state laws and the policies of their institution.
- Use of developmentally appropriate language when preparing children for procedures is essential.
- Children need to be praised for attempts at cooperation during a procedure and for accomplishing an expected task.
- Documentation of a procedure includes recording the preparation, key elements of the procedure, who performed the procedure, and how the child tolerated it.

- Standard Precautions are followed when collecting all specimens. Transmission-Based Precautions are used with patients known or suspected to have an infection that can be spread to others.
- Restraints are used only as a last resort to protect the child and others.
- Safety is of paramount concern for all children. Nurses must strictly observe safety principles when caring for children in a hospital setting.

REFERENCES

American Academy of Pediatrics. (2007). *Technical report: Reaffirmed. Mercury in the environment: Implications for pediatricians—2001.* Retrieved from http://aappolicy. aappublications.org/cgi/content/full/pediatrics;120/3 /683#SEC5.

American Academy of Pediatrics, Task Force on Sudden Infant Death Syndrome. (2008). *Policy statement: Reaffirmed. The changing concept of sudden infant death syndrome: Diagnostic coding shifts, controversies regarding the sleeping environment, and new variables to consider in reducing risk—2005.* Retrieved from http://aappolicy. aappublications.org/cgi/content/full/pediatrics;116/5/ 1245.

Axelrod, P. (2000). External cooling in the management of fever. *Clinical Infectious Disease, 31*(Suppl 5), 224-229.

Bahr, S., Senica, A., Gingras, L., & Ryan, P. (2010). Clinical nurse specialist-led evaluation of temporal artery thermometers in acute care. *Clinical Nurse Specialist: The Journal for Advanced Nursing Practice, 24*(5), 238-244.

Beckstrand, J., Ellett, M. L. C., & McDaniel, A. (2007). Predicting internal distance to the stomach for positioning nasogastric and orogastric feeding tubes in children. *Journal of Advanced Nursing, 59*(3), 274-289.

Boots, B., & Edmundson, E. (2010). A controlled, randomised trial comparing single to multiple application lidocaine analgesia in paediatric patients undergoing urethral catheterisation procedures. *Journal of Clinical Nursing, 19*, 744-748.

Brenner, M. (2007). Child restraint in the acute setting of pediatric nursing: An extraordinarily stressful event. *Issues in Comprehensive Pediatric Nursing, 30*(1-2), 29-37.

Carbone, E., Flanagan, C., Gibbons, S., et al. (2010). Is tympanic thermometry an accurate method compared to axillary thermometry for recording temperature in infants less than 6 months of age? *Journal of Pediatric Nursing, 25*(2), e2-e3.

Centers for Disease Control and Prevention. (2002). Guideline for hand hygiene in health care settings. *MMWR Morbidity and Mortality Weekly Report, 51*(RR16), 1-44.

Centers for Disease Control and Prevention. (2011). *Dental fluorosis.* Retrieved from www.cdc.gov/fluoridation/ safety/dental_fluorosis.htm#6.

Child Health Corporation of America (Nursing Falls Study Task Force). (2009). Pediatric falls: The state of the science. *Pediatric Nursing, 35*(4), 227-231.

Chorney, J., & Kain, Z. (2010). Family-centered pediatric perioperative care. *Anesthesiology, 112*(3), 65-74.

Davie, A., & Amoore, J. (2010). Best practice in the measurement of body temperature. *Nursing Standard, 24*(42), 42-49.

Devrim, I., Kara, A., Ceyhan, M., et al. (2007). Measurement accuracy of fever by tympanic and axillary thermometry. *Pediatric Emergency Care, 23*(1), 16-19.

El-Radhi, A., & Patel, S. (2007). Temperature measurement in children with cancer: An evaluation. *British Journal of Nursing, 16*(21), 1313-1316.

Etoubleau, C., Reveret, M., Brouet, D., et al. (2009). Moving from bag to catheter for urine collection in non-toilet-trained children suspected of having urinary tract infection: A paired comparison of urine culture. *The Journal of Pediatrics, 154*(6), 803-806.

Exergen Corp. (2005). *Exergen temporal artery thermometer: Instructions for use.* Retrieved from www.exergen.com// medical/PDFs/tat2000instrev6.pdf.

Farrington, M., Lang, S., Cullen, L., & Stewart, S. (2009). Nasogastric tube placement verification in pediatric and neonatal patients. *Pediatric Nursing, 35*(1), 17-24.

Finley, G., Stewart, S., Buffett-Jerrott, S., et al. (2006). High levels of impulsivity may contraindicate midazolam premedication in children. *Canadian Journal of Anesthesia, 53*, 73-78.

Goldman, L., Shannon, M., & Committee on Environmental Health. (2001). Technical report: Mercury in the environment: Implications for pediatricians (RE 109907). *Pediatrics, 108*(1), 197-205.

Holzhauer, J., Reith, V., Sawin, K., & Yen, K. (2009). Evaluation of temporal artery thermometry in children 3-36 months old. *Journal for Specialists in Pediatric Nursing, 14*(4), 239-244.

Huffman, S., Jarczyk, K., O'Brien, E., et al. (2004). Methods to confirm feeding tube placement: Application of research in practice. *Pediatric Nursing, 30*(1), 10-13.

Ireton, F. (2007). Tracheostomy suction: A protocol for practice. *Paediatric Nursing, 19*(10), 14-18.

MacLaren, J., & Kain, Z. (2008). Development of a brief behavioral intervention for children's anxiety at anesthesia induction. *Children's Health Care, 37*, 196-209.

Mainer, J. (2010). Nonpharmacological interventions for assisting the induction of anesthesia in children. *Cochran Nursing Corner, 92*(2), 209-210.

McGillivray, D., Mok, E., Mulrooney, E., & Kramer, M. (2005). A head-to-head comparison: "Clean-void" bag versus catheter urinalysis in the diagnosis of urinary tract infection in young children. *The Journal of Pediatrics, 147*(4), 451-456.

Metheny, N. (2009). Verification of feeding tube placement (blinded inserted). *AACN (American Association of Critical Care Nurses) Practice Alert.* Retrieved from www.aacn.org/WD/Practice/Docs/PracticeAlerts/ Verification_of_Feeding_Tube_Placement_05-2005.pdf.

Mularoni, P., Cohen, L., DeGuzman, M., et al. (2009). A randomized clinical trial of lidocaine gel for reducing infant distress during urethral catheterization. *Pediatric Emergency Care, 25*(7), 439-443.

National High Blood Pressure Education Program Working Group on High Blood Pressure in Children and Adolescents. (2004). The fourth report on the diagnosis, evaluation, and treatment of high blood pressure in children and adolescents. *Pediatrics, 114*(Suppl 2), 555-576.

National Institute of Health and Clinical Excellence. (2007). *Feverish illness in children: Assessment and initial management in children younger than 5 years* (Clinical Guideline). Retrieved from www.nice.org.uk/nicemedia/ live/11010/30525/30525.pdf.

Paes, B., Vermeulen, K., Brohet, R., et al. (2010). Accuracy of tympanic and infrared skin thermometer in children. *Archives of Disease in Childhood, 95*(12), 974-978.

Parrilla, C., Scarano, E., Guidi, M. L., et al. (2007). Current trends in paediatric tracheostomies. *International Journal of Pediatric Otorhinolaryngology, 71*(10), 1563-1567.

Perrott, D., Piira, T., Goodenough, B., & Champion, G. (2004). Efficacy and safety of acetaminophen vs. ibuprofen for treating children's pain or fever: A meta-analysis. *Archives of Pediatrics, & Adolescent Medicine, 158*(6), 521-526.

Pickering, T., Hall, J. E., Appel, L. J., et al. (2005). Recommendations for blood pressure measurement in humans and experimental animals. Part 1: Blood pressure measurement in humans: A statement for professionals from the Subcommittee of Professional and Public Education of the American Heart Association Council on High Blood Pressure Research. *Hypertension, 45*(1), 142-161.

Razmus, I., Wilson, D., Smith, R., & Newman, E. (2006). Falls in hospitalized children. *Pediatric Nursing, 32*(6), 568-572.

Rieker, M., & Krowchuk, H. (2007). Should parents be present during their child's anesthesia induction? *MCN: The Journal of Maternal/Child Nursing, 32*(2), 72-73.

Romino, S., Keatley, V., Secrest, J., & Good, K. (2005). Parental presence during anesthesia induction in children. *AORN Journal, 81*(4), 780-792.

Schell, K. (2006). Evidence-based practice: Noninvasive blood pressure measurement in children. *Pediatric Nursing, 32*(3), 263-267.

Siegel, J., Rhinehart, E., Jackson, M., Chiarello, & the Healthcare Infection Control Practices Advisory Committee. (2007). *2007 Guideline for isolation precautions: Preventing transmission of infectious agents in healthcare settings.* Retrieved from www.cdc.gov/ncidod/dhqp/pdf/ isolation2007.pdf.

Sparks, L., Setlik, J., & Luhman, J. (2007). Parental holding and positioning to decrease IV distress in young children: A randomized controlled trial. *Journal of Pediatric Nursing, 22*(6), 440-447.

Vaughan, M., Paton, E., Bush, A., & Pershad, J. (2005). Does lidocaine gel alleviate the pain of bladder catheterization in young children? *Pediatrics, 116*(4), 917-920.

Ward, M., & Lentzsch-Parcells, C. (2009). Fever: Pathogenesis and treatment. In J. Cherry, S. Kaplan, G. Demmler-Harrison, & W. Steinbach (Eds.), *Feigin & Cherry's textbook of pediatric infectious diseases* (6th ed., pp. 105-109). Philadelphia: Elsevier.

Wilson, M. (2005). Tracheostomy management. *Paediatric Nursing, 117*(3), 38-44.

Medication Administration and Safety for Infants and Children

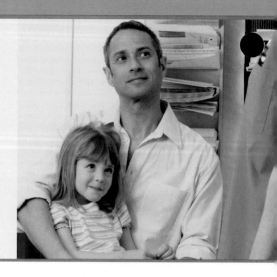

evolve WEBSITE

http://evolve.elsevier.com/James/ncoc

LEARNING OBJECTIVES

After studying this chapter, you should be able to:

- Describe different methods of administering medications to children.
- List the advantages and disadvantages of each route of administering medication to children.
- Describe the physiologic differences between children and adults that affect medicating a child.

- Describe psychosocial interventions for teaching and successful medication administration for each age-group.
- Describe quality and safety issues associated with medication administration in children.

Medicating infants and children is one of the nurse's most important responsibilities. The nurse plays a key role in administering medications, supporting the child and family during the experience, and teaching the child and parents about pharmacologic aspects of the child's care. Although physicians or nurse practitioners prescribe medications, the nurse or caregiver is responsible for their administration. The nurse has a legal responsibility to administer medications safely and accurately. Safe administration of medications to children requires an understanding of the dosages of the medications used for children and the expected actions, possible side effects, and signs of adverse reactions or toxicity. Nurses should use reliable sources of information (e.g., pharmacists, drug handbooks, hospital formularies) when administering medications and should ask the prescribing practitioner questions about orders that are unclear, inaccurate, or potentially incorrect before administering the medication.

Giving medications to children requires special skills. To gain the child's cooperation and to administer the medication in the least traumatic manner, the nurse needs to understand the physical characteristics and psychological needs of children at each developmental level. The nurse should use developmentally appropriate strategies to manage children's fears, prevent injury, and enhance coping.

It is vitally important to provide parents with information about medications used in their child's treatment and to encourage parents to support their child during experiences related to medications. Involving parents in the task of eliciting their child's cooperation not only makes the job easier but also gives the family a sense of self-management and control. If the parents will need to administer medications to their child at home, the nurse ensures that the parents receive complete instructions and correctly demonstrate medication administration techniques before the child is discharged.

Adherence to taking the full course of a medication to treat an acute illness or following a medication regimen for chronic illness management continues to be a challenge for children, adolescents, and their families (Matsui, 2007; Rapoff & Lindsely, 2007). Barriers to effective adherence to medications include cost, medication taste, inability to read or comprehend directions, misunderstanding about the correct dose or number of times to take the medication, and lack of understanding about the illness and need for the medication (Gerald, McClure, Mangan et al., 2009; Mears, Charlebois, & Holl, 2006).

Factors that improve medication adherence include allowing adequate time for the health care provider to educate the parent and child, continuity of care, availability of the health provider to answer questions about the medication, a medication schedule that fits the family's lifestyle, low cost, oral route, palatable taste for oral drugs, and low potential for side effects. Any medication regimen should consider the child's developmental needs. Further, a variety of administration, educational, and behavioral strategies need to be used; these include simple dosing schedules that correlate with daily routine, explanation of treatment goals, negotiation of treatment regimens, teaching ways to minimize side effects, supervised practice of skills by child and family, providing cues for monitoring adherence, promoting adherence through positive reinforcement, and encouraging self-management for older children and adolescents (Kamps, Rapoff, Roberts, et al., 2008; Rapoff & Lindsely, 2007).

PHARMACOKINETICS IN CHILDREN

An understanding of pharmacokinetics and pharmacodynamics guides appropriate interventions in children. Pharmacokinetics refers to the actions of a drug (e.g., movement, biotransformation) within the human body over time, and pharmacodynamics is the behavior of a drug as it interacts with the biochemical and physiologic milieu of the body. The pharmacokinetic actions of absorption, distribution, metabolism, and excretion are influenced by the physiologic environment in which the drug moves, and this environment differs between adults and children (Figure 14-1). The physiologic differences in body systems are most striking in the neonate.

Absorption
Oral Route
When a medication is given orally, several factors influence its absorption along the gastrointestinal (GI) tract. Because most medication absorption occurs in the small intestine, the drug must reach that location in a form suitable for maximum absorption. Four factors influence this process.

- Gastric acidity
- Gastric emptying time
- GI motility, or transit time through the GI tract
- Function of the pancreatic enzymes

Gastric Acidity. The gastric secretions of infants are less acidic than those of older children or adults. Secretions slowly increase in acidity during the first 2 years of life. Children, particularly infants and toddlers, tend to eat more frequently than adults and thus often have food and digestive enzymes present in their stomachs. Formula or milk can increase the alkalinity of gastric secretions, decreasing the absorption of medications that require a more acidic environment, and enhancing the absorption of medications that require a more alkaline milieu. These factors can greatly affect serum drug levels.

Gastric Emptying. Gastric emptying is intermittent and unpredictable in infants; it does tend to be slower than in older children. This slower pace can prolong the time it takes a medication to reach the intestinal absorption site.

Gastrointestinal Motility. Depending on whether an infant or young child has eaten recently, peristaltic activity in the intestine can be faster or slower than in an older child or adult. Infants up to 8

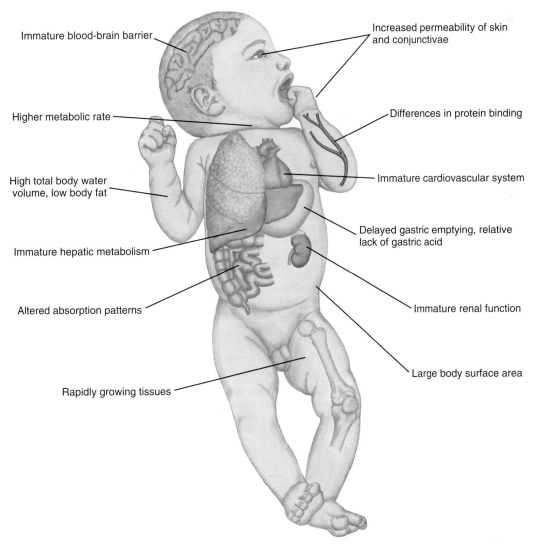

FIG 14-1 Physiologic differences between children and adults affect drug absorption, metabolism, distribution, and excretion. These differences are most significant for infants.

Labels on figure:
- Immature blood-brain barrier
- Higher metabolic rate
- High total body water volume, low body fat
- Immature hepatic metabolism
- Altered absorption patterns
- Rapidly growing tissues
- Increased permeability of skin and conjunctivae
- Differences in protein binding
- Immature cardiovascular system
- Delayed gastric emptying, relative lack of gastric acid
- Immature renal function
- Large body surface area

months of age tend to have prolonged motility. Certain adverse health conditions, such as diarrhea, can alter intestinal motility by increasing peristalsis. The longer the transit time in the intestine, the more medication that is absorbed. Conversely, a shortened transit time decreases medication absorption.

Enzyme Activity. Pancreatic enzyme activity also is variable in infants for the first 3 months of life as the gastrointestinal system matures. Medications that require specific enzymes for dissolution and absorption might not be converted to a suitable form for intestinal action.

Other Routes

Adequate absorption of medication administered intravenously (IV) depends on adequate peripheral perfusion. Medications given IV are immediately available for absorption into the child's bloodstream. When compared to an adult, a child's peripheral circulation is less reliable and more responsive to environmental changes. As a result, vasoconstriction or vasodilation can occur and alter the absorption of a parenteral medication. Also, the cardiovascular system is less able to accommodate large or rapid changes in volume, and fluid overload can result from poorly controlled IV infusions. A child has a smaller muscle mass than an adult; an infant's body weight is about 25% muscle, compared to an adult whose body weight is about 40% muscle. Thus, infants have fewer sites available for intramuscular (IM) injections. Further, blood flow to muscle tissue can be erratic in young children, and this can increase or decrease the absorption of IM medications.

Infants and young children have a thinner outer skin layer (stratum corneum) and a larger body surface area (BSA) to weight ratio. Infants have more skin surface area relative to weight than adults and thus the absorption of topical medications is much greater than adults. Skin pH varies with age and can affect the absorption of topical medications as well. Children also tend to be more prone to skin irritation, resulting in more frequent contact dermatitis and other allergic reactions. Irritated or open skin can enhance the absorption of topical medications.

Distribution

Distribution refers to the general and specific concentration of the medication in body fluids and tissues. Medications are distributed to body tissues through blood and body fluids.

Differences in Body Fluids

Fluid differences between children younger than 2 years and older children must be considered when the nurse determines dosages of medication. The body fluid content ranges from 75% of body weight in infants to 60% of body weight in children 2 years and older (see Chapter 16). Because of their greater fluid volume per weight, children need a higher dose per kilogram of a water-soluble medication to achieve the desired distribution effects.

A higher percentage of the young child's body fluid is located in the extracellular fluid compartment. During certain illnesses, this extracellular fluid can be lost rapidly, causing fluid depletion. It is important to adjust medication dosages accordingly in an ill infant or young child to avoid overdosing or underdosing.

Differences in Fat Percentages

Percentages of fat also change as the child grows. Fat makes up about 16% of an infant's weight, although total body fat varies from child to child. The percentage of fat per body weight is increased in a 1-year-old as compared to an infant, but then decreases in a preschool child. The percentage of body fat affects the distribution of fat-soluble medications in children. Because body fat must be saturated with a fat-soluble medication before the drug becomes detectable in the blood, dosages often must be varied to achieve desired effects.

Differences in Proteins

Medications bind to plasma proteins, mainly albumin, for distribution. Only free, unbound medication can be absorbed by the body. Because preterm and newborn infants have lower levels of plasma proteins than do older children, more unbound drug circulates. This alters the amount of medication needed to maintain a therapeutic drug level and may increase the infant's vulnerability to adverse drug effects.

Blood-Brain Barrier

The blood-brain barrier does not fully mature until a child is about 2 years old. This immaturity causes the barrier to be less selective, allowing the distribution of medications into the central nervous system. As a result, encephalopathy can occur with some medications.

The relative immaturity of the neurologic system also can lead to paradoxical effects from certain medications. For example, medications that normally cause sedation in adults may have the opposite effect in some children, causing hyperactivity.

Metabolism

Most medications are metabolized in the liver. Metabolic enzyme systems are less mature in newborn and premature infants, so they may not properly metabolize all the medication in a given dose. Older infants, toddlers, and preschoolers metabolize certain drugs (e.g., pain medications) more rapidly than adults. For this reason, larger dosages or more frequent administration of certain drugs might be needed for young children to achieve desired therapeutic outcomes.

Excretion

Most medications are excreted through the renal system. A newborn's renal system is immature with a lower glomerular filtration rate and less efficient renal tubular function. Adult levels of renal function are not reached until between 1 and 2 years of age. Infants and young children also are unable to concentrate urine as compared to older children or adults (see Chapter 20).

Because of renal immaturity, adequate quantities of a given medication may not be filtered out of circulating blood and excreted in the urine (the primary method of medication excretion). As a result, a medication can circulate longer and reach toxic levels in the blood. Fluid volume loss (dehydration) can also decrease a child's ability to excrete medications and can adversely affect serum drug levels.

Concentration

To safely administer medications to children, nurses need to know the concentration of certain medications in the bloodstream. Maintaining serum levels within a safe, therapeutic range maximizes the desired effect of a medication while reducing the risk of toxicity. With certain medications, the physician will order peak and trough serum levels to be measured in order to monitor medication concentration. The peak concentration is not necessarily the highest concentration, but the concentration of the medication after it has been distributed. A medication reaches its peak concentration at a specified time after the medication has been administered.

The medication trough is the level at which the serum concentration is lowest. Trough levels usually are obtained just before the next medication dose is scheduled to be administered. Knowing the peak and trough range for a specific medication will assist the nurse to accurately assess the child's response, and potential for toxic effects.

PSYCHOLOGICAL AND DEVELOPMENTAL FACTORS

Growth and developmental principles and differences among age groups must always be considered when medicating a child. Eliciting support from the parents often will help ease the child's concerns and fears.

Always approach children according to their developmental level, providing appropriate explanations about medication procedures. To decrease feelings of powerlessness, give the child as many choices as possible. For example, ask if a preschooler wants to hold the cup or have the nurse or a parent hold it while drinking the medicine.

Restraints are seldom necessary for administration of medications. It is appropriate to ask a staff member to assist the child to hold still during an injection because the child's movements could jeopardize safe administration of the medication (see Chapter 13). Parents may help to distract and comfort their child.

Honesty, praise, and reward are important elements of the medication administration process. The nurse should give honest explanations and tell the child if a medication may have an unpleasant taste, when a procedure will be painful or uncomfortable and approximately how long the pain will last, and what the child can do to help during medication administration (e.g., not move, hold the cup). Terminology that is familiar and understandable (e.g., "pinching" or "stinging") should be used.

Praising the child after the medication administration for attempts at cooperation is important and helps gain trust and cooperation for future procedures. Even if the child had difficulty during the process, comment on at least one positive behavior (e.g., "I see that you did your best to take your medicine").

Rewards following a procedure often serve to encourage the child and reinforce appropriate behavior. The reward should be safe and appropriate for the child's age. Stickers are usually a good choice for younger children. For an older child, providing time for a favorite activity, such as watching a video, may serve as a suitable reward.

Infants

Administering medications to young infants can be relatively easy because of their small size. However, use of appropriate administration techniques is essential to prevent aspiration of liquid, oral medications or adverse effects from injections (see Chapter 5). Giving medications safely to a squirming, older infant can pose a great challenge, requiring the nurse to obtain help from other staff members to hold the child. Parents need to be informed about all medications their infant is receiving. Cuddling and comforting the infant before and after the procedure are also important interventions.

Toddlers and Preschoolers

Older toddlers (2 to 3 years) are prone to magical thinking and might view the administration of medication (especially if the procedure is invasive) as punishment for "bad" thoughts (see Chapter 6). The nurse prepares toddlers with age-appropriate explanations, using play if possible. Allowing older toddlers to examine the equipment before the procedure may enhance cooperation. Toddlers can prefer to sit on the parent's lap when receiving medications. Helpful approaches for toddlers include praise and cuddling after procedures as well as giving rewards, such as stickers.

Preschoolers (3 to 5 years) continue to use magical thinking. They fear the unknown and they fear painful procedures (see Chapter 6). This age-group benefits greatly from therapeutic play and participation. The nurse should offer the child as much control over the procedure and as many choices as possible (e.g., "Do you want to take your medication with juice or milk?"). The preschoolers may be able to hold

PATIENT-CENTERED TEACHING
Medication Administration and Parent Roles

Parents want to know how they can help their children during a procedure for administering medication. They may become concerned if the child refuses to take a medication that is intended to help the child recover from an illness. Nurses should do the following to empower parents:

- Obtain information from parents before administering a medication to their child:
  - Child's medication allergies or sensitivities
  - The child's ability to take medications (e.g., can the child swallow pills?)
  - Methods parents use to administer the medication (e.g., mixing it with a small amount of flavored syrup or jelly)
- Give parents a thorough explanation about all medications before administration. Include why the child needs the medication, anticipated therapeutic effects, possible side effects, how the medication will be administered (route, etc.), and expected location (e.g., injection site).
- Encourage parents to ask questions and express any concerns they may have, such as that a medication might not be effective or that it might be making their child ill. Parents know their children and often are aware of subtle changes before health care team members see them.
- According to the child's developmental level, explain to the child why a certain medication is needed. Be firm that the child must take the medication, but offer allowable choices whenever possible, such as what juice the child can drink after an oral medication or which leg can be used for an injection.
- If preferred by the child, allow parents to administer certain medications (e.g., oral, otic, ophthalmic). Check five of the "six rights" of medication administration (right patient, right drug, right dose, right time, and right route) *before* you allow a parent to administer a medication.
- Show parents the most acceptable position for their child when administering a particular medication. Assist the child to maintain this position as needed.
- To increase cooperation, recommend the use of positive reinforcements such as rewards or stickers after the child has taken a medication.
- Complete the sixth right of medication administration—the right documentation—by documenting all required information in the child's medical record.

still for an invasive procedure, though it is best to have a staff member ready to assist. Adhesive bandages after an invasive procedure, such as an injection, are important to children in this age-group because many believe a Band-Aid will "make it better," an example of magical thinking.

School-Age Children

School-age children fear loss of control, pain, and injury. At this age, a child can understand more complex explanations (see Chapter 7) as to why they need to take medication in order to recover from illness. Offering the child as much choice as possible is of great importance. School-age children often cooperate fully, even with invasive procedures, but often need a source of distraction (e.g., squeezing a person's hand, listening to music, talking about a subject of interest) and support (see Chapters 13 and 15). School-age children still appreciate receiving praise and rewards.

Adolescents

Adolescents fear separation from peers and loss of control (see Chapter 8). Persons in this age-group understand adult explanations and can assist in making decisions about their nursing care. Often, however, adolescents exhibit a hyper-response to procedures that can seem inconsistent with their age. It is important to praise their cooperation, offer distractions, and help them find outlets for their frustrations (e.g., drawing, writing).

CALCULATING DOSAGES

The safe administration of medications to infants and children requires use of added safeguards that are above and beyond those for adult patients (American Academy of Pediatrics [AAP], 2007). Incorrect dosing, which includes errors in dosage calculations and dosing intervals, is the most common type of medication error in pediatrics (AAP, 2007). The nurse must always verify the accuracy of the ordered dose of medication before administration. First, the recommended dosage for the medication in mg/kg/day is checked and a calculation performed based on the child's weight to ensure that the right dose has been ordered. For example, the recommended dose for amoxicillin is 20 to 40 mg/kg/day; for a 10-kg child, the ordered dose should be between 200 and 400 mg per day. Second, the recommendation for the number of divided doses (e.g., every 4 hours, three times a day, every 12 hours) is confirmed. Last, the nurse ensures that route of administration is correct.

Dosages can also be calculated based on body surface area or BSA (milligrams per square meter [mg/m²]). Figure 14-2 shows how to use a nomogram to obtain the BSA for a child. To calculate a medication dose on the basis of BSA, use the following formula:

$$\text{Approximate dose} = \frac{\text{BSA of child}\,(m^2)}{1.7 \times \text{Adult dose}}$$

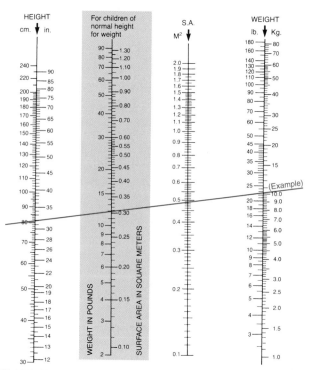

FIG 14-2 Nomogram for calculating BSA (body surface area); used for determining medication dosages for infants and children. (Nomogram in Custer, J., & Rau, R. [Eds.]. (2009). *The Harriet Lane handbook: A manual for pediatric house officers* [18th ed., p. 1032]. Philadelphia: Elsevier.)

MEDICATION ADMINISTRATION PROCEDURES

To avoid errors in medication administration, follow these general procedures:

- Adhere to the "six rights" of medication administration: right patient/child, right drug, right dose, right time, right route, and right documentation.
- Check the orders to be sure that all information is correctly transcribed. Note any allergies.
- Always double-check medication calculations before administration. Be sure the child's weight is accurately recorded.
- Double-check calculations of medications provided by the pharmacy in a unit dose form. Consult with the physician or pharmacist if there is any question about a dose.
- Ask another nurse to perform a second check for the following medications and any others as required by agency policy (Institute for Safe Medication Practices [ISMP], 2008):
  - Insulin (subcutaneous and IV)
  - Oral hypoglycemic agents
  - Dextrose hypertonic IV solutions (20% or greater)
  - Narcotics/opioids (transdermal, IV, and oral)
  - Medications administered via epidural/intrathecal route
  - Chemotherapeutic agents (oral and parenteral)
  - Digoxin or other inotropic medications
  - Anticoagulants
  - Anesthetic and moderate sedation agents (inhaled and IV)
  - Potassium chloride, hypertonic sodium chloride, and magnesium sulfate for injection

Medication Reconciliation

When admitting children to a hospital unit, the nurse obtains a list of all prescription and over-the-counter medications as well as any herbal preparations a child is taking at home. To ensure patient safety, the nurse compares the medications the child has been receiving at home to the list of medications prescribed for the child's hospital stay, identifying and communicating any discrepancies. This is referred to as medication reconciliation and is a process that is of paramount importance to preventing medication errors (Thompson, 2007). Further, the nurse assesses the parents' knowledge of all the medications (and herbal remedies) the child is taking. This includes the name of the medication, the dose, number of times a day the child is taking the medication, knowledge of side effects, the child's allergies, any adverse reactions the child might have experienced, and the time the medication was last administered. To facilitate medication reconciliation, parents are encouraged to bring all of their child's medications to the hospital or a clinic visit. However, one study found that this occurs only about half of the time and that the majority of parents were not able to provide complete information about their child's medication, adversely affecting the medication reconciliation process (Riley-Lawless, 2009).

At discharge, medication reconciliation includes providing clear, detailed written instructions to parents about all medications to be given at home and clearly communicating medication information to the next health care provider. The Joint Commission has recently updated its national patient safety goal for medication reconciliation to highlight critical risk points in the process (2010).

Children are at greater risk than adults for medication errors and adverse drug events causing harm to a child because of pharmacokinetics, dosages by weight or body mass, and narrow therapeutic-to-lethal ranges for many medications (Takata, Taketomo, & Waite, 2008). The Joint Commission (2008) has indicated that a significant percentage of pediatric adverse drug events are preventable. Recommendations to reduce the risk of pediatric medication errors include the following (The Joint Commission, 2010):

- Establish and implement standardized medications procedures and processes for drug administration.
- Limit the number of concentrations and dose strengths of high-alert medications.
- Use oral syringes to administer oral medications.
- Enable dose/dose range software programs to provide alerts for potentially incorrect dosages.
- Educate health care providers (nurses) about use of IV infusion pumps; recognize that medication errors can still occur.
- Use consistent physiologic monitoring (e.g., pulse oximetry) with age and size appropriate equipment for children under sedation.
- Use bar-coding technology that is adapted to pediatric processes and systems.
- On admission, weigh children in kilograms (kg) and use weight in kg for prescriptions, dose calculations, medical records, and staff communication.
- Use pediatric-specific medication formulations and concentrations.
- Comprehensive pediatric specialty training for all health care team members.

One of the major reasons for the increasing use of computer systems such as patient electronic medical records (EMRs) and computerized physician order entry (CPOE) is to reduce medication errors (Takata et al., 2008; Thompson, 2007). EMRs that include electronic medication administration records (EMARs) can improve communication of patient medication lists and other information, such as allergies, between different health care providers working in the same facility or in other settings (Agrawal & Wu, 2009). Use of web-based or computer dose calculators have been shown to reduce dosage calculation errors for pediatric patients (Conroy, Sweis, Planner et al., 2007). Although electronic systems have shown great potential to significantly reduce the incidence of medication errors, they have limitations and cannot eliminate all errors (Gerstle & Lehmann, 2007). These systems do not replace the responsibility of physicians and nurses for clear and complete medication orders, accurate dose calculations, and correct administration of medications to children.

Administering Oral Medications

The oral route is the most widely used method of administering medications. It is also one of the least reliable methods of administration because absorption is affected by the presence or absence of food in the stomach, gastric emptying time, GI motility, and stomach acidity. The oral route can be less predictable also because of medication loss to spillage, leaking, or spitting out.

Oral medications are available in liquid (elixir or suspension), tablet or capsule, chewable tablet, or sprinkle (powder) forms. If the child cannot swallow tablets or capsules, the nurse finds out whether the medication is available in a liquid form or as a chewable tablet. If not, the nurse determines if the tablet can be crushed or if the contents of a capsule can be emptied. It is not recommended to crush time-release medications (e.g., extended-release [XR], controlled-release [CR], sustained-release [SR]) as well as enteric-coated tablets.

Before administering oral medications, the nurse assesses the child's gag reflex and ability to swallow. The specific form of oral medication used should be tailored to the child's developmental level and ability

to successfully take a particular form. An assessment of the way the child takes medications at home will help determine the best form to use.

Preparation

When preparing to administer an elixir or a suspension, the nurse first ensures that the correct dose is drawn for administration. Physicians' orders often specify the dosage in milligrams (mg), *not* milliliters (mL), for liquid medications. It is important to calculate the mL dose properly on the basis of the number of mg per mL for the available liquid medication.

For volumes of 5 mL or less, a calibrated spoon or dropper, or a syringe designed for oral medication administration only, should be used. Pour larger volumes into calibrated plastic medicine cups, which generally hold up to 30 mL (1 oz.).

Mix a sprinkle, powder, or crushed tablet with a small amount (e.g., 1 to 3 teaspoons) of a nonessential food such as applesauce or pudding or with a liquid. Avoid mixing medications with necessary foods including formula, because this can alter the food's taste, and thus the child may refuse further intake of that food. Be sure to determine a medication's compatibility with food before mixing and administration.

Administration

The method for administering oral medications differs according to the child's age and developmental level. Infants usually receive elixir or suspension forms that are administered using an empty nipple or oral syringe. First, place the infant in an upright or semi-upright position, similar to the position used for feeding. Open the infant's mouth by applying gentle pressure to the chin or cheeks. If using a nipple, place the nipple in the infant's mouth and add the medication to the empty nipple when the baby begins to suck. If using an oral syringe, place the syringe gently in the infant's mouth along the side of the cheek and push the medication in slowly as the infant sucks (Figure 14-3). It may be necessary to hold an infant or young child in order to safely administer an oral medication. As seen in Figure 14-3, the nurse cradles the child's head between the nurse's nondominant arm and body, holds the child's hand with the nurse's nondominant hand, and then administers the oral medication using the dominant hand.

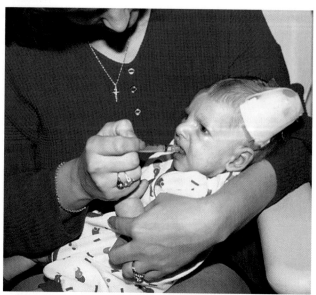

FIG 14-3 Administering an oral medication to an infant using an oral syringe. (Courtesy Parkland Health and Hospital System, Dallas, TX.)

Toddlers and preschoolers can easily take liquid medications from an oral syringe, a calibrated teaspoon, or a medicine cup. Allowing children to take their own medication, giving rewards as incentives, and providing choices that fit into the medication regimen enhance autonomy and cooperation.

Preschoolers and young school-age children can usually manage chewable tablets without difficulty. Many older, school-age children can swallow tablets or capsules; however, the nurse must assess a child's ability to swallow pills on an individual basis. If a child cannot swallow pills, the availability of other forms of oral medications, such as liquid suspensions or elixirs and powders, needs to be investigated.

Oral medications are given with the child in an upright or slightly recumbent position to facilitate swallowing and prevent aspiration. After administration of the medication, give the child a food or fluid item such as formula, juice, or an ice pop, if not contraindicated. Allow children to select what they would like to eat or drink after taking oral medications, whenever possible.

If a child vomits or spits up after administration of an oral medication, notify the physician. Another dose may need to be ordered depending on how long it has been since administration, the type of medication, and the amount of emesis.

Alternative Routes for Oral Medications

Oral medications can be administered directly into the GI tract through a feeding tube. If the medication is to be administered through a feeding tube, verify tube placement before administration (see Chapter 13) and, depending on the type of tube (e.g., transpyloric), determine whether the tube is the proper route for the ordered medication. Before and after the medication is administered, flush the tube with water to ensure that the medication has reached the GI tract and to prevent blockage in the tube.

Administering Injections

Injected medications are rapidly absorbed by diffusing into either plasma or the lymphatic system. Although injections result in faster and more reliable absorption than the oral route, injections are stressful and threatening to children and are not preferred. Injections are used most often for one-time doses of antibiotics (e.g., ceftriaxone for the initial treatment of severe infection), immunizations, insulin administration for diabetics, purified protein derivative (PPD) tuberculosis skin test, and allergy skin testing.

Appropriately preparing the child for an injection can reduce emotional and anticipatory concerns. Depending on the child's developmental level, explain the reason for the injection, any sensations the child might experience, and the length of time they are anticipated to last. Facilitate the child's understanding that an injection is not punishment but is needed to help the child get well or stay healthy. Practice distraction techniques such as deep breathing and singing with the child in advance.

Offer parents the option to stay with their child during the procedure or leave if they feel unable to cope with the stress. Many parents prefer to remain and help distract, comfort, and reassure their child who is receiving an injection.

To reduce the risk of injury, it is sometimes necessary to limit the child's movement before and during the administration of an injected medication. This can be accomplished by swaddling the child and/or obtaining the assistance of other health care professionals. Some parents may request to help hold their child while receiving an injection (Figure 14-4). Parents who feel confident in their ability to hold their child and prevent injury can be given this option. However, parents should not be required to restrain their child during a procedure.

Often children have great fears related to injections and perceive them to be very painful. Even with the best preparation and use of distraction techniques, it is hard for some children to cope with the pain of an injection although it may last for only seconds. Use of oral sucrose for infants and topical anesthetic agents, such as eutectic mixture of local anesthetics (EMLA) cream for all children, has been shown to be effective in reducing or even eliminating injection pain (see Chapter 15).

The child who must receive multiple injections might benefit significantly from therapeutic play during which the child uses a syringe to give "shots" to a doll. Therapeutic play is an effective approach to prepare a child for an injection (see Chapters 11 and 13). It may also help the child gain a sense of mastery over the experience of receiving injections, thus decreasing anxiety.

Documentation following an injection should include the amount of medication injected, the site used, and how the child tolerated the procedure. Federal vaccine regulations require nurses to record the vaccine manufacturer and lot number for each immunization given, as well as record and report any vaccine reactions.

Intramuscular Injections

Determine the injection site in advance, before initiating the injection procedure. The site should be soft and well vascularized with healthy, intact skin. The child's age, size, and muscle mass along with the volume and properties of the medication to be injected will influence the choice of the intramuscular (IM) injection site to be used. It is essential to accurately locate and inject at an appropriate IM site. This will help avoid injecting an IM medication into subcutaneous tissue or puncturing a blood vessel, nerve, or bone. The preferred IM injection sites in children are shown in Table 14-1.

Selection of the appropriate needle size and length will depend on the child's size, the amount of body fat (distance between skin surface and muscle), the injection site to be used, and the child's muscle mass at the IM site. It is important to always use the smallest size needle and the shortest length that that will safely and comfortably administer the

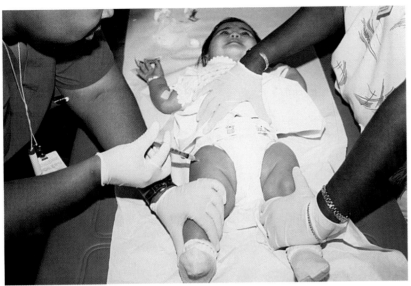
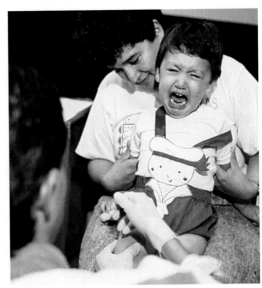

FIG 14-4 Two methods of holding a child for an IM injection at the vastus lateralis site. (*Left,* Courtesy Parkland Health and Hospital System Community-Oriented Primary Care Clinic, Dallas, TX. *Right,* Courtesy Cook Children's Medical Center, Fort Worth, TX.)

TABLE 14-1 PREFERRED INTRAMUSCULAR INJECTION SITES IN CHILDREN

SITE	KEY POINTS
Vastus lateralis 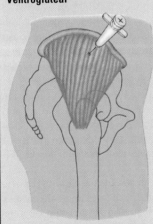	Location is the anterior lateral thigh. Well-developed muscle at birth. Often used for infants and children under 3 yr but acceptable site for all ages. Can tolerate larger fluid volumes. Not located near large nerves or blood vessels. Easy to access. Locate greater trochanter and knee joint; divide space into thirds; give the injection in the outer aspect of the middle third of the leg.
Ventrogluteal	Location is the gluteus medius muscle of the hip. Can be used for infants, children, and adolescents; often recommended for children 18-36 mo and walking. Can generally hold larger fluid volumes. Free of major nerves and vascular structures. Some reports of less pain than vastus lateralis site. Locate by placing heel of hand on greater trochanter with fingers pointed up and thumb pointed toward the groin. Place index finger over anterior superior iliac spine and middle finger along posterior iliac crest to form a **V** between the two fingers; give the injection in the center of the **V**.

Continued

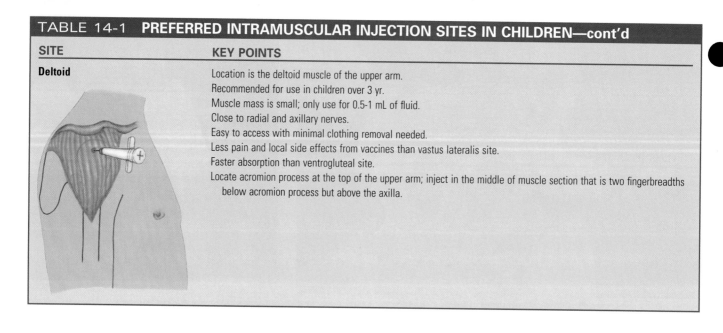

TABLE 14-1 **PREFERRED INTRAMUSCULAR INJECTION SITES IN CHILDREN—cont'd**

SITE	KEY POINTS
Deltoid	Location is the deltoid muscle of the upper arm.
	Recommended for use in children over 3 yr.
	Muscle mass is small; only use for 0.5-1 mL of fluid.
	Close to radial and axillary nerves.
	Easy to access with minimal clothing removal needed.
	Less pain and local side effects from vaccines than vastus lateralis site.
	Faster absorption than ventrogluteal site.
	Locate acromion process at the top of the upper arm; inject in the middle of muscle section that is two fingerbreadths below acromion process but above the axilla.

medication. In general, the needle size used for children will be 22 to 25 gauge and the length between $\frac{1}{2}$ and $1\frac{1}{2}$ inches. To inject a viscous medication, use of a larger gauge needle may be indicated.

⚡ SAFETY ALERT

Guidelines for Maximum Safe Volumes for Intramuscular Injections*

	SITE		
AGE	DELTOID	VENTROGLUTEAL	VASTUS LATERALIS
Premature	—	—	0.5 mL
Neonate	—	—	0.5-1 mL
Infant (1-12 mo)	—	—	1 mL
Toddler (13-36 mo)	0.5 mL	1 mL	1-1.5 mL
Young child (3-6 yr)	0.5-1 mL	1.5 mL	1.5-2 mL
Older child (6-14 yr)	0.5-1 mL	1.5-2 mL	1.5-2 mL
Adolescent (15 yr-adult)	1 mL	2-3 mL	2-3 mL

*Evaluate the individual child's muscle mass before injection.

Safe volumes for IM injections range from 0.5 mL for infants and young children to 3 mL for adolescents; however, each child's size and muscle mass must be individually assessed. After performing hand hygiene, don gloves, clean the skin at the injection site with an antiseptic swab or pad, and allow it to dry. Insert the needle at a 90-degree angle with a quick darting motion. Pull back gently on the plunger to aspirate for blood. If blood is noted, withdraw the needle and discard the needle and syringe. A new syringe and needle will be used to draw up medication again and attempt injection into a different site. If no blood is noted, give the injection slowly at a rate of 1 mL per 10 seconds. Remove the needle and apply gentle pressure at the site with a dry gauze pad; do not massage. If the child will receive several IM injections over time, it is important to rotate sites to prevent tissue irritation and possible muscle atrophy and wasting.

❓ CRITICAL THINKING EXERCISE 14-3

You need to immunize an infant with the hepatitis B vaccine. The dosage ordered for the infant is 2.5 mcg. The vaccine you have available has 5 mcg per mL. How many milliliters (mL) will you administer to infant via an intramuscular (IM) injection?

Subcutaneous Injections

A subcutaneous injection is given into the connective tissue that lies just below the dermis layer of the skin. This type of administration is used for medications that provide a sustained effect (e.g., heparin, insulin) or for certain immunizations. A subcutaneous injection should be given only into healthy tissue free from infection, bruising, and scarring. If circulation is impaired because of conditions such as shock or vascular disease, a subcutaneous injection should not be used because absorption will be altered.

Preferred subcutaneous injection sites for children are outer posterior aspects of the upper arms and the anterior aspects of the thighs (Figure 14-5). The abdomen, excluding a 2-inch radius around the umbilicus, is another site that is often used for children who require frequent subcutaneous injections (e.g., type 1 diabetics). Systematically rotating sites can facilitate consistent drug absorption. The site of each subcutaneous injection must be recorded in order to properly rotate sites.

Subcutaneous injections are typically given with a 25- to 27-gauge needle that is $\frac{3}{8}$ to $\frac{5}{8}$ inch long. Volumes for subcutaneous injections are usually 0.5 mL; maximum volume is 1 mL.

After performing hand hygiene, don gloves, clean the site in a circular pattern with an antiseptic swab, and allow the skin to dry. Gently pinch the tissue to raise the subcutaneous tissue from the muscle. The angle of needle insertion is usually 45 degrees; some nurses use a 90-degree angle with a $\frac{1}{2}$-inch needle. Insert the needle with the bevel up using a dart-like motion. Release the tissue and inject the medication. After removing the needle, gentle pressure can be applied to the site using a dry gauze pad; do not massage.

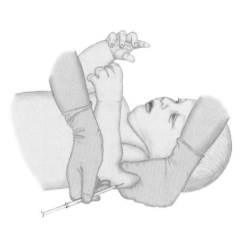

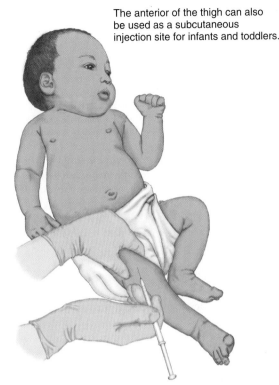

The anterior of the thigh can also be used as a subcutaneous injection site for infants and toddlers.

Use the dorsum of the upper arm of infants and toddlers for subcutaneous injections.

FIG 14-5 Two of the preferred subcutaneous injection sites for infants and toddlers.

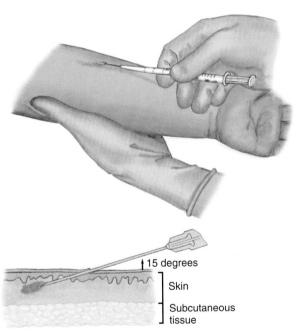

15 degrees

Skin

Subcutaneous tissue

FIG 14-6 Intradermal injection site and technique.

Intradermal Injections

Intradermal injections enter the dermis layer of skin, which is just below the epidermis, and usually on the inner aspect of the forearm or on the upper back. They are most often used for allergy testing or TB screening (PPD). The needle used is 25 or 27 gauge and ⅜- to

⅝-inch in length. The maximum volume injected is 0.1 mL. After performing hand hygiene, don gloves and clean the site in a circular pattern with an antiseptic swab and allow the skin to dry. Turn the bevel of the needle up and insert gently at a 5- to 15-degree angle, barely penetrating the skin (Figure 14-6). Inject the medication slowly to form a bleb or wheal.

Rectal Administration

Medications given rectally can have a localized effect on the GI tract such as prompting defecation. They also can have a systemic effect such as decreasing fever, though absorption of medication administered by the rectal route is not as reliable as the oral route. Per rectum medication administration is usually reserved for times when a child cannot eat or drink or is unable to tolerate oral intake because of nausea and vomiting. There is a risk of injury to the anal and rectal tissues. This route should not be used if the rectum is full of stool. Also, rectal medication is contraindicated in children with rectal disease or those who have had rectal surgery.

Rectal administration is stressful for children because they fear intrusive procedures. Carefully prepare the child and explain the reason the medication is being given via this route, the steps of the procedure, and what the child can do to help.

Position the child on the left side with the right leg slightly flexed, exposing the anal area sufficiently for visibility. Adequate draping is essential for preschool and older children. Distraction and deep-breathing exercises can help the child relax the external sphincter.

Perform hand hygiene and don gloves. Place water-soluble lubricant on the suppository. Advise the child to take a deep breath or bear down, if possible, to relax the sphincter. Then, depending on the size of the child's anus, use either the index finger or little finger to gently insert the suppository through the anus and past the internal sphincter (approximately 1.5 to 2.5 cm). After insertion, hold the infant or young child's buttocks together for at least 5 minutes. Instruct older children and adolescents not to expel the suppository for 5 to 10 minutes.

Vaginal Administration

The vaginal route is used primarily for school-age or adolescent girls who require topical treatment with an antiinfective agent for a vaginal infection. It is essential to explain the procedure, why it is indicated, and how the child can help.

Ask the child to void and then assist her into a supine position with the soles of her feet together and her knees resting on the bed (frog-leg position). Remember to use drapes and provide for privacy. After hand hygiene and donning gloves, gently spread the labia so that the vaginal orifice is visible. Lubricate the tablet, suppository, or applicator with a water-soluble lubricant. Have the patient take a deep breath and then gently insert the vaginal medication approximately 7.5 to 10 cm along the posterior wall of the vagina.

After the procedure is completed, the child may need to remain in a supine position for at least 10 minutes. Older school-age children and adolescents can be taught to instill their own vaginal medications.

Ophthalmic Administration

For children, most ophthalmic medications come in the form of drops or ointment. If these preparations are refrigerated, allow them to warm to room temperature before instillation. After performing hand hygiene and donning gloves, gently remove any exudates by wiping the child's eye with a sterile gauze pad (move from inner to outer canthus) using a different pad for each eye. Shake all suspensions well before instillation. Eyedrops are instilled into the conjunctival sac. Eye ointment is applied along the inside edge of the lower eyelid from the inner to the outer canthus (Procedure 14-1).

Otic Administration

When instilling medications into the ear (otic), the child is positioned supine with the head turned to allow access to the appropriate side (Procedure 14-2). If drainage is present, which may occur if the tympanic membrane is ruptured, gloves must be worn, following hand hygiene, to instill eardrops. First, gently clean any exudates from the outer ear with a sterile gauze pad. Never attempt to clean the ear canal by placing any item such as a cotton-tipped applicator (Q-tip) inside the ear. To avoid pain, otic solutions should be allowed to warm to room temperature before administration.

Nasal Administration

Generally, nose drops and sprays are used for localized treatment of the nasal passages. However, the mucous membranes inside the nose allow for fairly rapid systemic absorption of medications. A wide range of medications can be given to children intranasally, including antidiuretic hormone (DDAVP), fentanyl, ketamine, midazolam (Versed), and lorazepam.

Before administering nose drops to an infant, the nurse removes any excess mucus by gently suctioning the nares with a bulb syringe.

PROCEDURE 14-1   ADMINISTERING AN OPHTHALMIC PREPARATION

PURPOSE: To Treat an Eye Infection, Dilate Pupils for Diagnostic Testing, or Keep Eyes Moist

1. Explain the purpose for the medication or lubricating drops. Explain any expected sensations to the child in developmentally appropriate terms (e.g., "It will feel like there is something in your eye for just a minute"). Explain that the child might have blurred vision for a short time afterward. Tell the child how to help with the procedure ("Be sure to not rub your eyes"). Assistance in holding a young child might be necessary.
2. Gather needed equipment: Eyedrops or ointment, gloves, gauze pads, sterile saline solution for irrigation, and tissues. Use appropriate hand hygiene and don gloves.
3. Assist the child into a supine position with the neck slightly hyperextended (e.g., by placing a rolled towel or small blanket under the shoulder blades).
4. If the drops are to be instilled into the eye of an infant or young child, obtain assistance in holding the child's arms and head or use a mummy wrap if necessary.
5. If crusts or exudates are seen, use a sterile gauze pad that has been moistened with sterile saline and gently remove the crusts and drainage. Perform hand hygiene and don a new pair of gloves.
6. Instruct an older child to look upward and gently pull the lower lid down and away from the eye.
7. Place the drops into the space between the eye and lower lid, the conjunctival sac, taking care not to contaminate the end of the dropper.
8. Place a ribbon of ointment on the inside edge of the lower eyelid moving from the inner to the outer canthus, taking care to not contaminate the end of the ointment tube. If both drops and ointment are ordered, the drops should be administered first.

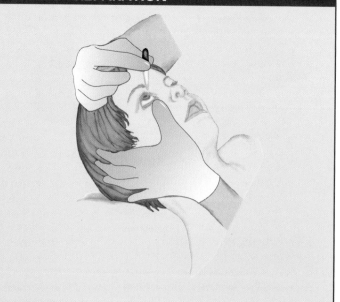

9. Have the child look down as the lower lid is released. Encourage the child to close both eyes gently and keep them closed for several seconds. Carefully blot any excess medication. Remove gloves and perform hand hygiene.
10. Praise the child for cooperation and assistance. Document all pertinent information, including how the child tolerated the procedure and responded to the medication, in the child's medical record.

PROCEDURE 14-2 ADMINISTERING OTIC DROPS

PURPOSE: To Treat Inflammation or Infection of the Ear Canal, Relieve Pain, or Prevent Otitis Externa

1. Explain any expected sensations to the child in developmentally appropriate terms (e.g., "It may sound like there is a butterfly flying inside your ear"). Describe how the child can help. Assistance in holding a young child might be necessary.
2. Gather the following equipment: Otic drops, gloves, sterile gauze pad, sterile cotton-tipped applicator, and cotton pieces. Use appropriate hand hygiene and don gloves. Ensure that the otic drops are at room temperature.
3. If drainage is noted in the ear, remove it from the external ear *only* with a sterile gauze pad or cotton-tipped applicator. Perform hand hygiene and don a new pair of gloves.
4. Position the child lying down with the affected ear up or sitting with the head turned so the affected ear is up.
5. Brace the administering hand against the child's head above the ear.
6. If the child is 3 years old or younger, pull the pinna of the ear down and toward the back of the head, holding near the lobe. If the child is older than 3 years, pull the pinna up and toward the back.
7. Insert the required number of drops, taking care not to contaminate the end of the drops container. Then gently massage or apply slight pressure to the tragus (anterior portion) with the index finger.
8. Place cotton loosely into the outermost portion of the canal, if ordered. Instruct the child not to remove the cotton or place anything inside the ear.
9. Keep the child on the unaffected side for 5 to 10 minutes after administration. If medication is to be administered in both ears, repeat the procedure in the other ear.
10. Remove gloves and perform hand hygiene.
11. Praise the child for cooperation and assistance. Document all pertinent information, including how the child tolerated the procedure and responded to the medication, in the child's medical record.

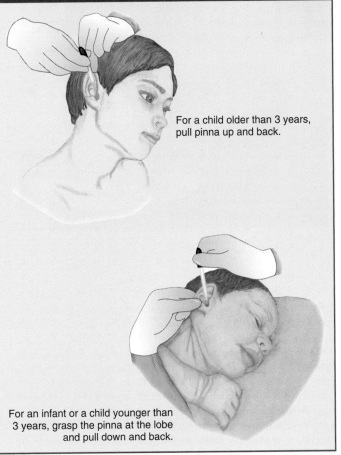

For a child older than 3 years, pull pinna up and back.

For an infant or a child younger than 3 years, grasp the pinna at the lobe and pull down and back.

To make eating more comfortable for a congested infant, saline nose drops are given followed by gentle suction, 20 to 30 minutes before feedings.

Nose drops can cause an uncomfortable sensation when administered, which can be stressful for young children. Provide a thorough explanation of what the child will feel, how the medication will make it easier to breathe through the nose, and what the child needs to do to help. Assistance with holding may be necessary for young children.

Place the child supine with the head in the midline position and the neck slightly hyperextended. After performing hand hygiene and donning gloves, instill the number of drops ordered into each naris. Keep the child's head in this same position for 1 minute. Instruct the child not to blow the medication out the nose. Praise all efforts at cooperation.

Topical Administration

Topical medications (creams, lotions, ointments, patches, and pastes) can produce local as well as systemic effects when absorbed through the skin. Adhesive, transdermal patches release medication on a continuous basis over a prescribed time period (hours or even days). They are changed at scheduled intervals, and thus the child is cautioned to keep the patch in place. The patch is applied to clean, dry skin free of bruises, abrasions, and irritation. The nurse must wear gloves during the application of a transdermal patch.

A variety of prescription and over-the-counter creams, lotions, and ointments are used to treat skin irritation, dryness, or infection. Once the procedure has been explained to the child, perform hand hygiene, don gloves, cleanse the skin to remove any exudates, scales, or other residue, and allow it to dry. Don a new pair of gloves and apply the ointment or cream per orders/instructions. Encourage the child to avoid touching the treated areas.

Inhalation Therapy

Respiratory medications, used frequently in children, are delivered by a nebulizer or a metered-dose inhaler, a hand-held device that delivers "puffs" of medication for inhalation (see Chapter 21). Although many inhaled medications have an unpleasant taste or smell, this route is a relatively nonthreatening form of medication delivery. Monitoring for desired therapeutic effects as well as systemic side effects is essential.

Nebulized medications are diluted in normal saline solution and administered with a hand-held, small-volume nebulizer. The nebulizer aerosolizes the medication for the child to inhale. Medication can be delivered through a facemask or through a plastic mouthpiece held between the lips or close to the face (Figure 14-7). Encourage the child to breathe deeply and slowly during the treatment.

Nebulized medication can be delivered along with supplemental oxygen to a hospitalized child with an acute episode of respiratory distress. Nebulized medications can also be delivered to an unconscious

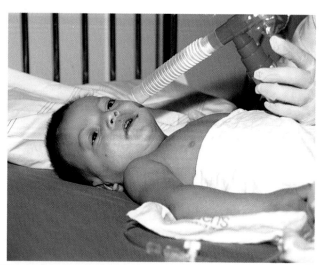

FIG 14-7 Administration of nebulized medication to an infant. (Courtesy Children's Medical Center, Dallas, TX.)

PROCEDURE 14-3 **USING A METERED-DOSE INHALER (MDI)**

PURPOSE: To Deliver Medication Directly to the Respiratory System

1. Verify the physician's order for the medication(s) to be administered and the number of puffs prescribed.
2. If one of the medications is an inhaled steroid, administer it last.
3. Explain the procedure to the child and parents. It is often helpful to demonstrate the use of the inhaler and to explain specifically what the child is expected to do.
4. Perform hand hygiene. Shake the inhaler well and remove the cap.
5. Hold the inhaler upright and attach to the spacer. Tell the child not to inhale too quickly or the spacer will whistle.
6. Ask the child to tilt the head back slightly, take a deep breath, and then exhale ("big breath out") slowly. Place the spacer mouthpiece in the child's mouth or the spacer mask over the face. The child might be more comfortable holding the spacer and helping you.
7. Tell the child that you will now depress the inhaler and release the medication into the spacer. Then direct the child to inhale ("big breath in") slowly, over 3 to 5 seconds, and deeply.
8. Encourage the child to hold his or her breath for about 10 seconds or until you finish counting slowly to 5.
9. Remove the inhaler and ask the child to exhale slowly through the nose.
10. Wait at least 1 to 2 minutes and then repeat the complete procedure if another puff is ordered. Praise the child for cooperating and helping.
11. Encourage the child to rinse his or her mouth with water. Rinse the inhaler adapter and spacer with cool water and allow it to dry. Perform hand hygiene.
12. Praise the child for cooperation and assistance. Document all pertinent information, including how the child tolerated the procedure and responded to the medication, in the child's medical record.

---

or intubated child by inserting the aerosol administration device in-line between the child and a bag-valve-mask device or ventilator.

Metered-dose inhalers offer a portable means of delivering inhaled medications. Many people, particularly children, have difficulty using a metered-dose inhaler correctly. The effectiveness of these medications is increased with the use of a spacer device. A spacer is a cylindrical piece of hard or expandable plastic that attaches to the inhaler on one side and a mouthpiece or facemask on the other side. The child depresses the inhaler, and the medication enters the spacer, allowing the child time to deeply inhale the medication that is now mixed with air (Procedure 14-3).

Initial and ongoing education of the parent and child is important to ensure the effectiveness of inhalation therapy. The techniques for using home nebulizers and metered-dose inhalers and spacers must be demonstrated by the health care provider and then a return demonstration given by the child and parents. Parents must also be taught how to clean and maintain a home nebulizer. Correct use of the metered-dose inhalers/spacers must be reviewed at each physician's office or clinic appointment.

INTRAVENOUS THERAPY

Intravenous (IV) therapy is widely used for children. Fluids and electrolytes, total parenteral nutrition (TPN), blood products, and medications can be delivered by the IV route. When used to administer medications, IV therapy produces consistent therapeutic blood levels. Some medications can only be given via the IV route. IV medications have a nearly immediate onset of action. The risks of IV therapy include fluid overload, adverse drug reactions, septicemia, and inflammation or infection at the IV catheter insertion site.

Intravenous Catheter Insertion

Typically, over-the-needle IV catheters, 22 to 26 gauge, are used for children's peripheral IV lines. Vein size and the kind of fluid to be infused guide catheter selection. Generally, the smallest catheter through which fluids and medications can be safely infused should be used.

Venous access sites in children are shown in Figure 14-8. The rate and type of fluid to be infused, the projected length of time the IV line

will be needed, and the availability of veins often determine site selection in children. The nurse also considers the child's developmental level. For example, placement of an IV line into a toddler's foot is often a poor choice because it inhibits walking, a newly learned skill. Inserting IV lines in a child's dominant hand is avoided so as not to interfere with activities of daily living. The hand, forearm, and antecubital sites are frequently used in infants and children. Scalp veins can be used for infant IV lines; they can be adequately secured to allow the infant to move without dislodging the IV catheter. Scalp veins have no valves and can be infused in either direction.

Before an IV catheter is inserted, explain the procedure to the child and parent. Include all available information about why the catheter is being placed, what the child will see and feel during each step of the procedure, where it will be inserted, how long it will be in place, what function(s) it will perform, and if additional equipment (e.g., an infusion pump) will be used. Reassure the parent that once the IV catheter is inserted and secured in place, they will be able to hold their child. Explain to the child how participating in play activities and self-care is still possible.

Assess the child's level of fear and anxiety and have the child practice coping strategies in advance. Pharmacologic interventions are essential to reduce or eliminate pain from IV catheter insertion. Topical anesthetic agents such as EMLA or other devices such as the J-Tip, which delivers buffered lidocaine to the skin, must be used. Nonpharmacologic interventions including guided imagery (e.g., putting on an imaginary "magic glove" that keeps the hand from hurting) and

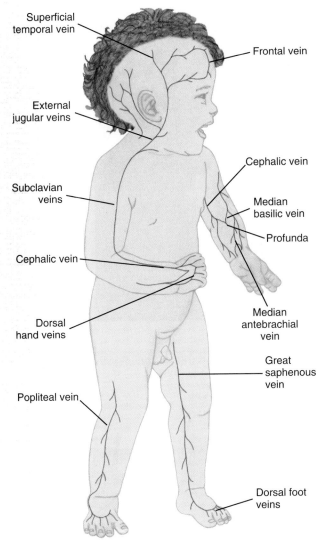

Superficial temporal vein

Frontal vein

External jugular veins

Cephalic vein

Subclavian veins

Median basilic vein

Profunda

Cephalic vein

Dorsal hand veins

Median antebrachial vein

Great saphenous vein

Popliteal vein

Dorsal foot veins

FIG 14-8 Venous access sites in children.

NURSING QUALITY ALERT

Using EMLA Anesthetic Cream

- Choose a site for the procedure where there is intact, healthy skin. Clean the site with soap and water, then dry. Perform hand hygiene and don gloves.
- Place a mound of EMLA cream (2.5 g; half of a 5-g tube) on the selected skin site and cover it with an occlusive, transparent dressing. Do not rub it into the skin.
- Leave the EMLA in place for a minimum of 1 hour and no longer than 4 hours.
- Perform hand hygiene, don gloves, take off the dressing, and remove all of the EMLA cream from the site.
- Begin the venipuncture procedure. The anesthetic (numbing) effect will last for 1 to 2 hours.
- If the child is receiving IV therapy in an ambulatory care setting, provide the parent with a prescription for EMLA and directions for use. The parent should apply the cream at least 1 hour before the child's appointment.
- Use EMLA with caution in infants younger than 12 months. Do not apply to mucous membranes. Prevent accidental ingestion by older infants and young children. Do not administer EMLA to any child with methemoglobinemia.

randomly assigned to an experimental group (being held in an upright position by a parent) and a control group (lying supine on an examination table with parent comforting and distracting), demonstrated that young children experienced significantly less procedural distress if the parent held their child in an upright position during IV insertion. However, there is still debate related to whether parental presence during pediatric invasive procedures maintains or alters the continuum of holistic patient care (Pruitt, Johnson, Elliott, & Polley, 2008).

Explain the procedure at each step to the child and parents. The nurse applies the tourniquet and selects the IV site, beginning with the most distal veins of the nondominant hand or forearm. The nurse then cleanses the skin at the chosen site and inserts the IV catheter (see Procedure 13-3, Venipuncture, for more detailed information). Catheter placement is confirmed by a blood return; a normal saline solution flush verifies that there is no infiltration. After the catheter is placed, secure it in place with tape and a sterile, transparent, occlusive dressing. The clear dressing allows for adequate visibility and ongoing monitoring of the insertion site. Alternative types of securement devices (such as the STATLOCK stabilization device) may be used. Tape the catheter extension tubing to the extremity, maintaining access to the plastic clamp.

It is common to attach a well-padded arm board to the child's extremity to prevent injury and keep the IV catheter intact (Figure 14-9). This is particularly important for active children. The extremity is placed in the anatomically correct position on the arm board and secured firmly but not so tight that circulation is impaired or nerve damage can occur. Placement also should allow some restricted use of the extremity. For example, an arm board for an IV near the wrist would be positioned to prevent the child from bending the wrist but allow use of the fingers and thumb. A clear plastic shield (such as an I.V. House UltraDome) placed on top of the IV insertion site adds further protection for the IV catheter while allowing the nurse to visualize the site.

The nurse documents in the child's medical record the location of the IV catheter; the antiseptic used to prep the site; the number of IV

distraction (e.g., music, videos, books) should be used as well (see Chapter 15 for further pain management information).

Determine if the child will be able to hold the arm (or foot) still during the procedure. This is of major importance to prevent injury and to successfully insert the IV catheter. In most cases with young children, the nurse will need another health care provider to hold the child and the extremity during the insertion procedure and until the IV catheter is completely secured.

This procedure should be performed in the treatment room of the hospital unit. The nurse should have all the needed equipment ready in advance: IV catheter of appropriate size, ordered IV solution, primed infusion set, primed extension tubing, 3 to 5 mL of bacteriostatic normal saline for injection in a syringe, strips of tape, sterile transparent occlusive dressing, a padded arm board, a clear plastic "IV house" shield, a tourniquet, antiseptic swabs (frequently 2% chlorhexidine or ChloraPrep is used), and gloves.

Parents often want to remain with the child during an IV insertion, if they feel able to cope with the stress of the situation. Parents should not be expected to restrain the child during the procedure. Sparks, Setlik, and Luhman (2007), using an experimental research design in which young children needing IV catheter insertion were

A padded arm board gently limits movement of the hand, and a plastic shield allows visibility yet keeps the IV site intact.

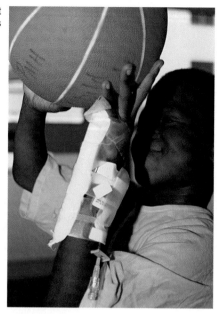

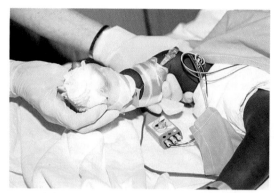

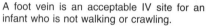

A foot vein is an acceptable IV site for an infant who is not walking or crawling.

FIG 14-9 IV sites in children are secured and well-protected to allow for activities and prevent dislodging the IV catheter. (Courtesy Parkland Health and Hospital System, Dallas, TX.)

insertion attempts; if blood return occurred; use and amount of normal saline flush; the condition of the skin at the site; the type, length, and gauge of the IV catheter; the date and time it was inserted; and how the child tolerated the procedure.

Intravenous Catheter Monitoring

The nurse should assess and document the IV catheter site of a child at least every hour, looking specifically for signs and symptoms of infiltration, phlebitis, and/or infection. By gently touching the site on top of the dressing, the nurse can detect warmth or coolness as well as any hardness of the vein. Observations are made for any redness, blanching, swelling, and/or exudates. If there is pain at the site, the nurse assesses the quality of the pain (sharp or dull) as well as the degree of pain using a pain scale. In accordance with hospital policy, the nurse documents in the child's medical record the IV site assessment findings. One way to assess for infiltration is by observing for symmetry in the size and shape of limbs or scalp as well as gently touching the site to determine whether it is soft or taut or whether the scalp site is boggy. If signs and symptoms of complications (e.g., edema, erythema, pain, blanching, coolness, purulent drainage, or red streaking of the skin above the vein) are noted, the IV infusion is discontinued and the physician is notified.

Because of the fragility of children's veins, the difficulty of finding new sites, and the stress of insertion, children's IV sites are to be changed only when clinically indicated (O'Grady, Alexander, Burns et al., 2011). IV fluid bags, in general, are changed every 24 hours. It is now recommended to change IV tubing no more frequently than every 96 hours but at least every 7 days (O'Grady et al., 2011) to minimize risk of intravascular infection. However, hospital policies do vary. IV bags and tubing should be changed more frequently (e.g., every 24 hours) when total parenteral nutrition, lipids, or blood products are administered (O'Grady et al., 2011).

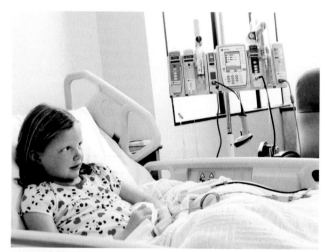

FIG 14-10 Alaris System IV infusion pump. (Courtesy Care Fusion, San Diego, CA.)

Intravenous Infusion Monitoring

To accurately control the infusion rate for IV fluid or medication administration, infusion pumps that deliver a preset volume at a set rate are used for infants and children (Figure 14-10). Infusion pumps are programmed with IV fluid limits to prevent accidental fluid overload. Many hospitals have policies that require a child's IV pump be set to infuse no more than a 2-hour fluid volume.

An additional safety feature used in some institutions is the burette, an in-line volume-control set with a graduated chamber and IV tubing (such as a Buretrol or SoluSet). A burette usually has a 100- to 150-mL capacity. The nurse fills the burette chamber with IV fluids for 2 hours according to the physician's orders and then sets the infusion pump rate to deliver only that amount over 2 hours. Medications can be mixed with an appropriate amount of IV fluid in the burette; the pump is then set at a rate to infuse the amount in the burette over the designated time period.

Infusion Rates and Methods

Physicians order hourly IV fluid infusion rates based on a child's daily maintenance fluid requirements, and additional fluid needs to replace deficits, if applicable. Box 14-1 illustrates how the nurse can use the formula to determine maintenance fluid requirements and corresponding IV rates based on a child's weight. The nurse verifies the IV rate with the physician's order and documents on the child's medical record the type of IV solution, the location of the site, the ordered rate (which should be the same as the rate set on the infusion pump), and the actual quantity of IV fluid that the child has received. *Even if the child is receiving IV fluids through an infusion pump, the nurse verifies the amount of fluid administered to the child at least hourly.* Pumps can malfunction, risking fluid overload if not meticulously monitored.

Administering Intravenous Medications

IV medications can be administered as a continuous infusion or intermittently. Methods for intermittently administering IV medications

BOX 14-1 DAILY MAINTENANCE FLUID REQUIREMENTS AND RATES

Formula for Calculating Daily Fluid Requirements*

CHILD'S WEIGHT	MAINTENANCE FLUIDS
10 kg or less	100 mL/kg/day
Over 10 to 20 kg	1000 mL/day + 50 mL/kg/day for each added kg over 10 kg to 20 kg
Over 20 kg	1500 mL/day + 20 mL/kg/day for each additional kg over 20 kg

Example 1:

Child's weight = 7.2 kg	Maintenance fluids
First 10 kg of body weight	7.2 × 100 mL/kg/day = 720 mL/day
Hourly rate	720 mL/day (24 hr) ÷ 24 = 30 mL/hr

Example 2:

Child's weight = 15 kg	Maintenance fluids
First 10 kg of body weight	10 × 100 mL/kg/day = 1000 mL/day
Added 5 kg of body weight	5 × 50 mL/kg/day = 250 mL/day
	1250 mL/day
Hourly rate	1250 mL/day (24 hr) ÷ 24 = 52 mL/hr

Example 3:

Child's weight = 23 kg	Maintenance fluids
First 10 kg of body weight	10 × 100 mL/kg/day = 1000 mL/day
Added 10 kg of body weight	10 × 50 mL/kg/day = 500 mL/day
Added 3 kg of body weight	3 × 20 mL/kg/day = 60 mL/day
	1560 mL/day
Hourly rate	1560 mL/day (24 hr) ÷ 24 = 65 mL/hr

*Holiday-Segar method from Custer, J., & Rau, R. (Eds.). (2009). *The Harriet Lane handbook: A manual for pediatric house officers* (18th ed.). Philadelphia: Elsevier.

are bolus and intermittent infusion. The appropriate method must be chosen to meet the needs of the child and to accommodate any restrictions posed by the medication and the volume of fluid.

When administering IV medications to children, the nurse must consider the compatibility of the medication with IV solutions, the type of IV tubing to be used, the recommended concentration for IV administration, the volume of the diluted medication, the suggested administration rate, and the amount of flush needed. Hospital policies and procedures may establish the type of administration to be used and the amount of flush needed. Reference information about the administration of specific IV medications can be obtained from pharmacists or the hospital formulary.

Intravenous Bolus Administration

Medications delivered by IV bolus (push) are given over a defined period of time (a few minutes), directly into the IV catheter through the port closest to the child's insertion site. The volume of medication infused is small, usually 5 mL or less, and the effects can be seen immediately. A number of medications are administered by this method, including opioids, antiepileptics, sedatives, corticosteroids, antiemetics, diuretics, and antibiotics. It is imperative that the nurse verify the administration rate for an ordered medication to ensure that it can be safely given IV push. It is recommended to use needleless systems to access IV tubing (O'Grady et al., 2011).

Before administering the medication, the nurse checks the IV site for any signs of infiltration or phlebitis and determines that the IV line is intact and patent. The nurse performs hand hygiene and dons clean gloves. The access port is then scrubbed thoroughly with an antiseptic swab, allowed to dry, and the sterile tip of the syringe containing the medication is connected to the port—actions designed to prevent catheter-associated intravascular (bloodstream) infections (O'Grady et al., 2011). The nurse occludes the IV line by pinching it just above the injection port while pushing the medication and then releases the tubing to allow IV fluids to infuse when not pushing the medication (Perry & Potter, 2011). If the medication is not compatible with the infusing IV fluid or if the medication is going into an intermittent infusion port, flush the tubing with approximately 2 to 3 mL of normal saline solution before and after administering the medication. Be sure to scrub the access port with an appropriate antiseptic (and allow to dry) each time the port is about to be entered.

Administer the IV medication *exactly* at the prescribed rate over the *required* time period per the physician's orders. Closely assess the child during and immediately after administration for intended as well as potential adverse effects of the medication. Reassess the child at frequent intervals.

Intravenous Intermittent Infusion Administration

Programmable infusion pumps are frequently used to facilitate safe intermittent infusion of IV medications for children via the "piggyback" method. These pumps have dual programming capabilities that allow a secondary line attached to an IV bag containing medication, diluted to the correct concentration, to run concurrently or sequentially with a primary infusion of IV fluids. It is essential that the nurse verify that the medication is compatible with the IV solution being used. Another type of IV pump often used with children is the syringe pump. The nurse places a syringe containing medication that has been mixed and properly diluted by the pharmacist, along with primed, low-volume tubing, into the pump. After connecting the tubing to the child's IV line, the nurse programs the pump to deliver the volume of medication in the syringe over a specified time period.

Some hospitals use "smart" pumps (see Figure 14-10) with preprogrammed drug libraries that assist in the prevention of medication errors by alerting the nurse if a medication dose or IV administration rate exceeds parameters recommended by the hospital pharmacy (Conroy et al., 2007). Thus, a "smart" pump that contains an individual child's profile (weight, list of ordered medications) would not "allow" the nurse to set the pump to administer an incorrect medication, the wrong dose, or an inappropriate rate. Though an IV pump is an excellent safety tool, the nurse must still adhere to the six rights of medication administration. For IV medications, the nurse verifies that the "right" dose includes that the medication is correctly diluted and is running at the recommended rate of infusion.

When performing intermittent infusion of IV medications, the nurse will often flush the IV tubing with fluid to complete the delivery of all the medication to the child. When the medication infusion is done, many pumps are set to sound an alarm so that the nurse can return to complete the flush. The volume needed for the flush varies according to the type of IV tubing used. All volumes including the IV medication, added fluids for dilution, and flush or flushes used need to be counted and documented as fluid intake. The total volume infused should be within safe limits for the child.

Before administering any IV medication, determine that the IV line is functioning properly and that the IV catheter site is free of complications. If the child does not have a running IV line but is receiving intermittent medication infusions, be sure to flush the IV catheter with normal saline to ensure patency, before attaching the secondary infusion set. Follow hospital policy regarding labeling and flagging the syringe or IV bag containing the medication. In addition to documenting the medication given in the child's medical record, all volumes of the different IV fluids infused are recorded as well.

> ### ❓ CRITICAL THINKING EXERCISE 14-4
>
> 1. The physician has ordered ampicillin 1.4 grams (g) IV every 4 hours for your patient.
> 2. The ampicillin for injection is available in a vial that has 2 g in 5 mL. How many mL will you need to withdraw from the vial for the 1.4-g dose?
> 3. You add the ampicillin you withdrew from the vial to a 50-mL IV bag of normal saline. The physician's order specifies to infuse this IV bag with ampicillin over 30 minutes. At what rate (in mL/hr) will you set the IV pump?

Venous Access Devices
Intermittent Infusion Ports

Intermittent infusion ports (saline or heparin locks) allow drugs to be administered IV without the need for a running IV line. The intermittent infusion port is an IV catheter that is placed, flushed with a normal saline or diluted heparin solution to maintain patency, and then locked with an adapter. The port is accessed when needed for fluid or medication infusion. When the port is accessed, meticulous procedures are used including hand hygiene and thorough cleansing of the port's hub with antiseptic solution to prevent catheter-associated bloodstream infections. IV site monitoring and site care are the same as for any IV catheter.

The frequency of flushing a saline or heparin lock is determined by hospital policy. Routine flushing with a normal saline or a heparinized saline solution to maintain patency is generally performed every 8 to 12 hours. The device is also flushed with normal saline before and after medication administration and may be flushed at the end of the procedure with a heparinized saline solution, if ordered or in accordance with hospital policy.

Central Venous Access Devices

Central venous access devices are catheters placed directly into major blood vessels. They are most often used to administer medications, blood products, IV fluids, and parenteral nutrition to children over a prolonged period of time. These devices can be tunneled or nontunneled central catheters and implanted infusion ports. All central venous access devices need routine care (dressing changes, flushing) according to hospital protocols. Although the insertion site is assessed several times per day, dressing changes are done on a scheduled basis; frequency varies. When a transparent dressing is used, some institutions recommended cleaning the site and changing the dressing every 7 days. In most cases, each lumen of a central venous line is flushed with heparinized saline at least every 24 hours and after medication administration or a blood draw.

Because these devices enter the central venous system, all procedures are done using strict aseptic technique. Central line–associated bloodstream infections are the most common type of nosocomial infection in pediatric ICUs (Costello, Morrow, Graham et al., 2008). Use by health care providers of groups or "bundles" of aseptic practices for central venous line insertion as well as dressing changes and port access have been shown to significantly decrease the incidence of infection (Costello et al., 2008). These practices include proper hand hygiene, 10-minute scrubs of access ports before use, and prompt removal of unneeded lines.

Tunneled central lines (such as Broviac or Hickman catheters) are surgically placed lines that are held in place by a Dacron cuff located in a subcutaneous tunnel. They are most commonly placed in an external jugular vein but may also be placed in the cephalic, axillary, subclavian, femoral, saphenous, or internal jugular veins. The tip of the tunneled catheter is threaded until it rests at the junction of the superior vena cava and right atrium. Short-term or non-tunneled central catheters are most frequently placed in the subclavian or femoral veins. These lines involve the placement of a large-gauge catheter that is then sutured in place.

An implanted venous access device (such as a Port-A-Cath or Infusaport) consists of a catheter that is connected to a port or reservoir. As with the tunneled catheter, the catheter tip rests at the junction of the superior vena cava and right atrium. The port is under the skin and is accessed with a non-coring needle placed through the skin into the port. The needle is then covered with a biooclusive dressing, and an extension set is attached to the end. When the port is no longer needed for infusions or obtaining blood specimens, it is flushed with a heparin solution, and the needle is withdrawn. The child with an implanted port can participate in typical childhood activities except those with a potential for high-impact contact with the chest (e.g., tackle football).

A peripherally inserted central catheter (PICC) line is often used for a child who needs IV access for a period longer than a peripheral IV catheter can be maintained. A PICC is a long catheter made of polyurethane or silicone that is threaded through an introducer placed in a peripheral vein of the upper arm (basilic, cephalic, or brachial vein). It is usually inserted by a specially trained nurse. The catheter is threaded so that the tip is located in the superior vena cava; the introducer is then removed. The catheter at the insertion site is covered with a bio-patch and then a transparent dressing. Placement is verified by x-ray examination. Several times per day, the insertion site and dressing are assessed for redness, moisture, drainage, or swelling, and catheter integrity is verified. Generally, the dressing is changed at 24 hours postinsertion to and then every 7 days if it remains dry and intact. These catheters can be usually left in place for several weeks to months and frequently are used for home antibiotic therapy. The major complications of this type of line are phlebitis, infection, thrombosis, and catheter occlusion.

ADMINISTRATION OF BLOOD PRODUCTS

Before administering blood products to a child, it is essential to prepare the child and family for the procedure. A child may be disturbed or frightened by seeing blood products in IV bags and tubing. The nurse explains to the child at a developmentally appropriate level, and to the parents, the reason the child needs to receive blood products; how long it will take; what the child will feel, see, and hear; and the type of blood products to be given. Information about the child's blood transfusion history including reactions is obtained from the family.

The nurse confirms the child's ABO blood type and Rh factor. Meticulous procedures must then be followed to ensure that the child receives a donor blood product that is ABO and Rh compatible and has been crossmatched specifically for the intended recipient. In most health care settings, it is required that two nurses (or a nurse and physician) identify the child and verify ABO/Rh type, donor number, and blood expiration date/time. The child needs a patent IV line; catheters as small as 23 to 25 gauge can be used, though the infusion rate may be slower for packed red blood cells (American Association of Blood Banks, 2010). Blood administration tubing is used that includes a filter to remove particulates from the blood and a "Y" connection that allows normal saline to be available for infusion. An IV pump is often used to facilitate precise regulation of the infusion rate and prevent too-rapid transfusion.

Children must be monitored closely during blood product administration for potential complications that include hemolytic (transfusion) reactions, allergic reactions, febrile reactions, circulatory overload, hypothermia, and electrolyte disturbances. Guidelines for nursing care include the following:

- Obtain baseline vital signs, including blood pressure, before administering blood products. Take vital signs every 15 minutes for the first 1 to 2 hours and then hourly until the infusion is complete.
- The rate of infusion of packed red blood cells is approximately 5 mL/kg/hr over no more than 4 hours.
- Monitor the child closely for signs and symptoms of an adverse reaction: fever or chills, headache, nausea, pain at the IV site, or difficulty breathing. The child should not be left alone while receiving blood products.
- If a reaction is suspected, stop the transfusion immediately and notify the physician. Infuse normal saline solution through new tubing to keep the IV line patent. Continue to monitor vital signs. Check urine output hourly and send samples of the child's blood and urine to the laboratory per physician orders.

CHILD AND FAMILY EDUCATION

It is a key nursing responsibility to educate and prepare children and families for medication administration at home, before discharge from the hospital, clinic, or physician's office. Studies have determined that parents make unintentional but frequent errors in giving the correct dose of oral medications to their children (Taylor, Robinson, MacLeod, et al., 2009; Yin, Mendelsohn, Wolf et al., 2010). Further, it has been shown that parents with lower health literacy (level of health information and understanding) make more dosing errors (Yin et al., 2010).

Teaching the family about medications begins with a thorough assessment of all medications the child is currently taking, including over-the-counter medications and herbal preparations. Any history of allergies to medications should be noted to prevent potential drug interactions. The nurse must provide thorough verbal and written information and instructions to the family regarding the medications to be given, the dosage, when to administer, therapeutic effects, and potential side effects and adverse reactions. The child and family members are encouraged to ask questions to guide additional instruction.

The nurse must emphasize taking all medications exactly as ordered. Information that needs to be highlighted includes finishing the full course of a prescribed antibiotic, not changing dosages without consulting the physician, and returning for follow-up appointments.

The nurse problem solves with the family to develop acceptable schedules for medication administration, to determine the best methods of administering oral medications (e.g., liquid or crushing and mixing with food), and to identify foods or fluids that might be mixed with the medication or given immediately after the medication is taken. The family is then provided a written schedule for medication administration.

The nurse also needs to demonstrate how to measure the correct dosage of a liquid medication using the administration device the parents will use at home (calibrated spoon or oral syringe) and then have the parents perform a return demonstration. If teaching a child or adolescent and parents to do subcutaneous injections (such as for insulin), supervised practice of the injection procedure and ongoing education is required.

It is essential to reinforce general safety information, such as keeping medications in a locked cabinet that is out of the reach of children and keeping all medications in their original pharmacy containers. The nurse evaluates interventions by asking questions of family members (scenarios work well) to determine their level of understanding about all aspects of the medication and the administration process. Careful observation of return demonstrations by the child and family helps the nurse to judge teaching effectiveness. All teaching provided and validation of understanding should be specifically documented in the child's medical record.

PATIENT-CENTERED TEACHING

Medication Administration at Home

Address the needs of parents to determine the best way to administer medication to their child at home before the child leaves the hospital or ambulatory care setting. This can help prevent medication errors and ensure that the child and family will follow the physician's orders for the home treatment plan. Provide the parents (and child according to the developmental level) the following information:

- Name of the medication (trade and generic)
- Why it has been prescribed for the child
- What the desired "therapeutic" effects are (e.g., how the medication is supposed to help the child)
- How to take the medication (how much, how often, how long to take it, techniques for administering the medication)
- Acceptable measuring device for home administration of oral medications (oral syringe, calibrated spoon, or small, calibrated medicine cup)
- How to use calibrated droppers or syringes to measure and give the right amount of medication
- Expected or potential side effects and what to do if they occur
- When the parents should notify a nurse or physician if the child had an adverse reaction
- Any dietary or activity restrictions

If the child will need to take medication during the school day, the physician must provide a written order that the parents give to the school nurse along with a parental permission form authorizing administration of the medication at school. The school nurse should also receive complete written information and instructions that include a description of the medication, the intended purpose of the treatment, potential side effects and adverse reactions, and when the medication should be given. Parents are required to provide the medication in the original pharmacy container. The school nurse also needs a complete list of all the medications the child is taking at home as well as at school.

KEY CONCEPTS

- Standardized dosage ranges for many medications have not been established for children.
- Children respond differently to medication than adults.
- The nurse must incorporate principles of growth and development when administering medications to children.
- The margin of safety for medication administration is narrow for children.
- Based on developmental level, different types of devices and techniques are used to administer oral medications to children.
- Injections are stressful to children and used for a limited number of medications and immunizations.
- Site selection for IV insertion is influenced by the rate and type of fluid to be infused and the accessibility of veins.

- Though an infusion pump is used to control the rate and quantity of IV fluids administered to children, the nurse must assess the actual fluid administered hourly.
- Infants and children must be closely monitored when receiving IV medications because of the immediate onset of action.
- Using "bundles" of aseptic practices, including hand hygiene and scrubbing the port's hub before accessing an IV line, can prevent catheter-related bloodstream infections.
- A child undergoes a comprehensive, baseline assessment before blood product administration.
- Education of the child and parents is important to ensure that medications are administered accurately and in accordance with the physician's orders and the treatment plan.

REFERENCES

Agrawal, A., & Wu, W. (2009). National patient safety goals: Reducing medication errors and improving systems reliability using an electronic medication reconciliation system. *Joint Commission Journal on Quality & Patient Safety, 35*(2), 106-114.

American Academy of Pediatrics. (2007). *Policy statement: Prevention of medication errors in the pediatric inpatient setting.* (Reaffirmed January of 2007). Retrieved from http://aappolicy.aappublications.org/cgi/content/full/pediatrics;112/2/431

American Association of Blood Banks. (2010). *Primer on blood administration.* Retrieved from www.bloodcenter.org/webres/File/Hospital%20.pdf%20forms/AABB%20Primer%20of%20Blood%20Administration.pdf.

Conroy, S., Sweis, D., Planner, C., et al. (2007). Interventions to reduce dosing errors in children: A systematic review of the literature. *Drug Safety, 30*(12), 1111-1125.

Costello, J., Morrow, D., Graham, D., et al. (2008). Systematic intervention to reduce central line-associated bloodstream infection rates in a pediatric cardiac inten care unit. *Pediatrics, 121*(5), 915-923.

Gerald, L., McClure, L., Mangan, J., et al. (2009). Increasing adherence to inhaled steroid therapy among schoolchildren: Randomized, controlled trial of school-based supervised asthma therapy. *Pediatrics, 123*(2), 466-474.

Gerstle, R., & Lehmann, C. (2007). Electronic prescribing systems in pediatrics: The rationale and functionality requirements. *Pediatrics, 119*(6), e1413-e1422.

Institute for Safe Medication Practices. (2008). *ISMP's list of high-alert medications.* Retrieved from http://ismp.org/Tools/highalertmedications.pdf.

Joint Commission. (2008). *Sentinel event alert: Preventing pediatric medication errors (Issue 39).* Retrieved from www.jointcommission.org/assets/1/18/SEA_39.PDF.

Joint Commission. (2010). *Topic library item: National patient safety goal on reconciling medication information (NPSG.3.06.01).* Retrieved from www.jointcommission.org/npsg_econciling_medication.

Kamps, J., Rapoff, M., Roberts, M., et al. (2008). Improving adherence to inhaled corticosteroids in children with asthma: A pilot of a randomized clinical trial. *Children's Health Care, 37*(4), 261-277.

Matsui, D. (2007). Current issues in pediatric medication adherence. *Pediatric Drugs, 9*(5), 283-288.

Mears, C., Charlebois, N., & Holl, J. (2006). Medication adherence among adolescents in a school-based health center. *Journal of School Health, 76*(2), 52-56.

O'Grady, N., Alexander, M., Burns, L., et al. (2011). *Centers for Disease Control and Prevention: Guidelines for the prevention of intravascular catheter-related infections.* Retrieved from www.cdc.gov/hicpac/pdf/guidelines/bsi-guidelines-2011.pdf.

Perry, A., & Potter, P. (2011). *Mosby's pocket guide to nursing skills and procedures* (7th ed.). Maryland Heights, MO: Elsevier

Pruitt, L., Johnson, A., Elliott, J., & Polley, K. (2008). Parental presence during pediatric invasive procedures. *Journal of Pediatric Healthcare, 22*(2), 120-127.

Rapoff, M., & Lindsely, C. (2007). Improving adherence to medical regimens for juvenile rheumatoid arthritis. *Pediatric Rheumatology, 5*(10), 1-7.

Riley-Lawless, K. (2009). Family-identified barriers to medication reconciliation. *Journal of Specialists in Pediatric Nursing, 14*(2), 94-101.

Sparks, L., Setlik, J., & Luhman, J. (2007). Parental holding and positioning to decrease IV distress in young children: A randomized controlled trial. *Journal of Pediatric Nursing, 22*(6), 440-447.

Takata, G., Taketomo, C., & Waite, S. (2008). Characteristics of medication errors and adverse drug events in hospitals participating in the California Pediatric Patient Safety Initiative. *American Journal of Health-System Pharmacists, 65*, 2036-2044.

Taylor, D., Robinson, J., MacLeod, D., et al. (2009). Therapeutic errors among children in the community setting: Nature, causes and outcomes. *Journal of Paediatrics and Child Health, 45*, 304-309.

Thompson, K. (2007). Medication reconciliation: Challenges and opportunities. *American Journal of Health-System Pharmacists, 64*, 1912.

Yin, H. S., Mendelsohn, A., Wolf, M., et al. (2010). Parents' medication administration errors: Role of dosing instruments and health literacy. *Archives of Pediatrics and Adolescent Medicine, 164*(2), 181-186.

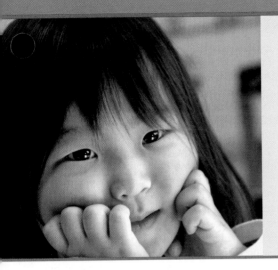
Pain Management for Children

⊖volve WEBSITE

http://evolve.elsevier.com/James/ncoc

LEARNING OBJECTIVES

After studying this chapter, you should be able to:
- Define *pain*.
- Discuss the gate control theory of pain.
- Discuss the myths and realities of pain and pain management.
- Discriminate between acute and chronic pain.
- Explain pain assessment in children according to developmental stages.

- Describe common pain assessment tools.
- Discuss nonpharmacologic and pharmacologic interventions that may be used for pediatric pain management.
- Use the nursing process to describe nursing care of the child in pain.

Assessing and treating **pain** in children can be difficult. Infants and children are often unable to communicate the presence, location, type, or intensity of pain. Parents may be hesitant to allow suitable pain management because of fears related to side effects from the use of **opioids,** including inaccurate fears regarding **addiction.** Additionally, nurses and other health care providers continue to have misconceptions about opioid pharmacokinetics and unwarranted concern about adverse effects of opioid use in infants and children (Griffin, Polit, & Byrne, 2008; Van Hulle Vincent & Gaddy, 2009).

Comprehensive research and knowledge gains over the past 10 to 15 years have greatly improved the assessment and treatment of pain in children. Yet, despite the increasing knowledge regarding safe and effective pain management in children, as well as widespread anecdotal experience, children remain at risk for unrecognized and undertreated pain. It is well documented that the youngest children have the greatest probability of receiving insufficient pain medications, that pain medication administration varies by age, and that pain medication is underused for many children (American Pain Society [APS], 2011a; Griffin et al., 2008).

Individual nurses vary in their ability to assess pain. Some of these differences have been linked to the lack of or inaccurate clinical knowledge regarding pain, inappropriate stereotyping of patients who require treatment for pain, and lack of nursing experience (Rieman & Gordon, 2007; Twycross, 2007a; Twycross, 2007b; Twycross, 2008). Additionally, consistent, appropriate use of pediatric pain assessment tools is not always seen among pediatric nurses (Griffin et al., 2008).

The behaviors of many health care professionals, including nurses, do not always correspond with the attitudes and beliefs they report concerning pain assessment and management (Twycross, 2007b).

⊖ Recent increases in quality pediatric pain research have led to more precise pain assessment and improved prescribing and administering of analgesics. Age-appropriate **adjuvants** are being used more frequently. The most current resources and strategies for pain management, however, are not always implemented, emphasizing the continuing need for educating all health care providers. Nurses, having frequent interaction with physicians and other health care providers, can facilitate a significant improvement in pain management for infants and children. They can also play a vital role in educating other health care providers, as well as parents and children, with regard to appropriate pediatric pain management.

DEFINITIONS AND THEORIES OF PAIN

There are many definitions of pain. The International Association for the Study of Pain (IASP), Subcommittee on Taxonomy (1979, p. 249) defines pain as "an unpleasant sensory and emotional experience associated with actual or potential tissue damage, or described in terms of such damage." In a commonly accepted definition, pain is whatever the person experiencing the pain says it is, existing whenever the person says it does (Pasero & McCaffery, 2011). The **pain threshold** will vary among individuals. Both definitions underscore the fact that pain is complex, multidimensional, subjective, and personal. The pediatric pain experience involves the interaction of behavioral, developmental, physiologic, psychological, and situational factors (APS, 2011a).

Gate Control Theory

Pain, or nociceptive, impulses travel between the initial site of injury and the brain, and certain mechanisms affect pain intensity. According to the gate control theory, proposed by Melzack and Wall in 1965, a gating mechanism at the level of the dorsal horn in the spinal cord can facilitate or dampen the transmission of pain signals. Stimulation of the larger afferent nerves, which carry benign sensations, can blunt the transmission of pain signals. The gating mechanisms are influenced by the relative activity in the sensory fibers. Input from the large fibers closes the gate, whereas input from the small fibers opens it. For example, rubbing an injured part activates large-fiber activity, which decreases the ability of small-fiber activity to open the gate, thus decreasing the pain. The theory further postulates that cognitive processes, such as attention, emotion, and memory, influence the gating mechanism and have an impact on the transmission of pain. The gate control theory lends support for the use of both physiologic and psychological interventions in pain management.

Acute and Chronic Pain

Nursing assessment and interventions will vary on the basis of the nature of the pain. Children may have acute or chronic pain. Acute pain usually has a sudden onset, is from an identifiable trauma, and continues for a limited time. Resolution generally occurs with healing of the trauma. Frequently, the acute pain experienced by children in health care settings is a result of invasive procedures (e.g., injections) or complications (e.g., tissue injury from IV infiltration). This is particularly evident for children with cancer and other chronic illnesses that require frequent medical care. Acute pain is also experienced with acute disease states, after surgery, and after trauma (such as falls, or nonaccidental injury from child abuse). Events that cause acute pain may persist, leading to the development of chronic pain.

Chronic pain continues for an unpredictable period beyond the expected recovery period, is unlikely to resolve quickly, and may adversely affect the child's daily activities of living. Causes and types of chronic pain vary widely. Children with conditions such as juvenile arthritis, sickle cell disease, and cancer have chronic, repeated exacerbations of acute pain. Neuropathic pain is one of the most complex types of chronic pain to treat. Chronic pain in childhood is much more prevalent than previously realized. A survey of the general pediatric population indicates that approximately 15% of children are living with chronic pain (Thompson, Knapp, Feeg et al., 2010).

Accurate assessment and successful treatment of chronic pain is very difficult. It remains a significant, unsolved challenge in pediatric pain management, leading to concerns regarding the long-term functional consequences of chronic childhood pain. The American Pain Society (2011b) has issued a position statement with the intent of increasing awareness and improving treatment of chronic pain in children. It advocates for increased education of all health professionals and more research on pediatric pain management.

Improvements in pain management have enabled children with pain related to chronic conditions to achieve a higher quality of life. They are able to enjoy a greater degree of normalcy by spending less time in the hospital and actively participating in school, play, and other activities of childhood (see Chapter 12). Nurses who work in the school, home health care, and hospice settings have added resources (e.g., knowledge, medication, equipment) that facilitate pain control, resulting in more comfortable, satisfying lives for these children and their families.

RESEARCH ON PAIN IN CHILDREN

Over the past three decades, there has been a proliferation of pediatric pain-related research which has led to clinical practice guidelines and additional standards of care for both acute and chronic pain (see publications from the World Health Organization [WHO], the American Pain Society [APS], the American Academy of Pediatrics [AAP], the American Society for Pain Management Nursing, and the International Association for the Study of Pain on the Evolve website).

The World Health Organization's three-step analgesic ladder was developed in the early 1980s to improve treatment for cancer pain. The ladder suggests nonopioid analgesics for mild pain, weak opioids for mild to moderate pain, and opioid analgesics for severe pain, along with accessory medications to prevent breakthrough pain (WHO, 2010). These guidelines are the basis for pain management of children and adults, particularly related to multidrug therapy. Beginning in 1999, the APS has developed and published clinical guidelines related to care of pediatric (and adult) patients with acute and chronic pain associated with sickle cell disease, cancer pain, juvenile chronic arthritis pain, acute pain, and fibromyalgia syndrome pain (APS, 2011c). The AAP and the APS issued a joint position statement in 2001 with recommendations for the assessment and management of acute pain in infants, children, and adolescents (APS, 2011b). Since 2001, the Joint Commission accreditation standards have continued to address both pain assessment and management by requiring health care agencies to provide pain management education and guarantee all hospitalized patients the right to developmentally appropriate, comprehensive pain assessment and management, from admission until discharge (Joint Commission, 2011).

One major area of concern is pain management for premature infants, neonates, and very young infants, particularly with regard to painful procedures. Based primarily on animal studies, researchers have speculated that pain experiences of neonates may result in long-term emotional, behavioral, and learning disabilities (AAP & Canadian Paediatric Society, 2006). There is also concern that prolonged exposure to pain or severe pain may increase neonatal morbidity (Mancuso & Burns, 2009).

Anand (2007) suggests that it is difficult to accurately assess and then manage pain in preterm neonates because they do not produce "specific" responses to acute pain on a consistent basis. Further, for these nonverbal patients, pain assessment is based solely on observed behavioral and physiologic responses to acute pain (such as facial expressions), and there is significant variability in the subjective interpretation of an infant's pain level by different practitioners (Anand, 2007).

Important determinants of the long-term outcomes of infant pain include timing, degree of injury, and the analgesic used. There are also concerns for older children in relation to their memories of painful experiences (Busoni, 2007). Long-term consequences of childhood pain may include negative reactions to painful events and poor acceptance of health care interventions later in life (Von Baeyer, Marche, Rocha, & Salmon, 2004).

Advances in research, knowledge, and clinical expertise have led to significant increases in academic literature, research studies, and practice guidelines and standards regarding pediatric pain management. However, improvements are still needed in the following areas: research on nurse-physician collaboration for pediatric pain management and barriers to suitable pain management; education of health care providers about appropriate, effective pain management; increased information about pain management in neonates and infants; and testing for the safety and efficacy, specifically in children, of new analgesics as they are introduced.

TABLE 15-1   PAIN AND PAIN MANAGEMENT IN CHILDREN: MYTHS AND REALITIES

MYTH	REALITY
Neonates do not feel pain because of incomplete myelinization in peripheral nerves and the CNS.	Myelinization is not necessary for pain perception. Central and peripheral structures required for nociception are present and functional early in gestation. Therefore, infants have the neurologic capacity for pain perception at the time of birth, even those born prematurely (Franck, Greenberg, & Stevens, 2000).
Children have no memory of pain.	Feeding and sleeping differences have been reported in studies of infants who experienced pain, which suggests that the procedure had consequences extending beyond the event (Anand, 2007).
There is a correct or standard amount of pain associated with a specific injury or procedure.	The amount of pain a child experiences varies and cannot be predicted because of individual cognitive, developmental, and emotional factors affecting the child (Page & Blanchette, 2009; Pasero & McCaffery, 2011).
Children can easily become addicted to narcotic analgesics.	There is no identified characteristic of childhood physiology or development that indicates any increased risk of physiologic or psychological dependence. The actual risk of addiction is very low (Pasero & McCaffery, 2011; Twycross, 2010).
Narcotic administration can easily cause respiratory depression.	No data support the belief that children are at higher risk for respiratory depression than adults. Respiratory depression is rare (Twycross, 2010; Walco & Goldschneider, 2008).

OBSTACLES TO PAIN MANAGEMENT IN CHILDREN

Obstacles to appropriate pain management in children include belief in myths, knowledge deficits, inaccuracy of pain assessment and pain assessment measures, insufficient awareness of pain management interventions, lack of confidence regarding efficacy of pain management, lack of communication with children and their parents, and personal attitudes and beliefs about pain (APS, 2011a; Rieman & Gordon, 2007; Twycross, 2007a).

The two beliefs of parents and nurses that are most likely to interfere with the provision of adequate pain relief in infants and children are fear of respiratory depression and fear of addiction. Table 15-1 lists and refutes other prevalent myths about pain and pain management in children.

One strategy used by pediatric institutions to provide a comprehensive pain management program is a pain management team. The team may be composed of nurses certified in pain management, advanced practice nurses (APNs), physicians, pharmacists, and other health care practitioners. The team educates patients, families, nurses, physicians, and other health care providers. Further, they offer pain management recommendations to the health care team based on the most current knowledge. Availability and personalization of education may provide motivation for changes in beliefs and attitudes among health care providers, as well as patients and families. Pain management team members can also train resource nurses from each hospital unit, to provide advice and support to their colleagues on best practices in pain management for children.

Nurses who recognize the importance of implementing appropriate pain management strategies need ongoing access to the most current information. The Internet can be a powerful tool for instant, up-to-date information. Nurses and families are cautioned to ensure that they obtain information from trustworthy websites. Box 15-1 lists some suggested Internet resources. Given the rapidity with which Internet information changes, it is essential to verify the appropriateness of the website and accuracy of the information presented.

ASSESSMENT OF PAIN IN CHILDREN

Pain in children is multidimensional and subjective (APS, 2011a). It is affected by the type and duration of pain, developmental level, emotional status, previous pain experiences, culture and ethnicity,

BOX 15-1   PAIN MANAGEMENT RESOURCES ON THE INTERNET

- American Academy of Pain Medicine: www.painmed.org
- American Pain Foundation: www.painfoundation.org
- American Pain Society: www.ampainsoc.org
- American Society for Pain Management Nursing: www.aspmn.org
- Center for Pediatric Pain Research: http://pediatric-pain.ca
- International Association for the Study of Pain: www.iasp-pain.org
- Special Interest Group on Pain in Childhood: International Association for the Study of Pain: http://childpain.org
- NIH (National Institutes of Health) Pain Consortium: http://painconsortium.nih.gov

personality type, gender, genetic variations, and parental response to the child's pain. These factors should all be taken into consideration when assessing an infant or a child in pain. Consequently, assessing pain in infants and children is more challenging than in adults. Infants and young children may not have the language or cognitive abilities to communicate their pain. Their crying and verbal responses occur for many other reasons including hunger, sleepiness, and anxiety. Accordingly, the nurse must use a combination of behavioral and physiologic signs together with an appropriate pain assessment tool to determine the pain level in infants and some children (Von Baeyer & Spagrud, 2007) (Box 15-2).

Vital signs data such as heart rate, blood pressure, respiratory rate, and oxygen saturation have been reported to provide information about neonatal acute pain. However, these physiologic signs are also affected by other factors such as illness, fever, and medications, and there is little evidence to support using changes in vital signs to assess pain (Herr, Coyne, Key et al., 2006).

Behavioral and some physiologic signs can play an important role in pain assessment of children who are giving a verbal report of pain that differs from their nonverbal behaviors. An example might be a child who gives a verbal report of little or no pain out of concern that someone will become angry or that pain medication might involve an injection. Visually, the nurse might see the child grimacing, perhaps with tears, lying rigidly in bed and not moving. Such nonverbal behaviors would lead the nurse to speak and interact gently with the child

BOX 15-2 INDICATORS OF PAIN ACCORDING TO DEVELOPMENTAL LEVELS

Neonate and Infant

- Usually demonstrate changes in facial expression, including frowns, grimaces, wrinkled brow, expression of surprise, and facial flinching
- May demonstrate increases in blood pressure and heart rate, and decrease in oxygen saturation
- High-pitched, tense, harsh crying
- Tend to demonstrate a generalized or total body response to pain that becomes more purposeful as the infant matures
- May thrash extremities and exhibit tremors
- Older infants may localize the pain, rubbing the painful area, or pull away and guard the involved part

Toddler

- Likely to demonstrate loud crying
- Able to verbalize words that indicate discomfort such as "ouch," "hurt," "boo-boo"
- May attempt to delay procedures perceived as painful
- May demonstrate generalized restlessness
- May guard the site
- May touch painful areas
- May run from the nurse

Preschooler

- May think the pain is punishment for something he or she said or did
- Likely to cry and struggle
- Able to describe the location and intensity of pain (e.g., "ear hurts bad")
- May demonstrate regression to earlier behaviors, such as loss of bladder and bowel control
- May demonstrate withdrawal
- May deny pain to avoid taking oral medicine or a possible injection
- May have been told to "be brave" and deny pain, even if pain is present

School-Age Child

- Able to describe pain and quantify pain intensity
- Fears bodily injury
- Has an awareness of death
- May demonstrate stiff body posture
- May demonstrate withdrawal
- May procrastinate or bargain to delay procedure

Adolescent

- Perceives pain at a physical, emotional, and cognitive level
- Understands cause and effect
- Able to describe pain and quantify pain intensity
- May have increased muscle tension
- May demonstrate withdrawal and decreased motor activity
- May use words such as "sore," "ache," or "pounding" to describe pain

Although older children may be able to verbalize their discomfort, they are often afraid of treatment that includes a painful procedure such as an injection. They may have also been told to "be brave" and not verbalize or demonstrate the pain they are experiencing. Increasingly, it is also seen that even children as young as 5 or 6 years may be fearful of taking pain medication because of the emphasis on "saying no" to drugs. Such an emphasis is meant to focus on illegal substances or inappropriate use of prescription medications. Despite this fact, some children translate this to mean they should not use any drugs, even appropriate and necessary pain medications. Nurses need to provide developmentally appropriate education to children and their parents to overcome barriers to pain assessment and management.

Pain assessment and treatment are influenced by the cultural beliefs and practices of children and their families. Working to understand the impact of cultural differences on pain management is a crucial aspect of pediatric nursing care (Al-Atiyyat, 2009; Briggs, 2008; D'Arcy, 2009; Kirmayer, 2008; Narayan, 2010). Transcultural nursing literature can assist nurses to understand the diversity in nonverbal expressions of pain (facial expressions and other body language), words used for pain, descriptions of pain, and rating of pain noted among different cultures. Evidence supporting the validity of pain assessment scales for children from different cultures needs to be examined as a basis for nursing practice.

Assessment According to Developmental Level
Neonates and Infants

The fact that neonates and young infants have immature central nervous systems that lack myelinization of pain fibers has led clinicians in the past to believe that they are incapable of perceiving pain. However, in recent years substantial research has demonstrated that neonates and infants do feel pain and that infants whose pain is not addressed can experience long-term, negative consequences (AAP & Canadian Paediatric Society, 2006; Anand, 2007; APS, 2011a; Golianu, Krane, Seybold et al., 2007). Franck, Greenberg, and Stevens (2000) noted the difference between the nociceptive processes for infants and adults: Infants may actually have a lower pain threshold and perceive pain more intensely than older children and adults because of immature control mechanisms in the nervous system that limit their ability to modulate the pain experience.

Assessing acute pain in neonates and infants is difficult and is primarily based on behavioral and certain physiologic indicators. Rapid changes in an infant's behavioral state and sleep/activity patterns signal the likelihood of pain. Behaviors that often serve as indicators of infant pain include crying, fist clenching, grimacing, wrinkling of the forehead, fussiness, and restlessness (Anand, 2007; Boyle, Freer, Wong et al., 2006). Facial expression is considered the most consistent cue available when judging pain in infants and children (Schiavenato, 2008). Facial expression, in combination with short latency to onset of cry and a long duration of the first cry cycle, typifies infants' reactions to painful procedures. Cries associated with pain are higher pitched, tense, and harsh; they may sound different from those associated with hunger, discomfort, and stress. Therefore, parents and nurses may be able to differentiate between the usual cries of infants and the cries of pain.

Motor movements associated with pain in the neonate and infant progress from a generalized body response to more purposeful movements. For example, infants ages 9 to 12 months can use their hands to push the nurse away if they perceive a painful action is about to begin. The responses of neonates to painful stimuli are sometimes described as total body responses (Figure 15-1). The infant's extremities may thrash about, and some infants exhibit tremors. Older infants may rub the painful area, pull away, or guard the involved body part.

about the actual level of pain to ensure appropriate pain management. Children who suffer from chronic pain may not demonstrate behavioral changes that are noticeable to the nurse, and they may be unable to accurately describe their pain level. It is important to assess the impact of pain on a child's daily life including sleeping, eating, attending school, social and physical activities (e.g., play or sports), and interactions with family and peers (APS, 2011b). Changes in these areas, such as being unwilling or unable to play with peers, may be subtle signs that a child is experiencing pain (Busoni, 2007).

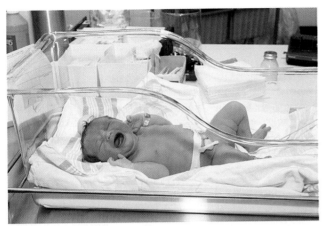

FIG 15-1 Infant total body response to pain with arms thrashing, tremors, and vigorous crying.

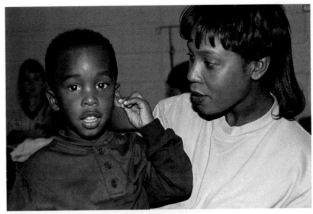

FIG 15-2 Toddlers and preschoolers may express pain by guarding or touching the painful area. The toddler pulling on his ear is a characteristic expression of ear pain from otitis media. (Courtesy University of Texas at Arlington College of Nursing, Arlington, TX.)

The responses of infants to pain are greatly determined by their state immediately before painful stimulation; pain scores are higher and behavioral changes are greater when infants are awake and active compared to when they are asleep (Badr, Abdallah, Hawari et al., 2010). Though preterm infants lack the autonomic functions and maturity to handle stress, it remains unclear if repeated exposure to pain results in heightened responses or desensitization (Badr et al., 2010). The nurse must be cognizant of this information to make a beginning assessment of pain through observation of an infant's facial expressions, motor response, and cry. Neonates who are experiencing prolonged or persistent pain may not exhibit the usual behavioral signs of pain seen in neonates who are experiencing acute pain and, instead, exhibit signs and symptoms of energy conservation (AAP & Canadian Paediatric Society, 2006; Anand, 2007).

Physiologic changes may be more difficult to assess and serve as just one part of a complete pain assessment. A nurse should suspect that an infant experiences pain before physiologic changes are observed. Increases in blood pressure, heart rate, and respiratory rate and decreases in arterial oxygen saturation have been associated with pain in neonates, although these changes can be linked to other alterations such as agitation. Crying may also affect the infant's physiologic responses. Distinguishing between pain and agitation is sometimes difficult. If an infant is simply agitated, yet is treated for pain, the cause of the agitation may remain untreated.

The behavioral and physiologic indicators discussed are components in several different pain assessment tools used for the preverbal or nonverbal child. The reliability and validity of these assessment tools have been studied extensively. In order to provide high-quality care, it is important that nurses use pain assessment tools rather than rely on personal, subjective appraisals of infant behavioral and physiologic indicators.

Toddlers

The toddler in pain tends to cry longer than the infant. As verbal abilities become more advanced, the toddler can vocalize displeasure when a painful experience occurs. The toddler may ask for parents, use words that indicate discomfort ("ouch," "hurt"), and even verbalize negative emotions about the nurse. The toddler may also try to delay the nurse's implementation of a procedure judged as painful. The older toddler can often localize the pain and point to the body part that hurts.

Generalized restlessness, guarding the site, and touching the painful area are signs of pain in the toddler (Figure 15-2). The toddler may

associate discomfort with a particular procedure, such as a dressing change, and may run from the nurse when approached. The toddler's facial expressions can indicate anger and fear. The child may avoid eye contact or look sad. In response to discomfort and pain, the toddler may also demonstrate regression to earlier, more comfortable behaviors such as lying on a parent's lap in a fetal position.

Preschoolers

Preschoolers are egocentric. Relating only to the present, they have difficulty associating discomfort with any positive outcome, and this can intensify their pain experience. For example, the preschooler will not understand that débriding a painful burn will ultimately have a positive effect. Children in this age-group are able to describe the location and intensity of pain.

Preschoolers tend to think pain will magically go away and that experiencing pain is punishment for some previous thought or deed. They also fear body mutilation, particularly of the genitals. Preschoolers may deny pain from a surgical incision, for example, in order to avoid an invasive procedure such as a pain medication injection. They may also cry and struggle in an attempt to escape from the procedure. Preschoolers can regress to earlier, more comfortable behaviors, such as thumb sucking, in response to pain, or they can withdraw and not participate in play activities.

School-Age Children

School-age children can describe pain and relate it to a specific body part, as well as quantify pain intensity. They are beginning to understand the need for painful procedures. They fear body harm and have

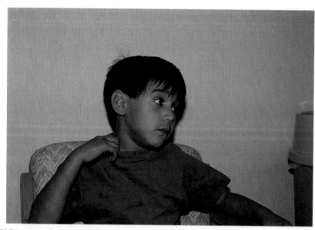

FIG 15-3 School-age children may become very quiet and withdrawn when ill or in pain. The child with asthma is not attentive or active; his mother knew that something was wrong because of his withdrawn behavior. (Courtesy Parkland Health and Hospital System Community-Oriented Primary Care Clinic, Dallas, TX.)

> **! NURSING QUALITY ALERT**
> *Assessing Pain in Children*
>
> - The use of a pain assessment tool is imperative in the assessment of pain in children and the evaluation of pain management interventions. The tool used is documented in the patient's medical record.
> - If the child is unable to express or quantify pain, use parents as one of the first resources to assist in assessing the child's pain and response to interventions.
> - Behavioral changes such as guarding, body positioning, crying, grimacing and other altered facial expressions, and changes in activity level, may or may not be seen in a child experiencing pain.
> - Physiologic changes are only one source of information when assessing pain in the neonate or infant. Other states, such as fear and anxiety, may also cause physiologic changes. Physiologic changes tend to occur during an acute pain experience and then return to normal; they may not be valid indicators of sustained or chronic pain.

---

an awareness of death. Therefore, they may appear to overreact to illness or injury. As in other age-groups, the school-age child remembers previous pain experiences, which will affect the current response. The child's culture, gender, and cognitive abilities will also affect the pain experience (Finley, Kristjansdottir, & Forgeron, 2009).

Nonverbal and behavioral cues are very important in assessing a school-age child's pain. The child may exhibit a stiff body posture, may withdraw, or may be found quietly sobbing (Figure 15-3). If the school-age child resists a treatment, cries loudly, or otherwise acts in an aggressive manner, the child may later deny the behavior. School-age children may also attempt to procrastinate or bargain to delay a painful procedure. As with younger children, the school-age child may demonstrate regressive behaviors when experiencing pain.

Adolescents

Adolescents can think abstractly and understand cause and effect. They can describe and quantify pain intensity and their feelings about pain. They can also discuss the strategies to help manage their pain. They are able to perceive and understand pain at a physical, emotional, and cognitive level. However, having these abilities does not mean the adolescent will use them. Adolescents are often confused by control issues and are uncertain of their roles as they move from childhood to adulthood. Regression may also occur at this age in relation to pain.

Because adolescents are egocentric, they tend to think that others focus on their behaviors and therefore, adolescents may suppress manifestations of pain. In addition, they may not report pain because they believe that the nurse knows when they hurt; subsequently, they expect to receive pain medication when they *need* it and not just when they ask for it. Adolescents tend to exhibit fewer outward signs of pain as compared to younger children. Signs observed may include increased muscle tension, withdrawal, and decreased motor activity. Hospitalized adolescents use words such as "sore," "like an ache," "pounding," and "miserable" to describe pain.

Assessment Tools

Consistent, appropriate use of a pain assessment tool is essential to pediatric pain management. A number of valid and reliable pain assessment tools are available to help the nurse make a more accurate pain assessment. Both self-report and behavioral instruments are

available. Examples of these tools are detailed in Table 15-2. Children benefit when pain assessment tools are used because they are given a simple and effective way to communicate the pain they are experiencing. Assessment tools provide more objective data, reducing the chance that discreet signs of pain will be overlooked. Unfortunately, they are not always used consistently and correctly in clinical settings. Using a tool in a way other than the developer intended may invalidate the pain assessment.

An assessment tool should be used that corresponds to the child's developmental abilities. The crucial factors concerning selection of a pain assessment tool are that it is appropriate for the child's developmental level and can facilitate the development of an effective pain management plan based on the information gathered from the assessment. Varieties of tools are available for infants and the preverbal or nonverbal child, such as those who are neurologically unresponsive, developmentally delayed, or unable to speak because of medical treatment such as intubation (Herr et al., 2006). Tools for infants and preverbal children usually are based on behavioral cues (e.g., facial expression, motor responses, intensity of cry). One such tool, the Face, Legs, Activity, Cry, Consolability (FLACC) scale, has been examined numerous times for reliability and validity. It has been shown to be an appropriate, effective tool for the preverbal or nonverbal child (Herr et al., 2006; Voepel-Lewis, Zanotti, Dammeyer, & Merkel, 2010) and is being used with increasing frequency.

Children verbalize words for pain by approximately 18 months of age, and cognitive development is sufficient for reporting the extent of pain by 3 to 4 years of age. Self-report tools are effective in children older than 3 years. The Oucher, the Poker Chip Tool, and the FACES Pain Rating Scale are examples of tools for preschoolers and school-age children. For some children, the African-American, Asian, First Nations (Canadian Indian), or Hispanic versions of the Oucher pain scale (Figure 15-4) may facilitate a more culturally sensitive assessment (Beyer, Villarruel, & Denyes, 2009). The Wong-Baker FACES Pain Rating Scale has been translated into 10 different languages. Matching the tool to the child's ethnicity and primary language can provide better information about pain experienced by children from diverse populations and promote better pain control (Wong-Baker FACES Foundation, 1983).

School-age children can understand concepts of order and number and can use numeric rating scales, word-graphic rating scales, and visual analog scales. Table 15-2 describes pain assessment tools and lists the age or developmental level of children appropriate for its use

TABLE 15-2   PAIN ASSESSMENT TOOLS

TOOL	DESCRIPTION	AGE
Adolescent and Pediatric Pain Tool (APPT) (see Figure 15-6)	Three-part tool composed of a body outline, an intensity scale, and a pain descriptor word list (Savedra, Tesler, Holzemer, & Ward, 1992).	8-17 yr
CRIES Pain Scale	Five behavioral categories: *C*rying, *R*equires oxygen for SaO$_2$ < 95%, *I*ncreased vital signs, *E*xpression, *S*leepless; 0-2 for each with total score from 0-10. A higher score indicates greater pain or distress (Krechel & Bildner, 1995).	Neonates; 0-6 mo
COMFORT Behavior Scale	Six categories are scored: Alertness, Calmness/Agitation, Respiratory response (if on ventilator) or Crying (if breathing spontaneously), Physical Movement, Muscle Tone, Facial Tension; 1-5 for each category with total score from 6-30. A higher score indicates greater pain or distress (Van Dijk, Peters, Van Deventer, & Tibboel, 2005).	Infants and children in critical care settings
FLACC	Five behavioral categories: *F*ace, *L*egs, *A*ctivity, *C*ry, *C*onsolability. Each scored from 0-2, resulting in a total score from 0-10. A higher score indicates higher pain or distress (Merkel, Voepel-Lewis, & Malviya, 2002).	Infants and preverbal or nonverbal children
FACES Pain Rating Scale (see Figure 15-5)	Six cartoon faces with neutral to gradually increasing painful expressions, corresponding to an analog scale with words ranging from a happy face (0; No Hurt) to a crying face (5 or 10; Hurts Worst). Accommodates a 0-5 or 0-10 system (Hockenberry & Wilson, 2009).	3 yr and older
Numeric Rating Scale (NRS)	Patient is asked to give a number that reflects the pain level: 0 = no pain; 1-3 = mild; 4-6 = moderate; 7-10 = severe (Pasero & McCaffery, 2011).	Child 9 yr and older
The Oucher (see Figure 15-4)	A poster with a 0-100 scale for older children and a six-picture photographic scale for young children who cannot count to 100; 0 is no pain and 100 is the greatest pain. Five versions available: Caucasian/white, Asian (boy or girl), First Nations (boy or girl), Hispanic, and African-American/black (Beyer, Villarruel, & Denyes, 2009).	3-12 yr
Poker Chip Tool	Four poker chips are used, with each chip representing a piece of hurt. One poker chip represents a little hurt, and four chips represent the most hurt the child could have (Hester, Foster, Jordan-Marsh et al., 1998).	4-12 yr
Visual Analog Scale (VAS)	Usually a 10-cm line with one end representing "no pain" and the opposite end "the worst pain" (Cline, Herman, Shaw, & Morton, 1992).	7-18 yr

(Figures 15-5 and 15-6). The same tool should be used each time a child is assessed to obtain consistent data and to avoid confusing the child. Whenever possible, the child should be taught how to use the rating tool before pain is experienced. This can be a part of pre-procedure or preoperative education for the child and family.

In assessing pain and obtaining the pain history, the nurse should first ask the child and family which word, or words, the child uses to indicate pain. A child may use words such as "owie" or "ouchie" when describing pain or hurt. A child's word(s) must be used consistently by the nurse in any future discussions with the child regarding pain. In interviewing the parents and family, the nurse should address the presence and involvement of different family members, cultural and/or spiritual beliefs, and practices regarding pain and pain relief. Box 15-3 describes how to obtain a pain experience history from both the child and parents. Information to be gathered includes the child's past experiences with pain, how the child reacts to pain, the person the child tells about pain, how the parents know when their child is in pain, and what works best to take the child's pain away.

NONPHARMACOLOGIC AND PHARMACOLOGIC PAIN INTERVENTIONS

Pain management for children needs to be "multimodal" using an effective combination of a quiet, calm environment and both nonpharmacologic and pharmacologic approaches (APS, 2011a). The nurse's assessment helps determine the suitable intervention. If pharmacologic interventions are determined to be the first and best option, nonpharmacologic interventions may always be presented as an adjuvant for the chosen analgesic. Doing so may offer the child a sense of accomplishment and control that can replace the sense of helplessness that often accompanies the presence of pain, illness, and hospitalization.

Nonpharmacologic Interventions

The nurse caring for a child in pain can provide nonpharmacologic interventions in addition to pharmacologic interventions. Use of nonpharmacologic interventions in preparing the child for procedures and treatments can help minimize or relieve pain by reducing anxiety and fear of the unknown (see Chapter 11). Nonpharmacologic interventions must be suitable for the child, considering stage of development, the child's personality, and the circumstances surrounding the child.

Parents play a very important role in assessing and providing pain management for their children. They are a resource for determining what methods of pain relief were effective in the past. They can help the nurse assess their child's current pain status and need for intervention. Repositioning, holding, touching, massage, warm or cold compresses, breathing techniques, distraction, guided imagery, and muscle relaxation are all techniques that can be used by the person the child usually trusts the most—a parent. Many techniques require preliminary instruction by the nurse or other qualified individuals but then are easily learned and put into practice by parents. This is also a mechanism to give parents "hands-on" involvement and a sense of control when their child is hospitalized. Infant kangaroo care (holding with skin-to-skin contact) is an example of an effective pain reduction intervention provided by the mother (Kashaninia, Sajedi, Rahgozar, & Noghabi, 2008).

Distraction can be one of the more effective adjuvants for pain management (Figure 15-7). It is also one of the simplest to accomplish. Distraction works by refocusing the child's attention from the pain to something else. For example, a child brought to the emergency department after an accident is invariably frightened. Even if the injury is minor, the fear and pain are real to the child. By using distraction, the nurse can decrease the child's anxiety and subsequently the pain is reduced. Some children experiencing pain may engage in activities on their own in an effort to ignore or "forget" their pain. It is important not to discount the pain a child is experiencing when a child is able to use distraction effectively to control pain.

The form of distraction used should be appropriate for the child's developmental level. Techniques include blowing bubbles, looking through a kaleidoscope, listening to music or stories, reading, playing number, video or board games, watching a video, and even doing multiplication tables or spelling words. Another distraction method used during a procedure or treatment involves allowing a child to help by handing, opening, or holding objects. This should be done only when it is safe and there is no danger of contamination of materials or of the treatment site.

If a child has a favorite doll or stuffed animal, it may be used to create a story or a game. Children love to talk about their pets, and the nurse can ask the child to tell a favorite story about the pet. Engaging a child in conversation that is meaningful to the child not only aids in pain control but also facilitates development of a therapeutic nurse-patient relationship. Although each child is different, cues or verbal instruction from the child and the parent can indicate whether the

---

PATIENT-CENTERED TEACHING

Pain Management for Children at Home

- Parents are given a pain assessment tool with instructions on accurate use. They should verbalize understanding about the tool and give a return demonstration using the tool with their child.
- The dose, route, and schedule for all pain medications are explained to the parents verbally and in writing. *All instructions should be in the appropriate language for the family, using clear, straightforward terminology that is at an educational level suitable for the parents.*
- Nonpharmacologic interventions that are appropriate and comforting for the child's pain (e.g., massage, warm or cold compresses, repositioning) are explained and demonstrated. Written instructions are provided as necessary.
- Parents are instructed to notify the primary health care provider if interventions for pain management are ineffective or if the child shows behavior or physiologic changes not consistent with the expected outcomes for the child.
- Parents are given a phone number where they can contact a nurse or other health care provider if they have any questions about their child's condition once the child is in the home setting.

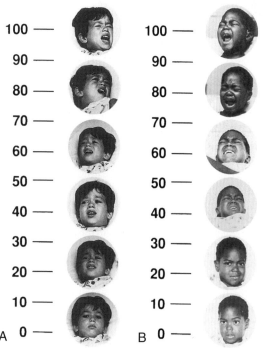

FIG 15-4 **A,** The Hispanic version of the Oucher pain scale. **B,** The African-American version. (**A,** Developed and copyrighted by Antonia M. Villarruel, RN, PhD, and Mary J. Denyes, RN, PhD, 1991. **B,** Developed and copyrighted by Mary J. Denyes, PhD, RN, FAAN [Wayne State University], and Antonia Villarruel, PhD, RN, FAAN [University of Pennsylvania] at the Children's Hospital of Michigan in 1990. Cornelia P. Porter, PhD, RN, and Charlotta Marshall, MSN, RN, contributed to the development of this scale.)

BOX 15-3 PAIN EXPERIENCE HISTORY

Child Form*
- What word(s) do you use to describe your pain?
- Tell me what pain is.
- What does a child with pain look like?
- How do you feel when you have pain?
- Have you ever had pain just like this before? Tell me about a time when you had pain.
- Is the pain you have now different than pain you have had before?
- Do you tell others when you hurt? Who do you tell?
- What helps the most to take your hurt away?
- What do you do for yourself when you are hurting?
- What do you want other people to do for you when you hurt?
- What don't you want other people to do for you when you hurt?
- Did anyone tell you that you might have pain? If yes, who told you and how did they tell you?
- Is there anything else at all you want to tell me about pain? (If yes, have child describe.)

Parent Form
- What word or words does your child use to describe pain?
- Describe the pain experiences your child has had in the past.
- Does your child tell you or others when in pain?
- How do you know when your child is in pain?
- How does your child usually react to pain?
- What do you do when your child is in pain?
- What does your child do when he or she is in pain?
- What works best to take away your child's pain?
- Is there anything special that you would like me to know about your child and pain? (If yes, describe.)

Modified from Hester, N. O., & Barcus, C. S. (1986). Assessment and management of pain in children. *Pediatrics: Nursing Update, 1*(14), 2-8; Cheng, S., Foster, R. L., Hester, N. O., & Huang, C. (2003). A qualitative inquiry of Taiwanese children's pain experiences. *Journal of Nursing Research (Taiwan Nurses Association), 11*(4), 241-250.
*Substitute the word *pain* or *hurt* with the word the child uses (e.g., "owie" or "ouchie").

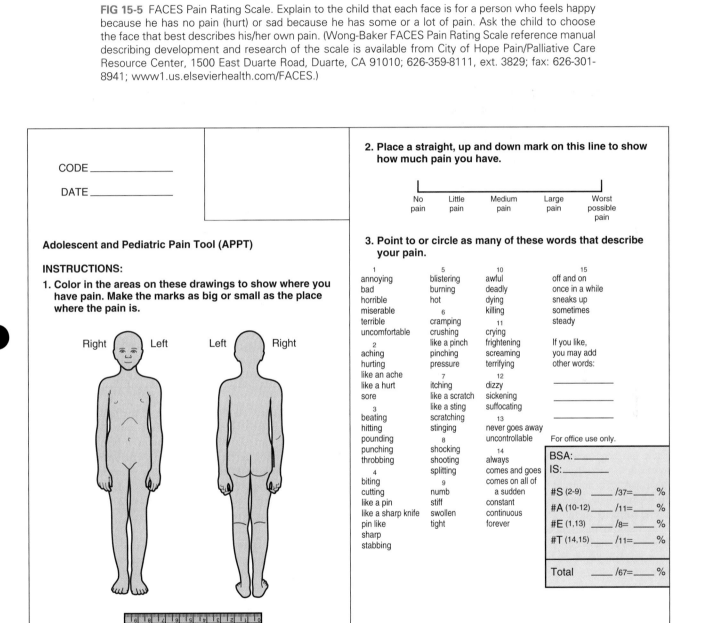

FIG 15-5 FACES Pain Rating Scale. Explain to the child that each face is for a person who feels happy because he has no pain (hurt) or sad because he has some or a lot of pain. Ask the child to choose the face that best describes his/her own pain. (Wong-Baker FACES Pain Rating Scale reference manual describing development and research of the scale is available from City of Hope Pain/Palliative Care Resource Center, 1500 East Duarte Road, Duarte, CA 91010; 626-359-8111, ext. 3829; fax: 626-301-8941; www1.us.elsevierhealth.com/FACES.)

FIG 15-6 Adolescent and Pediatric Pain Tool (APPT). Use with 8- to 17-year-olds. (From Savedra, M. C., Tesler, M. D., Holzemer, W. L., & Ward, J. A. [1992]. *Adolescent and pediatric pain tool: User's manual*. San Francisco: University of California, San Francisco, School of Nursing. Copyright 1989, 1992.)

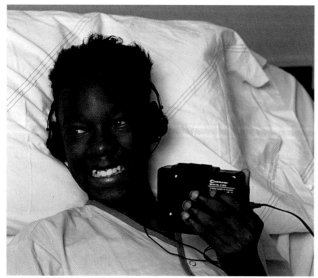

FIG 15-7 The boy listens to music, which serves as a distraction to refocus attention and reduce pain. (Courtesy Children's Medical Center, Dallas, TX.)

nurse should hold the child's hand, touch the child's head, or provide some other interventions that are appropriate and comforting for the child.

Once both the child and nurse can communicate personally, the nurse might say, "I see you have a baseball shirt." If the child expresses an interest in the game, the nurse can continue, "What is your favorite team?" The nurse should be comfortable with the topic because the child will sense a lack of genuine interest. If it is appropriate on the basis of the child's developmental level and degree of egocentricity, the nurse might interject a personal note such as "I enjoy going to baseball games with my family." This conversation could go on for 10 to 15 minutes, certainly long enough for minor procedures such as suturing a laceration, to be completed. The child will not be focusing as much on the procedure as on baseball. The topic must be of interest to the child in order to distract the child's attention away from pain.

There has been considerable research regarding the use of oral sucrose with or without nonnutritive sucking (NNS) on pacifiers as a nonpharmacologic adjuvant for neonatal and infant pain management. Several studies have provided evidence that giving oral sucrose alone and with NNS before and during a procedure are safe and effective interventions that reduce procedural pain in infants (Hatfield, 2008; Stevens, Yamada, Beyene et al., 2005; Thompson, 2005). However, other research indicates that oral sucrose may not be as effective as analgesic drugs (Slater, Cornelissen, Fabrizi et al., 2010).

Table 15-3 lists additional nonpharmacologic approaches to pain management for infants and children. It is important to remember that, regardless of the technique used; the nurse should evaluate its effectiveness and change the intervention if the chosen technique provides ineffective pain relief.

Pharmacologic Interventions

Reluctance to administer analgesics to infants and children stems from the fears of many nurses and physicians that analgesics will cause respiratory depression and/or lead to addiction. Some health care providers incorrectly believe that a child does not experience enough pain to justify analgesic administration. If a procedure, surgery, or trauma causes pain in an adult, it will cause pain in a child, and analgesic medications are necessary. However, it is important to ensure that the correct medication and dose are ordered and administered. In some cases, the analgesic is underdosed and the child still experiences untreated, unwarranted pain. Increased pain management experience and research have taught that a combination of medications (multi-drug therapy) is often far more effective than a single analgesic. However, no one analgesic or combination of analgesics will provide optional pain management for all patients or in all circumstances. The chosen analgesic therapy must have a prompt onset of action, a predictable duration of action, manageable side effects, and an appropriate reversal agent.

Administration of Analgesics

Analgesics can be administered by various routes—oral, rectal, intranasal, topical, transdermal, intravenous (IV), intramuscular (IM), subcutaneous, and epidural (see Chapter 14 for a discussion of the common routes). The least invasive route that provides optimum analgesia should always be chosen. Whenever possible, as soon as the child can tolerate oral nutrition, pain medication should be given by the oral route. Rectal medication should be avoided because this route can be very disturbing to children and is generally disliked. The IM route is used infrequently because many children are very afraid of injections ("shots").

> **! NURSING QUALITY ALERT**
> **Disadvantages of Intramuscular (IM) Analgesics**
>
> - Most children have a significant fear of pain associated with IM injections.
> - Fluctuations in tissue absorption lead to peaks and troughs in analgesia.
> - Children may not have enough suitable sites for IM injections.
> - Some medications can cause injury to tissues and nerves.
> - IM analgesics have a shorter duration of action than do oral analgesics.
> - IM analgesics are contraindicated in children with low platelet counts and bleeding disorders such as hemophilia.

Patient-Controlled Analgesia. One of the most effective ways of administering opioids is by use of a patient-controlled analgesia (PCA) pump. The pump administers an IV bolus of pain medication either with or without a continuous infusion of the same medication. The patient controls the infusion of the bolus. An underlying safety principle associated with PCA is that a sedated or sleeping patient will not be able to activate a bolus dose (Manworren, 2007) and therefore the risk of overdosing is reduced.

When the child needs pain medication, a small dose of the opioid medication is received after a button connected to the pump is pushed (Figure 15-8). After each dose, there is "lock-out" time during which the pump will not release the medication even if the button is pushed. The pump also has a maximum amount of medication that can be given over a designated period—usually 1 hour. If the maximum amount of medication for the designated time period has been reached, the pump will not release medication even if the button is pushed.

After checking to ensure that all doses are within appropriate range for the child, two registered nurses (RNs) must check the bag or syringe of medication before hanging it. After a PCA pump is programmed, it must then be double-checked by a second RN. Box 15-4 gives an example of orders for a PCA infusion. The opioid bag or syringe is locked into the PCA pump, and the pump itself is locked to the IV pole. Typically, the PCA tubing is special tubing that does not have IV access ports.

The child is monitored frequently to ensure that pain control is effective and that the equipment is functioning correctly. The nurse

TABLE 15-3   NONPHARMACOLOGIC PAIN-RELIEF TECHNIQUES

TECHNIQUE	DESCRIPTION	NURSING CONSIDERATIONS
Distraction	Related to the Gate Control Theory, use of distraction techniques "closes the gate" by focusing the child on the distraction rather than on the pain experience. Active methods are more effective than passive (Twycross & Dowden, 2009). Wide range of techniques (e.g., playing with toys, video games, blowing bubbles, watching videos, listening to music, singing, reading).	Relatively easy to use and often employed by nurses and other health care providers to help children cope with pain. Distraction must be developmentally appropriate for the child.
Regulated (controlled) breathing	Provides a focal point for distraction and produces relaxation. A simple mode for biofeedback.	Teach the child how to achieve a slow, rhythmic breathing pattern; teach parents the technique and how to help their child.
Guided imagery	The child is encouraged to remember or imagine the sounds, sights, and smells of an enjoyable item or experience such as playing in the water or a birthday celebration (Srouji, Ratnapalan, & Schneeweiss, 2010). The facilitator talks in a soft, calm voice while "guiding" the child's imagination. Can be coupled with relaxation techniques such as rhythmic breathing.	Facilitated by trained health care providers (e.g., nurse, child-life therapist). Studies have shown reductions in children's pain from a variety of causes (Ball, Shapiro, Monheim, & Weydert, 2003; Huth, Broome, & Good, 2004).
Biofeedback	Involves measurement of physiologic indicators (e.g., blood pressure, heart rate, skin temperature, sweating, and muscle tension) using specialized equipment. Alerts patients instantly to early signs of tension so they can commence relaxation techniques; the child learns to control physiologic responses based on the biofeedback. Has proven effective for treatment of headaches and other types of pain (Twycross & Dowden, 2009).	Requires trained personnel to administer and teach tension recognition and relaxation techniques.
Progressive muscle relaxation	Progressive, systematic, purposeful relaxation of one muscle group at a time through contraction and then relaxation of muscles; usually proceeds from head to toe. Often used effectively for migraine and tension headaches (Twycross & Dowden, 2009).	Teach the older child and adolescent the technique; encourage frequent practice.
Hypnosis	Focused, narrowed attention and an altered state of consciousness that facilitates relaxation. Used in association with painful procedures and treatments, postoperatively, or for chronic pain.	Hypnotists receive special training; children can be taught self-hypnosis.
Acupuncture	Based on traditional Chinese concepts of energy balance; insertion of very thin needles through the skin to stimulate anatomic points (meridians). Limited research in children (Twycross & Dowden, 2009). Effective for acute and chronic pain in children (Kundu & Berman, 2007).	Treatment is done by a trained acupuncturist; children may have concerns about the use of needles.
Topical heating and cooling	Application of cold or heat to a painful area provides pain relief and comfort; the mechanism of action is uncertain (McCaffery & Pasero, 1999). Effectively treats pain from disease states, injuries, and procedures (Twycross & Dowden, 2009).	Used by nurses, physical therapists, sports trainers, and other clinicians.
Massage	Purposeful manipulation of the body, providing tactile and kinesthetic stimulation. Evidence regarding benefits is varied; strongest effect is anxiety reduction (Beider, Mahrer & Gold, 2007).	Performed by massage therapists; nurses may provide basic massage.
TENS (transcutaneous electrical nerve stimulation)	Small amounts of electrical energy are delivered to the skin via electrodes. By interfering with the transmission of pain signals, TENS completely or partially blocks the sensation of pain in the stimulated area (Twycross & Dowden, 2009).	Usually administered by physical therapists. Used frequently for children and adults.
Techniques for neonates and infants	Several noninvasive techniques used during and/or after a painful procedure or experience include breastfeeding; oral sucrose; nonnutritive sucking on a pacifier; skin-to-skin contact (kangaroo care) with the infant positioned directly on the mother's chest; holding and rocking by a parent or caregiver; and tucking or swaddling where the infant is wrapped with the extremities close to the trunk (Srouji et al., 2010).	Nurses may use a variety of techniques separately or in combination to distract the infant and reduce the severity of the pain experience. Parents can be taught to use techniques.

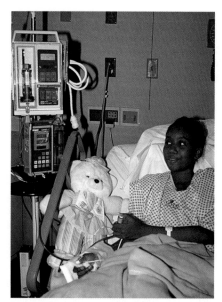

FIG 15-8 Patient-controlled analgesia (PCA) allows the child greater control over her own pain management. (Courtesy Children's Medical Center, Dallas, TX.)

BOX 15-4 **ASPECTS OF PATIENT-CONTROLLED ANALGESIA ORDERS**

Medication/concentration: _____

Mode: PCA only _____ PCA and basal infusion _____

Continuous infusion only _____

Dosages:

PCA bolus _____ mg (recommended starting dose is 0.02 mg/kg/dose for morphine)

Basal rate or continuous infusion _____ (recommended starting dose is 0.02 mg/kg/hr for morphine)

Lock-out: _____ minutes (usual is 6 to 10 min as needed)

1-hour limit: _____ mg PCA and basal rate combined (usual is 0.075 mg/kg for morphine)

---

should also carefully assess the child for signs of overmedication (especially depressed respiratory rate or inability to awaken) and the side effects that may accompany opioid administration. Vital signs should be assessed every 2 to 4 hours. Some institutions require hourly documentation of respiratory rate.

Additionally, many institutional policies require that children receiving PCA therapy be placed on continuous pulse oximetry, cardiac and respiratory monitoring, or both. Oxygen, a bag-valve-mask device, and IV naloxone (Narcan) should be readily available. Naloxone will reverse opioid-related analgesia and respiratory depression; it must be administered slowly until it is first noted that respiratory depression is reversed. It has a short half-life and may need to be repeated every 30 to 60 minutes. Many institutions mandate that naloxone must be given in the presence of a physician because too-rapid infusion can result in cardiac arrest.

Frequent pain assessment is essential, usually every 1 to 4 hours and with any bolus dose, in order to assess the effectiveness of PCA therapy in general and the bolus. Charting will include hourly documentation as to the number of bolus doses received and the number of bolus attempts made by the child. Total milligram dosages of the medication received will be noted every 1 to 4 hours and documented on the medication administration record.

Most hospitals permit use of PCA by children 5 to 7 years of age or older, when developmentally appropriate. For younger children or those not able to operate a PCA pump independently and control their own analgesia, family or health care providers have administered PCA by proxy (for the child). Because of adverse events that occurred with PCA by proxy, the Joint Commission in 2004 recommended that hospitals implement strict protocols for patient selection and institute a warning system that alerts unauthorized staff and families not to administer bolus doses for the patient. The American Society for Pain Management Nursing (2006) has issued recommendations for use of Authorized Agent–Controlled Analgesia (AACA) by carefully selected nurses or family members (nurse-controlled analgesia or caregiver-controlled analgesia). These include (1) developing stringent guidelines for selecting and educating nurses or appropriate family caregivers; (2) providing oral and written instructions that address how to assess when the child needs to receive a bolus and when the child should not receive a bolus; (3) selecting a single nurse or caregiver who will be with the patient consistently and can assess for medication effects and potential adverse consequences; and (4) documenting teaching and supervision of the person giving the AACA (Wuhrman, Coone, Dunwoody et al., 2007).

Topical Anesthetic Agents. Several non–injection-based, topical anesthetic agents are available for use before painful procedures. These agents have been found to effectively reduce in children the pain associated with invasive procedures such as injections, venipunctures, lumbar punctures, and bone marrow aspirations (Gilboy & Hollywood, 2009). Further, many pediatric institutions mandate that numbing agents be used for all IV catheter insertions, unless it is on an emergency basis.

Lidocaine-prilocaine 5% cream (eutectic mixture of local anesthetics [EMLA]) was the first agent that demonstrated efficacy for numbing the skin for invasive procedures. Additional topical agents used for children include 4% amethocaine gel (Ametop), liposomal lidocaine 4% or 5% cream (LMX4 or LMX5), and the Synera patch with 70 mg of lidocaine and 70 mg of tetracaine (Lander, Weltman, & So, 2006; Singer, Taira, Chisena et al., 2008).

A cream or patch is applied to intact skin with no open wounds, burns, abrasions, cuts, or inflammation. The technique for application and amount of time the agent must be in contact with the skin varies according to the agent used (see Chapter 14). Generally, an anesthetic cream is placed on the skin at the procedure site for 30 minutes to 2.5 hours and provides a numbing effect for 1 to 2 hours after removal. Parents may apply an agent at home before a scheduled procedure such as an immunization injection to prevent pain. Parents are instructed to wear gloves when applying anesthetic creams. Young children must be supervised so they do not remove the dressing, rub the cream in their eyes or ears, or eat the cream, which may look like cake frosting.

The main side effect seen with any of the topical anesthetic creams is skin redness or blanching, with normal skin color returning in a few hours. The child should be monitored for burning, swelling, itching, or a rash at the application site; if seen, this would necessitate immediate removal of the cream from the skin.

A vapocoolant spray, dichlorodifluoromethane/trichlorodifluoromethane vapocoolant (Fluori-Methane or cold spray), is used to provide immediate numbing of the skin for urgent procedures (Farion, Splinter, Newhook, & Gaboury, 2008; Overmyer, 2010). Cold spray is sprayed either directly on the skin at the site or on a sterile cotton ball, which is then applied to the site for 15 seconds. The onset of action is immediate and the numbing effect lasts approximately 15 seconds.

Needleless systems are also used to painlessly deliver anesthetic medication below the surface of the skin. Lidocaine hydrochloride 2% with 1:100,000 epinephrine topical solution (Numby Stuff) comes in an electrode patch and uses iontophoresis, a mild electric current, to push lidocaine and epinephrine into the skin to a depth of 10 mm. A newer approach is the J-Tip jet device, which delivers 1% buffered lidocaine into the skin at a depth of 5 to 8 mm via a carbon dioxide gas–driven plunger. Some studies have shown use of the J-Tip to reduce pain for children during IV catheter insertions, though its efficacy over other topical anesthetics is still being investigated (Auerbach, Tunik, & Mojica, 2009; Jimenez, Bradford, Seidel et al., 2006; Spanos, Booth, Koenig et al., 2008). These methods can only be used in health care settings.

Optimal care for children undergoing painful, invasive procedures requires the combined use of several different interventions. Though topical anesthetic agents significantly reduce or even remove pain, children can still experience fear and anxiety, which in turn causes distress for the entire family. Use of topical agents along with distraction or other nonpharmacologic methods, and parental presence, work together to alleviate pain and stress for the child and family (Gilboy & Hollywood, 2009). Nurses serve as patient advocates by encouraging parents, older children, and adolescents to participate in the selection of the agents and techniques to be used.

Acetaminophen and Antiinflammatory Drugs

Acetaminophen (brand name Tylenol) is the most commonly used analgesic for mild to moderate pain as well as the drug of choice for treating children's fevers in the United States. It has a minimal antiinflammatory effect. The short-term use of acetaminophen is safe, even in neonates. It does not have the gastric irritation and GI bleeding side effects. Usually related to overdosage, acetaminophen can cause hepatic damage. It is of critical importance to monitor the total amount of acetaminophen a child is receiving because it is often combined with other prescription and over-the-counter medications to treat pain, fever, and other symptoms associated with upper respiratory infections and influenza.

Nonsteroidal antiinflammatory drugs (NSAIDs) reduce pain, fever, and inflammation by inhibiting the production of prostaglandins. Ibuprofen, naproxen/naproxen sodium (Aleve, Naprosyn, Anaprox), and ketorolac (Toradol) are the NSAIDs that are frequently used to treat mild to moderate pain in children. NSAIDs often are the preferred drugs to treat bone and inflammatory pain associated with bone injuries, arthritis-like conditions, or certain types of cancer (see Chapter 26).

Though aspirin (acetylsalicylic acid) is an effective antiinflammatory drug, it is not recommended for use in children to treat pain or fever due to an association with Reye syndrome (see Chapter 28). In 1982, the U.S. Surgeon General advised against the use of aspirin to treat children with influenza or chickenpox; subsequently the incidence of Reye syndrome has sharply declined (Belay, Bresee, Holman et al., 1999).

Opioids

Opioids are natural or synthetic opium derivative analgesics that bind to central nervous system (CNS) opioid receptors and control pain by depressing pain impulse transmission. Opioids are the cornerstone drugs in the management of moderate to severe acute and chronic pain, including postoperative pain, posttraumatic pain, the pain of sickle cell vaso-occlusive crisis, and cancer pain. Opioids commonly used for children include codeine, fentanyl, hydrocodone, hydromorphone, methadone, morphine, and oxycodone. In pain management, *opioid* is the correct term for this class of medications. The antiquated

term "narcotic" is often associated with illegal drug use and trafficking; referring to analgesics as narcotics may deter patients and families from appropriate use of these analgesics.

Opioids can be administered by most routes. However, the oral route should be used when it is appropriate and the child is able to take and tolerate oral opioids. Sustained-release forms of morphine and oxycodone, which last 12 to 24 hours, are available. These are supplemented with a short-acting form of these analgesics for "break-through" pain, resulting in longer pain-free periods for children with moderate to severe, long-term pain (e.g., cancer pain). Short-acting liquid opioids may be used for children who cannot swallow tablets. When the oral route is contraindicated, intravenous or subcutaneous opioids (morphine, fentanyl, hydromorphone, methadone) may be given by bolus or continuous infusion. The intramuscular route should only be used when absolutely necessary, due to the great fear of injections seen in many children (American Medical Association, 2010).

The starting dose for opioids is determined according to the child's body weight, physiologic development, and medical situation. The goal

---

DRUG GUIDE

Acetaminophen

Classification
Analgesic, antipyretic.

Action
Unknown, thought to produce analgesia by blocking generation of pain impulses.

Indications
Mild pain or fever.

Dosages and Routes
By mouth or rectal suppository dosage 10 to 15 mg/kg/dose every 4 to 6 hr (every 6 to 8 hr for neonates). Maximum dose of 90 mg/kg/24 hr; not to exceed 4000 mg/day.

Absorption
Rapid and almost complete absorption from GI tract; less complete absorption from rectal suppository; peak effects in 1 to 1.5 hr.

Excretion
Ninety percent to 100% of drug excreted as metabolites in urine; excreted in breast milk; effects last 4 to 6 hr.

Contraindications
Hypersensitivity to acetaminophen or phenacetin; administration to patients with anemia or hepatic disease; cautious use in arthritic or rheumatoid conditions affecting children younger than 12 yr; thrombocytopenia.

Adverse Reaction
Negligible with recommended dosage; rash.

Nursing Considerations
May be crushed. Chewable tablets need to be thoroughly chewed and wet before swallowing. With high doses or long-term therapy, periodic tests of hepatic, renal, and hematopoietic function are advised. Caution the parents about giving other medications that also contain acetaminophen. No more than six doses in 24 hr should be given to children unless prescribed by a physician. Available in infant strength (drops). Be sure to advise parents to check the strength before administering acetaminophen (Tylenol) in liquid, chewable tablet, or tablet forms, to prevent overdosing.

DRUG GUIDE

Ibuprofen

Classification
NSAID, analgesic.

Action
Blocks prostaglandin synthesis.

Indications
Relief of mild to moderate pain. Chronic, symptomatic rheumatoid arthritis and osteoarthritis.

Dosages and Route
By mouth dosage 5 to 10 mg/kg/dose every 6 to 8 hr. Not to exceed 40 mg/kg/24 hr. Juvenile arthritis dosage 30 to 50 mg/kg/24 hr. Medication comes in liquid form for young children.

Absorption
80% absorbed from gastrointestinal (GI) tract; peak action in 1 to 2 hr.

Excretion
Excreted primarily in urine; some biliary excretion.

Contraindications
Contraindicated in children in whom urticaria, severe rhinitis, bronchospasm, angioedema, nasal polyps are precipitated by other NSAIDs; active peptic ulcer; bleeding abnormalities.

Precautions
Hypertension, history of GI ulceration, impaired hepatic or renal function, chronic renal failure.

Adverse Reactions
Heartburn, nausea, vomiting, epigastric or abdominal discomfort or pain, GI ulceration.

Nursing Considerations
Give with meals or milk to decrease GI intolerance. If the child is unable to swallow a tablet, administer the medication in liquid form. Ibuprofen that is not enteric coated can be crushed and mixed with a small amount of food or liquid before swallowing.

DRUG GUIDE

Ketorolac

Classification
NSAID, analgesic.

Action
Blocks prostaglandin synthesis.

Indications
Short-term management of moderate acute pain.

Dosages and Route
Children older than 6 months, IV dosage 0.5 to 1 mg/kg one time, up to 30 mg followed by 0.5 mg/kg/dose every 6 hr, up to a maximum of 60 mg/24 hr.

Absorption
Peak action in 15 min.

Excretion
Excreted in the urine; effects last 4 to 6 hr.

Contraindications
Contraindicated in patients in whom urticaria, severe rhinitis, bronchospasm, angioedema, nasal polyps are precipitated by other NSAIDs; active peptic ulcer; bleeding abnormalities, severe renal impairment.

Precautions
Cautious use with history of ulcers, impaired hepatic or renal function.

Adverse Reactions
Drowsiness, dizziness, nausea, GI pain, hemorrhage.

Nursing Considerations
Do not administer longer than 5 days. Monitor renal and liver function studies, signs and symptoms of GI upset or bleeding.

is to control pain as rapidly as possible, so the starting dose should be optimal (APS, 2011a). Weight-based starting doses have empirically been shown to be safe; however, they are not maximum doses. Opioids do not have a ceiling effect; further doses should be titrated based on the child's response. The dose should be titrated upward if pain is not significantly reduced or relieved, or titrated downward if a child experiences intolerable side effects.

The nurse should remember that opioids can produce sedation and respiratory depression, in addition to analgesia. Other adverse effects can include constipation, pruritus, nausea, vomiting, cough suppression, and urinary retention. Although children experiencing adverse effects must be closely monitored, most can tolerate these medications if their dosages are adjusted. Pruritus, nausea, sedation, and urinary retention tend to be time limited and will resolve spontaneously within 1 to 3 days. Until that time, antiemetics and antipruritics can be provided. Constipation does not resolve spontaneously. The nurse must remain vigilant and advocate for the use of laxatives and bowel stimulants to prevent constipation.

Hydrocodone is the most commonly given oral opioid for moderate pain. It is only available in combination with acetaminophen or ibuprofen, in tablet and liquid forms. As with all opioids, the nurse should carefully check dosing parameters for both the hydrocodone and the acetaminophen or ibuprofen prescribed. Oxycodone and codeine are also used to control moderate pain. These drugs come as single agents or in combination with acetaminophen. Oxycodone also is available as a sustained-release tablet.

Morphine is the preferred opioid for children. It reaches its peak effect 10 to 20 minutes after IV administration and 1 hour after oral administration. It can produce sedation along with the analgesia. If this occurs, maximum respiratory depression will happen 7 minutes after IV administration. Naloxone (Narcan) should be available to reverse sedation or respiratory depression, if necessary. For adequate pain management, titration of morphine is provided using an "as needed" dosage range (APS, 2004) in response to meticulous pain assessment. The physician order for titrated morphine must contain the safe dosage range and the time interval during which it may be given (APS, 2004). Hydromorphone (Dilaudid) is very similar to morphine. It is approximately six times more potent than morphine. It may be used as a first-line opioid for moderate to severe pain or as an alternative for patients who experience intolerable adverse affects from morphine.

DRUG GUIDE

Hydrocodone

Classification
Opioid analgesic.

Action
Binds to opiate receptors in the CNS to diminish pain.

Indications
Mild pain to moderate pain; acute pain

Dosage and Route
By mouth dosage 0.1 to 0.2 mg/kg every 3 to 4 hr. Maximum dosage dependent on acetaminophen or ibuprofen content of product.

Absorption
Onset 10 to 20 min; duration 4 to 6 hr.

Excretion
Excreted in the urine, half-life 3.5 to 4.5 hr.

Contraindications
Hypersensitivity to codeine, hydromorphone, or other morphine derivatives, addiction.

Precautions
Addictive personality, respiratory depression, hepatic disease, renal disease. Cautious use in head injuries, increased intracranial pressure, asthma, and other respiratory conditions.

Adverse Reactions
Nausea, vomiting, constipation, pruritus, dizziness, lightheadedness, confusion, hallucinations, mood changes, sedation, respiratory depression, dependence.

Nursing Considerations
Nausea is a common side effect; report if this is accompanied by vomiting. Because dizziness and lightheadedness may occur, supervision of ambulation and other safety precautions may be necessary. Assess respiratory status carefully; assess for CNS changes and implement appropriate safety measures.

DRUG GUIDE

Codeine

Classification
Opioid analgesic.

Action
Binds with opiate receptors in the CNS; alters both perception of and emotional response to pain.

Indications
Mild to moderate pain.

Dosage and Route
By mouth dosage 0.5 to 1 mg/kg/dose every 4 to 6 hr; maximum dose 60 mg/dose.

Absorption
Readily absorbed from GI tract, with peak action in 1 to 2 hr.

Distribution
Crosses placenta; distributed into breast milk.

Excretion
Effects last approximately 4 hr; excreted in urine.

Contraindications
Hypersensitivity to codeine, hydrocodone, or other morphine derivatives; hepatic or renal dysfunction, addiction.

Precaution
Use cautiously in very young children and those with an addictive personality.

Adverse Reactions
Primarily CNS symptoms: dizziness, lightheadedness, drowsiness, sedation, lethargy, euphoria, agitation, restlessness, respiratory depression. GI symptoms: nausea, vomiting, constipation. Genitourinary (GU) symptoms: urinary retention. Pruritus.

Nursing Considerations
May be given with food or milk to lessen GI upset. Nausea is a common side effect; report if this is accompanied by vomiting. Because dizziness and lightheadedness may occur, supervision of ambulation and other safety precautions may be necessary. Assess respiratory status carefully; assess for CNS changes and implement appropriate safety measures.

Available in combination with acetaminophen: Tylenol #2 = 15 mg codeine/300 mg acetaminophen, Tylenol #3 = 30 mg codeine/300 mg acetaminophen, Tylenol #4 = 60 mg codeine/300 mg acetaminophen.

Fentanyl and its analogs (sufentanil, alfentanil) have a shorter duration of action than morphine and are 50 to 100 times more potent. Because much less histamine is released, these agents may cause less pruritus. The short duration of effect makes IV use of these drugs appropriate when a brief, severely painful procedure is to be performed (e.g., bone marrow aspiration, inserting a chest tube, changing a burn dressing) and when children are critically ill. Fentanyl should be administered in a closely monitored setting. The fentanyl patch (Duragesic) is indicated for chronic pain; experience with its use in children is limited. Though administered to children as young as 2 years old, it is usually prescribed for adolescents. Transdermal fentanyl, 25 mcg/hr system, is approximately equal to 15 mg of IV morphine in 24 hours or 90 mg of oral morphine in 24 hours.

Methadone is metabolized very slowly and therefore has a prolonged duration of action. It is absorbed well after oral administration and is given via the IV route as well. Because of its long duration, it must be carefully titrated according to the patient's pain level; thus, diligent pain assessment is required. It is equal in potency to morphine.

Meperidine (Demerol) should be used only for short-term pain control (e.g., postoperatively) in children who have shown an allergy or intolerance to other opioids. The duration of analgesia is shorter than with morphine. Meperidine has been associated with convulsions and dysphoria after as few as two doses. It also has been known to cause hallucinations and agitation. Meperidine is infrequently prescribed for children.

Procedural Sedation

Procedural sedation is a medically controlled state of depressed consciousness that allows the patient to respond appropriately to verbal

DRUG GUIDE

Oxycodone

Classification
Opioid analgesic.

Action
Inhibits ascending pain pathways in the CNS, increases pain threshold, alters pain perception.

Indications
Moderate to severe pain. Acute or chronic pain.

Dosage and Route
By mouth starting dosage 0.1 to 0.2 mg/kg/dose every 4 to 6 hr; maximum starting dose 10 mg.

Absorption
Onset 10 to 20 min; duration 4 to 6 hr.

Excretion
Excreted in the urine, half-life 3.5 to 4.5 hr.

Contraindications
Hypersensitivity to oxycodone, codeine, or other morphine derivatives; hepatic or renal dysfunction, addiction.

Precautions
Addictive personality, respiratory depression, hepatic disease, renal disease. Cautious use in patients with head injuries, increased intracranial pressure, asthma, and other respiratory conditions.

Adverse Reactions
Nausea, vomiting, constipation, pruritus, dizziness, lightheadedness, confusion, hallucinations, mood changes, sedation, respiratory depression, dependence.

Nursing Considerations
Nausea is a common side effect; report if this is accompanied by vomiting. Because dizziness and lightheadedness may occur, supervision of ambulation and other safety precautions may be necessary. Assess respiratory status carefully; assess for CNS changes and implement appropriate safety measures. Titrate dosage up or down to maximize pain relief and minimize adverse effects.

DRUG GUIDE

Morphine

Classification
Opioid analgesic.

Action
Binds with CNS opiate receptors; alters physical and emotional response to pain.

Indications
Moderate to severe pain. Acute and chronic pain.

Dosages and Routes
By mouth or per rectum intermittent dosage 0.2 to 0.5 mg/kg/dose every 4 to 6 hr; extended-release dosage 0.3 to 0.6 mg/kg/dose every 8 to 12 hr. IV or subcutaneous intermittent dosage 0.05 to 0.1 mg/kg/dose every 2 to 4 hr; maximum dose 15 mg/dose. Continuous IV infusion dosage 0.01 to 0.05 mg/kg/hr.

Absorption
Variable absorption from the GI tract; peak action 60 min orally, 10 to 20 min IV.

Excretion
Excreted primarily in the urine; 7% to 10% excreted in bile. Effects last up to 7 hr.

Contraindications
Hypersensitivity to opioids, increased intracranial pressure, seizure disorders, chronic pulmonary disease, respiratory depression.

Precautions
Cautious use with cardiac arrhythmias, reduced blood volume, addictive personality.

Adverse Reactions
Primarily CNS symptoms: dizziness, lightheadedness, drowsiness, sedation, lethargy, euphoria, agitation, restlessness, respiratory depression. GI symptoms: nausea, vomiting, constipation. GU symptoms: urinary retention. Pruritus.

Nursing Considerations
Nausea is a common side effect; report if this is accompanied by vomiting. Because dizziness and lightheadedness may occur, supervision of ambulation and other safety precautions may be necessary. Assess respiratory status carefully and frequently; assess for CNS changes and implement appropriate safety measures. Monitor intake and output related to urinary retention and constipation. Begin with the lowest dosage and titrate dosage up or down to maximize pain relief and minimize adverse effects.

and tactile stimulation and to maintain oxygenation and airway control independently. The child retains protective airway reflexes (e.g., cough and gag reflexes). There is a continuum of sedation levels: minimum, moderate (referred to as conscious sedation), and deep (American Society of Anesthesiologists, 2009).

Procedural sedation is generally achieved through IV administration of a sedative-hypnotic (midazolam, propofol, nitrous oxide), an analgesic (opioid), or a dissociative (ketamine) medication or a combination of these medications (Krauss & Green, 2006). However, multiple routes can be used: IV, intranasal, rectal, IM, oral, or sublingual. Frequently used for sedation as well as induction of general anesthesia is midazolam (Versed), a short-acting sedative-hypnotic that may be given by multiple routes. Midazolam is often used for procedural sedation because it has minimal side effects, is short acting, and can be used without IV access. It has no analgesic properties; therefore, for painful procedures, it should be given in combination with an opioid.

Children receiving procedural sedation require the care of clinicians with advanced skills in airway management such as trained physicians, anesthesiologists, or nurse anesthetists. The level of sedation is not dose dependent. Children given recommended doses may remain alert and only experience reduced anxiety, or they may become moderately to deeply sedated. The nurse's role in administering and monitoring patients receiving sedation agents may vary by agency policies and state regulations. It is important that nurses participate in the frequent assessment and documentation of the child's vital signs, oxygen saturation, capnography (concentration of exhaled carbon

DRUG GUIDE
Hydromorphone

Classification
Opioid analgesic.

Action
Inhibits ascending pain pathways in the CNS, increases pain threshold, alters pain perception.

Indications
Moderate to severe pain, acute and chronic pain.

Dosages and Routes
By mouth or subcutaneous dosage 0.03 to 0.08 mg/kg/dose every 4 hr with maximum starting dose of 7.5 mg. IV intermittent dosage 0.015 mg/kg/dose every 3 to 6 hr. IV continuous infusion dosage 3 to 5 mcg/kg/hr.

Absorption
Onset 15 to 20 min; peak 0.5 to 1 hr; duration 4 to 5 hr.

Excretion
Excreted in the urine, half-life 3.5 to 4.5 hr.

Contraindications
Hypersensitivity, addiction.

Precautions
Addictive personality, respiratory depression, hepatic disease, renal disease. Cautious use in head injuries, increased intracranial pressure, asthma and other respiratory conditions, and impaired renal or hepatic function.

Adverse Reactions
Nausea, vomiting, constipation, pruritus, dizziness, lightheadedness, confusion, hallucinations, mood changes, sedation, respiratory depression, dependence, increased urine output, urinary retention, seizures, palpitations, bradycardia, tachycardia, hypotension, other changes in blood pressure.

Nursing Considerations
Nausea is a common side effect; report if this is accompanied by vomiting. Because dizziness and lightheadedness may occur, supervision of ambulation and other safety precautions may be necessary. Assess respiratory status carefully; assess for CNS changes and implement appropriate safety measures. Titrate dosage up or down to maximize pain relief and minimize adverse effects.

DRUG GUIDE
Fentanyl

Classification
Opioid analgesic.

Action
Opioid agonist with actions similar to morphine and meperidine, but action is faster and less prolonged.

Indications
Moderate to severe pain, particularly for brief procedures and when children are critically ill or high risk. Transdermal fentanyl is for moderate to severe chronic pain only; experience with children is limited.

Dosages and Routes
IM or IV intermittent dosage 1 to 2 mcg/kg/dose every 30 to 60 min. IV continuous infusion dosage 0.05 to 3 mcg/kg/hr. Transdermal patch dosage 25 mcg/hr system; used only in opioid-tolerant children older than 2 years.

Absorption
Absorbed rapidly after IV administration; 6 to 8 hr transdermally.

Excretion
Excreted in the urine. Lasts 30 to 60 min IV; 72 hr transdermally.

Contraindication
Hypersensitivity, addiction, patients who have received monoamine oxidase inhibitors within 14 days.

Precautions
Addictive personality. Use cautiously in children with head injuries, increased intracranial pressure, respiratory problems, hepatic and renal dysfunction.

Adverse Reactions
Nausea, vomiting, constipation, pruritus, dizziness, lightheadedness, confusion, hallucinations, mood changes, sedation, respiratory depression, dependence, increased urine output, urinary retention, seizures, palpitations, bradycardia, tachycardia, hypotension, other changes in blood pressure.

Nursing Considerations
Watch carefully for signs and symptoms of respiratory distress and depression. Have oxygen, resuscitative equipment, and naloxone available. Administer slow IV push to prevent chest wall rigidity.

dioxide), and level of consciousness both during and after procedural sedation.

Epidural Analgesia

Pain medication (usually an opioid, a local anesthetic, or both) can be administered through an epidural catheter inserted into the epidural space of the spinal canal and secured to the child's back with an occlusive dressing. Because the medication is administered directly to the nerves that transmit pain, smaller doses are required for pain control, with fewer side effects than are usually associated with systemic (IV) opioid administration. Epidural analgesia is used for children following abdominal, anal, and genitourinary surgeries and procedures; open-heart and thoracic surgeries; and orthopedic surgeries of the lower limbs.

Nursing care of the child with an epidural catheter is similar to that for a child receiving PCA therapy. The child is attached to a continuous cardiac monitor and pulse oximeter. It is essential that the nurse assess the child for adequate pain relief, the presence of adverse effects (particularly decreased respirations), and for complications related to the epidural catheter placement (Ellis, Martelli, LaMontagne, & Splinter, 2007). Possible side effects include constipation, nausea, vomiting, urinary retention, motor block, and sensory block. The child's dermatome level (the level of sensory blockade) and motor responses are checked at least every 4 hours. It is important to avoid any action that would pull or place tension on the catheter. The epidural catheter insertion site must be inspected frequently. If displacement (slippage), bleeding, leakage of cerebrospinal fluid, or a hematoma is noted, this must be reported to the child's physician or anesthesiologist immediately.

DRUG GUIDE

Methadone

Classification
Opioid analgesic.

Action
Depresses pain impulse transmission at the spinal cord level through interaction with opioid receptors, thus producing CNS depression.

Indications
Severe acute and chronic pain, opioid withdrawal.

Dosages and Routes
By mouth, subcutaneous, IM, or IV dosage 0.05 to 0.1 mg/kg/dose every 4 to 6 or 12 hr. Maximum single dose 10 mg.

Absorption
Variable absorption from the GI tract; peak action 60 min orally, 20 min IV.

Excretion
Excreted in the urine, crosses the placenta, excreted in breast milk. Half-life 15 to 30 hr.

Contraindications
Hypersensitivity to this drug, chlorobutanol injection, addiction.

Precautions
Cautious use with addictive personalities, increased intracranial pressure, respiratory depression, hepatic or renal disease.

Adverse Reactions
Sedation, dizziness, confusion, euphoria, seizures, respiratory depression, hypotension, bradycardia, palpitations, nausea, vomiting, constipation, urinary retention.

Nursing Considerations
Carefully and frequently assess level of sedation and respiratory status. Assess cough reflex. Monitor intake and output checking for urinary retention and constipation. Titrate dosage up or down to maximize pain relief and minimize adverse effects.

! NURSING QUALITY ALERT

Pain Management for Children

- The preferred route of administering analgesics to children is oral or IV.
- As soon as the child can tolerate oral intake, pain medication should be changed from the IV to the oral route.
- After starting with the recommended initial dose for opioids, the dose is adjusted (titrated) to achieve best pain management with the fewest side effects.
- Opioids do not have a dose limit. The maximum dose is the dose that causes unacceptable side effects.
- Infants and children receiving epidural opioids should be monitored by a cardiac and apnea monitor, and pulse oximetry.
- A cardiac and apnea monitor and a pulse oximeter may be required to monitor certain infants and children receiving IV opioids (e.g., neonates, children who are opioid naïve, children with a history of apnea or other respiratory difficulties). The risk of respiratory depression is greatest during the first 24 hours of administration.
- If respiratory depression occurs with opioid use, naloxone hydrochloride should be administered for reversal, if oxygen and stimulation of the child are ineffective.

KEY CONCEPTS

- Pain is whatever the experiencing person says it is, existing whenever the person says it does (Pasero & McCaffery, 2011).
- According to the gate control theory of pain, there is a gating mechanism in the spinal cord that facilitates or inhibits pain transmission. Stimulation of the larger afferent nerves can dull pain.
- Two prevalent myths, that children receiving pain medication are at high risk for respiratory depression and that they are at increased risk for addiction, are not supported by evidence and yet interfere with adequate pain management for infants and children.

- Pain assessment in infants and children takes a multidimensional approach. The child and parent are both interviewed and behavioral and physiologic changes are evaluated.
- A developmentally appropriate pain assessment tool is used to assess, implement, and document effective pain management for an infant, child, or adolescent.
- Both pharmacologic and nonpharmacologic measures should be used together in the treatment of pain in children.

REFERENCES

Al-Atiyyat, N. M. H. (2009). Cultural diversity and cancer pain. *Journal of Hospice & Palliative Nursing, 11*(3), 154-166.

American Academy of Pediatrics & Canadian Paediatric Society. (2006). Prevention and management of pain in the neonate: An update. *Pediatrics, 118*(5), 2231-2241.

American Medical Association. (2010). *Module 6 pain management: Pediatric pain management.* Retrieved from www.ama-cmeonline.com/pain_mgmt/printversion/ama_painmgmt_m6.pdf.

American Pain Society. (2004). T*he use of "as-needed" range orders for opioid analgesics in the management of acute pain: A consensus statement of the American Society for* Pain Management Nursing & the American Pain Society. Retrieved from www.ampainsoc.org/advocacy/range.htm.

American Pain Society. (2011a). *The assessment and management of acute pain in infants, children, and adolescents: A position statement from the American Academy of Pediatrics Committee on Psychosocial Aspects of Child and Family Health and American Pain Society Task Force on Pain in Infants, Children and Adolescents.* Retrieved from www.ampainsoc.org/advocacy/pediatric2.htm.

American Pain Society. (2011b). *Pediatric chronic pain: A position statement from the American Pain Society.* Retrieved from www.ampainsoc.org/advocacy/pediatric.htm.

American Pain Society. (2011c). *Publications: Clinical practice guidelines.* Retrieved from www.ampainsoc.org/pub/cp_guidelines.htm.

American Society for Pain Management Nursing. (2006). *Authorized and unauthorized ("PCA by proxy") dosing of analgesic infusion pumps.* Retrieved from www.aspmn.org.

American Society of Anesthesiologists. (2009). *Continuum of depth of sedation definition of general anesthesia and levels of sedation/analgesia.* Retrieved from www.asahq.org/For-Healthcare-Professionals/~/media/For%20Members/documents/Standards%20Guidelines%20Stmts/Continuum%20of%20Depth%20ofSedation.ashx.

Anand, K. (2007). Pain assessment in preterm neonates. *Pediatrics, 119*(3), 605-607.

Auerbach, M., Tunik, M., & Mojica, M. (2009). A randomized, double-blind controlled study of jet lidocaine compared to jet placebo for pain relief in children undergoing needle insertion in the emergency department. *Academic Emergency Medicine, 16*(5), 388-393.

Badr, L., Abdallah, B., Hawari, M., et al. (2010). Determinants of premature infant pain responses to heel sticks. *Pediatric Nursing, 36*(3), 129-136.

Ball, T., Shapiro, D., Monheim, C., & Weydert, J. (2003). A pilot study of the use of guided imagery for the treatment of recurrent abdominal pain in children. *Clinical Pediatrics, 42*(6), 527-532.

Beider, S., Mahrer, N., & Gold, J. (2007). Pediatric massage therapy: An overview for clinicians. *Pediatric Clinics of North America, 54*(6), 1025-1041.

Belay, E., Bresee, J., Holman, R., et al. (1999). Reye's syndrome in the United States from 1981–1997. *New England Journal of Medicine, 340*(18), 1377-1382.

Beyer, J., Villarruel, A., & Denyes, M. (2009). *The Oucher: User's manual and technical report.* Retrieved from www.oucher.org/downloads/2009_Users_Manual.pdf.

Boyle, E., Freer, Y., Wong, C., et al. (2006). Assessment of persistent pain or distress and adequacy of analgesia in preterm ventilated infants. *Pain, 124*(1-2), 87-91.

Briggs, E. (2008). Cultural perspectives on pain management. *Journal of Perioperative Practice, 18*(11), 466-471.

Busoni, P. (2007). Difficulties in controlling pain in children. *Regional Anesthesia and Pain Medicine, 32*(6), 505-509.

Cline, M. E., Herman, J., Shaw, E., & Morton, R. D. (1992). Standardization of the Visual Analogue Scale. *Nursing Research, 41*(6), 378-379.

D'Arcy, Y. (2009). Pain pointers: The effect of culture on pain. *Nursing Made Incredibly Easy, 7*(3), 5-7.

Ellis, J., Martelli, B., LaMontagne, C., & Splinter, W. (2007). Evaluation of a continuous epidural analgesia program for postoperative pain in children. *Pain Management Nursing, 8*(4), 146-155.

Farion, K., Splinter, K., Newhook, K., & Gaboury, I. (2008). The effect of vapocoolant spray on pain due to intravenous cannulation in children: A randomized controlled trial. *Canadian Medical Association Journal, 179*(1), 31-36.

Finley, G., Kristjansdottir, O., & Forgeron, P. (2009). Cultural influences on the assessment of children's pain. *Pain Research & Management, 14*(1), 33-37.

Franck, L. S., Greenberg, C. S., & Stevens, B. (2000). Pain assessment in infants and children. *Pediatric Clinics of North America, 47*(3), 487-512.

Gilboy, S., & Hollywood, E. (2009). Helping to alleviate pain for children having venipuncture. *Paediatric Nursing, 21*(8), 14-19.

Golianu, B., Krane, E., Seybold, J., et al. (2007). Non-pharmacological techniques for pain management in neonates. *Seminars in Perinatology, 31*, 318-322.

Griffin, R. A., Polit, D. F., & Byrne, M. W. (2008). Nurse characteristics and inferences about children's pain. *Pediatric Nursing, 34*(4), 297-307.

Hatfield, L. (2008). Sucrose decreases infant biobehavioral pain response to immunizations: A randomized controlled trial. *Journal of Nursing Scholarship, 10*(3), 219-225.

Herr, K., Coyne, P., Key, T., et al. (2006). Pain assessment in the nonverbal patient: Position statement with clinical practice recommendations. *Pain Management Nursing, 7*(2), 44-52.

Hester, N. O., Foster, R. L., Jordan-Marsh, M., et al. (1998). Putting pain measurement into clinical practice. In G. A. Finley & P. J. McGrath (Eds.), *Measurement of pain in infants and children* (Vol. 10). Seattle: International Association for the Study of Pain Press.

Hockenberry, M., & Wilson, D. (2009). *Wong's essentials of pediatric nursing* (8th ed.). St. Louis: Mosby.

Huth, M., Broome, M., & Good, M. (2004). Imagery reduces children's post-operative pain. *Pain, 110*(1-2), 439-448.

International Association for the Study of Pain (Subcommittee on Taxonomy). (1979). Pain terms: A list with definitions and notes on usage. *Pain, 6*(3), 249-252.

Jimenez, N., Bradford, H., Seidel, K., et al. (2006). A comparison of a needle-free injection system for local anesthesia versus EMLA for intravenous catheter insertion in the pediatric patient. *Anesthesia & Analgesia, 102*, 411-414.

Joint Commission. (2004). *Patient-controlled analgesia by proxy.* Retrieved from www.jointcommission.org/assets/1/18/sea_33.pdf.

Joint Commission. (2011). Facts about pain management. Retrieved from www.jointcommission.org/assets/1/18/Pain_Management.pdf.

Kashaninia, Z., Sajedi, F., Rahgozar, M., & Noghabi, F. (2008). The effect of kangaroo care on behavioral responses to pain of an intramuscular injection in neonates. *Journal of Specialists in Pediatric Nursing, 13*(4), 275-280.

Kirmayer, L. J. (2008). Culture and the metaphoric mediation of pain. *Transcultural Psychiatry, 45*(2), 318-338.

Krauss, B., & Green, S. (2006). Procedural sedation and analgesia in children. *Lancet, 367*, 766-780.

Krechel, S.W., & Bildner, J. (1995). CRIES: A new neonatal postoperative pain measurement score. Initial testing of validity and reliability. *Paediatric Anaesthesia, 5*(1), 53-61.

Kundu, A., & Berman, B. (2007). Acupuncture for pediatric pain and symptom management. *Pediatric Clinics of North America, 54*, 885-899.

Lander, J., Weltman, B., & So, S. (2006). EMLA and amethocaine for reduction of children's pain associated with needle insertion. *Cochrane Database of Systematic Reviews, 3*, CD004236.

Mancuso, T., & Burns, J. (2009). Ethical concerns in the management of pain in the neonate. *Paediatric Anaesthesia, 19*(10), 953-957.

Manworren, R. (2007). It's time to relieve children's pain. *Journal for Specialists in Pediatric Nursing, 12*(3), 196-198.

McCaffery, M., & Pasero, C. (1999). *Pain: Clinical manual.* St. Louis: Elsevier.

Melzack, R., & Wall, P. (1965). Pain mechanisms: A new theory. *Science, 150*(699), 971-979.

Merkel, S., Voepel-Lewis, T., & Malviya, S. (2002). Pain assessment in infants and young children: The FLACC scale: A behavioral tool to measure pain in young children. *American Journal of Nursing, 102*(10), 55-58.

Narayan, M. C. (2010) Culture's effects on pain assessment and management: Cultural patterns influence nurses' and their patients' responses to pain. *American Journal of Nursing, 110*(4), 38-49.

Overmyer, M. (2010). Analgesic spray offers clinical benefits, cost efficiency: Product is less expensive than topical creams and has immediate effect. *Urology Times, 38*(3), 14 & 16.

Page, L. O., & Blanchette, J. (2009). Social learning theory: Toward a unified approach of pediatric procedural pain. *International Journal of Behavioral Consultation and Therapy, 5*(1), 124-141.

Pasero, C. & McCaffery, M. (2011). *Pain assessment and pharmacologic management.* St. Louis: Mosby.

Rieman, M., & Gordon, M. (2007). Pain management competency evidenced by a survey of pediatric nurses' knowledge and attitudes. *Pediatric Nursing, 33*(4), 307-311.

Savedra, M. C., Tesler, M. D., Holzemer, W. L., & Ward, J. (1992). *Adolescent and pediatric pain tool: User's manual.* San Francisco: University of California, San Francisco, School of Nursing.

Schiavenato, M. (2008). Facial expression and pain assessment in the pediatric patient: The primal face of pain. *Journal for Specialists in Pediatric Nursing, 13*(2), 89-97.

Singer, A., Taira, B., Chisena, E., et al. (2008). Warm lidocaine/tetracaine patch versus placebo before pediatric intravenous cannulation: A randomized controlled trial. *Annals of Emergency Medicine, 52*(1), 41-47.

Slater, R., Cornelissen, L., Fabrizi, L., et al. (2010). Oral sucrose as an analgesic drug for procedural pain in newborn infants: A randomized controlled trial. *Lancet, 376*(9748), 1225-1232.

Spanos, S., Booth, R., Koenig, H., et al. (2008). Jet-injection of 1% buffered lidocaine versus topical ELA-MAX for anesthesia before peripheral intravenous catheterization in children: A randomized controlled trial. *Pediatric Emergency Care, 24*(8), 511-515.

Srouji, R., Ratnapalan, S., & Schneeweiss, S. (2010). Pain in children: Assessment and nonpharmacologic management. *International Journal of Pediatrics, 2010*, 1-11.

Stevens, B., Yamada, J., Beyene, J., et al. (2005). Consistent management of repeated procedural pain with sucrose in preterm neonates: Is it effective and safe for repeated use over time? *Clinical Journal of Pain, 21*(6), 543-548.

Thompson, D. (2005). Utilizing an oral sucrose solution to minimize neonatal pain. *Journal for Specialists in Pediatric Nursing, 10*(1), 3-10.

Thompson, L. A., Knapp, C. A., Feeg, V., et al. (2010). Pediatricians' management practices for chronic pain. *Journal of Palliative Medicine, 13*(2), 171-178.

Twycross, A. (2007a). Children's nurses' post-operative pain management practices: An observational study. *International Journal of Nursing Studies, 44*, 869-881.

Twycross, A. (2007b). What is the impact of theoretical knowledge on children's nurses' post-operative pain management practices? *Nursing Education Today, 27*, 697-707.

Twycross, A. (2008). Does the perceived importance of a pain management task affect the quality of children's nurses' post-operative pain management practices? *Journal of Clinical Nursing, 17*, 3205-3216.

Twycross, A. (2010). Managing pain in children: Where to from here? *Journal of Clinical Nursing, 19*(15-16), 2090-2099.

Twycross, A., & Dowden, S. (2009). *Managing pain in children: A clinical guide.* West Sussex, UK: Wiley-Blackwell.

Van Dijk, M., Peters, J., Van Deventer, P., & Tibboel, D. (2005). The COMFORT behavior scale: A tool for assessing pain and sedation in infants. *American Journal of Nursing, 105*(1), 33-36.

Van Hulle Vincent, C., & Gaddy, E. (2009). Pediatric nurses' thinking in response to vignettes on administering analgesics. *Research in Nursing & Health, 32*, 530-539.

Voepel-Lewis, T., Zanotti, J., Dammeyer, J., & Merkel, S. (2010). Reliability and validity of the Face, Legs, Activity, Cry, Consolability behavioral tool in assessing acute pain in critically ill patients. *American Journal of Critical Care, 19*(1), 55-61.

Von Baeyer, C. L., Marche, T. A., Rocha, E. M., & Salmon, K. (2004). Children's memory for pain: Overview and implications for practice. *Journal of Pain, 5*(5), 241-249.

Von Baeyer, C., & Spagrud, L. (2007). Systematic review of observational (behavioral) measures of pain for children and adolescents aged 3 to 18 years. *Journal of Pain, 127*(1-2), 140-150.

Walco, G., & Goldschneider, K. (2008). *Pain in children: A practical guide for primary care.* Totowa, NJ: Humana Press (Springer).

Wong-Baker FACES Foundation. (1983). *Translations of the Wong-Baker FACES Pain Rating Scale.* Retrieved from www.wongbakerfaces.org/wp-content/uploads/2010/12/FACES_translation1.pdf.

World Health Organization. (2010). *WHO's pain ladder.* Retrieved from http://who.int/cancer/palliative/painladder/en.

Wuhrman, E., Cooney, M., Dunwoody, C., et al. (2007). Authorized and unauthorized ("PCA by proxy") dosing of analgesic infusion pumps: Position statement with clinical practice recommendations. *Pain Management Nursing, 8*(1), 4-11.

The Child with a Fluid and Electrolyte Alteration

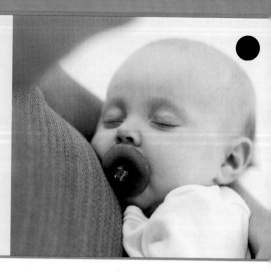

evolve WEBSITE

http://evolve.elsevier.com/James/ncoc

LEARNING OBJECTIVES

After studying this chapter, you should be able to:

- Identify the regulatory mechanisms that maintain fluid and electrolyte balance in the body.
- Compare those differences in body fluid and electrolyte composition and regulation between infants/children and adults that make infants and children more vulnerable to imbalances.
- Describe dehydration and acid-base imbalance.
- Differentiate among the various types of acid-base disturbances.

- Describe the processes and nursing care of a child with diarrhea or vomiting.
- Integrate assessment findings with nursing implementation to determine the success of therapy.
- Describe nursing interventions to prevent fluid and electrolyte imbalances.

CLINICAL REFERENCE

REVIEW OF FLUID AND ELECTROLYTE IMBALANCES IN CHILDREN

Characteristics unique to children affect their fluid and electrolyte balance. Infants and young children are more vulnerable than adults to changes in fluid and electrolyte balance. Under normal conditions, the amount of fluid ingested during a day should equal the amount of fluid lost through sensible water loss (e.g., urine output) and insensible water loss (through the respiratory tract and skin). Insensible water loss per unit of body weight is significantly higher in infants and children. The faster respiratory rates of infants and young children also result in higher evaporative water losses. Any condition that prevents normal oral fluid intake (e.g., vomiting) or results in fluid losses (e.g., diarrhea, hyperventilation, burns, hemorrhage) is especially significant because it depletes the body's store of water and electrolytes much more rapidly in infants and young children than in adults.

Body water is located in two major compartments: within the cell, in the intracellular compartment; and outside the cell, in the extracellular compartment. These two compartments are separated by the cell membrane, across which body fluid is continually exchanged. Extracellular fluid (ECF) is located in several places: in interstitial spaces (surrounding the cells [e.g., lymph fluid]), intravascularly (within the blood vessels or plasma), and transcellularly (e.g., cerebrospinal fluid, pericardial fluid, pleural fluid, synovial fluid, sweat, digestive secretions). A child is more likely to lose ECF than intracellular fluid (ICF). ECF is lost first when fluid loss occurs (e.g., through illness, trauma, fever). The intracellular compartment is more difficult to dehydrate.

In the neonate, approximately 40% of body water is located in the extracellular compartment compared with 20% in the adolescent and adult. In the infant, half of the ECF may be exchanged compared with an adult exchange of one sixth of the ECF in a similar time. Because approximately 50% of this ECF is exchanged daily in an infant, dehydration can occur very suddenly and rapidly if fluid intake is inadequate or fluid losses are excessive. Because of the infant's higher metabolic rate, the rate of water turnover is rapid. Depletion of ECF, often caused by gastroenteritis, is one of the most common problems among infants and young children. In adults and older children,

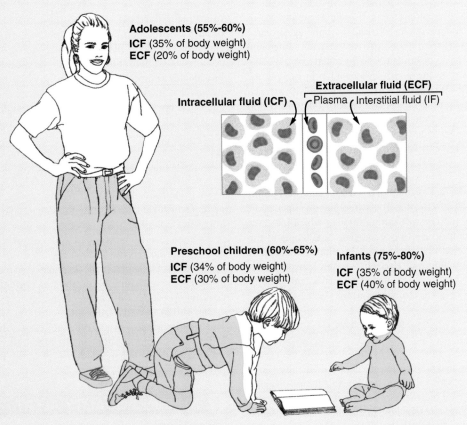

Adolescents (55%-60%)
ICF (35% of body weight)
ECF (20% of body weight)

Intracellular fluid (ICF)

Extracellular fluid (ECF)
Plasma Interstitial fluid (IF)

Preschool children (60%-65%)
ICF (34% of body weight)
ECF (30% of body weight)

Infants (75%-80%)
ICF (35% of body weight)
ECF (40% of body weight)

Because infants and younger children have a higher proportion of extracellular fluids than older children and adults, they are more susceptible to rapid fluid depletion.

PEDIATRIC DIFFERENCES RELATED TO FLUID AND ELECTROLYTE BALANCE

Infants

- Because of the higher percentage of water in the ECF, infants can lose fluids equal to their ECF within 2 to 3 days.
- Infants are less able to concentrate urine because of immature renal function.
- Infants have a higher rate of peristalsis than do older children.
- Infants have an immature lower esophageal sphincter, making them more prone to gastroesophageal reflux, which can lead to dehydration and electrolyte disturbances.
- Infants have a harder time compensating for acidosis because of their decreased ability to acidify urine.

Infants and Young Children

- Infants and young children have a higher metabolic turnover of water relative to adults because of a higher metabolic rate. (If losses are not replaced rapidly, imbalance occurs.)
- Infants and young children are unable to verbalize or communicate thirst.

Infants and Children

- In comparison with adults, infants and children have a proportionately greater body surface area in relation to body mass, resulting in a greater potential for fluid loss through the skin and gastrointestinal tract.
- Infants and children have a higher proportionate water content (premature infants have 90%, term infants 75% to 80%, preschool children 60% to 65%, and adolescents and adults approximately 55% to 60%), with a larger proportion of fluid in the extracellular space.
- The immune system of infants and children is not as robust as an adult's immune system, rendering young children more susceptible to infectious diseases, fever, gastroenteritis, and respiratory infections, all of which can result in fluid and electrolyte disturbances and fluid-volume deficit.
- Infants and children are at higher risk because of increased exposure to infections in a daycare or nursery setting.

because a greater proportion of fluid is located in the intracellular compartment, severe fluid depletion does not occur as rapidly. Maturity in body space distribution is usually reached around age 3 years.

Body fluids are basically composed of two elements, water and solutes. *Water* is the primary constituent, with the infant's weight being approximately 75% water to the adult's 55% to 60%. In general, the volume of total body water to total body weight decreases with increasing age. An inverse relationship exists between total body water and total body fat. Compared with adults, neonates, particularly premature infants, have a lower proportion of fat.

Solutes are composed of both electrolytes and nonelectrolytes. Most of the body's solutes are electrolytes, primarily sodium (Na^+), potassium (K^+), chloride (Cl^-), calcium (Ca^{2+}), and magnesium (Mg^{2+}). The primary electrolyte of the ECF is sodium; potassium and magnesium are the primary electrolytes in the ICF. The extracellular compartment contains more sodium and chloride during infancy, which increases the vulnerability of infants to electrolyte imbalances. Changes in the concentration of these electrolytes may result in cellular dysfunction and illness. Problems of fluid and electrolyte balance involve both water and electrolytes; thus treatment includes replacement of both, calculated according to serum electrolyte laboratory values.

ALTERATIONS IN ACID-BASE BALANCE IN CHILDREN

Alterations in acid-base balance can affect cellular metabolism and enzymatic processes. The body's ability to regulate this status is crucial. Children can have acid-base imbalance as a result of many pathologic conditions. The pH, or measure of acidity or alkalinity of body fluids, is regulated within a narrow range (normal blood pH is 7.35 to 7.45). Maintenance of serum pH within normal limits is crucial to maintaining cellular function, enzyme activity, and neuromuscular membrane potentials. Chemical buffers, the respiratory system, and the kidneys work together to keep the blood pH within normal range. Acid is constantly produced as a byproduct of metabolism. The body attempts to maintain blood pH within normal limits by reducing the buildup of acid. Chemical and cellular buffer systems minimize the effect of alterations in blood pH by neutralizing excess acids and bases that accumulate in body fluids. Two of the most significant buffers are bicarbonate and proteins. Bicarbonate, the most important buffer for plasma and interstitial fluids, is responsible for most ECF buffering and can exert its effects relatively quickly (within minutes).

When alterations in pH become too much for the buffer systems to handle, compensatory mechanisms in the respiratory and renal systems are activated. The respiratory system works rapidly to compensate for acid-base disturbances. If the blood pH drops below normal (causing **acidosis**), the respiratory rate and depth will increase, removing carbon dioxide and raising blood pH. Conversely, in the presence of alkalosis, the respiratory rate and depth decrease, thus lowering blood pH.

Kidneys regulate bicarbonate and remove hydrogen ions from the blood. If the blood is too alkaline, the kidneys conserve hydrogen ions, thus lowering blood pH. In the presence of acidosis, the kidneys excrete hydrogen ions and conserve bicarbonate, raising blood pH. Renal compensatory processes work more slowly than respiratory mechanisms—usually within 1 to 2 days. If compensatory mechanisms are ineffective, acid-base imbalances occur. When a dysfunction results in decreased hydrogen ion concentration in the blood, the arterial pH increases (causing alkalosis). When a dysfunction results in an increase in hydrogen ions, the arterial pH decreases (causing acidosis).

! NURSING QUALITY ALERT

Treatment Goals in Acid-Base Imbalance

The treatment of metabolic acid-base disturbance is oriented toward correcting the underlying problem. The treatment of respiratory imbalance is directed toward reestablishing alveolar ventilation.

OVERVIEW OF FLUID AND ELECTROLYTE DISORDERS

DISORDER	PRECIPITATING EVENTS	CLINICAL MANIFESTATIONS
Hyponatremia (sodium <135 mEq/L)	Fever Increased water intake without electrolytes Decreased sodium intake Diabetic ketoacidosis Burns and wounds SIADH Malnutrition Cystic fibrosis Renal disease Vomiting, diarrhea, nasogastric suction	Neurologic: Usually do not show signs until sodium reaches 125 mEq/L Behavioral changes: irritability, lethargy, headache, dizziness, apprehension Cardiovascular: Increased heart rate Decreased blood pressure Cold, clammy skin Muscle cramps (especially abdominal) Nausea
Hypernatremia (sodium >150 mEq/L)	Water loss or deprivation High sodium intake Diabetes insipidus Diarrhea Fever Hyperglycemia Renal disease	Intense thirst Oliguria Agitation, restlessness Flushed skin Peripheral and pulmonary edema Dry, sticky mucous membranes Nausea and vomiting Serum sodium 150 mEq/L: disorientation, seizures, hyperirritability when at rest

GI, Gastrointestinal; *SIADH,* syndrome of inappropriate secretion of antidiuretic hormone.

OVERVIEW OF FLUID AND ELECTROLYTE DISORDERS—cont'd

DISORDER	PRECIPITATING EVENTS	CLINICAL MANIFESTATIONS
Hypokalemia (potassium <3.5 mEq/L)	Stress Starvation Malabsorption Excessive loss of GI fluids through vomiting, diarrhea, sweat, nasogastric tube Administration of diuretics (especially furosemide, ethacrynic acid, thiazide diuretics) IV fluids without added potassium Administration of corticosteroids Diabetic ketoacidosis	Muscle weakness, paralysis Leg cramps Decreased bowel sounds, nausea Weak and irregular pulse, tachycardia or bradycardia, cardiac arrhythmias Hypotension Ileus Irritability, fatigue Decreasing blood pressure
Hyperkalemia (potassium >5 mEq/L)	Increased intake of potassium (e.g., salt substitutes) Decreased urine excretion Kidney failure Metabolic acidosis Hyperglycemia Potassium-sparing diuretics Dehydration (severe) Too-rapid IV administration of potassium Burns	Irritability, anxiety, increased restlessness Twitching, hyperreflexia Weakness, flaccid paralysis Nausea, diarrhea, abdominal cramps Bradycardia, irregular pulse Decreased blood pressure Cardiac arrest (concern if potassium >8.5 mEq/L) Apnea, respiratory arrest
Hypocalcemia (calcium <8.5 mg/dL, ionized calcium <4.5 mg/dL)	Inadequate intake of calcium Vitamin D deficiency Renal insufficiency Calcium losses (e.g., infection, burns) Alkalosis Administration of diuretics Hypoparathyroidism	Numbness and tingling of fingers, toes, nose, ears, circumoral area Hyperactive reflexes, seizures Muscle cramps, tetany Laryngospasm Lethargy and poor feeding in the neonate Positive Trousseau's and Chvostek's signs Hypotension Cardiac arrest
Hypercalcemia (calcium >11 mg/dL, ionized calcium >5.5 mg/dL)	Milk-alkali syndrome (chronic ingestion of calcium carbonate antacids or milk) Excessive IV or oral calcium administration Acidosis Prolonged immobilization Hypoproteinemia Renal disease Hyperparathyroidism Hyperthyroidism	Lethargy, weakness, anorexia Thirst Itching Behavioral changes: confusion, personality change, stupor Nausea, vomiting, constipation Bradycardia, cardiac arrest

ASSESSMENT OF FLUID DISTURBANCES

PARAMETER	FLUID VOLUME DEFICIT	FLUID VOLUME EXCESS
Weight	Loss: Percentage suggests degree of dehydration	Gain: Related to retention of interstitial and vascular fluid volume
Heart rate/pulse	Rapid, weak, thready	Rapid, bounding
Respirations	Normal	Moist breath sounds, dyspnea
Blood pressure	Normal to decreased (late sign of impending shock)	Increased
Skin and mucous membranes	Pale, cool, poor turgor, prolonged capillary refill (>2 sec), dry mucous membranes	Edema
Salivation or tearing	Decreased to absent	Normal
Sensorium changes	Thirst, irritability, lethargy; stupor or coma if associated metabolic acidosis	Fatigue

Data from Porth, C. (2011). *Essentials of pathophysiology* (3rd ed.). Philadelphia: Wolters Kluwer.

CLINICAL REFERENCE

COMMON LABORATORY AND DIAGNOSTIC TESTS FOR FLUID AND ELECTROLYTE IMBALANCE*

TEST	DESCRIPTION	INDICATIONS	NORMAL FINDINGS
Urine osmolality	24-hr urine collection or random test	Altered fluid status	300-900 mOsm/kg
Urine sodium	24-hr urine collection or random urine specimen	Altered fluid status, hyponatremia	50-130 mEq/L
Urine specific gravity	Random urine specimen	Altered fluid status	1.002-1.030
Urea nitrogen	Random blood specimen	Altered fluid status, renal function	5-18 mg/dL
Serum osmolality	Random blood specimen	Altered fluid status	275-295 mOsm/kg
		Measures solute concentration of blood	

*None of these studies have any specific nursing considerations, although the nurse may be required to collect and transport the specimen; there is no advance preparation for collection.

SELECTED LABORATORY VALUES FOR ACID-BASE DISTURBANCES

TEST	METABOLIC ACIDOSIS	METABOLIC ALKALOSIS	RESPIRATORY ACIDOSIS	RESPIRATORY ALKALOSIS
ABG: pH	<7.35	>7.45	<7.35	>7.45
$PaCO_2$ (mm Hg)	<40	>45	>45	<35
PaO_2 (mm Hg)	WNL or slightly decreased	Decreased	Decreased	Decreased
HCO_3^- (mEq/L)	<22	>26	WNL or slightly increased	Decreased
K^+ (mEq/L)	>4	Decreased	WNL	Slightly decreased
Na^+ (mEq/L)	Varies according to condition	Decreased	WNL	Slightly decreased
Cl^- (mEq/L)	Usually increased	Decreased	WNL	Slightly decreased

ABG, Arterial blood gas; HCO_3^-, bicarbonate; $PaCO_2$, partial pressure of carbon dioxide in arterial blood; PaO_2, partial pressure of oxygen in arterial blood; *WNL*, within normal limits.

ACID-BASE DISTURBANCES: PRINCIPAL CAUSES, CLINICAL MANIFESTATIONS, AND TREATMENT

CONDITION	PRINCIPAL CAUSES	COMPENSATORY MECHANISMS*	CLINICAL MANIFESTATIONS	PRINCIPAL TREATMENT METHODS
Metabolic acidosis	Ketoacidosis (DKA, alcohol-induced ketoacidosis) Increasing metabolic rates from fever, RDS, seizures Interference with normal metabolism: ketosis, tissue hypoxia Loss of bicarbonate from diarrhea, ileostomy, or fistula drainage Acute and chronic renal failure ECF expansion and decreasing HCO_3^- concentration	Hyperventilation causes decreased $PaCO_2$	Increasing heart rate, arrhythmias (fibrillation) Hyperventilation Kussmaul respirations Cold, clammy skin (mild to moderate acidosis) Warm, dry skin (severe acidosis) Level of consciousness changes from weakness, fatigue and confusion to stupor and coma	Identify and treat the underlying disorder Provide $NaHCO_3$, K^+ replacement, and mechanical ventilation as indicated

BPD, Bronchopulmonary dysplasia; *CHF*, congestive heart failure; *CNS*, central nervous system; *DKA*, diabetic ketoacidosis; HCO_3^-, bicarbonate; *KCl*, potassium chloride; *NaCl*, sodium chloride; $NaHCO_3^-$, sodium bicarbonate; $PaCO_2$, partial pressure of carbon dioxide in arterial blood; *RDS*, respiratory distress syndrome.

*Important items to remember when acid-base compensation occurs:
- Normal values from which to interpret blood gases: $PaCO_2$ 35 to 45 mm Hg; pH 7.35 to 7.45; bicarbonate 22 to 26 mEq/L.
- When metabolic compensation occurs, assume origin in respiratory alteration.
- When respiratory compensation and release of tissue buffers occur, assume metabolic origin.

ACID-BASE DISTURBANCES: PRINCIPAL CAUSES, CLINICAL MANIFESTATIONS, AND TREATMENT—cont'd

CONDITION	PRINCIPAL CAUSES	COMPENSATORY MECHANISMS*	CLINICAL MANIFESTATIONS	PRINCIPAL TREATMENT METHODS
Metabolic alkalosis	Volume depletion related to various conditions (vomiting, pyloric stenosis, gastric drainage, and diuretics) Increased alkali intake Medical conditions (cystic fibrosis)	Hypoventilation causes increased PaCO₂	Arrhythmias (atrioventricular with prolonged QT interval) Increasing heart rate Decreased respiratory rate and depth Change in level of consciousness from apathy and confusion to stupor Muscular weakness	Treatment depends on underlying cause; mild to moderate alkalosis usually does not require treatment Use of fluids with NaCl and KCl, along with isotonic saline solution, an H₂-receptor antagonist (e.g., cimetidine) to decrease gastric hydrochloric acid, acidifying agents, and potassium-sparing diuretics (e.g., spironolactone [Aldactone], mannitol)
Respiratory acidosis	Pulmonary disease (BPD, RDS, asthma, cystic fibrosis, croup) Airway obstruction Chest conditions (flail chest, pneumothorax) Acute and chronic respiratory failure Neuromuscular abnormalities (Guillain-Barré syndrome, toxins, drugs, paralysis) CNS depression from sedative overdose, trauma, anesthesia	Release of HCO₃⁻ and increased renal reabsorption of HCO₃⁻ and acid excretion	Increasing heart rate Arrhythmias with hypotension Increasing rate and depth of respirations, forceful use of accessory muscles with retraction and cyanosis Increasing intracranial pressure	Correction of ventilation problem: use of oxygen, intubation, mechanical ventilation, NaHCO₃⁻
Respiratory alkalosis	Hyperventilation from CNS stimulation such as emotions, fear, hysteria, pain, salicylate poisoning Decreased lung compliance and hypoxemia from conditions such as pulmonary edema, CHF, pneumonia, asthma, pulmonary emboli Pregnancy Compensation from metabolic acidosis Sepsis	Decreased renal reabsorption of HCO₃⁻	Dizziness, paresthesias, lightheadedness, diaphoresis Arrhythmias (changes in ST-T wave)	Mild to moderate respiratory alkalosis usually does not require specific treatment For hyperventilation-induced conditions, provide oxygen, rebreathing oxygen masks, breathing into a paper bag, psychological reassurance Institute mechanical ventilation if condition is severe Give sedatives or tranquilizers for anxiety-induced condition, acetazolamide to prevent motion sickness

DEHYDRATION

Dehydration, or fluid loss in excess of fluid intake, is one of the most common causes of hospitalization in infants and children because it results from occurrences of severe gastroenteritis, which is a major cause of morbidity and mortality (Diggins, 2008). Decreased fluid intake or increased fluid loss may cause dehydration. Dehydration produces both fluid and electrolyte deficiencies. Dehydration is classified as isonatremic, hyponatremic, or hypernatremic (Table 16-1), according to the status of the serum sodium concentration. In isonatremic dehydration, the most common type of dehydration in children, water and electrolytes are lost in approximately the same proportion as they exist in the body, and serum sodium levels remain within the normal range of 138 to 145 mEq/L. In hyponatremic dehydration, the electrolyte loss is greater than the water loss, resulting in a serum sodium concentration of less than 135 mEq/L. In hypernatremic dehydration, the water loss is greater than the electrolyte loss and the serum sodium concentration is more than 150 mEq/L.

TABLE 16-1 TYPES OF DEHYDRATION: ETIOLOGY, CLINICAL MANIFESTATIONS, AND LABORATORY VALUES

ISONATREMIC DEHYDRATION	HYPONATREMIC DEHYDRATION	HYPERNATREMIC DEHYDRATION
Etiology Vomiting, diarrhea, insensible fluid loss from respiratory and integumentary systems Decreased oral intake with increased activity	***Renal Losses*** Diuretics, hyperglycemia, nephritis, adrenal insufficiency ***Extrarenal Losses*** Vomiting, diarrhea, third spacing, burns, tube drainage ***Other*** CHF, SIADH, nephrosis; administration of large amounts of electrolyte-free solutions (plain water) during illness or postoperatively	***Renal Losses*** Osmotic diuretics, diabetes insipidus, diabetes mellitus ***Extrarenal Losses*** Vomiting, diarrhea ***Other*** Fever, increased sodium in formula, diet, or tube feeding; administration of hypertonic sodium IV fluids; burns; ineffective breastfeeding
Clinical Manifestations Mild thirst Skin turgor poor Dry skin Decreased urine output Dry mucous membranes Skin temperature cold Body temperature afebrile or febrile Lethargy	Increased thirst Skin turgor very poor Skin usually clammy Decreased urine output Mucous membranes dry to slightly moist Skin temperature cold Body temperature afebrile or febrile Very lethargic, possible seizures	Thirst very increased Skin turgor fair Skin texture thickened or "doughy" Decreased urine output Mucous membranes parched Skin temperature cold or hot Body temperature afebrile or febrile Lethargic, hyperirritable with stimulation
Laboratory Values Serum sodium: 138-145 mEq/L Urine sodium usually within normal limits Specific gravity slightly elevated Osmolality usually within normal limits Volume usually within normal limits or slightly decreased	***Renal Losses*** Serum sodium <135 mEq/L Plasma osmolality decreased Urine sodium increased Urine specific gravity decreased Urine osmolality decreased Urine volume increased	***Renal Losses*** Serum sodium >150 mEq/L Urine sodium increased Urine specific gravity decreased Urine osmolality decreased Urine volume increased
	Extrarenal Losses Serum sodium <135 mEq/L Urine sodium decreased Urine specific gravity increased Urine osmolality increased Urine volume decreased	***Extrarenal Losses*** Serum sodium >150 mEq/L Urine sodium decreased Urine specific gravity increased Urine osmolality increased Urine volume decreased
	Other Serum sodium <135 mEq/L Urine sodium decreased Urine specific gravity increased Urine osmolality increased Urine volume decreased	***Other*** Serum sodium >150 mEq/L Urine sodium decreased Urine specific gravity increased Urine osmolality increased Urine volume decreased

Data from Greenbaum, L. (2007). Electrolyte and acid base disorders. In R. Behrman, R. Kliegman, H. Jenson, & B. Stanton (Eds.), *Nelson textbook of pediatrics* (18th ed.). Philadelphia: Elsevier Saunders.
CHF, Congestive heart failure; *SIADH,* syndrome of inappropriate secretion of antidiuretic hormone.

Etiology and Incidence

Dehydration has many varied causes. Common alterations that may lead to dehydration reflect disturbances in the following systems:

- *Gastrointestinal tract:* Vomiting, diarrhea, pyloric stenosis, malabsorption
- *Endocrine system:* Fever, diabetes mellitus, cystic fibrosis
- *Skin:* Burns
- *Lungs:* Tachypnea
- *Kidneys:* Renal failure
- *Heart:* Congestive heart failure

Any age-group can be affected, but neonates and infants, as discussed previously, are especially vulnerable to the effects of dehydration. Gastroenteritis with resulting dehydration accounts for 1.5

million deaths worldwide in children and is the second leading cause of death globally in children (Bhutta, 2011).

Manifestations

Classifications of the severity of dehydration vary according to the published source. In general, for infants and young children with isonatremic dehydration, the fluid deficit is described as mild, moderate, or severe dehydration, depending on the percentage of body weight lost (Greenbaum, 2011; Yu, Lougee, & Murno, 2010):

- *Mild dehydration:* Less than 5% loss of body weight
- *Moderate dehydration:* 5% to 10% loss of body weight
- *Severe dehydration:* Greater than 10% of body weight
- The Centers for Disease Control and Prevention (2008) adds an additional category, minimal dehydration (<3% body weight loss) for treatment purposes

One milliliter of body fluid is approximately equal to 1 g of body weight, so a weight loss or gain of 1 kg (2.2 lb) in 24 hours represents a 1-L fluid loss or gain.

Older children have a lower total body water content and ECF volume than do infants and younger children. Therefore, an equivalent percentage of body weight lost from dehydration represents a more severe fluid depletion in the older child. Isonatremic dehydration in the older child is classified as *mild* if less than 3% of body weight is lost, *moderate* if 3% to 6% of body weight is lost, and *severe* if more than 6% of body weight is lost (Greenbaum, 2011).

The signs and symptoms associated with degree of isonatremic dehydration are listed in Table 16-2. As with impending shock, the most essential manifestations are changes in heart rate; general appearance, behavior, or sensorium; urine output; skin and mucous membrane qualities; and, in infants, fontanels. Sunken eyes and decreased tears are definitive signs of dehydration (Goldman, Friedman, & Parkin, 2008), but lack of tears is not an accurate sign in very young infants, who may not produce tears until approximately 2 to 3 months of age.

⚡ SAFETY ALERT

Signs of Impending Shock in the Dehydrated Child

Because of the child's ability to compensate and maintain an adequate cardiac output, changes in heart rate, sensorium, and skin color are earlier indicators of impending shock than is blood pressure.

Diagnostic Evaluation

Key factors to consider in determining the type and severity of dehydration in children include the following:

- A history of acute or chronic fluid loss
- Clinical manifestations
- Child's weight
- Serum electrolyte values for moderate to severe dehydration

Abnormal serum electrolyte values, which include decreased bicarbonate, decreased potassium, and decreased glucose, are not unusual in the dehydrated child, although in isonatremic dehydration the sodium level remains within normal limits (Porth, 2011). Serum pH levels provide information about acid-base balance in an infant or a child suspected of being acidotic or alkalotic. An elevated urine specific gravity (>1.020) suggests dehydration.

Therapeutic Management

Management is directed toward correcting the fluid and electrolyte imbalance and then treating the causative factors. In 2003, the Centers for Disease Control and Prevention (CDC) published evidence-based guidelines for addressing dehydration; these guidelines were accepted as policy in 2004 by the American Academy of Pediatrics (AAP) (CDC, 2003; AAP, 2004). Evidence-based systematic review has affirmed these guidelines as being the management of choice in infants and young children (Hartling, Bellemare, Wiebe, et al., 2006/2009).

TABLE 16-2   ASSESSMENT OF THE SEVERITY OF DEHYDRATION

CLINICAL SIGNS	MINIMAL OR NO DEHYDRATION	MILD TO MODERATE DEHYDRATION	SEVERE DEHYDRATION
Weight loss	<3%	<5%-10%	>10%
Vital signs			
Pulse	Normal	Normal to increased, weak	Tachycardic, bradycardic in most severe cases; thready
Respiratory rate	Normal	Normal to fast	Rapid and deep
Blood pressure	Normal	Normal	Markedly decreased as a sign of hypovolemic shock
General appearance	Well, alert; drinks normally, might refuse liquids	Fatigued, restless, irritable; thirsty and eager to drink	Apathetic, lethargic, unconscious; drinks poorly or unable to drink
Mucous membranes	Normally moist	Dry	Parched
Anterior fontanel	Normal	Sunken	Markedly depressed
Eyes	Normal, tears present	Slightly sunken, tears decreased	Markedly sunken, tears absent
Capillary refill	<2 sec; extremities feel warm	Prolonged; extremities cool	Prolonged, minimal; extremities cold; mottled or cyanotic
Skin turgor (see Figure 16-1)	Normal	Prolonged recoil	Tenting
Urine output	Mildly decreased	Decreased, concentrated urine	Minimal

Modified from Centers for Disease Control and Prevention. (2003). Managing acute gastroenteritis among children: Oral rehydration, maintenance, and nutritional therapy. *MMWR: Morbidity and Mortality Weekly Report, 52,* Table 1, p. 5. Retrieved from www.cdc.gov; Greenbaum, L. (2011). Deficit therapy. In R. Kliegman, B. Stanton, J. St. Geme, et al. (Eds.), *Nelson textbook of pediatrics* (19th ed., pp. 246-247). Philadelphia: Elsevier Saunders.

PATHOPHYSIOLOGY

Dehydration

In the early phases of dehydration, fluids, with some electrolytes, are lost from the ECF. If the fluid loss continues, loss of ICF can occur. Dehydration can lead to hypovolemic shock (see Chapter 11).

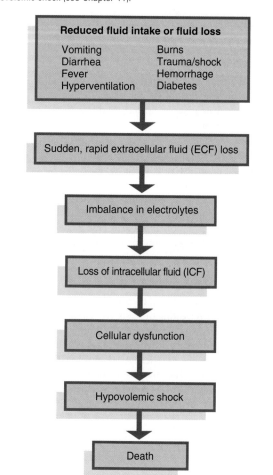

Reduced fluid intake or fluid loss

Vomiting	Burns
Diarrhea	Trauma/shock
Fever	Hemorrhage
Hyperventilation	Diabetes

↓

Sudden, rapid extracellular fluid (ECF) loss

↓

Imbalance in electrolytes

↓

Loss of intracellular fluid (ICF)

↓

Cellular dysfunction

↓

Hypovolemic shock

↓

Death

Minimal Dehydration

Treatment of minimal dehydration consists of continuing breastfeeding or age-appropriate diet, along with fluid replacement for each episode of fluid loss (stool, emesis) (Table 16-3). Regardless of the child's age, fluids are replaced with an oral rehydration solution (ORS), such as the World Health Organization's solution, Rehydralyte, Gastrolyte, Pedialyte, or Infalyte (CDC, 2008). The ORSs have changed from the days of homemade recipes (mixtures of water, salt, sugar, and cereals) to today's commercially available, lower-osmolality fluids. Because of their osmotic effect, the high carbohydrate content in fluids such as apple juice or colas may further aggravate diarrhea and cause additional fluid loss.

Electrolyte or sports drinks (e.g., Gatorade) have long been accepted oral rehydration formulations for older children. Recent studies, however, suggest that sports drinks are not the best solutions for rehydration and may in fact worsen diarrhea because of their high percentage of sugar and carbohydrates. These supplements greatly increase the osmotic load in the intestines and further aggravate diarrhea (CDC, 2008).

Mild to Moderate Dehydration

Treatment of fluid and electrolyte imbalances in children with mild to moderate dehydration should include rapid oral rehydration therapy (ORT) with an ORS in addition to replacing fluid losses. Suggested rehydration for children with mild to moderate dehydration is 50 to 100 mL/kg (based on the degree of dehydration) of ORS over 3 to 4 hours, with evaluation of the child's hydration status at least every 1 to 2 hours (Diggins, 2008; Yu et al., 2010). Breastfeeding infants should continue to breastfeed during oral rehydration; an age-appropriate diet should be offered to all other children once the hydration status has improved (CDC, 2008). The resumption of solid food promotes more rapid resolution of diarrhea (Bhutta, 2011).

Severe Dehydration

If the child is severely dehydrated or unable to take fluids by mouth and continuing fluid replacement is needed, parenteral fluid and electrolyte therapy is initiated. Initial therapy is aimed at treating or preventing shock. Either lactated Ringer's solution or 0.9% sodium chloride solution is the fluid of choice for parenteral rehydration and restoration of circulation. Sodium chloride (0.9%) solution may be ordered initially in boluses (20 mL/kg; 10 mL/kg in frail or ill infants) until the child's hydration status has improved (as assessed by improved level of consciousness), at which time ORT (100 mL/kg) can be initiated (Diggins, 2008). If the child cannot tolerate oral fluids, the remainder of the fluid replacement (maintenance requirement plus deficit less fluid amount already given) is provided IV over the next 24 hours (Greenbaum, 2011). If necessary, potassium is added to the IV solution once urine output is adequate, and additional fluid losses (by diarrhea or vomiting) are replaced as well. Box 16-1 lists daily fluid requirements by body weight and age-appropriate urine output.

⚡ SAFETY ALERT

Guidelines When Administering Potassium

- Do not administer potassium chloride if urine output is not age appropriate. See Box 16-1 for adequate urine output.
- *Never* give potassium by IV push.
- Give no more than 40 mEq/L, at a rate no faster than 1 mEq/kg/hr.
- Always check the dose and dosage calculations of potassium chloride. (Incorrect placement of a decimal point can result in a dose lethal to a child.)
- To avoid the risk of inadequate mixing, add potassium chloride to IV fluids with the plastic IV bag in the upright (noninfusion) position rather than in the down (infusion) position. (Inadequate mixing could result in the child's receiving an excessive amount of potassium chloride in the first few minutes.)
- Because of irritation of the vessel walls and potential phlebitis, IV solutions containing more than 30 mEq/L of potassium chloride should not be given through a peripheral IV line.

The type of dehydration determines the rate of administration of replacement fluids. For the child with hyponatremic or hypernatremic dehydration, lost fluids may be replaced more slowly, with the amount of replacement fluid tied to the change in serum sodium levels (Greenbaum, 2011). For hypernatremic dehydration, the goal is to decrease serum sodium concentration by no more than 12 mEq/L in each 24 hours (Greenbaum, 2011). Replacement may occur over several days. Potassium losses must also be replaced; this process should proceed slowly to avoid hyperkalemia. Potassium replacement should begin only after urine output is adequate (see Box 16-1) and should be

TABLE 16-3 ORAL REPLACEMENT AND REHYDRATION THERAPY IN CHILDREN WITH VOMITING OR DIARRHEA

MINIMALLY DEHYDRATED	MILD TO MODERATE DEHYDRATION	SEVERE DEHYDRATION
Oral Rehydration Therapy (ORT) Not necessary unless not taking other fluids well	50-100 mL/kg of oral rehydration solution (ORS) plus replace continuing losses rapidly over a 3- to 4-hr period	IV therapy: bolus (or multiple boluses) of 20 mL/kg of normal saline or lactated Ringer's solution; begin ORT for the remaining deficit (100 mL/kg over 2-4 hr) when child is stable and alert and can take oral fluids; alternatively, infuse 5% dextrose in half-strength normal saline solution, initially in a bolus of 20 mL/kg over 2 hr, then at a rate that replaces the remaining fluid deficit over the next 24 hr; keep IV line in place until child is drinking well
Continuing Losses 60-120 mL ORS for child weighing <10 kg, 120-240 mL for child weighing >10 kg to replace fluid loss from each episode of diarrhea or vomiting, **or** lost volume is measured and replaced (1 mL/g fluid loss)	60-120 mL ORS for child weighing <10 kg, 120-240 mL for child weighing >10 kg to replace fluid loss from each episode of diarrhea or vomiting, **or** lost volume is accurately measured and replaced (1 mL/g fluid loss)	60-120 mL ORS for child weighing <10 kg, 120-240 mL for child weighing >10 kg to replace fluid loss from each episode of diarrhea or vomiting, **or** lost volume is accurately measured and replaced (1 mL/g fluid loss); if unable to drink, administer replacement through nasogastric tube **or** infuse 5% dextrose and quarter or half-strength normal saline solution; potassium 20 mEq/L may be needed after urination established
Feeding Continue age-appropriate diet	Continue breastfeeding; resume age-appropriate diet as soon as dehydration is corrected	Continue breastfeeding if able to take oral fluids; resume age-appropriate diet as soon as dehydration is corrected and able to take oral foods
Reevaluate Hydration and Estimate Continuing Fluid Losses As necessary	Every 1-2 hr	Continuous evaluation; must evaluate after each bolus of IV solution

Modified from Centers for Disease Control and Prevention. (2003). Managing acute gastroenteritis among children: Oral rehydration, maintenance, and nutritional therapy. *MMWR: Morbidity and Mortality Weekly Report, 52,* 1-16. Retrieved from www.cdc.gov; Greenbaum, L.(2011). Deficit therapy. In R. Kliegman, B. Stanton, J. St. Geme, et al. (Eds.), *Nelson textbook of pediatrics* (19th ed., p. 247). Philadelphia: Elsevier Saunders

BOX 16-1 MAINTENANCE FLUID REQUIREMENTS AND MINIMUM URINE OUTPUT

Daily Fluid Requirements by Body Weight

≤10 kg:	100 mL/kg
10-20 kg:	1000 mL + 50 mL/kg for each additional kilogram between 10 and 20 kg
>20 kg:	1500 mL + 20 mL/kg for each additional kilogram over 20 kg

Minimum Urine Output by Age-Group

Infants and toddlers	>2-3 mL/kg/hr
Preschoolers and young school-age children	>1-2 mL/kg/hr
School-age children and adolescents	0.5-1 mL/kg/hr

administered with extreme caution. If the child is anuric, potassium is retained, causing elevated potassium levels.

Adjunctive Management

In addition to providing fluid resuscitation and replacement, there has been recent discussion relative to using antiemetics to reduce vomiting during ORT. The AAP has not supported the use of antiemetics; however, recent evidence suggests that using ondansetron (Zofran) reduces vomiting and allows for more rapid fluid replacement through ORT (Colletti, Brown, Sharieff, et al., 2010; Freedman, Steiner, & Chan, 2010).

NURSING CARE OF THE CHILD WITH DEHYDRATION

Assessment

Because dehydration can develop very quickly in infants and young children, the nurse must be alert for early signs of dehydration in children with conditions in which fluid losses are likely to occur, such as diarrhea, vomiting, burns, diabetes, trauma, and fever. The condition of infants and young children can change rapidly when fluid and electrolyte imbalances occur. It is particularly important to assess the following:

- *Intake and output:* Measure all fluid intake and losses accurately (including vomitus, urine, stools, nasogastric drainage, and wound drainage). The practitioner must also consider insensible water loss.

- *Urine output and specific gravity:* Output of less than 2 to 3 mL/kg/hr in infants and toddlers, 1 to 2 mL/kg/hr in preschoolers and young school-age children, and 0.5 to 1 mL/kg/hr in school-age children or adolescents or a specific gravity greater than 1.020 may indicate dehydration. Glucose, large amounts of protein, and radiographic dyes, however, elevate the specific gravity and may interfere with its accuracy.
- *Weight:* Weight is a crucial indicator of fluid status. Accurate measurements of the weight of the unclothed child, using the same scale at the same time of day, are essential. Changes in weight related to changes in IV lines or dressings should be identified by recording "with IV." Weight gain during illness may indicate fluid retention or pulmonary or generalized edema. The weight should be rechecked, and the child should be assessed for pulmonary crackles and periorbital edema.
- *Stools, vomitus:* Frequency, type, amounts, and consistency should be assessed and recorded.
- *Sweating:* Estimate from dampness of clothing and linen.
- *Serum electrolytes:* See p. 340.
- *Skin:* Assess color, temperature, turgor (Figure 16-1), moisture, and capillary refill.
- *Mucous membranes and presence of tears:* Dry or sticky mucous membranes and the absence of tears indicate dehydration. Absence of tears is not significant in an infant younger than 2 to 3 months because infants of this age often do not manufacture tears.
- *Anterior fontanel:* A sunken or depressed fontanel in infants indicates dehydration. Cranial suture lines may also become prominent with dehydration.
- *Vital signs:* Fever increases the metabolic rate and fluid requirements. With dehydration, the pulse is rapid, weak, and thready. An increase in the respiratory rate compensates for metabolic acidosis, which often accompanies dehydration. Blood pressure may be decreased in moderate and severe dehydration, but it is a late sign of hypovolemia.
- *Behavior:* Irritability, lethargy, confusion, or seizures may be present. The child's cry may be high pitched and weak.

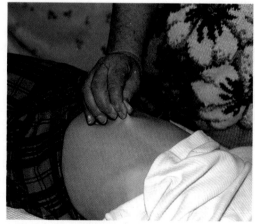

FIG 16-1 Testing skin turgor. Turgor refers to the elasticity of the skin, which is affected by the extent of hydration. The nurse tests turgor by gently grasping the skin. When the skin is released, it should instantly spring back into place; if it does not, tissue turgor is considered poor. (Courtesy University of Texas at Arlington School of Nursing, Arlington, TX.)

■ Nursing Diagnosis and Planning

- Deficient Fluid Volume related to gastric or intestinal infection or inflammation, hemorrhage, burns, or failure of fluid regulatory mechanisms.

Expected Outcome. The infant or child will display adequate fluid volume, as evidenced by age-appropriate urine output, age-appropriate urine specific gravity, elastic skin turgor and moist mucous membranes, serum pH and electrolyte levels within normal limits, and weight gain.

- Deficient Knowledge related to incomplete understanding of preventive measures for fluid loss.

Expected Outcomes. The parent or caregiver will describe how to appropriately administer fluids to prevent dehydration. The parent or caregiver will describe concerning signs and symptoms and seek medical assistance when needed.

■ Interventions

Teach parents how to prevent dehydration (see Patient-Centered Teaching: Dehydration box). Parents should be taught to give infants and young children extra fluids during hot weather, to avoid overdressing their children, and to encourage frequent rest periods during high-energy play times. During minor illness, providing additional fluids to a child with fever may prevent the development of more serious problems. Teach parents how to identify the early signs and symptoms of dehydration, and instruct them to seek professional help if these signs and symptoms should occur.

PATIENT-CENTERED TEACHING

Dehydration

Signs and Symptoms of Dehydration
Watch for the following signs and symptoms of dehydration:
- Fewer wet diapers (especially no wet diaper for more than 6 to 8 hours)
- No tears when your child is crying if older than 2 to 3 months
- Inside of mouth dry or sticky
- Irritability; high-pitched cry
- Difficulty in awakening
- Increased respiratory rate or difficulty breathing
- Sunken fontanel, sunken eyes with dark circles
- Abnormal skin color, temperature, or dryness

Because a young child's condition may worsen faster than an older child's, seek professional assistance early if your child is younger than 6 months old.

Also, teach parents how to replace fluids when the child is mildly dehydrated. Oral rehydration formulations, such as Rehydralyte, Infalyte, Gastrolyte, or Pedialyte, contain the appropriate concentration of electrolytes and should be used. Parents need to understand that giving plain water alone or in large amounts can be extremely dangerous and why it is dangerous. The infant or child needs to continue to eat as tolerated.

When caring for the hospitalized child with fluid and electrolyte imbalance, the nurse assumes the responsibility of continuously monitoring the child's condition and administering oral and IV fluids safely (see Chapter 14 for a discussion of IV therapy). When caring for children with conditions such as fever, burns, diarrhea, vomiting, or trauma, the nurse must continuously assess for signs of dehydration.

EVIDENCE-BASED PRACTICE

Assessing Dehydration

Level VI

It is an important part of contributing to evidence-based nursing practice for nurses not only to conduct research but also to participate in research carefully conducted by others. In the emergency department setting, finding a rapid, but accurate, way of assessing the severity of dehydration in young children (younger than 5 years old) would facilitate the initiation of an appropriate rehydration method. Researchers in a children's hospital in Toronto recruited experienced emergency triage nurses to assist with validating a four-descriptor dehydration assessment scoring method, which could improve the ability to detect the degree of dehydration in young children so that appropriate management could be quickly initiated. The scoring method had been developed several years previously, but not validated. Of the dehydration descriptors presented in Table 16-2, the researchers previously demonstrated that four are significant as a group for predicting degree of dehydration (none, some, moderate/severe). These four descriptors are general appearance, sunken appearance of the eyes, dryness of mucous membranes, and presence/absence of tears. Each of these dehydration descriptors was given a score of 0 to 2. For example, mucous membranes were scored a 0 if they were moist, a 1 if they were "sticky," and a 2 if they were dry. Each characteristic of dehydration was given a precise definition so that well-trained nurses could reliably and quickly assign a score.

Two hundred six children diagnosed with acute gastroenteritis participated in this Level VI prospective and observational study after informed consent by their parents. Health histories and physical examinations were performed, after which the triage nurse determined the dehydration score. The nurse did not communicate the score to the physicians treating the children, nor was the score documented in the chart, and the treatment the children received was based on physician assessment alone. The researchers concluded that the scoring system was valid for assessing degree of dehydration and that the individual scores strongly predicted the type of treatment the child received (ORT versus IV), as well as hospital length of stay.

Think about the ways in which nurses can participate in clinical research. What types of clinical problems might you identify that would be of interest to a nurse researcher? Think about how sources of error could be controlled in clinical research studies.

From Goldman, R., Friedman, J., & Parkin, P. (2008). Validation of the clinical dehydration scale for children with acute gastroenteritis. *Pediatrics, 122*(3), 545-549.

? CRITICAL THINKING EXERCISE 16-1

You have admitted a 9-month-old child who has been diagnosed with moderate dehydration to the emergency department. The physician has ordered ORT for this child based on a weight of 9.5 kg at 50 mL/kg over 4 hours. In addition, the physician has ordered replacement fluid of 120 mL for each episode of diarrhea or vomiting. Over the first 4 hours of observation, the child had two episodes of diarrhea. How many milliliters would the child be expected to receive over the 4-hour period?

■ **Evaluation**

- Is the child alert?
- Is urine output appropriate for age with a specific gravity within normal limits?
- Is the skin elastic and soft?
- Are the mucous membranes moist?
- Are serum pH and electrolyte levels within normal limits?

DIARRHEA

Diarrhea, one of the most common disorders in childhood, is defined as an increase in the frequency, fluidity, and volume of stools. Worldwide, approximately 2.5 billion children are affected by diarrhea annually, with prevalence highest in developing countries (Bhutta, 2011); deaths annually occur in children younger than 5 years old from complications related to diarrhea (Boschi-Pinto, Velebit, & Shibuya, 2008). Diarrhea accompanies many childhood disorders and may be acute or chronic, inflammatory or noninflammatory. Diarrhea caused by infection is usually called *gastroenteritis*. Viral gastroenteritis is the major cause of diarrhea in children older than 1 year. Rotavirus infection, the most common type of infectious diarrhea, accounted for one third to one half of hospitalizations of U.S. children younger than 5 years of age, due to the resulting fluid imbalances (CDC, 2009). Norovirus infection is seen frequently as well (Bhutta, 2011).

If not treated, acute diarrhea in infants and children can lead to dehydration, electrolyte imbalance, and hypovolemic shock. Acute diarrhea can be life threatening in infants and small children if gastrointestinal fluid losses are not adequately replaced.

Etiology and Incidence

There are many causes of both acute and chronic diarrhea (Table 16-4). Diarrhea with ensuing dehydration is a leading killer of children worldwide and is a major cause of morbidity, as well as a primary sign of many other conditions. Diarrhea can be either a short-term or a long-term condition.

PATHOPHYSIOLOGY

Diarrhea

- Increased motility and rapid emptying of the intestines result in impaired absorption of nutrients and water and in electrolyte imbalance. Water, sodium, potassium, and bicarbonate are drawn from the extracellular space into the stool, resulting in dehydration, electrolyte depletion, and metabolic acidosis.
- Diarrhea occurs when there is excess fluid in the small intestine. This condition can result from a number of processes:
  - Bacterial toxins stimulating active transport of electrolytes into the small intestine: cells in the mucosal lining of the intestines are irritated and secrete increased amounts of water and electrolytes.
  - Organisms invading and destroying intestinal mucosal cells, decreasing intestinal surface area, and impairing the intestine's capacity to absorb fluids and electrolytes.
  - Inflammation, which decreases the intestine's ability to absorb fluid, electrolytes, and nutrients. This condition occurs in malabsorption syndromes.
  - Increased intestinal motility, resulting in impaired intestinal absorption.

Manifestations

Diarrhea may manifest either quickly or insidiously. Its manifestations include the following:

- *Integumentary:* Dry, hot skin; changes in skin texture and turgor; dry mucous membranes
- *Small intestine:* Cramps, nausea, vomiting; large-volume stools, light in color, loose to watery in texture; stools that tend to be soupy, greasy, or foul-smelling

TABLE 16-4   CAUSES AND MANIFESTATIONS OF DIARRHEA IN INFANTS AND CHILDREN

CAUSES OF DIARRHEA	MANIFESTATIONS
Intestinal infection:	Watery stools containing mucus and possibly blood
Bacterial (*Campylobacter jejuni,** *Salmonella,** *Shigella,** *Escherichia coli*)	Pain, cramps, nausea, vomiting, fever (101.6° F [>38.7° C]) with bacterial infection); risk of dehydration, electrolyte imbalance, and shock
Viral (rotavirus,* cause of more than 50% of cases of acute diarrhea in children; norovirus, enteric adenovirus)	
Parasitic (*Giardia lamblia,** *Cryptosporidium,** high incidence of both in daycare centers)	
Fungal overgrowth	
Food intolerance (lactose intolerance, overfeeding, introduction of new foods)	Diarrhea, increased mucus in stools, flatus, pain after ingestion of lactose or offending food
Malabsorption (cystic fibrosis, disaccharide deficiencies, celiac disease)	Diarrhea, cramps, distention, steatorrhea occurring after meals
	Anorexia, weight loss, fatigue
Medications (antibiotics, chemotherapy)	Diarrhea after administration of medications, which usually stops when medications are discontinued
Colon disease (ulcerative colitis, Crohn disease, enterocolitis)	Inflammation and ulceration of intestinal walls, increased motility
	May have 10-20 stools per day
	Abdominal pain, fever, chills, anorexia, weight loss
Irritable bowel syndrome	Diarrhea alternating with constipation or normal bowel function
	Pain, distention, nausea may be present
Intestinal obstruction (including intussusception)	Partial obstruction may result in diarrhea caused by increased intestinal motility
	Pain, nausea, and sometimes bloody stool; may note mucus in stools
Emotional stress (anxiety, fatigue)	Increased motility
Infectious disease (otitis media, upper respiratory infection, urinary tract infection)	Diarrhea frequently accompanies other infections

*Most common causative organisms.

- *Large intestine:* The urge to defecate with insignificant stool present; mushy, jellylike, or even bloody fecal matter; stool that is usually dark in color; stool that is rarely foul-smelling
- *Other:* Increased heart and respiratory rates, decreased tearing, fever

Diagnostic Evaluation

Most infectious causes of diarrhea are self-limiting, making comprehensive testing of minor cases of diarrhea impractical. Because of the different possible causes, the diagnostic workup is frequently geared toward ruling out infectious agents and anatomic and physiologic reasons, such as allergies, food intolerance, and bowel problems. Tests to be performed after an initial history has assessed for food intolerance, stress, or school- or work-related problems include the following:

- *Stool:* Cultures (for bacteria, ova, parasites), pH, red blood cells, leukocytes, glucose (Clinitest), blood (guaiac test or Hemoccult), various immunoassays for viral causes, such as rotavirus or norovirus
- *Blood tests:* Especially blood cell counts, electrolytes, blood urea nitrogen, glucose, and blood cultures (if an infectious agent is suspected)
- *X-ray films:* Check for possible bowel abnormalities

Therapeutic Management

The treatment of diarrhea is aimed at maintaining and restoring fluid and electrolyte balance and returning the bowel to normal function. Preventing the spread of infection to others is an important component of care, with meticulous hand hygiene (washing with soap and water) being critical. Parents must be informed of specific fluid intake

requirements and signs of dehydration, which would signal a worsening of the child's condition. Treatment of diarrhea and prevention of dehydration include replacing fluids, continuing feedings, and close monitoring and observation. Infants should continue to be given breast milk or regular-strength formula.

The continued feeding of a normal diet can prevent dehydration, reduce stool frequency and volume, and hasten recovery. It does not prolong diarrhea, and there is evidence that it may reduce the duration of diarrhea (CDC, 2008). If adding milk to the diet increases diarrhea, transient lactose intolerance may be considered, although it is not as common as was once thought. Common foods that are especially well tolerated during diarrhea are bland but nutritional foods, including complex carbohydrates (e.g., rice, wheat, potatoes, cereals), yogurt containing live cultures, cooked vegetables, and lean meats. This recommendation is a change from the formerly recommended BRAT diet, which consisted of bananas, rice, applesauce, and toast. The BRAT diet can be tolerated but is low in energy, density, fat, and protein.

Preventing dehydration is a primary issue in the management of the infant or child with diarrhea. ORS is given to replace each loose stool. In addition to continuing an age-appropriate diet, children weighing less than 10 kg should have losses replaced with 60 to 120 mL of ORS for each episode of diarrhea. Children weighing more than 10 kg should receive 120 to 240 mL of ORS (CDC, 2008; Hartling et al., 2006/2009). For infants with mild to moderate diarrhea who have not become dehydrated, fluid loss replacement is started at home.

If an infant or a child has become mildly to moderately dehydrated and requires a visit to a clinic or an emergency room, ORT is recommended as described previously and in Table 16-3. At the end of each hour of rehydration, hydration and replacement losses should be assessed. Initial rehydration may require limiting the intake to smaller volumes (sips) to reduce any incidence of associated vomiting (e.g., 5 mL every 2 to 5 minutes) with a gradual increase in volume as tolerated. Nasogastric administration of ORS may be necessary to provide slow, steady, continuous administration to rapidly hydrate the child and prevent hospitalization.

Feeding of solids or formula is started as soon as the child is rehydrated. Children should be encouraged to eat frequently—every 3 to 4 hours. Parents should be instructed that, although stool output may increase, feeding will not prolong diarrhea and the child will be absorbing necessary nutrients and calories. For a child with severe dehydration and continuing losses, ORT is not recommended. Such children are usually admitted to a hospital for observation and IV therapy.

If bacteria, parasites, or fungi cause the diarrhea, other types of medication along with antibiotics may be ordered. The use of antidiarrheal medication is not recommended in children because of the binding nature of these products and the potential for toxicity (Grimwood & Forbes, 2009). Antidiarrheal medications have not been found to shorten the course of the diarrhea, and in cases where the diarrhea is caused by pathogens, they may increase fluid and electrolyte loss by interfering with the body's attempt to rid itself of the organism and allowing the pathogen to remain in the body longer.

Prognosis

Most children with diarrhea and subsequent dehydration usually have a relatively quick recovery, provided that the cause of the diarrhea is determined and therapy is started as soon as possible. Oral rotavirus vaccine is recommended by the CDC for prevention of diarrhea caused by rotavirus. There are two approved rotavirus vaccines: RV5 and the newly released RV1. Each is effective for preventing rotavirus, although their dosage scheduling is different. RV5 rotavirus vaccine is given to infants at ages 2, 4, and 6 months, whereas the RV1 vaccine is given at 2 and 4 months only (CDC, 2009).

NURSING CARE OF THE CHILD WITH DIARRHEA

■ Assessment

When a child is admitted to a hospital setting, the child's condition and hydration status should be the first area of assessment. The primary concern about dehydration is the potential for shock. The child and family should be questioned about possible food allergies, intolerance to foods, foods eaten over the past 24 hours, and outbreaks of diarrhea in the nuclear or extended family or daycare setting. If diarrhea is present, stools should be assessed for amount, color, consistency, and time (ACCT) and odor. When assessing and monitoring for ACCT, note the quantity and quality of the stool, its color (e.g., green, brown, clear, blood tinged), consistency (watery, loose), the presence of mucus, and the length of time since the stool's consistency has changed.

Other continuing assessments include monitoring intake and output; assessing the current weight and comparing it with the last known weight; assessing for thirst, along with skin turgor and texture and mucous membranes; and monitoring the child's level of activity. The nurse also monitors electrolyte values, if ordered. If diarrhea is severe, it may be necessary to apply a urine bag to measure urine output and to obtain urine to measure specific gravity. Skin integrity must be monitored, especially if a urine bag is to be used. Observe the skin in the perineal area for color, texture, lesions, or drainage with each diaper change. Assess family members' knowledge of the transmission of infection by questions or testing. Observe family members as they use Contact Precautions. Ask family if any members have cramping or diarrhea.

■ Nursing Diagnosis and Planning

The following nursing diagnoses and expected outcomes may be appropriate in the treatment of diarrhea in a child:
- Deficient Fluid Volume related to increased stool output.

Expected Outcomes. The child will maintain fluid balance within normal limits, as evidenced by age-appropriate urine output, capillary refill time less than 2 seconds, elastic skin turgor, moist mucous membranes, and weight gain.
- Impaired Skin Integrity related to exposure to stool.

Expected Outcomes. The child will have no sign of skin breakdown, as evidenced by intact perineal and perianal skin, or will exhibit signs of healing on affected or excoriated areas.
- Risk for Infection (in others) related to lack of knowledge about transmission prevention.

Expected Outcomes. Family members will show no signs of infection and demonstrate correct precaution technique (Contact Precautions).
- Imbalanced Nutrition: Less than Body Requirements related to decreased intake and inability of body to absorb fluids.

Expected Outcome. The child will tolerate the diet, as evidenced by weight gain and no recurrence of diarrhea.

■ Interventions

The child with diarrhea should be weighed unclothed on admission and daily on the same scale and at the same time each day to precisely determine changes in weight. To accurately determine fluid losses with each episode of diarrhea in untrained infants and children, weigh the diaper after each voiding and liquid stool and compare to the weight of the same type of diaper dry (each gram of excess diaper weight is equal to 1 mL of fluid output). Measuring amounts of liquid stool may be required for the older child. Accurate accounting of losses is necessary to maximize the effectiveness of the ORT and to prevent deficits and imbalances in electrolytes. Document the child's intake, as well as output.

Signs of dry mucous membranes, decreased tearing, and sunken fontanel (if appropriate) or eyes are often the first indicators of dehydration and should be immediately reported. Vital signs should be measured every 4 hours, or as needed. Determining the causes of diarrhea may include obtaining stool cultures and other tests to determine specific management approaches.

Infants and young children may have skin excoriation resulting from continual contact with loose stools. Nursing intervention includes providing meticulous skin care. Gently wash the area with warm water and mild soap after each loose stool and pat dry. Apply an ointment to protect the child's skin and, if ordered, a medicated cream to heal the skin. Some children benefit from exposing damaged skin to the air for small periods of time to promote healing. Turning every 2 hours keeps pressure off the skin and facilitates circulation to the affected area.

Nursing interventions, along with the prescribed therapy, work together to achieve the expected outcomes of managing any dehydration, decreasing the number of stools, and returning the bowel to normal function. ORT may be initiated in a hospital setting after IV rehydration. Administer the ORS as ordered, increasing the volume as tolerated. If the child refuses or is unable to tolerate the ORS, nasogastric therapy may be considered.

Most cases of diarrhea in children can be managed at home. Parent teaching needs to be clear, concise, and specific (see Patient-Centered Teaching: Caring for a Child with Diarrhea box). Education about

PATIENT-CENTERED TEACHING

Caring for a Child with Diarrhea

Diet

Diet depends on the age of the child and the severity of the diarrhea.

Mild Diarrhea (Mushy Stools) in Children of Any Age

Continue with an age-appropriate diet. Continue breastfeeding, formula, or milk. Encourage increased intake of fluids. Avoid fruit juices, because they may worsen diarrhea. Provide a variety of nutritious foods, including foods containing complex carbohydrates, such as rice, potatoes, bread, and cereals. Avoid fatty or spicy foods.

Moderate Diarrhea (Watery or Frequent Stools) in Children Younger than 1 Year

Continue breastfeeding or formula and age-appropriate diet. Provide additional fluids by using Infalyte, Pedialyte, Rehydralyte, or other similar commercially prepared oral rehydration solutions if urine output begins to decrease. If the diarrhea is severe and the child is uncomfortable with cow's milk–based formulas, soy formula (e.g., Isomil, ProSobee) may be considered. Feed infants older than 6 months with such bland foods as applesauce, strained carrots, rice cereal, and yogurt with live cultures. Watch closely for signs of dehydration and report these immediately to your health care provider.

Moderate Diarrhea (Watery or Frequent Stools) in Children Older than 1 Year

Continue age-appropriate diet with foods that are nutritional, bland, and high in starch. Suggested foods include breads, crackers, rice, mashed potatoes, noodles, yogurt with live cultures, cooked vegetables, and lean meats. Avoid beans, spices, and fatty foods. Avoid sports drinks, colas, and apple juice. Give additional fluids in the form of Infalyte, Pedialyte, or Rehydralyte. Watch closely for signs of dehydration and report these immediately to your health care provider.

Preventing the Spread of Infection

Infectious diarrhea is highly contagious. Some of the infectious agents can live on toys, water fountains, and other inanimate objects for several days. Thorough handwashing after diaper changing or using the toilet is crucial to prevent others in the household from getting diarrhea. All family members should be taught the importance of thorough and frequent handwashing. Diapers should be changed on a surface designated for that purpose, *not* on the kitchen counter where food is prepared. Changing areas should be cleaned with disinfectant after each diaper change.

Skin Care

To prevent breakdown of the sensitive skin in the diaper area, diarrhea stools should be completely washed off with mild soap and water after each bowel movement. (Washing the child under running water in the bathtub makes the job easier. The tub should be cleaned with disinfectant before anyone else uses it.) The skin should be patted dry and a layer of A+D ointment or other protective or "barrier" ointment applied.

Changing diapers immediately after bowel movements is important to prevent skin breakdown. The use of commercial baby wipes should be avoided because they may further irritate and cause additional breakdown of the skin. To prevent overflow of diarrhea from the diaper, diapers should be applied snugly.

When to Call the Physician

Call the physician immediately if any of the following occurs:
- The child does not urinate for longer than 6 hours.
- Crying produces no tears, or the mouth becomes dry.
- The infant's fontanel appears sunken.
- The child's behavior or mental status changes.
- Blood or pus appears in the diarrhea, or the diarrhea becomes severe and lasts longer than 24 hours.
- Severe abdominal cramps occur.
- The child has a fever (>102° F [>39° C]).

Oral Rehydration Therapy

Giving plain water alone or in large amounts can be extremely dangerous because it does not contain needed electrolytes. Instead, commercially available oral rehydration solutions should be given.

Data from Centers for Disease Control and Prevention. (2011). Updated norovirus outbreak management and disease prevention guidelines. *MMWR Morbidity and Mortality Weekly Report, 60*(RR03), 1-15; National Digestive Diseases Information Clearinghouse. (2011, January). *Diarrhea.* NIH Publication 11-2749. Retrieved from http://digestive.niddk.nih.gov.

appropriate oral replacement fluids should include avoidance of sugary drinks, apple juice, sports beverages, and colas. Fluids should be offered in small amounts to prevent gastric distention and at room temperature to prevent increased peristalsis stimulation.

Additional education needs to occur regarding prevention of illness in the nuclear and extended family or daycare setting. In most instances, preventing infection transmission includes handwashing with soap and water. Handwashing is considered to be more effective against organisms that commonly cause diarrhea in children than antibacterial hand sanitizer (CDC, 2011). Instruction in careful handwashing technique before and after caring for the sick child will prevent spread of infection or reinfection. Proper disposal of and cleaning of contaminated articles and surfaces decreases spread of infection.

■ **Evaluation**

- Are weight, urine output, and specific gravity within normal limits for age?
- Is the capillary refill time less than 2 seconds?
- Is skin turgor elastic, and are mucous membranes moist?

- Have signs of excoriation, redness, blisters, pruritus, and infection been reduced or eliminated?
- Are family members free of infection?
- Do family members correctly practice Contact Precautions technique on a consistent basis?
- Can the child retain food and fluids?
- Are normal bowel elimination patterns present?
- Has the child maintained or shown an increase in weight?

? CRITICAL THINKING EXERCISE 16-2

Mrs. Peters calls the clinic about 8-month-old David. She states that David has had diarrhea for 2 days and that she does not know what to do. She also states that her neighbor said she should stop breastfeeding and give David clear liquids. Mrs. Peters tells you that she is afraid she may have done something to cause David to get sick.

1. What questions should you ask Mrs. Peters about her infant?
2. What teaching can you do to help Mrs. Peters?

VOMITING

Vomiting is the forcible ejection of stomach contents through the mouth. It involves a complex reflex associated with sweating, salivation, and often tachycardia (all symptoms of autonomic nervous stimulation). Other terms that may be used to differentiate vomiting episodes include *spitting up* (or *chalasia*, which is a normal process during infancy), *regurgitation* (associated with gastroesophageal reflux or overfeeding), and, if severe, *projectile vomiting* (usually indicative of obstruction, tumor, pyloric stenosis, or increasing intracranial pressure). Isolated incidents of vomiting are usually of little concern. The consequences of persistent or prolonged vomiting, however, can be serious.

Etiology

Vomiting, which occurs frequently in children, is usually a sign of some other underlying problem or disease. Vomiting has many possible causes. Some of them are infections, obstructions, motion sickness, metabolic alterations, and psychological alterations. If vomiting occurs in association with diarrhea, it may be related to gastroenteritis. Vomiting can also result from allergic reactions or occur as a side effect of medications (e.g., chemotherapy), as a toxic effect of medications or ingested substances, and from certain eating disorders.

Manifestations

Sour milk curds without green or brown color and undigested food from the stomach are manifestations of vomiting. Green emesis usually indicates the presence of bile and possible intestinal obstruction below the ampulla of Vater. A fecal odor indicates lower intestinal obstruction or peritonitis. Emesis may be blood tinged, or the color may be bright red or look like coffee grounds. Bright red blood indicates that the blood has not been in contact with gastric juices.

The force of vomiting varies. Regurgitation, a backward flow of undigested food, could be caused by overfeeding. Forceful vomiting could indicate some obstruction. Projectile vomiting may indicate obstruction (see Chapter 19), tumor, or increased intracranial pressure. Continuous vomiting in a young child, in the absence of diarrhea, can contribute to metabolic alkalosis.

PATHOPHYSIOLOGY

Vomiting

Vomiting is under the control of the emetic center, located in the reticular core of the medulla (in the brainstem). The emetic center receives stimuli from one of three sources:

- From the vagal and sympathetic afferent nerves, such as the stimulation of irritation, distention, obstruction, or inflammation
- Chemically, from drugs (e.g., ipecac, opioids), cerebral hypoxia, inner ear disturbances, or increased intracranial pressure
- From the higher cortical centers, with stimuli such as sights, odors, and fright or fear

The mechanism of vomiting occurs in the presence of several complex reflexes:

- Autonomic nervous system discharge, which causes salivation, sweating, pallor, and an increased heart rate
- Contraction of the stomach antrum and duodenum
- Relaxation of the remainder of the stomach, esophagus, and sphincters
- Closure of the glottis and soft palate
- Contraction of the diaphragm and abdominal muscles, which increases intraabdominal pressure and compresses abdominal contents, thus propelling them into the esophagus and out the mouth

Diagnostic Evaluation

Vomiting in children is usually of brief duration and not severe. If vomiting continues and the child starts to look deficient in fluid or electrolytes, however, the following tests may be indicated:

- Complete blood cell counts and electrolyte studies, blood urea nitrogen, glucose levels, and urine tests
- Radiographic studies (if an obstructive or neurologic process is suspected)
- Blood cultures (if an infectious disease is suspected)
- Arterial blood gas determinations

Therapeutic Management

The primary focus of managing vomiting is detecting and treating the cause, with the secondary intent of preventing complications. ORT, as indicated for the treatment of diarrhea (see Table 16-3), is also appropriate for the vomiting child. Even with continued vomiting, most children can maintain hydration with small frequent feedings of an ORS and an age-appropriate diet as tolerated (Colletti, Brown, Sharieff et al., 2010), and therefore the vomiting can be managed at home. Adequate fluid intake and replacement of continuing losses from emesis are necessary. The practitioner and parents must estimate the volume of emesis and replace it. Reevaluation and continuing loss replacement should be done every 1 to 2 hours for a mild to moderately dehydrated child. As the vomiting decreases in frequency, the amount and interval between feedings can increase. If the vomiting is severe or prolonged in neonates and young infants, however, IV therapy may be initiated.

Most children will respond well to treatment, but some will need antiemetics. Freedman, Steiner, and Chan (2010) found that administration of ondansetron (Zofran) in an emergency department setting facilitated the success of oral rehydration and decreased vomiting episodes, need for intravenous fluid resuscitation, and time spent in the emergency department. To rid the mouth of the hydrochloric acid, and to freshen the mouth, the parent should rinse the child's mouth and brush the child's teeth after each time the child vomits.

NURSING CARE OF THE VOMITING CHILD

■ Assessment

Major concerns with vomiting are dehydration and fluid and electrolyte imbalance; therefore, it is essential that hydration status be carefully assessed, including accurate assessment of intake and output, weight, fontanels in infants, general behavior, dryness of mucous membranes, skin turgor, eyes, and urine output. Ask the parent to describe the type and force of vomiting (e.g., "spitting up" as opposed to regurgitation, forceful vomiting, or projectile vomiting) and the character (using the acronym ACCT: amount, color, consistency, time) of the vomitus. Because vomiting is often associated with gastric distention, the relationship, if any, with infant feeding should be assessed (e.g., poor feeding techniques, failure to bubble or burp, regurgitation with burp or "wet burp," improper positioning). Inquire about any other signs or symptoms the child may have.

■ Nursing Diagnosis and Planning

The following nursing diagnoses and expected outcomes may be appropriate in the treatment of the vomiting child:

- Deficient Fluid Volume related to increased loss of gastrointestinal contents.

Expected Outcomes. The child will maintain fluid balance within normal limits, as evidenced by age-appropriate fluid intake, and will

> ⚠ **NURSING QUALITY ALERT**
>
> *Caring for the Child Who Is Vomiting*
>
> Nursing care of the child who is vomiting is directed toward the following:
> - Observing and reporting vomiting
> - Assessing for associated problems, such as dehydration
> - Implementing measures to reduce the vomiting
> - Recording accurate intake and output
> - Evaluating the effectiveness of therapy
> - Preventing aspiration

have age-appropriate urine output, a capillary refill time of less than 2 seconds, elastic skin turgor, and moist mucous membranes.

- Imbalanced Nutrition: Less Than Body Requirements related to vomiting.

Expected Outcomes. The child will maintain electrolyte and acid-base balance within normal limits, as evidenced by adequate amount of calories absorbed, steady weight gain or lack of weight loss, and decreased vomiting episodes.

■ Interventions

The vomiting child should be placed in an upright or side-lying position to prevent aspiration. Nursing interventions are frequently determined by the cause of the vomiting and therefore may be very specific. For example, if the vomiting is found to be caused by incorrect feeding techniques, the nurse's role is to educate the family regarding appropriate feeding techniques (e.g., adequate bubbling and burping and positioning after the feeding) and preparation of formulas. Once the cause of vomiting has been determined, nursing interventions are directed toward ensuring a continued reduction in the vomiting and preventing dehydration. Advise the parent to offer an ORS (see Table 16-3) in small, frequent feedings to avoid gastric distention and to continue age-appropriate diet as tolerated. The parent can gradually increase the amount of fluids and foods as vomiting episodes decrease. Another important consideration is education for the child and family about avoiding certain foods (e.g., fatty, acidified, or seasoned foods) and minimizing stimuli such as stress, anxiety, or unfavorable-smelling foods, which might lead to nausea and subsequent vomiting. Decreased stimuli and avoidance of food or activities that might tend to upset the stomach, either directly or by association, may be helpful in decreasing nausea and vomiting. If the child repeatedly vomits or vomits large volumes, or if the child begins to exhibit signs of dehydration, the parent should notify the physician.

■ Evaluation

- Is the child taking age-appropriate amounts of fluid without vomiting?
- Is the child's urine output age appropriate?
- Is the child's skin turgor elastic, with a capillary refill time of 2 seconds or less?
- Does the child have moist mucous membranes?
- Is the child tolerating an age-appropriate diet?

■ KEY CONCEPTS

- Infants and children are at a much greater risk than adults for fluid and electrolyte disturbances.
- The three mechanisms by which acid-base balance is maintained are chemical buffering, respiratory control of carbon dioxide, and renal regulation of bicarbonate and secretion of hydrogen ions.
- The two major forms of acid-base disturbance are acidosis and alkalosis, either of which may be respiratory or metabolic.
- The treatment of metabolic disturbances is directed toward correcting the underlying problem. Interventions for respiratory alterations are implemented toward reestablishing alveolar ventilation.
- Dehydration may be classified as isonatremic (the most common form), hyponatremic, or hypernatremic.
- Assessment of intake and output, vital signs, and level of activity (or sensorium) is crucial in appropriately managing the child with a fluid or electrolyte disturbance.
- Diarrhea can lead to loss of bicarbonate (and subsequently to acidosis).
- Oral rehydration therapy is indicated for the child with diarrhea, dehydration of any degree, and vomiting.

REFERENCES

American Academy of Pediatrics (AAP). (2004). Statement of endorsement: Managing acute gastroenteritis among children: Oral rehydration, maintenance and nutritional therapy. *Pediatrics, 114*(2), 507.

Bhutta, Z. (2011). Acute gastroenteritis in children. In R. Kliegman, B. Stanton, J. St. Geme, et al. (Eds.), *Nelson textbook of pediatrics* (19th ed., pp. 1323-1339). Philadelphia: Elsevier Saunders.

Boschi-Pinto, C., Velebit, L., & Shibuya, K. (2008). Estimating childhood mortality due to diarrhea in developing countries. *Bulletin of the World Health Organization, 86*(9), 710-717.

Centers for Disease Control and Prevention. (2003). Managing acute gastroenteritis among children: Oral rehydration, maintenance, and nutritional therapy [Electronic version]. *MMWR Morbidity and Mortality Weekly Report, 52*, 1-16.

Centers for Disease Control and Prevention. (2008). *Information for healthcare providers: Guidelines for management of acute diarrhea.* Retrieved from www.cdc.gov.

Centers for Disease Control and Prevention. (2009). Prevention of rotavirus gastroenteritis among infants and children: recommendations of the Advisory Committee on Immunization Practices (AICP). *MMWR Morbidity and Mortality Weekly Reports, 58*(RR02), 1-25.

Centers for Disease Control and Prevention. (2011). Updated norovirus outbreak management and disease prevention guidelines. *MMWR Morbidity and Mortality Weekly Report, 60*(RR03), 1-15.

Colletti, J., Brown, K., Sharieff, G., et al. (2010). The management of children with gastroenteritis and dehydration in the emergency department. *Journal of Emergency Management, 38*(5), 686-698.

Diggins, K. (2008). Treatment of mild to moderate dehydration in children with oral rehydration therapy. *Journal of the American Academy of Nurse Practitioners, 20*, 402-406.

Freedman, S., Steiner, M., & Chan, K. (2010). Oral ondansetron administration in emergency departments to children with gastroenteritis: an economic analysis. *PLoS Medicine, 7*(10), e1000350. Retrieved from www.plosmedicine.org.

Goldman, R., Friedman, F., & Parkin, P. (2008). Validation of the clinical dehydration scale for children with acute gastroenteritis. *Pediatrics, 122*(3), 545-549.

Greenbaum, L. (2011). Deficit therapy. In R. Kliegman, B. Stanton, J. St. Geme, et al. (Eds.), *Nelson textbook of pediatrics* (19th ed., pp. 245-249). Philadelphia: Elsevier Saunders.

Grimwood, K., & Forbes, D. (2009). Acute and persistent diarrhea. *Pediatric Clinics of North America, 56*(6), 1343-1361.

Hartling, L., Bellemare, S., Wiebe, N., et al. (2006/updated and reaffirmed 2009). Oral versus intravenous rehydration for treating dehydration due to gastroenteritis in children. *Cochrane Database of Systematic Reviews, 3*, CD004390. Retrieved from www.thecochranelibrary.com.

Porth, C. (2011). *Essentials of pathophysiology* (3rd ed.). Philadelphia: Wolters Kluwer.

Yu, C., Lougee, D., & Murno, J. (2010). Diarrhea and dehydration. *American Academy of Pediatrics, PEDS Curriculum* (Module 6). Retrieved from www.aap.org.

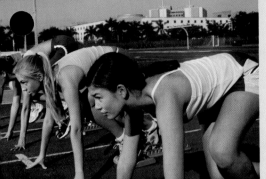

The Child with an Infectious Disease

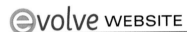 WEBSITE

http://evolve.elsevier.com/James/ncoc

LEARNING OBJECTIVES

After studying this chapter, you should be able to:

- Analyze the infectious process.
- Compare the modes of transmission of infectious diseases.
- Analyze the pathophysiology, clinical manifestations, complications, and nursing management of childhood infectious diseases.

- Analyze the pathophysiology, clinical manifestations, complications, and nursing management of sexually transmissible infections.
- Use the nursing process to describe the nursing care of a child with an infectious disease.

CLINICAL REFERENCE

REVIEW OF DISEASE TRANSMISSION

Microorganisms exist throughout the environment. Most are harmless residents and a normal part of human flora. An organism that invades body tissue, causing tissue damage and disease, however, is a pathogen. For pathogens to invade a host, they must breach the normal host defenses, by either attaching to or penetrating the host. The power of these pathogens, known as their virulence, depends on their ability to overcome the host defense mechanisms. Thus a highly virulent organism can cause disease with relative ease.

Microorganisms can have one of several relationships with the host: commensalism, mutualism, or parasitism. Those that cause infectious

MICROORGANISMS AND HOST RELATIONS

- Commensalism: Host provides shelter and food for the organism; organism retains the ability to exist independently (e.g., nonpathogenic bacteria living in human intestines).
- Mutualism: Host provides shelter and food for the organism; both benefit.
- Parasitism: Host provides shelter and food; the parasite benefits, but the host may be harmed (e.g., a tapeworm living at the expense of its human host).

disease are classified into five types: bacteria, viruses and rickettsiae, fungi, protozoa, and helminths.

Exogenous pathogens are transmitted from outside the body to the host by various mechanisms. Exogenous organisms exist in contaminated air, food, water, and body fluids and on objects contaminated by these substances. *Endogenous pathogens* are found within the human body. Microorganisms (normal flora) exist on the skin and in the nose, mouth, gastrointestinal tract, and urogenital tract. For example, *Staphylococcus epidermidis* inhabits the skin, and *Escherichia coli* are found in the intestines. These microorganisms are beneficial and play an important role in the body's defenses. They help prevent virulent pathogens from colonizing by maintaining an acidic pH environment to discourage pathogen attachment, taking up epithelial space to prevent growth of pathogens, and stimulating the immune system. However, situations may arise in which these normally benign organisms become virulent and harmful to the host.

Chain of Infection

For a pathogen to maintain its infectious state, it must be transmitted to another host. Certain factors and conditions must be present for a disease (infection) to begin. These components and their relations are often referred to as a chain of infection. The major variables in the chain of infection include the agent (organism), reservoir

TRANSMISSION OF PATHOGENS
Direct

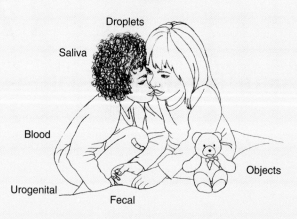

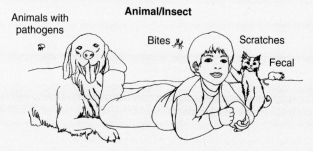

Animal/Insect

(environment in which the agent exists and multiplies), portal of exit (route by which the agent leaves the host), transmission mode, portal of entry (route by which the agent enters the new host), and host susceptibility (internal and external environmental factors that increase or decrease the likelihood the host will develop disease). Changes in any one variable result in a change in the presence, intensity, and frequency of the entire infectious-disease process.

Transmission of Pathogens

Infection transmission occurs through several modes, or routes. For example, pathogens from the respiratory tract are shed through sneezing, coughing, and talking. If the pathogens survive in the air, they can infect others who inhale them (airborne route). Because this mode of transmission is relatively uncontrollable, infections can easily be spread in crowded conditions.

Pathogens may also be shed through fecal matter. When personal hygiene is poor and hand hygiene is not routinely practiced, pathogens have ample opportunities to enter through the mouth (fecal-oral transmission). Unclean hands can also contaminate food, which is then ingested.

Sexual activity involving direct mucosal contact is the most common means of transmission of sexually transmissible infections (STIs) (direct contact transmission). If the mother's birth canal is infected, newborn infants can be infected by direct contact during birth. Saliva is another avenue of transmission, as is direct contact with infected skin. Pathogens can also be present in breast milk and can infect a nursing infant.

A tick, mosquito, mite, or animal can inject pathogens into the skin and blood of the host. Organisms carried in this way are considered to be vector borne. For example, a certain species of mosquito carries the malaria parasite; likewise, certain bats carry the rabies microorganism.

Contamination by blood of an infected host can occur through transfusions, blood products, and the use of contaminated needles

(direct inoculation). A pregnant woman can transmit such pathogens through the placenta. Other modes of transmission also exist, such as through spores found in soil (e.g., tetanus).

Epidemiologic Investigations

Epidemiology is the study of the distribution of health and illness within a population and the factors that determine the population's health status. Nurses may not realize that they are contributing to this process when they gather patient history information as part of the nursing-assessment process. The data nurses collect help the entire health care team identify, treat, and prevent disease processes as well as promote health. Moreover, the specific steps of the epidemiologic process mirror the steps in the nursing process and include defining the condition; determining the condition's natural history; identifying critical control points; and designing, implementing, and evaluating control strategies.

INFECTION AND HOST DEFENSES

The first stage of infection begins with colonization of the host by the pathogen. Microorganisms invade either by adhering to tissues or by invading cells. Initially, replication of the pathogen does not cause tissue damage, and colonization can occur without development of a clinical infection. As the host "recognizes" the invasion, the defense system—the immune response—is activated. The two components of the immune response are the innate, nonspecific immune response and the adaptive, specific immune response: cell mediated and humoral (see Chapter 18).

The first lines of defense in the innate immune system are the skin and intact mucous membranes. The skin serves as a barrier, preventing colonization of most pathogens. The acid secreted in sweat and by sebaceous glands inhibits pathogenic invasion. Smooth muscle contraction and ciliary actions, such as those seen in bladder and bowel emptying and coughing and sneezing, remove pathogens mechanically. Physical and chemical barriers are provided through mucus production by goblet cells in mucous membranes. Nevertheless, the innate system may be unable to prevent the invasion. *Phagocytosis,* the process by which phagocytes digest and thereby destroy foreign microorganisms, can be overwhelmed. Large numbers of pathogens or their toxins can inhibit phagocytosis. When this process occurs, the adaptive immune system is activated. This system "recognizes" and responds to pathogens by destroying them. The adaptive immune system "imprints" on these pathogens so that if the body encounters them again, the response will be rapid and specific.

IMMUNITY

Immunity is the body's resistance to the effects of harmful agents. It occurs as an antigen-antibody reaction that takes place whenever a foreign agent or its toxins enter the bloodstream. Immunity can be either active or passive. Active immunity occurs as a result of immune system stimulation from exposure to antigens, either naturally or through vaccine administration. Passive immunity is a form of infection protection acquired through the administration of serum containing antibodies.

Some childhood diseases have been significantly reduced and some nearly eliminated through the administration of vaccines producing active or passive immunity. A variety of preparations of disease-specific vaccines and preparations can artificially accomplish active or passive immunity (see Chapter 4).

Infectious diseases are a major reason health care is sought for infants and children. Although most infections are not life threatening, fatal complications can develop, especially in infants or children with an immature or compromised immune system. Moreover, a child's illness directly affects the family and caregivers. Absence from work for the parent of a sick child can jeopardize job security, and the accompanying missed income can be devastating for both single- and two-income families.

Nurses play a major role in preventing pediatric infectious diseases and decreasing the incidence of disability and death in both community and hospital settings. Regardless of their clinical setting, nurses must be able to confidently recognize the sometimes subtle signs and symptoms of infectious diseases in children and initiate appropriate treatment and nursing care. Nurses must also provide education about accessing appropriate community resources and limiting exposure of other children and community members.

In addition, because of the growing number of uninsured and underserved children in the United States, nurses may be the first and sometimes only health care professionals to evaluate and treat children in community-based settings. School nurses are frequently required to notify parents and caregivers when their children have been exposed to infectious diseases. Figure 17-1 illustrates an example of a notification letter from a school nurse written to inform parents and caregivers about an exposure to erythema infectiosum (fifth disease). Regardless of the particular type of infection, underlying principles of nursing care are similar.

VIRAL EXANTHEMS

Viruses are small parasitic organisms with unique characteristics that cause them to be quite different from other organisms. They contain only one type of nucleic acid—either deoxyribonucleic acid (DNA) or ribonucleic acid (RNA). This prevents them from reproducing on their own. Instead, a host cell is needed to allow the virus to replicate.

The replication process begins with the virus first attaching itself to a host cell. After the initial attachment, a virus must invade the interior of the cell. Replication of the virus's nucleic material begins after the envelope and capsule (capsid) are shed and the nucleic material of the virus is released into the cell; the host cell then assists in the formation of the necessary nucleic material. New capsules are then formed and released into the host's cells. The infected host cell can respond to the viral invasion by cell death (lysis) and destruction, or the infected cells can remain alive and continue to function while new viral particles are slowly released. This slow release occurs in an asymptomatic person who is a carrier of the virus. Some viruses are selective about the cells to which they attach. For example, the human immunodeficiency virus (HIV) prefers to attach to the T cell (see Chapter 18).

A virus can also invade a host and remain dormant until a trigger stimulates the virus to begin replicating. Many triggering factors are not fully understood. However, some triggers have been identified. An example of this triggering effect is the effect of stress in herpes simplex (a viral disease), resulting in the formation of cold sores.

Nursing Considerations for the Child with a Viral Exanthem Infection

An exanthem is an eruption or rash on the skin. Several childhood infectious diseases are characterized by rashes with distinctive characteristics. Nurses need to be aware that rashes have more than one characteristic and should obtain a detailed history of the characteristics of the rash, including its onset, initial location, and progression, as well

as any associated physical signs or symptoms. Specific characteristics of the rash should be documented, including color, elevation, pattern or shape, size (in centimeters), location and distribution on the body, and any drainage. Vital signs, including temperature, should be taken and recorded. Also record the child's general state of health, recent exposures to illnesses, and any prescribed or over-the-counter medications and treatments taken and their results. Perform a general physical assessment to look for associated signs of inflammation, which may include abnormal enlargement or tenderness of the spleen, liver, or lymph nodes.

Children with typical uncomplicated viral exanthems are usually cared for at home. Hospitalization is indicated when complications occur or the exanthema is known to be associated with severe disease. Nurses who care for hospitalized children with an infectious disease should not also care for high-risk (immunosuppressed) children to prevent any possible cross transmission by the nurse.

Whether the child is cared for in the hospital or at home, any specific isolation measures will be determined by the child's specific infectious disease process (see Patient-Centered Teaching: How to Care for the Child with a Viral Exanthem box on p. 359).

Rubeola (Measles)

Causative agent:	RNA virus
Incubation period:	8 to 12 days from exposure to onset of symptoms
Infectious period:	Ranges from 3 to 5 days before the appearance of the rash to 4 days after appearance of the rash
Transmission:	Transmitted between individuals by direct contact with infectious droplets or less frequently by airborne spread
Immunity:	Natural disease or live attenuated vaccine
Season:	Late winter and spring

Manifestations

The measles virus enters the body and slowly spreads. Respiratory symptoms appear after an average of 10 days. Typically, children have a prodrome period with fever that rises gradually and the "three Cs" (coryza [profuse runny nose], cough, and conjunctivitis) that lasts between 1 and 4 days. Children are usually quite ill during this time. Koplik spots appear approximately 2 days before the appearance of the rash (Figure 17-2). Koplik spots are small, blue-white spots with a red base that cluster near the molars on the buccal mucosa. These spots last approximately 3 days, after which they slough off. As prodromal symptoms reach a peak, the exanthem appears and is characterized by a deep-red, macular rash that usually begins on the face and neck and spreads down the trunk and extremities to the feet. The rash blanches easily with pressure and will gradually turn a brownish color. The duration of the rash is approximately 6 to 7 days.

A partially immune child, such as an infant younger than 9 months who has passively acquired maternal antibodies or a child given immune gamma globulin, may contract modified measles. The prodromal period is shorter and the symptoms are minimal, with few to no Koplik spots. The rash progression follows the pattern of regular measles.

Complications

Although considered a relatively rare disease since vaccine became available, approximately 10 million cases of measles occur each year, and 197,000 children die each year from the measles (Centers for Disease Control and Prevention [CDC], 2009b). Because of respiratory

Text continued on p. 359

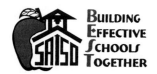

San Angelo Independent School District
HEALTH SERVICES
Ph: (915) 657-4049 Fax: (915) 657-4087

Susan Schultz, RN, BSN
Coordinator of Health Services

Dear Parent/Guardian:

Several students in our school district have been diagnosed as having Fifth Disease (Erythema Infectiosum). This is caused by a virus and can cause outbreaks, particularly among children, because the individual is infectious before symptoms appear. Symptoms are mild and it is usually recognized by a rash appearing on the cheeks resembling a "slapped cheek." There may also be a lacy rash on the trunk, arms and legs. Sometimes these characteristics are preceded by a low-grade fever, which lasts 5-7 days. No treatment is necessary. Children are no longer contagious and do not need to be excluded from school once the rash occurs.

Fifth Disease is generally a very mild disease. Please contact your primary care provider immediately if:

1. The rash becomes itchy

2. Your child develops a fever over 101°

3. You feel your child is getting worse

4. You have other concerns or questions

If you, a family member or a friend are pregnant and are exposed to a child with Fifth Disease, contact your obstetrician.

Please contact the nurse at your school if you have further questions or concerns.

Sincerely,

Susan Schultz, RN

Susan Schultz, RN, BSN
Coordinator, Health Services

Dr. Joe E. Gonzales, Superintendent • 1621 University • San Angelo, TX 76904

FIG 17-1 Sample notification letter from school nurse informing parents and caregivers about an exposure to an infectious disease. (Courtesy Susan Schultz, RN, BSN, Coordinator, Health Services, San Angelo Independent School District, San Angelo, TX.)

◎ NURSING CARE PLAN

The Child with an Infection in the Community Setting

Focused Assessment

Obtain a complete history, focusing on the following:

- Child's usual state of health
- Any signs or symptoms of developing disease (prodrome)
- Vital signs, especially body temperature
- Description of any skin lesions or rashes, including color, pattern, or shape; size, location, and distribution on the body; presence of any drainage or erythema; and any changes since initial eruption
- Any other family members, classmates, or playmates (friends) showing signs or symptoms
- Any other associated signs or symptoms (arthralgia, malaise, pain, vomiting, headaches)
- History of exposure to illness or environmental vectors
- Medications or treatments tried and their effects

Planning

Nursing Diagnosis

Risk for Infection (cross contamination of self or others) related to insufficient knowledge of how to avoid the spread of infectious disease.

Expected Outcomes

The child's contacts will remain free from symptoms of infection.

The child will demonstrate absence of infection, as evidenced by vital signs within normal parameters, resolving lesions with no evidence of complications, and age-appropriate behavior.

The family and child (if age-appropriate) will:

- State symptoms of infectious disease and symptoms of secondary bacterial infections and appropriate disease-containment procedures.
- Verbalize understanding of written health promotion information, including contact information for local community agencies and resources.

Intervention/*Rationale*

1. Teach the family and child (if old enough) the symptoms of secondary bacterial infections and complications of infectious diseases that should be promptly reported to their primary medical caregiver (e.g., redness, warmth, swelling, tenderness or pain, new onset of drainage or change in drainage from wound, increase in body temperature, malaise, abdominal pain, vomiting or diarrhea, enlarged glands, changes in skin lesions including sores or wounds that do not heal). Provide the phone number or numbers to call if complications occur.

   Promptly recognizing and reporting signs and symptoms of secondary bacterial infections can decrease complications.

2. Teach the family and/or child about the underlying concepts of infection transmission (e.g., airborne, fecal-oral, direct contact), including how and to whom the infection should be reported.

   Understanding promotes cooperation with infectious disease containment issues, policies, and procedures (e.g., child with chickenpox may not return to daycare or school until the sixth day after onset of rash or sooner if all lesions have dried and crusted).

3. Emphasize the importance of and encourage the child and family to complete the full course of any prescribed medication unless experiencing adverse side effects.

   Not taking a complete course of antibiotics may result in incomplete resolution of disease and contributes to antibiotic resistance.

4. Model and teach the child and family infection prevention behaviors, such as frequent and meticulous hand hygiene, disposal of used dressings to prevent spread of infectious disease to others, proper disposal of tissues, and covering the mouth when coughing or sneezing. (Follow Standard Precautions guidelines during any contact with blood, mucous membranes, nonintact skin, or any body substance except sweat; use goggles, gloves, and gowns when appropriate; help the family access these if needed.)

   Demonstration and active participation are more effective teaching strategies than verbal instruction alone (parents will retain better if they "use" the instruction). Nurses must assume all people are carrying bloodborne pathogens such as HIV or hepatitis B or C virus (HBV, HCV). Standard Precautions apply to everyone. Alcohol-based gels may provide as effective hand hygiene as washing with soap and water in most instances.*

5. Review the child's plan of care, including provision of rest, proper nutrition, fever control, recognition of the development of secondary infection, and when the child can resume normal activities. Provide written information about any instructions for treatment, medication administration, and any scheduled follow-up visits with the child's primary health care provider.

   Providing written information assists with adherence to the plan after discharge.

6. Provide health promotion information and education (e.g., routine immunization schedule) for the family and child.

   Refer the family and child to local community agencies (health departments, clinics) as appropriate. Maintenance of an ongoing relationship with a primary care provider provides continuity of care and methods for access to care for the well and sick child as needed.

Evaluation

Have any of the child's contacts contracted the disease?

Is the child free from infection, afebrile, and exhibiting age-appropriate behavior?

Have the parents and/or child verbalized an understanding of the infectious process and disease-containment procedures?

Are the family and/or child cooperative with written contact information and accessing follow-up and preventive health care and appropriate community resources?

Can the child and family members describe and demonstrate proper hand hygiene?

Planning

Nursing Diagnosis

Ineffective Health Maintenance related to insufficient knowledge about how to obtain needed information about infectious disease and its management.

Expected Outcomes

The child and family will follow an agreed-upon infection control plan.

The child and family will meet goals for health maintenance.

Intervention/*Rationale*

1. Teach the family or child skin and wound assessment and ways to monitor for signs and symptoms of infection, complications, and healing.

   Early assessment and intervention help prevent serious problems from developing (e.g., sexually transmissible infections [STIs] in the adolescent girl can result in sterility). Providing information and encouragement promotes understanding and adherence to the treatment plan, thus preventing secondary infection or adverse consequences from infection.

2. Teach adolescents health-promoting and health-seeking behaviors to reduce the risk of contracting an STI; this includes a description of the direct contact transmission mode and recognition of complications.

   Providing information and establishing a nonjudgmental environment encourage future health-seeking behaviors. Long-term complications (e.g., sterility, chronic abdominal pain from untreated STIs) can be avoided with early detection, treatment, and appropriate follow-up care.

Continued

◎ NURSING CARE PLAN

The Child with an Infection in the Community Setting—cont'd

Intervention/*Rationale*—cont'd

3. Screen for STIs as appropriate (e.g., a prepubescent girl with signs and symptoms of an STI). For prevention, teach children that it is not all right for someone to look at or touch their private parts.
   Signs and symptoms of problems with the genital area (itching, rash, vaginal or penile discharge) should always be explored by the nurse with a complete history of symptoms to rule out sexual abuse, especially in prepubescent children. Sexual abuse of a child is a reportable offense and must be ruled out.

4. Provide health promotion information and education (e.g., Papanicolaou [Pap] smears for sexually active adolescents). Refer the family or child to local community agencies (e.g., health departments, clinics) as appropriate.
   Maintenance of an ongoing relationship with a primary care provider provides continuity of care and methods for access to care for health promotion and disease prevention.

Evaluation

Do the child and family follow the agreed-on infection control plan? Are they able to meet goals for health maintenance?

Planning
Nursing Diagnosis

Risk for Ineffective Thermoregulation related to infection.

Expected Outcome

The child will be afebrile and exhibit age-appropriate behavior.

Intervention/*Rationale*

1. Teach the family and/or child normal temperature parameters (e.g., What is a fever?) and temperature-monitoring techniques (see age-appropriate guidelines in Chapter 13).
   Consistently monitoring and promptly recognizing and reporting fever higher than normal parameters allow for early intervention and can decrease the potential for disability or death.

2. Teach the family the signs and symptoms of hyperthermia and the complications that should be promptly reported to their primary medical caregiver (e.g., visual disturbances, headache, nausea, vomiting, muscle flaccidity, absence of sweating, delirium, coma). Provide the phone number(s) to call if complications occur.
   Understanding promotes cooperation and adherence to the child's treatment and care plan.

3. Teach the family about specific comfort measures (cool environment, light clothing) and medication administration (antipyretics) for fever. Teach parents the appropriate use of antipyretics (see Chapter 13). Use acetaminophen or ibuprofen as directed for fever control. Avoid aspirin products because of the possibility of developing Reye syndrome (see Chapter 28). Check all over-the-counter medicines to be sure they do not contain aspirin or salicylate. Provide written information that explains the various preparations available (drops, suspension, chewable tablets, suppositories) and the appropriate dose and administration intervals for their child. For example: The dosage of acetaminophen for a 2- to 3-year-old child is 160 mg. Any one of the following can be given every 4 to 6 hours as needed for fever or discomfort:
   Concentrated drops (80 mg in 0.8 mL) = 0.8 mL + 0.8 mL = 1.6 mL
   Suspension liquid (80 mg in ½ tsp) = 1 tsp
   Children's chewable (80 mg each) = 2 tablets
   Suppository (80 mg each) = 2 suppositories
   Appropriate teaching promotes cooperation and adherence to the child's treatment and care plan and can also prevent innocent administration of readily available, potentially lethal over-the-counter medication to a child with a viral illness. Providing information and creating awareness of self-care

steps the family or adolescent can take to maintain or regain health promotes positive health-seeking behaviors. Because of the many different formulations of both of these over-the-counter medications, parents are frequently confused and inadvertently give the wrong dose, sometimes resulting in overdosing or underdosing and inadequate fever control.

4. Teach the importance of and specific techniques for maintaining adequate hydration (monitoring the child's intake and output, frequently offering cool liquids, ice pops).
   Maintaining adequate hydration will help maintain a normal body temperature. An elevated temperature is associated with increased metabolism and fluid use.

5. Provide written health promotion information and education about fever control and when to access the health care system.
   Maintenance of an ongoing relationship with primary care provider provides continuity of care and methods for access to care for well- and sick-child care as needed.

Evaluation

Has the child maintained a body temperature within normal parameters? Is the child's behavior within normal parameters for age?

Planning
Nursing Diagnosis

Fatigue related to discomfort associated with the infectious disease.

Expected Outcomes

The child will experience an increase in comfort level and energy, as evidenced by verbalization of decreased discomfort, a relaxed body posture, ability to rest appropriately, decreased crying and irritability, and an interest in age-appropriate activities.

Intervention/*Rationale*

1. Teach and provide written information for comfort measures (cool environment; lightweight, cool clothing); treatments (monitoring the child's temperature); or medication administration (antipruritics, antipyretics).
   Appropriate teaching promotes cooperation and adherence to the child's treatment and care plan. Maintaining adequate hydration will help maintain a normal body temperature. An elevated temperature is associated with increased metabolism and fluid use.

2. Encourage energy conservation during the healing process of an infectious disease; children usually pace their own activity levels when ill. Provide age- and energy-appropriate activities depending on the child's level of wellness.
   Energy conservation promotes the healing process and provides comfort to children with discomfort, pain, or fever. Using nonpharmacologic techniques, such as distraction, provides pain relief.

3. Teach the child's family personal hygiene principles to promote the healing process and maintain health after the infectious disease process. Keep the child's skin clean, and change linens and clothing frequently. Wash clothes and linen in mild detergent, and double rinse.
   Clean clothing helps prevent the spread of secondary infections. Double rinsing reduces the potential irritants in the clothing, thereby minimizing irritation in children with pruritus related to skin manifestations.

Evaluation

Has the child experienced relief from discomfort by demonstrating a relaxed body posture, an interest in age-appropriate play, and verbalization of an increased comfort level?

◎ NURSING CARE PLAN

The Child with an Infection in the Community Setting—cont'd

Planning

Nursing Diagnosis

Social Isolation related to the confinement for the duration of the communicable disease.

Expected Outcomes

The child and family will describe the reasons for isolation and incorporate the resulting restrictions into their home management.

The child will participate in age-appropriate activities within the restrictions imposed.

The family will contact community agencies for assistance if appropriate.

Intervention/Rationale

1. Encourage the family and child to maintain contact with friends and family by telephone, mail, or e-mail while the child is isolated.
   Maintaining contact with family and friends helps the family adjust to activity limitations, reduces boredom, and provides emotional support.

2. Provide written information to family about age- and energy-appropriate activities.
   Providing age-appropriate activities prevents boredom and promotes normal growth and development.

3. Provide information about community resources for respite and/or sick child care.
   Providing resources for family provides caregiver relief and could result in the family's primary wage earner (especially in single-parent families) returning to work with less loss of income and decrease in the financial burden on the family.

Evaluation

Can the child and family describe the reasons for the isolation, and have they incorporated the appropriate restrictions?

Is the child engaging in age-appropriate activities?

Is the family able to maintain contact with family and friends?

Have support systems been mobilized, both within the family and in the community?

*Smith, B. (2010). Infection control. *Advance for Nurses.* Merion Publications CEU. Retrieved from http://nursing.advance.web.com/Editorial/Content/PrintFriendly.aspx.

PATIENT-CENTERED TEACHING

How to Care for the Child with a Viral Exanthem

- For elevated temperature, the child's activity should be restricted to age-appropriate, quiet activities and bed rest. As the fever decreases, the activity level can be gradually increased to a normal level.
- Generally, fever can be controlled with acetaminophen or ibuprofen (no aspirin products because of the possible risk of developing Reye syndrome), sponge baths, decreased clothing, decreased environmental temperature, and increased fluid intake. Bed linens may need to be changed frequently during periods of high fever. Over-the-counter antipyretic acetaminophen comes in several different formulations. Read the label carefully and ask your primary health care provider if you have any questions regarding medication administration. Seizure precautions should be taken if your child has had a seizure previously.
- The amount of skin irritation and discomfort will vary. Lukewarm baths with colloid preparations (Aveeno), oatmeal, or baking soda (½ cup in tub of water) may help relieve itching. Soothing lotions (Lubriderm, Curel, Moisturel) may also provide comfort. Avoid the use of topical corticosteroids unless ordered by your primary health care provider. Use superfatted soaps for sensitive skin (Dove, Basis, Neutrogena, Aveeno). Fingernails should be short. If the child continues to scratch, cotton mittens or socks can be applied to the child's hands. Integrity of the skin must be maintained to prevent any secondary infections. If secondary infections occur, antibiotic therapy may be necessary.

- Administer antihistamines or antipruritics as prescribed.
- Dress your child in lightweight clothing that is not irritating. Avoid wool and scratchy materials.
- Coughing can be managed with cool humidification of the room and antitussives.
- For arthralgia, antiinflammatory medications may be used. Involvement of weight-bearing joints may warrant bed rest.
- Some viral exanthems cause photophobia. In such cases, keeping the room dimly lit or providing sunglasses for the child may be helpful. If the child has conjunctivitis, secretions or crusts should be removed with tepid water and a clean cloth to prevent contamination.
- Fluid intake is important for successfully managing febrile stages of the disease. Encourage your child to drink cool liquids frequently. If the child's mucous membranes are involved, soft, bland foods may be beneficial.
- As your child progresses through the stages of illness, diversional activities will be necessary during the period of isolation. Choose activities that your child likes and can participate in without becoming unduly tired.
- Call your physician if your child develops any severe symptoms, such as high fever, dry mouth, decreased urine output, persistent cough, seizures, or nonresponsiveness.

involvement, secondary infections such as otitis media, bronchopneumonia, and laryngotracheobronchitis (croup) can occur, especially in infants and younger children. Rarely, central nervous system (CNS) complications such as encephalitis develop during the prodromal period and can lead to long-term sequelae such as brain death. Measles can cause premature birth and miscarriage in pregnant women (Cherry, 2009c).

Therapeutic Management

The treatment of measles is symptomatic, whether the child is hospitalized or remains at home. If hospitalized, the child will require Airborne Isolation Precautions. During the febrile period, the child should be restricted to quiet activities and bed rest. Fluids are encouraged, and humidification and antitussives are used to relieve the cough (Cherry, 2009c).

First day   Third day

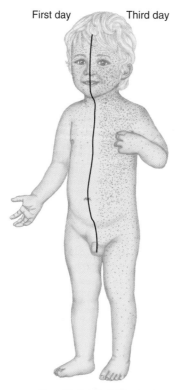

- Preceded by Koplik spots on buccal mucosa
- Begins behind ears, at hairline, and on upper neck and spreads downward toward feet
- Red, maculopapular rash that gradually turns brownish
- Duration: 6 to 7 days

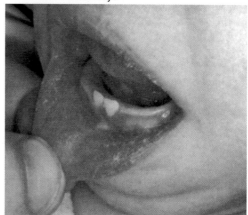

Measles Rash Distribution

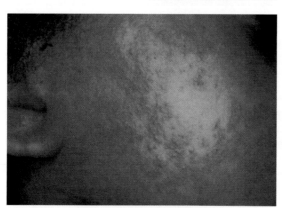

Measles Rash, Dark Skin

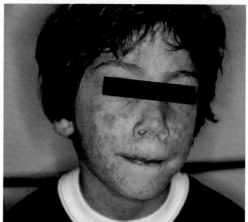

Measles Rash, Light Skin

FIG 17-2 Rubeola (measles) lesions and rash distribution. (Reprinted from Fegin, R., & Cherry, J. [Eds.]. [2009]. *Textbook of pediatric infectious diseases* [6th ed.]. Philadelphia: Saunders; from Paller, S. A. [2012]. *Hurwitz clinical pediatric dermatology: A textbook of skin disorders of childhood and adolescence* [4th ed.]. Philadelphia: Saunders.)

Low levels of vitamin A are associated with many measles cases and an increase in measles severity. Vitamin A deficiency is rare in the United States but is common in developing countries, causing the American Academy of Pediatrics to recommend vitamin A supplementation in certain more severe cases of measles (Cherry, 2009c).

Children can be protected against measles and other vaccine-preventable diseases by receiving all their routine immunizations during their routine well-child checkups. Two doses of measles, mumps, and rubella (MMR) vaccine are required to be fully protected.

The first MMR is recommended routinely at 1 year of age. The second dose of MMR is recommended at 4 to 6 years but may be administered during any visit if at least 4 weeks has elapsed since the first dose and both doses are administered beginning at or after 12 months of age. Children who have not previously received their second MMR dose should complete the schedule no later than their 11- to 12-year health maintenance visit (CDC, 2008a).

In 2005, the U.S. Food and Drug Administration (FDA) licensed a combination measles-mumps-rubella-varicella vaccine. Recent studies reveal that there is a very slight increased risk of fever and febrile seizures 7 to 10 days after vaccination in children ages 12 to 24 months compared to the separate MMR and varicella vaccines. Nurses should educate parents about the risk before vaccination (Klein, Fireman, Yih et al., 2010).

Rubella (German Measles, 3-Day Measles)

Causative agent: RNA virus
Incubation period: 14 to 21 days
Infectious period: Ranges from 7 days before onset of symptoms to 14 days after appearance of the rash
Transmission: Airborne particles or direct contact with infectious droplets, transplacental transmission; small number of infants with congenital rubella continue to shed the virus for months after birth
Immunity: Natural disease or live attenuated vaccine
Season: Late winter and early spring

Manifestations

Rubella is usually a mild disease for children and adults. The virus enters the host, producing a rash after approximately 14 to 16 days. Young children are often asymptomatic until the appearance of the rash. Older children may report profuse nasal drainage, diarrhea, malaise, sore throat, headache, low-grade fever, polyarthritis, eye pain, aches, chills, anorexia, and nausea. Children of all ages usually have impressive posterior cervical, posterior auricular, and occipital lymphadenopathy.

The rash manifests as a pinkish rose maculopapular exanthem that begins on the face, scalp, and neck (Figure 17-3). It spreads downward to include the entire body within 1 to 3 days. As the rash spreads to the trunk, the rash on the face begins to fade. Petechiae (spots), which are red or purple color and pinpoint in size, may occur on the soft palate. Their appearance is sometimes referred to as Forschheimer's sign.

Complications

The availability of rubella vaccine has effectively eliminated rubella in the United States (CDC, 2010d). Rubella has relatively few complications. The most common are arthritis and arthralgia, which occur more often in adult women than in children or adolescents. Mild thrombocytopenia may also occur but is usually self-limiting and of short duration. A rare complication is encephalitis, which is usually less severe than measles-related encephalitis.

The importance of recognizing and respecting this viral illness is not the morbidity of the disease itself but rather the consequences that can occur to a fetus during maternal infection. The most devastating form of rubella is congenital rubella that occurs after maternal infection, usually during the first 12 weeks of pregnancy. One of the most common manifestations of congenital rubella is intrauterine growth retardation. These infants typically weigh less than 2500 g and continue to have failure to thrive in infancy. Mortality is highest during the first year. Common causes of death include pneumonia, heart defects, encephalitis, and immune deficiency (Cherry, 2009g).

Therapeutic Management

Treatment is generally supportive and symptomatic, with the disease being self-limiting. Recommendation for exclusion of affected children from school or child care is 7 days after the rash begins. Infants with

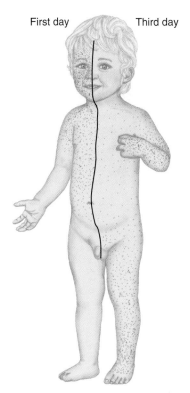

First day   Third day

German Measles Rash Distribution

- Begins on face, neck, and scalp and spreads downward to entire body; fades on face as it spreads to trunk
- Pinkish, maculopapular rash
- Reddish, pinpoint petechiae may occur on soft palate (Forschheimer's sign)

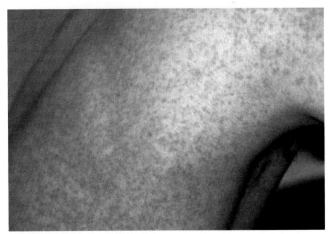

FIG 17-3 Rubella (German measles) lesions and rash distribution. (From Paller, S. A. [2012]. *Hurwitz clinical pediatric dermatology: A textbook of skin disorders of childhood and adolescence* [4th ed.]. Philadelphia: Saunders.)

congenital rubella are presumed contagious until age 1 year or nasopharyngeal and urine cultures for the rubella virus are repeatedly negative. Primary prevention of rubella can be accomplished through administration of the rubella vaccine in combination with measles and mumps vaccine (MMR), as previously discussed.

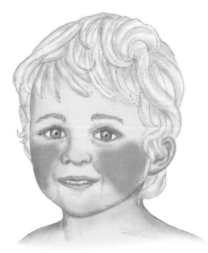

Erythema Infectiosum: "Slapped Cheek" Appearance

- Presents with fiery-red, edematous rash on cheeks—"slapped cheek" appearance
- Followed in 1-4 days by erythematous, maculo-papular, lacy rash on trunk and extremities

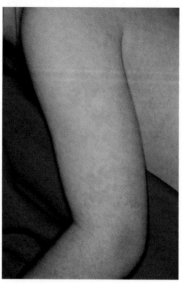

FIG 17-4 Erythema infectiosum lesions and rash distribution. (From Paller, S. A. [2012]. *Hurwitz clinical pediatric dermatology: A textbook of skin disorders of childhood and adolescence* [4th ed.]. Philadelphia: Saunders.)

⚡ SAFETY ALERT

Congenital Rubella

The rubella virus can cross the placenta and infect the fetus, causing fetal death or abnormalities.

Erythema Infectiosum (Fifth Disease, Parvovirus B19)

Causative agent: Parvovirus B19
Incubation period: 4 to 14 days but can be up to 21 days
Infectious period: Shedding of virus occurs between days 5 and 12 of the infection; usually from the prodromal period until the rash appears
Transmission: Airborne particles, respiratory droplets, blood, blood products, transplacental transmission
Immunity: Natural disease is thought to provide antibodies for immunity
Season: Winter and spring

This disease is most common in children ages 5 to 14 years but may also occur in adults.

Manifestations

Fifth disease is a relatively mild systemic disease. Typically the child may appear well but has an intense, fiery red, edematous rash on the cheeks, which gives a "slapped cheek" appearance (Figure 17-4), or a history of a rash that "comes and goes." Before the appearance of the rash, many children are asymptomatic or have nonspecific symptoms such as headache, runny nose, malaise, and mild fever. Approximately 1 to 4 days after the facial rash appears, an erythematous, maculopapular rash appears on the trunk and extremities. The rash fades with a central clearing area, resulting in a lacy appearance. The rash may last 2 to 39 days and reappear when aggravated by environmental factors, such as heat, exercise, warm baths, rubbing of the skin, and stress.

Complications

Because the disease is mild, complications are not usually reported, especially in children. Patients with sickle cell disease or beta-thalassemia are at risk for anemia and aplastic crisis. Patients with a poor immune system are also at risk for anemia. Because pregnant women are at risk for intrauterine infection, the nurse should obtain a careful history, with an emphasis on identifying any pregnant family members, teachers, or friends to prevent intrauterine infection and death. Many school districts notify pregnant staff if they have been exposed to a child with fifth disease and recommend that they contact their health care provider. Parvovirus B19 occurs in approximately 1 in 400 pregnancies. There is a 15% increase in the risk of miscarriage if infected in the first 20 weeks of pregnancy (Duncan, 2008).

Therapeutic Management

The disease is generally benign and self-limiting. Treatment is symptomatic and supportive.

Roseola Infantum (Exanthem Subitum)

Causative agent: Human herpesvirus 6 (HHV-6)
Incubation period: Unknown but estimated to be 9 to 10 days
Infectious period: Unknown but thought to extend from the febrile stage to the time the rash first appears
Transmission: Most likely by contact with secretions (saliva, cerebrospinal fluid [CSF]) of asymptomatic close contacts
Season: Throughout the year without a distinctive seasonal pattern

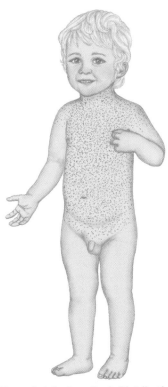

- Rash appears several hours to 2 days after fever subsides
- Erythematous maculopapular or macular rash may be surrounded by whitish ring
- Blanches with pressure
- Predominantly on neck and trunk
- Usually persists for 24-48 hours

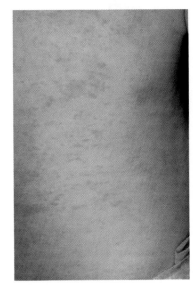

Roseola Infantum Rash Distribution

FIG 17-5 Roseola infantum lesions and rash distribution. (From Paller, S. A. [2012]. *Hurwitz clinical pediatric dermatology: A textbook of skin disorders of childhood and adolescence* [4th ed.]. Philadelphia: Saunders.)

Manifestations

HHV-6 appears to be the major causative agent, although other viruses have been implicated as well. Most clinical cases of roseola occur in children 6 to 18 months old. The child has a sudden high fever (103° to 106° F [39.4° to 41.1° C]), malaise, and irritability but may remain active and alert. An intermittent or constant fever may persist for 3 to 5 days. The child may also have a mild cough, runny nose, abdominal pain, headache, vomiting, and diarrhea (Shelov, 2010). After 3 to 5 days the fever subsides, and within several hours to 2 days a rash appears. The rash consists of rose-pink maculopapules or macules that blanch with pressure (Figure 17-5). The rash occurs predominantly on the neck and trunk and may be surrounded by a whitish ring. It normally persists for 24 to 48 hours before fading.

Complications

Complications associated with roseola are uncommon. Febrile seizures (see Chapter 28) may occur.

Therapeutic Management

Treatment is symptomatic. Family members should be taught about fever control and management.

Antipyretic medications, decreased clothing, cooler environmental temperatures, and increased fluid intake all assist with fever control. Temperature monitoring, medication administration (prescription and over-the-counter medications), and other comfort measures should be discussed. The nurse verifies that the child's family has access to a thermometer and knows how to use it. In addition, parents should be given information regarding the absolute avoidance of any form of aspirin (including over-the-counter medications containing salicylates) because of the potential risk of developing Reye syndrome (see Chapter 28). Anticipatory guidance should include alerting the parent to the possibility of febrile seizures and teaching about seizure precautions (especially if the child has a history of previous febrile seizures).

Parents' understanding of the care necessary for their child is important, particularly measures to control and prevent the spread of infection. Teach the parents how to recognize the signs and symptoms of complications so they can seek medical treatment when warranted. Providing parents with written instructions that they can refer to at home may prove helpful.

Enterovirus (Nonpolio) Infections (Coxsackieviruses, Group A and Group B), Echoviruses, and Enteroviruses

Causative agents:	RNA viruses including 23 group A coxsackieviruses (types A1 to A24, except type A23), six group B coxsackieviruses (types B1 to B6), 31 echoviruses (types 1 to 33, except types 10 and 28), and four enteroviruses (types 68 to 71)
Incubation period:	Usually 3 to 6 days
Infectious period:	Unknown, but fecal viral excretion and transmission can continue for several weeks after the onset of infection
Transmission:	Spread by fecal-oral and possibly by oral-oral (respiratory) routes
Season:	In temperate climates infections are most common in the summer and fall, but no seasonal pattern is evident in the tropics

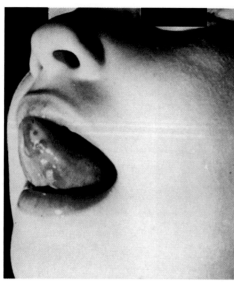

FIG 17-6 Coxsackievirus mouth lesions. (Reprinted from Fegin, R., & Cherry, J. [Eds.]. [2009]. *Textbook of pediatric infectious diseases* [6th ed.]. Philadelphia: Saunders.)

Manifestations

Common presentations in both infants and children include nonspecific febrile illnesses with a wide variety of respiratory, gastrointestinal, cardiac, neurologic, skin, oral, and eye signs and symptoms.

A frequently seen pattern of illness in young children is hand-foot-and-mouth disease, caused by coxsackievirus A16 or other enteroviruses. Inflammation and lesions in the mouth (Figure 17-6), on the palms of the hands, and on the soles of the feet are the hallmarks of this syndrome, along with mild fever; some children experience small lesions on the buttocks (Schmitt, 2010). Lesions become vesicular over the course of several days and usually resolve by 1 week. If lesions are particularly widespread in the oropharynx, the child may refuse to eat or drink; the potential for dehydration exists in very young children.

Complications

Although each of these groups of symptoms can be associated with different enteroviruses, complications can occur from specific strains. Young infants with a history of prematurity are at higher risks for complications and death. Serious complications such as myocarditis, hepatitis, and encephalitis are often the cause. Mortality rates are highest for coxsackievirus B and lowest for coxsackievirus A (Cherry, 2009b).

Therapeutic Management

Currently, no specific therapy exists for enteroviral infections, but clinical trials are evaluating the effectiveness of pleconaril for neonates with severe disease (Cherry, 2009b). However, enteric Contact Precautions are indicated for any affected hospitalized infant or child. Parents and caregivers should be given educational information regarding the importance of hand hygiene and personal hygiene, especially after diaper changes and trips to the bathroom.

Management of hand-foot-and-mouth disease is symptomatic. The parent can provide comfort and pain relief with acetaminophen and frequent administration of cool liquids. Milk-based ice cream

is especially palatable. Extensive oropharyngeal lesions that prevent adequate oral intake can be treated with a salt and water mouth rinse or a topical solution of equal parts lidocaine gel, diphenhydramine liquid, and a liquid antacid (mixed by prescription) either applied directly to lesions or used as a mouthwash.

Nursing Considerations

The nurse needs to obtain a detailed history of the onset of symptoms with a focused assessment on the particular body systems involved. Children with an enterovirus infection can be challenging because of the wide variety and degree of signs and symptoms. Supportive care is similar to that of any child with a viral exanthem. Parents and caregivers should be given educational information about disease transmission, school or daycare attendance policies, and any available community resources (sick-child care).

Varicella-Zoster Infections (Chickenpox, Shingles)

Causative agent:	Varicella-zoster virus
Incubation period:	10 to 21 days
Infectious period:	1 to 2 days before the onset of rash until all lesions are dried (crusted over), usually 5 to 7 days
Transmission:	Direct contact, droplet, airborne particles
Immunity:	Natural disease of varicella; same virus causes zoster, and child may contract zoster at a later time; varicella vaccine
Season:	Late winter through early spring

Primary infection with the varicella-zoster virus causes chickenpox. Prior to 1995, when the vaccine became available, chickenpox was one of the most common childhood diseases in children 5 to 9 years old. Approximately 4 million cases of varicella and 100 deaths occurred each year in the United States (Freed, 2009). Zoster (shingles), which is the reactivation of the latent varicella-zoster virus, occurs most frequently in the elderly population but can occur in children as well, especially adolescents and young adults. Generally varicella and zoster in children are not life threatening.

Manifestations

Varicella. During the 24 to 48 hours before the appearance of lesions, symptoms may include a slightly elevated body temperature, malaise, and anorexia. A rash generally first appears on the trunk and scalp (Figure 17-7), followed by the appearance of lesions, which quickly become teardrop vesicles with an erythematous base. The vesicles then become pustular, after which they begin to dry and develop a crust. The lesions appear in crops over the course of usually 3 to 4 days and can be seen to be in different stages of development. The number of lesions varies from child to child, but children in the household with secondary cases generally have more extensive rashes than does the child with the primary case. The lesions may appear on the mucous membranes in the mouth, genital area, and rectum. Second attacks are rare and are more common in immunocompromised children. Breakthrough attacks in immunized children are also rare, and the disease presentation is mild, with few lesions (Martin, Güris, Chaves et al., 2007).

Herpes Zoster (Shingles). During the primary infection with varicella, the varicella-zoster virus enters the sensory nerve ending and the dorsal root ganglion and establishes a latent infection. Activation of the infection causes herpes zoster (shingles). Zoster manifests with tenderness along the involved nerve and surrounding skin for approximately 2 weeks before the appearance of the lesions. If

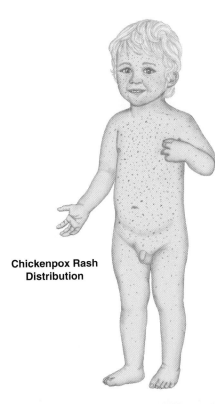

- Macular rash 24-48 hours after slight fever, malaise, anorexia
- Lesions appear in "crops," first on trunk and scalp, then moving sparsely to extremities; may appear in mucous membranes (mouth, genital area, rectum)
- Generally three successive eruptions over 3-4 days
- Lesions begin as a macular rash, develop into a red papular rash, then move quickly into tear-drop vesicles with erythematous base; vesicle becomes pustular and begins drying, and a crust develops
- Rash varies from child to child

**Chickenpox Rash
Distribution**

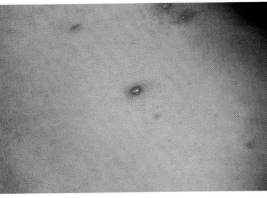

Shingles

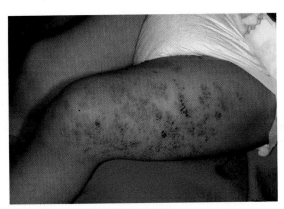

Chickenpox

FIG 17-7 Chickenpox and shingles lesions and rash distribution. (From Paller, S. A. [2012]. *Hurwitz clinical pediatric dermatology: A textbook of skin disorders of childhood and adolescence* [4th ed.]. Philadelphia: Saunders.)

pain is present, its intensity can range from an unpleasant, abnormal sensitivity to touch to burning, tingling, itching, sharp knifelike prickling, or even deep pain. Unilateral crops of lesions appear along the nerve. These lesions progress through the same stages as varicella. There may be enlargement and tenderness of the lymph nodes in the same region.

Risk factors for shingles are a history of chickenpox, age over 50 years, weakened immune system, stress or trauma, and being treated for cancer. Zoster is thought to be an infection of elderly people, but there are cases when children can get zoster. Most commonly, there was an undiagnosed case of varicella early in infancy or the infant was exposed in utero (Cherry, 2009h).

Complications

The most common complication of varicella-zoster virus infection is secondary bacterial infection of the skin lesions. Staphylococci and group A beta-hemolytic streptococci are the usual causative agents. CNS complications have been associated with mild to severe varicella infections. Encephalitis with ataxia, tremor, and nystagmus may occur in the first week. The prognosis is generally positive unless CNS involvement is severe—usually manifested by convulsions and coma. Children with these complications may have future CNS difficulties, including seizures, intellectual disability, or behavior disorders. If a patient is immunocompromised, varicella can be severe or even fatal (Cherry, 2009h).

Varicella pneumonia, a common complication in adults, rarely occurs in children. Reye syndrome has been known to occur after varicella infection (see Chapter 28), particularly if aspirin is given. Corneal involvement can occur if lesions involve the eye.

Complications of herpes zoster are rare but may involve the same difficulties with secondary infections that occur with varicella.

Parents should be given educational information regarding the absolute avoidance of any form of aspirin (including over-the-counter medications containing salicylates) because of the potential risk for developing Reye syndrome.

Therapeutic Management

Treatment is symptomatic and supportive for the healthy child. Frequent bathing in an oatmeal bath and use of antihistamines can relieve itching. Acetaminophen to control fever is the best option because aspirin must be avoided. Although oral acyclovir is not routinely recommended for healthy children with varicella, it can be considered for use in severe cases, people with chronic illnesses, those receiving long-term aspirin therapy, or children on short-term corticosteroid treatment. For immunocompromised children, acyclovir is given intravenously (IV) because the oral route is less reliable for these children (Cherry, 2009h). The decision to use these medications, along with the duration and route, is individually determined by the primary health care provider. Response to antiviral drugs is good provided that the treatment is started early in the illness, because antiviral drugs have a limited "window of opportunity" (Cherry, 2009h).

In the hospital setting, children with varicella or zoster infections should be placed in a private room with strict isolation (Airborne and Contact Transmission Precautions). The nurse assigned should not simultaneously care for immunocompromised clients to decrease the risk of varicella transmission.

Because of the effectiveness of the vaccine, varicella-zoster immune globulin is no longer being produced in the United States. Human varicella immune globulin is a new product from Canada that can be used with approval from local and central institutional review boards (Cherry, 2009h). The CDC recommends that varicella vaccine can be given to healthy, nonimmune children (1 year of age or older) immediately after exposure and before 3 to 5 days; in some cases this will reduce the severity of the disease.

Primary prevention of varicella includes screening and administering the vaccine at routine well-child visits (see Chapter 4). Varicella vaccine is recommended at any visit on or after the first birthday for healthy susceptible children without a reliable history of actual disease or immunization and without contraindications to receiving the vaccine. A booster dose is given between 4 and 6 years of age. Susceptible children 13 years or older should receive two doses of vaccine given at least 4 weeks apart (CDC, 2008a).

Nursing Considerations

Care of children with varicella in the community can be challenging, because the condition is very contagious. A single case can quickly spread to others who are not immune, so prevention is essential. The nurse needs to educate parents of children with varicella about skin care to prevent secondary bacterial infections and emphasize the importance of absolute avoidance of any form of aspirin (including over-the-counter medications containing aspirin).

In the hospital setting, all contaminated materials must be bagged and labeled before reprocessing. Hands should be washed after contact with the child and before contact with another patient. Hospitalized children who have been exposed to varicella should be kept in strict isolation for 8 to 21 days after the onset of rash in the infected individual. At birth, neonates with mothers who have active varicella infections should be placed in strict isolation. In addition, Airborne Precautions and Contact Precautions should be in effect for children with herpes zoster infections.

SAFETY ALERT

Varicella and the Immunocompromised Child

Immunocompromised children who contract varicella may have large hemorrhagic lesions. Primary varicella pneumonia is a frequent complication. Some children may develop an acute form of varicella with disseminated intravascular coagulation (DIC) that is fatal, often before antiviral therapy can be started.

OTHER VIRAL INFECTIONS

Mumps

Causative agent:	Paramyxovirus
Incubation period:	Usually 16 to 18 days but may extend to 25 days
Infectious period:	From 7 days before swelling to 9 days after onset
Transmission:	Airborne droplets, salivary secretions, possibly urine
Immunity:	Natural disease or live attenuated vaccine
Season:	Late winter and spring

Manifestations

Prodromal manifestations include fever, myalgia, headache, and malaise. The classic clinical sign of parotid glandular swelling (parotitis) often follows these, although a substantial number of individuals have no such swelling. When parotid swelling occurs, it may be accompanied by fever.

Complications

Mumps generally affects the salivary glands but can involve multiple organs. The most common complication is aseptic meningitis, with the virus identified in the CSF. Signs of CNS involvement include nuchal rigidity, lethargy, and vomiting. Children with these manifestations usually completely recover. A less common CNS complication is meningoencephalomyelitis manifested by fever, headache, nausea, vomiting, nuchal rigidity, and changes in sensorium. These complications are treated symptomatically and generally have an uneventful recovery period.

The potential complication of most concern to parents is orchitis (inflammation of a testis). Orchitis is a complication frequently seen in adolescent boys; however, sterility is uncommon. Rarely, mumps can cause ovarian or breast inflammation in postpubertal girls. Although infrequent, mumps can cause sensorineural hearing impairment.

Therapeutic Management

Uncomplicated mumps may require only symptomatic care. Droplet Precautions are indicated until 9 days after the onset of the parotid swelling. Parents should be given educational information regarding the absolute avoidance of any form of aspirin (including over-the-counter medications containing salicylates) because of the potential risk of developing Reye syndrome.

Orchitis requires bed rest, intermittent application of ice packs, emotional support, and diversional activities. CNS complications require neurologic evaluations and vital sign measurement as indicated by the child's condition when the complications require hospitalization.

Nursing Considerations

The nurse needs to obtain a history of the onset of symptoms, examine the child's ears and throat, and perform a neurologic assessment. The child's vital signs (including temperature), usual state of health, and characteristics of the lymph nodes in the neck should be documented. In boys, an examination of the testes should be included in the initial assessment.

Typically, children with mumps are not hospitalized unless they have complications. Therefore, good hand hygiene technique should be taught to the child, the family, and close contacts to prevent transmission. Hospitalized children are placed in isolation according to the facility's policies (usually Droplet Precautions).

Primary prevention of mumps can be accomplished through administration of the mumps vaccine in combination with measles and rubella vaccine (MMR), as previously discussed.

Cytomegalovirus (CMV)

Causative agent:	Human cytomegalovirus (CMV)
Incubation period:	Unknown, except for 3 to 12 weeks after blood transfusions and 4 weeks to 4 months after organ (tissue) transplantation
Transmission:	Saliva, urine, blood, semen, cervical secretions, breast milk, organ transplants
Immunity:	None, although CMV immune globulin, used only in seronegative transplant clients, has had moderate effectiveness
Season:	Can occur during any season

CMV infection is a common cause of congenital infection in infants and is a leading cause of hearing loss and intellectual disability in the United States. A child may become infected with the virus during the prenatal, perinatal, or postnatal period. Only infections in utero cause permanent infection. Approximately one third of women with primary CMV infections transmit CMV to the fetus. The prevalence in the United States is 1 in 150 live births (Stowell, Forlin-Passoni, & Cannon, 2010). Only 10% of infants with congenital CMV infection have symptoms evident at birth; some infants who appear asymptomatic at birth later manifest signs of CMV. Asymptomatic infants have a better prognosis, but 10% to 15% may still develop disabilities (Stowell et al., 2010). The most common disability is hearing loss (Stowell et al., 2010). Among children, CMV is the leading nongenetic cause of deafness. Signs and symptoms in the infant can include jaundice, lethargy, seizures, enlarged spleen and liver, petechial rash, respiratory distress, microcephaly, and intracerebral calcifications. The child can continue to shed the virus for up to 5 years.

During the postnatal period, the infant may acquire CMV from a maternal or nonmaternal source. The virus can be transmitted through the breast milk of an infected mother. Blood transfusions, which can be numerous in the premature infant, can also be a source of CMV infection. Children who are not infected congenitally or perinatally often acquire the virus during their toddler or preschool years. Because of sexual activity, the teen years may be another period of acquisition. Affected adolescents are generally asymptomatic but can have a mononucleosis-like syndrome with fever, hepatosplenomegaly, mild hepatitis, and absence of heterophil antibody.

Therapeutic Management

The treatments for CMV are directed at early detection of disabilities and appropriate interventions. Hearing aids, cochlear implants, and speech therapy are used to treat hearing loss. Assessments to detect learning disabilities and early intervention with physical, speech, and cognitive therapy play an important role. Recently, studies have shown that children who receive treatment with the antiviral drug ganciclovir develop fewer developmental delays, but more research is needed (Stowell et al., 2010). Treatment with CMV immune globulin as well as antivirals is being studied to treat pregnant women with CMV. Using CMV-negative donors for neonatal transfusions can reduce the risk of exposure associated with bloodborne viral transmission. Several investigational vaccines are currently being researched, but presently education about congenital CMV and promoting good hygiene practices is the best source of prevention.

Nursing Considerations

The nurse needs to obtain a history of the child's symptoms and possible exposures. Children with congenitally acquired CMV may develop a wide range of manifestations, so nursing care will vary according to the child's specific needs. When developmental delays, intellectual disability, neurologic deficits, or hearing losses occur, the nurse can help coordinate the health care team's efforts to meet the child's needs. Parents will need support and education in caring for a child with developmental deficits. The nurse will play a key role in identifying the need for referral and any resources available in the community, including parental support groups.

Epstein-Barr Virus (Infectious Mononucleosis)

Causative agent:	Epstein-Barr virus (EBV, a herpeslike virus)
Incubation period:	4 to 7 weeks
Infectious period:	Unknown; the virus is commonly shed before clinical onset of disease until 6 months or longer after recovery; asymptomatic carriers are common
Transmission:	Saliva, intimate contact, blood
Immunity:	Natural disease
Season:	Can occur during any season

The primary sites of infection in infectious mononucleosis are the epithelial cells and the B lymphocytes. EBV has been well recognized as the causative agent in infectious mononucleosis. It has also been associated with other diseases, especially outside North America. It has been identified as a cofactor in Hodgkin disease; in Burkitt lymphoma, often seen in Africa; and in cases of nasopharyngeal carcinoma, seen in China and Southeast Asia. EBV alone cannot cause the lymphomas or the carcinoma, but it acts in association with other factors.

Manifestations

Infectious mononucleosis typically occurs in otherwise healthy individuals, most commonly in older children and young adults. Clinical signs include fever, exudative pharyngitis, lymphadenopathy, and hepatosplenomegaly. The severity of the clinical signs can range from asymptomatic and mild to severe and fatal. Some children develop a maculopapular rash. Children may report malaise, headache, fatigue, nausea, and abdominal pain. The acute illness usually lasts 2 to 4 weeks and is followed by a gradual recovery. EBV can remain dormant after the infection and recur during times of suppressed immunity. The prognosis is generally excellent if no complications occur.

Complications

Common complications, which are rare, include exanthems and hepatitis. More serious complications involve the pulmonary, neurologic, and hematopoietic systems. The risk of splenic rupture associated with EBV infection occurs most frequently during the first to third weeks of the illness. Patients with a palpable spleen are at a higher risk for rupture. Swelling of the pharynx and tonsils can be severe enough to compromise respiration. The outcome of these complications depends on the severity of the infection and the course of the complications.

Therapeutic Management

The illness is generally self-limiting; therefore, treatment is supportive. Antivirals have little effect on the illness. Complications are addressed with appropriate medical treatment. Use of steroids to treat acute tonsillar swelling and other symptoms of infectious mononucleosis is controversial. A recent evidence-based report (Dickens, Nye, & Rickett, 2008) suggests that evidence is insufficient to support use of corticosteroids, with the possible exception of risk for abrupt airway compromise. Strenuous physical activity and contact sports should be avoided during the acute illness and as long as the spleen is enlarged to minimize the risk of splenic rupture.

Nursing Considerations

The history should include presenting signs and symptoms. Physical examination of the pharynx should be performed, with documentation of any redness or swelling. Note any rashes, including a description of their distribution and appearance. The spleen and liver should be evaluated for enlargement. The child's body temperature should be recorded and nutrition and hydration status evaluated.

Because EBV infection is self-limiting, nursing care is mainly supportive. Most children are cared for at home. Hospitalization with Standard Precautions for hydration therapy may be necessary if the child is unable to swallow. Care in both settings involves bed rest, hydration, and relief of discomfort.

Education and reinforcement regarding the importance of avoiding contact sports, including roughhousing at home with family and friends, should be given to older children or adolescents to help them understand the risks involved (see Patient-Centered Teaching: How to Care for the Child with Infectious Mononucleosis box).

PATIENT-CENTERED TEACHING

How to Care for the Child with Infectious Mononucleosis

- Prolonged rest is indicated during the acute stage of the illness.
- Acetaminophen may be useful in controlling discomfort caused by fever and enlarged tonsils.
- Activity restrictions include no contact sports of any type, including no roughhousing at home with siblings or friends, to protect the child's enlarged spleen from rupture. With improvement in clinical signs, the child should be allowed to gradually resume normal activities as tolerated.
- The parents and child need to be prepared for a slow and gradual recovery. Fatigue may continue, necessitating a gradual return to school activities.
- Hydration should be monitored and encouraged.
- In children with a sore throat, soothing liquids, bland foods, and milkshakes may be better tolerated than a regular diet.
- Anxiety related to missed schoolwork should be anticipated. Homebound school programs should be arranged if the child will be absent from school for a prolonged period.
- The parents should have an understanding of the disease and the usual course of recovery. They may need support in exploring options for caring for their child during a lengthy recovery period, including referrals for alternative child-care arrangements, to decrease lost income and maintain job security.

Rabies

Causative agent:	Rhabdovirus (RNA virus)
Incubation period:	5 days to more than 1 year; incubation can extend to 6 years, but the average is 2 months
Infectious period:	10 days (if the animal is still healthy, rabies is unlikely); however, bats may harbor the virus for a longer period
Transmission:	Bites with contaminated saliva, scratches from claws of infected animals, airborne transmission in laboratory settings and in bat-infested caves, transplantation of corneas from undiagnosed donors
Immunity:	Human diploid cell vaccine (HDCV), purified chick embryo cell vaccine (PCECV), and rabies vaccine absorbed (RVA)
Season:	Can occur during any season

Rabies is caused by a virus that can infect any warm-blooded animal. In the United States, the reservoir consists of skunks, bats, raccoons, foxes, squirrels, and woodchucks. Over the past few decades, most cases of rabies have been caused by bats. Dogs and cats may also be reservoirs, but the use of animal vaccines makes them a less common source of infection.

Manifestations

The rhabdovirus results in a slowly developing infection. The virus travels up the axons of the motor or sensory neurons to the brain. For this reason, bites that occur on the feet or lower extremities are associated with longer incubation periods than are bites on the face. Incubation periods are shortened in children.

When left untreated, the virus will cause vague signs and symptoms. The child may report not feeling well. The child may have a sore throat, headache, fever, discomfort at the site of the bite, hyperactivity, anxiety, muscle spasms, or convulsions. The decreased ability to swallow results in drooling or aspiration, which explains the use of the term *hydrophobia* in connection with rabies. Once the disease has established itself, it is fatal. Once symptoms appear, the disease generally lasts 5 to 6 days before progressing to death.

Therapeutic Management

The focus of rabies management is preventive and includes educating adults and children to avoid touching and petting strange animals, especially those in unusual settings exhibiting strange behaviors. When an animal bites a child, a determination must be made regarding whether to treat that child. Factors to be considered include the geographic area, type of animal, circumstances of the bite, and the animal's vaccination record. If the animal is available, it can be observed for 10 days or killed for microscopic examination of the brain.

The bite wound should be cleaned with copious amounts of soap and water. Human rabies immune globulin (HRIG) is given. One half of the dose is infiltrated locally around the wound, and the other half is administered intramuscularly. Rabies vaccination should be administered as early as possible after exposure, preferably within 24 hours. Additional doses of the vaccine are given into the deltoid muscle on days 3, 7, 14, and 28 after the first vaccine. Rabies vaccine is the only vaccine that can be given after exposure and result in successful vaccination.

Nursing Considerations

A complete history of the event should be obtained, including the type of animal involved, identification of the animal as wild or domestic, immunization record of the animal, and the present location of the animal (if known). This information will determine the course of action. The wound should be examined and a description noted in the child's record.

For the child who will undergo a complete series of vaccinations, the nurse may use a variety of distraction techniques (e.g., counting, singing). Allowing the child to administer injections to a doll may help relieve some anxiety associated with multiple injections. For the older child, an explanation of the injection process and reasons for treatment may be adequate.

Primary prevention of rabies includes anticipatory guidance focusing on teaching children to avoid petting or touching unknown animals. Responsible pet care, including vaccination, and stray animal control will assist in decreasing the risk of exposure (CDC, 2010d).

For the child who develops rabies, nursing actions are supportive, including support of the child and family through the dying process (see Chapter 12). The child is placed in strict isolation, and Standard Precautions are instituted. The family will need support in preparing for the child's inevitable death and in coping with feelings of guilt.

BACTERIAL INFECTIONS

Bacteria are abundant in the environment, yet relatively few cause diseases that have an impact on human beings. Bacteria are organisms that contain both DNA and RNA. They lack a nuclear membrane but have a complex cell wall. The properties of the cell wall determine the bacterium's classification as either gram positive or gram negative. Gram-positive bacteria have a thicker wall that helps resist bile activity, drying, and other environmental factors. Gram-positive bacteria can cause chronic inflammation of dermal tissue, fever, and shock. Gram-negative bacteria have a thinner cell wall.

Outside the cell wall, many bacteria have flagella, which help propel the bacteria through their environment. They may also have pili—rigid projections that assist in attachment to the host cell or other bacteria. Capsules help hide the bacteria's presence from the host and make phagocytosis by the host cell more difficult.

Bacteria excrete toxins. Exotoxins are highly poisonous substances that cause cell damage by cell lysis, inhibition of protein synthesis, or interference with passage of nerve impulses. Endotoxins, which are a portion of the gram-negative cell, cause fever, shock, and disseminated intravascular coagulation (DIC).

Pertussis (Whooping Cough)

Causative agent:	*Bordetella pertussis* (a gram-negative bacillus)
Incubation period:	6 to 20 days
Infectious period:	Catarrhal stage (1 to 2 weeks) until the fourth week
Transmission:	Direct contact or respiratory droplets from coughing
Immunity:	Bacteria or vaccine, both of which provide varying degrees and duration of immunity against pertussis
Season:	Can occur during any season

Manifestations

The three stages of pertussis are catarrhal, paroxysmal, and convalescent (Box 17-1). Diagnosis is through positive nasopharyngeal culture.

Complications

The most frequently seen complication of pertussis is pneumonia. Other respiratory complications may occur to varying degrees, ranging

---

BOX 17-1   STAGES OF MANIFESTATION OF PERTUSSIS

Catarrhal
- Duration: 1 to 2 weeks
- Symptoms: Symptoms of upper respiratory tract infection (rhinorrhea, lacrimation, mild cough, low-grade fever).

Paroxysmal
- Duration: 2 to 4 weeks or longer
- Symptoms: Increased severity of cough. Repetitive series of coughs during a single expiration, followed by massive inspiration with a whoop (older children may not manifest this). Cyanosis, protrusion of tongue, salivation, distention of neck veins. Coughing spells may be triggered by yawning, sneezing, eating, or drinking. Coughing may induce vomiting.

Convalescent
- Duration: 1 to 2 weeks
- Symptoms: Episodes of coughing, whooping, and vomiting that decrease in frequency and severity. Cough may persist for several months.

---

from atelectasis to interstitial or subcutaneous emphysema to pneumothorax. Hypoxemia can lead to CNS involvement. Malnutrition and dehydration may result from extensive vomiting and can be quite dangerous, especially for infants. Other complications include otitis media, ulcers of the frenulum of the tongue, epistaxis, hernia, and rectal prolapse. Infants younger than 6 months old are at greatest risk for complications and are more likely to acquire pertussis because they do not receive maternal immunity and may be incompletely immunized. Neonatal mortality rates are between 1% and 3% (Cherry, 2009e).

Therapeutic Management

Primary prevention of pertussis can be accomplished through administration of the pertussis vaccine in combination with tetanus and diphtheria (DTaP). Because of waning immunity in the adolescent population, the American Academy of Pediatrics in 2005 recommended a booster, called Tdap, for children ages 11 to 12 who completed a primary series of DTaP. This replaces the first of the recommended 10-year Td boosters (CDC, 2010c).

Erythromycin, azithromycin, or clarithromycin (depending on age), if given during the catarrhal stage, will eliminate the organism from the nasopharynx within a few days, thereby reducing communicability. Infants and young children who are exposed to pertussis should continue their routine schedule of immunization. Erythromycin, azithromycin, or clarithromycin is also given to all close contacts, which include most children older than 13 years, because the immunity conferred by the childhood immunization declines by early adolescence.

Hospitalization and supportive care for the infant may be necessary to monitor airway patency, whereas older children can usually be cared for at home. Respiratory status is monitored with a cardiopulmonary monitor and pulse oximeter. Droplet Precautions are observed.

Nursing Considerations

The nurse obtains a complete immunization history and any recent known exposures to illnesses. Often pertussis goes unrecognized in adolescents and adults, leading to an increased risk of exposure. This is why it is vital for families and caregivers of young infants to be immunized against pertussis. Documentation also includes the parent's description of any respiratory events before admission and indicators such as coughing, secretions, cyanotic episodes, and the child's activity level. Assessment of the child's respiratory, fluid, nutrition, output, and neurologic status should be done.

The child's respiratory status needs monitoring with a cardiopulmonary monitor and pulse oximeter. If the child is hospitalized, the limits of the monitor should be checked frequently. Explain any monitoring devices to the child (if age appropriate) and parents to help alleviate anxiety. Suction and oxygen equipment should be readily available. Supplemental oxygen therapy could be ordered if the child's oxygen saturation falls below an acceptable range (especially during any coughing episodes). If the child needs oxygen therapy, instruct the parent about any oxygen equipment and the timing and possible length of treatment. Some children will need additional oxygen only during the paroxysmal spells.

Because the child's coughing paroxysms may be triggered by noises or frightening experiences, a quiet environment and a calm, reassuring approach should be used when caring for the child and supporting the parents. Paroxysmal episodes should be monitored for any drop in oxygen saturation levels. Parents and children will need additional support and reassurance that assistance is near and ready if needed during the child's coughing spells because these episodes can be extremely frightening.

The infant's nutritional status should be closely monitored. Small, frequent feedings may benefit infants if the feeding process becomes exhausting. If the child's intake becomes insufficient, nutritional support (gavage or parenteral nutrition) may be needed to prevent dehydration or weight loss. If the child has vomiting episodes when coughing, frequent oral care will be necessary.

Nursing care activities should be clustered, if possible, to allow the child and parent to rest. Diversional activities should be age appropriate. Parents may need emotional support to deal with feelings of guilt, especially if they chose not to immunize their child.

Scarlet Fever

Causative agent:	Group A beta-hemolytic streptococci
Incubation period:	1 to 7 days (average of 3 days)
Infectious period:	Acute stage until 24 hours after antimicrobial therapy has begun
Transmission:	Airborne (inhalation or ingestion), direct contact
Immunity:	None
Season:	Late fall, winter, and spring

Manifestations

Abrupt fever, vomiting, headache, abdominal pain, pharyngitis, and chills may characterize the onset of scarlet fever. The fever reaches a peak by the second day and returns to normal within 5 to 6 days. Within 24 hours a fine red papular rash appears in the axillae, groin, and neck, which feels like sandpaper to the touch. The rash then spreads peripherally to cover the entire body (Figure 17-8). The rash will blanch on pressure except in areas of deep creases (Pastia's sign). *Desquamation*, peeling of the skin, begins on the face at the end of the first week, and flaking proceeds down the trunk. This process may continue for up to 6 weeks. The tongue is initially coated with a white, furry covering with red, projecting papillae (so-called white strawberry tongue). By the fourth day the papillae slough off, leaving a red, swollen tongue (so-called strawberry tongue). The tonsils are edematous and may be covered with a gray-white exudate, which may spread to the pharynx. Petechial hemorrhages cover the soft palate.

Complications

Complications generally result from extension of the streptococcal infection. They may include sinusitis, otitis media, mastoiditis, peritonsillar abscess, bronchopneumonia, meningitis, osteomyelitis, rheumatic fever, and glomerulonephritis.

Therapeutic Management

Rapid streptococcal screening in an office setting, usually with laboratory confirmation (generally by a throat culture) if the rapid screen is negative is recommended for children with sore throats because of the similarity of symptoms between viral and group A beta-hemolytic streptococcal sore throats. The preferred treatment for any streptococcal infection is penicillin. Children allergic to penicillin can be given erythromycin. Supportive care for symptoms is indicated. Children with streptococcal infections (throat, skin) may return to school or daycare 24 hours after beginning antibiotics when they are no longer considered contagious. Droplet Precautions should also be observed until the child has been on antibiotics for 24 hours.

Nursing Considerations

The nurse should obtain and document a complete history of symptoms. The nurse also assesses the child's throat, tongue, rash, nutritional and fluid intake, vital signs, and level of general wellness. Any history of sensitivity to penicillin should be thoroughly explored and prominently noted on the child's records.

Generally, children with scarlet fever are cared for at home. Comfort measures include encouraging fluids (especially cool, nonacidic liquids) and administering antipyretics for fever control.

Analgesics may be given for discomfort, and antipruritic comfort measures may be necessary. Parents should understand the typical course of disease and any treatment measures, including the importance of completing the full course of any antibiotics prescribed (to prevent growth of resistant bacteria). Bed rest and quiet activities may be beneficial during the acute stage (see Patient-Centered Teaching: How to Care for the Child with Scarlet Fever box).

PATIENT-CENTERED TEACHING

How to Care for the Child with Scarlet Fever

- The entire course of antibiotic therapy (usually 10 to 14 days) must be taken to destroy all the bacteria and decrease the risk of complications. If a partial course of antibiotics is given (antibiotic stopped by parent when child is feeling better), the bacteria can become resistant and fail to be eradicated with subsequent attempts.
- Cool drinks and liquid refreshments (ice pops, milkshakes) may be soothing and help maintain hydration.
- Acetaminophen, ibuprofen, throat lozenges, antiseptic throat spray (e.g., Chloraseptic), and cool mist may be used to relieve discomfort.
- Encouraging quiet activities will help prevent fatigue.
- In providing oral care, acidic preparations should be avoided. Saline rinses may provide comfort and promote hygiene.
- A soft, bland diet should be offered.
- Call your primary health care provider if your child develops drooling or great difficulty swallowing or acts very sick. After 48 hours of antibiotic therapy, your child should not have a fever.
- Your child is no longer contagious after 24 hours of antibiotic therapy. The rash is not contagious.

First day   Third day

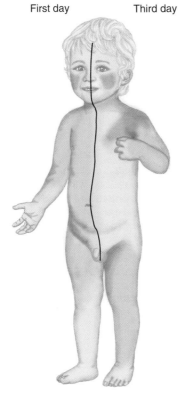

Scarlet Fever Rash Distribution

- Red, fine, papular rash appears within 24 hours of fever and other symptoms; in dark skin, rash is often seen as punctate papular elevations
- Begins in axillae, groin, and neck and spreads to cover entire body
- Desquamation begins on face at end of first week, and flaking proceeds down trunk; may continue up to 6 weeks
- Tongue: initially has a white, furry coat with red, projecting papillae (white strawberry tongue); by the fourth day, the white sloughs off , leaving a red, swollen tongue (strawberry tongue)

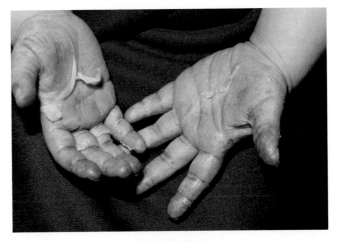

Desquamation

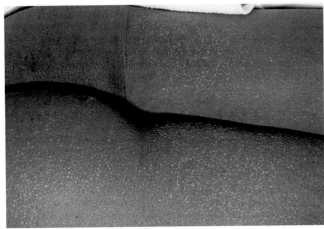

Rash, Light Skin

Rash, Dark Skin

FIG 17-8 Scarlet fever rash distribution and appearance. Note the characteristic skin peeling. (From Paller, S. A. [2012]. *Hurwitz clinical pediatric dermatology: A textbook of skin disorders of childhood and adolescence* [4th ed.]. Philadelphia: Saunders.)

Children with severe symptoms and complications may, however, need hospitalization and supportive care. In such cases, vital signs, especially body temperature, should be monitored.

Methicillin-Resistant *Staphylococcus aureus* (MRSA)

Causative agent: *Staphylococcus aureus* (gram-positive cocci)
Transmission: Contact
Immunity: None
Season: No seasonal pattern

Methicillin-resistant *S. aureus* (MRSA) was first identified in the 1960s and became increasingly prevalent in hospital settings. It is estimated that the incidence of MRSA is 60% in American intensive care unit (ICU) settings and continues to rise at a rate of 2% per year (Hinckley & Allen, 2008). MRSA is categorized as either hospital-acquired or community-acquired. The first case of community-acquired MRSA (CA-MRSA) was documented in 1998, and its incidence has tripled over the past decade. It is believed that the new community strains mutated from community-based methicillin-susceptible

S. aureus (Hinckley & Allen, 2008). Currently, CA-MRSA has surpassed hospital-acquired MRSA (HA-MRSA) as the source of most skin and soft tissue infections. In 2007, 82% of MRSA infections in children 15 years and younger were CA-MRSA (Jancin, 2010). The criteria necessary for diagnosing CA-MRSA are being diagnosed in an outpatient setting or within 48 hours of hospital admission, no present use of medical devices, and no history of prior MRSA infection (So & Farrington, 2008).

Manifestations

HA-MRSA is often the cause of medical device–related infections, pneumonia (including ventilator-associated pneumonia), and catheter-related bloodstream infections. The most common CA-MRSA infections are skin and soft tissue infections (furuncles, carbuncles, and abscesses) and, less commonly, urinary tract infections (UTIs), pneumonia, and bacteremia. Some of the more serious and potentially fatal complications include osteomyelitis, endocarditis, and necrotizing fasciitis.

Some risk factors for MRSA include a history of a chronic illness, immunocompromised status, participating in close-contact team sports, and attendance at a daycare center (So & Farrington, 2008).

Therapeutic Management

A clinical practice guideline for the treatment of adults and children with MRSA contains evidence-based treatment recommendations (Liu, Bayer, Cosgrove et al., 2011). HA-MRSA is difficult to treat as it is resistant to beta-lactam and cephalosporin antibiotics; therefore, treatment, after incision and drainage of a cutaneous lesion or abscess, includes IV vancomycin or linezolid, among others (Liu et al., 2011). For more severe infections or bacteremia, IV vancomycin is used; follow-up blood cultures monitor the resolution of the bacteremia. Infectious endocarditis (see Chapter 22) is a risk (Liu et al., 2011).

For most skin and soft tissue infections acquired in the community, incision and drainage with culture and sensitivity is the option of choice, and antibiotic administration is not considered necessary unless there is severe disease present, the infection progresses rapidly, or the wound does not respond to incision and drainage alone (Liu et al., 2011). If necessary, CA-MRSA can be treated with a 5- to 10-day course of oral clindamycin, sulfamethoxazole-trimethoprim, tetracycline, or linezolid. Patients who are colonized are instructed to disinfect their body using chlorhexidine gluconate and nasal mupirocin (So & Farrington, 2008).

Nursing Considerations

Education on proper hand hygiene is of utmost importance in reducing the spread of MRSA. Athletes should avoid sharing of personal equipment and towels. Coaches must ensure that all equipment is properly cleaned. Protocols to ensure the early identification of cases are vital to prevent the spread of MRSA in the hospital setting.

Clostridium difficile

Causative agent:	*Clostridium difficile* (gram-positive anaerobic bacterium)
Transmission:	Contact (fecal-oral)
Incubation period:	Unknown
Immunity:	None
Season:	No seasonal pattern

C. difficile has become an increasingly common cause of diarrheal disease in infants and children. In the past it was only associated with

the health care setting and antibiotic use, but in recent years it is becoming more commonly seen in previously health infants and children. In 2005, the CDC reported an increase of cases in children who were previously thought to be at minimal risk for *C. difficile*–associated disease (CDAD) (Bell, 2010). Children ages 1 through 4 are most often affected. Recent data show that there has been a steady increase in CDAD, with a 56% increase from 2001 through 2006 in a study of 22 U.S. children's hospitals (Bell, 2010).

Manifestations

Though some patients can be asymptomatic, many have watery diarrhea, abdominal cramps, fever, and possible systemic toxicity. *C. difficile* is associated with antibiotic administration in young children, and its growth results from reduction of the normal bowel flora. Symptoms usually begin while the child is receiving a course of antibiotics, but may occur after the course is complete. Complications are more common with immunocompromised patients or those with inflammatory bowel disease and include intestinal perforation and toxic megacolon, both of which can be fatal (AAP, 2009c).

Therapeutic Management

Diagnosis of *C. difficile* is through identification of the specific toxin in the stool. Infants younger than 12 months of age are commonly colonized with *C. difficile* in their gastrointestinal tract and are usually asymptomatic. Therefore, infants that age are not usually tested for *C. difficile*. The initial treatment is cessation of the antibiotic course (if applicable), which is effective in approximately a quarter of the cases. Almost all antibiotics have the potential to cause CDAD, but clindamycin, third-generation cephalosporins, and penicillin are more often associated with CDAD. The antibiotics used for treatment of CDAD include oral metronidazole for mild to moderate disease and vancomycin for more severe disease. Resistance to either of these agents is rare (Bell, 2010).

Nursing Considerations

Patients are placed on contact precautions in the hospital setting. Proper hand hygiene is crucial. Because the *C. difficile* spores are not killed by alcohol-based hand sanitizer, it is recommended that health care workers use soap and water for hand hygiene after contact with a patient who has CDAD. Parents of young patients are cautioned about proper cleaning techniques (use of bleach-based products).

Neonatal Sepsis

Causative agent:	Multiple organisms depending on stage of onset (early, late, or late late) (Bateman & Seed, 2010); include streptococci, *Escherichia coli*, *Staphylococcus aureus*
Incubation period:	Unknown
Transmission:	Placental, perinatal, postnatal from mother or environment

Neonatal sepsis occurs when bacteria or their poisonous products, known as *endotoxins*, gain access to the bloodstream, causing systemic signs and symptoms. Evaluation of the newborn for the presence of bacterial sepsis is a common occurrence in the newborn nursery and presents challenges for the health care team in both the evaluation and treatment procedures. The challenges are the result, in part, of the varied and frequently nonspecific subtle signs and symptoms of the infant with neonatal sepsis.

Annual incidence of neonatal sepsis has been reported as 0.56 cases per 1000 children in the United States (Czaja, Zimmerman, & Nathens, 2009). Before antibiotic use, the mortality rate from bacterial sepsis was 95% to 100%, but early recognition of signs and symptoms, vigorous initiation of antibiotic therapies, and supportive care have reduced the mortality rate. However, the infant's survival remains highly variable and dependent on the organism and underlying or associated conditions. Because of the widespread screening and treatment of group B streptococcus (GBS), there has been a decrease in the incidence of early-onset sepsis (EOS). Unfortunately, this is not the case with premature or low birth weight infants; the incidence of EOS has increased in this population (Bateman & Seed, 2010). Preterm infants are at an increased risk for sepsis because they have an immature immune system and lack vernix, which is a protective barrier against bacteria. Preterm infants often require treatment with invasive medical equipment, which increases their risk of sepsis (Cherry, 2009d).

Manifestations

The early signs and symptoms of sepsis may be vague and nonspecific. Often, the mother or nurse first recognizes that something is wrong or "just not right" but is unable to describe any one specific physical sign or symptom. The infant may have respiratory or gastrointestinal symptoms. Additional clinical manifestations of sepsis include temperature instability, lethargy, changes in mood or eating patterns, abnormal Moro reflex, change in muscle tone or activity, persistent pulmonary hypertension or other cardiac signs (see Chapter 22), fluid and electrolyte and acid-base imbalances, signs of neurologic irritation (high-pitched cry, tremors, seizures, decreased responsiveness, bulging fontanel), skin manifestations (petechiae, purpura, rashes), jaundice or hepatosplenomegaly, and hyper- or hypoglycemia.

Therapeutic Management

The treatment approach used for evaluation of infants for neonatal sepsis is generally called a *sepsis (or septic) workup*. The exact management plan or treatment approach varies with each infant, but all are based on assessment of clinical signs, careful history, and appropriate laboratory findings. Diagnostic tests, including cultures (blood, urine, nasopharyngeal, CSF [if indicated]) and additional blood tests (complete blood count [CBC] with white blood cell count [WBC] and complete differential count, C-reactive protein [CRP]) are obtained, and a lumbar puncture is always performed in the symptomatic neonate and may be done in asymptomatic infants if the infant's condition warrants. Neonates with suspected sepsis or meningitis are started on antibiotics as soon as the appropriate cultures and IV access are obtained. Ampicillin and an aminoglycoside, usually gentamicin, make up one of the combinations that have proved to be highly effective against a majority of causative organisms. Once the pathogen or pathogens and their sensitivities are identified, antimicrobial therapy is modified accordingly. Aminoglycoside levels should be monitored to avoid toxic levels and long-term side effects (hearing impairment).

Late-onset sepsis (LOS) often has a more varied treatment that is dependent on the infant's environment and may also include a third-generation cephalosporin. Antimicrobial therapy is continued for 7 to 10 days depending on the culture results and the infant's response to treatment (Cherry, 2009d).

A major recommendation for prevention is universal screening of pregnant women for vaginal and rectal group B streptococcal colonization at 35 to 37 weeks. Approximately 21% of women test positive for group B streptococcus (Cherry, 2009d). Some women for whom screening is positive for group B streptococcus, or who have diagnosed group B streptococcal bacteriuria, will require intrapartum penicillin prophylaxis to reduce exposure for the newborn. The complete CDC and AAP recommendations are available online at www.cdc.gov/mmwr/preview/mmwrhtml/rr5111a1.htm.

Supportive measures make up a large part of the treatment of all septic infants. Once neonates are symptomatic, they should be treated in an intensive care nursery, with full cardiopulmonary monitoring and respiratory and cardiac support as needed. Monitoring the effectiveness of any therapy is an essential part of the supportive care for the neonate with sepsis. Constant environmental temperature control is essential because the neonate's thermal regulation system is immature. Respiratory support with supplemental oxygen, blood gas and oxygen saturation determinations with subsequent intubation, and mechanical ventilation may be necessary. In addition, vital signs (blood pressure, centrally if indicated), blood glucose levels, and hydration status (urine output, hourly if indicated) must also be assessed, documented, and reported to the primary care provider when normal parameters are exceeded so supportive treatment can be rapidly initiated.

Nursing Considerations

The nurse carefully and thoroughly reviews the maternal history (including labor and delivery) to identify any risk factors for the development of sepsis. All infants considered at risk should be closely observed for the development of the often subtle signs and symptoms of sepsis. Thorough documentation of the infant's behavior during each shift allows nurses to determine whether the behavior they observe is different or abnormal for that infant. The nurse should immediately notify the physician if any changes are observed in the infant's respiratory status, muscle tone, activity level, or temperature or if the infant lacks interest in or does not tolerate feedings. Infants at risk for sepsis should be closely observed to ensure early recognition and treatment. Extra measures may be necessary to warm or cool the infant to minimize the harmful effects of temperature extremes.

⚡ SAFETY ALERT

The Infant with Neonatal Sepsis

The infant's condition can deteriorate rapidly from apparently normal to fulminant septic shock and death, especially if the causative agent is group B streptococcus. When diagnostic tests are ordered, the nurse should evaluate the results and bring any abnormal values to the immediate attention of the infant's physician. Monitoring culture results promptly and notifying the physician of any positive results and antibiotic sensitivities can help ensure prompt institution of specific therapy.

❗ NURSING QUALITY ALERT

Monitoring Temperature

The infant's temperature is monitored closely because both hypothermia and hyperthermia may be signs of sepsis, although hyperthermia is rare.

In most cases, early identification and treatment can prevent the complications of sepsis. Diagnostic tests should be completed before antibiotic therapy is initiated. Antimicrobial therapy cannot be specific for the invading organism until the cultures have grown and antimicrobial sensitivities have been determined. Early in the clinical course of sepsis, the infant may be unable or unwilling to take oral feedings. Adequate fluid and caloric intake should be ensured by administering gavage feedings or IV fluids as ordered. The importance of proper infection control methods and appropriate use of medical devices such as catheters is emphasized. Awareness that the effects of severe sepsis last well beyond the hospitalization is vital. Many infants require more than one readmission, which places them at risk for acquiring additional morbidities such as nosocomial infections (Czaja et al., 2009).

Rare Viral and Bacterial Infections

Table 17-1 presents several rarely seen viral and bacterial infections. Many of these have been nearly eliminated as a result of vigorous vaccination and immunization programs.

FUNGAL INFECTIONS

Fungi are free-living organisms that can be found throughout the environment. Some species of fungi are part of the normal human flora, especially those in the mouth, intestine, vagina, and skin. A fungus is transmitted through inhalation or penetration of tissue as a result of trauma. Fungi grow quite slowly, so clinical symptoms may appear only after a prolonged period. They are aerobic, can grow in a wide range of temperatures, and are resistant to most antibiotics. They exist in two forms: molds and yeasts.

Infections caused by fungi are classified into four groups:
1. Opportunistic: caused by a defect in host immunity
2. Systemic: involving deep tissues and organs
3. Subcutaneous: limited to deep subcutaneous tissue
4. Superficial: limited to skin, hair, and nails

TABLE 17-1 RARE VIRAL AND BACTERIAL INFECTIONS

DISEASE	TRANSMISSION	MANIFESTATIONS	COMPLICATIONS	THERAPEUTIC MANAGEMENT AND NURSING CONSIDERATIONS
Smallpox Variola virus	Transmitted through droplets via direct and prolonged face-to-face contact with an infected person; less commonly, smallpox transmitted through contact with contaminated objects Most contagious when lesions rupture	Prodrome of fever, malaise, headache, muscle pain, prostration, and often nausea, vomiting, and backache Fever of 101° F (38.3° C) but can be higher Lesions appear as red spots in the mouth and on the tongue, develop into sores and break After a few days a generalized vesicular rash appears (Figure 17-9) Lesions progress into pustules, then form scabs; complete scabbing of pustules by end of second week	May be fatal	Supportive care Infection control and prevention (CDC, 2009c): Isolate exposed individuals as soon as fever appears Place patient in negative air pressure room with Airborne and Contact Precautions Wear N95 respiratory protection Only vaccinated health care workers can care for patients Vaccinate all exposed contacts
Poliomyelitis Poliovirus	Fecal-oral, oral-oral (respiratory)	Fever, malaise, anorexia, nausea, headache, sore throat, and generalized abdominal pain, which begin as mild symptoms, then grow more intense Flaccid paralysis, especially of lower extremities	Cervical involvement, called bulbar polio, affects the respiratory and vasomotor centers, resulting in potential damage to respiratory centers and inability to breathe	No specific treatment Respiratory paralysis is treated with mechanical ventilation Physical therapy helps maintain muscle integrity and prevent contractures Prevention through routine immunization Risk for postpolio syndrome
Diphtheria *Corynebacterium diphtheriae* (a gram-positive, nonmotile bacillus)	Contact with carrier or disease, droplets	Nasal manifestations initially resemble the common cold, then gradually begin to include discharge of foul-smelling mucopurulent material Low-grade fever is common Hallmark sign: thin, gray membrane on the tonsils and pharynx, causing "bull neck," or neck edema Respiratory compromise due to a narrowing of the upper airway	Upper airway obstruction Myocarditis Peripheral neuropathies	IV diphtheria antitoxin and antibiotics (e.g., erythromycin or penicillin G) within 3 days of the onset of symptoms Prevention through routine immunization and boosters at regularly recommended intervals (CDC, 2010d)

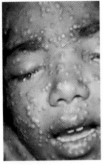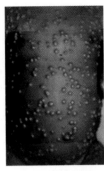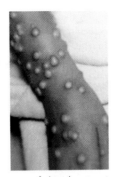

FIG 17-9 Lesions of variola are at the same stage of development on all body parts. (Reprinted from Centers for Disease Control and Prevention. [2002]. *Evaluating patients for smallpox.* Atlanta: Author.)

Common fungal infections include tinea capitis, tinea pedis, and candidal infections (see Chapter 25).

RICKETTSIAL INFECTIONS

Rickettsiae are small, parasitic bacteria that are transmitted to human beings by blood-sucking arthropods. A vertebrate is not necessary for the survival of the bacteria, and the host arthropod (usually a tick) appears not to be affected adversely by the rickettsiae. Replication of the rickettsiae in the new host cell causes cell death, which may be accompanied by vasculitis with thrombosis, increased permeability, tissue edema, hemorrhage, circulatory failure, and meningoencephalitis. Rickettsial diseases cannot be transmitted from person to person.

Rocky Mountain Spotted Fever

Causative agent:	*Rickettsia rickettsii*
Reservoir:	Wild rodents, dogs
Vector:	Tick (wood, dog, Lone Star)
Incubation period:	2 to 14 days (average of 7 days)
Transmission:	Bite of infected tick
Season:	April through October

Manifestations

The onset of Rocky Mountain spotted fever (RMSF) is marked by nonspecific signs and symptoms such as headache, fever, anorexia, and restlessness. Generally, on the third day a characteristic maculopapular or petechial rash appears. This rash begins on the extremities (usually the wrists, palms, ankles, and soles) and spreads to the rest of the body. As the rash progresses, hemorrhagic and necrotic lesions can appear. Approximately 60% of cases have a history of a tick bite or exposure to tick-infested habitats. Children under the age of 15 account for two thirds of all cases, with a peak age of 5 to 9 years (CDC, 2008b). The mortality rate of RMSF is 5% to 7%. This rate is increased in cases in which diagnosis is delayed beyond 1 week (Cherry, 2009f).

Therapeutic Management

With early detection and treatment in children (within 5 days of the beginning of the illness), the likelihood of positive resolution increases. Doxycycline is the recommended treatment with a fluoroquinolone as an alternative. Treatment usually lasts 7 to 10 days. Doxycycline is used with caution in children under 8 years because of staining of the teeth

(Cherry, 2009f). If vascular damage has already occurred, however, the drugs may not alter the course of the disease. There is no vaccine available at this time to prevent RMSF (Cherry, 2009f).

Nursing Considerations

The assessment of children with symptoms indicating RMSF should include obtaining a complete history of skin eruptions, medications taken, exposure to infectious diseases, and recent hiking or other activities in wooded areas. Any rashes or skin lesions should then be examined, with documentation of distribution and morphology. The child's vital signs, especially body temperature, should also be assessed and noted.

Hospitalized children will require supportive care for their symptoms. Straws should be used, and the mouth should be flushed if tetracycline is administered because it can stain the teeth. Parents should be cautioned to give the full course of any antibiotic to decrease the risk of complications and ensure that the disease is eradicated. Education regarding the control measures for prevention of tick-borne infections is vital (Box 17-2).

BORRELIA INFECTIONS

Borrelia is a genus of spiral bacteria that are transmitted to human beings by arthropods. The diseases caused by *Borrelia* are relapsing fever and Lyme disease.

Relapsing Fever

Relapsing fever is spread from person to person by lice or ticks. The bacteria are introduced into a bite wound when the bite is rubbed. This infection is spread when people fail to wash thoroughly and do not change clothes.

Tick-borne relapsing fever (*Borrelia hermsii, B. turicatae*) results from tick exposures in rodent-infested cabins in western mountainous areas of the United States, including state and national parks. *B. turicatae* infections occur less frequently, with the majority of cases in Texas.

Manifestations

The abrupt onset of high fever (up to 106.7° F [41.5° C]), shaking chills, sweats, headache, muscle and joint pains, and progressive weakness characterize relapsing fever. The symptoms resolve within a week, reoccur 1 to 2 weeks later, and continue to reoccur until treated. When the fever resolves, there are two classic phases: the chill phase, which includes high fever and possible confusion, and the flush phase, in which the fever decreases rapidly, causing the child to sweat profusely (CDC, 2008c).

Therapeutic Management

Several antibiotics provide effective treatment. These include penicillin, tetracycline, erythromycin, and chloramphenicol for children older than 8 years and penicillin or erythromycin for younger children.

Nursing Considerations

Assessment should include a complete history of rash onset and characteristics, medications taken, and living environment, including available bathing and washing facilities. Fever, headache, and arthralgia should be treated with antipyretics and analgesics. Antibiotics should be given as ordered. Education includes personal hygiene, the use of pediculicides, and eradication methods.

Lyme Disease

Causative agent:	*Borrelia burgdorferi* (spirochete)
Vector:	Tick (Figure 17-10)
Incubation period:	3 to 32 days
Transmission:	Bite of infected tick (person-to-person transmission not possible)
Season:	April to October

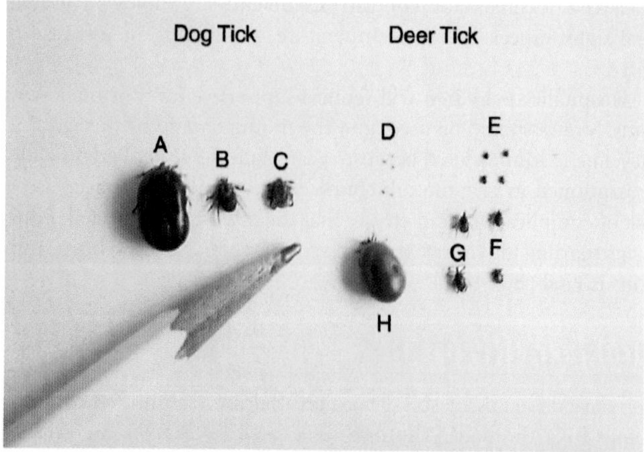

Of the tick-borne diseases seen in the United States, Lyme disease is seen most frequently (Eppes, 2011). The main cause of transmission in the northern or eastern United States is the deer tick, while the western black-legged tick transmits the disease to those on the Pacific Coast (CDC, 2007). Lyme disease is a multisystem illness that affects the skin and the musculoskeletal, cardiovascular, and nervous systems.

Manifestations

The manifestations of Lyme disease can be divided into three stages (early localized, early disseminated, and late disseminated). In the first stage (early localized), the skin lesions are most prominent; in the second stage (early disseminated), cardiac and neurologic findings are prominent; and in the third stage (late disseminated), arthritis is the main manifestation (Cherry, 2009a).

In the early localized stage of Lyme disease, local reactions to an infected tick bite occur, along with vague, flulike symptoms (headache, chills, fatigue, and vague muscle aches and pains). An erythematous macule or papule forms at the site of the tick bite within 3 to 30 days (Figure 17-11). This rash can enlarge to 16 to 68 cm in diameter, with a clearing in the center (erythema migrans, or "bull's eye" rash). It may itch, prickle, or burn. The rash generally lasts for 3 to 4 weeks, during which time it gradually fades.

In the early disseminated stage (generally 1 to 4 months after the bite), neurologic symptoms may be the first to occur. CNS symptoms may include severe headaches with myelitis, nausea, vomiting, facial nerve paralysis (Bell's palsy), forgetfulness or decreased concentration, and cerebral ataxia. General lymphadenopathy and joint and muscle pain may also be present. Lyme arthritis generally affects the large joints, with the knee being the most often involved. Children infrequently manifest carditis. The signs and symptoms generally resolve over a few days, but many individuals have recurrences. Skin lesions may recur but are smaller and more diffuse than the initial ones.

Symptoms of late disseminated Lyme disease (occurring months to years after the initial infected tick bite) occur intermittently and include chronic arthritis, profound fatigue, and chronic neurologic manifestations. The debilitating effects frequently affect a child's ability to participate in normal activities (e.g., sports) because of extreme fatigue or cardiac complications.

Therapeutic Management

Primary prevention of Lyme disease includes anticipatory guidance and information about routine preventive measures to avoid insect bites. Early identification and treatment with antibiotics results in a

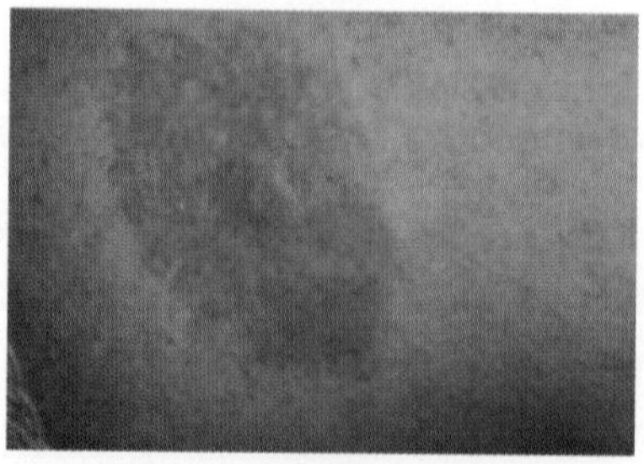

FIG 17-10 Dog (wood) ticks and deer (black-legged) ticks compared with a pencil. Dog ticks: **A,** engorged female; **B,** female; **C,** male. Deer ticks: **D,** larvae; **E,** nymphs; **F,** males; **G,** females; **H,** engorged female. (Courtesy Lyme Disease Foundation, www.lyme.org.)

FIG 17-11 Characteristic lesion of Lyme disease. (Reprinted from Larson, W. G., Adams, R. M., & Maibach, H. I. [1991]. *Color text of contact dermatitis*. Philadelphia: Saunders.)

rapid resolution of symptoms, especially in the early stages of the infection. A course of doxycycline, amoxicillin, or cefuroxime is commonly used for oral treatment. The length of treatment is usually 14 to 21 days, although a shorter 10-day course may be as effective. If the patient has neurologic or cardiac symptoms, intravenous ceftriaxone or penicillin may be used (CDC, 2009a). In addition, disease identified in early stages and treated with antibiotics does not progress to the more debilitating stages. The characteristic rash of Lyme disease linked to other symptoms leads to a diagnosis except in cases where the child has atypical manifestations of the disease (e.g., one septic joint, usually the knee).

Nursing Considerations

Assessment should include a complete history of rash onset and characteristics; medications taken; recent exposures to infectious diseases; and recent hiking, working (forestry, farming, outdoor construction or maintenance), or vacationing (camping [e.g., Boy Scouts or Girl Scouts], hunting) in a known endemic area or heavily wooded area. Because ticks must be attached for longer than 24 hours to transmit the disease, parents must be vigilant in inspecting the skin after exposure to a wooded area. Proper use of insect repellents such as DEET should also be stressed. Fever, headache, and arthralgia should be treated with antipyretics and analgesics. Parents should have a complete understanding of the course of treatment, including the importance of administering medications and antibiotics as prescribed. The importance of completing the entire course of antibiotic treatment should be stressed. Generally, affected children will be treated at home. Parental and caregiver education is important to prevent further exposures and to facilitate early recognition of disease symptoms.

HELMINTHS

Helminths are worms that live as parasites. The three groups with the greatest impact on human beings are tapeworms, flukes, and roundworms (Table 17-2). Children are more commonly infected than adults, primarily as a result of frequent hand-to-mouth activity and the likelihood of fecal contamination. Transmission may occur by oral-fecal ingestion, ingestion of contaminated tissue from another host, skin penetration, or the bite of a blood-sucking insect.

Therapeutic Management

Treatment consists of the administration of oral medications effective against a specific helminth. Treatment is provided to the entire family. Anticipatory guidance to prevent reinfestation and education about the prevention of the spread of disease (basic enteric isolation procedures) for the family and primary caregivers, along with personal hygiene and sanitary practices, are also necessary (see Patient-Centered Teaching: How to Prevent Parasitic Infections box).

PATIENT-CENTERED TEACHING

How to Prevent Parasitic Infections

- Handwashing (including under the fingernails) with soap and water should be done before eating or handling of food and after using the toilet.
- Placing hands in the mouth and nail biting should be discouraged.
- Toilets or other appropriate bathroom facilities should be used for elimination.
- Toilets or bathroom facilities should be cleaned with agents containing bleach.
- Scratching the anal area with bare hands should be discouraged.
- Dogs and cats should be kept at a distance from play areas and sandboxes, and the latter need to be covered when not in use.
- Shoes should be worn when outside.
- All fruits and vegetables should be washed before being eaten.
- Diapers should be changed frequently and disposed of properly (out of children's reach).
- Swimming facilities that allow diapered children should be avoided.
- Only bottled water should be used during camping outings.

Nursing Considerations

A thorough history, including the child's general wellness, personal hygiene practices, and the availability of running water and bathing and laundry facilities, along with nutritional intake, should be obtained.

Most parasites are identified in fecal smears obtained from stool specimens. If the family or caregiver is to bring a stool specimen in for laboratory testing, the nurse needs to provide specific, clear instructions and provide a container if needed. Sample size and number, as well as proper storage, should be clearly explained. Stool

TABLE 17-2	**COMMON HELMINTHS**			
CLASS AND TYPICAL AGENT	**TRANSMISSION**	**MANIFESTATIONS**	**DIAGNOSIS**	**TREATMENT**
Roundworm (Ascaris lumbricoides)	Ingestion of eggs from contaminated soil or food, transfer to mouth from fingers, toys, or other vectors	Abdominal pain or distention, abdominal obstruction, vomiting with bile staining, pneumonitis	Fecal smear	Mebendazole, albendazole
Pinworm (Enterobius vermicularis)	Ingestion or inhalation of eggs, transfer from hands to mouth	Nocturnal anal itching, sleeplessness	Cellophane tape test and microscopic examination	Pyrantel pamoate, mebendazole, albendazole
Tapeworm (Taenia saginata)	Ingestion from handling or eating infected beef or pork	Asymptomatic, segments of worms seen in stool, abdominal pain, nausea, anorexia, weight loss, insomnia	Fecal smear or microscopic examination	Praziquantel
Hookworm (Necator americanus)	Skin penetration from direct contact with contaminated soil	Dermatitis, anemia, pneumonitis, blood loss, malnutrition	Fecal smear or microscopic examination	Mebendazole, albendazole, pyrantel pamoate

specimens that have not been contaminated with urine are ideal. Obtaining urine-free specimens may be difficult, especially in infants or very young children. Plastic wrap can be placed over the toilet bowl or a potty chair, or specimens can be collected from a diaper using a clean tongue blade and placing in a container. The container should be marked with the child's name and the date and time of collection. It should then be refrigerated until it is delivered to the laboratory.

Education for the parents and primary caregivers should focus on medication administration, primary prevention of future reinfestations, and resource identification with referral to available community and social services for any basic living needs (running water, bathing facilities). The rationale for evaluating and treating the entire family for infection and the usual mode of transmission must be discussed to prevent future reinfestation or cross contamination of family members. Anticipatory guidance regarding primary prevention and teaching about prevention (personal hygiene and health habits) should be covered with the child's family. The nurse should help the family identify any resources (access to care, social services) necessary and initiate referral if appropriate.

SEXUALLY TRANSMISSIBLE INFECTIONS

The rates of infection of many sexually transmissible infections (STIs), or infections transmitted through sexual activity, are highest among adolescents. Those adolescents at highest risk are male homosexuals, sexually active heterosexuals, younger sexually active adolescents, and IV drug users. The CDC estimates that one in four women between the ages of 14 and 19 years has an STI (as cited in Holland-Hall, 2008). Often, adolescents lack knowledge of methods for preventing STIs. Moreover, the use of drugs and alcohol in this population increases the risk for unsafe and unprotected sex. Adolescents' inherent developmental stage and sense of invulnerability lead to risky behavior and risk taking (see Patient-Centered Teaching: Sexually Transmissible Infections box).

Neonates are at risk for transplacental transmission of STIs from an infected mother or from direct contamination during the birthing process. Sexual abuse should be suspected in children who acquire STIs after the neonatal period (see Chapter 29).

Chlamydial Infection

Causative agents:	*Chlamydia trachomatis, Chlamydophila psittaci, Chlamydophila pneumoniae*
Incubation period:	7 to 21 days
Transmission:	During birth if mother is infected; through sexual activity

Chlamydial infections are the most prevalent STIs in the United States. *Chlamydia* affects up to 20% of sexually active adolescents and young adults (AAP, 2009b). Therefore, the CDC recommends screening all sexually active females under the age of 26 (CDC, 2009d). Infants are infected during the birthing process. Half of all infants born vaginally to infected mothers will develop the disease. Chlamydial infection can cause morbidity in the infant and is responsible for neonatal eye infections and interstitial pneumonia.

Manifestations

Many people with a chlamydial infection have few or no symptoms. As a result, the disease may go undiagnosed until complications develop.

Neonatal conjunctivitis develops anywhere from a few days to several weeks after birth and manifests with a watery discharge that

---

PATIENT-CENTERED TEACHING
Sexually Transmissible Infections

- STIs are infections that can be transmitted through body fluids (semen, vaginal fluids, blood) and contact with infected mucous membranes (mouth, vagina, anus).
- Not all STIs have symptoms. Many people with chlamydia (an STI) do not have any symptoms. Transmission of an STI that you do not know you have to someone else is possible.
- STIs can be painful, ugly, and dangerous to those who have them. Some can even cause sterility, neurologic (brain) damage, cancer, or death.
- STIs can infect anyone, regardless of race, religion, sexual preference, social status, or gender.
- Because many STIs can be transmitted through sexual intercourse, through oral sex, and skin-to-skin contact, even the most careful individuals can be susceptible to infections.
- Some STIs, such as gonorrhea, chlamydia, and syphilis, can be cured fairly easily by completing a course of medication. Others, such as herpes, genital warts, and human immunodeficiency virus (HIV), cannot be cured, although some treatments are available to reduce their symptoms.
- Abstinence is the only 100% effective way to prevent both pregnancy and STI transmission.
- Abstinence means never engaging in any form of sexual contact with a partner.
- Deciding if and when to have sex is an important issue to think about.
- No one should ever be pressured to have sex.
- If you choose to have sex, a male or female condom can reduce (not eliminate) your chances of acquiring or passing on an STI.
- Some symptoms that might mean you have an STI are unusual discharge, swelling, pain, sores, or a rash in your genital area; unusual nonmenstrual bleeding; pain when you urinate or have a bowel movement; or a sore throat for several weeks.
- If you are sexually active and note any of these symptoms, see your primary health care provider as soon as possible. Detecting and treating an STI early will decrease the chances of permanent damage.

---

becomes purulent. Eyelids are edematous, and the conjunctiva may become inflamed. Mucoid rhinorrhea may be associated with the infection. Many infants with conjunctivitis will develop infection of the nasopharynx, which can progress to pneumonia. These infants may have a history of a cough and congestion. Long-term abnormalities of pulmonary function may result in chronic respiratory problems.

Urethritis with dysuria, urinary frequency, or mucopurulent discharge may indicate chlamydial infection. Any identification of this organism in young children indicates possible sexual abuse.

Therapeutic Management

In infants with conjunctivitis or pneumonia, a 14-day course of oral erythromycin is recommended; for incomplete eradication, a subsequent course of erythromycin may be necessary. For uncomplicated genital tract infection, a single dose of azithromycin is effective for children and adolescents, and a 7-day course of doxycycline may also be used for older children (older than 8 years) and teenagers (AAP, 2009b). Follow-up for a repeat culture is indicated if symptoms persist, because reinfection is common.

It is important that the nurse counsel the patient about the need to treat all sexual partners contacted in the last 60 days and to abstain from sexual intercourse for 7 days and until all symptoms have resolved (Holland-Hall, 2008).

Gonorrhea

Causative agent:	*Neisseria gonorrhoeae* (gram-negative diplococcus)
Incubation period:	2 to 7 days
Transmission:	Intimate contact (perinatally, through sexual abuse, by sexual intercourse)

Gonorrhea may be transmitted three different ways:

Perinatally: Transmission can occur during birth of a neonate whose mother is infected or with premature rupture of the membranes. The neonate can acquire the disease through aspiration of vaginal secretions, which leads to sepsis; through direct contact through the conjunctiva; or through direct contact through attachment of a fetal scalp electrode.

Sexual abuse: Any child with a positive culture and without a prior history of voluntary sexual behavior should be considered a potential sexual abuse victim until proven otherwise. Transmission through sexual play with children has been documented but is rare. Almost all children diagnosed with gonorrhea at age 1 year or older have experienced sexual abuse.

Voluntary sexual activity: This route of transmission remains the primary route of infection among adolescents. Sexual abuse should not, however, be excluded as a possibility.

The United States Preventive Services Task Force (USPSTF) recommends screening even asymptomatic high-risk females.

Manifestations

Ophthalmia neonatorum is the most common type of gonorrheal infection in the infant, manifesting 1 to 4 days after birth. A thick, purulent discharge from the eyes may be present and, if not treated promptly, will progress to corneal ulceration, rupture, and blindness. Ophthalmia neonatorum has been controlled through prophylactic treatment with an ophthalmic antibiotic given immediately after birth. In older children, ophthalmic infection can be the result of self-inoculation from the genital site.

Girls with gonorrheal infection may have a purulent vulvovaginitis, whereas boys often have urethritis. A history of purulent discharge with burning during urination is often elicited. Adolescent girls may exhibit cervicitis, urethritis, perihepatitis, and salpingitis. One serious complication of gonorrhea is pelvic inflammatory disease (PID), which is an infection of the female upper genital tract. PID can lead to ectopic pregnancy, infertility, and chronic pelvic pain (Abatangelo, Okereke, Parham-Foster et al., 2010).

Therapeutic Management

Because hepatitis B, HIV, syphilis, and *Chlamydia* infection are also often present in individuals with gonorrhea, testing should take place for those diseases. Both penicillin and fluoroquinolones are no longer used as a treatment because of an increased incidence of resistance in the United States. Currently, cefixime, ceftriaxone, and cefotaxime for newborns are recommended. Patients should also be treated with azithromycin or doxycycline for presumed *Chlamydia* infection. Adolescents co-infected with syphilis are treated appropriately as well. Sexual partners should be treated.

Herpes Simplex Virus

Causative agent:	Herpes simplex virus, type 2 (see Chapter 25)
Incubation period:	2 to 14 days
Transmission:	Direct sexual contact with an infected person

Herpes simplex virus (HSV), type 2, is the predominant cause of genital herpes infection. Genital herpes is one of the most frequently seen STIs in the United States. It is especially problematic because an infected mother can transmit it to her newborn during vaginal delivery, causing multisystem disease. Women with active HSV infection may be advised to have a cesarean delivery as labor and delivery approach.

Manifestations

At the initial infection, lesions occur in the genital area, usually on the vulva, perineum, or perianal area. However, lesions may also occur in the vagina and on the cervix, areas where they cannot be seen. Pain and tenderness in the affected area may coincide with lesion eruption. Vesicles erupt, rupture, and then ulcerate over the course of 1 to 7 days. The virus is shed for 2 to 3 weeks. Occasionally, flulike symptoms (fever, malaise, dysuria, enlarged lymph nodes) can accompany vesicular eruption. After the acute phase has passed, the virus can remain dormant in the nerve ganglia, where it can reappear later in response to stressful triggers.

Therapeutic Management

Viral culture from vesicular fluid can confirm the diagnosis. There is no cure for HSV 2, but administration of acyclovir (Zovirax) can diminish symptoms and reduce shedding time. Infected neonates are treated with parenteral acyclovir; those with ocular involvement receive a topical ophthalmic drug as well. Adolescents are treated for 7 to 10 days with oral acyclovir, valacyclovir, or famciclovir. Infected individuals should refrain from all sexual contact until the lesions have healed completely. Because shedding time in an initial infection is prolonged, abstinence is recommended for several weeks. Current research shows that patients diagnosed with HSV are at significant risk for acquiring HIV (CDC, 2010b).

> **? CRITICAL THINKING EXERCISE 17-1**
>
> Adolescents with an STI may seek out school- or community-based health care. Their symptoms may be vague, with generalized feelings of malaise or fever; or specific, with reports of painful urination or vaginal or penile discharge. Often they hope that the nurse will ask about sexual activity because they feel they cannot trust other adults. What challenges does the nurse face when caring for these adolescents?

Human Papillomavirus

Causative agent:	Human papillomavirus (HPV); there are in excess of 130 types
Incubation period:	4 weeks to many months
Transmission:	Direct sexual contact, perinatal contact during delivery

Human papillomavirus is responsible for the common wart and for genital warts (condylomata acuminata). Anogenital warts may be contracted primarily through direct sexual contact, and having multiple sex partners increases the risk. Children with anogenital warts should be investigated for sexual abuse. A person can get common warts through autoinoculation from other body sites. A break in skin integrity is necessary for infection to occur. Genital HPV infection has become endemic in the United States. The CDC estimates that at least half of all sexually active women will develop HPV, with adolescence through young adulthood being the period of greatest risk (Alexander, Dempsey, Gillison, & Palefsky, 2010b).

Manifestations

Anogenital warts begin as small papules that grow into soft, clustered lesions. They are found in moist areas, such as the labia minora, vagina, cervix, anus, rectum, and glans penis. Common warts are frequently found on fingers, palms of the hands, and soles of the feet. Most common warts in children resolve within several years. Adolescents usually clear low-risk types in 4 to 5 months and high-risk types in 8 to 10 months, but warts may persist longer.

HPV types such as HPV-6 and HPV-11 are associated with genital warts and do not cause cancer. Of the more than 130 types, approximately 35 have been associated with neoplastic lesions. HPV-16 and HPV-18 cause approximately 70% of cervical cancers (Alexander et al., 2010b).

Therapeutic Management

In many instances, genital warts resolve spontaneously. Treatment, which is often difficult, can include topical gels or creams such as imiquimod, cryotherapy, electrocautery, laser treatment, and various types of surgical removal. For sexually active individuals, transmission can be decreased by the use of condoms. Screening for cervical cancer with a Papanicolaou (Pap) test can detect cervical cancer in an early form and prevent progression to cervical cancer. The CDC (2010a) recommends that women have yearly Pap tests starting at age 21 or 3 years after their first sexual encounter, whichever occurs first.

There are two licensed vaccines against HPV in the United States. In 2006, the quadrivalent HPV-6/11/16/18 vaccine (Gardasil, Merck) was approved by the FDA for females and males ages 9 to 26. More recently, in 2009, a bivalent vaccine (Cervarix, GlaxoSmithKline) against HPV-16 and HPV-18 was approved for females ages 10 to 25. The CDC's Advisory Committee on Immunization Practice recommends that females ages 11 to 12 be immunized with either the quadrivalent or bivalent vaccine. Both vaccinations are given in a three-dose series (Alexander, Dempsey, Gillison, & Palefsky, 2010a). Newly issued guidelines (Friedman, Bell, Kahn et al., 2011) recommend that adolescent males be routinely considered for quadrivalent vaccine to prevent genital warts, and that the cost for the immunization be covered by Medicaid and the Vaccines for Children program.

Bacterial Vaginosis

Causative agent:	Specific cause is not clearly identified; however, the normal vaginal flora is replaced by an overgrowth of organisms such as *Gardnerella vaginalis, Mycoplasma hominis,* or anaerobic bacteria; a corresponding decrease in the concentration of lactobacilli occurs (AAP, 2009a)
Incubation period:	Unknown
Transmission:	Presumed to be transmitted through sexual contact because it is uncommon in females who are not sexually active

Bacterial vaginosis can occur alone or concurrently with infections that result in vaginal discharge, such as trichomoniasis, and it is a common diagnosis in adolescent girls who are sexually active.

Manifestations

Bacterial vaginosis is characterized by a profuse, white, malodorous (having a fishy smell) vaginal discharge that sticks to the vaginal walls.

Bacterial vaginosis may be asymptomatic and is not usually associated with abdominal pain, skin rashes, itching, or painful urination. Because other STIs may occur simultaneously, sexually active adolescents with bacterial vaginosis should be tested for coexisting STIs. Bacterial vaginosis is a risk factor for pelvic inflammatory disease.

Bacterial vaginosis in a prepubertal girl is commonly caused by poor hygiene, a vaginal foreign body, or other infections.

Syphilis

Causative agent:	*Treponema pallidum*
Incubation period:	Acquired primary infection: 10 to 90 days (average 21 days)
Transmission:	Intimate contact, transplacentally, or sexually

Congenital syphilis can be transmitted transplacentally by an infected mother at any time during pregnancy or birth. Acquired syphilis is contracted through sexual contact. In children, syphilis diagnosed after the neonatal period can almost always be linked to sexual abuse.

Manifestations

If untreated during pregnancy, congenital syphilis can cause stillbirth or neonatal death. Infants with congenital syphilis may be asymptomatic or may exhibit signs and symptoms within the first 3 months of life. The classic signs are rhinitis, a maculopapular rash, and hepatosplenomegaly. Diagnostic radiographs may show osteochondritis, periosteitis, or metaphyseal changes, especially in the long bones of the femur and humerus. Late manifestations are a result of the scarring from the systemic disease process. The bones, teeth, eyes, and eighth cranial nerve are involved. The teeth are notched (Hutchinson's teeth), and hearing loss can occur suddenly at approximately 8 to 10 years of age. Acquired syphilis is divided into three stages and has the same clinical course in children as in adults. The primary stage is characterized by one or more painless ulcers which heal spontaneously. One to 2 months later in the secondary stage there is a generalized rash that includes the palms and soles. The final stage is latent syphilis, in which there are no clinical manifestations (AAP, 2009d).

Therapeutic Management

Syphilis responds well to a single dose of benzathine penicillin G intramuscularly (the preferred treatment for children and adults). Aqueous crystalline penicillin G or procaine penicillin is effective with congenital syphilis. Acquired syphilis can be treated with benzathine penicillin G. Tetracycline and doxycycline for 14 days are options for the child older than 8 years but should not be used in younger children because of the greater risk of permanent tooth staining. In addition, the effectiveness of drugs other than penicillin and tetracycline remains unproven. When follow-up cannot be guaranteed, particularly for penicillin-allergic children younger than 8 years, skin testing for penicillin allergy can be considered (AAP, 2009d).

Education regarding potential long-term effects of partially or untreated syphilis must be discussed. Resources should be available and care should be accessible to ensure completion of treatment and eradication of disease.

Trichomoniasis

Causative agent:	*Trichomonas vaginalis* (flagellated protozoan)
Incubation period:	5 to 28 days (average of 1 week)
Transmission:	Perinatal contact during delivery, sexual activity

Manifestations

Infections with *Trichomonas* are frequently asymptomatic. Only up to 50% of females with trichomoniasis will exhibit symptoms. Most males with the infection are asymptomatic. When symptoms occur, they may include dysuria, vaginal itching and burning (in females), and a frothy, yellowish green, foul-smelling discharge. Infected mothers can transmit the disease to their newborn infants during birth. Children with a positive culture for *Trichomonas* should be investigated for possible sexual abuse.

Therapeutic Management

A single dose of metronidazole (Flagyl, Protostat) or tinidazole is the treatment of choice for adolescents; they have an approximate cure rate of 90% to 95%. For prepubertal girls, metronidazole is given in two or three divided doses. Sexual partners should also be treated, and patients are counseled to avoid sexual contact until they and their partners are asymptomatic.

Education regarding the potential presence of other STIs should be thoroughly discussed, especially with the adolescent client, in a respectful and confidential manner.

Bacterial vaginosis responds well to oral metronidazole or to vaginal gels and creams (5- and 7-day administration schedules). Use of clindamycin cream, which is oil based, may alter the effectiveness of latex condoms for at least 72 hours after the last application (AAP, 2009a). Male partners do not need to be treated, but patients should be aware of the risk of recurrence.

Nursing Considerations

Prevention, early identification, and treatment are the goals of nursing care associated with any STI. The nurse plays a key role in educating

---

EVIDENCE-BASED PRACTICE

To Vaccinate or Not

HPV is one of the most frequently seen STIs in the United States, with one quarter of 14- to 19-year-olds acquiring HPV. Though some cases of HPV are asymptomatic, many can cause genital warts or lead to several different types of cancer later in life. With the licensing of two HPV vaccinations, pediatric primary care providers are able to prevent not only genital warts and the painful procedures used to treat them, but also certain types of cancer, such as cervical, vaginal, anal, and penile cancers, as well as those of the head and neck.

The U.S. FDA approved the first quadrivalent vaccination in June 2006 and a second, bivalent vaccine in October 2009. Recent data from the CDC (2010) show that only 44.3% of adolescent females had started the three-dose series and a mere 26.7% of female adolescents completed the vaccination series. These statistics demonstrate that adolescents and their parents are frequently not following the CDC's Advisory Committee on Immunization Practices (ACIP) recommendation for routine vaccination of females ages 11 to 12 with catch-up vaccination for those 13 through 26 years.

There are many arguments both for and against HPV vaccination of children; providers are in a position to assist parents in making an informed decision by educating them on HPV and the HPV vaccination.

Many parents report that they receive information regarding the HPV vaccination through the TV, news, and the Internet. Often these sources provide erroneous information, especially concerning adverse side effects, which can lead to declining HPV vaccination rates. The concern regarding the safety of the vaccine is very important in parents' decision whether or not to vaccinate their child.

Rivera Medina et al. (2010) completed a blind, randomized controlled study (Level II evidence) that examined the safety of the HPV bivalent vaccine. Two thousand twenty-seven girls from several different countries, ages 10 to 13 years, were randomly assigned to an experimental (HPV vaccine) or control (hepatitis A vaccine) group and were followed for 1 year after vaccine administration. Researchers documented information about mild and serious (new chronic diseases or significant adverse events that required a visit to an emergency department or physician) effects related to the vaccines. Both groups reported mild local or systemic reactions; only the control group had one serious event (UTI) considered to be directly related to the vaccine. Their research supported other studies that concluded the vaccine is safe for this population (Rivera Medina et al., 2010).

Another parentally perceived barrier to receiving the HPV vaccination is the cost ($360 for the three-dose series) and whether it will be covered by their health insurance carrier. The cost is covered by Medicaid and those eligible for the Vaccines for Children program.

There are, however, persuasive arguments for vaccinating children against HPV. First and foremost is the protection against HPV-related cancers. Both vaccinations are 100% effective against the HPV types included in the vaccine. With high immunization rates, there will be a significant decrease in morbidity and mortality. Approximately 3700 women in the United States die each year from cervical cancer alone (Alexander, Dempsey, Gillison, & Palefsky, 2010b). Recent economic studies show that there is a significant savings related to health care costs. Despite parental concerns that the vaccine will promote sexual activity in adolescents, data show that a significant number of high school students already report having sexual intercourse (Vamos, McDermott, & Daley, 2008), despite various approaches to sex education.

Pediatric primary care providers bear the responsibility for educating parents and adolescents by providing accurate, up-to-date information. Several studies have indicated that the most important reason parents cite when deciding whether to vaccinate their daughters is a health care provider's recommendation. As a health care provider, you will need to decide when is the appropriate time to vaccinate patients and to have productive conversations about their sexuality and the importance of safe sex.

When providing evidence-based information to parents and their children, think about what you would recommend:

If a parent asks you about the HPV vaccination, what information would you provide?

Would you recommend the vaccination to children and adolescents ages 9 through 26?

Alexander, K., Dempsey, A., Gillison, M., & Palefsky, J. (2010b). The disease burden of HPV. *Infectious Diseases in Children*, 4-11. Vindico Medication Educations.

Centers for Disease Control and Prevention. (2010). National, state, and local area vaccination coverage among adolescents 13-17 years: U.S., 2009. *MMWR Morbidity and Mortality Weekly Report, 59*(32), 1018-1023.

Rivera Medina, D., Valencia, A., de Velasquez, A., et al. (2010). Safety and immunogenicity of the HPV-16/18 AS04-adjuvanted vaccine: A randomized, controlled trial in adolescent girls. *Journal of Adolescent Health, 46*, 414-421.

Vamos, C., McDermott, R., & Daley, E. (2008). The HPV vaccine: Framing arguments for and against mandatory vaccination of all middle school girls [Electronic version]. *Journal of School Health, 78*(6), 302-309.

young people about STIs. Often, the school nurse is the health care professional whom adolescents feel they can trust; therefore, school nurses may be the care providers in the best position to educate this population. Establishing rapport with the teenager by using a nonjudgmental approach and reassurance of confidentiality is key. The nurse must be aware of symptoms and assist in identifying those adolescents who are at risk for STIs. Encouraging abstinence in those who are not sexually active and condom use in sexually active adolescents is a way to prevent STIs. The nurse may be the one to assume responsibility for helping the adolescent obtain proper medical treatment and gain an understanding of the importance of completing the entire course of medication, as well as treatment of partners.

An issue that has become increasingly concerning is the number of young adolescents who practice oral sex. Research on this subject suggests that approximately 7% of young adolescents have been either active or passive participants in oral sex, and many of these teens do not understand or believe that they are at risk for STIs from this behavior. Many adolescents report earlier initiation of oral sex as compared to vaginal sex (Markham, Peskin, Addy et al., 2009). Health providers need to assess adolescents for oral sex participation and provide appropriate information about the risks involved in the same way information is provided about vaginal sex.

KEY CONCEPTS

- Infectious diseases can be transmitted by direct contact with another infected person, by contact with animal or insect carriers, by ingestion of contaminated food or water containing the pathogens, and by contact with a contaminated object.
- Vaccines can be live or attenuated, killed or inactivated toxoids, human immune globulin, or animal serums or antitoxins.
- Assessment of the child with an infectious disease includes a thorough history (recent exposure, other family members or friends exhibiting signs or symptoms, environmental causes) and documentation of the type, configuration, and distribution of any

lesions; the child's temperature; and any associated signs and symptoms.
- Children with infectious diseases usually can and should be cared for at home.
- STIs can be transmitted to neonates from exposure to organisms during delivery, but children who acquire an STI after the neonatal period should always be evaluated for possible sexual abuse.
- Abstinence is the only 100% effective way to prevent both pregnancy and STI transmission. Sexually active individuals need to use barrier protection to prevent STIs.

REFERENCES

Abatangelo, L., Okereke, L., Parham-Foster, C., et al. (2010). If pelvic inflammatory disease is suspected empiric treatment should be initiated. *Journal of the American Academy of Nurse Practitioners, 22,* 117-122.

Alexander, K., Dempsey, A., Gillison, M., & Palefsky, J. (2010a). HPV vaccines. *Infectious Diseases in Children,* 14-19.

Alexander, K., Dempsey, A., Gillison, M., & Palefsky, J. (2010b). The disease burden of HPV. *Infectious Diseases in Children,* 4-11.

American Academy of Pediatrics. (2009a). Bacterial vaginosis. In L. K. Pickering, C. J. Baker, D. W. Kimberlin, & S. Long (Eds.), *Red Book 2009 report of the Committee on Infectious Diseases* (28th ed.). Elk Grove Village, IL: Author.

American Academy of Pediatrics. (2009b).*Chlamydia trachomatis.* In L. K. Pickering, C. J. Baker, D. W. Kimberlin, & S. Long (Eds.), *Red Book 2009 report of the Committee on Infectious Diseases* (28th ed., pp. 255-259). Elk Grove Village, IL: Author.

American Academy of Pediatrics. (2009c). *Clostridium difficile.* In L. K. Pickering, C. J. Baker, D. W. Kimberlin, & S. Long (Eds.), *Red Book 2009 report of the Committee on Infectious Diseases* (28th ed., pp. 263-265). Elk Grove Village, IL: Author.

American Academy of Pediatrics. (2009d). Syphilis. In L. K. Pickering, C. J. Baker, D. W. Kimberlin, & S. Long (Eds.), *Red Book 2009 report of the Committee on Infectious Diseases* (28th ed., pp. 638-651). Elk Grove Village, IL: Author.

Bateman, S., & Seed, P. (2010). Procession to pediatric bacteremia and sepsis: Covert operations and failures in diplomacy. *Pediatrics, 126,* 137-150.

Bell, E. (2010). Changing *C. difficile*–associated disease. *Infectious Diseases in Children, 23,* 6-9.

Centers for Disease Control and Prevention. (2007). *Lyme disease.* Retrieved from www.cdc.gov/ncidod/dvbid/lyme/index.htm.

Centers for Disease Control and Prevention. (2008a). *Catch-up immunization schedule for persons aged 4*

months-18 years who start late or who are more than 1 month behind. Retrieved from www.cdc.gov.

Centers for Disease Control and Prevention. (2008b). *Rocky Mountain spotted fever: statistics.* Retrieved from www.cdc.gov/ticks/diseases/rocky_mountain_spotted_fever/statistics.html.

Centers for Disease Control and Prevention. (2008c). *Tickborne relapsing fever.* Retrieved from www.cdc.gov/ncidod/dvbid/RelapsingFever/index.html.

Centers for Disease Control and Prevention. (2009a). *Lyme disease.* Retrieved from www.cdc.gov/niosh/topics/lyme.

Centers for Disease Control and Prevention. (2009b). *Overview of measles disease.* Retrieved from www.cdc.gov/measles/about/overview.html.

Centers for Disease Control and Prevention. (2009c). *Questions and answers about infection control and isolation of smallpox patients.* Retrieved from www.cdc.gov.

Centers for Disease Control and Prevention. (2009d). *Sexually transmitted diseases surveillance, 2008.* Retrieved from http://cdc.gov/std/stats08/chalamydia.htm.

Centers for Disease Control and Prevention. (2010a). *Cervical cancer screening guidelines.* Retrieved from www.cdc.gov/cancer/cervical/guidelines.htm.

Centers for Disease Control and Prevention. (2010b). *Genital herpes: CDC fact sheet.* Retrieved from www.cdc.gov/std/Herpes/STDFact-Herpes.htm.

Centers for Disease Control and Prevention. (2010c). Pertussis: prevention. Retrieved from www.cdc.gov/pertussis/about/prevention.html.

Centers for Disease Control and Prevention. (2010d). Summary of notifiable diseases—United States, 2008. *MMWR Morbidity and Mortality Weekly Report, 57*(54), 1-94.

Cherry, J. (2009a). Borrelia. In R. Fegin, J. Cherry, G. Demmler-Harrison, & S. Kaplan (Eds.), *Textbook of pediatric infectious diseases* (6th ed.). Philadelphia: Elsevier.

Cherry, J. (2009b). Enteroviruses and parechoviruses. In R. Fegin, J. Cherry, G. Demmler-Harrison, & S. Kaplan (Eds.), *Textbook of pediatric infectious diseases* (6th ed.). Philadelphia: Elsevier.

Cherry, J. (2009c). Measles virus. In R. Fegin, J. Cherry, G. Demmler-Harrison, & S. Kaplan (Eds.), *Textbook of pediatric infectious diseases* (6th ed.). Philadelphia: Elsevier.

Cherry, J. (2009d). Perinatal bacterial diseases. In R. Fegin, J. Cherry, G. Demmler-Harrison, & S. Kaplan (Eds.), *Textbook of pediatric infectious diseases* (6th ed.). Philadelphia: Elsevier.

Cherry, J. (2009e). Pertussis and other *Bordetella* infections. In R. Fegin, J. Cherry, G. Demmler-Harrison, & S. Kaplan (Eds.), *Textbook of pediatric infectious diseases* (6th ed.). Philadelphia: Elsevier.

Cherry, J. (2009f). Rickettsial and ehrlichial diseases. In R. Fegin, J. Cherry, G. Demmler-Harrison, & S. Kaplan (Eds.), *Textbook of pediatric infectious diseases* (6th ed.). Philadelphia: Elsevier.

Cherry, J. (2009g). Rubella virus. In R. Fegin, J. Cherry, G. Demmler-Harrison, & S. Kaplan (Eds.), *Textbook of pediatric infectious diseases* (6th ed.). Philadelphia: Elsevier.

Cherry, J. (2009h). Varicella-zoster disease. In R. Fegin, J. Cherry, G. Demmler-Harrison, & S. Kaplan (Eds.), *Textbook of pediatric infectious diseases* (6th ed.). Philadelphia: Elsevier.

Czaja, A., Zimmerman, J., & Nathens, A. (2009). Readmission and late mortality after pediatric severe sepsis. *Pediatrics, 123,* 849-857.

Dickens, K., Nye, A., & Rickett, K. (2008). Should you use steroids to treat infectious mononucleosis? *Journal of Family Practice, 57,* 754-755.

Duncan, D. (2008). Recognizing slapped cheek syndrome. *Practice Nursing, 9,* 436-438.

Eppes, S. (2011). Lyme disease (*Borrelia burgdorferi*). In R. Kliegman, B. Stanton, J. St. Geme, et al. (Eds.), *Nelson textbook of pediatrics* (19th ed., pp. 1025-1029). Philadelphia: Elsevier Saunders.

Freed, G. (2009) Then and now: Varicella vaccine [Electronic version]. *Contemporary Pediatrics, 26,* 28-29.

Friedman, L., Bell, D., Kahn, J., et al. (2011). Human papillomavirus vaccine: An updated position statement of the Society for Adolescent Health and Medicine. *Journal of Adolescent Health, 48,* 215-216.

Hinckley, J., & Allen, P. (2008). Community-associated MRSA in the pediatric primary care setting. *Pediatric Nursing, 34*, 64-71.

Holland-Hall, C. (2008). Sexually transmitted infections in teens. *Contemporary Pediatrics, 25*, 56-65.

Jancin, B. (2010). Majority of MRSA is now community acquired. *Infectious Diseases in Children, 23*, 7.

Klein, N., Fireman, B., Yih, W., et al. (2010). Measles-mumps-rubella-varicella combination vaccine and the risk of febrile seizures [Electronic version]. *Pediatrics, 126*, e1-e8.

Liu, C., Bayer, A., Cosgrove, S. E., et al. (2011). Clinical practice guidelines by the Infectious Disease Society of America for the treatment of methicillin-resistant *Staphylococcus aureus* infections in adults and children: Executive summary. *Clinical Infectious Diseases, 52*(3), 285-292.

Markham, C., Peskin, M., Addy, R., et al. (2009). Patterns of vaginal, oral, and anal sexual intercourse in urban seventh-grade population. *Journal of School Health, 79*, 193-200.

Martin, M., Güris, D., Chaves, S. S., et al. & Advisory Committee on Immunization Practices, Centers for Disease Control and Prevention (CDC). (2007). Prevention of varicella: Recommendations of the Advisory Committee on Immunization Practices (ACIP). *MMWR Morbidity and Mortality Weekly Report, 56*(RR4), 1-40.

Schmitt, B. (2010). *Hand-foot-mouth disease.* Retrieved from www.healthychildren.org.

Shelov, S. (2010). *Roseola infantum.* Retrieved from www.healthychildren.org.

So, T., & Farrington, E. (2008). Community-acquired methicillin-resistant *Staphylococcus aureus* infection in the pediatric population. *Journal of Pediatric Health Care, 22*(4), 211-217.

Stowell, J., Forlin-Passoni, D., & Cannon, M. (2010). Congenital cytomegalovirus: An update [Electronic version]. *Contemporary Pediatrics, 27*, 38-51.

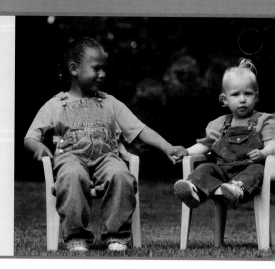

evolve WEBSITE

http://evolve.elsevier.com/James/ncoc

LEARNING OBJECTIVES

After studying this chapter, you should be able to:

- Describe how the immune system attempts to maintain homeostasis of the internal and external environment and what happens when it overfunctions or underfunctions.
- Explain how neonates acquire active and passive immunity.
- Delineate how to prevent the spread of organisms in children with an immune deficiency.

- Describe how to prevent, test for, care for, and support children with human immunodeficiency virus and their families throughout the entire spectrum of illness.
- Outline critical information needed by families with children receiving long-term corticosteroid therapy.
- Describe nursing interventions to help prevent the sudden death of a child having an anaphylactic reaction.

CLINICAL REFERENCE

REVIEW OF THE IMMUNE SYSTEM

The body's network of first-line, or external, defenses—intact skin and mucous membranes and processes such as sneezing, coughing, and tearing—helps keep it free of disease. When a foreign substance penetrates first-line defenses, the immune (lymphoreticular) system, or internal defense system, provides secondary and tertiary protection through nonspecific and specific responses. The immune system is able to distinguish the body's own cells, or self, from foreign substances, or nonself; activate a response to detect and destroy foreign substances; suppress a response against the self; and memorize and store information.

Foreign substances, or antigens, possess unique configurations on their cell surfaces that mark them as foreign. The immune system first responds to the invader through nonspecific immune functions. If the antigen survives the action of the nonspecific response, the immune system initiates specific immune functions. It begins producing proteins called antibodies or immunoglobulins. Each antibody is specific for a particular antigen, contains sites that are complementary, and can combine, or bind, with the antigen. This combination of antigen and antibody is called the antigen-antibody complex or immune complex.

The immune complex prevents the antigen from binding with receptors on vulnerable cells.

The major organs and tissues of the immune system include the bone marrow, thymus, spleen, lymph nodes, and lymphoid tissue. Both the circulatory system and the lymphatic system connect these organs and tissues to one another. Specific types of cells are also important to the immune system.

Nonspecific Immune Functions

The body's innate immune system consists of nonspecific immune functions, which are protective barriers activated in the presence of an antigen but not specific to that antigen. Among these nonspecific immune functions are chemical barriers, such as bactericides and fungicides and enzymes in body secretions; interferon, a protein produced in response to viruses; and inflammation, increased capillary permeability, vasodilation, phagocytosis (cell eating), and elimination of cell products.

During an inflammatory response, vasodilation of small capillaries at the site of the organism invasion increases the circulation to the site. The resulting alteration in microvascular pressure facilitates movement of plasma cells into tissue, where they accumulate. Neutrophils

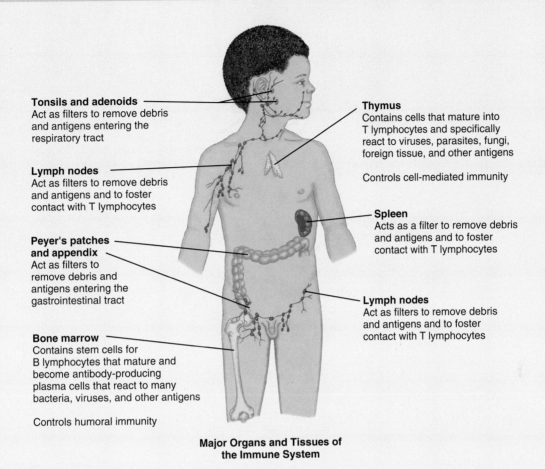

Tonsils and adenoids
Act as filters to remove debris and antigens entering the respiratory tract

Lymph nodes
Act as filters to remove debris and antigens and to foster contact with T lymphocytes

Peyer's patches and appendix
Act as filters to remove debris and antigens entering the gastrointestinal tract

Bone marrow
Contains stem cells for B lymphocytes that mature and become antibody-producing plasma cells that react to many bacteria, viruses, and other antigens

Controls humoral immunity

Thymus
Contains cells that mature into T lymphocytes and specifically react to viruses, parasites, fungi, foreign tissue, and other antigens

Controls cell-mediated immunity

Spleen
Acts as a filter to remove debris and antigens and to foster contact with T lymphocytes

Lymph nodes
Act as filters to remove debris and antigens and to foster contact with T lymphocytes

Major Organs and Tissues of the Immune System

are the first phagocytes that arrive at the site. Complement is a series of serum proteins involved in enzyme action and antigen death. Antigens activate the complement system, and this system acts as an inflammation stimulator to attract neutrophils to the site. Complement also promotes the increase in circulation and vascular permeability involved with the inflammatory response (Porth, 2011).

Phagocytosis can occur alone or as part of the inflammatory response. Phagocytes ingest the antigen and either survive or die. In dying, the phagocytes release additional chemicals that draw more phagocytes to the area.

Increased capillary permeability and vasodilation result in redness and edema. The products of phagocyte antigen death include toxins that give rise to fever, pain, and purulence. As the antigens are destroyed, the toxins are cleared from the lymph nodes, which often become enlarged. If the immune response is effective, the inflammation subsides.

Specific Immune Functions

If the antigen survives within the phagocyte, two types of specific immune functions can recognize and destroy it: humoral and cell mediated. Both responses are closely related.

Lymphocytes, which are a subclassification of leukocytes (white blood cells), function in both types of immune response. Lymphocytes circulate in the blood and the lymphatic system. They make up 53% to 57% of white blood cells during the first year of life, when specific immunity develops rapidly, but they make up only 25% to 30% after 12 months of age. Two classes of lymphocytes are involved in the immune response: B lymphocytes (B cells) and T lymphocytes (T cells).

B cells, which promote the humoral response, originate in the bone marrow or liver but mature in the lymphoid tissue, becoming plasma cells. When exposed to antigens, some of the plasma cells produce antibodies, whereas others become memory cells. Antibodies are classified as immunoglobulins G, M, A, D, and E, often abbreviated IgG, IgM, IgA, IgD, and IgE. Immunoglobulins bind to antigens and facilitate their destruction.

T cells, which are responsible for the cell-mediated response, originate in the bone marrow and mature in the thymus, where they react specifically to viruses, fungi, parasites, foreign tissue, and other antigens. The three major types of T cells are helper T cells, cytotoxic T cells, and regulatory T cells.

Natural killer cells, or large granular lymphocytes that resemble T lymphocytes, can recognize and directly destroy infected or malignant cells. They are not antigen-specific cells (Buckley, 2007).

The Humoral Response

The humoral response involves chiefly B cells, although the cooperation of helper T cells is almost always necessary. Macrophages ingest antigens and introduce them into the circulation. In response, the B cells and helper T cells interact. The helper T cells secrete substances that cause B cells to multiply and differentiate into plasma cells, which produce vast quantities of antibodies specific to the antigen. These antibodies combine with the antigens to form immune complexes. The antibodies promote phagocytosis and destroy the antigens. Destruction and elimination of antigens eventually result in a decrease in the chemical factors that enhance the humoral response, "turning off" the response when it is no longer needed (Porth, 2011).

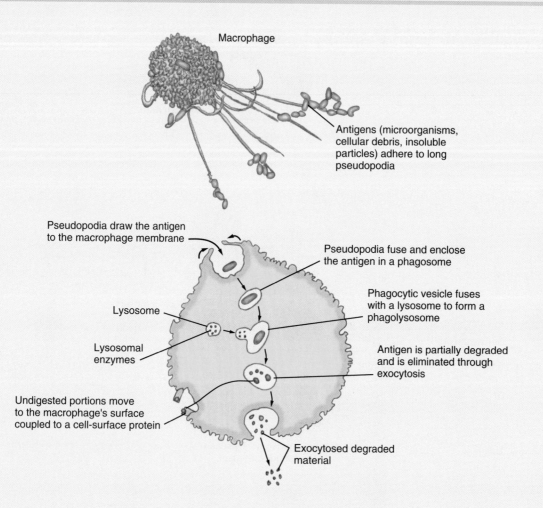

Macrophage

Antigens (microorganisms, cellular debris, insoluble particles) adhere to long pseudopodia

Pseudopodia draw the antigen to the macrophage membrane

Pseudopodia fuse and enclose the antigen in a phagosome

Lysosome

Phagocytic vesicle fuses with a lysosome to form a phagolysosome

Lysosomal enzymes

Antigen is partially degraded and is eliminated through exocytosis

Undigested portions move to the macrophage's surface coupled to a cell-surface protein

Exocytosed degraded material

CELLS INVOLVED IN THE IMMUNE RESPONSE

CELL TYPE	NONSPECIFIC IMMUNE RESPONSE (INNATE IMMUNITY)
Granulocytes	
Neutrophils	First leukocytes to respond to tissue damage. Ingest and destroy antigens, especially bacteria, by phagocytosis. Increase in number during acute inflammation, bacterial infection, and necrosis. Immature neutrophils are called bands. Increased bands (shift to the left) indicate infection.
Eosinophils	Help control the inflammatory response. Neutralize histamine. Increase in number during hypersensitivity reactions and kill parasites directly.
Basophils	Secrete histamine, heparin, and serotonin in inflammation and immediate hypersensitivity reactions. Basophils located in tissue rather than in blood are called mast cells, which activate the inflammatory allergic response.
Agranulocytes	
Monocytes/macrophages	Monocytes, immature macrophages, are large phagocytic agranulocytes. Monocytes ingest and introduce antigens into the circulation for recognition by B and T lymphocytes. Macrophages engulf bacteria and cellular debris to finish the cleanup process started by the neutrophils.
Natural killer (NK)	Recognize and directly kill viruses, tumor cells, and other abnormal cells

Data from Banasik, J. (2005). Inflammation and immunity. In L. Copstead & J. Banasik (Eds.), *Pathophysiology* (3rd ed., pp. 203-243). St. Louis: Elsevier Saunders; Porth, C. (2011). *Essentials of pathophysiology* (3rd ed., pp. 321-341). Philadelphia: Wolters Kluwer.

CELLS INVOLVED IN THE IMMUNE RESPONSE—cont'd

CELL TYPE	SPECIFIC IMMUNE RESPONSE (ADAPTIVE IMMUNITY)
B lymphocytes	Found primarily in lymphoid tissue. Noncirculating, short-lived cells responsible for humoral immunity. B lymphocytes contain receptor sites that recognize specific foreign substances. Differentiate into plasma cells capable of secreting antibodies against bacteria. First responder to viral infection. Some become memory cells for long-term recognition of specific antigens.
T lymphocytes	Mature in the thymus then migrate to lymphoid tissue. Responsible for cellular immunity. Interact with specific antigens on cell surfaces and directly attack invading microorganisms. Respond to viruses, fungi, parasites, and foreign tissue. T cell regulatory functions mobilize or deactivate the other cells in the immune system.
Helper (CD4+) T cells	Recognize antigens that have been processed and presented to them. CD4+ cells secrete cytokines that stimulate B cells to manufacture antibodies. Helper T cells facilitate function of most other cells in the immune system.
Regulatory T cells	Inhibit the immune response. Help keep the immune system cells in check.
Cytotoxic (CD8+) T cells	Kill target cells directly. Particularly effective with viruses and malignant cells.

PEDIATRIC DIFFERENCES IN THE IMMUNE SYSTEM

The Organs of the Immune System Mature during Infancy and Childhood

- Lymphoid tissue increases in mass during infancy and early childhood. It reaches adult size by 6 weeks of age, grows larger during the prepubertal years, and involutes at puberty.
- The thymus reaches its peak mass before puberty and then involutes.
- The spleen reaches its full size during adulthood.
- The number of Peyer's patches increases until the adult mean is exceeded during adolescence.

Immaturity of the Immunologic System Places the Infant and Young Child at Greater Risk for Infection

- The infant has a limited capacity to mount an antibody response. The ability to respond to infections develops gradually as the infant acquires immunity actively and passively.
- Because of the immaturity of the inflammatory response in neonates, the more common signs and symptoms of infection (e.g., fever) are less pronounced, making diagnosis more difficult.
- Neonates' diminished nonspecific immune response allows a more rapid spread of infection, leading potentially to sepsis.
- The term newborn infant receives an adult level of IgG as a result of transplacental transfer from the mother. This level begins to disappear during the first 6 to 8 months, causing a physiologic drop in IgG.
- Premature infants are more susceptible to neonatal infections because of lower levels of transplacental transfer of IgG from the mother and a more severe physiologic drop in IgG.

- IgM, IgE, and IgD are normally in low concentration at birth. IgM, IgE, IgA, and IgD do not cross the placenta. The immunoglobulins approach adult levels at different ages*:
  - *IgM:* 1 year
  - *IgA:* 6 to 7 years
  - *IgG:* 7 to 8 years
  - *IgE:* 6 to 7 years
- Absolute lymphocyte counts reach a peak during the first year. Helper T cells reach adult levels by 6 years of age.
- Passive placental transfer of IgG may affect infants' response to active immunization (i.e., pertussis or diphtheria).
- Immature or inexperienced immune cells affect the reliability of delayed hypersensitivity skin reactions. For this reason, allergy skin tests are not routinely used with infants.

Disorders of the Immune System Manifest Differently in Children than in Adults

- Primary immunodeficiencies typically manifest in the first 6 months of life.
- HIV infection, the major secondary immunodeficiency in children, typically (1) infects an infant through the mother, not sexually; (2) is diagnosed by measuring an aspect of the virus, not antibodies as in adults; and (3) has a shorter latency period in infants, with several different AIDS-defining illnesses.

*Buckley, R. (2007). The T-, B-, and NK-cell systems. In R. Kliegman, R. Behrman, H. Jenson, & B. Stanton (Eds.), *Nelson textbook of pediatrics* (18th ed., pp. 873-879). Philadelphia: Elsevier Saunders.

The Cell-Mediated Response

A cell-mediated response is initiated by macrophages presenting antigens to T lymphocytes. Once activated, helper T cells secrete substances that facilitate macrophages to destroy antigens as well as stimulate the production and circulation of additional macrophages. One set of T cells, called cytotoxic T cells, tracks down and kills viruses, tumor cells, and other pathogens directly. Regulatory T cells, interacting with other immune components, draw the immune response to a close (Porth, 2011).

Development of Immunity

By 8 weeks of gestational age, B cell differentiation begins. The normal fetus can produce IgM by 20 to 24 weeks of gestation. The neonate's immune protection comes from prenatal transfer of maternal antibodies (IgG) and breast milk transfer of IgA. Gradually, the normal newborn infant's own humoral and cell-mediated responses to infections begin; immunity is acquired both actively and passively.

Active Acquired Immunity

When the body reacts to an antigen through either a humoral or a cell-mediated response, it is developing active immunity. Active immunity is long lived and measured in months, years, or even a lifetime; it follows exposure to environmental antigens or vaccines. Immediately after exposure, there is a latency period when antibody levels are low. When the body recognizes the antigen as foreign, it makes antibodies. The first antibodies produced are predominantly IgM and subsequently IgG. After a second exposure to the antigen, antibodies appear at a faster rate, and the latency period is shortened or nonexistent. The antibody levels remain high and persist for much longer periods. The predominant antibody in a secondary response is IgG.

Infants receive specific live or attenuated vaccines on a recommended schedule to induce immunity against the antigens in the vaccine (see the recommended schedule at www.aap.org/immunization/izschedule.html).

Passive Acquired Immunity

Passive immunity results from antibody transfer from one person to another. Transfer of antibodies from a woman to her fetus is an example of passive immunity. The fetus receives maternal IgG antibodies across the placenta and becomes protected against many infections. Most maternal antibodies dissipate in the infant by 6 to 9 months of age, but some persist for up to 18 months. The duration depends on the level of a particular antibody in the maternal plasma. Protection against measles, for example, may last through the second year of life, whereas protection against certain bacterial infections may last only 1 to 2 months. The reason neonates are so susceptible to infections by bacteria such as *Escherichia coli* is that the respective antibodies do not cross the placenta.

Other sources of passive acquired immunity include administration of immune globulin to produce temporary protection after an exposure and certain other disease-specific antibodies (e.g., rabies).

COMMON LABORATORY AND DIAGNOSTIC TESTS OF IMMUNE FUNCTION

Immunodeficiencies

A variety of laboratory tests evaluate immune system function. Laboratory evaluation determines intactness of its major functions: B-cell immunity, T-cell immunity, and phagocytosis. Many values vary significantly with age, especially during infancy. Among these are the differential in the complete blood cell count, the amount of various immunoglobulins, the lymphocyte surface antigen count (e.g., CD4+ count), and the total lymphocyte count.

Allergy

Measurement of eosinophilia and IgE levels, along with a radioallergosorbent test (RAST) and skin testing, is helpful in diagnosing allergic reactions.

IMMUNOGLOBULIN FUNCTION AND PEDIATRIC IMPLICATIONS

IMMUNOGLOBULIN TYPE*	PERCENT (%) OF TOTAL Ig*	FUNCTION AND PEDIATRIC SIGNIFICANCE	LOCATION
IgG	80-85	Comprises approximately 80% of circulating immunoglobulin Contains most antibodies against bacteria, viruses, and fungi in blood and body spaces Crosses the placenta; provides maternal antibody protection to infants Responsible for Rh reactions IgG response is longer and stronger than that of the other immunoglobulins	Appears in all internal body fluids; present in majority of B cells
IgM	5-10	Earliest immunoglobulin produced in response to bacterial and viral infections Responsible for transfusion reactions in the ABO blood typing system Does not cross placenta, so values are low in neonates However, IgM is produced early in life, and level increases after 9 mo of age Presence in cord or infant blood may mean infection in utero or in newborn period	Appears mostly in the circulation Attached to B cells; released into plasma during immune response
IgA	10-15	Prevents infection across mucous membranes (local immunity) Especially important in antiviral protection Passes to neonate in breast milk	Appears in body secretions (nasal and respiratory secretions, saliva, tears, breast milk)
IgE	0.004	Leads to release of histamines, producing an allergic response Elevation may indicate allergy in children Plays a role in defense against parasites	Found on the surface membranes of basophils and mast cells Produced by plasma cells in mucous membranes and tonsils and in lymphoid tissue
IgD	0.2	Poorly understood Thought to influence B-cell differentiation	Appears in small amounts in serum Attached to B cells

Data from Tosi, M. (2004). Immunologic and phagocytic responses to infection. In R. Fegin, J. Cherry, G. Demmler, & S. Kaplan (Eds.), *Textbook of pediatric infectious diseases* (5th ed., pp. 25-27). Philadelphia: Elsevier Saunders.
*Normal immunoglobulin values differ for age.

COMMON LABORATORY AND DIAGNOSTIC TESTS OF IMMUNE FUNCTION

TEST	FUNCTION	NURSING CONSIDERATIONS
Serum immunoglobulins (IgG, IgM, IgA, IgE)	Tests humoral immunity function Measures levels of immunoglobulins by separating them through immunoelectrophoresis	Immunization and toxoids received in the past 6 mo and blood transfusions, tetanus antitoxin, and gamma globulin received can affect results and should be noted on the laboratory requisition.
Lymphocyte surface antigen	Determines the types and subtypes of lymphocytes present in blood Names of lymphocyte surface antigens are based on "clusters of differentiation" (CDs). CD antigens on a lymphocyte allow its identification. The two most frequently found surface antigens and the cell types they identify: CD4+: helper T cells CD8+: regulatory T cells	To determine the number of a particular type of cell, a CBC must also be done.
Serum antibody titer to commonly received antigens in vaccines (e.g., tetanus, diphtheria)	Used to evaluate humoral immune function	Tests antibody level to specific antigens
Skin tests to *Candida*, tuberculosis	Used to evaluate cell-mediated immune function	Administered intradermally Size of induration is measured at daily intervals for 3 days
Differential WBC count	Part of the CBC, describes the relative amount of the five types of WBCs (leukocytes) in the blood: neutrophils, eosinophils, basophils, monocytes, and lymphocytes. The differential WBC count is expressed in number per cubic millimeter (mm^3) and as a percent of the total number of WBCs.	Helps identify infection, immune status, and allergy
Allergy skin tests	On administration of minute amounts of antigen into the skin, tests either immediate or delayed-type hypersensitivity	Because anaphylactic reactions can occur even in the presence of minimal allergen exposures, emergency equipment and medications should be immediately available
RAST	Measures the quantity and increase of antigen-specific IgE present in the serum. Exact quantities of antibodies to pollens, foods, and so forth can be tested.	More expensive than traditional allergy skin testing but provides precise information without risk for hypersensitivity reaction

Data from Pagana, K., & Pagana, T. (2009). *Mosby's manual of diagnostic and laboratory tests* (4th ed.). St. Louis: Elsevier Mosby.
CBC, Complete blood cell count; *WBC*, white blood cell.
Refer to Evolve website for normal values.

LABORATORY AND CLINICAL SCREENING TESTS FOR ALLERGY

TEST	FINDINGS SUGGESTIVE OF ALLERGY
CBC, differential	Excess eosinophils (>5% of WBCs)
Total eosinophil count	>450 µL eosinophils
Nasal smear	Excess eosinophils (>4% in young children, >10% in adolescents)
Serum IgE	Elevated for age
RAST, antigen-specific IgE	Increase in antigen-specific IgE in the serum
Skin testing	Urticarial wheal appears on skin within 20 to 30 min after administration of selected potential allergens; reaction can be immediate or delayed and can even include anaphylaxis

CBC, Complete blood cell count; *RAST*, radioallergosorbent test; *WBC*, white blood cell.

Immunologic alterations typically are chronic, lasting from months to years and interfering with a child's life. Physical signs range from simple, such as impaired skin integrity, to complex, such as overwhelming infection. Intervals of wellness, relapses, and sometimes a decline in health should be expected. Repeated office visits and hospitalizations, disruptions in family routines, altered social interactions, and emotional and financial strain often are coupled with anxiety about the future.

Initially, the nurse helps the family adjust to a new, often devastating diagnosis. Care during the acute phase of the illness may be critical in nature, as underlying organisms are diagnosed and treated and fevers and pain are controlled. Once the acute crisis has resolved, the nurse prepares the family for discharge by teaching home management and identifying community resources and referrals for continuing support. The nurse also teaches the family how to prevent the spread of microorganisms through infection control practices at home and describes parameters for when to call the health provider. The nurse discusses ways to maintain the child's skin integrity, the body's first line of protection against microorganisms, and recommends a diet that supports immune cell growth. The nurse must keep abreast of current information because the field of immunology continues to evolve. Nurses also play a vital role in advocating for children with conditions such as human immunodeficiency virus (HIV) infection.

Despite all efforts, rehospitalization is often inevitable. The family is an integral part of the multidisciplinary team, keeping the physicians, nurses, and social workers informed of changes in the child's condition, administering medications, providing respiratory care, and often making difficult decisions about continued treatment and comfort.

HUMAN IMMUNODEFICIENCY VIRUS INFECTION

HIV infection is an acquired cell-mediated immunodeficiency disorder that causes a wide spectrum of manifestations in children, ranging from no signs or symptoms to mild and moderate to severe signs and symptoms. Because of improved medical approaches to this condition, HIV infection is viewed as a chronic condition with ongoing challenges. Acquired immunodeficiency syndrome (AIDS) is the most advanced manifestation of this infection.

Etiology

HIV, present in an infected individual's blood or body fluids, can enter an uninfected adult's or adolescent's body in several ways, including sharing of needles or syringes, engaging in unprotected sexual activity with an infected person where body fluids are shared, or receiving an infected blood product. Infected women can transmit the virus to a fetus across the placenta during pregnancy, to the infant at delivery, and to the young child through breastfeeding. Since 1994, when it became practice to administer zidovudine (ZDV) to mothers prenatally and intrapartally and to the newborn infant, the incidence of perinatal transmission has decreased markedly (Centers for Disease Control and Prevention [CDC], 2010). Increases in prenatal counseling and testing and a combination antiretroviral regimen during pregnancy, combined with specific obstetric interventions designed to prevent transmission during labor, have reduced the transmission risk to less than 2% (CDC, 2010). The risk of children acquiring HIV infection through sexual abuse still exists.

Incidence

The incidence of HIV infection in infants and children in the United States is approximately 200 children annually, and this has been stable

for several years (CDC, 2009a). Ninety-one percent of cases of HIV infection are the result of perinatal transmission (CDC, 2010). In the United States, more than 10,000 children younger than 19 years of age are living with HIV/AIDS (CDC, 2009a). This brings challenges for children, families, and health professionals alike.

Heterosexual intimacy and infection through intravenous drug use are the most common transmission modes of HIV for women and adolescent girls. In the United States, African-American children younger than age 13 years are disproportionately affected, followed by Hispanic children (CDC, 2009a).

Manifestations

Box 18-1 lists findings associated with general immunodeficiency. Children with HIV manifest most or all of these signs. HIV infection in children and adults differs in several ways (Working Group on

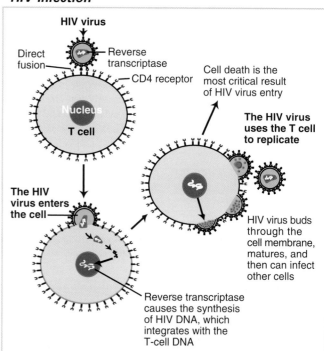

PATHOPHYSIOLOGY

HIV Infection

HIV is a retrovirus composed of RNA and an enzyme, reverse transcriptase, which plays a key role in viral replication. HIV gains entry into a CD4+ cell by direct fusion of the viral envelope to CD4+ receptors on the cell surface. This fusion allows the viral RNA and other enzymes to enter the CD4+ cell. Within the CD4+ cell, reverse transcriptase causes the synthesis of HIV DNA. This integrates with the CD4+ cell's DNA. The virus then uses the CD4+ cell to make more copies of itself. The new viruses assemble at the host cell's surface. As they bud through the cell membrane, the viruses mature, are released, and can infect other CD4+ cells. The most critical result of HIV entry into the CD4+ cell is cell incapacitation and death.*

Because CD4+ cells primarily enhance cell-mediated immunity, severely infected infants and children will exhibit symptoms of viral or fungal infection. In addition, CD4+ helper cells interact with the humoral immune response. Immunoglobulins become nonfunctional, making the child extremely vulnerable to bacterial infections.

*Kumar et al. as cited in Porth, C. (2011). *Essentials of pathophysiology* (3rd ed.). Philadelphia: Wolters Kluwer.

BOX 18-1 CLINICAL FINDINGS ASSOCIATED WITH IMMUNODEFICIENCY

Frequently Present, Highly Indicative Signs
- Repeated or persistent respiratory tract infection
- Repeated or persistent otitis media or sinusitis
- Severe bacterial infections
- Opportunistic infections, such as PCP or cryptosporidiosis
- Poor response to appropriate therapy

Frequently Present, Somewhat Suggestive Signs
- Skin lesions
- Failure to thrive or grow
- Chronic diarrhea
- Thrush
- Hepatosplenomegaly
- Anemia, thrombocytopenia, neutropenia
- Small or absent lymph nodes, tonsils, and adenoids

? CRITICAL THINKING EXERCISE 18-1

It has become the standard of care to include HIV testing of all women, along with other tests done prenatally to identify possible communicable disease. HIV testing is done on an "opt out" basis, meaning that the test will be done unless the pregnant woman chooses not to be tested. What might be the primary goal for this type of testing? What are the major issues that need to be considered if a woman decides to decline testing when it is offered?

Antiretroviral Therapy and Medical Management of HIV-Infected Children, 2008; Yogev & Chadwick, 2011):

- The progression of HIV infection to AIDS is faster in infants and children younger than 5 years of age. One factor contributing to the rapid progression in children is a higher viral load.
- Signs in children may include physical and developmental failure to thrive.
- Children have early opportunistic infections (e.g., chronic oral candidiasis), a greater number of bacterial infections from childhood illnesses, and lymphoid interstitial pneumonitis (LIP), a condition in which the child may be asymptomatic or may have parotid gland enlargement, hypoxia, and digital clubbing.
- *Pneumocystis jiroveci* (formerly *carinii*) pneumonia (PCP) in children with perinatally acquired HIV infection can occur early in infancy.

The CDC classifies the clinical manifestations of HIV infection as not symptomatic (Category N), mildly symptomatic (Category A), moderately symptomatic (Category B), or severely symptomatic (Category C) in children younger than 13 years (Panel on Antiretroviral Therapy and Medical Management of HIV-Infected Children, 2011). Mild signs of the illness may be nonspecific and include lymphadenopathy, hepatomegaly, splenomegaly, dermatitis, parotitis, and recurrent or persistent upper respiratory infection, sinusitis, or otitis media. In moderate disease, some signs are considered to be important if they persist or recur, particularly anemia, neutropenia, or thrombocytopenia; diarrhea; fever for longer than 1 month; herpes simplex; and oral candidiasis in children older than 6 months. Other signs of moderate infection include bacterial meningitis, pneumonia, or sepsis (one episode); cardiomyopathy; complicated chickenpox;

herpes zoster; hepatitis; nephropathy; LIP; and toxoplasmosis onset before age 1 month (Panel on Antiretroviral Therapy and Medical Management of HIV-Infected Children, 2011, pp. 32-33). In general, in addition to LIP the most common indicators of AIDS in children younger than 13 years are serious confirmed bacterial infections (multiple or recurrent), PCP and other opportunistic infections, encephalopathy, lymphomas and Kaposi sarcoma, and severe nutritional deficits with fall-off on growth percentiles (wasting syndrome) without evidence of being caused by another disease process (Panel on Antiretroviral Therapy and Medical Management of HIV-Infected Children, 2011).

Diagnostic Evaluation

Because most HIV infections in infants and children occur as a result of perinatal transmission, HIV-positive pregnant women must be identified, educated, and treated. Early identification and treatment of women reduce the HIV transmission rate and enable early diagnosis and treatment for infected infants. Recommendations for preventing HIV transmission to neonates now includes universal testing of all pregnant women (unless they "opt out") and HIV counseling. Women who are found to be at risk for HIV are tested a second time at 36 weeks' gestation. If a woman does not receive HIV counseling and treatment during pregnancy, counseling and treatment as soon as possible after delivery facilitates optimal management of the newborn (Panel on Treatment of HIV-Infected Pregnant Women and Prevention of Perinatal Transmission, 2010).

Diagnosing HIV-Exposed Infants

Diagnosing HIV through traditional HIV antibody measurement by enzyme-linked immunosorbent assay (ELISA) or Western blot assay is not accurate for a positive or negative diagnosis in infants younger than 18 months because of the presence of maternal antibodies. Instead, virologic assay tests are used. These include deoxyribonucleic acid polymerase chain reaction (HIV DNA PCR) or ribonucleic acid (HIV RNA) assay.

For infants who have been exposed to HIV, virologic testing is performed when the infant is 14 to 21 days old, at 1 to 2 months, and again at 4 to 6 months; health care providers should consider performing virologic studies immediately after birth for infants known to be at risk for exposure (Panel on Antiretroviral Therapy and Medical Management of HIV-Infected Children, 2011).

Two positive virologic assays obtained on two separate occasions establish a positive diagnosis. Two negative virologic assays from separate specimens taken at ≥1 month of age and again at ≥4 months of age in nonbreastfed infants can establish negative HIV status; some specialists will follow up with an antibody test at between 12 and 18 months to confirm (Panel on Antiretroviral Therapy and Medical Management of HIV-Infected Children, 2011). Two negative HIV antibody tests from separate specimens can rule out HIV infection in a child older than 6 months. HIV antibody measurement may be used if the child is older than 18 months. For all these tests, infants must not show any clinical signs of HIV infection (Panel on Antiretroviral Therapy and Medical Management of HIV-Infected Children, 2011).

Ongoing Diagnostic Monitoring

CD4+ lymphocyte counts and HIV RNA assays assess an infected young child's immune status, response to therapy, risk for disease progression, and need for PCP prophylaxis after 1 year of age. Low CD4+ counts or decreased percentage indicate reduced immune function. CD4+ counts are measured at diagnosis and every 3 to 4 months thereafter, except in adolescents who have stable immune function; counts in stable and medication-adherent adolescents can be done less frequently. Monitoring may occur more often for infants younger than 12 months old, when a deterioration in physical condition is suspected, and when making decisions to treat or change treatment (Panel on Antiretroviral Therapy and Medical Management of HIV-Infected Children, 2011). Although the CD4+ lymphocyte counts vary by age in children younger than 5 years old, the CD4+ cell percentage does not, and so the percentage is considered to be a more accurate assessment for childhood disease progression in children of this age-group (Panel on Antiretroviral Therapy and Medical Management of HIV-Infected Children, 2011).

The amount of virus in peripheral blood is called the *viral burden.* The HIV viral burden is measured by plasma HIV RNA copy number and is determined by use of a quantitative HIV RNA assay. The HIV RNA copy numbers work in tandem with the CD4+ percentage to provide independent information about prognosis and guide treatment decisions. HIV RNA copy number is assessed immediately after positive virologic diagnosis of HIV and every 3 to 4 months subsequently, or more often, depending on the child's clinical and treatment status (Panel on Antiretroviral Therapy and Medical Management of HIV-Infected Children, 2011). Infants who are infected perinatally initially have a high viral burden; this burden decreases gradually over several years. A high viral burden (>299,000 copies/mL) in infants younger than 12 months of age may be related to more rapid disease progression (Panel on Antiretroviral Therapy and Medical Management of HIV-Infected Children, 2011).

Therapeutic Management

The goals of management are directed toward rapidly decreasing the viral load to below detectable levels with the lowest risk of drug toxicity, preserving immune function, facilitating normal growth and development, and preventing medication resistance (Panel on Antiretroviral Therapy and Medical Management of HIV-Infected Children, 2011). Viral suppression that is ineffective can result in medication resistance, so a dosage schedule that is the least complex to manage, while providing maximum benefit with fewest toxic effects, results in improved adherence to a medication regimen.

If a mother's HIV status is unknown when she begins labor, HIV antibody testing should be done and her infant treated as if there were a known HIV exposure. If maternal antibody test results are negative, treatment for the infant may be discontinued (Panel on Treatment of HIV-Infected Pregnant Women and Prevention of Perinatal Transmission, 2010).

HIV-Exposed Infants

In addition to giving intravenous (IV) ZDV to the mother during labor, all infants of known HIV-positive mothers should receive oral ZDV therapy within 6 to 12 hours after birth. This should continue for 6 weeks or until the infant is positively diagnosed with HIV, at which time the regimen is changed to a combination of medications (Panel on Antiretroviral Therapy and Medical Management of HIV-Infected Children, 2011; Panel on Treatment of HIV-Infected Pregnant Women and Prevention of Perinatal Transmission, 2010).

In general, to decrease the risk of transmission to an infant during labor, HIV-positive women who have a high viral load (HIV RNA copies exceeding 1000 copies/mL) near delivery should be considered for cesarean section at 38 weeks (Panel on Treatment of HIV-Infected Pregnant Women and Prevention of Perinatal Transmission, 2010). Discussion about treatment options and recommendations should not be threatening. The mother makes the final decision about the use of antiretroviral medications. Women who decide not to accept treatment with ZDV or other drugs should not face punitive action or denial of care (Panel on Treatment of HIV-Infected Pregnant Women and Prevention of Perinatal Transmission, 2010).

Because HIV-exposed infants, whether infected or uninfected, are more prone to acquiring opportunistic infections from an HIV-infected mother, prophylaxis of opportunistic infections is an important focus (CDC, 2009b). HIV-exposed infants are at particular risk from *Pneumocystis jiroveci* pneumonia (PCP), certain strains of tuberculosis, bacterial and viral infections, and fungal infections, such as *Candida.* The CDC (2009b) strongly recommends testing HIV-exposed infants for tuberculosis at 3 months of age, or if exposed to contagious TB. If positive, antituberculosis medications are initiated. The CDC also recommends that varicella-zoster immune globulin be given to unimmunized infants within 96 hours of exposure to varicella or zoster infection.

Perhaps the most serious infection acquired by HIV-exposed infants is *Pneumocystis jiroveci* pneumonia. The CDC (2009b) strongly recommends that all HIV-exposed infants receive PCP prophylaxis with trimethoprim-sulfamethoxazole beginning at 4 to 6 weeks of age until the infant reaches 1 year. HIV-exposed infants for whom HIV infection has been ruled out may have PCP prophylaxis discontinued once HIV-negative status has been confirmed. After 1 year of age, infected children receive PCP prophylaxis according to CD4+ percentage or count, and prophylaxis may be discontinued with close monitoring if the child has been determined to have an acceptable percentage or count for 3 consecutive months (CDC, 2009b).

HIV-Infected Infants and Children

The Panel on Antiretroviral Therapy and Medical Management of HIV-Infected Children, available from www.aidsinfo.nih.gov, updates treatment recommendations regularly.

Treatment Considerations. Treatment is directed toward suppressing viral load with medications or combinations of medications that are in an acceptable and palatable form for children, that have the greatest effect while minimizing toxicity, that have an administration routine that maximizes the child's and family's quality of life, and that reduce the risk for medication resistance. Other goals of management for infants and children infected with HIV include facilitating optimal growth and development, providing ongoing support for the child and family, and referring the child for clinical trials as they become available (Panel on Antiretroviral Therapy and Medical Management of HIV-Infected Children, 2011). Infants and children who are HIV infected should be cared for by a multidisciplinary team of providers (physicians, nurses, social workers, pharmacists, dentists, nutritionists, psychologists, and outreach workers) led by specialists in pediatric HIV management (Panel on Antiretroviral Therapy and Medical Management of HIV-Infected Children, 2011).

More potent and improved antiretroviral medications have benefited HIV-infected children who have immunologic or clinical symptoms of HIV infection. These benefits include enhanced survival, improvements in growth and development, and reduced opportunistic infections and other complications related to HIV infection. Highly active antiretroviral therapy (HAART) has dramatically affected HIV-infected children's health, although its rigorous treatment schedules are challenging for children and families to maintain. There are also associated short- and long-term toxicities, which can have an impact on children (Panel on Antiretroviral Therapy and Medical Management of HIV-Infected Children, 2011).

Considerations of drug resistance and adherence are of primary importance. Before a medication routine is initiated, all infants and children with HIV should be tested for antiretroviral drug resistance. The rationale for this is that infants can acquire a drug-resistant strain of HIV from their HIV-infected mother or can develop drug resistance while receiving prophylaxis in anticipation of a diagnosis (Panel on Antiretroviral Therapy and Medical Management of HIV-Infected Children, 2011). Drug resistance testing should also be done when consideration is being given to changing a medication regimen. Resistance testing can help the specialist decide on antiretroviral drugs that are most appropriate for an individual child (Panel on Antiretroviral Therapy and Medical Management of HIV-Infected Children, 2011).

One of the most important factors to consider when deciding on a treatment approach is the child's and the caregiver's ability to adhere to the prescribed regimen, because failure to follow the regimen can result in the development of drug resistance and subsequent treatment failure. Adherence issues need to be addressed before a decision to start therapy is made, and adherence needs to be assessed and discussed at each visit (Panel on Antiretroviral Therapy and Medical Management of HIV-Infected Children, 2011). The Panel on Antiretroviral Therapy and Medical Management of HIV-Infected Children (2011) describes multimethod strategies for improving adherence, which include choosing a medication regimen that fits as much as possible into the child's and family's lifestyle, use of adherence aids (e.g., pillboxes, alarm watches, stickers), and providing ongoing teaching, support, and encouragement. A multidisciplinary team including physicians, nurses, pharmacists, and sometimes peers is the most helpful to families. Strategies focus on both the child and the caregiver and must address any social issue that is affecting the family's adherence to the prescribed regimen.

The Panel strongly recommends that the provider verify adherence by at least one means other than viral load monitoring at each visit. This can include strategies such as having the parent or child make available a medication log (self-report), doing pill counts or checking the refill history with a pharmacist, or using a modified form of direct observation (m-DOT) (Panel on Antiretroviral Therapy and Medical Management of HIV-Infected Children, 2011). Adherence during adolescence can be even more challenging, so regimens may need to be reevaluated at that time.

Treatment Initiation. Currently, 20 antiretroviral agents have been approved for treatment of children with HIV infection; 15 of those are available in pediatric form (Panel on Antiretroviral Therapy and Medical Management of HIV-Infected Children, 2011). Drug classes include nucleoside analog reverse transcriptase inhibitors (NRTIs, NtRTIs), nonnucleoside reverse transcriptase inhibitors (NNRTIs), protease inhibitors (PIs), entry inhibitors, and integrase inhibitors. The preferred drug combination for initial treatment of infants and children with HIV infection includes the following (Panel on Antiretroviral Therapy and Medical Management of HIV-Infected Children, 2011, p. 47):

- *For children 14 days to younger than 3 years of age:* Two NRTIs plus lopinavir/ritonavir.
- *For children 3 years of age or older:* Two NRTIs plus lopinavir/ritonavir or two NRTIs plus efavirenz (not for adolescent girls).
- *For children 6 years of age or older:* Two NRTIs plus efavirenz (not for adolescent girls) or two NRTIs plus lopinavir/ritonavir, or two NRTIs plus atazanovir and low-dose ritonavir.
- Two NRTIs plus an NNRTI (nevirapine, but only if not used for primary prophylaxis) can be used at any age as an alternative.

Doses for infants and children are individualized according to age and growth considerations. Doses for adolescents are determined by multiple factors, including the adolescent's size, weight, age in relation to adult dosing, risk of pregnancy, use of contraceptives, and Tanner stage (see Chapter 8).

For perinatally infected infants, ZDV is discontinued as soon as HIV status has been confirmed, and combination therapy is started. In the past, treatment of asymptomatic HIV-infected infants with normal immunologic status was controversial; current recommendations call for aggressive treatment for all infants younger than 1 year of age irrespective of clinical or virologic status (Panel on Antiretroviral Therapy and Medical Management of HIV-Infected Children, 2011). Because of a more rapid disease progression in children than in adults and the fact that laboratory studies are less precise in predicting disease progression, children are treated aggressively. Table 18-1 presents current recommendations for initiating antiretroviral therapy in infants and children infected with HIV. Treatment is based on a combination of symptoms, CD4+ percentage, and viral load as determined by HIV RNA copy number.

Additional Issues Related to the Child with Human Immunodeficiency Virus Infection

Multigenerational Problems. One of the unique aspects of perinatal HIV infection is the multigenerational nature of the disease, in which both the mother and child may be infected. The transition to motherhood is challenging under normal circumstances, but may be exacerbated when the mother has HIV.

When considering the special needs of the mother-infant dyad, the nurse needs to be aware of mothers' concerns both during pregnancy and after delivery in order to provide optimal nursing care. Shannon, Kennedy, and Humphreys (2008) conducted a longitudinal study that explored maternal concerns during pregnancy and during the period of time mothers were awaiting the infant's diagnosis. They described the pregnant mothers in their sample as being far more concerned about their infant's health, and whether the infant would contract HIV, than about their own health. Other issues of concern prenatally included feelings about whether they would be able to cope with an ill infant, disclosure of their condition to others, and financial concerns regarding the infant's possible need for treatment (Shannon et al., 2008). While awaiting final results of virologic testing, Shannon and colleagues described changes in mothers' concerns according to each point of diagnostic result. After final diagnosis, some mothers still expressed uncertainty about a negative diagnosis, that it was really true. Additional concerns after diagnosis focused on maintaining health to be able to care for their infants, guardianship issues, possible abandonment, and financial concerns (Shannon et al., 2008).

Another important but difficult area to be addressed is future planning. This can include exploring the efficacy of standby guardianship, kinship care, or foster and adoptive placement. In addition, for children with advanced HIV disease, families have to make difficult decisions about an infected child's continuing care. Should aggressive treatment continue, or should the goal of treatment be to make the child comfortable? These decisions are best made in consultation with a multidisciplinary team that can identify areas of concern and develop strategic approaches that incorporate family culture, beliefs, available physical and emotional resources, and knowledge.

Disclosure. Initial reactions to an HIV diagnosis may include confusion, anger, denial, and despair. Informing a child about a shared HIV status may be intimidating in light of the parent's and child's physical, emotional, and social experiences. Unlike disclosure about other chronic illnesses children and adolescents may experience, disclosure about HIV status brings fear of social stigma (Butler, Williams, Howland et al., 2009). Now that children with HIV are surviving into adolescence, the issue of disclosure becomes a vital part of their health care management, particularly considering the prevalence of

TABLE 18-1 CONSIDERATIONS FOR INITIATING ANTIRETROVIRAL MEDICATIONS IN INFANTS AND CHILDREN WITH HIV

AGE-GROUP	CRITERIA FOR INITIATION	TREATMENT RECOMMENDATIONS
<12 mo	Regardless of clinical symptoms, immune status, or viral load	Treat
1 yr to <5 yr	AIDS or significant HIV symptoms*	Treat
	Meet age-related CD4+ threshold for initiating treatment irrespective of symptoms or plasma HIV RNA level[†]	Treat
≥5 yr	Asymptomatic or mild symptoms[‡] and CD4+ ≥25% and plasma HIV RNA ≥100,000 copies/mL	Treat
	Asymptomatic or mild symptoms[‡] and CD4+ ≥25% and plasma HIV RNA <100,000 copies/mL	Consider[§]
	AIDS or significant HIV symptoms*	Treat
	CD4+ count ≤500 cells/mm^3	Treat
	Asymptomatic or mild symptoms[‡] and CD4+ count >500 cells/mm^3 and plasma HIV RNA ≥100,000 copies/mL	Treat
	Asymptomatic or mild symptoms[‡] and CD4+ count >500 cells/mm^3 and plasma HIV RNA <100,000 copies/mL	Consider[§]

Conditions for initiating treatment for children who have been deferred include the following:

- Increasing HIV RNA levels (e.g., HIV RNA levels approaching 100,000 copies/mL);
- Rapidly declining CD4 count or percentage to values approaching the age-related threshold for consideration of therapy;
- Development of clinical symptoms; and
- The ability of caregiver and child to adhere to the prescribed regimen.

From Panel on Antiretroviral Therapy and Medical Management of HIV-Infected Children. (2011, August 11). *Guidelines for the use of antiretroviral agents in pediatric HIV infection* (p. 38). Retrieved from www.aidsinfo.nih.gov.

*CDC Clinical Category C and most B conditions (except for single episode of serious bacterial infection) irrespective of CD4+ percentage or count or plasma HIV RNA level.

[†]Age-related CD4+ percentage for treatment initiation in children 1 to <5 years = <25%; CD4+ count for children ≥ 5 years = <500 cells/mm^3.

[‡]CDC Clinical Category A or N or the following Category B condition: single episode of serious bacterial infection.

[§]Clinical and laboratory data should be reevaluated every 3 to 4 months.

◎ NURSING CARE PLAN

The Child with HIV Infection in the Community

Focused Assessment

- Regardless of setting (home, school, day care), assess development and well care, particularly immunization status (Table 18-2)
- Assess adherence to the anti-HIV medication regimen
- Obtain a history of recent exposure to any communicable disease and whether the child is adhering to medication prophylaxis against opportunistic infections
- At each well or ill visit, ask the caregivers about any fever, nausea, vomiting, diarrhea, ear pulling, or changes in appetite, sleep pattern, or behavior that might suggest a secondary infection.
- Assess the family's understanding about the HIV-related spectrum of illness, including immunologic status and treatment options.
- Inquire how the family is coping financially and emotionally, and whether referral may be needed for additional support.
- At hospital admission, focus the assessment on the following:
  - *Hydration status:* Intake, output, skin turgor
  - *Respiratory status:* Signs of respiratory distress, adventitious or diminished breath sounds, oxygen saturation
  - *Mucous membranes:* White patches on tongue or inside cheeks, blisters on the lips, or lesions on the tonsils or soft palate
  - *Skin:* Lesions (especially in diaper area; blotchy, red, flat areas, blistering, dryness, rashes or vesicles)
- Pain by self-report using an age-appropriate pain scale

Planning

Nursing Diagnosis

Deficient Knowledge about the natural history of pediatric HIV infection, potential complications associated with HIV infection, and current treatment modalities related to emotional reaction to the diagnosis.

Expected Outcome

The family will demonstrate knowledge acquisition, as evidenced by explaining what has been taught about HIV infection and playing an active role in determining the plan of care for the child.

Intervention/Rationale

1. Determine the family's knowledge about HIV infection, treatment modalities, and home care (*Patient-Centered Teaching: How to Care for the Child with an HIV Infection box*).

   Teaching needs to begin at the family's level of understanding. It is important to note that because the majority of HIV-infected children are infected perinatally, the nurse may also be educating parents about their own disease process.

2. Teach the family about HIV infection, its signs and symptoms, progression, and treatment.

   Knowledge and understanding of HIV may increase cooperation and adherence to the often-complicated treatment regimens that are necessary to achieve viral suppression and will also serve to reduce anxiety.

NURSING CARE PLAN

The Child with HIV Infection in the Community—cont'd

Intervention/Rationale—cont'd

3. Identify the family's areas of concern (e.g., a new diagnosis, fear of transmission by casual contact within the family).

   Addressing family concerns decreases misinterpretation. First, educate about the lack of transmission by household contact and correct any myths or misperceptions that may exist.

4. Use teaching strategies that will maximize potential for success (e.g., medication sheet that details medication name, dosage, how often to give, why the child is on the medication, and hints for administering unpalatable tasting medication).

   Written information may assist the family to ensure that the correct medication regimen is being followed.

5. Educate the family about what signs or problems necessitate calling the health care provider for management advice.

   Early identification of potential problems may prevent serious complications from developing.

Evaluation

Can the family describe the natural history of HIV, systems affected by HIV, current treatment modalities, and care for the child at home?

Can the family administer the correct dosages of medications at the appropriate times?

Does the family readily participate in developing and carrying out a plan of care for the child?

Does the family contact health care providers when the child is ill and in need of services?

Planning

Nursing Diagnosis

Anxiety (primary caregiver) related to fear of disclosure.

Expected Outcomes

The family will share the diagnosis with those family members, health care professionals, and school staff who need to know.

The family will move through the stages of disclosure and feel comfortable sharing their feelings about the diagnosis with appropriate people.

The family will answer the child's questions honestly and share the diagnosis when the time is right.

Intervention/Rationale

1. Listen quietly when the family talks about the diagnosis of HIV. Note their stage of disclosure (secrecy, exploratory, readiness, or full disclosure).

   Sharing the diagnosis occurs on a continuum, with secrecy at one end and full disclosure at the other. Families initially may want to keep their feelings about the diagnosis private. However, a time may come when they wish to talk; the nurse should develop rapport and gain trust.

2. Maintain confidentiality concerning the HIV diagnoses. Ask the primary caregiver what individuals know about the diagnosis and what specific information they have. Encourage the family to share the diagnosis with health care professionals.

   Health care professionals who plan and coordinate care need to know the diagnosis to facilitate an optimal treatment plan.

3. Help family members decide who needs to know the child's diagnosis and offer them education and support in the process of disclosure. Encourage peer support groups when the family is ready.

   Do not assume that all family or friends accompanying the child to the clinic or hospital know the child's or parent's diagnosis. Although many people would like to know the diagnosis, only a few need to know. Ask families to

consider the following when choosing whom to tell: the child's age, clinical condition, and health care requirements; the likelihood that bloody injuries will occur; and the use of Standard Precautions.

4. Encourage the family to be honest with the child and to explain the reason for physicians' visits and procedures.

   When to tell the child the diagnosis is a personal choice, but families need to understand that children will worry more if no one talks with them or if they sense dishonesty; ethical considerations make it important that adolescents be aware of their diagnosis (Butler et al., 2009).

5. Encourage the family to listen to the questions the child is asking and to answer the questions briefly, using words the child can understand. Look for readiness cues that indicate the child wants to know more.

   It is important for families to understand what their children are asking and to answer their questions, keeping responses short and simple.

6. Encourage the family to speak with a health care professional when the child asks questions that are difficult to answer. Suggest that the parent seek counseling to help find the appropriate language for answering the child.

   Role playing is a useful technique that allows families to practice potential responses to difficult questions. The nurse can offer to accompany them if they decide to share the diagnosis.

7. Promote normal routines at home.

   Children with HIV infection can go to school, church, and parties; play sports and games; and develop or maintain friendships.

Evaluation

Is the family able to share the diagnosis with all appropriate health care professionals and at least one significant person?

Does the family appear to be moving through the stages of disclosure and seeking out support from peers?

Is the family able to seek social and health services for which they qualify on the basis of their HIV/AIDS status?

Can family members answer the child's questions in a developmentally appropriate way?

Planning

Nursing Diagnosis

Ineffective Family Therapeutic Regimen Management: Nonadherence related to lack of support systems or denial of the illness.

Expected Outcomes

The mother who is infected with HIV will keep her own health care appointments and those of her child.

The family will work toward accepting the diagnosis.

The family will view themselves as valued members of the health care team.

The child/family will adhere to the medication regimen.

Intervention/Rationale

1. Use language that shows respect. Offer information in a language that can be understood by the child and family. Use a translator as needed.

   Families affected by HIV do not want their children called innocent victims or AIDS babies, nor do they want to be judged as promiscuous or substance abusers. Labels can create barriers, which can result in nonadherence with health care recommendations.

2. Encourage the HIV-infected mother to keep her own health care appointments.

   HIV-infected women often neglect their own health care needs as they attend to those of their children.

Continued

⊙ NURSING CARE PLAN

The Child with HIV Infection in the Community—cont'd

Intervention/*Rationale*—cont'd

3. Accept the parents' use of denial during periods of emotional respite. Refer for counseling to assist with the grieving process.

   The diagnosis of HIV brings a series of losses, including the loss of the future and all that the future holds for a child. Denial is a coping mechanism.

4. Maintain realistic hope when possible.

   With new prophylaxis agents for HIV-positive pregnant women and their infants, HIV infection develops in fewer than 2% of all perinatally HIV-exposed babies, and antiretroviral treatments have been successful in preserving immune function in infected infants.

5. Refer the family to social services for assistance with finances, transportation, food, housing, clothing, medical care, and respite care as needed.

   Many families simply lack the basic resources for adherence to a treatment regimen. Problems that affect the caregiver's ability to manage the therapeutic plan include inadequate or inconsistent housing or transportation and personal HIV disease. In some instances, substance use or abuse or mental illness can affect adherence. Guilt about passing HIV on to a child can interfere with providing the structure and discipline necessary for establishing a successful regular medication regimen.

6. Teach the family how to give antiretroviral agents at home, keep a log, and adjust the schedule to accommodate school schedules, if necessary.

   Give suggestions about helpful devices, such as daily or weekly pill boxes that can be prefilled, alarm watches, and pictorial medication reminders.* The antiretroviral regimen may include a combination of medications in addition to other medications a child may be taking. A daily log or other medication reminder device helps families keep track.

7. Monitor medication adherence every visit.

   A multifaceted approach works best in adherence issues. Palatability of the medication, ability to meld the medication schedule with existing routines, denial, guilt, and embarrassment about the diagnosis are all barriers to appropriate cooperation with the medication regimen.

8. Suggest ways to make medications more palatable to children:

   Encourage early pill taking.

   Mix medication with chocolate syrup or follow with chocolate candy.

   Give ice or ice pop before giving the medication.

   Use an oral syringe to place the medication back in the mouth away from taste buds.

   Avoid mixing medications in food or drink, fighting with the child, and skipping medication doses.

   Making the medication and medication routine palatable to children and families enhances adherence.

9. Liquid formulations of HIV medications may be foul tasting or have a gritty texture.

   Unlike short-course medications, these medications must become part of the family's everyday routine for years.

Evaluation

Is the mother able to take care of herself?

Has the patient or caregiver been able to move from denial to anger to acceptance of the diagnosis?

Are the primary caregivers active, participatory, and valued members of the health care team?

Does the child/family adhere to the medication regimen?

*Panel on Antiretroviral Therapy and Medical Management of HIV-Infected Children. (2011, August 11). *Guidelines for the use of antiretroviral agents in pediatric HIV infection.* Retrieved from www.aidsinfo.nih.gov.
IVIG, Intravenous immune globulin.

TABLE 18-2   RECOMMENDATIONS FOR ROUTINE IMMUNIZATION OF HUMAN IMMUNODEFICIENCY VIRUS–INFECTED CHILDREN IN THE UNITED STATES

VACCINES	HIV INFECTION	COMMENTS
Hepatitis B	Yes	Post-vaccination testing 1 to 2 mo after last dose; revaccinate (three doses) if anti-hepatitis B surface antigen (anti-HBS) level is <10 mIU/mL
Hepatitis A	Yes	Beginning at 12 months; two doses should be separated by at least 6 mo
DTaP	Yes	Tdap should be given to adolescents as a booster dose at 11 to 12 yr (5 yr after the primary series)
IPV	Yes	
MMR	Yes	May be given to children who are not severely immune depressed (CD4+ <15% or <200 cells/μL); administer close to the first birthday and 1 mo later
Hib	Yes	
Rotavirus	Consider risk/benefit	No safety or efficacy data available
Pneumococcal	Yes	Pneumococcal polysaccharide vaccine (PPSV) should be given to children 2 yr or older, ≥2 mo after last PCV dose; older children and adolescents may receive one dose of PPSV if not previously immunized and one booster dose of PPSV if they had the PPSV series previously
Influenza	Yes	Use trivalent inactivated vaccine (TIV) only; immunize eligible close contacts
Varicella	Consider risk/benefit	May be given to children with CD4+ percentages ≥15% or count ≥200 cells/μL; give first dose near the first birthday and second one 3 mo later; do not give to immunosuppressed children (CD4+ percentage <15% or count <200 cells/μL)
Meningococcal (MCV)	Yes	Children who receive meningococcal polysaccharide vaccine (MPSV) should receive a booster of MCV 3 to 5 yr after the MPSV if meningococcal infection continues to be a risk
Human papillomavirus vaccine (HPV)	Yes	HIV-infected females older than age 9 yr, three-dose schedule

Data from Centers for Disease Control and Prevention. (2009). Guidelines for the prevention and treatment of opportunistic infections among HIV-exposed and HIV-infected children. *MMWR: Morbidity and Mortality Weekly Report, 58*(RR-11), 161-165.
NOTE: Always check the most current immunization schedule.

PATIENT-CENTERED TEACHING

How to Care for the Child with an HIV Infection

Review the following information and health practices at the time of initial testing and subsequent visits.

Transmission

HIV can be spread by the following:
- Unprotected sexual activity
- Sharing of needles
- An infected mother to her baby
- Breastfeeding
- Open wounds (if there is blood-to-blood contact)

HIV cannot be spread by the following:
- Sharing knives, forks, spoons, or cups
- Using the same toilet seats, bathtubs, or showers
- Coughing or sneezing
- Hugging, holding, or touching people

Prevention

The best way to prevent the spread of HIV is to do the following:
- Abstain from sex and from sharing needles, or
- Use latex condoms with nonoxynol 9, and
- Wash needles in a 1:10 bleach solution

The best way to prevent pregnancies is to do the following:
- Abstain from sex, or
- Use a latex condom
- Use contraception
- Undergo tubal ligation

If infected with HIV, follow these precautions:
- Do not breastfeed
- Do not donate blood, sperm, or organs

Testing

- The most common HIV tests used for older children and adults are the ELISA and the Western blot assay, which measure levels of antibodies to the virus.
- The most common HIV tests used for infants and children younger than 18 months are the HIV DNA PCR and HIV RNA quantitative assays, which detect the presence of the virus itself.
- CD4+ counts or percentage indicate how well the immune system is working.

Illness (AIDS)

Children with HIV infection might initially be asymptomatic. Mild and moderate symptoms include the following:
- Persistent upper respiratory and ear infections
- Thrush
- Skin conditions
- Vomiting and diarrhea
- Enlarged liver, spleen, lymph nodes, and parotid gland
- Growth and development problems
- LIP: a rare lung disease

Some severe symptoms of the illness include the following:
- Opportunistic infections, such as PCP and cytomegalovirus (CMV)
- Recurrent bacterial infections, such as sepsis, meningitis, and pneumonia
- Severe developmental delay or neurologic symptoms
- Wasting syndrome/failure to thrive

Medications
- Resistance testing
- Adherence to schedule (keep a written record of missed doses)
- Proper administration
- Safe and proper storage
- Side effects

Home Care

Offer a high-calorie, high-protein diet if growth is a problem:
- Mix formula as directed.
- Do not add extra water or cereal to formula.
- Give supplemental vitamins and minerals as ordered.

Practice basic infection control measures and follow Standard Precautions, including the following practices:
- Avoid touching blood.
- Do not share toothbrushes, pierced earrings, razors, or nail clippers.
- Use a barrier when caring for a cut or a bloody nose.
- Cover open sores.
- Leave scabs alone.
- Wipe up blood spills with a paper towel, wash the area with soap and water, rinse with bleach and water, and air dry.
- Wrap disposable materials soiled with blood in newspaper, tie off in a plastic bag, and throw away in a plastic-lined trash can.
- Wash hands with soap and water if you touch blood.
- Rinse blood-soiled clothing with hydrogen peroxide or cold water and then wash as usual.
- Allow blood to air dry on dry-clean-only clothing.

Keep your child's immunizations up to date. Your child should also receive the following:
- Pneumococcal vaccine at 2 years of age, if not given during infancy
- Flu shot each fall
- Immune globulin after measles exposure
- Varicella-zoster immune globulin after chickenpox exposure
- Tetanus immune globulin for tetanus-prone wounds

Call the physician if any of the following symptoms occur:
- Fever higher than 101° F (38.3° C)
- Vomiting and diarrhea
- Decreased appetite, difficulty swallowing, drooling
- Rashes, bumps, lumps, or sores on the skin
- Coughing or chest congestion
- Ear pain, pulling on the ears, or drainage from the ears
- Wounds that will not heal
- Exposure to measles or chickenpox

Give prophylaxis against PCP and antiretroviral drugs as ordered.

---

adolescents who engage in sexual activities. The American Academy of Pediatrics (AAP) Committee on Pediatric AIDS has issued a policy statement regarding disclosure of illness status to HIV-infected children and adolescents (AAP, 1999/2005). Basing their recommendations on research that suggests more positive emotional status in both

children and parents who have disclosed, the AAP recommends that disclosure be considered in light of the child's cognitive and psychosocial development and clinical status, as well as the multitude of factors affecting parents' decision to disclose. Although health care professionals respect the wishes of parents regarding disclosure, it is

NURSING CARE PLAN
The Adolescent with HIV Infection

Focused Assessment

- Assess the adolescent's knowledge of the disease and disease process
- For the adolescent who was infected perinatally, assess growth and development
- Inquire about the adolescent's risk-taking behaviors, especially those that could potentially transmit the virus to others
- Pay particular attention to the adolescent's adherence to any antiretroviral therapy; use confirmatory methods for assuring adherence in addition to self-report
- Assess the adolescent's understanding of the importance of regular medical follow-up
- Obtain information about any specific concerns

Planning

Nursing Diagnosis

Deficient Knowledge about the effect of HIV on adolescents, current treatment options available, and preventing transmission of virus to others.

Expected Outcomes

The adolescent and family will explain in their own words what has been taught about HIV infection, including potential treatment regimens, goals of preserving or restoring immune function, and issues related to adolescent risk taking and adolescent sexuality.

The adolescent and family will adhere to a mutually agreed-on treatment regimen.

Intervention/Rationale

1. Document the adolescent's and family's knowledge of HIV infection and associated concerns and emphasize the necessity for regular well care, developmental monitoring, nutritional support, medication adherence, and immunizations.

   Teaching needs to be geared toward the adolescent's cognitive and emotional readiness to learn about HIV, its treatment, and prevention of complications.

2. Identify the adolescent's specific concerns and address them first.

   Acknowledging the adolescent's concerns may help allay fears and anxiety and help begin to develop a trusting relationship.

3. Educate the adolescent about potential symptoms and problems to report to the health care provider.

   Early identification of problems may prevent development of serious complications.

4. Establish readiness to adhere to medication regimen. Include the adolescent in decision making about a treatment routine that will maximize adherence (e.g., compatibility with daily routine, minimum number of required pills and capsules, fewest side effects).

   Adherence to medication regimens is critical to prevent development of viral resistance. Doses for adolescents may be according to Tanner stage of puberty (see Chapter 8), weight, or adult dose. Because of usual developmental issues of adolescence, the adolescent may deliberately not take medication or forget to do so because of lifestyle issues.

5. Discuss high-risk behaviors that could result in transmission of HIV to others (e.g., sexual activity, IV drug use) and methods of prevention of transmission.

   Frank discussions may empower the adolescent to assume responsibility for reducing the risk for transmission to others by encouraging safer behaviors in sexual practices and drug use.

6. Offer participation in peer support groups.

   The adolescent may benefit from sharing thoughts and feelings about living with HIV, difficulties in taking medications, and so on with others.

7. Encourage school attendance and promote normal routines at home.

   When possible, promoting normalcy assists in meeting developmental needs, as well as preventing social isolation.

8. Refer the adolescent and family to an appropriate transition team that will manage transition into adult HIV care.

   HIV infection has become a chronic condition, and many HIV-infected adolescents will need a period of time to transition from pediatric to adult care. Transition issues are similar to those of any adolescent with a chronic condition who must be on a lifelong medication regimen.

Evaluation

Can the adolescent and family explain what HIV is and its treatment goals?

Can the adolescent describe appropriate measures to reduce disease transmission to others?

Does the adolescent state adherence with the prescribed therapeutic regimen?

---

important to create a continuing supportive environment in which disclosure issues can be discussed and adequate preparation for eventual disclosure can occur (AAP, 1999/2005). The AAP recommendations for disclosure strongly emphasize encouraging disclosure to school-age children and state the ethical responsibility of pediatricians to fully disclose HIV status to affected adolescents (AAP, 1999/2005). Parents and other guardians of an HIV-infected child should be counseled by a knowledgeable health care professional about disclosure to the child. This counseling may need to be repeated throughout the course of the child's illness.

Butler and colleagues (2009) conducted a study that followed 395 children from nondisclosure to disclosure status to assess whether their quality of life was negatively impacted by the disclosure and to estimate the average age of disclosure. The study found that the mean age for disclosure in this sample of children was 11 years; interestingly, the average age for disclosure decreased in the years after the relative beginning of the AIDS epidemic in the early 1980s. The researchers found only minimal change in quality-of-life measurements from pre- to

postdisclosure and suggest that both fear and the social stigma previously associated with HIV may be diminishing to the point that disclosure at a younger age would not be detrimental to the child's psychological well-being (Butler et al., 2009).

HIV and School Settings. As the population of children living with HIV/AIDS gets older, there are more HIV-infected children and adolescents in school systems. Parents of these children strive to maintain normal in-school and out-of-school routines as much as possible. Children who have HIV are protected by the federal Individuals with Disabilities Education Act and may not be discriminated against in the school. The National Association of State Boards of Education (NASBE) in 2001 produced an excellent guide to education policy and HIV infection that asserts that HIV is not a significant risk to others in the school setting when school personnel follow appropriate guidelines, and affirms the right of children and adults with HIV to fully participate in both the education and extracurricular programs at school. This document is in current use. Most states have written policies based on this document, and these state-specific policies can be accessed through the NASBE. Privacy provisions are clearly stated and maintain that no one is required to disclose HIV status, nor will HIV antibody testing be required for any reason (National Association of State Boards of Education, 2001). Strict confidentiality and health record keeping and storage procedures will be followed for all in the school setting according to the law, and a person's HIV status will not appear in educational records without consent. Schools will operate according to the standards promulgated by the U.S. Occupational Safety and Health Administration for the prevention of bloodborne infections. (For a complete copy of this guide, "Someone at School has AIDS," go to www.nasbe.org.) Because most HIV medications are now given once or twice daily under most circumstances, it is no longer necessary for school nurses to be involved in the administration of a child's medications.

CORTICOSTEROID THERAPY

Corticosteroids, given as part of a treatment regimen, act as natural products of the adrenal glands, reducing local and systemic inflammatory symptoms.

Incidence

Topical steroids are applied to the skin or mucous membranes to reduce edema and redness and to counteract itching. They may be used to treat ophthalmic reactions and skin conditions such as eczema. Hydrocortisone cream is one example of a topical steroid. Systemic steroids reduce the inflammatory symptoms of generalized allergic reactions (e.g., asthma, hives, severe contact dermatitis). Systemic steroids are also given increasingly to treat malignant or autoimmune disorders. An example of a systemic steroid is prednisolone (see Drug Guide).

Inhaled corticosteroids produce a very strong local action and can control symptoms in children with asthma and allergic rhinitis. An example of an aerosol steroid is beclomethasone (see Chapter 21). Studies have varied as to whether long-term use of inhaled corticosteroids results in growth delay, with the general consensus being that there may be an initial period of growth delay but little effect on eventual height (National Heart, Lung, and Blood Institute & National Asthma Education and Prevention Program, 2007; Weldon, 2009). Inhaled corticosteroids may also have a possible long-term effect on bone density, although not as much an effect as long-term use of oral steroids (Weldon, 2009).

Pathophysiology

Corticosteroids have many different effects but are usually prescribed for their antiinflammatory or immunosuppressive properties. As antiinflammatories, they inhibit chemical mediators and the occurrence of edema, capillary dilation, phagocytic activity, and the migration of leukocytes associated with the inflammatory response. As immunosuppressives, they decrease monocyte and macrophage differentiation and block lymphokine production, leading to T-cell inhibition.

The side effects of steroids vary widely with the child and the medication. Generally, the higher the dose and the longer the medication is taken, the more serious are the side effects. More knowledge about reactions and a broader selection of steroids and alternatives have significantly reduced untoward reactions in recent years.

Manifestations

Clinical manifestations of excess topically administered steroids include skin atrophy, delayed wound healing, telangiectasis or dilation of the cheek blood vessels, striae, and excess absorption leading to any of the clinical manifestations of systemic use.

DRUG GUIDE

Prednisolone (Pediapred, Prelone)

Classification
Corticosteroid

Action
Decreases inflammation; suppresses the immune response; affects bone marrow and the metabolism of proteins, carbohydrates, and fats.

Indications
Given for severe allergic and inflammatory conditions (e.g., asthma, eczema, juvenile arthritis), immunosuppression, and some autoimmune disorders.

Dosages and Route
Pediatric, oral: 0.5 to 2 mg/kg daily in divided doses; comes in syrup (15 mg/5 mL) or tablets (1 mg, 5 mg, 25 mg).

Absorption
Rapid absorption from the gastrointestinal tract.

Excretion
Half eliminated in 2 to 4 hr; metabolized in the liver and excreted in the urine.

Contraindications
Do not give if the child has a systemic fungal infection or is sensitive to any of the ingredients.

Precautions
Children taking prednisolone are more prone to infection. Avoid exposure to measles or chickenpox while on prednisolone; immunize the child with live-virus vaccines (measles, mumps, rubella; varicella) before beginning corticosteroid treatment. Avoid giving with nonsteroidal antiinflammatory drugs or aspirin because it may increase the risk for gastrointestinal bleeding.

Adverse Reactions
Gastrointestinal distress, cushingoid state (moon face, buffalo hump), delayed wound healing, skin eruptions, carbohydrate intolerance, fluid retention, growth delay in children. Acute adrenal insufficiency can occur when the child is under stress or if the medication is withdrawn abruptly. Do not discontinue this medication without tapering the dose.

Nursing Considerations
Teach the parent to have the child take the medication with food or milk. Store the medication in a cool, dry location. Teach the parent to notify the physician if the child exhibits any of the following: fever, other signs of infection, fatigue, muscle weakness, sudden weight gain, severe gastric irritation, slow wound healing, or growth delay, or if the child is experiencing increased stress.

Some clinical manifestations of excess steroid administered systemically include the following:

- Edema, particularly in the face
- Gastrointestinal irritation, even bleeding
- Bruising and delayed wound healing
- Susceptibility to infections
- Growth limitations
- Hypertension
- Loss of muscle mass
- Increased appetite and weight gain
- Amenorrhea
- Pancreatitis
- Joint pain and osteoporosis (may lead to bone fractures)
- Cataracts

Diagnostic Evaluation

The diagnosis of corticosteroid excess is suspected when clinical manifestations appear and it is confirmed by administering a bolus of adrenocorticotropic hormone (ACTH) to the child. ACTH challenges the adrenal gland to respond to pituitary stimulation. If serum cortisol levels do not rise after administration of ACTH, adrenal suppression (cortisone excess) is present.

Therapeutic Management

Every effort is made to prevent corticosteroid excess by observing the following:

- Short-term, high-dose therapy (for 1 week or less) is preferred over long-term therapy if there is a strong indication for the use of steroids.
- If long-term use is necessary, alternate-day administration may be prescribed.
- At the time of an acute infection or surgery, supplementary steroids are indicated for children who have received them over a long period.
- Because of immunosuppression, killed-virus vaccines are substituted for live-virus vaccines for children receiving high-dose or long-term steroids.

Children and adolescents who are receiving long-term oral or inhaled corticosteroids need to be meticulous about taking recommended calcium and vitamin D. In addition, height velocity should be assessed on a regular basis (Weldon, 2009).

NURSING CARE OF THE CHILD RECEIVING CORTICOSTEROIDS

■ Assessment

Assessment of a child receiving long-term steroid therapy includes measuring height, weight, and blood pressure at each visit. In addition, the nurse observes the child for facial puffiness, abdominal pain, increased appetite, blurred vision, and increased thirst or urination. Families may report recent illnesses, bruising, or delayed wound healing.

■ Nursing Diagnosis and Planning

The nursing diagnoses and expected outcomes that may be appropriate after assessment of a child receiving corticosteroid therapy are as follows:

- Ineffective Family Therapeutic Regimen Management: Nonadherence related to associated complications.

Expected Outcome. The child will take all medications as directed.

- Disturbed Body Image related to changes caused by treatment.

Expected Outcome. The child will share feelings about any changes in appearance.

- Risk for Infection related to immunosuppression.

Expected Outcome. The child will be afebrile and free of signs of secondary infections.

- Risk for Injury (adrenal insufficiency, delayed wound healing) related to insufficient knowledge.

Expected Outcomes. The child will not experience injury as a result of too-rapid withdrawal of medication or delayed wound healing. The parent can explain the reason for not withdrawing the medication abruptly.

- Risk for Delayed Development related to growth suppression and muscle wasting.

Expected Outcome. The child will continue to grow according to his or her own height and weight curve.

■ Interventions

The nurse should provide the family with written instructions that specifically state what to do if a dose is missed and when to decrease dosages. In general, if a dose is missed, the child should take it as soon as it is remembered; if it is almost time for the next dose, the child should skip the dose altogether. The nurse should emphasize not to discontinue corticosteroid therapy abruptly. The child needs to take the medication with foods or milk to minimize the risk for gastrointestinal bleeding. Because the child's appetite may be increased, encouraging low-calorie snacks throughout the day is appropriate. (The nurse should remind the family that salt may increase fluid retention.) Liquid forms of systemic corticosteroids can seem unpalatable to children. In this instance, the child may prefer a crushed tablet that has been put in a very small amount of a sweet food, or the liquid can be mixed with a sweet drink. Be sure to tell parents to mix the medication in 1 teaspoon or less of food or only a small amount of liquid to ensure that the child receives all the medication.

Changes in appearance are temporary and reversible. The nurse can compare changes in appearance and weight gain at each visit and encourage expression of the child's feelings. Weight and height monitoring of the child receiving long-term corticosteroid therapy is important; fluid retention can mask muscle wasting and growth suppression.

Corticosteroids can also mask infections. The family should be instructed to call the physician in the event of temperature elevation, cough, runny nose, ear tenderness, decreased appetite, nausea, vomiting, diarrhea, or behavioral change, or even if the child just "does not seem right." The child's skin should be checked routinely for bruising and signs of wound infection, and lesions that do not resolve as expected should be reported. The family should not treat the child with over-the-counter products without consulting the physician. The child receiving long-term therapy should avoid others who are sick; parents should promptly report any exposure to a communicable disease, such as measles or chickenpox, to the health care provider.

Because of possible impact on growth and bone density, the child should have a diet high in calcium-rich foods. Most young children receive vitamin D supplements, which enhance the absorption of calcium; children who are taking corticosteroids may need to be evaluated for increased requirements for calcium and vitamin D.

Potential environmental hazards and accident prevention strategies based on the child's developmental age should be emphasized. If the child gets a cut, the parent may hold gentle pressure to the site for 3 to 5 minutes to stop the bleeding and prevent hematoma formation. The child should wear a medical-alert bracelet stating the key clinical manifestations of corticosteroid excess or adrenal insufficiency.

⚡ SAFETY ALERT
The Child Taking Oral Corticosteroids

Long-term corticosteroid therapy causes adrenal insufficiency because exogenous (outside the body) use reduces the need for endogenous (within the body) production. Abrupt cessation of corticosteroid use without allowing for a gradual increase in adrenal production can cause insufficiency.

- Taper the dose to allow for a gradual return of adrenal function.
- Carefully monitor the child during the tapering process for the following: fatigue, muscle weakness, joint pain, dizziness, anorexia, nausea.
- Supplemental glucocorticoids might be necessary during times of increased stress to prevent adrenal insufficiency.

▪ Evaluation

- Is the child taking corticosteroids as directed?
- Is the child able to express feelings about any changes in appearance?
- Does the child remain afebrile and free of any signs of secondary infection?
- Are any wounds healing at a normal rate?
- Is the child displaying any signs of adrenal insufficiency, and can the parent explain why the medication should not be withdrawn abruptly?
- Is the child growing at a rate appropriate for age as measured on a standard growth chart?
- Is the child obtaining an appropriate amount of calcium and taking recommended vitamin D supplements?

IMMUNE COMPLEX AND AUTOIMMUNE DISORDERS

Immune Complex Disorders

Immune complexes are clusters of interlocking antigens and antibodies. Under normal conditions, immune complexes are removed from the blood. In some circumstances, however, immune complexes continue to circulate. Eventually they become trapped in the tissues of the kidneys, lungs, skin, joints, or blood vessels. There they set off reactions that lead to tissue inflammation and damage.

Deposition of immune complexes is considered to be a precipitator for several different conditions in childhood. Both Kawasaki disease (see Chapter 22) and acute poststreptococcal glomerulonephritis (see Chapter 20) are thought to be caused by immune complex deposition in tissue.

Autoimmune Disorders

Sometimes the immune system's ability to differentiate self from nonself breaks down and the body begins to make antibodies against its own cells, tissues (particularly connective tissue), and organs. Such antibodies are known as autoantibodies. Autoantibodies are common in conditions such as rheumatic fever (see Chapter 22), juvenile arthritis (see Chapter 26), and systemic lupus erythematosus.

It is still unclear what initiates an autoimmune response. Several theories have been proposed:

- Activation of immature B cells that do not develop antigen-specific receptors
- Alteration of normal tissue cells by infection or another process, which causes them to become antigenic
- Similarity between the structures of some infectious organisms and self-antigens, causing a cross-reaction
- Genetic predisposition of defective immune regulation

The response is exacerbated by a malfunction of helper T and suppressor T cells when there are too many helper cells and not enough suppressor cells to turn off the immune response. Some autoimmune disorders also manifest with increased tissue deposits of immune complexes.

SYSTEMIC LUPUS ERYTHEMATOSUS

Systemic lupus erythematosus (SLE) is a chronic, multisystem autoimmune disease characterized by inflammation of the connective tissue. SLE varies in severity and is marked by remissions and exacerbations.

Etiology

Although the etiology of SLE is not known, genetic, environmental, hormonal, and immune response factors are likely to be responsible. Environmental factors can include exposure to the sun, ultraviolet light, stress, fatigue, viruses, bacteria, certain medications, and some food additives.

Incidence

The overall prevalence of SLE is 3.3 to 8.8 per 100,000 (Kamphuis & Silverman, 2010). The condition is relatively rare in young children and has an average age of onset between 11 and 12 years. In young children, the female-to-male ratio is 4-5 : 1; after puberty, this ratio increases to 9 : 1. More African-American, Hispanic, Native American and Asian children are affected than white children (Kamphuis & Silverman, 2010).

PATHOPHYSIOLOGY

Systemic Lupus Erythematosus

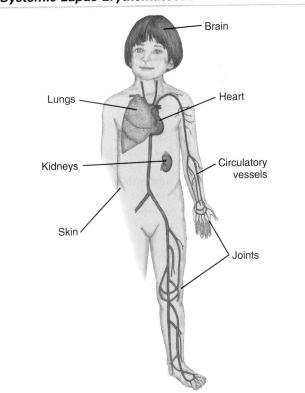

Body Systems Affected by SLE

Many abnormalities in the immune system are associated with SLE. Autoantibodies, referred to as antinuclear antibodies (ANAs), act against DNA and other cell nucleus components. Abnormal immune complex formation and nonspecific activation of B lymphocytes cause an increase in immune globulins, a process that triggers autoantibodies. This response is exacerbated by a reduction in the number of suppressor T cells. These autoantibodies produce inflammation and damage tissues and organs, including the skin, joints, heart, lungs, kidneys, brain, and circulatory vessels.

A child with SLE also might have weight loss, growth impairment, headache, and memory problems. Occasionally, children will have Raynaud's phenomenon, in which the digits of the hands and feet suddenly change color (mottled to white to blue) in response to cold. The most serious complications of SLE include renal disease and neurologic problems.

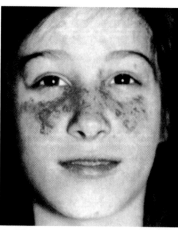

FIG 18-1 The butterfly rash of systemic lupus erythematosus. (From Kliegman, R., Stanton, B., St. Geme, J., Schor, N., & Behrman, R. [Eds.]. [2011]. *Nelson textbook of pediatrics* [19th ed., p. 842], Philadelphia: Elsevier.)

Manifestations

Malaise, arthralgia, and recurrent fever of unknown etiology frequently are among the early manifestations of SLE, and these manifestations can be easily confused with signs of other childhood illnesses. Neurologic manifestations, such as headaches, mood disorders, cognitive disorders, and seizure disorders, are often seen in children with SLE (Muscal & Brey, 2010). In general, signs and symptoms depend on what organs the immune complexes affect and can include the following (Klein-Gitelman, 2010):

- Malar butterfly rash: A fixed, red, flat or raised rash over the cheeks and the bridge of the nose (Figure 18-1)
- Discoid rash: Red, round, raised patches that spread
- Photosensitivity: Skin rash from sun exposure
- Oral and nasal ulcers: Usually painless lesions
- Arthritis: Painful, swollen joints with edema
- Pleuritis, pericarditis, or peritonitis
- Renal disorder: Protein, casts, or red blood cells in urine
- Neurologic disorders: Headaches, personality changes, seizures, or psychosis
- Hematologic disorders: Anemia, leukopenia, lymphopenia, or thrombocytopenia
- Immunologic disorders
- Positive antinuclear antibody (ANA) assay

Diagnostic Evaluation

Conforming with the American Rheumatism Association 1982 criteria for diagnosis, the presence of four or more of the clinical manifestations just listed, regardless of whether they occur simultaneously, is suggestive of SLE. In addition, a number of tests can be used to diagnose and monitor the progress of SLE. A positive ANA test, the presence of anti-DNA antibody, and the presence of antiphospholipid antibody are highly suggestive of SLE. Blood urea nitrogen levels, gamma globulin levels, and the erythrocyte sedimentation rate might be elevated. Complement levels (C3 and C4) can be decreased. Pathologic changes compatible with SLE may be confirmed by electrocardiography, computed tomography, and magnetic resonance imaging and by skin and renal tissue biopsy specimens demonstrating immune complexes.

Therapeutic Management

The treatment of SLE is tailored to the organ system or systems affected and is aimed at preventing exacerbations and complications. The goal of treatment is to use the least amount of pharmacologic intervention needed. Helping the child and family develop long-term coping strategies is important.

Systemic corticosteroids are most often given to control the inflammatory response. When steroid treatment is not effective or renal progression is rapid, cyclophosphamide (Cytoxan) might be considered. Nonsteroidal antiinflammatory drugs, excluding ibuprofen, are sometimes used to treat arthritis, serositis, and febrile attacks. Because they can cause liver damage, they are used with caution and careful monitoring. Children with renal and neurologic disorders generally receive anticonvulsant and antihypertensive therapy, whereas those with skin lesions and joint problems take antimalarial drugs such as hydroxychloroquine (Plaquenil). Killed-virus vaccines rather than live-virus vaccines are used in affected children. A low-salt diet may reduce fluid retention and prevent elevated blood urea nitrogen levels; a low-protein diet helps preserve renal function.

The long-term prognosis for children with SLE is positive; the 5-year survival rate is close to 100% (Klein-Gitelman, 2010). Close monitoring is essential for positive outcomes. Adverse outcomes can include delayed growth and onset of puberty, decreased bone mass, atherosclerosis, and decreased quality of life (Klein-Gitelman, 2010).

NURSING CARE OF THE CHILD WITH SYSTEMIC LUPUS ERYTHEMATOSUS

▪ Assessment

During a period of disease exacerbation, a child with SLE can become acutely ill. The nurse monitors the child's vital signs, mobility, activity level, and pain and completes a neurologic examination that assesses for decreased sensation, weakness in the extremities, and changes in behavior. Of equal importance is evaluation of the effect of living with a chronic illness on a young child's self-image and interaction with peers.

▪ Nursing Diagnosis and Planning

The nursing diagnoses that apply to the child with SLE are as follows:
- Disturbed Body Image related to changes secondary to the disease process and treatments.

Expected Outcome. The child will share feelings about altered appearance or function.
- Powerlessness related to memory and emotional alterations.

Expected Outcome. The child and family will seek assistance in managing memory or emotional problems.
- Activity Intolerance related to the effects of the disease process.

Expected Outcome. The child will participate in activities to the extent possible.
- Chronic Pain related to arthritis and numbness of the hands and feet.

Expected Outcome. The child will be free of pain, demonstrating an acceptable level on an age-appropriate pain assessment tool and the ability to gain appropriate rest and participate in age-appropriate activities.
- Ineffective Family Therapeutic Regimen Management: Nonadherence related to associated complications and developmental level.

Expected Outcome. The child will take all medications as directed and describe the medication plan and any medication side effects.

▪ Interventions

The nurse needs to help the child and family understand the importance of drug therapy and activity restriction during acute exacerbations. Avoiding triggers that cause exacerbations is essential (e.g., avoiding exposure to sun or avoidable sources of infection). Wearing an appropriate sunscreen is a necessity (sun protection factor above 15, waterproof, para-aminobenzoic acid free, ultraviolet A and ultraviolet B protective). Raynaud's phenomenon can be prevented by dressing warmly in cold weather, paying particular attention to hat, gloves, and warm socks. An adolescent will have difficulty achieving a balance between the need to take risks and be accepted by peers and the realities of a chronic illness (see Chapter 12). The teenager with a chronic illness needs to participate as fully as possible in activities at home, at school, and in the community. Documenting episodes of fatigue along with associated activities allows young people to gain some control. They can then use this information to make sensible decisions about participation in extracurricular activities. The adolescent should be encouraged to plan an appropriate and convenient medication self-administration schedule and should be able to describe the side effects of the prescribed medications.

Anger about the diagnosis and alienation from peers are common. Wearing makeup can mask rashes and improve appearance. Keeping a diary also helps the young person vent anger. An affected peer who is in remission can offer support, as can national SLE organizations (see Evolve website). The Internet is also a source of support and information.

■ Evaluation

- Does the child share feelings about her (or his) appearance or function?
- Do the child and family seek assistance as needed for related memory or emotional problems?
- Does the child participate in sports and extracurricular activities without becoming overly fatigued?
- Is the child free of pain as documented on an age-appropriate pain assessment tool?
- Is the child taking all medications as directed, and can the child describe the medication plan and side effects of the medications?

ALLERGIC REACTIONS

Allergy is the immune response to an antigen called an allergen that causes a hypersensitivity reaction in various body systems. This hypersensitivity reaction, which occurs with a second exposure to an antigen, can be immediate or delayed. The classification of allergic reactions often reflects the pathophysiologic features of each type (Table 18-3). In most children with allergies, there is a genetic link. Common allergic conditions include allergic rhinitis, hives, eczema, asthma, colic, and migraines (Table 18-4).

Allergic rhinitis is an immediate hypersensitivity reaction to allergens trapped by the hairs and mucus that line the inside of the nose (see Chapter 21). Anaphylaxis is a life-threatening allergic response. Allergic reactions are related to the antibody IgE.

ANAPHYLAXIS

Anaphylaxis, a severe, immediate hypersensitivity reaction to an excessive release of chemical mediators, affects the entire body.

Etiology

Food allergy is a major cause of anaphylaxis in children (Leonard, 2010). Other causes include penicillin or other antibiotics, insect stings, immunizations, allergy immunotherapy (desensitization), chemotherapeutic agents, blood products, and diagnostic contrast media. Peanuts (including peanut butter) and tree nuts (e.g., cashews, almonds, walnuts, pecans, pistachios) are particularly potent substances, causing anaphylaxis in increasing numbers. Other frequently seen food allergies include milk, eggs, wheat, shellfish, and other fish. Anaphylactic reactions to products containing latex have increased in incidence, especially among children with spina bifida (see Chapter 28) and children with abnormalities of the urinary tract.

Incidence

Approximately 6% to 8% of children in the United States have severe allergic reactions to foods (Leonard, 2010). In many cases, previous exposure to the allergen is undocumented, so the child has anaphylaxis presumably on first documented exposure. In the child who is allergic to foods, the allergen usually is small particles of food protein (National Institute of Allergy and Infectious Diseases [NIAID], 2010). For children with allergies to peanuts or other nuts, an anaphylactic reaction can occur with exposure to nut oils, surfaces contaminated with nuts, shell fragments, or cooking and serving utensils used previously for nut products.

The incidence of anaphylaxis in the United States from all causes is considered to be 50 per 100,000 (Sampson & Leung, 2011).

PATHOPHYSIOLOGY

Anaphylaxis

Anaphylaxis occurs when an allergen binds with IgE on mast cells and basophils, causing degranulation and release of histamines and other chemical mediators. Histamine action precipitates respiratory signs of bronchoconstriction with bronchospasm and edema (especially laryngeal edema) from increased vascular permeability. Other systems most affected during an anaphylactic response include gastrointestinal (itchiness and tingling along the gastrointestinal tract, vomiting, diarrhea, pain) and integumentary (urticaria). Anaphylaxis can lead to circulatory collapse and death if not promptly managed. An allergen that has previously provoked a response, or one that has not, can cause anaphylaxis.

TABLE 18-3 CLASSIFICATION OF ALLERGIC REACTIONS

TYPE	PATHOPHYSIOLOGY	EXAMPLES
I. Immediate (anaphylactic) hypersensitivity	IgE attaches to mast cells and basophils, causing rupture and release of all contents (i.e., histamines).	Allergic rhinitis, acute anaphylaxis, hives, eczema, asthma
II. Cytotoxic hypersensitivity	An allergen (e.g., red blood cell) stimulates IgE or IgM to react and mobilize complement to destroy the allergen.	Transfusion reaction after receiving incompatible blood
III. Arthus hypersensitivity (immune complex)	Immune complex is formed and can destroy tissues.	Serum sickness, glomerulonephritis
IV. Delayed cell-mediated hypersensitivity	An allergen reacts with T lymphocytes, and these lead other cells to produce damage.	Contact dermatitis (e.g., poison ivy)

TABLE 18-4 COMMON ALLERGIC CONDITIONS IN CHILDREN

ALLERGENS	MANIFESTATIONS	DIAGNOSIS
Inhalants		
Pollen, dust, mold, dander	Sneezing; red, itchy nose, eyes, pharynx, and palate; edematous nasal passages; tongue clicking; runny or congested nose; mouth breathing; chronic cough; dark circles under eyes; nose wrinkling; pale, boggy nasal mucous membranes	Allergic rhinitis
Applicants		
Heat, cold, wool, cosmetics, solutions for hair permanents, sunscreens, plants, grasses	Well-defined red, raised skin or mucosal lesions	Hives Contact dermatitis
Foods		
Milk, wheat, eggs, strawberries, tomatoes, oranges, chocolate, nuts, shellfish	Intestinal cramping, nausea, vomiting, diarrhea Bronchospasm Red patches on cheeks, face, wrists, neck, hands, extremities; swelling; itching; weeping; scales and crust Well-defined red, raised skin or mucosal lesions Vascular headaches	Colic Asthma Eczema Hives Migraines Possible anaphylaxis
Medicines		
Penicillin, cephalexin, immunizations, allergy immunotherapy, chemotherapy	Redness, swelling, pain Weakness, restlessness, edema, laryngospasm, cardiovascular collapse	Local inflammation Anaphylaxis
Insects		
Stings of bees, wasps, hornets	Redness, swelling, pain Weakness, restlessness, edema, laryngospasm, cardiovascular collapse	Local inflammation Anaphylaxis

Manifestations

The onset of anaphylaxis is sudden, usually occurring within seconds to minutes after exposure to an allergen. Initial symptoms of impending anaphylaxis include the following:

- Sneezing
- Tightness or tingling of the mouth or face, with subsequent swelling of the lips and tongue
- Severe flushing, urticaria, and itching of the skin, especially on the head and upper trunk
- Rapid development of erythema
- A sense of impending doom

These symptoms might be followed by gastrointestinal and respiratory symptoms, which include nausea, vomiting, diarrhea, and cramping, as well as rhinorrhea, stridor, wheezing, and hoarseness.

The most serious features of anaphylaxis are laryngospasm, edema, cyanosis, hypotensive shock, vascular collapse, and cardiac arrest. Several hours after the initial phase of anaphylaxis resolves, a second, or biphasic, reaction can occur. This second reaction can be as severe as the initial reaction, affects similar body systems, and can occur hours up to several days after the initial episode.

Diagnostic Evaluation

Anaphylaxis occurs suddenly, allowing no time for diagnosis. The etiology is determined later by obtaining a history of the exposure. Serum studies may reveal an elevated IgE for the agent of exposure. In some cases the allergen can be confirmed by skin tests or radioallergosorbent test (RAST). For children with food allergy, a combination of skin prick testing, allergen-specific serum IgE levels, and atopy patch test best confirm a diagnosis of food allergy (NIAID, 2010).

Therapeutic Management

Treatment of anaphylaxis must begin immediately because it may be only a matter of minutes before shock occurs. In the community setting, immediately activate the emergency response system. Injectable epinephrine is the first drug of choice in the acute treatment of anaphylaxis. In addition to epinephrine, oral diphenhydramine, a histamine inhibitor (e.g., ranitidine, cimetidine), and/or corticosteroids may be indicated.

Epinephrine (0.01 mg/kg/dose of 1:1000 concentration) is administered to children with suspected anaphylaxis. Children with known severe allergic reactions need to have an EpiPen or other preloaded, automatic delivery system available at all times. The EpiPen (0.3 mg) is appropriate for children who weigh more than 25 kg, and the EpiPen Jr. (0.15 mg) can be administered to children who weigh 10 to 25 kg (NIAID, 2010).

In a hospital or emergency setting, managing anaphylactic shock includes the following:

- Ensure an adequate airway, possibly by endotracheal intubation (see Chapter 10).
- Administer epinephrine. If reaction is caused by an insect sting, place a tourniquet proximal to the site of the sting and administer epinephrine in the uninvolved extremity and in the area of reaction, with repeat dosing within 5 to 10 minutes.
- Administer oxygen if available.
- Administer corticosteroids and antihistamines as ordered.
- Keep the child warm and lying flat or with feet slightly elevated.
- Start an IV line.

Children who have had life-threatening insect sting anaphylaxis and demonstrate venom-specific IgE antibodies on skin studies or

RAST are candidates for venom immunotherapy. All children experiencing episodes of anaphylaxis in the community should be transported by ambulance to an emergency facility (see Chapter 10) and kept for observation at least 4 to 6 hours after the episode is resolved to ensure prompt intervention should a biphasic reaction occur.

NURSING CARE OF THE CHILD WITH ANAPHYLAXIS

■ Assessment

The child should be monitored closely for airway obstruction and vascular collapse during the acute phase of anaphylaxis. Assessment includes noting airway patency, respiratory rate and effort, heart rate, peripheral pulses, capillary refill time, oxygen saturation, urine output, and level of consciousness. After emergency efforts, the nurse can try to determine the cause of the attack by correlating when the symptoms first occurred with foods ingested, medications administered, and the possibility of an insect sting.

■ Nursing Diagnosis and Planning

The nursing diagnoses that apply to the child with anaphylaxis and to the family are as follows:

- Ineffective Breathing Pattern and Decreased Cardiac Output related to an excessive hypersensitive reaction to an allergen.

Expected Outcome. The child will maintain a patent airway and adequate cardiac output (short term).

- Deficient Knowledge about allergens and prevention through risk reduction related to inexperience.

Expected Outcome. The child and family will describe the child's allergic reaction and initiate a management plan for avoiding allergens and treating reactions (long term).

■ Interventions

Initially, the nurse maintains an adequate airway by administering oxygen and assisting with aerosol treatments and intubation as necessary. A laryngoscope, an intubation tray, and a tracheostomy kit should be available, and the code cart should be nearby. In the case of an insect sting or injected medication, a tourniquet applied to the affected extremity just proximal to the site might help confine the allergen. It is important to have IV access, with a large-bore needle, in at least one site, preferably two, for medication administration. The nurse administers IV fluids, epinephrine, corticosteroids, and antihistamines as ordered and informs the physician of the child's improvement or deterioration. Extra fluids (crystalloids or colloids) and plasma expanders should be administered if the child shows signs of vascular collapse (see Chapter 10). Because epinephrine causes vasoconstriction and an increase in cardiac output, a child receiving the drug might have heart palpitations and tachycardia. This is frightening and aggravated by the emergency nature of the situation. The nurse should offer gentle reassurance to the child and provide the family with frequent reports about the child's condition.

After an initial anaphylactic episode, the nurse should assure the child and family that they were not at fault for the anaphylactic reaction and discuss how to prevent recurrences. Any child who has experienced anaphylaxis should have and learn to use an injectable epinephrine. The EpiPen Jr. for children (weighing less than 25 kg) delivers 0.15 mg of epinephrine through a spring-loaded injector, and the EpiPen (for children weighing more than 25 kg) provides 0.3 mg of epinephrine. The dosage chosen by the provider is based on the child's weight. Teach the parent or child to hold the injector against the skin of the upper outer region of the child's thigh for 10 seconds after administering the injection to deliver the medication completely. The EpiPen can be injected through clothing. A medical-alert bracelet alerts others to the child's allergy.

Caring for the child at school presents an additional challenge (see Patient-Centered Teaching: Communicating with the School about Peanut Allergies box). The school nurse must be aware of and communicate to appropriate others information about any child who has had anaphylaxis. Policies about storage of and access to the EpiPen in the school setting differ in each school district. Some school districts train nonmedical personnel to administer the epinephrine if the child goes on a field trip; other school districts require a parent of a child who cannot self-administer epinephrine to accompany the child on a field trip. It is necessary for the school nurse to notify teachers and school nutrition personnel if a child or children in the school have allergies to peanuts or other foods. In some instances, the child may be so highly allergic that lunch needs to be eaten in the school health office, away from even the odor of peanut butter. Most commercial fast-food establishments post signs if pastries or other foods contain peanuts or other allergenic substances.

PATIENT-CENTERED TEACHING

Communicating with the School about Peanut Allergies

If your child has had a severe reaction to peanuts or other nuts, it is important for you to talk to your health care provider about whether the child should have medication available at home and school.

Epinephrine, the medication that relieves a severe allergic reaction, is available in an easy-to-use automatic injector, which older children can self-administer and teachers or other school personnel can be taught to administer.

Important things to remember when using automatically injected epinephrine are as follows:

1. If using an EpiPen, the injection can be given through the child's clothing.
2. After starting the injection, you must continue to hold the EpiPen against the child for at least 10 seconds for all the medication to be delivered.

Your child should have an allergy action plan readily available at school. You can obtain a sample action plan from www.foodallergy.org.

Talk to the school nurse about the severity of your child's reaction and work with the nurse to create a way your child can avoid contact with peanuts while not singling the child out for special attention.

Many school districts have policies that prohibit sharing of food or eating food on school buses. Other practices available at certain schools include peanut-free classrooms and a peanut-free area in the school cafeteria. Your school nurse can help you decide what modifications are appropriate for your child.

■ Evaluation

- Is the child awake and alert with adequate oxygenation and a patent airway?
- Are the child's vital signs within normal limits for age?
- Is the family taking appropriate steps to reduce the risks of another anaphylactic reaction (see Patient-Centered Teaching: How to Prevent Insect Stings box)?
- Do the child, family, and other appropriate adults demonstrate the proper use of the insect sting kit?

PATIENT-CENTERED TEACHING

How to Prevent Insect Stings

- Select clothes with white or khaki colors, not dark or brightly decorative ones.
- Wear fitted clothes with long sleeves, pants, and shoes.
- Use unscented soaps, lotions, and deodorants.
- Apply insect skin protection.
- Avoid orchards, flowers, blooming trees, and shrubs.
- Stay away from picnic areas.

- Keep out of the garden.
- Keep car windows closed while driving.
- Place screens on all windows.
- Cover all garbage cans.
- Move away slowly from approaching insects.

KEY CONCEPTS

- The immune system maintains homeostasis of the internal and external environment through nonspecific functions (inflammation, phagocytosis) and specific functions (humoral and cell-mediated immunity). Any derangement results in an immunologic imbalance whereby the immune system either underfunctions or overfunctions.
- When the immune system underfunctions, susceptibility to infections is increased (immunodeficiency). When the immune system overfunctions, it produces antibodies against cells of the body in autoimmune disease or against external sensitizing agents, forming the basis for allergies.
- Children with acquired or congenital immunodeficiency are vulnerable to bacterial and viral infections. The best way to prevent the spread of organisms is to practice appropriate hand hygiene routinely and to follow basic infection control practices on the basis of three principles: (1) prevent contact with organisms, (2) create barriers if contact is unavoidable, and (3) kill organisms if contact is made.
- HIV infection is the best-known acquired immunodeficiency disease. It causes a wide spectrum of illness in children, ranging from no symptoms to mild and moderate symptoms to severe symptoms.

- Standard treatments for HIV infection include a modified immunization program, antiretroviral therapy, PCP prophylaxis, and aggressive use of antibiotics.
- For children with HIV, nurses have the challenging tasks of respiratory management, promoting normal growth and development, preventing infections, and providing comfort. In addition, nurses must support families in dealing with a stigmatizing illness that is chronic in nature.
- Children who acquired HIV when they were born are now reaching teen years. Nurses must discuss issues of infection transmission and medication adherence with these teens.
- Corticosteroids have immunosuppressive and antiinflammatory properties. Tapering the dose during both long-term and short-term therapy regimens allows for the gradual return of adrenal function.
- Emergency treatment takes priority in an anaphylactic reaction because it is only a matter of minutes before the child will go into shock. In a community setting, epinephrine is administered to children with a known prior anaphylactic episode and the emergency service system is activated. Initially, the goal is to maintain an adequate airway, sometimes necessitating endotracheal intubation. This is followed by the administration of epinephrine.

REFERENCES

American Academy of Pediatrics Committee on Pediatric AIDS. (1999, reaffirmed 2005). Disclosure of illness status to children and adolescents with HIV Infection. *Pediatrics, 103,* 164-165.

Banasik, J. (2005). Inflammation and immunity. In L. Copstead, & J. Banasik (Eds.), *Pathophysiology* (3rd ed., pp. 203-243). St. Louis: Elsevier Mosby.

Buckley, R. (2007). The T-, B-, and NK-cell systems. In R. Kliegman, R. Behrman, H. Jenson, & B. Stanton (Eds.), *Nelson textbook of pediatrics* (18th ed., pp. 873-879). Philadelphia: Elsevier Saunders.

Butler, A., Williams, P., Howland, L., et al., & Pediatric AIDS Clinical Trials Group 219C study team. (2009). Impact of disclosure of HIV infection on health-related quality of life among children and adolescents with HIV infection. *Pediatrics, 123,* 935-943.

Centers for Disease Control and Prevention. (2009a). Diagnosis of HIV infection and AIDS in the United States and dependent areas, 2009. *HIV Surveillance Report, 21.* Retrieved from www.cdc.gov.

Centers for Disease Control and Prevention. (2009b). Guidelines for the prevention and treatment of opportunistic infections among HIV-exposed and HIV-infected children. *MMWR: Morbidity and Mortality Weekly Report, 58*(RR-11), 1-176.

Centers for Disease Control and Prevention. (2010). *One test two lives.* Retrieved from www.cdc.gov.

Kamphuis, S., & Silverman, E. (2010). Prevalence and burden of pediatric onset SLE. *Nature Reviews of Rheumatology, 6,* 538-546.

Klein-Gitelman, M. (2010). *Pediatric systemic lupus erythematosus.* Retrieved from http://emedicine.medscape.com.

Leonard, S. (2010). *Food allergy: What you need to know.* Retrieved from www.medscape.com.

Muscal, E., & Brey, R. (2010). Neurologic manifestations of systemic lupus erythematosus in children and adults. *Neurologic Clinics of North America, 28,* 61-73.

National Association of State Boards of Education. (2001). *Someone at school has AIDS: A complete guide to education policies concerning HIV infection.* Retrieved from www.nasbe.org.

National Heart, Lung, and Blood Institute & National Asthma Education and Prevention Program. (2007). *Expert panel report 3: Guidelines for the diagnosis and management of asthma.* Retrieved from www.nhlbi.nih.gov.

National Institute of Allergy and Infectious Diseases. (2010). *Guidelines for the diagnosis and management of food allergy in the United States.* Retrieved from www.niaid.nih.gov.

Panel on Antiretroviral Therapy and Medical Management of HIV-Infected Children. (2011, August 11). *Guidelines for the use of antiretroviral agents in pediatric HIV infection.* Retrieved from www.aidsinfo.nih.gov.

Panel on Treatment of HIV-Infected Pregnant Women and Prevention of Perinatal Transmission. (2010, May 24). *Recommendations for use of antiretroviral drugs in pregnant HIV-1 infected women for maternal health and intervention to reduce prenatal HIV transmission*

in the United States. Retrieved from www.aidsinfo.nih.gov.

Porth, C. (2011). *Essentials of pathophysiology* (3rd ed.). Philadelphia: Wolters Kluwer.

Sampson, H., & Leung, D. (2011). Anaphylaxis. In R. Kliegman, B. Stanton, J. St. Geme, et al. (Eds.), *Nelson textbook of pediatrics* (19th ed., pp. 816-819). Philadelphia: Elsevier Saunders.

Shannon, M., Kennedy, H., Humphreys, J. (2008). HIV-infected mothers' foci of concern during the initial testing of their infants. *Journal of the Association of Nurses in AIDS Care, 19*(2), 114-126.

Weldon, D. (2009). The effects of corticosteroids on bone growth and bone density. *Annals of Allergy Asthma and Immunology, 103,* 3-11.

Working Group on Antiretroviral Therapy and Medical Management of HIV-Infected Children. (2008, February). *Guidelines for the use of antiretroviral agents in pediatric HIV infection.* Retrieved from www.aidsinfo.nih.gov.

Yogev, R., & Chadwick, E. (2011). Acquired immunodeficiency syndrome (human immunodeficiency virus). In R. Kliegman, B. Stanton, J. St. Geme, et al. (Eds.), *Nelson textbook of pediatrics* (19th ed., pp. 1157-1177). Philadelphia: Elsevier Saunders.

The Child with a Gastrointestinal Alteration

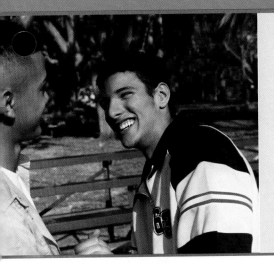

evolve WEBSITE

http://evolve.elsevier.com/James/ncoc

LEARNING OBJECTIVES

After studying this chapter, you should be able to:

- Describe the development of the gastrointestinal system and its relation to selected congenital defects.
- Describe the anatomy and physiology of the gastrointestinal system in the infant and child.
- Describe the common diagnostic and screening tests used to detect alterations in gastrointestinal function.
- Discuss and demonstrate an understanding of the structural and functional alterations in the gastrointestinal system.
- Discuss and demonstrate an understanding of the pathophysiology, etiology, clinical manifestations, diagnostic evaluation, and therapeutic management of malabsorption and infectious problems affecting the gastrointestinal system.

- State expected nursing diagnoses for gastrointestinal alterations.
- Use the nursing process to develop nursing care plans and teaching guidelines for the child with gastrointestinal alterations.
- Develop home care guidelines for the child with gastrointestinal alterations.
- Implement child and family teaching.
- Develop nursing implications for common medications used with the child with gastrointestinal alterations.
- Demonstrate critical thinking skills to manage a given patient care situation.

CLINICAL REFERENCE

REVIEW OF THE GASTROINTESTINAL SYSTEM

Upper Gastrointestinal System

The upper gastrointestinal (GI) system includes the mouth, esophagus, and stomach. Its primary functions are to take in food and fluids, begin the digestive process, and propel food into the intestines, where nutrients are absorbed. The mouth, or buccal cavity, is the entrance to the GI tract. Here food is broken up and mixed with saliva. This process starts the digestion of carbohydrates. The submandibular, parotid, and sublingual glands secrete saliva in response to the smell, taste, or thought of food. The tongue contains taste buds that distinguish salt, sweet, sour, and bitter sensations. The tongue is essential for swallowing.

At birth, the esophagus measures approximately 10 cm in length; it lengthens to 18 to 25 cm by adulthood. The upper third of the esophagus consists of striated voluntary muscle; the lower two thirds consist

of smooth muscle. The upper esophageal sphincter (UES) prevents the reflux of esophageal contents into the pharynx and lungs and prevents esophageal distention during respiration; the lower esophageal sphincter (LES, or cardiac sphincter) prevents the reflux of gastric contents into the lower esophagus.

Swallowing is under both voluntary and involuntary control. As food is chewed, it forms a small bolus, or mass; the tongue propels the bolus toward the oropharynx. The presence of this mass in the oropharynx stimulates the medulla, causing the soft palate to rise. The nasal passages close, the pharyngeal muscles contract, the larynx closes, and respiration is inhibited. As a result of these processes, food is propelled to the esophagus. Through peristalsis, the bolus moves on to the LES, the muscle relaxes, and the bolus enters the stomach.

The stomach lies in the epigastric, umbilical, and left hypochondrial regions of the abdomen. It is a muscular pouch, shaped somewhat like a gourd, where the bolus is received. As the LES and the pylorus

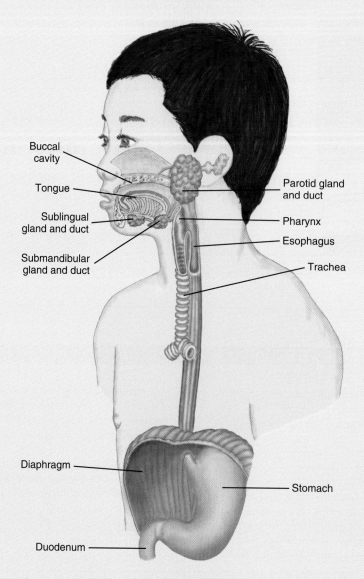

Buccal cavity

Tongue

Sublingual gland and duct

Submandibular gland and duct

Parotid gland and duct

Pharynx

Esophagus

Trachea

Diaphragm

Stomach

Duodenum

Anatomy of the Upper Gastrointestinal Tract

contract, the stomach muscles churn the contents. The contents mix with the digestive juices to form chyme. The chyme moves on to the pylorus and into the duodenum.

A mucous-bicarbonate barrier in the stomach provides a thick layer of mucus and a buffer zone to neutralize acid. Stomach acids diffuse slowly through this layer toward the gastric wall. They are neutralized by bicarbonate ions from the surface epithelial cells. Thus a neutral pH is maintained at the gastric epithelial surface.

Lower Gastrointestinal System

The lower GI system includes the duodenum, liver, gallbladder, pancreas, jejunum, ileum, cecum, appendix, ascending colon, transverse colon, descending colon, sigmoid colon, rectum, and anus. The primary functions of the lower GI tract are to digest and absorb nutrients, detoxify and excrete unwanted waste, and aid in fluid and electrolyte balance.

The duodenum, the first part of the small intestine, extends from the pylorus to the jejunum. Partially digested chyme from the stomach enters the duodenum, where pancreatic enzymes and bile are excreted to further break down fats, carbohydrates, and proteins. The pancreas is an oblong gland lying behind the stomach that secretes enzymes to digest food and secretes glucagon and insulin to control motility and absorption.

The liver, the largest organ in the body, is located under the right diaphragm. The liver lies predominantly in the right upper quadrant, with the left lobe extending into the left upper quadrant. It is divided into two lobes separated by the falciform ligament. Within each lobe are numerous lobules, which form the functional units of the liver.

The liver is unique in that it is supplied with blood from two sources: (1) the hepatic artery, which supplies oxygenated blood; and (2) the hepatic portal vein, which supplies deoxygenated blood

COMMON LABORATORY AND DIAGNOSTIC TESTS FOR GI DISORDERS

TEST	DESCRIPTION	NORMAL FINDINGS	INDICATIONS	PREPARATION AND NURSING CONSIDERATIONS
Stool				
Culture and sensitivity	Organisms from a small sample of stool are grown in culture media.	Normal GI flora	To identify infectious organisms and determine their antibiotic sensitivity.	No patient preparation is necessary. The sample is delivered to the laboratory immediately; it must be kept free from contamination.
Reducing substances (Clinitest)	Stool is diluted with water and then tested for undigested carbohydrates with Clinitest tablets.	Negative	Used to diagnose malabsorption syndromes.	No preparation is necessary. The test is done by the nurse, who checks for a color change in the solution.
Occult blood (guaiac, Hematest)	Stool is smeared on filter paper and prepared with solution.	Negative	Used in inflammatory conditions and bowel necrosis.	No preparation is necessary. The test is done by the nurse; a blue color is positive.
Ova and parasites (O&P)	Stool is examined microscopically for presence of parasites or their eggs.	Negative	To identify enteric parasites in child with diarrhea or abdominal pain.	No patient preparation is necessary. Sample must be free from water or urine contamination. The sample is delivered to the laboratory either fresh or in preservatives. Barium, antacids, mineral oil, and antibiotics may interfere with results. One to three samples are collected.
Urine				
Urobilinogen	Dipstick or laboratory analysis is performed to determine bile byproducts in urine.	Negative	Levels determined in hepatic dysfunction and obstruction.	No preparation is necessary. The test is done by the nurse.
Blood				
Liver function tests	Serum levels are measured to give an indication of liver function.	AST: child <9 yr, 15-55 U/L; child >9 yr, 5-45 U/L ALT: 5-45 U/L Total bilirubin: 0.2-1.0 mg/dL Ammonia: 29-70 mcg/dL in children; 90-150 mcg/dL in newborns	Studies are performed when liver problems are suspected.	No preparation is necessary. Venipuncture is performed.
Endoscopy				
Fiberoptic upper GI endoscopy	Study allows direct viewing of the lining of the esophagus, stomach, and proximal duodenum. It also provides a means to obtain material for biopsies and cultures.	Normal mucosa	Used to rule out various upper GI tract disorders.	Preparation includes teaching, keeping the child on NPO status for at least 6 hr before the examination, providing conscious sedation, and monitoring the child's respiratory function during sedation.
Colonoscopy	The colon is viewed directly by a fiberoptic scope and camera inserted rectally.	Normal mucosa and patent bowel	Performed to detect mucosal changes and abnormalities in the lumen of the colon.	Preparation includes teaching, keeping the child on NPO status, bowel cleansing, and providing conscious sedation.

Key: *ALT,* alanine transaminase; *AST,* aspartate transaminase; *GI,* gastrointestinal; *NPO,* nothing by mouth.

Continued

COMMON LABORATORY AND DIAGNOSTIC TESTS FOR GI DISORDERS—cont'd

TEST	DESCRIPTION	NORMAL FINDINGS	INDICATIONS	PREPARATION AND NURSING CONSIDERATIONS
Endoscopy—cont'd				
Biopsy (gastric, jejunal, rectal, liver)	A small piece of tissue is removed for analysis.	No abnormal tissue	Study determines the amount of mucosal inflammation and the absence of ganglion cells.	Preparation includes teaching, bowel cleansing, and providing sedation or anesthesia if the procedure is done percutaneously (liver).
Radiologic Examinations				
Abdominal flat plate	Anterior and posterior radiographs are obtained.		Radiographs demonstrate stool and gas patterns, inflammation, and patency of the GI tract. It is commonly performed in cases of abdominal pain, imperforate anus, intussusception, and appendicitis.	Usually no preparation is necessary other than teaching.
Barium swallow examination	Radiopaque contrast medium or air (or both) is swallowed.	Normal swallowing, no anatomic defects	Study identifies esophageal abnormalities, swallowing difficulties, and sphincter function.	Preparation includes teaching and keeping the child on NPO status for 2-4 hr before the examination. Adequate fluids are essential after the examination to prevent barium impaction.
Upper GI examination	Radiopaque contrast material is swallowed or inserted by NG tube.	Normal gastric emptying and no other abnormalities	Study outlines the stomach and pyloric canal and can be used to determine gastric emptying time.	Preparation includes teaching and keeping the child on NPO status for 4 hr before the examination. Adequate fluids are essential after the examination to prevent barium impaction.
Barium enema, air-contrast barium enema examination	Radiopaque contrast material or air (or both) is placed in the large intestine via the rectum.	Patent bowel and no abnormalities	Study used to identify abnormalities on the surface of the bowel lumen and to determine bowel patency. It also provides hydrostatic reduction of intussusception.	Preparation includes teaching, keeping the child on NPO status, and bowel cleansing. Adequate fluids are essential after the examination to prevent barium impaction.
CT scan	Oral radiopaque contrast material often used. May also use IV or rectal contrast.	Normal anatomy without evidence of inflammation	Used to identify inflammatory conditions and appendicitis.	No patient preparation other than teaching. Sedation may be used if child unable to remain still. Can be completed in less than 15 min.
Other				
Ultrasound	Study uses sound waves noninvasively to image anatomy and inflammation.	No abnormalities	Performed to identify anatomic abnormalities and inflammatory conditions.	Preparation includes teaching. For pelvic ultrasound, a full bladder is needed to improve imaging of pelvic organs.
Breath hydrogen test	Carbohydrate solution is given by mouth and exhaled. Breath samples are collected over 3 hr.	Less than 20 ppm above baseline	Used to diagnose maldigestion or malabsorption syndromes. Inadequately digested carbohydrate produces hydrogen when acted on by GI flora.	Nursing preparation entails teaching about the procedure. The child prepares by fasting for $4\frac{1}{2}$ hr. The study is noninvasive. A facemask may be worn to collect expired air.

Key: *CT,* computed tomography; *NG,* nasogastric.

with absorbed nutrients from the GI tract. The liver has numerous functions, including phagocytosis, bile production, detoxification, glycogen storage and breakdown, and vitamin storage. The production of bile is essential for the absorption of fat and the excretion of the end products of blood cell breakdown. The primary function of the gallbladder, a saclike structure attached to the underside of the right lobe of the liver, is to store bile for secretion into the duodenum when stimulated by the presence of fat in its lumen.

The jejunum and ileum form the remainder of the small intestine. Absorption of all nutrients and vitamins occurs here through the villi and microvilli by the processes of diffusion and active transport. Absorption of vitamin B_{12} occurs only in the terminal ileum.

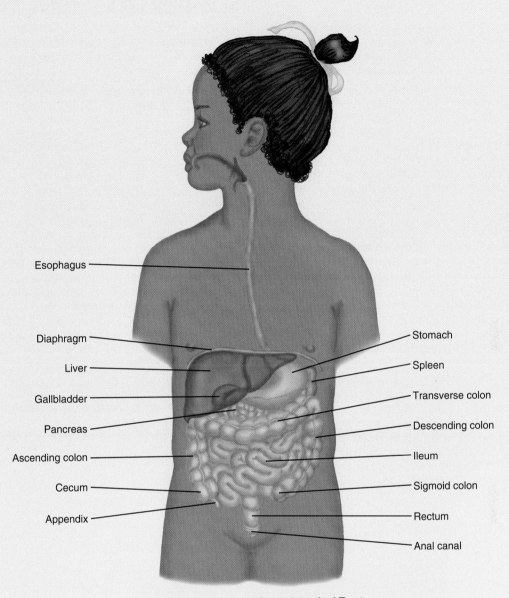

Anatomy of the Lower Gastrointestinal Tract

Esophagus

Diaphragm

Liver

Gallbladder

Pancreas

Ascending colon

Cecum

Appendix

Stomach

Spleen

Transverse colon

Descending colon

Ileum

Sigmoid colon

Rectum

Anal canal

MAJOR DIGESTIVE ENZYMES

LOCATION	ENZYME	FUNCTION
Mouth	Amylase	Converts complex carbohydrate to simple carbohydrate.
Stomach	Pepsin	Converts proteins to proteases.
Small intestine	Enterokinase	Activates trypsin.
	Peptidases	Convert peptides to amino acids.
	Sucrase, maltase, lactase	Convert disaccharides to monosaccharides.
Pancreas	Trypsin	Converts peptides to amino acids.
	Lipase	Converts fat to fatty acids and glycerol.
	Amylase	Converts carbohydrates to disaccharides.
Liver, gallbladder	Bile	Emulsifies fat, allowing the lipase to function.
		Increases fat and fat-soluble vitamin absorption.

The large intestine starts with the cecum. This blind pouch, 2 to 3 inches long, begins at the ileocecal valve, which prevents reverse peristalsis into the small intestine. Attached to it is the appendix, a wormlike tube about 3 inches long. The open end of the cecum attaches to the remainder of the colon, which is divided into four sections: the ascending, transverse, descending, and sigmoid colon. One major function of the large intestine is water reabsorption, which occurs mostly in the cecum and ascending colon. Intestinal bacteria ferment the remaining carbohydrates and aid in the synthesis of vitamins B and K. Final breakdown of bile occurs here. Mucus secretion and peristalsis of wastes are also important functions.

The rectum is the last 7 to 8 inches of the intestine, and the anal canal refers to the last 1 to 2 inches. Stool is stored in the rectum until distention of the rectal walls initiates the defecation reflex—the final stage of the GI processes.

Prenatal Development

The primitive gut is formed from the endoderm in the first 4 weeks of embryonic development. The primitive gut then gives rise to the following three sections of the GI tract, each having an individual blood supply and rate of development:

- Foregut: From the pharynx to the duodenum, including the liver, pancreas, and biliary tract
- Midgut: From the duodenum to the transverse colon
- Hindgut: Descending colon, rectum, and anal canal

Problems in the development of each of these three sections give rise to specific malformations and disease states. Anatomically, development is complete at birth, but physiologically, the neonate's GI tract is immature.

Fetal swallowing, intestinal motility, and defecation are detectable in the second trimester of gestation, but the most rapid and extensive development of the GI system occurs in the third trimester. The newborn must be able to adapt from total parenteral nutrition to total enteral nutrition because the placenta no longer performs nutrient exchange and waste removal.

PEDIATRIC DIFFERENCES IN THE GI SYSTEM

- Infants have minimal saliva.
- Swallowing is not under voluntary control until 6 weeks.
- Infants and children have less stomach capacity:

AGE	STOMACH CAPACITY (mL)
Newborn	10-20
1 wk	30-90
2-3 wk	75-100
1 mo	90-150
3 mo	150-200
1 yr	210-360
2 yr	500
10 yr	750-900
16 yr	1500
Adult	2000-3000

- The stomach lies transversely and is horizontal in the infant's abdomen; the abdomen is round in infants and toddlers.
- Peristaltic waves may reverse in infancy, causing regurgitation and vomiting. Peristalsis is faster; food remains in the stomach for a shorter period.
- Hydrochloric acid concentration is low until school age.
- Fever increases the rate of propulsion.
- The immature neonatal liver is not yet efficient in its detoxifying ability, which results in less vitamin and mineral breakdown than in older children.
- The large intestine is relatively short, with less epithelial lining to absorb water from a fecal mass. As a result, stools have a soft consistency and peristalsis is more rapid.

Children with GI alterations and their families have many special needs. Some GI problems begin at birth, with life-threatening consequences. Some require the parents to accept their child's altered appearance. Other problems develop after birth and provide long-term challenges in management and treatment. Sudden, unexpected surgery may be necessary. GI alterations cause anxiety and affect nutrition, elimination, respiratory status, skin integrity, body image, family processes, growth and development, and educational needs.

Upper and lower GI conditions can be categorized as follows:
- Developmental problems, such as cleft lip and palate, hernias, esophageal atresia, tracheoesophageal fistula, imperforate anus, and abdominal wall defects
- Problems affecting motility, such as gastroesophageal reflux, constipation, encopresis, and irritable bowel syndrome
- Inflammatory or infectious conditions, including ulcers, gastroenteritis, appendicitis, inflammatory bowel disease, and necrotizing enterocolitis
- Obstructive disorders, such as pyloric stenosis, intussusception, and Hirschsprung disease

- Malabsorption conditions, such as lactose intolerance and celiac disease
- Hepatic disorders, such as hepatitis, biliary atresia, and cirrhosis

Disorders that involve the liver and biliary tract may be the result of congenital malformations or acquired infection. Because the liver is important to metabolism, alterations in its function can affect many body systems, including the cardiovascular, integumentary, renal, neurologic, hematologic, and immunologic systems. These disorders can also have significant effects on growth and development. Nursing care may involve nutritional support, infection control, developmental stimulation, family support, and intensive physiologic care during a period of crisis.

DISORDERS OF PRENATAL DEVELOPMENT

Cleft Lip and Palate

Cleft lip, cleft palate, and cleft lip and palate are separate anomalies that are closely related in etiology, pathophysiology, and nursing care.

These distinct problems are all abnormal openings in the lip or palate. The defects may occur unilaterally (on either side) or bilaterally and are the most common congenital craniofacial deformity.

Incidence

The incidence ranges from 1 in 700 to 1000 births for cleft lip and palate and 1 in 2000 for cleft palate alone (Cleft Palate Foundation, 2007; March of Dimes, 2007; Zarate, Martin, Hopkin et al., 2010). Cleft lip is seen predominantly in male infants and cleft palate in female infants. The prevalence of cleft lip and/or palate is higher in Asians and Native Americans and has a lower frequency in African-Americans. The etiology of cleft lip and palate malformations is thought to be multifactorial, including both genetic and environmental factors (Rojas-Martinez, Reutter, Chacon-Camacho et al., 2010). While there appears to be a genetic pattern or familial risk involved, environmental factors such as maternal smoking have been found to be associated with an increased risk of oral cleft defects (Lebby, Tan, & Brown, 2010). Many infants who are affected with cleft lip and palate have other associated defects.

Manifestations and Diagnostic Evaluation

Cleft lip has the following manifestations: a notched vermilion border, variably sized clefts that involve the alveolar ridge, and dental anomalies (usually deformed, supernumerary, or absent teeth). Cleft palate includes nasal distortion, midline or bilateral cleft with variable extension from the uvula and soft and hard palates, and exposed nasal cavities.

The diagnosis of cleft lip and cleft palate is based on observation at birth and complete examination in the neonatal period. Diagnosis may also be made in utero with ultrasound. Cleft lip is readily diagnosed through inspection of the lip. The first sign of cleft palate may be formula coming from the nose. A gloved finger placed in the mouth to feel the defect of the palate or visual examination with a flashlight confirms the diagnosis.

Therapeutic Management

Management is based on the severity of the defect. A number of professionals are involved in this process, including surgeons; nurses; geneticists; psychologists or psychiatrists; ear, nose, and throat specialists; audiologists; and occupational and speech therapists. Orthodontists and plastic surgeons become involved in the lengthy management. Pediatricians provide ongoing child health care.

The first intervention involves modifying feeding techniques as needed to allow adequate growth. Use of special feeding techniques, obturators, and unique nipples and feeders can usually accomplish this goal and allow early discharge home with parents (Figure 19-1). These modified techniques can decrease the energy required for the infant to take in adequate nutrition. Before surgical repair, removable orthopedic devices such as a Latham device may be used to expand and realign parts of the palate or decrease the size of a wide lip cleft.

Cleft lip repair is usually performed by age 3 to 6 months. Early repair may improve bonding and makes feeding much easier. The surgical technique involves the use of a staggered suture line to minimize scarring. Some cosmetic modifications may be needed again at age 4 to 5 years.

Cleft palate repair is individualized and based on the degree of deformity and size of the child. Closure is completed between ages 6

PATHOPHYSIOLOGY

Cleft Lip and Palate

Cleft lip and cleft palate occur from embryonic developmental failures related to multiple genetic and environmental factors. These developmental failures result in an abnormal opening in the lip, palate, and, sometimes, nasal cavity. Cleft lip results when the medial nasal and maxillary processes fail to join at 6 to 8 weeks of gestation. Cleft palate results from failure of the primary palatal shelves, or processes, to fuse at 7 to 12 weeks of gestation.

Each of these abnormalities appears as a distinct malformation, but they may also appear together. Achieving suction during feedings may be impossible, and fluids may enter the nose, putting the child at risk for aspiration, feeding difficulties, and respiratory distress.

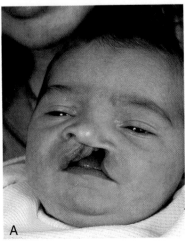 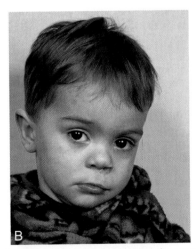

Child born with a cleft lip and palate, before **(A)** and after **(B)** repair. Repair of facial clefts usually requires multiple surgeries at different stages in the child's growth. Early repair of a cleft lip facilitates parent-infant bonding and improves feeding. Children generally experience good outcomes with today's surgical, orthodontic, and speech therapy techniques. (Courtesy Children's Medical Center, Dallas, TX.)

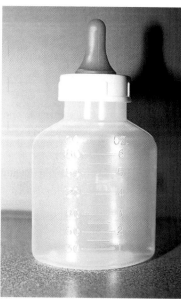

FIG 19-1 Before and after repair of a cleft lip or palate, special feeding techniques are essential for adequate nutrition. A feeder with compressible plastic sides allows gentle squeezing of the sides of the bottle to help eject the breast milk or formula. A slightly longer nipple allows the milk to be swallowed with less chance of milk entering the nasopharynx and without stimulating the gag reflex.

and 24 months. Most teams recommend repair by 1 year of age. Earlier closure facilitates speech development.

Concurrent treatment of altered dentition, recurring otitis media, speech dysfunction, emotional issues, and cosmetic concerns completes the ongoing therapy. Children with cleft palate are at high risk for developing chronic otitis media, which can cause long-term hearing loss.

Esophageal Atresia with Tracheoesophageal Fistula

Esophageal atresia (EA) and tracheoesophageal fistula (TEF) are congenital malformations in which the esophagus terminates before it reaches the stomach and/or a fistula is present that forms an unnatural connection between the esophagus and the trachea. Figure 19-2 portrays the most common type of EA with a distal TEF.

Etiology and Incidence

The cause of TEF and EA is unknown. Esophageal atresia with or without TEF occurs in 1.2 to 4.67 in 10,000 live births, with no difference by gender (National Birth Defects Prevention Network, 2009). Nearly half of infants born with esophageal atresia have other associated anomalies of the cardiac, GI, and central nervous systems. Prematurity and low birth weight are frequent concomitant problems that have a significant impact on long-term prognosis.

Manifestations

- Failure to pass suction catheter, nasogastric (NG) tube at birth
- Excessive oral secretions, coughing, choking
- Vomiting
- Abdominal distention
- Airless, scaphoid abdomen (atresia without fistula)

Diagnostic Evaluation

A history of maternal polyhydramnios is a significant prenatal clue. If TEF is suspected prenatally, diagnosis can be made at the ideal

---

PATIENT-CENTERED TEACHING

Home Care of the Child with Cleft Lip or Palate

Your infant may require a special feeding method to maximize growth while waiting for surgery, and you may need to practice the feeding method to be used after surgery until the incision heals. The feeding method you use will be based on what works for your child and what your physician recommends. In general, the following apply:

- Breastfeeding may be possible if your child has a small cleft lip or palate.
- A soft plastic, compressible bottle will prevent your child from having to suck vigorously because the breast milk or formula can be squeezed into the mouth, if needed.
- A longer nipple may allow the milk to be swallowed without entering the nose. It must not be so long that it causes gagging. Enlarging the nipple hole or "cross-cutting" a nipple may also be effective.
- A syringe with a rubber tip may also be used, especially after surgery.
- Feed your child slowly and provide short periods of rest for swallowing; children usually develop a feeding pattern of sucking, swallowing, and resting that helps them become more efficient eaters.
- Try to keep your child in an upright position during feedings to allow gravity to assist in the feeding and decrease the chance that your child might choke.
- Burp your child frequently because excess air is often swallowed.

Before surgical repair, devices may be placed in your child's mouth to help line up the cleft in the palate for better surgical repair or to decrease the size of the lip cleft. These devices may require special care and cleaning. Consult your cleft team and nurses for specific instructions about your child's device.

After surgery, elbow restraints ("no-no's") may be used so that your baby cannot touch the stitches. The following are recommendations:

- Do not apply the restraints too tightly. They should be loose but still prevent elbow bending.
- Remove "no-no's" every 2 hours for 10 to 15 minutes and play games with your child that encourage movement of the elbows. Look for any skin irritation every time you remove an elbow restraint.
- Remove only one elbow restraint at a time.

Position your child for sleep on the back, so the child does not rub the stitches on the linens. An infant seat may be used.

Do not brush your child's teeth for 1 to 2 weeks after surgery. Feeding a small amount of water after meals will help keep the teeth clean. Clean your child's lip as recommended by your physician. If ordered, you may use a cotton swab and a gentle rolling motion down the suture line and then apply antibiotic ointment using the same technique.

Make use of the many support professionals in following your child for speech, hearing, dental, or orthodontic problems.

Contact the American Cleft Palate-Craniofacial Association and the Cleft Palate Foundation at www.cleftline.org for further information.

---

time—in the delivery room. Atresia should be suspected if an NG tube cannot be passed 10 to 11 cm beyond the gum line. This suspicion is confirmed with an abdominal radiograph that will identify a proximal esophagus dilated with air (atresia) or abdominal distention (fistula). The radiologist can identify the specific type of defect after instilling less than 1 mL of a water-soluble contrast medium into the NG tube and documenting its movement into the tracheal tree and the proximal pouch. This is then withdrawn from the pouch to minimize the risk of aspiration. Bronchoscopy and endoscopy are also used to identify and assess fistulas. The infant needs to have diagnostic testing for commonly associated cardiac and other congenital anomalies because these often are seen with this type of anomaly (Kahn & Orenstein, 2011a).

NURSING CARE PLAN

The Child with a Cleft Lip or Palate

Focused Assessment

- During examination of the newborn with cleft lip and/or cleft palate, assess and document:
  - Degree of involvement
  - Infant's ability to suck, swallow, and breathe without distress
  - Infant's ability to handle normal secretions
- Assess and document:
  - Parent's initial reactions to the infant's appearance
  - Parent's interactions with the infant (i.e., touching, holding, examining)

Planning

Nursing Diagnoses

Imbalanced Nutrition: Less Than Body Requirements related to inability to suck and to the surgical repair.

Deficient Knowledge about feeding techniques and surgery related to unfamiliarity with the information.

Expected Outcomes

The child will drink the desired amount of fluid within 30 minutes.

The child will be content during and after feeding.

The child will gain weight and height according to the normal growth curve.

The parents will express satisfaction with progress of feedings.

The parents will understand expected preoperative and postoperative feeding techniques.

Intervention/Rationale

1. Describe the degree of cleft lip and/or palate and impairment of sucking.
   Infants with cleft lip alone or simple cleft dental arch may be successful with breastfeeding or bottle feeding without modifications.
2. Keep care and teaching simple and as closely related to normal infant feeding as possible.
   Nutrition, parent-infant relationship, and adherence may be improved if normal techniques can be used.
3. Provide alternative assistive feeding devices as needed and ordered.
   Some infants may be able to breastfeed successfully. Techniques and equipment vary among institutions. Use what is available and effective for each child. Encourage breastfeeding first because breastfeeding confers added immune protection.
4. Burp the infant frequently, and hold the infant in a more upright position.
   Burping minimizes air swallowing and GI flatus and minimizes risk of aspiration.
5. Document the feeding program in written form for parents to use at home, and provide the plan to other health professionals.
   Documentation provides consistency at home and at other times when the family is in contact with numerous medical professionals treating the child.
6. Provide emotional support and positive reinforcement to parents as they learn to feed their child.
   Self-care and bonding are improved when parents can assume total care.
7. Keep an accurate record of the child's growth by using a growth chart.
   A chart identifies growth changes early, when intervention can be most effective.
8. Explain preoperative and postoperative procedures: oral feedings withheld for 6 hours, placement of IV lines, use of arm restraints, appearance of repair in the immediate postoperative period (see the Patient-Centered Teaching: Home Care of the Child with Cleft Lip or Palate box).
   Explanation decreases parental anxiety and encourages involvement.

9. Postoperatively:
   a. Keep straws, pacifiers, spoons, or fingers away from the child's mouth for 7 to 10 days. Do not take temperatures orally.
      Avoiding contact with the incision site reduces stress on surgical repair and prevents accidental tearing of very fine sutures.
   b. Advance the child's diet as ordered and tolerated from clear liquids to a normal soft diet within 48 hours.
      A normal diet minimizes nutritional deficits and stress on the child. No foods that can tear surfaces are offered.
   c. After repair of a cleft lip, resume preoperative feeding techniques.
      Little evidence shows that sucking causes excess suture stress.
10. After repair of a cleft palate, provide short nipples that do not rest on palatal sutures; give baby food or baby food mixed with water.
    Prevents direct contact with surgical site.

Evaluation

Is the infant following the appropriate growth curve?

Is the infant happy and content during and after feedings?

Do the parents express satisfaction with the feeding technique used and the time required to complete a feeding?

Can the parents explain and demonstrate expected preoperative and postoperative care?

Planning

Nursing Diagnosis

Interrupted Family Processes related to the emotional reaction to an infant with a visible defect.

Expected Outcomes

The parents will demonstrate positive behaviors toward the infant.

The parents will access appropriate support.

Intervention/Rationale

1. Encourage parents to discuss their fears, concerns, and negative emotions.
   Grief, anxiety, confusion, guilt, denial, and anger are not uncommon and should be expressed.
2. Encourage touching and holding.
   Contact encourages bonding and prevents a delayed attachment.
3. Make appropriate referral to a cleft lip and palate team of nurses, physicians, and other specialists as soon as possible.
   A health care team can provide accurate information and begin to outline a plan of action.
4. Express acceptance of the baby by modeling feeding and close physical contact.
   These interventions assist parents with the adaptation process.
5. Refer parents to community resources and parent groups (see Evolve website).
   Sharing with others in similar situations facilitates acceptance and adaptation.
6. Encourage parents to share concerns about long-term care and emotional and financial stress.
   Long-term concerns require extensive follow-up and can strain many families' resources. Identifying concerns early can increase problem-solving options.

Evaluation

Can the parents identify their infant's positive characteristics?

Do the parents hold, cuddle, and make eye contact with the infant?

Have the parents sought personal, community, or organizational support?

NURSING CARE PLAN

The Child with a Cleft Lip or Palate—cont'd

Planning

Nursing Diagnoses

Impaired Skin Integrity related to the surgical repair.

Risk for Infection related to the surgical repair and aspiration.

Expected Outcomes

The repair site will heal without complications.

The infant will show no signs of infection as evidenced by a clean and intact suture line, absence of fever, and clear breath sounds.

Intervention/Rationale

1. Clean the lip repair site according to physician protocol. Many physicians recommend cleaning with sterile water by using a cotton swab or saline after feeding and as ordered. Use a rolling motion vertically down the suture line. Have parents demonstrate this cleaning technique.

   The procedure decreases the medium for bacterial growth, decreases crusting, and minimizes scarring.

2. Apply antibiotic ointment as ordered.

   Antibiotic ointment prevents infection, crusting, and scarring.

3. Use elbow restraints (no-no's) to keep the child from touching the repair site. Continue for 6 to 8 days. Remove every 2 hours for 10 to 15 minutes. Remove restraint from only one elbow at a time, with a parent or nurse in constant attendance.

   Elbow restraints prevent accidental rupture or tear of sutures. Periodically removing restraints promotes contact with the child, decreases anxiety, and allows the nurse to assess skin integrity and circulation.

4. Do not brush the child's teeth for 1 to 2 weeks.

   Avoiding brushing prevents accidental tear of palatal sutures.

5. Keep the child in a supine position or in an infant seat.

   Careful positioning prevents contact of suture lines with bed linens.

6. Observe for redness, swelling, excessive bleeding, drainage, respiratory distress, or fever.

   Signs of infection must be identified early because additional inflammation can increase scarring.

7. To clean the palate repair site, rinse the child's mouth with water after feedings.

   Rinsing after feeding removes food and residual sugars from suture lines, reducing the risk of infection.

8. Encourage the parents to hold and cuddle the child as the child desires.

   Crying puts additional stress on the suture line.

9. Maintain lip protective devices if ordered.

   Protective devices prevent separation of lip suture lines.

Evaluation

Is the suture site clean, dry, and without redness, heat, or drainage?

Is the suture site intact and healing without crusting or excessive scarring?

Is the infant afebrile and demonstrating clear breath sounds?

Planning

Nursing Diagnosis

Acute Pain related to the surgical incision and elbow restraints.

Expected Outcome

The child will be free from pain as evidenced by ability to sleep, eat, and respond in a positive way.

Intervention/Rationale

1. Describe and document pain with appropriate tools (see Chapter 15).

   Infants and young children do not react to pain in typical adult ways, so alternative observations are needed to validate assessment findings. Parents are the best resource to validate the nurse's assessment of their infant.

2. Provide comfort measures, especially holding, rocking, and parental voices.

   Comforting increases parental involvement, relieves discomfort, and reduces stress on sutures caused by crying.

3. Provide analgesics and sedatives on a regular basis as ordered. Pain should decrease significantly after 24 to 48 hours.

   Administering medication on a regular basis can prevent peaks of pain that cannot be managed appropriately.

4. Report pain not managed by usual means.

   Pain may indicate hematoma formation or other complications of the repair.

Evaluation

Does the child participate in age-appropriate activities?

Is the child responding well to pain medication?

Does the child appear relaxed and content at rest?

Does the parent describe a child who is not in pain?

Planning

Nursing Diagnosis

Ineffective Health Maintenance related to the need for long-term care.

Expected Outcomes

The parents will seek continued follow-up care to evaluate and manage long-term complications.

The child will demonstrate normal speech and hearing.

Intervention/Rationale

1. Make appropriate and early referrals for any problems with speech impairment or language-based learning disabilities.

   Speech and language learning impairments are common complications of cleft lip and palate. Early intervention minimizes harm.

2. Monitor for recurrent or chronic otitis media. Schedule frequent hearing tests.

   Because of craniofacial deformities, otitis media can occur frequently and must be treated to prevent language and learning problems.

3. Encourage early speech attempts. Arrange speech therapy as needed.

   Cleft palate can make speech difficult to understand, and the child may feel self-conscious about speech errors. Practice improves development.

4. Encourage good dental care.

   With abnormalities of teeth and the alveolar ridge, malocclusion and dental caries are a major concern.

Evaluation

Do the parents continue to seek follow-up care (ear, nose, and throat [ENT]; speech therapy; dental)?

Does the child demonstrate age-appropriate speech?

Does the child have normal hearing?

Does the child have normal dentition?

◎ NURSING CARE PLAN

The Child with a Cleft Lip or Palate—cont'd

Planning

Nursing Diagnosis

Anxiety (parental) related to special care needs and surgery.

Expected Outcomes

The parents will express concerns and fears.
The parents will express control over special care needs.

Intervention/Rationale

1. Use a calm, reassuring, accepting approach with the infant and family.
   Being calm and accepting encourages communication and reinforces to parents that their child is worthwhile.
2. Explain all procedures and their rationale, including sensations likely experienced by their child.
   Uncertainty and loss of control contribute to increased levels of anxiety.

3. Listen actively to parents and their concerns. Encourage verbalization of feelings, perceptions, and fears.
   Talking and sharing may decrease anxiety.
4. Encourage parents to stay with their child in the immediate preoperative and postoperative periods.
   Staying with the child encourages parent participation and control over as much as possible.

Evaluation

Do the parents express concerns and fears?
Do the parents seek information to decrease anxiety?
Do the parents demonstrate ability to care for their child?

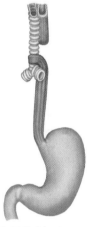

Esophageal Atresia with Distal TEF

Incidence: 85%-88%
Clinical Manifestations: Feeding causes regurgitation and coughing. Constant flow of saliva. Gastric distention.
Diagnostic Findings: Contrast reveals blind pouch. Air on abdominal radiograph.
Surgical Treatment: One-stage surgical repair to ligate fistula and anastomose esophagus.

FIG 19-2 Most common type of esophageal atresia and tracheoesophageal fistula (TEF).

PATHOPHYSIOLOGY

Esophageal Atresia and Tracheoesophageal Fistula

Tracheoesophageal fistula is the result of an embryonal failure to differentiate the foregut into the trachea and esophagus and the incomplete fusion of them into distinct organs. The failure occurs between the fourth and fifth week of pregnancy and can be manifested in several ways (see Figure 19-2 for most common type).

The presence of a fistula between the esophagus and trachea causes oral intake to enter the lungs or large amounts of air to enter the stomach. Coughing, choking, and severe abdominal distention can occur. Eventually aspiration pneumonia and severe respiratory distress will develop in the untreated child, and death may occur without surgical intervention. Esophageal atresia occurring by itself causes respiratory distress attributable to aspiration of saliva and any oral fluids that may be given before diagnosis.

Therapeutic Management

Keeping the infant supine with the head of the bed elevated decreases the chance of gastric secretions entering the lungs. An NG tube must be in place and aspirated every 5 to 10 minutes to keep the proximal pouch clear of secretions. Intravenous (IV) fluids are essential. Normal newborn care is appropriate, with special attention to keeping the infant warm and oxygenated.

Surgical repair is the mainstay of treatment. Initial repair includes ligation of the fistula and end-to-side anastomosis of the atresia to decrease the severity of stricture formation. If the gap between the two parts of the esophagus is too large, primary anastomosis may not be possible. Newest advances use traction suture ends to stimulate rapid growth of the esophageal ends over a 7- to 10-day period, allowing primary anastomosis. If a staged repair is necessary, a gastrostomy tube (G tube) and cervical esophagostomy are placed. Later, anastomosis, colon interposition, and dilation can be expected. Evaluation and treatment of esophageal motility dysfunction, gastroesophageal reflux, strictures, bronchitis, and pneumonia may occur as the child grows.

▌ NURSING CARE OF THE INFANT WITH TRACHEOESOPHAGEAL FISTULA

■ Assessment

The infant with TEF is at constant risk for aspiration. Assessment for respiratory distress in the immediate period after birth is essential. The nurse must examine the infant for excessive oral secretions, choking, and cyanosis. Difficulty swallowing, regurgitation, vomiting, and unexplained cyanosis after an initial feeding in the infant who is not diagnosed at birth are important assessment findings that must be reported to the physician immediately. Abdominal distention should be measured and the infant continually assessed for distress (vital signs, respiratory effort, nasal flaring, retractions, cyanosis). A newborn assessment should be completed, with special attention to identifying any concomitant congenital defects.

Family assessment of anxiety levels, fears, concerns, and knowledge level will provide important information for planning nursing care and teaching.

■ Nursing Diagnosis and Planning

The nursing diagnoses and expected outcomes appropriate after assessment of the infant with TEF include the following:

- Risk for Aspiration related to TEF.

Expected Outcome. The infant will not aspirate, as evidenced by control of oral secretions without coughing, cyanosis, or adventitious breath sounds.

- Imbalanced Nutrition: Less Than Body Requirements related to possible feeding difficulties.

Expected Outcomes. The infant will gain weight and follow growth chart at appropriate level.

- Risk for Impaired Skin Integrity related to G-tube and esophagostomy.

Expected Outcome. The infant will maintain skin integrity, as evidenced by intact skin around the G-tube and esophagostomy.

- Risk for Infection related to surgical repair.

Expected Outcomes. The infant will have surgical site, G-tube site, and esophagostomy free from infection, as evidenced by clean, intact skin without drainage, exudate, or redness.

- Acute Pain related to surgical repair.

Expected Outcome. The infant will be free from pain, as evidenced by resumption of normal activities, ease of comforting, and relaxed facial features.

- Anxiety (parental) related to neonatal surgical emergency.

Expected Outcome. The parents will express feelings and concerns.

- Deficient Knowledge related to home care needs and follow-up care.

Expected Outcomes. The parents will demonstrate procedures for safe G-tube feedings and site care.

⚡ SAFETY ALERT

Assessing and Managing the Child with Esophageal Atresia and Tracheoesophageal Fistula

> Any child who exhibits the "three Cs" of coughing, choking with feedings, and cyanosis should be suspected of having a tracheoesophageal fistula (TEF). Esophageal atresia and TEF represent a critical neonatal surgical emergency. While the baby is awaiting transfer to a neonatal unit and surgery, management centers on prevention of aspiration.

■ Interventions

Nursing interventions are different in the preoperative and postoperative periods. In the immediate period after birth, placing the newborn in a radiant warmer and administering humidified oxygen are essential to relieve respiratory distress. The child is prepared for surgery, remains on nothing by mouth (NPO) status, and is hydrated with IV fluids. Maintaining thermoregulation and fluid balance is essential, so monitoring temperature and other vital signs, using radiant warmers, and keeping accurate intake and output records are important.

■ **Minimizing Aspiration Risk.** The risk of aspiration must be minimized. A chalasia board that helps keep the child at a 30-degree angle while supine can be useful to decrease reflux. Placing a suction catheter in the proximal pouch and mouth will keep secretions to a minimum. Constant assessment of respiratory status is essential. Even after surgical repair, these children are prone to gastroesophageal reflux.

■ **Postoperative Care.** In the immediate postoperative period, monitoring respiratory status, supporting fluid balance and nutrition, maintaining thermoregulation, providing pain relief, monitoring for infection, and promoting bonding with parents take priority. The child will probably have a chest tube in place; patency must be maintained, suction monitored, and output documented. Respiratory rate and effort and the presence of abnormal breath sounds should be documented. Thermoregulation can significantly affect respiratory status in the newborn, so monitoring and maintaining temperature with a radiant warmer may be necessary. IV fluids, antibiotics, and parenteral nutrition may be ordered. The nurse must maintain patency of the IV line; monitor intake and output; and assess for signs of fluid and electrolyte alterations, including sunken fontanel and increased urine specific gravity measurements. Daily weights and measurement of head circumference can aid in assessing growth. Pain medications must be administered as needed on the basis of objective pain assessment measures.

If a cervical esophagostomy has been performed as the first stage of a surgical repair, it is kept covered with gauze to absorb saliva and provide skin care. Frequent cleaning and assessing for redness, breakdown, or exudate are essential because the skin in this wet area can easily become macerated and infected. Referral to an enterostomal therapist can be helpful in teaching parents esophagostomy care.

■ **Gastrostomy Tube Use.** In the immediate postoperative period, the gastrostomy tube is left open to drainage in order to allow gastric contents and air to escape; this promotes comfort and decreases risk of pressure at the anastomosis. A pacifier satisfies sucking needs, provides early training in swallowing, makes later feeding easier, and provides comfort through distraction. Pacifiers should not be offered until the child can manage oral secretions.

Numerous types of G-tubes are available for placement, either percutaneously (PEG tube) or during surgery. Among these are traditional gastrostomy tubes, which are anchored in place by an air- or saline-inflated balloon, as well as more innovative tubes that use a variety of means for anchoring. The skin-level gastrostomy button (MIC-KEY) allows secure connection of extension tubing to the gastrostomy site and is easy for parents to use (Figure 19-3). Tube selection is usually made by the physician, but long-term successful care and use of the tube are nursing and parental responsibilities.

■ **Home Care.** Parents should be taught the techniques of G-tube feeding and care (see Patient-Centered Teaching: Home Care of the Child with a Gastrostomy Tube). Skin care at the site may include using half-strength hydrogen peroxide to remove crusty drainage, rotating the tube, and using a skin barrier product, as well as other ostomy skin care products. Redness, exudate, pus, heat, or leakage of formula should be reported.

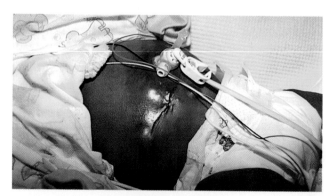

FIG 19-3 The skin-level gastrostomy button is good for children who require long-term gastrostomy feeding. It is relatively flat, reduces skin breakdown, increases comfort, and is fully immersible in water. (Courtesy Parkland Health and Hospital System, Dallas, TX.)

PATIENT-CENTERED TEACHING

Home Care of the Child with a Gastrostomy Tube

Your child's gastrostomy tube will require special care depending on the type of tube that is used. Your nurse and physician will help you learn the following skills:

- For a new gastrostomy, clean the site daily with soap and water. If crusty drainage appears, use half-strength hydrogen peroxide to clean. Apply antimicrobial ointment if indicated. Gently rotate or turn the tube every day.
- After 1 to 2 weeks, tub baths may be used to clean the site. Stomahesive Protective Powder may be used to decrease moisture.
- Keep the tube open during the initial postoperative period.
- While the site is healing, make sure the tube is stabilized. Proper stabilization technique will vary depending on the type of gastrostomy tube.
- When the tube is well healed, it can be secured as directed for specific tube type (tape or OpSite may be used).
- Use skin barriers around the stoma to prevent skin breakdown.
- Report any drainage, leakage of formula, redness, or pain to your physician.
- Ask your enterostomal therapist for help in making the best choices for your child.

Remember to use a pacifier or very small amounts of fluid in a bottle to allow your baby to practice sucking and swallowing. This should be done every day.

Parent education and support are critical components. Home care between stages of repair requires extra support from community health care providers and demonstration of parental proficiency in skin care, suctioning, gastrostomy feedings, and cardiopulmonary resuscitation (Castilloux, Noble, & Faure, 2010). These should include discussing feelings and anxieties, providing information about home care, practicing special techniques, providing stimulation to the infant, and using appropriate resources such as enterostomal therapists and dietitians.

▪ Evaluation

- Can the child coordinate sucking and swallowing?
- Is the child tolerating oral feedings without choking, coughing, or becoming cyanotic?
- Is the child growing according to the growth chart?
- Is the surgical site clean, dry, intact, and free of redness, drainage, or exudate?
- Is the skin intact and without breakdown around the gastrostomy tube and esophagostomy?
- Is the child resting contently without pain medication?
- Can the parents explain the need for the surgical procedure?
- Do parents demonstrate appropriate care of the gastrostomy tube?
- Have parents assumed all care responsibilities?

Upper Gastrointestinal Hernias

A hernia is an abnormal protrusion of part of an organ or tissue through the structures that normally contain it. Hernias can be either congenital or acquired. Some hernias can be reduced, whereas others become incarcerated and the protruding organ segment cannot be returned by manipulation to the anatomically correct location. A medical emergency occurs when a hernia becomes strangulated and blood supply is cut off. This condition can occur suddenly and requires immediate treatment. The most common hernias of the upper GI tract are discussed in Table 19-1.

Other Developmental Disorders

Table 19-2 on pp. 421-422 discusses other developmental disorders of the upper and lower GI tracts.

MOTILITY DISORDERS

Gastroesophageal Reflux Disease

Gastroesophageal reflux (GER) is regurgitation of gastric contents back into the esophagus. GER is a normal physiologic phenomenon; all adults and infants periodically experience reflux, especially after meals. GER disease (GERD) is a more severe and chronic form. Reflux can be divided into two types: physiologic GER and pathologic GERD (Box 19-1).

Etiology

Many factors contribute to the development of GERD. Neurologic impairment, such as cerebral palsy, Down syndrome, and head injury, may affect the transmission of neural signals to the lower esophageal sphincter (LES). Delayed gastric emptying of a liquid meal because of distention may contribute. Partial or incomplete swallowing dysfunction or drugs such as theophylline or caffeine can also trigger LES relaxations. Increased intraabdominal pressure incurred while straining, crying, coughing, or slumping tends to promote increased episodes of GER. These postural effects are most likely primary contributing factors in infants. Obesity and hiatal hernias also promote GERD. Finally, during the first 6 months of life, the LES pressure undergoes maturational development. Because infants have a short abdominal LES, they have GER more often. As the infant grows, the LES matures and the reflux improves. The prognosis is likely related to the severity of symptoms. Reflux from maturational causes will likely resolve by 1 to 2 years of age.

Incidence

Approximately 50% of healthy infants have signs of GER (Grossman & Liacouras, 2008), with most experiencing regurgitation accompanied by crying. The peak incidence of GER occurs at approximately 4 months of age and decreases thereafter, so that only 5% of children experience symptoms by the time they reach 1 year old (Grossman & Liacouras, 2008). GERD has been associated with neurologic or

BOX 19-1 TYPES OF GASTROESOPHAGEAL REFLUX

Physiologic (GER)

- Painless emesis after meals
- Parents may not be concerned or may think it is normal
- Rarely occurs during sleep
- No failure to thrive
- 40% asymptomatic by 3 months
- 70% asymptomatic by 18 months
- Pharmacologic and medical management very effective

Pathologic (GERD)

- Failure to thrive
- Aspiration pneumonia and/or asthma
- Apnea, coughing, and choking
- Frequent emesis, abdominal pain, and crying
- May require surgery and pharmacologic treatment

TABLE 19-1 **UPPER GI HERNIAS**

DESCRIPTION	CLINICAL MANIFESTATIONS	THERAPEUTIC MANAGEMENT	NURSING MANAGEMENT
Hiatal Hernia			
Protrusion of a portion of the stomach through the esophageal hiatus of the diaphragm	Vomiting Coughing, wheezing, short periods of apnea Failure to thrive	Medical management similar to that for the child with reflux. Surgical repair of defect.	Monitor intake and output. Document vomiting. Observe for respiratory distress. Provide routine postoperative care for GI surgery. Teach parents about surgery and medical treatment of reflux.
Congenital Diaphragmatic Hernia (CDH)			
Opening in the diaphragm through which abdominal contents herniate into the thoracic cavity during prenatal development Results in some degree of pulmonary hypoplasia, determined by the timing and size of the herniation Mortality rate: 50%-80%; 40% if extracorporeal membrane oxygenation (ECMO) used Degree of pulmonary hypoplasia determines outcome Incidence: 1 in 2200-5000 live births	Clinical findings depend on severity of defect. • Abdominal organs in chest (by fetal ultrasonography) • Diminished or absent breath sounds on affected side • Bowel sounds that may be heard over the chest • Cardiac sounds that may be heard on the right side of the chest • Respiratory distress developing soon after birth: dyspnea, cyanosis, nasal flaring, tachypnea, retractions • Scaphoid abdomen	If diagnosed prenatally, mother moved to tertiary care center before delivery. In utero surgery may be performed. Neonatal emergency NG intubation with suction. Ventilate with high-frequency ventilation. Manage acidosis with bicarbonate and ventilation. ECMO. Liquid ventilation. Manage pulmonary hypertension; inhaled nitric oxide may be used. Surgical reduction of hernia after physiologically stable; may wait 6-18 hr after birth. Respiratory support and ECMO until lungs functioning after surgery.	Identify clinical findings and report immediately. Place child in semi-Fowler position on affected side with head of bed elevated. Maintain patency of NG tube. Monitor IV fluids. Maintain mechanical ventilation, ECMO, chest tubes. Assess oxygenation. Do not use facemask or bag-valve-mask for ventilatory support because air can enter stomach and further impair respiratory function. Provide minimal stimulation. Provide routine postoperative care. Monitor for signs of infection, respiratory distress, and feeding difficulties; report to physician. Support family mourning loss of perfect child. Provide clear, truthful information to parents. Encourage parents to see and touch the infant. Use prescribed feeding techniques. Provide referral to support groups. Provide discharge teaching.

developmental problems in children, and in children with asthma or cystic fibrosis (Grossman & Liacouras, 2008).

Manifestations and Diagnostic Evaluation

Vomiting or spitting up after a meal, hiccupping, and recurrent otitis media related to pooled secretions in the nasopharynx during sleep are the hallmarks of GERD. In addition, the infant with pathologic GERD can experience weight loss, failure to thrive, irritability, discomfort, and abdominal pain. Severe GERD can result in hematemesis or melena and anemia. Frequently, respiratory illness or asthma is associated with GERD, and the child may experience coughing, choking, asthma, wheezing, pneumonia, apnea, or bradycardia.

A variety of chronic and acute illnesses have been associated with GERD. GERD should be confirmed only after other major conditions have been ruled out. In infants, signs and symptoms obtained through a comprehensive feeding and nutritional history can establish the diagnosis (Kahn & Orenstein, 2011b). Diagnostic tests in older children or those infants and children not amenable to treatment include barium swallow examination, upper GI study, fiberoptic endoscopy, esophageal manometry, ambulatory pH studies, gastroesophageal scintigraphy (radionuclide scan), ultrasound, and chest computed tomography (CT).

Therapeutic Management

Therapy for GERD is based on the severity of symptoms and includes dietary alterations, positional changes, medications, and surgery. Early treatment may prevent or lesson complications such as failure to thrive, esophagitis, and strictures. Many infants suspected of functional GER are treated conservatively with pharmacologic support. The American Academy of Pediatrics supports the North American Society for Pediatric Gastroenterology, Hepatology, and Nutrition (NASPGHAN) positioning guidelines for managing the child with gastroesophageal reflux.

Diet. Small, frequent feedings with frequent burping are often tried as the first line of treatment. These smaller feedings can help to

TABLE 19-2 DEVELOPMENTAL GI DEFECTS

IMPERFORATE ANUS	GASTROSCHISIS	OMPHALOCELE	UMBILICAL HERNIA
Pathophysiology, Etiology, and Clinical Manifestations			
Incomplete development or absence of the anus in its normal position in the perineum Defect can be high (above the levator ani muscle) or low (below the levator ani muscle) Symptoms include failure to pass meconium stool, absence of anorectal canal, presence of an anal membrane, external fistula to the perineum Condition is diagnosed during the newborn examination with radiography, ultrasound, or CT scan used to determine the level of the lesion and associated anomalies	Embryonal weakness in abdominal wall causes herniation of intestines on one side of umbilical cord during early development, most commonly on right side Viscera are outside the abdominal cavity and are not covered with the sac	Large herniation of intestines into umbilical cord Viscera are outside the abdominal cavity but inside translucent sac, covered with peritoneum and amniotic membrane	Imperfect closure of umbilical ring allows intestines to push outward at umbilicus during straining and crying Viscera are inside the abdominal cavity and under the skin The hernia is usually 1-3 cm and easily reduced
Incidence			
1 in 4000-5000 live births More common in male infants	1 in 4000 live births	1 in 5000-10,000 live births	Most common in low birth weight and African-American infants
Associated Anomalies			
Genitourinary, sacral, or additional GI anomalies	Prematurity Malrotation of intestines Decreased abdominal capacity Higher incidence of Meckel diverticulum Atresia, stenosis and other anomalies rare	Malrotation of intestines Decreased abdominal capacity Atresia and stenosis common Higher incidence of Meckel diverticulum Cardiac, genitourinary, or chromosomal anomalies in $\frac{1}{3}$ to $\frac{1}{2}$ of cases Associated with Beckwith syndrome (hypoglycemia, macrosomia, macroglossia)	Commonly occurs in children with Down syndrome, hypothyroidism, Hurler syndrome
Morbidity and Mortality			
Prognosis depends on the level of the lesion Complete continence may be impossible	Mortality rate 10%-15%	Mortality rate 20%-30% Common complications include sepsis and intestinal obstruction	Minimal
Therapeutic Management			
Anal stenosis is treated with repeated dilations All other defects require surgical intervention High defects may require a colostomy and bowel pull-through procedure	IV and NG tubes are placed immediately. Total parenteral nutrition (TPN) is provided Synthetic material (Silastic) is used to cover the intestines If defect is large, it is closed surgically after all contents have been returned to the abdominal cavity, which may take days or weeks Even if the defect is small, immediate surgical repair may be done in several stages If the condition is diagnosed prenatally, an abdominal delivery (C-section) is recommended Necrotic bowel may need to be removed surgically	IV and NG tubes are placed. TPN is provided. Silastic is used to cover the sac if ruptured or if the defect is large. Surgical correction is similar to gastroschisis. C-section delivery if diagnosed prenatally.	Most umbilical hernias disappear spontaneously by age 1 yr. No surgical repair is necessary unless the hernia causes symptoms, persists past age 5 yr, becomes strangulated, or enlarges.

Continued

TABLE 19-2 DEVELOPMENTAL GI DEFECTS—cont'd

IMPERFORATE ANUS	GASTROSCHISIS	OMPHALOCELE	UMBILICAL HERNIA
Nursing Care			
Report any skin dimples or the presence of stool in the urine or vagina	Thermoregulation is critical because significant heat loss can occur through the exposed intestines	Same as for gastroschisis	Binding is not effective in reducing or minimizing the bulge
Determine anal patency if meconium is not passed in the first 24 hr after birth	Use warmers and monitor the child's temperature		Monitor for changes in size of hernia
Assess for other GI or genitourinary anomalies	Use sterile technique in dealing with the defect; immediately cover it with warm, moist, sterile gauze and wrap with plastic to keep moist		Assess for changing bowel sounds and presence of an irreducible mass, which may indicate strangulation
Facilitate bonding	Minimize movement of the infant and handling of the intestines		
Provide appropriate postoperative care, including care of the colostomy	Assess for circulatory compromise, obstruction, sepsis		
	Monitor temperature, pulses, capillary refill time, skin color, changes in respiratory patterns, heart rate		
	Observe for respiratory distress from high intraabdominal pressure as the intestines return to the peritoneal cavity		
	Fluid volume management is a crucial nursing responsibility		
	Monitor intake and output and daily weights, assess fontanels, monitor electrolytes, and maintain IV line		
	Postoperatively, monitor and manage ileus, which commonly lasts for 2-4 wk		
	Maintain NG tube for decompression, monitor bowel sounds and stools, measure abdominal girth		
	Maintain TPN to sustain growth		
	Offer pacifier to meet sucking needs		
	Provide emotional support for parents as they deal with the loss of the "perfect child"		
	Encourage parents to provide care so they can talk to, touch and hold the infant, when appropriate		
Teaching and Home Care			
Teach parents colostomy care	Encourage parents to hold, cuddle, and bond with infant as soon as possible	Same as for gastroschisis	Teach parents signs of strangulation: vomiting, pain, irreducible mass at umbilicus
Demonstrate anal dilation (use only prescribed dilator, insert no more than 1-2 cm, and use a water-soluble lubricant)	Provide developmental stimulation during long-term hospitalization		Contact physician immediately if strangulation is suspected
Refer parents for counseling and support (March of Dimes Birth Defects Foundation, www.marchofdimes.org)	Assist parents in dealing with feelings of guilt and disappointment		
Provide guidance for toilet training	Use pictures to help parents understand the defect		
	Contact national support groups and community resources (e.g., March of Dimes)		
	Teach parents signs of bowel obstruction: vomiting, pain, irritability, anorexia, firm abdomen		
	Provide follow-up from nutritional support personnel as needed		

minimize the frequency of reflux, but may be impractical for the caregiver. Severe restrictions in feeding may also adversely affect the child's weight gain. NASPGHAN guidelines support the trial of hydrolyzed or amino acid formula in formula-fed babies with recurrent regurgitation and vomiting. Breastfed infants may benefit from a trial of withdrawal of cow's milk protein and eggs from the maternal diet. Feedings thickened with rice cereal (1 tbsp/oz) may decrease the frequency of daily regurgitation and emesis (Kahn & Orenstein, 2011b). Thickened feedings do tend to decrease crying and increase weight gain in infants (Kahn & Orenstein, 2011b). Concentrated, high-calorie formulas and NG tube feedings provide nutritional supplementation for the child with failure to thrive. Caffeinated, carbonated, acidic, spicy, and fatty foods all lower LES pressure and should be eliminated.

Positioning. Much attention has been given to the best positioning for GER. Although prone positioning more effectively reduces reflux, current recommendations from the American Academy of Pediatrics and the NASPGHAN are that infants younger than 12 months should be placed supine to sleep to reduce the risk of sudden infant death syndrome (SIDS), even if an infant is diagnosed with GERD. The only exception to this recommendation would be if the risk of death from aspiration or other complications of GERD greatly outweighed the increased risk from the prone positioning (Vandenplas, Rudolph, Di Lorenzo et al., 2009). When infants are awake, however, use of prone position with monitoring or the upright carried position can decrease reflux (Grossman & Liacouras, 2008; Kahn & Orenstein, 2011b). Elevating the head of the bed improves the condition of older children with GERD.

Medications. Although the U.S. Food and Drug Administration (FDA) has not approved many medications used in the treatment of GERD for children, their use in children is common and many are now available over the counter. Medications are often added to the treatment protocol. These medications include antacids for symptom relief, proton pump inhibitors (e.g., omeprazole and lansoprazole), histamine (H_2)-receptor antagonists (e.g., cimetidine, ranitidine) to decrease acid secretion, and prokinetic agents (e.g., cisapride, bethanechol, metoclopramide) to accelerate gastric emptying and improve esophageal and intestinal peristalsis. Antidopaminergic agents (e.g., domperidone and metoclopramide) facilitate gastric emptying.

Treatment of Acute Bleeding. Bleeding is a complication of long-standing GERD and esophagitis. Stomach lavage (washing) with an NG tube is commonly performed to evacuate blood and blood clots during an episode of upper GI bleeding. The use of iced saline lavage to stop bleeding is no longer advocated. Radiologic procedures or surgery to coagulate bleeding vessels may be needed.

Surgery. Up to 15% of infants with GERD require fundoplication. A 270- to 360-degree wrap to the stomach fundus is made around the distal esophagus. This procedure tightens the LES and prevents gastric reflux. Gas bloat syndrome may develop because of the child's inability to burp, and a gastrostomy tube may be temporarily needed for gastric decompression. Continuance of the pharmacologic treatment regimen may be needed after surgery.

NURSING CARE OF THE INFANT WITH GASTROESOPHAGEAL REFLUX DISEASE (GERD)

■ Assessment

The nurse initially obtains a thorough history related to feedings (amount, frequency, formula changes, positioning); the frequency, pattern, and characteristics of vomiting/emesis (i.e., projectile, painful, bloody); and respiratory illness/symptoms including pneumonia,

PATHOPHYSIOLOGY

Gastroesophageal Reflux

The LES, a zone of tonically contracted smooth muscle surrounding the distal esophagus, is innervated by vagal nerves and receives signals from multiple organs. A defect in this neural control may result in a dysfunctional LES with periods of transitory spontaneous relaxation. These periods of relaxation allow gastric contents to reflux back into the esophagus.

In addition, the esophagus traverses both the abdominal and thoracic cavities, with the LES positioned strategically between the two. Most of the LES is abdominal. The greater the length of intraabdominal esophagus, the more competent this valve becomes. Any condition that shortens the abdominal segment of the LES will increase the likelihood of reflux.

asthma, apnea, wheezing, choking, coughing or cyanosis. Unusual postural habits (head cocking, arching, arm thrashing) that may indicate discomfort due to esophagitis are assessed. The infant is observed during feedings to assess feeding behaviors, comfort (pain) level, dysphagia, and regurgitation. Auscultation for adventitious breath sounds is done, and the infant is assessed for signs of respiratory distress including retractions. The infant's length, weight, and head circumference are plotted on standard growth charts based on age. The nurse monitors the parent-child interactions and feeding styles. Parents are encouraged to discuss their feelings and concerns about caring for their infant with GERD.

■ Nursing Diagnosis and Planning

The following nursing diagnoses and expected outcomes may be appropriate after assessing the infant with GERD:

- Risk for Aspiration related to GERD.

Expected Outcome. The infant will maintain a patent airway without signs of respiratory distress.

- Deficient Fluid Volume related to decreased intake and frequent vomiting.

Expected Outcomes. The infant will swallow and retain each feeding with regurgitation of less than 10 mL. The infant will not become fluid volume deficient.

- Imbalanced Nutrition: Less Than Body Requirements related to dysphagia and reflux.

Expected Outcome. The infant will gain weight and grow according to standardized growth charts.

- Deficient Knowledge related to disease process, total care, and medications.

Expected Outcomes. The parents will explain GERD and demonstrate appropriate techniques for feeding, medication administration, and cardiopulmonary resuscitation (CPR). The parents will state correct purpose, dosage, schedule, and side effects for prescribed medications.

- Anxiety (parents) related to long-term care of the infant with GERD.

Expected Outcomes. The parents will exhibit effective coping mechanisms. Adequate support systems are in place.

■ Interventions

It is critically important that the infant be carefully monitored for any signs of respiratory distress or periods of apnea using a cardiac and/or apnea monitor plus frequent observation and vital signs checks by the nurse. Proper positioning (upright or prone, if awake) and minimal handling after feedings can decrease reflux and aspiration risk. Pacifier use reduces crying and encourages swallowing.

■ **Minimizing Reflux.** Multiple measures that should be used to minimize reflux include small feedings (1-3 oz) every 2 to 3 hours, use of breast milk or predigested formulas that are thickened with rice cereal (1-3 tsp/oz), frequent burping, and medications. Bottle nipples are cross-cut to enlarge the opening for thickened formula. The infant with frequent reflux and vomiting must be thoroughly assessed for signs of fluid volume deficit (dehydration), including sunken fontanel, no tears when crying, dry mucous membranes (mouth), poor skin turgor, and low urine output (fewer wet diapers).

Weight should be checked daily to assess stability and gains. Weight, length, and head circumference are periodically measured and plotted on charts to monitor nutritional status and growth.

■ **Family Education and Support.** Family education and support are vital. The nurse begins educating the parents so they learn what GERD is and how this chronic disease is managed. It is explained that different formulas, feeding routines, and medications may be tried before it is determined what will work best for their infant. The possibility of surgical treatment is discussed. Parents are taught the purpose, dosage, schedule, and side effects for each medication prescribed. The nurse shows parents how to monitor and care for their infant and then encourages them to practice assessment, positioning, formula preparation, feeding techniques, and medication administration with supervision until they demonstrate proficiency. Training for parents in infant CPR is mandatory. Parents of infants with GERD may feel overwhelmed by the complex health care needs of their infant and anxiety regarding their ability to care for their child on a long-term basis. The nurse encourages open communication so parents will share their concerns and fears. Referrals to community agencies and services can significantly increase parental competency. Support from other parents of children with GERD can improve coping.

■ **Evaluation**

- Is the infant's airway patent, without choking, coughing, cyanosis, or retractions?
- Can the infant swallow without incurring respiratory distress?
- Can the infant retain feedings with regurgitation of less than 10 mL?
- Is the infant adequately hydrated?
- Is the child growing according to growth charts?
- Is the child receiving medications as prescribed at the correct times and in the correct dosage?
- Can the parents explain GERD and the reasons for positioning and dietary modifications?
- Are parents using correct feeding techniques?
- Have the parents demonstrated the ability to provide total care for their infant?
- Have the parents expressed concerns and feelings related to caring for their infant?
- Do parents have adequate support systems and demonstrate effective coping strategies?

Constipation and Encopresis

Constipation is defined as a delay or difficulty in defecation that has been present for 2 or more weeks. A major concern with constipation is the development of encopresis, or fecal incontinence. Encopresis is repeated and involuntary defecation in a child older than 4 years who has normal colon and rectal anatomy. With encopresis, children often report that soiling occurs without warning. Parents find the situation frustrating, and soiling often becomes a major issue between parent and child. Often encopresis causes children to feel ashamed or

embarrassed, and they may avoid situations in which embarrassment might be heightened, such as spending the night with a friend or even going to school. If the condition persists over a long period, it usually affects the child's self-esteem and may impair social relations. Parents can experience a range of emotions including guilt, shame, disgust, or anger, and they may project these feelings onto the child.

PATHOPHYSIOLOGY

Constipation and Encopresis

When stool passes into the rectum, distention of the walls stimulates mass peristaltic movements in the bowel. This process is called the defecation reflex. If defecation is not desired, the external sphincter contracts and voluntary retention of stool occurs. As the stool remains in the rectum, the rectum relaxes and the defecation reflex wanes. Water reabsorption from the colon continues, resulting in hard, dry stool that is difficult to pass. The eventual passage of that stool may result in pain or anal fissures. If retention of stool continues, more fissures may develop or become worse, so that eventually even soft stool may produce pain. A cycle of pain develops in which the stool is retained to avoid pain but the retention leads to even more difficult defecation. Over time, the rectum becomes enlarged. An enlarged rectum can result in failure to control the external sphincter, which in turn results in encopresis.

Etiology and Incidence

Constipation can have many causes, such as changes in diet, dehydration, lack of exercise, emotional stress, certain drugs, pain from anal fissures, or excessive milk intake. If the child has no neurologic or anatomic disorders, encopresis is usually the result of recurrent fecal impaction and an enlarged rectum caused by chronic constipation. Factors predisposing to encopresis include inadequate or inconsistent toilet training or some type of psychological stress, such as starting school or the birth of a sibling.

Constipation can affect any child at any time. At least 3% of all visits to the pediatrician and at least 25% of pediatric gastroenterologist visits are constipation related (Greenwald, 2010). Encopresis affects an estimated 1.5% to 7.5% of children ages 6 to 12 years, with three to six times more boys than girls affected (Hardy, 2009). The incidence of encopresis is higher in lower socioeconomic classes and among children with learning disabilities.

Manifestations

Constipation. The principal symptoms of constipation are absence of stool, abdominal pain and cramping without distention, and palpable, movable fecal masses with large amounts of stool in an enlarged rectum. The child may also experience diarrheal overflow, normal or decreased bowel sounds, malaise, anorexia, headache, nausea, vomiting, and anal fissures.

Encopresis. Children with encopresis have evidence of soiled clothing and fecal odor without apparent awareness. Anal irritation leads to scratching or rubbing of the anal area. Social withdrawal and avoidance of extended contact with others (e.g., overnight stays, camp) are common. Urinary incontinence and urinary tract infections may also be present.

Diagnostic Evaluation

Abdominal radiographs may demonstrate an enlarged rectum with large amounts of stool and gas. The definitive diagnostic procedure is a rectal examination. This is rarely performed because of its emotional impact on the child and the possibility of pain from anal fissures. A thorough history is usually sufficient for the diagnosis.

Therapeutic Management

The best form of treatment is preventing development of a chronic problem through appropriate diet, exercise, and regular toileting habits. Education about "normal" bowel function can prevent a psychogenic component from compounding the problem. The focus of management is to remove the impaction, retrain the rectum so the child is aware when it is full, and help the child overcome the pain-retention cycle.

Treatment usually involves the following phases (Croffie & Fitzgerald, 2008; Culbert & Barez, 2007):

1. Disimpaction (critical for success of management)
   a. Enemas until impaction is cleared; use Fleet, 1 oz/5 kg; if the child is larger than 20 kg, use an adult size.
   b. Stool softener or laxative (osmotic and stimulant) including mineral oil, lactulose, magnesium hydroxide, GlycoLax, senna, and bisacodyl.
2. Education/demystification
   a. Extensive discussion with child and family about causes of constipation (diagrams are helpful) and discussion about feelings, social consequences, and embarrassment. The child and family need to be assessed for readiness to change.
3. Maintenance
   a. Mineral oil (14 to 45 mL) twice a day for children with low risk of vomiting or aspiration.
   b. Lactulose (10 g/15 mL), 1 or 3 mL/kg twice daily, or polyethylene glycol 3350 (1 to 2 g/kg/day).
   c. Dietary changes, including limiting milk intake, increasing water and fiber intake, and increasing residue.
4. Changing the retention habit
   a. Sitting on the commode for 5 to 10 minutes approximately 20 to 30 minutes after meals.
   b. Keeping a behavioral chart with positive rewards (daily stars may be helpful).
   c. Avoiding negative reinforcement.
   d. Using biofeedback, a potentially useful tool to reteach the feeling of rectal fullness,
   e. Increasing physical exercise, relaxation activities, and the use of stress reduction approaches to decrease anxiety

The goal is for the child to pass two or three soft stools per day without pain within the first month following treatment. Medications are withdrawn slowly over a 3- to 6-month period after the fear of pain is gone or significantly diminished.

For infant constipation, rectal stimulation is discouraged. For example, rectal thermometers and glycerin suppositories should not be used. Barley cereal can be substituted for rice cereal. Ingestions of fructose (prune juice) or lactulose can help. High-fiber fruits and vegetables will also decrease constipation.

NURSING CARE OF THE CHILD WITH CONSTIPATION OR ENCOPRESIS

■ Assessment

Obtain a thorough history of the soiling events including frequency, intensity, and duration. Because parent-child relationships are often strained, interview the parents and child separately to reduce the child's embarrassment. The nurse can explain to parents that a medical history and examination will be performed to rule out organic causes of the chronic constipation, such as Hirschsprung disease.

■ Nursing Diagnosis and Planning

The following nursing diagnoses and expected outcomes may be appropriate after assessing for constipation or encopresis in the child:

- Constipation or Bowel Incontinence related to inconsistent patterns of elimination, anxiety, or pain during elimination.

Expected Outcome. The child will have normal bowel function, as evidenced by the passage of soft stools without pain or incontinence, maintenance of a well-balanced diet high in fiber and sufficient fluid intake, and decreased reliance on laxatives.

- Compromised or Disabled Family Coping related to persistent stress, guilt, and embarrassment about the child's elimination difficulty.

Expected Outcomes. The family will function effectively as a unit, openly discuss problems, and develop a plan to achieve control over incontinence.

- Social Isolation related to embarrassment, peer teasing, and odor from bowel incontinence.

Expected Outcomes. The child will verbalize positive, realistic feelings about self and verbalize appropriate ways to achieve control over bowel incontinence.

- Impaired Skin Integrity related to poor hygiene in anal area, bowel incontinence, and lack of knowledge.

Expected Outcome. The child will maintain skin integrity, as evidenced by clean, intact skin.

■ Interventions

Because constipation and encopresis represent a continuum of the same problem, a variety of approaches can be tried as needed to treat the problem. Simple constipation may resolve with only dietary changes or changing a habit of retention. Severe encopresis may require that multiple interventions be continued for 3 to 6 months.

■ Overcoming Withholding. Before bowel retraining can begin, the child's bowel must be evacuated of all hard stool and impactions. This goal is best accomplished with the use of an appropriate size Fleet or isotonic enema every 12 hours until the impaction is cleared, usually within 48 hours. As indicated, parents are taught to administer enemas at home. During this time, the child should be monitored for hypernatremia or hyperphosphatemia, which could result from repeated use of Fleet enemas (see Chapter 13 for a discussion of enema administration).

After bowel cleansing has been achieved, the child older than 1 year may be started on mineral oil or another maintenance laxative. Lactulose may be used in infants at least 6 months old but younger than 12 months. Mineral oil is best tolerated when it is given chilled or mixed with cold drinks. The oil can be mixed with ice cream or chocolate milk, blended with ice cubes and fruit juice, or chilled to help disguise the taste. Mineral oil should not be given if the child is vomiting, as aspiration could lead to hydrocarbon pneumonia. The child may leak oil from the rectum when dosages are high, thus parents and children need to be aware that leakage does not constitute encopresis. At the end of this intervention, the child should be passing soft stool without pain or incontinence. Parents should be advised to adjust doses of laxatives based on characteristics of stool.

■ Dietary Changes. Dietary modifications are used as a part of the treatment. Increasing water and fiber intake by offering granola bars, dried fruits, whole-grain cereals, and fresh vegetables with low-fat dip can increase the bulk in stool and make it easier to pass. Decreasing sugar and milk intake also helps keep stools soft. It may be advised to supplement with fat-soluble vitamins when mineral oil is being used because the oil can theoretically interfere with vitamin absorption in the small intestine.

■ **Changing the Retention Habit.** To help reestablish a normal bowel habit, the child should sit on the toilet for 5 to 10 minutes after breakfast and dinner. This routine will allow the normal gastrocolic reflex to assist with defecation and will eliminate the need to be involved with retraining during school hours. Star charts and small prizes may be helpful in rewarding success. These interventions are continued for at least 3 to 6 months, during which the rectum will resume its normal size and the child will relearn to attend to the defecation reflex. If fecal impaction occurs at any time, enemas are again administered and the dosage of mineral oil is adjusted.

■ **Emotional Support.** The child and parents are encouraged to express their feelings of success and failure with the ongoing program. To minimize the damage to the child's self-esteem, the nurse encourages self-care as much as possible. To decrease embarrassment, school-age children should have a complete change of pants and underwear at school if leakage occurs. Age-appropriate support groups may be available in a center with a large patient population or encopresis clinic.

Though teaching is a major intervention, encouraging the child and parents to share feelings of embarrassment and other concerns is equally important. The child is provided developmentally appropriate anatomic information to assist with understanding the cause of the problem. Drawings and books may be effective ways to begin providing information and prompting the child to share feelings. Relieving the child of shame and embarrassment may improve cooperation with the plan of care.

■ **Home Care.** Because this condition is managed at home, parents require extensive education. The parents need to understand the correct way to administer enemas (see Chapter 13), adjust the child's diet, give medications, and initiate bowel retraining. They also need support in implementing and documenting the child's successes and setbacks. The child and parents need encouragement to continue the program, even when the successes seem few. This problem develops over time and takes time, patience, and perseverance to resolve.

■ **Evaluation**

- Is the child passing soft stools without pain?
- Does the food diary indicate a well-balanced, high-fiber diet?
- Is the child experiencing any incontinence?
- Are enemas, laxatives, or mineral oil still needed?
- Is the child experiencing success with bowel control as a result of implementation of a family-designed plan?
- Does the child more readily participate in age-appropriate activities and express increasing control over bowel incontinence?
- Is the skin in the anal area clean and intact?

Recurrent Abdominal Pain/Irritable Bowel Syndrome

Recurrent abdominal pain is not unusual in children older than age 6 years, and in many cases the cause is unknown or unexplained (functional pain). Some children experience symptoms that resemble the characteristic symptoms of irritable bowel syndrome (IBS) seen in some adolescents and adults (Sreedharan & Liacouras, 2011). It is possible that irritable bowel syndrome manifests in infancy as colic (Croffie & Fitzgerald, 2008).

Etiology and Incidence

The exact etiology of IBS is not understood, but it is believed to be triggered by factors such as stress, emotional events, or infection. The condition tends to occur in families with a history of other bowel disturbances or infantile colic. The condition tends to resolve by late adolescence but is sometimes present in adults as IBS. IBS is the most common diagnosis in children with recurrent abdominal pain. Patients have altered bowel habits and can fluctuate between periods of diarrhea and constipation. Some present as either diarrhea predominant or constipation predominant (Quartero, Meiniche-Schmidt, Muris et al., 2005).

Manifestations and Diagnostic Evaluation

Manifestations of IBS include diffuse abdominal pain unrelated to meals or activity; alternating constipation and diarrhea, with undigested food and mucus present in the stool; and normal growth.

The diagnosis is made on the basis of elimination of major GI pathologic conditions, including Crohn disease, giardiasis, lactose intolerance, and genitourinary abnormalities. Abdominal ultrasound, stool for ova and parasites (O&P) and cultures, abdominal radiography, and a complete gynecologic assessment age appropriate (if age-appropriate) are often ordered.

Therapeutic Management and Nursing Considerations

No definitive treatment exists for this poorly understood functional bowel problem. Management is aimed at identifying and reducing triggers and reducing bowel spasms, which decreases symptoms. The primary nursing intervention should be reassurance that it is a self-limiting, intermittent problem.

PATHOPHYSIOLOGY

Irritable Bowel Syndrome

The precipitating factors in irritable bowel syndrome are unknown but result in two distinct problems. The first is disorganized contractility, which causes spasmodic peristaltic rushes and lulls. This disorganization causes alternating diarrhea and constipation with intermittent abdominal pain. The second component is excess mucus production in the lumen of the bowel. This produces maldigestion and the passage of incompletely digested food and nutrients.

Unless lactose intolerance is suspected, no dietary modifications are required other than the maintenance of a healthy, well-balanced, moderate-fiber, lower-fat diet. The child is instructed to eat slowly, to avoid caffeine products, and not to drink carbonated beverages. For children with diagnosed lactose intolerance, supplemental lactase can be provided (Croffie & Fitzgerald, 2008).

Medications are sometimes used to treat the symptoms of IBS. Antispasmodic medications may help to improve IBS symptoms including abdominal pain in some children (Quartero et al., 2005). Antidepressants may also be used in severe cases. Alternative and complementary therapies, such as cognitive-behavioral therapy, guided imagery, relaxation, and biofeedback, may be helpful (Sreedharan & Liacouras, 2011; Zijdenbos, de Wit, van der Heijden et al., 2009).

Family and psychosocial assessments may reveal a family that is worried about a serious life-threatening disease and is quite focused on the child's bowel habits. The family may not be reassured by the normal findings on a physical and developmental examination.

The primary nursing interventions are teaching and reassurance. Health promotion activities such as exercise, balanced nutrition, and school activities can have a positive influence on the disease. Because of the associated psychosocial component, referral to mental health and family counseling services can be beneficial for some children, particularly if other measures have not been effective. The child and family are encouraged to express feelings and concerns that will assist in evaluating the interventions.

INFLAMMATORY AND INFECTIOUS DISORDERS

Ulcers

A peptic ulcer is an area of sharply circumscribed loss of the mucosa, submucosa, or muscular tissue occurring in areas of the digestive tract exposed to acid and pepsin. Peptic ulcers can be primary or secondary, gastric or duodenal. Primary or idiopathic ulcers occur in the absence of underlying systemic disease, tend to be chronic, and are usually located in the duodenum. Secondary ulcers tend to be acute in onset, occur in conjunction with serious illnesses or use of nonsteroidal antiinflammatory drugs (NSAIDs), and are found more often in the stomach.

PATHOPHYSIOLOGY

Ulcers

A thick mucous-bicarbonate barrier, a layer of mucus that provides a buffer zone for acid neutralization, lines the stomach and duodenum. Stomach acids diffuse slowly through this layer toward the gastric wall but are encountered and neutralized by slowly diffusing bicarbonate ions liberated from surface epithelial cells. The establishment of a neutral pH at the gastric epithelial surface provides protection from the combined effects of acid and pepsin. Ulcers result when any imbalance in the process occurs and erosions develop on the surface of the gastric or duodenal mucosa.

Etiology

Known factors that can alter the mucous-bicarbonate barrier in the stomach and duodenum of children include the following:

- Excessive acid secretion caused by Zollinger-Ellison syndrome or gastrinoma and hyperparathyroidism.
- Bile salts break down the adherent mucous structure of the gastric duodenal lining and expose the mucosa to acid.
- Prostaglandins augment both the mucous gel lining and bicarbonate secretion. Deficiencies in mucosal prostaglandins may cause impairment of the mucous-bicarbonate barrier.
- Duodenal ulcers show a familial tendency. Genetic factors together with environmental factors, may predispose children to ulcer formation. An association between ulcer activity and type O blood has also been noted.
- *Helicobacter pylori* (*H. pylori*) is a gram-negative spiral bacterium that has been identified in the gastric antrum of children with duodenal ulcers. It acts by weakening the gastric mucosal barrier and allowing acid and peptic digestion of the susceptible mucosa.
- Physiologic stress accounts for most of secondary ulcers encountered during infancy and early childhood. They tend to be acute and occur in seriously ill children.
- Medications such as aspirin, nonsteroidal antiinflammatory agents, and indomethacin, as well as tobacco and alcohol, are known to affect the gastroduodenal mucosa adversely.
- Diet does not seem to influence the development of ulcer disease in children. Although certain foods may cause indigestion, no convincing data show that dietary factors cause, perpetuate, or reactivate ulcers, especially duodenal. Colas, teas, and chocolate do, however, increase acid secretions and may be contributing factors.

- The importance of psychological factors is questionable. They likely influence exacerbations or complications but not initial ulcer activity.

Incidence

The true incidence of primary peptic ulcer disease in children is unknown because ulcers often spontaneously heal before a diagnosis is made. Only five to seven children are diagnosed with a gastric or duodenal ulcer per 2500 hospital admissions each year (Blanchard & Czinn, 2011). *H. pylori* infection has been found in approximately 80% of children with duodenal ulcers (Blanchard & Czinn, 2011). Secondary ulcers in children occur as a result of NSAID use or the physiologic stress associated with a critical illness such as severe burns, sepsis, shock or an intracranial lesion (Blanchard & Czinn, 2011).

Manifestations and Diagnostic Evaluation

Manifestations of ulcer disease in children are burning, cramping pain when the stomach is empty, awakening during the night or early morning with abdominal discomfort, and vomiting in children younger than 6 years. Hematemesis and melena are common in infants and young children.

Fiberoptic upper endoscopy is the diagnostic tool of choice for all children, including neonates. Endoscopy provides direct visual observation of the lining of the esophagus, stomach, and proximal duodenum and also is a means for obtaining biopsy or culture material. Ultrasound may be performed to rule out gallstones, tumors, or mechanical obstruction. The fecal occult blood test may be performed to check for GI bleeding.

Therapeutic Management

Medical management is the most common treatment for ulcer disease in children. Factors considered in ulcer treatment include drug safety, symptom relief, child and parent adherence to the prescribed regimen, and the prevention of complications or ulcer recurrence. A bland diet with milk and small, frequent feedings was long thought to be the mainstay of ulcer therapy. However, the protein and calcium in milk actually stimulate more acid secretions than they buffer. A regular diet low in caffeine is now generally prescribed because caffeine is a potent stimulant of acid secretion and exacerbates GERD. A diet high in fiber and polyunsaturated oils may also play a role in ulcer prevention.

Medications are now considered the first line of treatment. They include antibiotics, proton pump inhibitors, H_2-receptor antagonists, and mucosa protective agents. Four- to 6-week treatment using a combination of a proton pump inhibitor, an appropriate antibiotic, and bismuth salts is considered to be optimal therapy for eradicating *H. pylori* (Blanchard & Czinn, 2011). Vaccines to prevent *H. pylori* infections are currently under development.

Surgery is indicated for the management of ulcer complications such as hemorrhage, perforation, or obstruction. Vagotomy, pyloroplasty, ligation of a bleeding vessel, or closure of a perforation may be performed.

If the child is actively bleeding, an NG tube is inserted to remove blood, decompress the stomach, and estimate blood loss. IV fluids, oxygen, blood replacement, and vasoactive drugs such as vasopressin (Pitressin) may be given. Balloon tamponade with a Sengstaken-Blakemore tube may be indicated. Blood or clots are removed with room-temperature gastric lavage. The use of iced saline lavage to stop GI bleeding is no longer advocated because it increases bleeding and clotting times and prolongs the prothrombin time. It also imposes a risk of hypothermia on an already compromised child.

Nursing Considerations

Nursing assessment of the child with peptic ulcer disease begins with a thorough history, including a family history of ulcer disease, past episodes of abdominal pain, or recent stressful events in the home, school, or community. A complete assessment of pain includes a description of the nature of the pain and its location; its relationship to meals, defecation, or voiding; episodes of nocturnal pain; and medications used to effectively relieve the pain. The child is examined for the presence of epigastric tenderness, nausea, vomiting, abdominal distention, hematemesis, melena, or recent changes in appetite or eating habits.

All stools and emesis fluid should be checked for the presence of blood. Bowel sounds are auscultated for 5 minutes. If vomiting is present, the child is assessed for signs of dehydration. If bleeding is observed, the child is monitored for changes in vital signs and the physician is notified immediately. Finally, the nurse assesses family members for their understanding of the disease, the presence of a viable support system, and their ability to participate in their child's care.

Providing Information. The major focus of nursing interventions is teaching. The nurse reviews with the family pathophysiology, medication administration, and diet, and assesses the child for complications.

Preparing the child for diagnostic tests is an important nursing intervention. Because fiberoptic endoscopy is often performed, the child must be prepared for conscious sedation. Keeping the child on NPO status for at least 6 hours, maintaining an IV line, and monitoring vital signs and respiratory function during the procedure are nursing responsibilities. Upper GI examinations and ultrasonography may also be performed.

Home Care. Ulcers are managed almost exclusively in the home environment, so teaching, follow-up, and home health referral are essential. The correct use of medications and dietary modifications are parental responsibilities that may require educational materials, emotional support, help with time organization, and encouragement to continue even when symptoms are relieved. The nurse emphasizes to the parent that the medications must be given for the full prescribed course and should not be stopped when symptoms improve. The child should not be given aspirin and any other nonsteroidal antiinflammatory drug because they may cause bleeding. Parents are instructed to not use any over-the-counter or other drugs without contacting the physician first. Dietary modifications, such as avoiding foods with caffeine, carbonated beverages, and acidic foods, may relieve symptoms. Parents are taught to call the physician if the child exhibits "coffee-ground" vomitus, tarry stools, increased pain, diarrhea, vomiting, or unexplained weight loss.

Infectious Gastroenteritis

Infectious gastroenteritis is caused by a group of viruses, bacteria, and parasites capable of causing serious communicable diarrhea, massive fluid and electrolyte loss, sepsis, and death (for further discussion of fluid and electrolyte alterations, see Chapter 16).

Etiology

Ingestion of contaminated food or water and person-to-person contamination are the most frequent causes of infectious gastroenteritis in the United States. High-risk groups include children in daycare centers, preschools, and long-term care facilities and those who are immunocompromised. *Giardia* is the most common pathogen seen in children in daycare settings (Parashar, Gibson, Bresee, & Glass, 2006). Rotavirus is the most common viral cause of gastroenteritis in all children and accounts for 29% of all deaths due to diarrhea among

---

PATIENT-CENTERED TEACHING
Care of the Child with an Ulcer

Parents and older children need to understand the pathophysiology, causes, diagnosis, and therapeutic management of ulcers. When educating the parent and older child, follow these guidelines:

- Emphasize the relation of the ulcer to acute illness.
- Help the older child identify sources of excess stress that can be modified.
- Teach stress-reduction activities such as relaxation and exercise and refer parents to support groups.

Directions for administering medications include the following:

- Do not administer antacids within 1 hour of other antiulcer medications.
- Do not stop medications when symptoms improve; continue for the full prescribed course.
- Do not use aspirin or other nonsteroidal antiinflammatory drugs because they may cause bleeding.
- Do not use over-the-counter medications without your physician's knowledge.
- Do not add other drugs because your child's metabolism and absorption may be altered by ulcer medications.

Help parents make changes in diet as prescribed by teaching the following:

- If your child has a poor appetite, provide a well-balanced diet with many choices.
- Seek assistance from dietary services as needed.
- Provide meals and snacks every 2 to 3 hours.
- Make sure your child avoids coffee, chocolate, and caffeine and any other foods that might cause discomfort.

Instruct parents to call their physician if their child experiences any of the following problems:

- "Coffee-ground" vomitus
- Weight loss
- Tarry stools
- Increased pain
- Diarrhea
- Vomiting

---

children under age 5 years (Bhutta, 2011). Vaccination against rotavirus has been recommended for infants in the United States since February of 2006, and has been an effective method in reducing hospitalization and mortality rates for gastroenteritis (Bhutta, 2011; Desai, Esposito, Shapiro et al., 2010). In many cases the pathogen causing gastroenteritis is not identified (Table 19-3).

Incidence

Gastroenteritis is one of the most common outpatient infectious diseases in children. The World Health Organization and UNICEF estimate that nearly 2.5 billion episodes of diarrhea occur annually in children younger than 5 years of age in developing countries (Bhutta, 2011). Though the number of deaths from diarrheal illnesses is declining, it is estimated that 1.5 million childhood deaths still occur worldwide each year (Bhutta, 2011).

Manifestations

Gastroenteritis likely manifests with diarrhea of varying amount and consistency, vomiting, and abdominal pain. In addition, the child may experience tenesmus and fever. Dehydration is a severe consequence

TABLE 19-3   CHARACTERISTICS OF INFECTIOUS GASTROENTERITIS

CHARACTERISTICS	CLINICAL MANIFESTATIONS	DIAGNOSTIC FINDINGS	TREATMENT
Shigella (Enteroinvasive with Cytotoxin)			
Incubation period 1-2 days Most common in summer Fecal-oral spread Remains communicable for 1-3 wk	Symptoms last 5-10 days Diarrhea begins as watery, progresses to bloody, with mucus Severe abdominal pain High fever Neurologic symptoms: headache, nuchal rigidity, convulsions Risk for sepsis, hemolytic uremic syndrome, rectal prolapse, DIC (disseminated intravascular coagulation)	Blood, mucus, WBCs (white blood cells) in stool Positive stool culture in some cases	Supportive care Trimethoprim-sulfamethoxazole (TMP-SMX), 8-10 mg/kg/day for 3-5 days *or* Ampicillin, 50-100 mg/kg/day for 3-5 days Contact Precautions Identify source of infection if possible
Salmonella (Enteroinvasive)			
Incubation 1-3 days Most common in summer and fall Usually foodborne Infectious for duration of illness and variable period afterward	Symptoms last 2-5 days Rapid onset Secretory diarrhea Abdominal pain, nausea, and vomiting are common	Blood and PMNs (polymorphonuclear leukocytes) in stool Positive stool culture	Supportive care Antibiotics may be given in certain cases (TMP-SMX, Ampicillin) Contact Precautions Identify source of infection if possible
Escherichia coli (Enteroinvasive with Enterotoxin)			
Incubation period 1-3 days Most common in summer Foodborne most common	Symptoms for 3-7 days or longer Green, watery, secretory diarrhea May cause hemorrhagic colitis Fever	Blood and PMNs in stool	Supportive care Contact Precautions TMP-SMX and quinolones for severe cases Monitor renal function, hemoglobin, and platelets
Campylobacter			
Incubation 2-5 days Most common in infants and adolescents	Symptoms for 2-10 days Consumption of contaminated foods or water Severe abdominal pain Foul-smelling, watery diarrhea Fever	Blood and PMNs in stool	Supportive care Possible treatment with erythromycin or quinolones Contact Precautions
Giardia lamblia			
Incubation period 1-2 wk Most common cause of parasitic diarrhea Spread in contaminated food and water	Symptoms for days to weeks Afebrile Abdominal distention, cramps, and flatulence Variable diarrhea	Ova and parasites found in stool Parasites found on duodenal biopsy	Metronidazole (Flagyl) for 7 days Contact Precautions Treat all unknown water sources with chlorine/iodine before drinking
Rotavirus			
Incubation 1-3 days Common in winter months Fecally contaminated food	Symptoms usually last 3-7 days Vomiting, diarrhea, low-grade fever History of preceding or concurrent respiratory illness	Virus in stool detected by enzyme immunoassay	No pharmacologic treatment Supportive care; maintain hydration and electrolyte balance Contact Precautions Rotavirus vaccine at 2, 4, and 6 mo of age; series needs to be complete by 32 wk of age
Clostridium difficile			
Antibiotic associated Most common nosocomial diarrhea	Fever for 24-48 hr Diarrhea develops after antibiotic treatment	Blood and PMNs in stool	Cholestyramine used to enhance mucosal recovery and decrease length of diarrhea Possibly treated with vancomycin or metronidazole (Flagyl) for 10 days
Norwalk			
Incubation 1-2 days Common in winter in schools and other group settings Fecal-oral route of transmission	Symptoms last 1-2 days Nausea, vomiting, diarrhea Headache, low-grade fever, muscle aches, chills	Virus in stool	No pharmacologic treatment Contact Precautions

of gastroenteritis and occurs mainly in children younger than 2 years. A history of travel to other regions of the world can provide clues to the causative organism.

PATHOPHYSIOLOGY

Infectious Gastroenteritis

As the pathogen adheres to the mucosa of the intestine, it is no longer affected by peristaltic waves and is not removed from the site. Epithelial invasion occurs, causing an inflammatory response and epithelial cell death. This leads to ulcerations, pseudomembranes, bleeding, and possibly sepsis. As the pathogens multiply, they may produce toxins. Enterotoxins (e.g., cholera, *Shigella*) cause fluid and electrolyte shifts that result in increased secretion into the intestine and simultaneous decrease in absorption caused by edema. The absorptive capacity of the colon is exceeded, and massive diarrhea and dehydration result. Cytotoxins (e.g., *Salmonella*) produce local edema, malabsorption, and dehydration. Some pathogens are also capable of producing neurotoxins (e.g., *Shigella*) that act outside the GI tract.

Diagnostic Evaluation

A definitive diagnosis can be made when a stool culture yields a pathogen, but these cultures are expensive and result in many false-negative findings. Ova and parasites are more reliably found. Usually only children who appear to be in a toxic condition or have bloody stools, abdominal pain, or tenesmus undergo a diagnostic workup. The presence of white blood cells (WBCs) and blood in the stool can support the presumptive diagnosis on the basis of clinical findings. Blood cultures may also be needed in the acutely ill infant and young child. An unprepared sigmoidoscopy can be useful in determining the amount of mucosal involvement, obtaining more reliable samples for culture, and diagnosing the disease.

Therapeutic Management

The priority therapy is to replace water and correct acid-base or fluid and electrolyte disturbances with IV fluids or oral (PO) electrolyte replacement liquids. The rate of replacement may be as high as 50 to 100 mL/kg over a 4- to 6-hour period (1 to 2.5 times maintenance requirements). Because diarrheal fluid is high in sodium, potassium, and bicarbonate, oral rehydration solutions should be used to match losses (see Chapter 16). Hospitalization for treatment is not uncommon, especially for the infant or small child, to allow for continued assessment and management of symptoms or sepsis. Antimicrobial therapy is useful in cases of infection with *Shigella* and *Giardia*, and in some cases of infection with *Clostridium difficile* and *Escherichia coli* (*E. coli*), but not for rotavirus infection. The FDA licensed a rotavirus vaccine for use among infants in 2006. The Advisory Committee on Immunization Practices (ACIP) recommends that all infants be immunized with three doses of the vaccine at 2, 4, and 6 months of age.

NURSING CARE OF THE CHILD WITH INFECTIOUS GASTROENTERITIS

■ Assessment

Obtain an adequate history of the event, including the length of symptoms, the frequency and consistency of stools, and the presence of blood or mucus in stools. Noting the amount, color, consistency, and time (ACCT) of each stool or episode of vomiting is a consistent way to document findings. The concurrent appearance of symptoms in other members of the family can be helpful in the diagnosis. Any travel to other countries or wilderness areas should be recorded. Evaluating formula and food preparation at home and in daycare facilities, as well as examining sanitation and hygiene in these places, can provide valuable information.

The child may appear moderately to severely dehydrated with hyperactive bowel sounds and severe diarrhea, which is often bloody. Blood in the stool usually appears after the maximal fluid loss has occurred and can be useful in determining the stage of illness. The presence of abdominal pain, vomiting, tenesmus, and fever should be assessed. Headache, nuchal rigidity, irritability, and seizures are important symptoms of the neurotoxic effects of *Shigella*.

Assessment of hydration status is critical. Low urine output, high urine specific gravity, poor skin turgor, dry mucous membranes, crying without producing tears, a sunken or depressed fontanel in infants, and skin tenting can occur quickly with the large amount of fluid lost through diarrhea. Loss of bicarbonate from severe diarrhea and dehydration makes metabolic acidosis a major concern. The compensatory mechanisms of increased respiratory rate and effort are important to document.

■ Nursing Diagnosis and Planning

The following nursing diagnoses and expected outcomes may be appropriate for the infant or child with gastroenteritis:
- Deficient Fluid Volume related to severe diarrhea.

Expected Outcomes. The child will be adequately hydrated without electrolyte disturbance, as evidenced by moist mucous membranes; good skin turgor; urine output appropriate for age; return to normal weight; and normal serum sodium, potassium, and bicarbonate levels. The child will have soft, formed stools without diarrhea, blood, or mucus.
- Risk for Infection related to exposure of family members and others to infectious agents.

Expected Outcome. The child will not transmit pathogens to others.
- Acute Pain related to hyperactive motility.

Expected Outcome. The child will be free from abdominal pain, as evidenced by a return to normal activity and no reports of pain.
- Deficient Knowledge related to inadequate information about the disease and its control.

Expected Outcomes. The parents will describe how to prevent transmitting the condition to others and will use Standard Precautions and Contact Precautions when handling the child's excretions.
- Imbalanced Nutrition: Less Than Body Requirements related to malabsorption.

Expected Outcomes. The child will resume a normal diet and will regain weight lost during the acute phase within 1 week after symptoms abate.
- Risk for Impaired Skin Integrity related to skin contact with feces and the necessity for frequent cleansing.

Expected Outcome. The child will maintain skin integrity, as evidenced by clean, dry, intact skin without redness, drainage, or breakdown.

■ Interventions

■ **Maintaining Fluid Balance.** Critical nursing interventions are related to the fluid volume deficit. Oral or parenteral rehydration with correction of acid-base imbalances is essential to establish homeostasis. Accurate intake and output and weight measurements are important. Monitoring skin turgor, urine output, and serum electrolyte levels provides evaluation criteria in this area (see Chapter 16 for a further discussion of fluid and electrolyte alterations).

■ **Decreasing Risk.** Providing safety, assessing neurologic symptoms, and monitoring for seizures are also priorities for the child with *Shigella* infection. Preventing the spread of infection remains a critical nursing intervention. Thorough hand hygiene is a must. Contact Precautions must be strictly enforced for all staff and family members to minimize the risk of spreading the infection. These precautions must be maintained at home for up to 2 weeks; the time period may be less if antibiotics are given. Pain and fever may be treated with acetaminophen. Symptomatic treatment with antidiarrheal medications is not recommended because they tend to increase the length of symptoms. Parents and children need to be taught these interventions and given information about the disease process during this period. Depending on the organism causing the gastroenteritis, follow-up by the public health department may be necessary. Organisms such as *Salmonella* and *E. coli* can be found in food and present a significant public health concern. A dietary recall for possibly contaminated foods can be important in establishing the cause and minimizing the risk of spread to the public.

■ **Home Care.** The most important intervention that can be implemented at home is proper rehydration to prevent the need for hospitalization and IV therapy (see Chapter 16 for a discussion of oral rehydration fluids and care for the child with dehydration).

Dietary changes for vomiting and diarrhea may not be necessary if the child does not demonstrate dehydration. Breast milk may be offered as needed, and formula should be given full strength. Oral rehydration therapy (ORT) may also be used in addition to usual diet to replace GI losses and prevent dehydration (see Chapter 16). Vomiting does not prevent oral rehydration because the child can be successfully rehydrated with 5 to 10 mL of rehydrating solution every 2 minutes. When diet is continued, foods with fats and high sugar concentrations should be avoided. Complex carbohydrates, starches, lean meats, and vegetables should be encouraged. *Lactobacillus,* which can be found in yogurt or as a supplement, assists in reducing diarrhea by restoring normal bowel flora.

Children who demonstrate mild or moderate dehydration may require ORT at a rate of 50 to 100 mL/kg rapidly over a 3- to 4-hour period in addition to replacing fluid losses from vomiting or diarrhea (Centers for Disease Control and Prevention [CDC], 2003). Regular diet may be resumed as just described once the fluid deficit has been corrected. Once a dehydrated child has been rehydrated, resuming an age-appropriate diet enhances recovery (CDC, 2003). Severe dehydration may require parenteral therapy and hospitalization.

Preventing the spread of infection is also essential for home care (see the Patient-Centered Teaching: Care of the Child with Infectious Gastroenteritis box). Good hand hygiene; the disinfection of contaminated linens, clothes, and diapers; and the use of surface disinfectant sprays are important preventive measures.

■ Evaluation

- Has the child returned to preinfection weight within 1 week after symptoms subside?
- Does the child have good skin turgor, moist mucous membranes, and a urine specific gravity of less than 1.030?
- Does the child have a serum sodium level of 135 to 145 mEq/L and a serum potassium level of 3.5 to 5 mEq/L?
- Is the child passing soft, formed stools without diarrhea, blood, or mucus?
- Are other family members free from infectious diarrhea, and is the family following the appropriate precautions to prevent transmission?
- Is the child reporting abdominal pain?

PATIENT-CENTERED TEACHING

Care of the Child with Infectious Gastroenteritis

If your child has infectious gastroenteritis, you must do the following:

- Wash your hands frequently and thoroughly and insist that your child do so as well. Always wash your hands after changing diapers.
- Allow your child to use a separate bathroom if available.
- Continue to follow these measures for several weeks because bacterial diarrhea may be communicable for several weeks after symptoms disappear.
- Administer oral fluids with appropriate rehydration solutions (e.g., Rehydralyte) in small, frequent amounts (every 30 minutes). If your child is vomiting, administer 1 tsp of fluid every 5 to 10 minutes. Give one half cup for each watery stool.
- Do not give your child fruit juices, cola, sports drinks, tea, or sugary drinks.
- Continue to feed your child, but avoid high-fat or high-sugar foods. Breast milk and formula may be continued.
- Do not give over-the-counter medications without notifying your physician.

Call your physician if the following pertain:

- Your child is younger than 6 months.
- Your child has a fever.
- Diarrhea worsens.
- Diarrhea has blood in it.
- Vomiting increases or your child cannot keep down any fluid.
- Your child reports severe abdominal pain.
- Your child shows signs of dehydration, such as no tears, sunken eyes, or decreased urination.

- Does the child guard the abdomen during palpation?
- Are parents and staff at the daycare facility practicing infection control procedures, if appropriate?
- Can the child tolerate an age-appropriate regular diet?
- Is the child's skin intact and free from areas of irritation and breakdown?

Appendicitis

Appendicitis is the inflammation and infection of the vermiform appendix, a small lymphoid, tubular, blind sac at the end of the cecum. It is the most common cause of emergency surgery in children and adolescents.

Etiology and Incidence

Common causes of obstruction and subsequent appendicitis include lymphoid swelling related to viral infection, impacted fecal material, foreign bodies, and parasites. In most cases no definitive cause can be identified at the time of surgery.

Appendicitis occurs with equal frequency in both sexes, with most cases occurring during adolescence and early adulthood. Appendicitis is uncommon in children younger than 4 years, but in young children it is associated with a high frequency of perforation by the time of the first visit, most likely related to the difficulty in establishing the diagnosis.

Manifestations and Diagnostic Evaluation

The cardinal symptom of appendicitis is pain, progressing in intensity and localizing to the right lower quadrant at McBurney point (Figure 19-4). Associated signs and symptoms include nausea and vomiting,

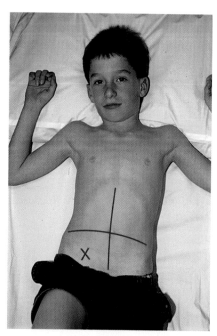

FIG 19-4 McBurney point is midway between the right anterior superior iliac crest and the umbilicus. It is usually the location of greatest pain in the child with appendicitis. (Courtesy University of Texas at Arlington College of Nursing, Arlington, TX.)

anorexia, diarrhea or constipation, and fever and chills. If the appendix perforates, the child will initially experience relief of pain. Other signs and symptoms will worsen, so that the child will appear acutely ill with high fever and signs of dehydration.

The diagnosis is usually made on the basis of classic abdominal findings of pain localizing at McBurney point, guarding, rebound tenderness, nausea, vomiting, and fever. A WBC count of 15,000 to 20,000/mm³ can support the clinical findings. A quick, safe, and accurate diagnosis can usually be made with ultrasound or with limited computed tomography (CT), which shows an enlarged, incompressible appendix that may be fluid filled and locally inflamed, and may be used to predict the severity of the disease (Toorenvliet, Wiersma, Bakker et al., 2010).

PATHOPHYSIOLOGY

Appendicitis

Obstruction of the appendix allows normal mucus secretions to accumulate in the appendix, producing distention. Distention eventually causes occlusion of the capillaries and engorgement of the walls of the appendix. Micro-abscesses form and can progress to abscesses and fistulas. Perforation occurs as a result of tissue breakdown and swelling. Bowel contents then contaminate the mesenteric bed and peritoneum, leading to peritonitis and sepsis.

Therapeutic Management

The definitive treatment for appendicitis and suspected appendicitis is appendectomy. Preoperatively the child is managed with fluid therapy, immobilization, pain control interventions, NPO status, antibiotics, and antipyretics, if indicated. The procedure may be done laparoscopically or through an open abdominal approach, particularly if perforation is suspected.

NURSING CARE OF THE CHILD WITH APPENDICITIS

■ Assessment

The nursing assessment will reveal a history of pain, fever, vomiting, and diarrhea or constipation. The physical examination discloses abdominal tenderness and guarding. The child may assume a supine position with the right leg flexed to decrease tension on the abdominal wall. The nurse must be keenly aware of the symptoms of perforation including a sudden relief from pain followed by an increase in pain, rigid abdomen, and early shock symptoms. Behavioral changes and refusal to eat are important indicators in infants and toddlers.

Assess anxiety in the child and family members, who are most likely facing unexpected surgery. Because of the pain, the child may be uncooperative with abdominal assessment. The parents may have financial concerns related to the unplanned surgery.

■ Nursing Diagnosis and Planning

The following nursing diagnoses and expected outcomes may be appropriate after assessing the child with appendicitis:
- Acute Pain related to abdominal inflammation and surgical incision.

Expected Outcome. The child will be free from pain, as evidenced by resumption of normal activity and movement with no reports of pain.
- Risk for Infection related to rupture and surgery.

Expected Outcomes. The child will have a clean, dry surgical incision that is free from redness, heat, or exudate, and the child will be afebrile with a WBC count of 5000 to 15,000/mm³.
- Deficient Fluid Volume related to vomiting or diarrhea.

Expected Outcome. The child will be well hydrated, as evidenced by moist mucous membranes, good skin turgor, and hourly urine output appropriate for age (see Chapter 16).
- Anxiety related to unplanned surgery.

Expected Outcomes. The parent or child will express feelings about surgery and will verbalize the need for emergency hospitalization.

! NURSING QUALITY ALERT

Assessing Appendicitis in the Young Child

Because symptoms of appendicitis can be vague and develop slowly over approximately a 12-hour period, the condition can be quite difficult to assess in young children. The complaint that "my tummy hurts" often is the only initial symptom. Appendicitis should be suspected if pain, anorexia, or nausea and vomiting, and fever occur simultaneously. If pain occurs before vomiting, appendicitis should be suspected. However, if vomiting precedes abdominal pain, gastroenteritis is more likely. The young child will usually refuse to play, preferring instead to lie down. Often, the child will lie in a knee-chest position to be comfortable. One way of helping the child describe the area of pain focus is to ask the child to stand on tiptoes and then drop to flat feet. The pain location elicited from this maneuver usually will be in the right lower quadrant.

■ Interventions

■ Uncomplicated Appendicitis. On admission, vital signs should be taken to monitor for sepsis or shock. The nurse institutes comfort measures including topical cold application, pain medications, and positions of comfort. Enemas or laxatives should not be administered.

No heat should be applied to the abdomen because it may increase the chance of perforation as a result of vasodilation. IV fluid therapy is started to prepare the child for surgery and correct any existing fluid, electrolyte, and acid-base disturbances related to vomiting and diarrhea.

If the procedure is performed by laparoscopy, the nurse can expect the child to be discharged within 24 hours. Open surgery may be followed by a few days of recovery in the hospital. After either operation, the child will be on NPO status until bowel function has returned.

■ **Ruptured Appendix.** The child with a ruptured appendix needs specialized care. If perforation is suspected, prepare the child for NG tube insertion. The NG tube provides decompression before surgery and allows gastric content drainage postoperatively. The child will need IV antibiotics, which may be started preoperatively. For the child with a perforation, IV antibiotics are continued and hospitalization may last 5 days or longer, if complications occur. After the NG tube is removed, the diet should be advanced gradually as tolerated so that the child can tolerate a normal diet without vomiting or diarrhea.

Depending on the extent of the peritonitis, the child may have postoperative incisional drains. These drains may be attached to suction, and aseptic technique and maintenance of patency are essential. The nurse carefully documents the drainage amount each shift. The wound is often left open and treated with sterile wet-to-dry or wet-to-moist (saline-soaked gauze) dressings and wound irrigation with antibacterial solutions.

Round-the-clock opioid analgesics provide relief from incisional pain and from pain caused by dressing changes (see Chapters 14 and 15). Continued reassessment of abdominal pain is essential for evaluating the presence of a wound infection, abscess, or fistula.

Monitor vital signs, including temperature, every 2 to 4 hours. Intermittent NG suction will likely be continued postoperatively until bowel sounds return. Positioning the child to facilitate drainage and minimize the spread of infection into the upper abdomen should be done by elevating the head of the bed or having the child lie on the operative side.

■ **Home Care.** After surgery and discharge, parents must be prepared to assume responsibility for the child's care. The surgical incision and any drain sites must be assessed for redness, drainage, dehiscence, or suture infections. Report any problems to the physician. Parents should advance the child's diet slowly, beginning with liquids and soft foods and progressing to the child's normal diet if tolerated without nausea or vomiting. Teach parents to watch for vomiting, abdominal pain, or distention as possible signs of bowel obstruction or peritoneal infection.

■ Evaluation

- Does the child report pain?
- Does the child demonstrate guarding on abdominal palpation?
- Has the child returned to normal activity level?
- Is the surgical incision clean, dry, and free from redness, heat, purulent drainage, or dehiscence?
- Is the child afebrile, with a WBC count of 5000 to 15,000/mm^3?
- Is the child tolerating an age-appropriate regular diet without vomiting, diarrhea, or increased abdominal pain?
- Are the child and parents able to express relief from anxiety?

Inflammatory Bowel Disease

Inflammatory bowel disease is a chronic inflammatory condition of the small or large intestine. It includes two distinct conditions; ulcerative colitis and Crohn disease. Ulcerative colitis affects only the colon and involves both the mucosal and submucosal layers of the intestine. Crohn disease can occur anywhere in the GI tract, from the mouth to the anus, and is transmural, involving all layers of the intestine.

Etiology

The exact cause of inflammatory bowel disease is not known. Several triggers have been identified, including viral and other infectious agents, food allergies, vasculitis, increased intestinal permeability, immunologic dysfunction, and genetic factors. Increasing evidence demonstrates a connection between inflammatory bowel disease and the effects of stress on the immune response.

Incidence, Manifestations, and Diagnostic Evaluation

The incidence, manifestations, and diagnostic evaluation for both ulcerative colitis and Crohn disease are summarized in Table 19-4.

Therapeutic Management

Management for inflammatory bowel disease is multidimensional and includes medication, dietary and nutritional support, and symptomatic treatment. Pharmacologic treatment includes antiinflammatory, antibacterial, antibiotic, and immunosuppressive drugs. The principal medications used to treat inflammatory bowel disease include the following:

- 5-Aminosalicylic acid (5-ASA) medications such as sulfasalazine or mesalazine
- Corticosteroids such as prednisone
- Immune-modulating agents such as azathioprine, methotrexate, 6-mercaptopurine (6-MP), and cyclosporin A
- Tumor necrosis factor–alpha (TNF-α) antibody (infliximab).
- Antibiotics such as metronidazole (Flagyl) and ciprofloxacin (quinolones)

5-ASA and 6-MP are first-line immunosuppressants that allow selected children with Crohn disease to avoid steroids and associated side effects. Infliximab (Remicade) has been approved for treatment of ulcerative colitis and Crohn disease in children. It binds to TNF-α to decrease inflammation and increase intestinal healing. It has been shown to be effective in moderate to severe acute disease and in children who do not gain results from corticosteroids (Jacobstein & Baldassano, 2008). It is well tolerated and safe with generally mild reactions that respond rapidly to intervention (Muniyappa, Gulati, Mohr, & Hupertz, 2009).

Nutritional intervention is part of a holistic approach for children with Crohn disease and is a useful component with no side effects. Total parenteral nutrition (TPN) may be needed during acute flare-ups. Exclusive enteral nutrition with an elemental formula via nasogastric tube or gastrostomy promotes healing of the mucosa and can control the disease in some children with Crohn disease as effectively as prednisone (Conklin & Oliva-Hemker, 2010; Grossman & Baldassano, 2011a).

Crohn disease is best managed before permanent structural changes have developed. Malnutrition is a common problem and can involve protein, fat, carbohydrate, and vitamin deficiencies, leading to growth failure. Nutritional support and teaching are essential. Surgery is not curative, but partial bowel resections may be necessary to treat abscesses, fistulas, or chronic recurrent obstruction.

For ulcerative colitis, it can be useful to avoid milk products and consume a hypoallergenic, low-fiber, low-fat, low-residue, high-protein, elemental diet. Surgical intervention for ulcerative colitis includes partial or total colectomy with creation of a colostomy or ileostomy. Optimally, a total colectomy is combined with an endorectal pull-through where the distal ileum is pulled down and sutured to the

TABLE 19-4 CROHN DISEASE AND ULCERATIVE COLITIS

CROHN DISEASE	ULCERATIVE COLITIS
Pathophysiology	
Affects entire GI tract, most common in the terminal ileum	Involves only colon, starting at the rectum and moving upward
Transmural involvement	Mucosa and submucosa only
Cobblestone appearance of mucosa	Mucosa lacking in most cases
Fistulas common	Fistulas rare
Remissions and exacerbations	Remissions uncommon
Diagnostic Evaluation: Colonoscopy, Rectoscopy, Barium Enema, Biopsy	
"Skip" lesions with deep fissures and granulomas	Inflammation and superficial ulceration; "cutoff" demarcation between areas of inflamed and normal colon
Biopsy reveals nonspecific chronic inflammation	
Incidence	
5 per 100,000 in United States and increasing	15 per 100,000 in United States
Equal gender distribution	Equal gender distribution
Not seen in infants; peaks in teens, early 20s	Peaks between ages 15 and 40 yr
Clusters in families	Clusters in families
Associated with higher standard of living	Affects whites more than others
Clinical Manifestations	
Abdominal pain	Abdominal pain unusual
Diarrhea, nonbloody	Diarrhea, occasionally with hemorrhage and anemia
Fever	
Palpable abdominal mass	No masses
Anorexia and severe weight loss	Moderate weight loss
Significant growth impairment	Mild growth impairment
Perianal and anal lesions	Perianal and anal lesions rare
Fistulas and obstructions	Fistulas and obstructions rare
Extraintestinal symptoms (arthralgia, arthritis)	Risk of toxic megacolon
Morbidity	
Regions of affected bowel increase over time	Remissions and exacerbations
50%-70% will eventually require surgery for obstruction or fistula	10% chance of cancer after 10 yr
Surgery does not cure disease	Removal of colon can cure the disease

distal rectum, allowing the child to maintain continence (Grossman & Baldassano, 2011b).

NURSING CARE OF THE CHILD WITH INFLAMMATORY BOWEL DISEASE

■ Assessment

Recurrent or chronic diarrhea is the primary finding in the nursing history of a child with inflammatory bowel disease (IBD). The major assessment findings are related to this diarrhea and the associated malabsorption that occurs. Weight loss, dehydration, anorexia, growth failure, vitamin deficiencies, and anemia are common. The severity of the GI symptoms and the amount and length of steroid use will have a significant influence on a child's growth rate. With ulcerative colitis, remissions and exacerbations of symptoms are common. Frank bleeding is also possible.

Intermittent cramping discomfort exacerbated by eating is common in Crohn disease. The child with Crohn disease may have oral lesions and perianal skin breakdown. Inflammatory changes also can occur outside of the GI system with arthralgia and arthritis, especially of the lower extremities, causing discomfort and mobility problems.

Depression, anxiety, fears about social interactions, and low self-esteem occur and are most likely related to the need to have quick access to restrooms at all times and to be close to home if an accident occurs. The chronic nature of this condition and its unknown prognosis can lead to family stress and tax the family's financial resources and support systems. Assessment should include questions about family and peer support, resources, and knowledge of the disease.

■ Nursing Diagnosis and Planning

The following nursing diagnoses and expected outcomes may be appropriate for the child with inflammatory bowel disease and the child's family:

- Imbalanced Nutrition: Less Than Body Requirements related to chronic malabsorption.

Expected Outcomes. The child will have acceptable bowel patterns, as evidenced by passing no more than four stools per day and being free from nocturnal diarrhea. The child will receive adequate nutrition, as evidenced by normal hemoglobin values and normal growth that follows the growth curve.

- Acute Pain related to cramping.

Expected Outcome. The child will be free from abdominal pain, as evidenced by resumption of normal activity and no reports of pain.

- Chronic Low Self-Esteem related to chronic diarrhea and colostomy.

Expected Outcome. The child will have a positive self-concept, as evidenced by leading an active lifestyle without depression.

- Delayed Growth and Development related to malnutrition, chronic illness, and steroid use.

Expected Outcome. The child will meet normal developmental milestones, as evidenced by progress on standard developmental screenings.

- Disturbed Body Image related to weight loss, water retention from steroid therapy, and colostomy or ileostomy.

Expected Outcomes. The child will state reasons for changes in body appearance and will share concerns about changes with family and support personnel.

- Anxiety related to chronic diarrhea and risk for surgery.

Expected Outcomes. The child will express concerns about the future and will ask for support as needed.

- Deficient Knowledge related to management of chronic disease.

Expected Outcome. The child will explain day-to-day management of disease and will demonstrate ability for self-care that is age-appropriate.

■ Interventions

Nursing interventions focus on maintaining pharmacologic interventions, developing long-term nutritional management, educating, and providing emotional support.

PATHOPHYSIOLOGY

Inflammatory Bowel Disease

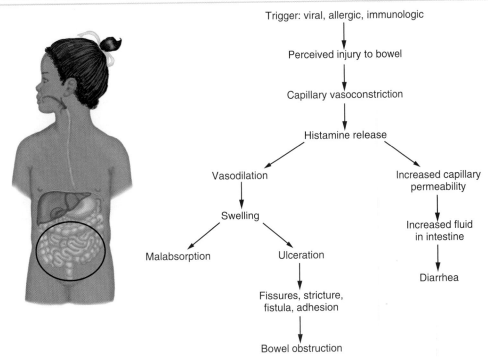

Trigger: viral, allergic, immunologic

Perceived injury to bowel

Capillary vasoconstriction

Histamine release

Vasodilation

Swelling

Malabsorption

Ulceration

Fissures, stricture, fistula, adhesion

Bowel obstruction

Increased capillary permeability

Increased fluid in intestine

Diarrhea

A triggering factor, whether viral, allergic, or immunologic, causes the bowel to "respond" as if to an injury and results in capillary vasoconstriction and histamine release within the bowel. The histamine has two effects on the bowel. The first is vasodilation, which results in swelling that can cause malabsorption by distorting the surface area of the villi. Swelling then produces cell death and ulceration, which can progress to the development of fissures, strictures, fistulas, adhesions, and bowel obstruction. The second effect of histamine release is increased capillary permeability, which results in increased fluid in the intestine and subsequent diarrhea. Crohn disease affects all layers of the bowel; ulcerative colitis affects the mucosa and submucosa only.

■ **Medications.** Teaching appropriate administration of medications is an important nursing role. Enemas are used before critical diagnostic tests and may serve as a method of medication administration. Any child who will be taking steroids (see Chapter 18) needs to understand the importance of regular administration as well as the risks associated with immunosuppression. Steroids should be given with food or antacids to prevent GI distress. The steroids, although beneficial in suppressing symptoms, may actually exacerbate the growth delays associated with inflammatory bowel disease.

■ **Nutritional Management.** Nutritional support varies with the disease and the child's tolerance of changes. In general, maintaining a low-fiber, low-residue, low-fat, milk-free, elemental diet provides some relief, although strict restrictions do not alleviate symptoms. A balanced, nutritious diet is recommended, as are vitamin, iron, and folate supplements.

During acute flare-ups or surgery, TPN and lipids may be needed to restore a seriously malnourished child. These interventions do not change the course of the inflammation in the bowel but provide essential nutritional support. Elemental diets, which can be absorbed without significant digestion, may be used during acute episodes of Crohn disease to allow the bowel to rest. NG or gastrostomy tube feedings during the night may be necessary to prevent further growth impairment (see Chapter 13).

Continued assessments of nutritional status, growth patterns, and development are important elements of nursing care for children with this chronic problem. Assessing the number of stools, nutritional status, weight, developmental milestones, and pain will help evaluate the child's response to treatment.

■ **Family Education and Support.** Because Crohn disease is a long-term health problem that requires numerous medical, pharmacologic, and surgical interventions, family support and financial resources can be strained to the limit. Appropriate community resources can provide education and assistance. The Crohn's and Colitis Foundation of America (CCFA) supplies educational materials and family information on local resources (including financial) and support groups (see Evolve website). Long-term nursing care can be improved by providing consistent caregivers and encouraging the child to form relationships. Self-care and management should be major goals in working with children with inflammatory bowel disease, as with other chronic diseases. A team approach that includes medical, nutritional, educational, rehabilitative, and psychological support is essential for success.

Another important resource for children with inflammatory bowel disease is camp programs such as Camp Oasis sponsored by the CCFA. With a dozen camps held each summer across the United States, children with IBD join together to learn more about their disease, create friendships with people who understand them, and gain self-confidence (CCFA, 2010).

■ **Home Care.** Home care is a mainstay of treatment as parents and child assume responsibility for care. Teaching parents to administer steroids, including providing information on their inherent side effects and the importance of not discontinuing their use abruptly, should be a high priority. Also, techniques of enema administration and skin care for perianal lesions must be taught. Nutrition diaries can provide useful information. TPN may be administered at home, and parents need complete instructions and referral to a home nursing care agency to obtain equipment, supplies, and support.

In addition, helping children and parents know when to seek medical care is important. Sudden exacerbations of symptoms, weight loss, blood loss, and severe abdominal pain should be reported promptly to health care professionals. Stress management and the avoidance of triggers can help minimize the symptoms of the disease and its impact on the child.

▪ Evaluation

- Is the child free from nocturnal diarrhea?
- Is the child passing fewer than four stools per day?
- Is the child gaining weight appropriately and following the growth chart?
- Is the child's hemoglobin value between 11 g/dL and 16 g/dL?
- Does the child report abdominal pain?
- Does the child participate in age-appropriate activities without evidence of depression?
- Is the child's development normal for age?
- Is the child able to share body image concerns with appropriate family members?
- Has the child or family sought external support through appropriate referral groups?
- Do the child and parent demonstrate appropriate skills for day-to-day management and make appropriate future plans for long-term management of disease?
- Do the child and family seek help when exacerbations occur?
- Does the child manage self-care appropriately for age?

OBSTRUCTIVE DISORDERS

Hypertrophic Pyloric Stenosis

Pyloric stenosis results when the circular area of muscle surrounding the pylorus hypertrophies and obstructs gastric emptying. This condition is one of the most common surgical disorders of early infancy.

Etiology and Incidence

The exact cause of pyloric stenosis remains unknown, but muscular hypertrophy is not present at birth. Pyloric stenosis may be associated with other GI anomalies such as malrotation, short bowel syndrome, esophageal and duodenal atresia, anorectal anomalies, hiatal hernia, and GER. Heredity and family predisposition seem to increase the risk of pyloric stenosis.

The incidence of pyloric stenosis is about 3 in every 1000 live births (National Birth Defects Prevention Network, 2009). Children and offspring of an affected parent are at highest risk. Male infants are affected more often than female infants, and term infants are affected more often than premature infants. The incidence is also higher in white infants than in African-American or Asian infants.

Manifestations

Progressive projectile, nonbilious vomiting in a previously healthy infant is the major manifestation of pyloric stenosis. The vomitus may become blood tinged if esophageal irritation occurs. A movable, palpable, firm, olive-shaped mass is felt in the right upper quadrant. This mass is most easily palpated when the stomach is empty and the infant

is relaxed. Deep gastric peristaltic waves from left upper quadrant to right upper quadrant may be visible immediately before vomiting. The infant will be irritable and hungry a short time after being fed. If the condition progresses, the infant may become dehydrated and experience metabolic alkalosis.

PATHOPHYSIOLOGY

Hypertrophic Pyloric Stenosis

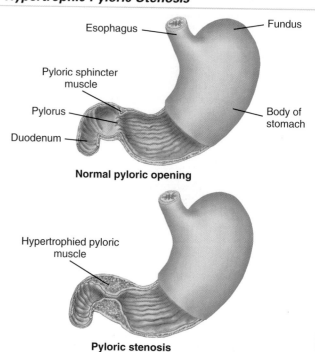

Pyloric spasms cause milk curds to be propelled against a narrowed pyloric channel and subsequently irritate its sensitive mucosal lining. Edema of the pyloric mucosa results. This edema further reduces the size of the pyloric canal and creates resistance to the flow of milk. To promote gastric emptying and compensate for this resistance, the pylorus contracts with more force and gradually enlarges. This enlarged pyloric muscle slowly begins to constrict the pyloric channel, and when the mucosal edema subsides, the resistance to flow still remains. A vicious cycle develops and progresses to a high-level obstruction of the pyloric canal.

Diagnostic Evaluation

The diagnosis is made on the basis of a history of vomiting, visible peristaltic waves, and a palpable pyloric mass. When the mass cannot be palpated, radiography and ultrasonography are helpful. A flat plate of the abdomen will show a narrow pylorus with a dilated stomach and the absence of gas distal to the pylorus. Ultrasonography can confirm the presence of a pyloric mass. A barium swallow examination will disclose the long, narrow pyloric canal and detect delayed gastric emptying. Laboratory findings may indicate metabolic alkalosis as a result of vomiting, including decreased serum potassium and sodium levels, increased pH and bicarbonate, and a decreased chloride level. Indirect bilirubin may be elevated.

Therapeutic Management

Because pyloric stenosis is usually diagnosed early, few infants are seen in advanced stages of dehydration, malnutrition, and alkalosis. If present, these conditions must be corrected before surgery. An infant who is slightly dehydrated with a total serum or plasma carbon dioxide (CO_2) level of 25 mEq/L or less, or an infant who is moderately dehydrated with a CO_2 of 26 to 35 mEq/L is managed with replacement IV fluids and electrolytes, and an NG tube for stomach decompression. Once the stomach is empty, most infants will stop vomiting. Surgery is usually delayed 24 to 48 hours until fluid and electrolyte deficits and the acid-base imbalances are corrected. Severely dehydrated and malnourished infants with CO_2 levels above 35 mEq/L may need a 3- to 5-day course of IV fluids, electrolyte replacement, and infusions of plasma or packed red blood cells (RBCs) before surgical repair.

A pyloromyotomy, an incision of the pyloric muscle to release the obstruction, is the definitive treatment. Pyloromyotomy is not considered an emergency procedure but is usually performed without delay in well-hydrated infants. The surgery is performed laparoscopically.

! NURSING QUALITY ALERT

Gathering Information from a Parent about Infant Vomiting

Eliciting a description of the amount and characteristics of vomiting can be difficult because descriptive terms are nonspecific and estimation of emesis amounts is very inconsistent. Useful questions include the following:

- Could you wipe the vomitus off the child with a diaper or cloth?
- Did it require a change of clothes for the infant or caregiver?
- If it was on a bed or sheet, how big a circle did it make?
- If it was on the floor, how big a circle did it make?
- Did it happen after every feeding?
- Did it look like what was just eaten, or was it curdled?
- What color was it?
- Did it appear to be under force and projected away from the child?

Encouraging the parents to keep a written record of answers to these questions can provide essential assessment information.

NURSING CARE OF THE CHILD WITH HYPERTROPHIC PYLORIC STENOSIS

■ Assessment

Hypertrophic pyloric stenosis is suspected in infants with a history of *projectile vomiting*, especially after meals. A thorough nursing history includes the infant's feeding schedule with the type, amount, and frequency of fluid taken. Determine and document the relation of feedings to vomiting. Vomiting is assessed for frequency, amount, color, and consistency, as well as projection.

Assess for signs of dehydration, such as the absence of tears, a weak cry, a depressed fontanel, poor skin turgor, and dry mucous membranes. Signs of potassium, sodium, and chloride depletion should be noted. The abdomen is checked for distention, tenderness, bowel sounds, the presence of a pyloric mass, and gastric peristaltic waves. Family members are evaluated for their understanding of the disorder, a viable support system, and the ability to participate in their child's care.

■ Nursing Diagnosis and Planning

The following nursing diagnoses and expected outcomes are appropriate after assessment of the child with hypertrophic pyloric stenosis:

- Deficient Fluid Volume related to vomiting.

Expected Outcomes. The infant will have a balanced intake and output, be free of signs of dehydration, and have a urine output greater than 2 to 3 mL/kg/hr.

- Imbalanced Nutrition: Less Than Body Requirements related to persistent vomiting.

Expected Outcomes. The infant will tolerate regular feedings and will continue to show growth according to a growth chart.

- Impaired Skin Integrity and Risk for Infection related to surgical incisions.

Expected Outcome. The infant will have clean, dry, intact incisions without redness or exudate.

- Deficient Knowledge related to insufficient information about the need for surgery or about pyloric stenosis.

Expected Outcomes. The parents will describe pyloric stenosis and the expected preoperative and postoperative care. Parents will assume total care of the infant before discharge.

- Acute Pain related to surgery.

Expected Outcomes. The child will not exhibit guarding to palpation and will be calm and content in parent's arms. The parent will be confident that the infant is pain free.

- Anxiety (parental) related to need for hospitalization and surgery.

Expected Outcomes. The parent will express feelings about the surgery and will list the reasons the infant needs to be hospitalized.

■ Interventions

■ Preoperative Care. Preoperatively, the infant is on NPO status and is stabilized with IV fluids and electrolytes. Measuring the vital signs, weighing the infant daily, and monitoring laboratory values and intake and output are essential nursing interventions. Intake and output should include all IV and PO fluids, blood products, emesis, urine output, stools, and NG drainage. The dehydrated infant is kept warm and quiet. The nurse should provide oral care because membranes are more susceptible to breakdown in their dehydrated state.

The head of the bed is elevated to reduce the risk of aspiration and blankets or towel rolls are used to maintain desired position. The NG tube should be patent and properly positioned. The nurse records the amount, color, and type of drainage. Frequent assessment for respiratory distress is performed.

The nurse explains procedures and plans to parents. Parents are encouraged to participate by holding and caring for their infant.

■ Postoperative Care. Postoperatively, the care can vary according to the individual preferences of the surgeon. Most surgeons remove the NG tube immediately and order feedings within the first 4 to 6 hours after surgery if bowel sounds are present. Because gastric peristalsis is normally depressed for 12 to 18 hours after the pyloromyotomy, other surgeons delay feedings for 24 hours and leave the NG tube in place.

Feeding is started with small amounts of an oral electrolyte solution, such as Pedialyte, and the amount is slowly increased. Formula is offered in half-strength concentrations and advanced to full strength within 48 hours after surgery. If the child is receiving breast milk, dilution is not necessary. Feedings are not advanced until the child can tolerate the previous amount without vomiting. IV fluids are continued until the infant is taking and retaining sufficient amounts of formula or breast milk. Many infants have some vomiting during the early postoperative period, but it is usually temporary and without complications. Ad lib feedings within 6 hours postoperatively are now being recommended to decrease time to full diet and discharge, but these protocols vary by institution (Askew, 2010).

Postoperative nursing care follows the same guidelines as preoperative care, with accurate monitoring of all vital signs, laboratory values, respiratory status, and hydration. In addition, the nurse assesses the small surgical or laparoscopic incisions for redness, swelling, or drainage. Parents participate as much as possible in their infant's care, however, they may need educational and emotional support from the nurse in the unfamiliar environment of the hospital.

■ **Home Care.** Because symptoms normally abate in the immediate postoperative period, parents may find taking care of their infant much easier than before surgery. They need to be instructed, however, to report any excessive vomiting, abdominal tenderness, fever, and incisional redness and drainage. If the child is discharged before the diet has been advanced to full strength, written instructions for advancing the diet are essential.

■ Evaluation

- Does the child have a flat fontanel, good skin turgor, moist mucous membranes, a urine specific gravity of less than 1.030, and a sodium level within normal limits?
- Is the child tolerating oral feedings without vomiting?
- Has the child's weight returned to preillness level within 1 week?
- Is the surgical site clean, dry, intact, and without drainage or redness?
- Can the parents explain the need for surgery and routine preoperative and postoperative care?
- Is the child calm, content, and free from pain?
- Have the parents assumed all care responsibilities at home without assistance?

Intussusception

Intussusception is an invagination of a section of the intestine into the distal bowel that causes bowel obstruction. In children, this condition most often occurs as a section of terminal ileum telescopes into the ascending colon through the ileocecal valve. It is the most common cause of intestinal obstruction in children between the ages of 3 months and 6 years (Kennedy & Liacouras, 2011). Although relatively rare, it is a pediatric emergency with classic assessment findings.

Animation—Intussusception

PATHOPHYSIOLOGY

Intussusception

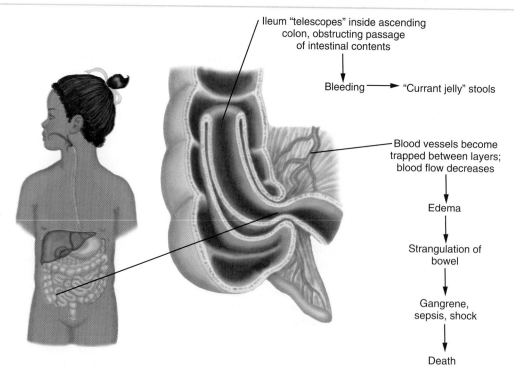

Ileum "telescopes" inside ascending colon, obstructing passage of intestinal contents

Bleeding ⟶ "Currant jelly" stools

Blood vessels become trapped between layers; blood flow decreases

Edema

Strangulation of bowel

Gangrene, sepsis, shock

Death

As the bowel telescopes inside itself, obstruction develops. In addition, the mesenteric vessels become trapped between the walls of the two layers, and ischemia occurs. This pressure on the bowel leads to bleeding and "currant jelly" stools. Mesenteric ischemia also causes edema and possible strangulation or infarction of the bowel, which can progress to perforation, peritonitis, sepsis, shock, and death.

Etiology and Incidence

In young children, the cause of intussusception is unknown. Contributing factors include a preexisting upper respiratory tract infection or other viral infection. A pathologic condition within the colon, such as a mass or an anatomic defect, is the most likely cause in children older than 6 years.

Intussusception generally affects infants and young children, with 80% of cases occurring before age 2 years and rarely before age 3 months. This incidence is 1 to 4 per 1000 births and it is more commonly seen in boys than girls (ratio is 3 : 1). Children with cystic fibrosis are at increased risk for intussusception (Kennedy & Liacouras, 2011).

Manifestations and Diagnostic Evaluation

Intussusception occurs in children who are well nourished and without a history of GI problems. Paroxysms of pain occur, subside, and recur during the first several hours and then progress to a more constant severe pain. The child may vomit. The following are classic signs of intussusception:

- Passage of bloody mucus ("currant jelly") stool and diarrhea, which may not occur until the postoperative period
- A sausage-shaped abdominal mass

Symptoms of shock and sepsis are present if obstruction has been present for longer than 12 to 24 hours. The child may be listless. Older children may have pain without other symptoms.

Abdominal radiographs may show abnormal gas patterns related to the bowel obstruction or a soft tissue mass. Ultrasonography is useful in identifying the location of the intussusception and the amount of edema in the area. A definitive diagnosis can be made and treatment provided simultaneously with a barium enema or air enema examination.

Therapeutic Management

The goal of treatment is to restore the bowel to its normal position and function as quickly as possible and preferably within the first 24 hours of the appearance of symptoms. In children who do not show symptoms of shock or sepsis, hydrostatic reduction is performed with a barium, isotonic saline, or air enema under fluoroscopic or ultrasonic guidance, with a 80% to 95% success rate (Kennedy & Liacouras, 2011). If reduction fails or findings indicate damage to the bowel, immediate surgery is performed. If the intussusception is detected and reduced within 24 hours, morbidity is minimal. Laparoscopy is now being used if the enema fails to reduce the intussusception except where bowel necrosis is present. There is a 10% recurrence rate after hydrostatic reduction and a 2% to 5% recurrence rate after reduction surgery (Kennedy & Liacouras, 2011).

NURSING CARE OF THE CHILD WITH INTUSSUSCEPTION

▪ Assessment

The nursing history typically reveals a previously healthy infant who suddenly began crying and flexing the legs in severe pain. This problem may resolve, only to recur a short time later and become more constant. The nurse should assess any child for a bowel obstruction with signs of vomiting, nausea, abdominal distention, and hypoactive or hyperactive bowel sounds. A palpable abdominal mass and passage of "currant jelly" stools will help confirm the diagnosis. The child's hydration status is assessed on admission. Fever, an increased heart rate, changes in level of consciousness or blood pressure, and respiratory distress should be reported immediately as they can indicate sepsis or peritonitis.

▪ Nursing Diagnosis and Planning

The following nursing diagnoses and expected outcomes may be appropriate for the child with intussusception and the child's family:

- Risk for Ineffective Tissue Perfusion (GI) related to bowel compression.

Expected Outcome. The child will have a patent bowel, as evidenced by the passage of soft, formed, Hematest-negative stools.

- Acute Pain related to bowel obstruction and surgery.

Expected Outcome. The child will be free from abdominal pain, as evidenced by age-appropriate play and activity, and no guarding during palpation.

- Deficient Fluid Volume related to vomiting and diarrhea.

Expected Outcomes. The child will be able to tolerate age-appropriate food and fluids without vomiting or recurrence of symptoms and will be free from fluid and electrolyte disturbances, as evidenced by return to normal weight, moist mucous membranes, good skin turgor, and normal serum sodium level and hematocrit.

- Deficient Knowledge related to possibility of surgery and the need for immediate intervention.

Expected Outcomes. The parents will verbalize an understanding of the need for immediate intervention and will explain the mechanisms of intussusception and hydrostatic reduction.

- Anxiety (parental) related to the child's hospitalization or possible surgery.

Expected Outcomes. The parents will express concerns and fears and will seek appropriate support as needed.

- Disturbed Sleep Pattern related to colicky abdominal pain.

Expected Outcome. The child will return to normal sleep patterns.

▪ Interventions

▪ **Initial Care.** Once the diagnosis is made, immediate plans are made to admit the child to the hospital for hydrostatic reduction. Prompt assessment for dehydration, shock, and sepsis is essential, including documenting mental status, capillary perfusion, and urine output. The child is given IV fluids, and an NG tube is inserted if distention is present. During reduction, pain medications or sedation may be needed to decrease spasm. After reduction, clear liquids are started and the diet is advanced gradually as tolerated.

▪ **Postreduction Care.** The nurse observes for the passage of barium, and notes the characteristics of the stool. The child is assessed for symptoms of bowel obstruction indicating a recurrence of intussusception. Resumption of a normal diet and activities, and the passage of stool without blood indicate a successful outcome. If hydrostatic reduction is unsuccessful, the child must be prepared for abdominal surgery or laparoscopy. Since intussusception can resolve spontaneously in some cases, the nurse continues to monitor the child for return of normal bowel function, eliminating the need for surgery.

Postoperatively, the child is kept on NPO status until bowel function returns. Intermittent NG suction, IV therapy, pain medications, maintenance of respiratory function, frequent assessment, and meeting developmental needs remain nursing responsibilities.

▪ **Family Education and Support.** During this difficult time for parents, relieving their anxiety by providing appropriate information is an essential nursing action. This includes describing the pathophysiology of intussusception, the process for hydrostatic reduction, and the expected recovery care for their child, including IV fluids, intermittent NG suction, and frequent vital sign checks and assessments. In addition, emotional support can be provided to the parents by encouraging participation in their child's care, listening to their concerns, and encouraging expression of their feelings during this stressful time.

To help parents visualize telescoping of the bowel with intussusception, the nurse can use a hospital glove, pressing one finger (representing the terminal ileum) into the inflated glove (the distal colon) and causing it to go inside itself. The same approach can show how hydrostatic reduction works. The nurse presses on the glove (the distal portion) with one hand, showing how the telescoped portion is pushed back into its normal position.

■ **Evaluation**

• In the preoperative period, does the child have moist mucous membranes, good skin turgor, and a urine specific gravity of less than 1.030?
• Is the child passing soft, formed, Hematest-negative stools?
• Does the infant guard the abdomen during palpation?
• Is the child demonstrating age-appropriate activity levels, sleep patterns, and play?
• Is the child tolerating age-appropriate food and fluids without vomiting or recurrence of symptoms?
• Can the parents explain the rationale for hydrostatic reduction?

• Are all the parents' questions answered to their satisfaction?
• Are the parents able to resume care of their infant without stress or anxiety?

Volvulus

Volvulus is a condition caused by a malrotation or twisting of the bowel that results in a bowel obstruction. It is the result of a defect in fetal development; the midgut, which normally rotates 270 degrees around the superior mesenteric artery, fails to rotate and fixes itself to the abdominal wall.

Affected infants usually manifest pain, bilious vomiting, and other signs of bowel obstruction. Surgery is essential to prevent bowel ischemia. The nursing care is similar to that for the child with intussusception who requires surgical treatment.

Hirschsprung Disease

Also known as congenital aganglionosis or megacolon, Hirschsprung disease is the result of an absence of ganglion cells in the rectum and, to varying degrees, upward in the colon. Hirschsprung disease is the major cause of lower bowel obstruction in newborns (Fiorino & Liacouras, 2011).

Animations—Volvulus and Volvulus, Pediatric

PATHOPHYSIOLOGY
Hirschsprung Disease

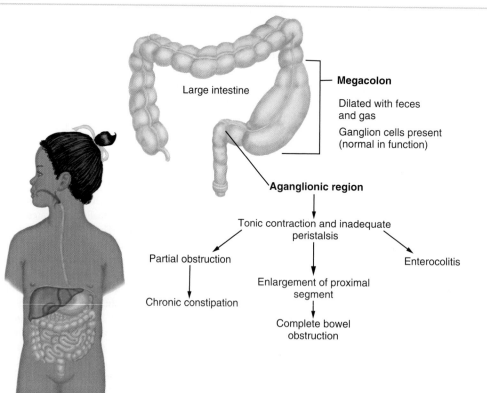

Ganglia provide parasympathetic innervation of the colon. In Hirschsprung disease, ganglia are absent from a variable length of colon extending proximally from the anus. Adequate peristalsis cannot occur in the affected colon, leading to a tonic contraction of the lumen. This produces a functional bowel obstruction, chronic constipation, and the passage of ribbon-like stools. It can lead to a complete bowel obstruction. Because of the constriction of the lumen, huge amounts of feces and gas collect proximal to the aganglionic portion, resulting in a gross enlargement of this segment (megacolon). The enlarged segment of colon is actually normal in its function.

Etiology and Incidence

The disease is a result of embryonic failure of migration of the hindgut ganglion cells to the most caudal portion of the GI tract, the rectum. The initiating factor in this failure is unknown.

Hirschsprung disease occurs in 1 in 5000 live births, with a 4 : 1 male to female ratio (Fiorino & Liacouras, 2011). It has a strong hereditary component and a higher incidence in children with Down syndrome.

Manifestations and Diagnostic Evaluation

Delayed passage or absence of meconium stool in the neonatal period is the cardinal sign of Hirschsprung disease. Any child who does not pass meconium within the first 24 hours and who is prone to constipation or stool infrequency in the first month after birth is suspected of having Hirschsprung disease. The neonate, infant, or older child may exhibit signs of bowel obstruction, abdominal pain and distention, vomiting, and failure to thrive. Chronic constipation beginning in the first month of life results in pellet-like or ribbon-like stools that are foul smelling.

A rectal examination reveals a tight internal sphincter and the absence of stool, followed by an often explosive release of gas and feces related to the sudden but transient increase in rectal size. Barium enema examination demonstrates an abrupt change in the size of the colon from a distended ganglionic proximal portion to the contracted, narrowed appearance in the aganglionic distal portion, with a transitional zone of tapered bowel between them (Mattei, 2008). Significantly, the child will not evacuate barium after the examination. The definitive diagnosis is made by suction rectal biopsy. During biopsy, a small core or punch sample that contains all layers of the bowel mucosa is removed. Absence of ganglionic cells in the sample confirms the diagnosis of Hirschsprung disease. Some children may require a full-thickness biopsy performed under anesthesia by a surgeon. Anal rectal manometry (ARM) is helpful in the diagnosis of ultrashort-segment Hirschsprung disease, also known as anal achalasia. This is a test in which a catheter with a balloon is inserted into the rectum to test the nerves and sphincter pressure of the anus. Children with Hirschsprung disease will have a nonrelaxing internal anal sphincter.

Therapeutic Management

Hirschsprung disease can involve the entire colon (total colonic Hirschsprung), a very short segment of the colon, or any amount in between. Treatment involves removing the aganglionic portion of the intestine in a one- or two-step surgical intervention. A one-step laparoscopic or transanal pull-through procedure is being used successfully with increasing frequency (Mattei, 2008). For neonates, a two-step surgical procedure is often used. First, to relieve the obstruction, a temporary colostomy is performed with the most distal section of normal bowel. Once the infant weighs 8 to 10 kg (18 to 22 lb), the final step, a pull-through procedure, is performed. All aganglionic portions of the bowel are excised, the normal bowel is reattached to the anal canal, and the colostomy is closed. Normal bowel function usually returns shortly after surgery. For children diagnosed after infancy, the type of surgical procedure and the time period between the steps of the pull-through procedure may vary. Medical interventions such as botulinum toxin (Botox) injections to the internal anal sphincter (IAS) muscle are used to decrease the resting IAS pressures. Rectal irrigations to remove air and stool, may be needed to relieve symptoms associated with entercolitis prior to surgery.

■ Assessment

The child with Hirschsprung disease will have constipation that has been present since the neonatal period and frequent passage of foul-smelling pellet-type and ribbon-like stools. Nutritional status should be assessed because malnutrition can develop as a result of extreme distention or enterocolitis. Thin extremities, abdominal distention, and a history of poor feeding should be noted.

If the child is acutely ill on presentation, enterocolitis must be suspected and reported immediately as this is a life-threatening complication. The nurse documents the assessment of bowel sounds and abdominal distention, the frequency of vomiting and diarrhea, and changes in abdominal circumference. Temperature readings must be obtained by a route other than rectal.

Family concerns and coping methods are assessed. This disease can drain family and financial resources during the diagnosis and surgical treatment. Mild disease may not be diagnosed until the child is older and appears as chronic constipation. Assessing the older child's feelings about chronic constipation and its treatment is important.

■ Nursing Diagnoses and Planning

The following nursing diagnoses and expected outcomes may be appropriate for the child with Hirschsprung disease:

- Constipation related to aganglionic bowel and inadequate peristalsis.

Expected Outcome. The child will pass soft, formed stools without retention.

- Risk for Deficient Fluid Volume or Excess Fluid Volume related to surgical preparation.

Expected Outcome. The child will be free from fluid or electrolyte disturbances related to presurgical bowel cleansing.

- Impaired Skin Integrity related to colostomy and surgical repair.

Expected Outcomes. The surgical and colostomy sites will be clean and free from exudate, redness, or drainage. The colostomy site will be intact without bleeding or skin irritation.

- Risk for Infection related to surgical repair.

Expected Outcome. The child will be afebrile without signs of infection at the site.

- Imbalanced Nutrition: Less Than Body Requirements related to GI surgery.

Expected Outcomes. The child will have normal bowel sounds, will pass stool, and will tolerate a regular diet.

- Acute Pain related to surgical incisions.

Expected Outcomes. The child will be free from pain and will be able to participate in usual activities of daily living.

- Deficient Knowledge related to incomplete information about the need for surgery, irrigation, or care of the ostomy.

Expected Outcomes. The parents will state the necessity for rectal irrigations or surgical intervention. The parents and child will assume responsibility for care of the ostomy and rectal irrigations, if indicated.

- Disturbed Body Image related to colostomy and irrigations.

Expected Outcomes. The child and family will express feelings about irrigations, ostomy care, and the impact the condition has had on the child's body image.

- Anxiety (parental and child) related to the loss of the perfect child or need for surgery.

Expected Outcomes. The parents and child will express fears and concerns and seek support as needed.

■ Interventions

■ **Preparing the Child for Surgery.** The nurse closely monitors and records the child's bowel elimination pattern. Isotonic saline enemas are administered preoperatively until the return is clear (see Chapter 13). An alternative bowel cleansing regimen is to administer a polyethylene glycol–electrolyte lavage solution (GoLYTELY) orally or through the NG tube. This regimen is used only in children older than 5 years and is given at a dosage of 25 to 40 mL/kg/hr. Sodium phosphate (Fleets Phosphosoda) is another alternative requiring ingestion of only approximately 200 mL at one time for children older than 5 years. After bowel cleansing, keep the child on NPO status until surgery. IV fluids are provided as needed and strict intake and output records are maintained.

■ **Preventing Infection and Maintaining Skin Integrity.** Neomycin 1.0% solution given by rectum or stoma is administered preoperatively to sterilize the bowel for surgery. IV antibiotics also contribute to bowel sterilization as well as prevention of surgical incision site infection. The nurse monitors vital signs regularly and measures the child's abdominal circumference each time. Tympanic, temporal, oral, or axillary methods for taking the temperature are used avoiding trauma to the rectal mucosa. The surgical site is checked for redness, swelling, and purulent drainage.

If the child has a colostomy, the stoma site is inspected for bleeding and impaired skin integrity. After the pull-through procedure, the nurse observes the anal site carefully for redness, discharge, and the presence of stool. To prevent skin breakdown, meticulous skin care of abdomen and perineum, is provided. Dressing changes are performed to keep incisions clean and dry. Ostomy sites are cared for by using appropriate-size, hypoallergenic ostomy supplies and appliances. The nurse encourages the parents and child to begin ostomy care as soon as possible.

■ **Maintaining Nutritional and Hydration Status.** Postoperatively, the child is on NPO status until bowel sounds return or the child passes flatus. The NG tube is set to intermittent suction until peristalsis returns. The nurse monitors the child for signs of dehydration and acid-base disturbances. To prevent dehydration, the child remains on IV fluids until tolerating oral fluids well. Then, the diet is advanced from clear liquids to a regular diet as ordered.

■ **Reducing Pain.** Pain medications are administered as ordered along with other complementary interventions to provide effective pain management. Most school-age children can use patient-controlled analgesia (PCA) for effective pain control (see Chapter 15). The nurse encourages the use of nonpharmacologic pain control measures such as repositioning, back rubs, music, holding, rocking, massage, and quiet talking. If pain control is not achieved as anticipated, the child must be assessed for complications such as a bowel obstruction or an infection.

■ **Providing Education and Relieving Anxiety.** Before the time of scheduled surgery, the parents may need to manage rectal irrigations at home. The parents must learn the procedure and observe for distention and signs of obstruction. Parents are prompted to express any concerns they may have about the need for irrigations or their ability to perform them. The nurse teaches the parents and child about the surgery and recovery process. If the child is to have a colostomy, the child and parents are given the opportunity to see and manipulate the equipment before surgery.

Postoperatively, preschoolers and young school-age children are encouraged to draw pictures, use dolls, and engage in play to express concerns about body appearance, irrigations, and the colostomy. The nurse provides time for the child and family to share their fears, concerns, and questions; active listening is a critical nursing intervention. Colostomy care is taught in the immediate postoperative period, so the parents can participate in the child's care with assistance by the nurse. For the older child, self-care of the colostomy is initiated as soon as possible. Referral to an enterostomal therapist is recommended. The nurse also can refer the family to support groups for children with ostomies and other community resources (see Evolve website).

■ Evaluation

- Does the child pass soft, formed stools without retention after completion of the surgical correction?
- Has the child tolerated the bowel cleansing regimen without signs of fluid and electrolyte imbalance, as evidenced by moist mucous membranes, good skin turgor, and an hourly urine output appropriate for age?
- Is the child afebrile, and are surgical sites free from redness, purulent drainage, excess heat, and dehiscence?
- Is the colostomy or anal pull-through area free from bleeding and skin breakdown?
- Are bowel sounds active and present in all four quadrants, and is the child tolerating an age-appropriate diet without vomiting or diarrhea?
- Does the child appear to be free of pain, as evidenced by the ability to sleep comfortably and participate in appropriate play activities when awake?
- Can the parents and child demonstrate all procedures needed for appropriate home care?
- Is the child able to express feelings about body changes related to treatments or procedures?
- Are the parents calm and able to resume all care of their child without anxiety?

MALABSORPTION DISORDERS

Lactose Intolerance

An inability to tolerate lactose, the sugar found in dairy products, is the result of an absence or deficiency of lactase, an enzyme found in the secretions of the small intestines that is required for the digestion of lactose. The two types of lactose intolerance are congenital and developmental. Congenital lactose intolerance, which is rare, appears at birth, with a complete absence of lactase. Developmental lactose intolerance is a deficiency of lactase that appears in early to late childhood.

Etiology and Incidence

Most cases of lactose intolerance are the result of inadequate levels of lactase. The exact reason for this deficiency is unknown. The condition is likely to be more severe during and after other illnesses affecting the GI mucosa, such as viral gastroenteritis or food poisoning.

The condition appears to have an ethnic association, with a 50% to 90% incidence in Asians, American Indians, Arabs, Jews, African-Americans, and southern Europeans (National Digestive Diseases Information Clearinghouse, 2009).

Manifestations and Diagnostic Evaluation

Manifestations of lactose intolerance include diarrhea that is frothy but not fatty, abdominal distention, cramping abdominal pain, and excessive flatus. The symptoms are not usually seen until lactase activity begins to decrease after age 3 years or during other GI illnesses. If the child has congenital lactose intolerance, symptoms will be seen immediately and may be severe.

A history of improvement after a lactose-free diet has been implemented provides a presumptive diagnosis. A finding of 1+ or higher on the Clinitest stool test (0 to 4+ range) can indicate intestinal malabsorption of sugar. Lactose tolerance testing (breath hydrogen test) involves giving the patient an oral lactose load and then measuring blood glucose levels and the amount of hydrogen in breath samples. Lower than expected blood sugar levels and elevated levels of hydrogen content in breath samples point to poor absorption of lactose in the small intestines.

Therapeutic Management

The treatment for lactose intolerance is removal of lactose from the diet. In most cases, total elimination is unnecessary. Removing milk as the beverage of choice can provide enough relief from symptoms. Additional dietary changes may be necessary to provide adequate sources of calcium and, in the infant, protein and calories. Formulas that do not contain lactose (Isomil, Nursoy, Nutramigen, Prosobee, and other soy-based formulas) may be given to the infant suspected of having lactose intolerance. Breastfeeding mothers are urged to eliminate lactose products from their diet.

PATHOPHYSIOLOGY

Lactose Intolerance

An absence or a deficiency of lactase leads to inability to digest lactose and the subsequent accumulation of lactose in the lumen of the small intestines. This causes water to be drawn into the colon, resulting in watery osmotic diarrhea containing undigested lactose. In addition, GI bacteria break down lactose and release hydrogen, which causes excess gas production, bloating, and abdominal pain.

These dietary changes can be supplemented with the use of commercial lactase preparations (Lactaid, Dairy Ease, Lac-Dose) that can be taken with lactose-containing food to provide adequate lactase levels and variable relief from symptoms.

NURSING CARE OF THE CHILD WITH LACTOSE INTOLERANCE

■ Assessment

Assessment will reveal a healthy-looking child with episodic abdominal pain and occasional diarrhea without any nutritional deficiencies or other health problems. The child and family may or may not be able to correlate symptoms with food intake. With a congenital absence of lactase, the condition is likely to be more severe and diarrhea is a major concern. The neonate or infant may be extremely dehydrated, with severe diarrhea and weight loss.

■ Nursing Diagnosis and Planning

The following nursing diagnoses and expected outcomes may be appropriate for the infant or child with lactose intolerance:
- Acute Pain related to bloating and flatus.

Expected Outcomes. The child will be free from abdominal pain, as evidenced by developmentally appropriate play and activity. The child will have normal bowel sounds with a soft abdomen that is not painful during palpation.
- Diarrhea related to maldigestion.

Expected Outcome. The child will have soft, formed stools.
- Deficient Knowledge related to incomplete understanding about needed dietary changes.

Expected Outcomes. The child will take in a minimum of 800 mg of calcium per day, as reported in the dietary history. The child and family will state foods to be avoided or provided in small amounts. The child will receive adequate calcium sources in diet and appropriate lactase products.

■ Interventions

The principal nursing intervention is teaching. Symptoms are often relieved after a lactose-free diet is followed for a short period. Foods containing small amounts of lactose may then be added gradually to assess the child's reaction. If small amounts of milk are tolerated, food or lactase preparations are given simultaneously with milk. These simple changes can offer instant relief.

After diagnosis and initial management, this condition is often perceived to be only a minor nuisance. Emotional support for the family, however, may be needed. Referring the family to self-help and information groups and encouraging family members to share successes and concerns are important nursing interventions.

■ Evaluation

- Is the child happy, content, and free of excess gas and bloating?
- Can the parent state what foods are essential to avoid?
- Are the child's stools normal and formed?
- Does the food diary indicate an intake of at least 800 mg of calcium daily for a child age 1 to 10 years?
- Does the parent express satisfaction with control of the child's condition?

PATIENT-CENTERED TEACHING

Care of the Child with Lactose Intolerance

- Your child must avoid all high-lactose foods (e.g., milk, ice cream). If you are unsure about whether a food contains lactose, examine labels for presence of milk or milk products.
- You can use soy-based, lactose-free formulas as needed for your infant (Isomil, Nursoy, Nutramigen, Prosobee). If you are breastfeeding, limit your own intake of dairy products.
- Soy-based beverages (Silk) are available in most grocery stores.
- You or your older child can obtain calcium through other foods besides milk. They include egg yolks, green leafy vegetables, dried beans, cauliflower, and molasses. Calcium supplements are also available.
- Once your child's symptoms have disappeared, you can gradually add yogurt, hard cheeses, and small amounts of milk to assess tolerance.
- If you are having difficulty determining what foods are lactose free or need help finding recipes that use lactose-free foods, ask for a dietary consultation.

Celiac Disease

Celiac disease, also known as gluten enteropathy or tropical sprue, results from the inability to digest gluten. *Gluten* is a general term that refers to the storage proteins found in wheat, barley, and rye. This is a lifelong deficiency requiring dietary modification to prevent chronic maldigestion and malabsorption.

Etiology and Incidence

The etiology of celiac disease (CD) is not fully understood, but it is considered to be an autoimmune disease that occurs in genetically susceptible patients (Tully, 2008). Patients with celiac disease have been found to carry either the *HLA-DQ2* or *HLA-DQ8* genes. However, there are also many people who carry one of these genes who do not develop CD despite recurrent gluten exposure. This suggests that the etiology of CD is multifactorial including both environmental and genetic factors (Silano, Agostoni, & Guandalini, 2010). Delaying the introduction of gluten into the infant's diet and breastfeeding before and during that introduction can delay the appearance of symptoms in at-risk individuals (Radlovic, Mladenovic, Lekovic et al., 2010; Silano et al., 2010).

The incidence of celiac disease varies in different regions. In the United States the incidence is approximately 1 in 1000 live births. The incidence is much higher in Europe. Siblings and children of affected individuals are at highest risk for the disease (Bardella, Elli, Velio et al., 2007).

Manifestations

The major manifestations in the child with celiac disease include diarrhea and growth failure. The child's growth usually is below the 25th percentile on growth charts.

The child may also have abdominal distention, vomiting, anemia, irritability, anorexia, muscle wasting, edema, and folate deficiency. Symptoms are not seen until 3 to 6 months after the introduction of grains to the diet, usually at age 9 to 12 months. The child in celiac crisis exhibits profuse, watery diarrhea and vomiting.

Diagnostic Evaluation

The immunoglobulin A (IgA) antitissue transglutaminase (tTG) antibody test or the IgA antiendomyseal antibody test has replaced antigliadin antibody testing in children with celiac disease. If children have a demonstrated IgA deficiency, the IgG antitissue transglutaminase test is used (Hoffenberg, Utterson, & Hoffenberg, 2008). Jejunal biopsy will unequivocally identify ulcerations in the GI tract. Monitoring the reaction to a gluten-free diet supports the diagnosis. Symptoms are often relieved in 1 week by removal of gluten from the diet.

Further diagnostic testing may include the breath hydrogen test to identify the amount of carbohydrate malabsorption occurring. This test is not specific for CD. D-Xylose testing indicates the amount of

PATHOPHYSIOLOGY

Celiac Disease

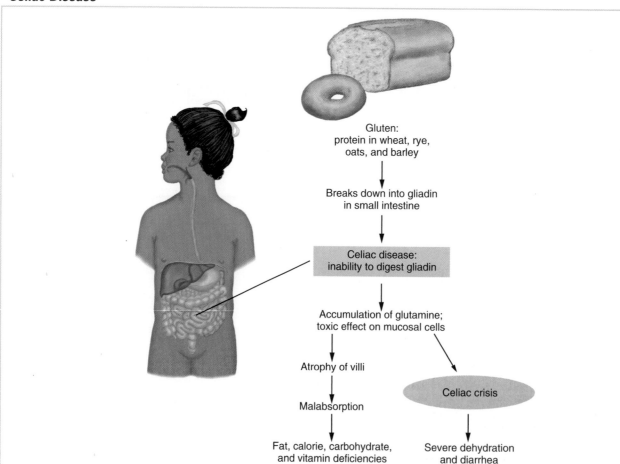

Gluten: protein in wheat, rye, oats, and barley

↓

Breaks down into gliadin in small intestine

↓

Celiac disease: inability to digest gliadin

↓

Accumulation of glutamine; toxic effect on mucosal cells

↓   ↓

Atrophy of villi   Celiac crisis

↓   ↓

Malabsorption   Severe dehydration and diarrhea

↓

Fat, calorie, carbohydrate, and vitamin deficiencies

Gluten—the protein found in rye, oats, barley, and wheat—breaks down into gliadin and other byproducts. Celiac disease results from an inability to digest gliadin. This results in the accumulation of glutamine in the intestine, which has a toxic effect on the mucosal cells. This leads to atrophy of the villi and a marked decrease in the absorptive surface. Malabsorption of fats, carbohydrates, and vitamins develops. Celiac crisis is a result of sudden accumulation of glutamine and the subsequent destruction of the mucosal cells, causing severe diarrhea and dehydration.

mucosal damage, allowing the remaining absorptive surface to be estimated.

Therapeutic Management

Dietary management is the mainstay of treatment. All wheat, rye, barley, and oats should be eliminated from the diet and replaced with corn and rice. To correct deficiencies, vitamin supplements, especially with fat-soluble vitamins and folate, may be needed in the early period of treatment.

Dietary restrictions are likely to be lifelong, although small amounts of grains may be tolerated after the ulcerations have healed. Adolescents have difficulty maintaining a gluten-free diet without having an unbalanced diet high in protein and fat. An adolescent on a strict gluten-free diet still has a risk for dietary imbalance; supplements and support from dietary services are essential for maintenance.

Occasionally the nurse is the first to see a child in celiac crisis. Celiac crisis causes profuse, watery diarrhea and vomiting, which can quickly lead to severe dehydration and metabolic acidosis. The cause of the crisis, usually an infection or a hidden source of gluten, must be identified. The child is given IV fluids to correct fluid, electrolyte, and acid-base imbalances, albumin to treat shock, and corticosteroids to decrease severe mucosal inflammation.

NURSING CARE OF THE CHILD WITH CELIAC DISEASE

▪ Assessment

Assessment of the infant with celiac disease usually reveals an irritable, malnourished infant who exhibits failure to thrive by 9 to 12 months. Any child with diarrhea, especially one with foul-smelling, fatty stools and significant growth delays, should be suspected of having CD. A noticeable decline in the child's rate of growth as charted on the growth curve, associated with the addition of grains to the diet, is essential supportive evidence.

Abdominal assessment reveals distention and ascites with an increasing girth. Observations by the nurse may identify other signs of malnutrition, such as thin, edematous extremities, pallor, and muscle wasting. Anemia is a common finding.

The child with severe diarrhea, foul-smelling stools, vomiting, poor perfusion, edema, or changes in vital signs (shock or metabolic acidosis) should be referred for emergency care of celiac crisis.

▪ Nursing Diagnosis and Planning

The following nursing diagnoses and expected outcomes may be appropriate for the infant or child with celiac disease:

- Imbalanced Nutrition: Less Than Body Requirements related to malabsorption.

Expected Outcome. The child will have soft, formed stools without diarrhea.

- Acute Pain or Chronic Pain related to abdominal distention.

Expected Outcome. The child will be free from abdominal pain, as evidenced by age-appropriate play and activity level.

- Delayed Growth and Development related to malnutrition.

Expected Outcome. The child will return to and follow a normal growth pattern according to a growth chart.

- Deficient Knowledge related to dietary changes.

Expected Outcomes. The family will offer appropriate foods to the infant or child, as evidenced by a food diary. The child and family will state the need for lifelong dietary changes and seek emotional and educational support as needed.

- Deficient Fluid Volume related to celiac crisis.

Expected Outcome. The child will be adequately hydrated, as evidenced by moist mucous membranes and good skin turgor.

▪ Interventions

The most significant nursing intervention is teaching parents and the child to modify the child's diet. Pain will likely be quickly relieved by eliminating gluten in the diet. Involvement of nutritionists in teaching and follow-up care is important. Careful and consistent monitoring will be necessary to ensure that the infant or child resumes normal growth and development. When the child has normal stools without diarrhea and resumes a normal growth pattern, teaching will have been effective.

PATIENT-CENTERED TEACHING

Care of the Child with Celiac Disease

- You must eliminate all wheat, rye, barley, oats, and hydrolyzed vegetable protein from your child's diet. This includes most pasta, baked products, and many breakfast cereals.
- You may be able to find gluten-free substitutes at specialized stores.
- You can substitute corn, rice, or millet as grains. These can be obtained as flour for baking.
- Your child should take vitamin supplements, especially folate and fat-soluble vitamins, because these vitamins will be hard to provide in your child's diet.
- You will need to read all labels on foods and medications carefully to avoid any unknown additives.
- When your child is old enough to understand, you will need to help your child make appropriate food choices. This can be difficult for an older child or adolescent because popular foods often contain ingredients that will make your child's condition worse. Encourage your child to talk with a nutritionist to plan a diet that is appropriate and not too different from the diet of peers.
- ⊖ Support groups are available to provide information and resources (see Evolve website).

⊖ Because celiac disease is a lifelong condition, support groups, camp programs, and other community resources can assist the child and family to manage the disease and sustain essential dietary modifications. The American Celiac Society is an excellent source of information and support (see Evolve website). The nurse should refer the family to this group and other support organizations. The child and parents are encouraged to share their fears and concerns about the chronic nature of the disease and its impact on the family as a unit as well as each family member's life.

▪ Evaluation

- Does the child have soft, formed stools without diarrhea or signs of dehydration?
- Is the child participating in age-appropriate activities?
- Has the child resumed a normal growth pattern according to a growth chart?
- Is the family able to verbalize an understanding of the child's dietary and emotional needs?
- Does a food diary indicate an intake of approximately 100 kcal/kg for the infant and for the child up to age 3 years?
- Do the parents use available support and education groups?
- Do the parents express satisfaction with the way they are coping with dietary changes?
- Does the child have good skin turgor, moist mucous membranes, and a urine output appropriate for age (see Chapter 16)?

HEPATIC DISORDERS

Viral Hepatitis

Hepatitis is an acute or chronic inflammation of the liver caused by several different viruses, toxins, and disease states. Although each type of hepatitis is unique, assessment findings and treatment have many similarities.

Etiology

The most common causes of viral hepatitis are hepatitis A, B, C, D, and E viruses (see Table 19-5). Children can also have hepatitis caused by rubella, cytomegalovirus (CMV), herpes simplex virus, and Epstein-Barr virus.

In children, hepatitis A virus (HAV) is highly contagious and spreads readily in households and daycare centers. Infection with hepatitis B virus (HBV) can be transmitted perinatally. The incidence of HBV infection transmitted by blood transfusions has decreased in recent years as a result of improved blood product screening procedures. Contaminated body fluids splashed into the mouth or eyes can produce HBV infection. HBV can survive in the dried state for 1 week or longer, thus percutaneous contact with contaminated objects can transmit infection.

Incidence

The incidence of acute hepatitis B infection in the United States has declined by approximately 82% since 1990 in all age-groups, with the greatest reduction of cases seen in children under 15 years of age (CDC, 2009). This is the direct result of the universal immunization of children against HBV, which began in 1991 (CDC, 2009). However, perinatal exposure to hepatitis B-positive mothers is still a significant cause of infection in young children (Yazigi & Balistreri, 2011). Acute hepatitis A incidence has decreased 92% since routine vaccination of children in the United States was recommended beginning in 1999 (CDC, 2009). Because the virus may be excreted for 2 to 3 weeks before the appearance of clinical signs and for 2 to 3 weeks afterward, outbreaks are common wherever good hand hygiene is not practiced.

TABLE 19-5   DIFFERENTIATION OF VIRAL HEPATITIS

TYPE/ETIOLOGY	TRANSMISSION	INCUBATION	CLINICAL MANIFESTATIONS	RECOVERY PROGNOSIS
Hepatitis A virus (HAV)	Person to person; fecal-oral route Ingestion of contaminated food or water	15-50 days (average, 28 days) Most contagious 1-2 wk before and 1 wk after symptoms	Jaundice, fever, fatigue, anorexia, nausea, vomiting, abdominal pain, dark urine, clay-colored stools, joint pain 70% of children under 6 yr are asymptomatic with no jaundice	Self-limited disease, rarely fatal No chronic carriers Recovery provides lifelong immunity
Hepatitis B virus (HBV)	Percutaneous or mucosal contact with infectious blood or body fluids (e.g., semen, saliva) via injection (drug abuse), sexual intercourse, needle sticks, blood transfusions, and birth	45-180 days (average, 90 days)	Same symptoms as HAV Severity from mild illness to severe, acute or chronic illness Most children <5 yr are asymptomatic; 30%-50% of children ≥5 yr have initial symptoms	Generally a full recovery Infected infants (90%) and children <5 yr (30%) will develop chronic carrier state 30%-90% of children <10 yr develop chronic hepatitis and are predisposed to cirrhosis and hepatocellular cancer
Hepatitis C virus (HCV)	Primarily by large or repeated percutaneous exposure to infectious blood via injection (drug abuse), blood transfusions, needle sticks, and birth	14-720 days (average, 30-360 days)	Same symptoms as HAV Most persons with chronic HCV infection are asymptomatic Treatment for children 3-17 yr is combination therapy with interferon and ribavirin	75%-85% progress to chronic infection; 60%-70% develop chronic liver disease Chronic HCV is leading indication for liver transplantation in the United States
Hepatitis D virus (HDV)	Percutaneous or mucosal contact with infectious blood or body fluids	30-60 days; coincides with HBV infection	Over half of children have chronic hepatitis Occurs only as co-infection with HBV, increasing severity of disease HBV vaccination reduces risk Uncommon in the United States	More likely to develop fulminating hepatitis than other strains
Hepatitis E virus (HEV)	Fecal-oral Ingestion of contaminated water	15-60 days (mean 40 days).	Same symptoms as HAV Outbreaks in countries with poor sanitation and contaminated water supply; rare in the United States	High incidence of mortality in pregnant women Children usually asymptomatic

Data from: Centers for Disease Control and Prevention (2009). *Viral hepatitis: For health professionals.* Retrieved from www.cdc.gov/hepatitis.

Manifestations

In infants and preschool-age children, HAV infection usually causes no symptoms or mild, nonspecific symptoms such as anorexia, malaise, and easy fatigability. In adults, the disease causes the more severe symptoms of nausea, jaundice, and malaise. Because most children with HAV infection have minimal to no symptoms, the disease may not be diagnosed until an outbreak of hepatitis occurs. Thus spread of HAV infection can occur before the initial case is identified.

PATHOPHYSIOLOGY

Viral Hepatitis

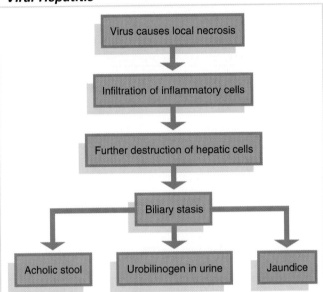

Hepatitis viruses cause necrosis of the parenchymal cells of the liver. The inflammatory response causes swelling and blockage of the drainage system in the liver. Biliary stasis and further destruction of the hepatic cells occur. Because the liver cannot excrete bile into the intestine, bile appears in the blood (causing hyperbilirubinemia), urine (as urobilinogen), and skin (causing hepatocellular jaundice).

Hepatitis infection may result in asymptomatic or mild illness, with complete regeneration of liver cells occurring within 2 to 3 months. More severe forms of hepatitis include fulminant hepatitis, in which hepatic necrosis and death can occur within 1 to 2 weeks and subacute or chronic hepatitis, which can result in permanent scarring of the liver and impaired liver function. Chronically infected individuals are carriers of the disease and are at increased risk for developing chronic liver disease (e.g., cirrhosis, chronic persistent hepatitis) or liver carcinoma later in life.

HBV infection may cause a wide range of clinical manifestations, from asymptomatic infection to acute fulminant hepatitis, which can be fatal. Symptomatic acute hepatitis occurs in two stages: the anicteric (without jaundice) phase and the icteric (jaundiced) phase.

During the anicteric phase, manifestations include anorexia, nausea and vomiting, right upper quadrant or epigastric pain, fever, malaise, fatigue, depression, and irritability. The anicteric phase lasts approximately 5 to 7 days. During the icteric phase, manifestations include jaundice, urticaria, dark urine, and light-colored stools. The child begins to feel better as jaundice becomes more apparent. Acute fulminating hepatitis is marked by bleeding abnormalities, encephalopathy, ascites, and acute hepatic failure. Fulminant hepatitis is caused primarily by HBV and HCV.

The symptoms and clinical changes should return to normal within 3 months of onset. If not, a chronic state should be suspected. Infection with HBV, HDV, and HCV can result in chronic hepatitis and cirrhosis. Chronic HBV infection can also cause hepatic carcinoma.

Diagnostic Evaluation

A history of exposure to jaundiced individuals, confirmed outbreaks in daycare centers, or percutaneous exposure to blood or body fluids should raise the suspicion of hepatitis. Although no liver function test is specific for hepatitis, aspartate transaminase (AST), alanine transaminase (ALT), bilirubin levels, and sedimentation rate can indicate liver damage caused by hepatitis. Serum bilirubin levels peak 5 to 10 days after jaundice appears. A history of exposure and the course of the disease are essential in making the appropriate diagnosis.

Blood tests to diagnose hepatitis include identification of the antigens (e.g., HBsAg, HBeAg, HBcAg), antibodies (e.g., anti-HAV, anti-HBcAg, anti-HCV), and genetic material (e.g., HCV RNA) associated with the disease. In hepatitis A, immunoglobulin M (IgM) anti-HAV antibodies are present at the onset of illness and are diagnostic (Feigin, Cherry, Demmler-Harrison, & Kaplan, 2009). They usually disappear within 6 months, but may persist for 12 months. Children with hepatitis B are diagnosed by the presence of antigen (HBsAg) and IgM antibodies to HBcAg. HCV serologic assays (e.g., polymerase chain reaction) are used to diagnose hepatitis C (Feigin et al., 2009).

Liver biopsy may be needed to evaluate the chronic active forms of the disease and to determine the extent of liver damage in advanced or fulminant cases. Liver fibrosis increases with the duration of HCV infection.

Therapeutic Management

Acute viral hepatitis has no specific treatment. In uncomplicated viral hepatitis, treatment is mainly supportive because the disease is self-limiting. Treatment is aimed at maintaining comfort and adequate nutritional balance. A low-fat, balanced diet can be helpful if the child has nausea and anorexia. Hospitalization is rarely needed. All nonessential medications should be discontinued and chemotherapy, corticosteroids, and alcohol should all be avoided during infection.

In fulminant hepatitis, intensive care may be needed to provide hemostasis, nutritional and fluid support, neurologic assessment, and management until the liver has time to recover.

Hepatitis A. Control of further spread is essential. Because HAV can survive on contaminated objects for weeks, good hand hygiene and thorough disinfection of diaper-changing surfaces are imperative. Children and adults who have had direct contact with a person infected with HAV should receive immune globulin (IG) as soon as possible after exposure. Immunization is currently recommended for all children beginning at age 1 year, as well other high-risk groups (CDC, 2009). Cases of hepatitis should be promptly reported to local public health officials. Testing for IgM anti-HAV antibodies should be done in suspected cases of infected daycare center employees and household contacts of infected persons (American Academy of Pediatrics, 2009).

Hepatitis B. Children with acute or chronic HBV infection should be cared for with scrupulous Standard Precautions. The most effective means of preventing HBV infection is immunization. Immunization against HBV is recommended to start at birth; all children should receive this vaccine as early in childhood as possible. Other persons who should receive HBV immunization include IV drug users, health care and residential facility workers, household contacts and sexual partners of HBV carriers, inmates of correctional facilities, and

TABLE 19-6 HEPATITIS PROPHYLAXIS

VIRUS	PREVENTION OF SPREAD	IMMUNIZATION	POSTEXPOSURE PROPHYLAXIS
HAV	Hand hygiene, PPE (personal protective equipment); gloves Identifying infected food handlers	Given as two injections at age 1 yr and at least 6 mo later Recommended for all children at age 1 yr and specific populations in high-risk areas	Within 2 wk, give hepatitis A immune globulin (HAIG), 0.02 mL/kg intramuscular (IM)
HBV	Standard Precautions PPE; gloves, mask, eye/face shield Safe injections (OSHA Bloodborne Pathogens Standard, 2009)	Three injections at birth, age 1-2 mo, and age 6-18 mo Recommended for all infants, children, and adolescents	For neonates of infected mothers, give hepatitis B immune globulin (HBIG) within 12 hr of birth followed by immunization HBIG, 0.06 mL/kg, within 24 hr of any percutaneous exposure
HCV	Standard Precautions PPE; gloves, mask, eye/face shield Safe injections (OSHA Bloodborne Pathogens Standard, 2009)	None	None

Data from: Centers for Disease Control and Prevention (2009). *Viral hepatitis: For health professionals.* Retrieved from www.cdc.gov/hepatitis.

international travelers. HBV immune globulin (HBIG) is effective in preventing HBV infection if given within 2 weeks after exposure. Hepatitis D can be prevented by preventing HBV (Table 19-6).

NURSING CARE OF THE CHILD WITH VIRAL HEPATITIS

▪ Assessment

The nursing history may identify a source of infection. In children, flulike symptoms of fever, malaise, anorexia, fatigue, and nausea may be the only indications of viral hepatitis. Abdominal assessment may disclose right upper quadrant tenderness and hepatomegaly. Stools will be pale and clay colored, and urine may be dark and frothy. Jaundice, if present, is best assessed in sclera, nail beds, and mucous membranes, and usually follows a cephalocaudal progression. In HBV infection, arthralgias may be the presenting symptom.

Fulminant hepatitis will likely manifest as acute hepatic failure with associated encephalopathy, bleeding, fluid retention, ascites, and an icteric (jaundiced) appearance.

▪ Nursing Diagnosis and Planning

The following nursing diagnoses and expected outcomes may be appropriate after assessing the child with viral hepatitis and the child's family:

- Imbalanced Nutrition: Less Than Body Requirements related to anorexia.

Expected Outcomes. The child will be able to tolerate an age-appropriate diet without weight loss, vomiting, or abdominal pain and will return to a normal activity level.

- Risk for Infection related to exposure of family members to infectious agents.

Expected Outcomes. The family will practice good hand hygiene and other necessary isolation procedures and will remain free from infection.

- Risk for Injury related to fulminant hepatitis.

Expected Outcomes. The child will return to preillness weight and activity level.

- Deficient Knowledge related to incomplete information about home care and long-term prognosis.

Expected Outcomes. The parents will verbalize a basic understanding of hepatitis and the importance of treatment and prevention.

▪ Interventions

Unless fulminant hepatitis develops, children are usually treated at home, so parental education is crucial. Teaching parents the importance of a nutritious, low-fat diet as tolerated by the child, adequate rest, and general supportive care is important. The child with hepatitis is often anorexic. Several small meals and snacks throughout the day are better tolerated than regular portions at mealtimes.

Fatigue and malaise can last for several weeks. Plenty of rest and sleep are important for recovery. Because HAV is not infectious within 1 week after the onset of jaundice, the child may return to school at that time if feeling well enough.

▪ **Child and Parent Teaching.** Teach the parents the danger signals that could indicate a worsening of the child's condition: changes in neurologic status, bleeding, and fluid retention. Jaundice may worsen before it resolves, and parents should be prepared for this possibility. Also, teach parents not to give their child any over-the-counter medications because impaired liver function may result in inadequate metabolism and excretion of the medication. Caution adolescents not to drink alcohol during the illness or recovery period.

Preventing the spread of infection is an essential intervention for HAV. Prevention should include the use of Contact Precautions for at least 1 week after the onset of jaundice and meticulous hand hygiene. Hand hygiene is the most important preventive measure. Family members are taught how to institute appropriate precautions and clean exposed household surfaces with a bleach solution. Diapers should not be changed on or near surfaces used for preparing or serving food. The nurse explains to family members the ways in which HAV (fecal-oral route) and HBV (parenteral route) are spread to others. Recommendations for hepatitis A and hepatitis B vaccination are discussed and immunizations are provided to family members as indicated (see www2.aap.org/immunization/IZschedule.html).

If the child has HBV infection, especially neonatal HBV, the parents are informed about the possibility for development of a chronic carrier state, cirrhosis, and hepatocellular cancer later in life. If a child or adolescent with HBV infection has a history of illicit IV drug use, the nurse has the responsibility of teaching about the risk of transmission of hepatitis and other infections via contaminated needles. Referral to a substance abuse program is advisable.

▪ **Home Care.** Children with hepatitis are almost always managed at home. Nursing interventions include teaching parents hand hygiene skills, the use of gloves, and disinfection of contaminated surfaces and articles. Parents must learn to monitor their child for complications associated with hepatitis; provide a well-balanced, low-fat diet; and watch other family members for signs and symptoms of infection. As indicated, all family members and especially any siblings/children should be immunized against hepatitis A and B.

■ Evaluation

- Has the child maintained a weight within 5% of the preillness weight?
- Is the child free of vomiting?
- Is the child participating in age-appropriate activities and play?
- Do family members practice good hand hygiene and adhere to procedures?
- Has the spread of hepatitis to other family members been avoided?
- Have all family members been immunized as appropriate?
- Can the parents describe the symptoms of hepatitis to watch for in other family members?

Biliary Atresia

Biliary atresia refers to the obstruction or absence of the extrahepatic bile ducts. At birth, the liver itself is normal without inflammation, but the structural problem leads to significant cellular damage and eventual liver failure and death.

Etiology and Incidence

The cause of biliary atresia is unknown. Because the problem originates during the prenatal period, viruses, toxins, and chemicals cannot be ruled out. The condition is unlikely to recur within the same family.

Extrahepatic biliary atresia occurs in 1 in 10,000 to 15,000 births, with a slightly higher incidence in female infants than in male infants (NASPGHAN, n.d.). It is the number one indication for liver transplantation in children (NASPGHAN, n.d.).

Manifestations

The child with biliary atresia appears healthy at birth. Manifestations that develop shortly afterward include acholic stools (light in color because of the absence of bile pigment), bile-stained urine, and hepatomegaly.

Diagnostic Evaluation

Investigation of liver function (bilirubin, aminotransferases [ALT, AST]) and clotting studies (prothrombin time [PT], partial thromboplastin time [PTT]) is important in establishing the diagnosis. Any newborn with conjugated hyperbilirubinemia should be thoroughly evaluated. To rule out inborn errors of metabolism (e.g., galactosemia and alpha$_1$-antitrypsin deficiency), which can produce similar initial findings, metabolic screening is performed. Hepatitis B and other viral titers are also measured to rule out neonatal hepatitis. Urine and stool samples should be examined and urobilinogen levels checked to determine the degree of obstruction.

Percutaneous liver biopsy can provide a definitive diagnosis if bile plugs, edema, and fibrosis are found in the presence of normal hepatic lobular structure (Benchimol, Walsh, & Ling, 2009). Cholangiography may be used to ascertain the extent of atresia.

Therapeutic Management

During and after exploratory laparotomy, the size of the lesion can be identified and drainage can be attempted. If no correctable lesion is found, a hepatic portoenterostomy (Kasai procedure) will be performed to allow bile to drain from the liver. This procedure allows bile to flow directly into the intestine through an anastomosis of the jejunum to the porta hepatis, the point at which the hepatic ducts join to form the common bile duct. The Kasai procedure does provide some long-term benefits, but hepatic dysfunction will persist. The main goal of the procedure is to allow growth and development of the child until liver transplantation can be performed.

Medical management involves treating the child's malnutrition and providing symptom relief. Medium-chain triglyceride (MCT) oil may be added to formula to increase calories or TPN can be administered to provide essential nutrition. Vitamin malabsorption must be attended to so night blindness (vitamin A), neuromuscular degeneration (vitamin E), rickets (vitamin D), and hypoprothrombinemia (vitamin K) are prevented. Assessment for and treatment of portal hypertension with its concomitant problems of ascites and variceal bleeding must be instituted. Controlling bleeding, restricting salt intake, and using diuretics are essential in managing portal hypertension.

Nursing Considerations

During the early phase of disease, in the first months of life, the infant with biliary atresia will appear jaundiced, with mild hepatosplenomegaly and increased abdominal girth. As the disease progresses, the child may appear thin, with failure to thrive, marked jaundice, and evidence of rickets caused by chronic vitamin D deficiency. Pruritus becomes a major problem; the child may develop skin infections or xanthomas (lipid deposits in the skin) as a result of retention of cholesterol in the skin.

After the Kasai procedure, the child needs to be assessed for evidence of portal hypertension, which may include the development of ascites and GI bleeding. Even after repair, acholic stools and bile-stained urine are not uncommon.

Psychosocial and family assessment must be a high priority. Biliary atresia is a life-threatening, chronic illness that requires surgical intervention, involvement of numerous health care providers, repeated hospitalizations, and eventually an extended wait for a liver transplant. The nurse gathers information about family structure and stability, financial resources, available support systems, and the feelings of the child and family about the management and progression of the disease.

Nursing interventions are directed toward six major areas: nutritional support, skin care, developmental stimulation, continued assessment, education, and emotional support.

Nutritional Support. Providing adequate calories, aiding in vitamin supply and absorption, and preventing hepatic encephalopathy are important goals. Calorie counts, daily weights, and abdominal girths are important assessment parameters that provide the data necessary to improve nutritional support. Concentrating calories with the use of Polycose and providing MCT supplements which do not require the presence of bile salts to digest, can significantly improve the child's nutritional status. NG tube feeding or TPN may be necessary at times. Supplements of vitamins A, D, E, and K, as well as calcium, phosphate, and zinc, are essential for adequate nutrition. Protein intake may need to be limited to avoid the development of hepatic encephalopathy. Plotting weight, length, and head circumference on growth charts monthly provides data to evaluate treatment effectiveness.

Skin Care. Bile acid binders, such as cholestyramine, aid in the excretion of bile salts and decrease pruritus and the development of xanthomas (Chang & Golkar, 2008). Colloidal oatmeal baths (Aveeno) can relieve severe itching. Preventing skin breakdown from severe scratching is essential. Wearing gloves during sleep and applying soothing lotions and creams for dry skin may prevent infection.

Developmental Stimulation. Teaching parents activities to provide developmental stimulation and accessing resources available through physical and occupational therapy are essential nursing

PATHOPHYSIOLOGY
Biliary Atresia

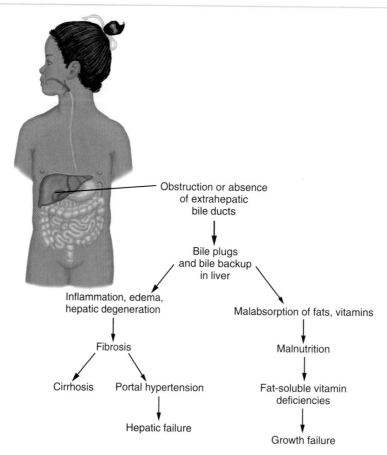

Obstruction or absence
of extrahepatic
bile ducts

Bile plugs
and bile backup
in liver

Inflammation, edema,
hepatic degeneration

Malabsorption of fats, vitamins

Fibrosis

Malnutrition

Cirrhosis   Portal hypertension

Fat-soluble vitamin
deficiencies

Hepatic failure

Growth failure

Obstruction of the extrahepatic bile ducts causes obstruction of the normal flow of bile out of the liver and into the gallbladder and small intestines. As a result, bile plugs form, causing bile to back up in the liver. This process causes inflammation, edema, and hepatic degeneration. Eventually the liver becomes fibrotic, and cirrhosis and portal hypertension develop, leading to liver failure. The gradual degeneration of the liver causes jaundice, icterus, and hepatomegaly. Because bile is not present in the intestines, fat and fat-soluble vitamins cannot be absorbed. This condition leads to malnutrition, deficiencies in fat-soluble vitamins, and growth failure.

responsibilities. As the child awaits a liver transplant, efforts should be made to facilitate achievement of developmental milestones related to gross and fine motor skills, and social and emotional abilities. Routine screening tests can document developmental growth and be used to evaluate interventions.

Continued Assessment. Continuous monitoring for the development of portal hypertension is vital. The parents must be taught to watch for GI bleeding, severe edema, and ascites. If any of these conditions are noted, the physician must be notified immediately; sodium intake restrictions, diuretics, IV albumin, and hospitalization may be required.

Family Education and Support. The family has many educational needs. The nurse helps family members understand the disease process, manage nutritional changes, provide skin care, assess for signs of complications, and enhance the child's development. Parents are given information about resources that are available. Organizations such as the Children's Liver Foundation provide programs, educational materials, and referral to support groups for children with liver disease and their families (see Evolve website).

The nurse plays a critical role by listening to parental concerns, providing information and support, and encouraging parents to participate in their child's daily care. Further, the nurse helps the parents focus on and prepare for their child's future liver transplant and related long-term care and treatment. Because transplantation usually occurs within the first 2 years of life, age-appropriate explanations for the toddler are also indicated.

The child and family should be prepared for the possible death of the child. Biliary atresia is a life-threatening condition and some children succumb to the disease before liver transplantation is able to be performed. Further, management of the disease requires numerous hospitalizations, many diagnostic tests, and an extensive daily care regimen. All of this places immense stress on families. Critical nursing interventions include arranging for and providing educational and emotional support to the child as well as to the parents so that they can effectively care for their child.

Home Care. The parents must be able to assume all home care responsibilities. They need to monitor nutritional intake, mix special formulas, manage NG feedings, provide skin care, give medications, and track their child's growth and development. Their ability to assess for GI bleeding, ascites, edema, and skin infections is critical so that treatment of complications can begin promptly.

Cirrhosis

Cirrhosis is a chronic, degenerative condition of the liver that results in the development of bands of fibrous tissue, firm nodules, and connections between the central and portal areas of the liver. This scarring causes irreversible damage to the liver.

PATHOPHYSIOLOGY

Cirrhosis

Stasis of bile causes inflammation and hepatomegaly. If this continues, destruction of the liver begins. As the liver attempts to heal itself, fibrotic regeneration and nodules develop and function is impaired. This scarring can cause altered hepatic blood flow and decreased liver cell function. Changes in hepatic blood flow can cause scarring and collapse of the hepatic vasculature, increased vascular resistance, and eventually portal hypertension. As the liver cells decrease in function, more cells die, and the liver cannot produce necessary proteins or bile, causing malabsorption and malnutrition. As liver cells continue to die, the cycle is repeated.

Etiology

Cirrhosis in children usually results from chronic liver disease, such as HBV infection, chronic hepatitis, or biliary atresia. Sickle cell disease, inborn errors of metabolism such as alpha$_1$-antitrypsin deficiency and disturbances in copper metabolism, cystic fibrosis, and Wilson disease are other possible causes of pediatric liver cirrhosis.

Incidence

Cirrhosis is uncommon in children, but as the life span of children with chronic disease continues to lengthen, the incidence of liver cirrhosis will rise.

Manifestations

The symptoms are often nonspecific, vague, and slow to develop. They result from either liver cell failure or portal hypertension. Liver cell failure results in jaundice, intense pruritus, steatorrhea, abdominal distention, edema, anemia, bleeding tendencies, anorexia, frequent infections, and poor growth. Portal hypertension may manifest as splenomegaly, esophageal varices, or GI bleeding. Both liver cell failure and portal hypertension contribute to the development of ascites.

Diagnostic Evaluation

Because the most likely cause of cirrhosis in children is chronic biliary obstruction, evaluation is based on the history of preexisting conditions. A presumptive diagnosis of cirrhosis can be made based on the presence of clinical manifestations of chronic liver disease and a history of hepatitis or biliary atresia. The results of liver function tests such as bilirubin, aminotransferases, ammonia, albumin, cholesterol, and prothrombin time, can support the diagnosis. A liver biopsy that identifies fibrous scarring and changes of hepatic vasculature is indicative of cirrhosis.

Therapeutic Management

No effective treatment is available to halt the progression of cirrhosis. Infections should be treated and obstructions repaired. Supportive care that includes rest, nutritional support, fluid management, and relief of symptoms, is provided. Management of life-threatening complications including bleeding varices, ascites, and hepatic encephalopathy, takes priority. Definitive therapy is a liver transplant. Liver function is carefully monitored to determine when the child will need liver transplantation.

Nursing Considerations

General appraisal will likely reveal a child with a history of failure to thrive and chronic biliary obstruction or HBV infection. The child may have varying degrees of distress and discomfort. Many children will have vague symptoms or be asymptomatic. The earliest findings of cirrhosis are likely to be anorexia, nausea, indigestion, fatigue, and right upper quadrant (RUQ) pain or fullness. Monitoring height and weight with a growth chart, gathering information on a typical day's food intake, and assessing sleep habits and activity levels can provide essential supportive evidence.

Abdominal palpation will likely reveal splenomegaly and RUQ tenderness or hepatomegaly. Distended superficial veins, edema, and tight, shiny skin can be seen. Jaundice and pruritus may be detected, especially if the cirrhosis is the result of biliary obstruction. A complete skin assessment, including nail beds and sclera, can identify jaundice at its earliest stages. The skin should be examined for breakdown or infection caused by intense scratching. The amount and location of edema is also noted. Skin assessment may also reveal bruises related to thrombocytopenia and pale color related to anemia. A stool specimen may be useful in identifying the degree of bile obstruction and malabsorption.

The most critical assessment needs to be centered on detecting signs of the three major complications of cirrhosis: ascites, varices, and encephalopathy. The child with significantly increased abdominal girth, edema, bloody emesis, or changes in level of consciousness should be referred for emergency medical care related to these life-threatening complications.

The goal of nursing care is to sustain the child in optimal condition until liver transplantation can be achieved. The care can be divided into four areas: nutritional support, skin care, prevention of complications, and developmental and parental support.

Nutritional Support. Providing optimal nutrition that allows the child to grow and develop is a major nursing intervention. The diet needs to be high carbohydrate, high calorie, normal protein, and low fat. These changes put minimal stress on the liver while meeting the child's growth requirements. Protein may need to be limited if encephalopathy develops. Restricted sodium intake can help prevent edema. Multivitamin supplements containing vitamins A, D, E, and K are essential. Vitamin K injections can be administered, if indicated. Because of anorexia, creative food options, NG tube feedings, and TPN may be needed. Monitoring the child's weight on a daily and a weekly basis as well as recording intake and output provides critical information about edema and growth. Support from dietary personnel is valuable when working with these children and their families.

Skin Care. Pruritus can be intense for the child with cirrhosis. Continued assessment for open lesions, scratch marks, bleeding, and ease of bruising is vital. Colloidal oatmeal baths and topical antipruritic lotions such as calamine, may provide temporary relief. Medications to treat pruritus are not usually given due to impaired liver function. Keeping the nails trimmed short or wearing cotton gloves during sleep can minimize injury to the skin from scratching.

Prevention of Complications. It is critical that the nurse prevent exposure of the child to infections as well as continuously monitor and immediately report fever or other signs of infection.

If the child is noted to be edematous, the nurse gives diuretics and albumin as ordered, and maintains a low-sodium diet. The child who develops acites will likely be hospitalized for treatment: tracking intake and output and weight, maintaining fluid balance, and monitoring abdominal girth and distention are key nursing interventions.

Stool guaiac tests and careful observation will aid the nurse in identifying bleeding as soon as possible. To prevent bleeding, injections are avoided, the child is protected from injury, and vitamin K is given as ordered. For the hospitalized child, nursing care involves transfusing blood or blood products safely, maintaining fluid balance, monitoring pulse and blood pressure, administering oxygen therapy, and assisting with endoscopic sclerotherapy or the placement of a Sengstaken-Blakemore tube for compression of bleeding esophageal varices.

Encephalopathy occurs as a result of excess ammonia in the blood due to incomplete breakdown of protein by the liver. The nurse must frequently assess the child for changes in behavior and level of consciousness to detect encephalopathy. Per orders, limiting protein in the diet, giving lactulose to decrease the GI bacteria that produce ammonia, and administering antibiotics are important nursing responsibilities. Also, careful consideration must be given before any drugs are administered to the child with cirrhosis. Impaired liver function adversely affects the metabolism of many drugs; sedatives, opioids, acetaminophen (Tylenol), and alcohol are strictly avoided.

Developmental and Parental Support. Children with cirrhosis are chronically ill and require much time and effort to maintain optimal health. Providing developmental stimulation on a daily basis is essential, and parents need education and support services to achieve this. In addition, parents need to be educated about the disease, its prognosis, the feasibility of a liver transplant, and the risk of complications. As the parents cope with the potential loss of their child, community resources and national support groups, such as the Children's Liver Foundation, are helpful.

Home Care The focus of nursing related to home care is education. Because the child will be cared for at home unless a serious complication arises or the child is hospitalized for a liver transplant, parents need complete information and instructions. Developing plans for meals and snacks that meet the child's special, daily nutritional needs can be difficult, and dietary personnel can provide invaluable assistance to parents. Nurses must teach parents how to prevent infection by sheltering their child from sources of infection and following hand hygiene and other disinfection protocols. The most critical nursing intervention is to educate parents so they can identify signs of complications such as GI bleeding, encephalopathy, and severe edema, and know when they must immediately contact the physician. When the child with cirrhosis remains generally healthy, the family can facilitate progression of the child's developmental skills and prepare for liver transplantation.

KEY CONCEPTS

- The GI system is formed in the first 4 weeks of embryonic development; this is when congenital defects occur.
- The anatomy of the GI tract is complete at birth but physiologically immature.
- Evaluating distress in small children must include a thorough history, physical assessment, pain assessment, and parent's perception of the child's pain.
- Fluid balance can rapidly shift in the child with vomiting, diarrhea, or anorexia; the nurse must thoroughly assess for changes frequently.
- Gastroesophageal alterations place the child at risk for respiratory distress. Assessment of respiratory function and maintenance of airway patency are critical interventions.
- Medications are essential in managing many GI diseases; the nurse must be knowledgeable of dosages, indications, side effects, and teaching needs.
- The emotional needs of the parents whose children have congenital anomalies need to be addressed.
- Postoperative nursing care of children following GI surgery is focused on fluid balance, pain control, nutrition, parental involvement, and the child's developmental level.
- Parental anxiety can have a significant effect on the child with GI alterations and must be addressed.
- Correct use of Standard Precautions is essential to preventing the spread of GI infections.
- Some GI malabsorption disorders can be managed by dietary changes.
- Educating parents to care for their children with GI alterations at home is a priority nursing action.
- Referral to community resources is a vital aspect of nursing care for children with GI alterations.

REFERENCES

American Academy of Pediatrics. (2009). *Red book: 2009 report of the committee on infectious diseases* (28th ed.). Elk Grove Village, IL: American Academy of Pediatrics.

Askew, N. (2010). An overview of infantile hypertrophic pyloric stenosis. *Pediatric Nursing, 22*(8), 27-30.

Bardella, M., Elli, L., Velio, P., et al. (2007). Silent celiac disease is frequent in the siblings of newly diagnosed celiac patients. *Digestion, 75,* 182-187.

Benchimol, E., Walsh, C., & Ling, S. (2009). Early diagnosis of neonatal cholestatic jaundice: Test at 2 weeks. *Canadian Family Physician, 55*(12), 1184-1192.

Bhutta, Z. (2011). Acute gastroenteritis in children. In R. Kliegman, B. Stanton, J. St. Geme, et al. (Eds.), *Nelson* *textbook of pediatrics* (19th ed., pp. 1323-1338). Philadelphia: Elsevier.

Blanchard, S., & Czinn, S. (2011). Peptic ulcer disease in children. In R. Kliegman, B. Stanton, J. St. Geme, et al. (Eds.), *Nelson textbook of pediatrics* (19th ed., pp. 1291-1294). Philadelphia: Elsevier.

Castilloux, J., Noble, A., & Faure, C. (2010). Risk factors for short- and long-term morbidity in children with esophageal atresia. *Journal of Pediatrics, 156*(5), 755-760.

Centers for Disease Control and Prevention. (2003). Managing acute gastroenteritis among children, oral rehydration, maintenance, and nutritional therapy. *MMWR Morbidity and Mortality Weekly Report, 52*(RR-16), 1-16.

Centers for Disease Control and Prevention. (2009). Surveillance for acute viral hepatitis—United States, 2007. *MMWR Morbidity and Mortality Weekly Report, 58*(SS-3), 1-30.

Chang, Y., & Golkar, L. (2008). The use of naltrexone in the management of severe generalized pruritus in biliary atresia: Report of a case. *Pediatric Dermatology, 25*(3), 403-404.

Cleft Palate Foundation. (2007). *About cleft lip and palate.* Retrieved from www.cleftline.org.

Conklin, L., & Oliva-Hemker, M. (2010). Nutritional considerations in pediatric inflammatory bowel disease. *Expert Review of Gastroenterology and Hepatology, 4*(3), 305-317.

Croffie, J., & Fitzgerald, J. (2008). Constipation and irritable bowel syndrome. In C. Liacouras & D. Piccoli (Eds.), *Pediatric gastroenterology* (pp. 30-41). St. Louis: Elsevier.

Crohn's and Colitis Foundation of America. (2010). *Welcome to Camp Oasis*. Retrieved from www.ccfa.org/kidstees/camp.

Culbert, T., & Barez, G. (2007). Integrative approaches to childhood constipation and encopresis. *Pediatric Clinics of North America, 54*(6), 927-947.

Desai, S., Esposito, D., Shapiro, E., et al. (2010). Effectiveness of rotavirus vaccine in preventing hospitalization due to rotavirus gastroenteritis in young children in Connecticut, USA. *Vaccine, 28*(47), 7501-7506.

Feigin, R., Cherry, J., Demmler-Harrison, G., & Kaplan, S. (2009). *Feigin and Cherry's textbook of pediatric infectious diseases* (6th ed.). Philadelphia: Elsevier Saunders.

Fiorino, K., & Liacouras, C. (2011). Congenital aganglionic megacolon (Hirschsprung disease). In R. Kliegman, B. Stanton, J. St. Geme, et al. (Eds.), *Nelson textbook of pediatrics* (19th ed., pp. 1284-1287). Philadelphia: Elsevier.

Greenwald, B. (2010). Clinical practice guidelines for pediatric constipation. *Journal of the American Academy of Nurse Practitioners, 22*(7), 332-338.

Grossman, A., & Baldassano, R. (2011a). Crohn disease. In R. Kliegman, B. Stanton, J. St. Geme, et al. (Eds.). *Nelson textbook of pediatrics* (19th ed., pp. 1300-1304). Philadelphia: Elsevier.

Grossman, A., & Baldassano, R. (2011b). Chronic ulcerative colitis. In R. Kliegman, B. Stanton, J. St. Geme, et al. (Eds.). *Nelson textbook of pediatrics* (19th ed., pp. 1295-1300). Philadelphia: Elsevier.

Grossman, A., & Liacouras, C. (2008). Gastroesophageal reflux. In C. Liacouras & D. Piccoli (Eds.), *Pediatric gastroenterology* (pp. 74-85). St. Louis: Elsevier.

Hardy, L. (2009). Encopresis: a guide for psychiatric nurses. *Psychiatric Nursing, 23*(5), 351-358.

Hoffenberg, E., Utterson, E., & Hoffenberg, A. (2008). Celiac disease. In C. Liacouras & D. Piccoli (Eds.), *Pediatric gastroenterology* (pp. 24-29). St. Louis: Elsevier.

Jacobstein, D., & Baldassano, R. (2008). Inflammatory bowel disease. In C. Liacouras & D. Piccoli (Eds.), *Pediatric gastroenterology* (pp. 131-141). St. Louis: Elsevier.

Kahn, S., & Orenstein, S. (2011a). Esophageal atresia and tracheoesophageal fistula. In R. Kliegman, B. Stanton, J.

St. Geme, et al. (Eds.), *Nelson textbook of pediatrics* (19th ed., pp. 1262-1263). Philadelphia: Elsevier.

Kahn, S., & Orenstein, S. (2011b). Gastroesophageal reflux disease. In R. Kliegman, B. Stanton, J. St. Geme, et al. (Eds.), *Nelson textbook of pediatrics* (19th ed., pp. 1266-1269). Philadelphia: Elsevier.

Kennedy, M., & Liacouras, C. (2011). Intussusception. In R. Kliegman, B. Stanton, J. St. Geme, et al. (Eds.), *Nelson textbook of pediatrics* (19th ed., pp. 1287-1289). Philadelphia: Elsevier.

Lebby, K., Tan, F., & Brown, C. (2010). Maternal factors and disparities associated with oral clefts. *Ethnicity & Disease, 20*(1), S1-146-149.

March of Dimes. (2007). Cleft lip and cleft palate. Retrieved from www.marchofdimes.com.

Mattei, P. (2008). Hirschsprung's disease. In C. Liacouras & D. Piccoli (Eds.), *Pediatric gastroenterology* (pp. 74-85). St. Louis: Elsevier.

Muniyappa, P., Gulati, R., Mohr, F., & Hupertz, B. (2009). Use and safety of rifaximin in children with inflammatory bowel disease. *Journal of Pediatric Gastroenterology and Nutrition, 49*(4), 400-404.

National Birth Defects Prevention Network. (2009). *Congenital malformations surveillance report*. Retrieved from www.nbdpn.org.

National Digestive Diseases Information Clearinghouse. (2009). *Lactose intolerance*. Retrieved from http://digestive.niddk.nih.gov/ddiseases/pubs/lactoseintolerance/index.htm.

North American Society for Pediatric Gastroenterologist, Hepatology, & Nutrition [NASPGHAN]. (n.d.) *Biliary atresia*. Retrieved from www.naspghan.org/user-assets/Documents/pdf/diseaseInfo/BiliaryAtresia-E.pdf.

Occupational Safety and Health Administration (OSHA) (2009). Bloodborne pathogens and needlestick prevention. Retrieved from www.osha.gov/SLTC/bloodbornepathogens/index.html.

Parashar, U., Gibson, C., Bresee, J., & Glass, R. (2006). Rotavirus and severe childhood diarrhea. *Emerging Infectious Diseases [serial on the Internet]*. Retrieved from www.cdc.gov/ncidod/EID/vol12no02/05-0006.htm.

Quartero, A., Meiniche-Schmidt, B., Muris, J., et al. (2005). Bulking agents, antispasmodic and antidepressant medication for the treatment of irritable bowel syndrome. *Cochrane Database of Systematic Reviews*, 2005, Issue 2. Art. No.: CD003460.

Radlovic, N., Mladenovic, M., Lekovic, Z., et al. (2010). Influence of early feeding practices on celiac disease in infants. *Croatian Medical Journal, 51*(5), 417-422.

Rojas-Martinez, A., Reutter, H., Chacon-Camacho, O., et al. (2010). Genetic risk factors for nonsyndromic cleft lip with or without cleft palate in an Mesoamerican population: Evidence for IRF6 and variants at 8q24 and 10q25. *Clinical and Molecular Teratology, 88*(7), 535-537.

Silano, M., Agostoni, C., & Guandalini, S. (2010). Effect of the timing of gluten introduction on the development of celiac disease. *World Journal of Gastroenterology, 16*(16), 1939-1942.

Sreedharan, R., & Liacouras, C. (2011). Functional abdominal pain (nonorganic chronic abdominal pain). In R. Kliegman, B. Stanton, J. St. Geme, et al. (Eds.), *Nelson textbook of pediatrics* (19th ed., pp. 1346-1349). Philadelphia: Elsevier.

Toorenvliet, B., Wiersma, F., Bakker, R., et al. (2010). Routine ultrasound and limited computed tomography for the diagnosis of acute appendicitis. *World Journal of Surgery, 34*(10), 2278-2285.

Tully, M. (2008). Celiac disease. In R. J. Young & L. Philichi (Eds.), *Clinical handbook of pediatric gastroenterology* (pp. 27-33). St. Louis: Quality Medical.

Vandenplas, Y., Rudolph, C., Di Lorenzo, C., et al. (2009). Pediatric gastroesophageal reflux clinical practice guidelines: Joint recommendations of the North American Society for Pediatric Gastroenterology, Hepatology, and Nutrition (NASPGHAN) and the European Society for Pediatric Gastroenterology, Hepatology, and Nutrition (ESPGHAN). *Journal for Pediatric Gastroenterology and Nutrition, 49*(4), 498-547.

Yazigi, N., & Balistreri, W. (2011). Viral hepatitis. In R. Kliegman, B. Stanton, J. St. Geme, et al. (Eds.), *Nelson textbook of pediatrics* (19th ed., pp. 1393-1405). Philadelphia: Elsevier.

Zarate, Y., Martin, L., Hopkin, R., et al. (2010). Evaluation of growth in patients with isolated cleft lip and/or cleft palate. *Pediatrics, 125*(3), e543-e549.

Zijdenbos, I., de Wit, N., van der Heijden, G., et al. (2009). Psychological treatments for the management of irritable bowel syndrome. (2009). *Cochrane Database of Systematic Reviews*, 2009, Issue 1. Art. No.: CD006442.

The Child with a Genitourinary Alteration

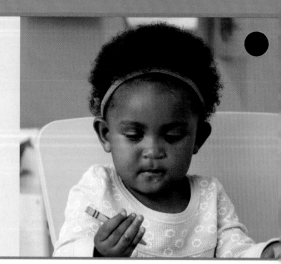

evolve WEBSITE

http://evolve.elsevier.com/James/ncoc

LEARNING OBJECTIVES

After studying this chapter, you should be able to:

- Describe the anatomy and physiology of the infant's and child's genitourinary system.
- Describe the most common diagnostic and screening tests used to assess alteration in genitourinary function.
- Discuss frequently seen alterations in the genitourinary system.
- Use the nursing process to assess, plan, and provide nursing care to children with common genitourinary alterations.
- Develop home care guidelines for the child with a genitourinary alteration.

CLINICAL REFERENCE

REVIEW OF THE GENITOURINARY SYSTEM

The urinary system consists of the kidneys and ureters, or the upper urinary tract, and the bladder and urethra, or the lower urinary tract. A child's genitourinary system differs in structure and function from an adult's in several ways.

Structure

The bean-shaped kidneys are located one on each side of the spinal column. In an adolescent or adult, the kidney is approximately the size of a fist; the infant's kidney is small but proportionally larger. The upper portion of the left kidney lies near the 12th rib, with the right kidney slightly lower. The *hilum*, the indentation in the kidney, is the area where the blood vessels, lymphatics, nerves, and *ureter* enter the kidney.

A thin, fibrous capsule encases the kidney. The outer region of the kidney is the cortex, and the inner region is the medulla; both can be observed with the kidney dissected longitudinally. The cortex contains the glomeruli and tubules, whereas the medulla contains the renal pyramids and portions of the tubules. The renal pelvis, located in the area of the hilum, is an extension of the upper end of the ureter.

The ureters extend downward from the kidney and enter the bladder wall. As the bladder fills with urine, it compresses the distal ureters, preventing urine reflux. The bladder is a muscular vessel with a rich blood supply. The bladder capacity for an infant or a child is approximately equal to 10 mL/kg of body weight. The urethra leads from the bladder and contains an internal sphincter and an external sphincter, which control urination. Boys have a longer urethra than do girls.

The *nephron* is the kidney's functional unit. It consists of the Bowman's capsule, glomerulus, proximal tubule, loop of Henle, distal tubule, and collecting duct. Each kidney contains approximately 1 million nephrons.

Blood enters the kidney through the renal arteries, which branch off the abdominal aorta. The renal artery divides and subdivides, eventually culminating in the afferent arterioles, which feed into the glomerular capillaries. The glomerular capillaries empty into the efferent arterioles.

Peritubular capillaries surround the proximal tubule, the loop of Henle, and the distal tubules. The capillaries drain into the venous system. Blood returns to the heart through the renal vein, which enters the inferior vena cava.

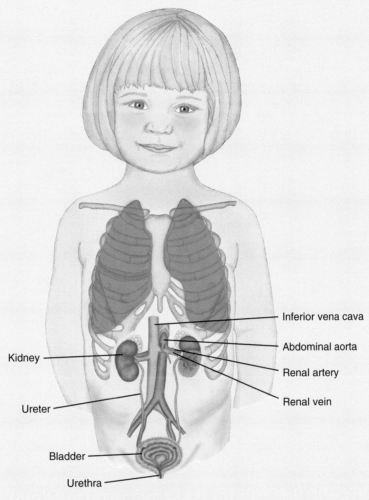

Inferior vena cava

Abdominal aorta

Renal artery

Renal vein

Kidney

Ureter

Bladder

Urethra

Anatomy of the Genitourinary System

PEDIATRIC DIFFERENCES IN THE GENITOURINARY SYSTEM

- In a healthy infant, the kidneys operate at a functional level appropriate for body size; however, function is reduced when the infant is under stress.
- By 6 to 12 months of age, kidney function is nearly like that of the adult.
- In premature infants, the reabsorption of glucose, sodium, bicarbonate, and phosphate is reduced.
- The young infant's kidneys cannot concentrate urine as efficiently as those of older children and adults because the loops of Henle are not yet long enough to reach the inner medulla, where concentration and reabsorption occur.* After the first few weeks of life, the ability of the kidneys to acidify the urine reaches adult levels. With acidosis, however, there is only a small increase in acid secretion, and susceptibility to acidemia rises.
- The neonate's bladder, which is in the lower abdominal cavity, gradually sinks into the pelvic cavity during early childhood.
- Young children have shorter urethras, which can predispose them to UTIs.
- Children usually achieve complete bladder control by approximately 4 to 5 years of age.
- Unlike adults, most children with acute renal failure regain normal function.

*Banasik, J. (2005). Renal function. In L. Copstead & J. Banasik (Eds.), *Pathophysiology*. St. Louis: Elsevier Saunders.

Function

The kidneys maintain fluid and chemical balance through glomerular filtration, tubular reabsorption, and secretion. The kidneys also have important hormonal functions:

- Production of *renin*, which helps with the regulation of blood pressure. Release of renin is stimulated primarily by decreased pressure in the afferent arterioles of the glomerulus.
- Production of *erythropoietin*, which stimulates red blood cell (RBC) production by the bone marrow.
- Metabolism of vitamin D to its active form, which is important in calcium metabolism.

Adequate renal function is important to the function of other body systems. When assessing a child for a possible genitourinary dysfunction, the nurse should consider such nonspecific assessment data as altered growth, skeletal anomalies, hypertension, skin lesions, and immune dysfunctions.

Genitourinary alterations in children encompass a wide range of conditions, from a single acute urinary tract infection (UTI) to end-stage renal disease (ESRD). The effects of illness on the child and family depend on the nature of the illness and on its severity and prognosis. Nursing care also varies. A child in an acute phase of nephrotic syndrome is sometimes hospitalized. Less severe genitourinary disorders may be treated at home. Therefore, the nurse can teach administration of an intravenous (IV) antibiotic or monitor adherence to a treatment plan.

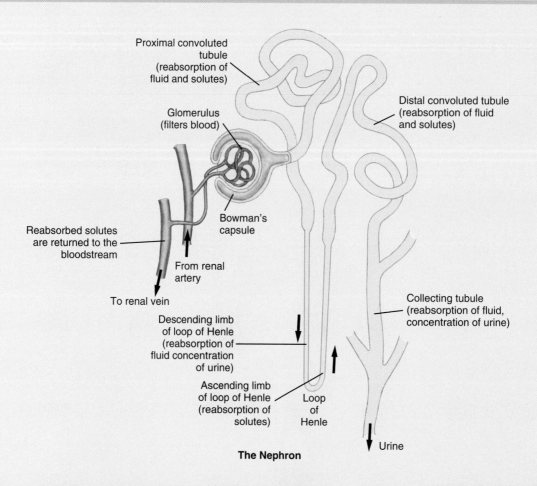

The Nephron

Proximal convoluted tubule (reabsorption of fluid and solutes)

Glomerulus (filters blood)

Bowman's capsule

Reabsorbed solutes are returned to the bloodstream

From renal artery

To renal vein

Descending limb of loop of Henle (reabsorption of fluid concentration of urine)

Ascending limb of loop of Henle (reabsorption of solutes)

Loop of Henle

Distal convoluted tubule (reabsorption of fluid and solutes)

Collecting tubule (reabsorption of fluid, concentration of urine)

Urine

COMMON LABORATORY AND DIAGNOSTIC TESTS FOR GENITOURINARY DISORDERS

TEST	DESCRIPTION	NORMAL FINDINGS	INDICATIONS	NURSING CONSIDERATIONS
Urinalysis				
Specific gravity	Measurement of concentration of urine	1.002-1.030	Provides information regarding hydration and renal concentration ability	Specific gravity is higher if protein or glucose is present
pH	Determines acidity and alkalinity	4.5-8.0	Increases in urinary infections	Affected by diet
Protein	Detection of protein in urine	Negative or trace	May be first indication of renal disease	Early-morning specimens preferable because they are more concentrated
Glucose	Detection of glucose in urine	Negative	Screens or confirms diabetes and monitors effectiveness of diabetes control; may be present in child with weight loss, dehydration, infection, renal disease	Nonspecific, needs further evaluation
Ketones	Formed in liver and completely metabolized; alteration in carbohydrate metabolism leads to excessive ketone production	Negative	Mainly associated with diabetes; may be present with fever, anorexia, diarrhea, fasting, starvation, prolonged vomiting	Children are more prone to development of ketouria
Leukocyte esterase	Enzyme released during WBC breakdown	Negative	May be present when WBCs in urine	Indicates possible UTI

UTI, urinary tract infection; *WBC,* white blood cell.

COMMON LABORATORY AND DIAGNOSTIC TESTS FOR GENITOURINARY DISORDERS—cont'd

TEST	DESCRIPTION	NORMAL FINDINGS	INDICATIONS	NURSING CONSIDERATIONS
Urinalysis—cont'd				
Nitrites	Produced by select bacteria	Negative	May be present when bacteria in urine	In infant and child, bacteria may not be present in bladder long enough to produce sufficient nitrites to yield positive results
WBCs	Microscopic finding of WBCs in urine	0-2/high-power field	Seen with infection	Urine culture indicated
RBCs	Microscopic finding of RBCs in urine	0-2/high-power field	Trauma, stones, infection, glomerulonephritis	Normal in menstruating females
Bacteria	Microscopic presence of bacteria in urine	None	UTI	Urine culture indicated
Casts	WBC casts and RBC casts originate in kidney tubules	None	Pyelonephritis, glomerulonephritis, renal infarction, collagen disease, interstitial inflammation of kidney	Helps in diagnosis
Urine Culture and Sensitivity				
	Presence of bacteria or other pathogens	Negative or ≤100,000 colonies/mL of urine from clean-catch or sterile bag specimen	Isolation and identification of pathogens in urinary tract; identification of antibiotic sensitivity	Diagnoses UTI See Chapter 13 for specimen-collection guidelines
Serum Studies				
BUN	End product of protein metabolism	Newborn: 3-12 mg/dL Infant/child: 5-18 mg/dL Adult: 10-20 mg/dl	Gross indicator of renal function	Increases in renal insufficiency
Serum creatinine	Byproduct of muscle metabolism; production is constant as long as muscle mass remains constant	Newborn: 0.3-1.0 mg/dL Infant: 0.2-0.4 mg/dL Child: 0.3-0.7 mg/dL Adolescent: 0.5-1.0 mg/dL Adult female: 0.5-1.1 mg/dL Adult male: 0.6-1.2 mg/dL	Increases in renal insufficiency	Should be assessed before giving nephrotoxic agents
Serum osmolality	Measurement of concentration of blood, determined by solute in blood	275-295 mOsm/kg	Indication of fluid and electrolyte balance	Helpful in evaluating hydration status, liver disease, antidiuretic hormone function
Radiography				
Kidney, ureter, bladder (KUB), flat plate film	Abdominal radiograph	Normal abdominal structures	Diagnoses renal stones; done before renal studies	No discomfort
Cystoscopy				
	Bladder and urethra examined with cystoscope—a tubular, lighted, telescopic lens	Normal appearance	Examination of bladder and lower tract; visualization of tumor and stones; removal of small stones; biopsy of bladder or tumors; fulguration of bladder tumors and posterior urethral valves	Usually performed with child under general anesthesia; little pain involved; encourage fluids; assess ability to void after procedure

BUN, blood urea nitrogen; *RBC,* red blood cell.

Continued

COMMON LABORATORY AND DIAGNOSTIC TESTS FOR GENITOURINARY DISORDERS—cont'd

TEST	DESCRIPTION	NORMAL FINDINGS	INDICATIONS	NURSING CONSIDERATIONS
Imaging Studies				
CT scan	Computerized calculations revealing a pattern of shades	Normal appearance	Renal tumors	Sedation may be required; child lies on back and should be still; oral contrast material may be administered; child is usually on NPO status because of sedation or oral contrast material
Voiding cystourethrogram (VCUG)	Contrast dye instilled in bladder; child or infant voids after bladder is full; serial films taken	Negative for reflux and dilation of posterior urethra, complete bladder emptying	Detects reflux of urine into ureters and its severity; detects bladder emptying problems; detects urethral problems	Can be done in nuclear medicine department to decrease radiation exposure; procedure is invasive; provide support and diversionary activities for child
Dimercapto-succinic acid (DMSA) renal scan	Injection of radioactive agent technetium-99m (^{99m}Tc)-DMSA to allow visualization of kidney structures and function; serial films taken	Prompt uptake and excretion of radioactive agent	Evaluates blood flow and renal function; assesses renal scarring; identifies pyelonephritis	Minimal radiation exposure; child must remain still for procedure
Renal ultrasonography	Noninvasive; high-frequency sound waves directed at kidneys, ureters, and bladder	Normal size, shape, position, function of kidneys	Assesses position, size, and contour of kidneys, ureters, bladder; detects obstruction and stones; localizes for renal biopsy	Child lies on abdomen; if for transplanted kidney, child lies on back
Urodynamic Studies				
	Invasive test involving urethral and rectal catheters and perineal surface electrodes; measures urine flow, bladder capacity, sensation, sphincter function, bladder pressures; measures voluntary and involuntary contractions	Normal bladder function	Voiding dysfunction, abnormal urinary tract	Inform child and family of procedure; provide support for child throughout procedure; provide diversionary activities

CT, computed tomography; *NPO,* nothing by mouth.

ENURESIS

Children with difficulties in urinary control are defined as having *enuresis.* Nocturnal enuresis occurs at nighttime during sleep, whereas diurnal enuresis occurs during the day, or in waking hours. *Primary enuresis* is defined as a child never having experienced a period of dryness, whereas *secondary enuresis* occurs when a 6- to 12-month period of dryness has preceded the onset of wetting.

Etiology

Although there is no single cause for enuresis, several risk factors have been implicated. Physical factors include decreased bladder capacity, underlying urinary tract abnormalities, neurologic alterations, obstructive sleep apnea, constipation, UTI, pinworm infestation, diabetes mellitus, and voiding dysfunction. Emotional factors related to increased stress can contribute to secondary enuresis. These factors include family disruption, inappropriate pressure during toilet training, inadequate attention to voiding cues, and decreased self-esteem. Sexual abuse must be considered in a child with secondary enuresis.

Incidence

Primary nocturnal enuresis is common, affecting approximately 15% to 20% of children at 5 years of age and decreasing spontaneously thereafter (Elder, 2011f). It occurs more frequently in boys and in children with a family history of bed-wetting. Most children eventually outgrow bed-wetting without therapeutic intervention. Some children have diurnal (daytime) enuresis without nocturnal enuresis. Waiting until the last minute to void and not being able to access a bathroom quickly may be a factor in diurnal enuresis, but the main cause is an overactive bladder, a condition in which the child experiences bladder spasms or increased urgency (Elder, 2011f). Primary enuresis often resolves spontaneously.

PATHOPHYSIOLOGY

Enuresis

Control of urination is related to the maturity of the central nervous system. By 5 years of age, most children are aware of bladder fullness and are able to voluntarily control voiding. Children usually achieve daytime urinary control first, with nighttime dryness occurring later. Girls seem to master this earlier than boys. Children who have primary nocturnal enuresis may have delayed maturation of this portion of the central nervous system.

A child with secondary nocturnal enuresis or with problems of daytime control and complaints of dysuria, urgency, or frequency should be evaluated for other conditions. Bladder infections can give rise to such symptoms. Excessive calcium loss in the urine can irritate the bladder and cause painful urination, urgency, frequency, or wetting. Secondary enuresis accompanied by excessive thirst and weight loss may indicate the onset of diabetes mellitus. Children whose bladders are very sensitive to urine volume may have uninhibited bladder contractions. Moderate to large amounts of urine in the bladder give rise to strong contractions of the bladder muscle. An anatomic abnormality in these cases is rare.

Manifestations

Nocturnal Enuresis

Children with a continuing history of bed-wetting are not able to sense bladder fullness and do not awaken to void. Because physical maturation varies, nocturnal enuresis is not a matter for excessive concern unless the child is older than 6 years or has markedly decreased self-esteem.

Diurnal Enuresis

Children with urgency, frequency, and inappropriate wetting during the day may be seen rushing to the bathroom or tightly crossing their legs. Often these children cannot sit still and they exhibit a constant odor of urine.

Diagnostic Evaluation

The diagnosis of enuresis is based on the history and clinical symptoms. Urinalysis and urine culture can rule out possible UTI. Urine specific gravity and glucose measurement test for underlying diabetes. In addition, the child's urine should be checked for excessive calcium, and a pinworm evaluation should be done to exclude infestation.

If the child has daytime enuresis, voiding dysfunction with urge incontinence is explored. Measures of urine flow and bladder capacity and bladder ultrasonography may be indicated. Children with UTIs should have a workup for underlying structural abnormalities.

Therapeutic Management

Treatment of primary nocturnal enuresis may begin with general interventions, such as explaining theories underlying the problem in terms the child can understand. The child is reassured that, with assistance, the problem can resolve. Commonsense approaches of limiting fluids after supper and voiding just before bedtime are encouraged. Diet modifications include avoiding extraneous sugar and caffeine intake after 4 PM, because these can act as bladder stimulants as well as diuretics (Elder, 2011f). Also, the child can be trained to use imagery: thinking about what a full bladder feels like and picturing waking up and going to the bathroom. This imagery is done as the child lies in bed before drifting off to sleep. The child should keep a record of the number of dry and wet nights to measure progress.

Reward systems assume that bed-wetting is a voluntary behavior and have had varying results for the child with primary nocturnal enuresis. The child may be given a roll of favorite stickers to mark the dry nights on the calendar. The family decides on a special reward or outing when the child has achieved a certain number of consecutive dry nights.

Behavioral conditioning with use of alarms has been successful in the older child with nocturnal enuresis. A device worn on the child's pajamas contains a moisture-sensitive alarm. As the child starts to void, the alarm goes off, awakening the child. The alarm system may need to be used consistently over 15 weeks for resolution.

Desmopressin acetate (1-deamino-8-D-arginine vasopressin [DDAVP]) has also been helpful because of its antidiuretic effect. Desmopressin acetate is given as a tablet and is taken at bedtime. Pharmacologic treatment is not recommended for children under 6 years of age.

Voiding frequently to keep urine volume in the bladder low may benefit children who are affected by uninhibited bladder contractions during the day. The use of an anticholinergic such as oxybutynin chloride, which relaxes the smooth muscle of the bladder, can be helpful for children with diurnal enuresis related to underlying bladder instability or small bladder capacity. Biofeedback may also help children with diurnal enuresis, particularly those with dysfunctional voiding.

NURSING CARE OF THE CHILD WITH ENURESIS

■ Assessment

The nurse should obtain a full set of vital signs and assess the child and parent for their understanding of enuresis, including the interventions they have already tried. The nurse asks the child and parent to describe voiding and bowel elimination patterns, establishing whether the enuresis is primary or secondary. The nurse should also ask whether the child participates in social activities with peers, such as sleepovers, and whether the child is concerned about the problem of wetting. Therapy is much more successful for the older child than for the younger child, who may not be bothered by bed-wetting. The nurse should assist the child in obtaining a urine specimen. The physical examination includes assessment for signs of sexual abuse or visible genital abnormalities. It also is important to observe the lower spine for the presence of a dimple or hair tuft that might suggest spina bifida occulta (see Chapter 28).

■ Nursing Diagnosis and Planning

The nursing diagnoses and expected outcomes that may be appropriate after assessment of the child with enuresis are as follows:

- Situational Low Self-Esteem related to bed-wetting or urinary incontinence.

Expected Outcome. The child will demonstrate positive self-esteem, as evidenced by a realistic description of the problem and positive self-statements.

- Impaired Social Interaction related to bed-wetting or urinary incontinence.

Expected Outcome. The child will participate in age-appropriate activities such as sleepovers and overnight camp.

- Compromised Family Coping related to negative social stigma and increased laundry load.

Expected Outcomes. The family will identify strengths and will describe positive problem-solving strategies.

- Risk for Impaired Skin Integrity related to prolonged contact with urine.

Expected Outcome. The child will have no rashes or redness in the perineal area.

■ Interventions

Enuresis can be a frustrating problem for both the child and family. The nurse can help by providing them with correct information about causes and therapeutic approaches. It is important that the family choose the treatment that will best meet its needs. Follow-up to determine the effectiveness of treatment is essential because becoming dry can be a long process, and the nurse is instrumental in providing support to the child and family over the entire course of therapy.

■ Evaluation

• Is the child able to describe ways to manage the condition?
• Is the child verbalizing a decrease in stress related to the enuresis, and does the child make positive self-statements?
• Is the child showing an increased interest in peer activities?
• Is the family able to identify its strengths and demonstrate appropriate problem solving?
• Is the child having increased dry nights?
• Does the child's skin remain intact and is it free from redness and rashes?

? CRITICAL THINKING EXERCISE 20-1

Mr. Sampson brings his son, Thomas, in for his 5-year-old well-child visit. As the nurse is obtaining a history, Mr. Sampson expresses concern that Thomas wets the bed at night. He has been fully toilet trained for 1 year and does not have daytime urine accidents. Thomas refuses to wear a diaper at night because he "doesn't want to be a baby." As a result, he consistently sleeps in wet sheets and clothing.
1. What additional data would be helpful to obtain from Mr. Sampson?
2. What suggestions for an initial approach to the problem should the nurse give Mr. Sampson?

URINARY TRACT INFECTIONS

Urinary tract infections (UTIs), which are characterized by the presence of bacteria in the urine along with systemic signs of infection, are commonly seen in children. In fact, UTIs result in significant morbidity in infants and children. These infections can have long-term complications that include renal scarring with decreased renal function, high blood pressure, and, rarely, end-stage renal disease.

Etiology

UTIs, except in newborn infants, are caused by bacteria ascending from outside the urethra into the bladder and from there into the upper urinary tract. Bacteria in the blood, which seed in the kidney, can cause UTIs in newborn infants.

Fecal bacteria cause most UTIs. *Escherichia coli* are the bacteria implicated in 75% to 90% of all UTIs in girls (Elder, 2011d). Other bacteria known to cause UTIs are group B streptococci, *Klebsiella pneumoniae*, *Proteus* species, *Enterobacter* species, enterococci, and *Staphylococcus* species. Viruses and fungi, specifically *Candida* species, can rarely cause infections.

The following conditions predispose the infant or child to UTI:
• *Urinary tract obstructions, which can be congenital or acquired.* These include strictures, ureteropelvic narrowing, or other urinary tract anomalies. *Hydronephrosis* is dilation of the renal pelvis, usually caused by ureteropelvic junction obstruction.

Phimosis, which is a narrowing of the prepuce opening, prevents the foreskin from being retracted.
• *Voiding dysfunction resulting in urinary stasis.* Conditions contributing to incomplete bladder emptying include neurogenic bladder and bladder instability. Constipation that causes pressure on the bladder can inhibit complete bladder emptying.
• *Anatomic differences.* Young girls have a short urethra, which expedites bacterial transit.
• *Individual susceptibility to infection.* Some infants and children have UTIs without any structural abnormality and may be more prone to bacterial adherence to epithelial cells in the urinary tract.
• *Reflux.* A primary contributing factor to upper UTI, or pyelonephritis, is vesicoureteral reflux (VUR).
• UTIs in toddler-age girls are more frequent during toilet training, most probably as a result of urinary retention or incomplete bladder emptying (Elder, 2011d). It is generally accepted, however, that bacterial colonization of the prepuce of uncircumcised infants can increase the risk of UTI in infant boys younger than 1 year.
• Sexually active adolescent girls are at risk for UTIs.

Incidence

The overall prevalence of UTIs in the United States is 3% to 5% in girls and 1% in boys. In girls, the first UTI generally occurs before 5 years of age with an increase in the number of cases seen during infancy and toilet training. For boys, most UTIs occur during the first year of life with a higher incidence in uncircumcised infants (Elder, 2011d). Symptoms of a UTI may be missed in children with coexisting gastrointestinal or respiratory symptoms, so UTI should be considered as a cause in any child with significant illness, especially if febrile (National Institute for Health and Clinical Excellence [NICE], 2007). It is important to diagnose UTIs quickly, as an ascending UTI can result in renal scarring. VUR is a frequently seen underlying anatomic abnormality in children with UTIs.

UTIs are more prevalent in white, Asian, and Hispanic children and less prevalent in African-American children (Shaikh, Morone, Lopez et al., 2007). Breastfeeding has been found to significantly reduce the risk of UTIs in both boys and girls because of the protective factors observed in human milk that prevent microbial attachment to the mucosa (Marild, Hansson, Jodal et al., 2004).

PATHOPHYSIOLOGY
Urinary Tract Infections

Fecal bacteria colonize the perineal area or under the prepuce of uncircumcised infant boys. Bacteria adhere to epithelial cells in the urinary tract and then ascend through the urethra into the bladder, causing a bladder infection, or *cystitis*. In most circumstances, the bladder is emptied on a regular basis, which decreases the opportunity for bacterial growth. In children with incomplete bladder emptying, bacteria grow in the residual urine.

Bacteria ascending from the bladder into the ureters and up into the renal parenchyma cause pyelonephritis. Pyelonephritis is more frequently seen in children with VUR but can occur in its absence.

Scarring, as an inflammatory consequence of pyelonephritis, is more frequently seen in infants younger than 1 year and is a significant cause of hypertension during childhood. Scarring causes decreased arterial perfusion to the kidney, mimicking volume depletion. This triggers the renin-angiotensin mechanism to increase aldosterone release and cause sodium and fluid retention. The subsequent increase in circulating blood volume results in hypertension.

Manifestations

Clinical manifestations of UTI vary widely; factors include the child's age, sex, underlying anatomic or neurologic abnormalities, and frequency of recurrence. Signs in the young child and infant are more vague and nonspecific. Fever (100.4° F [38° C]) without a known focus for infection in infants and young children 2 to 24 months of age suggests a UTI. Suprapubic tenderness may be an accompanying sign in an infant. Signs and symptoms in a verbal child include abdominal pain, frequency, urgency, and dysuria (Shaikh et al., 2007).

An abdominal mass can suggest hydronephrosis in an infant (Elder, 2011c). Other signs and symptoms of hydronephrosis are similar to those for an infant with a UTI (Box 20-1).

Diagnostic Evaluation

Bacteria in the urine establish a diagnosis of UTI. Symptoms of UTI in the absence of bacteriuria can be caused by perineal inflammation, vaginitis, pinworms, or chemical irritation from bubble baths.

Routine urinalysis that demonstrates hematuria, presence of white blood cells (WBCs), and positive nitrites can suggest a UTI. Urinalysis should be performed on a first morning urine specimen to be most accurate.

Urine culture is the single determining diagnostic study for a UTI. Any bacterial growth of a single-strain bacterium exceeding 100,000 colony-forming units/mL in a clean-catch urine specimen establishes a diagnosis of UTI. Obtaining a sterile urine sample is difficult in

PATHOPHYSIOLOGY

Vesicoureteral Reflux

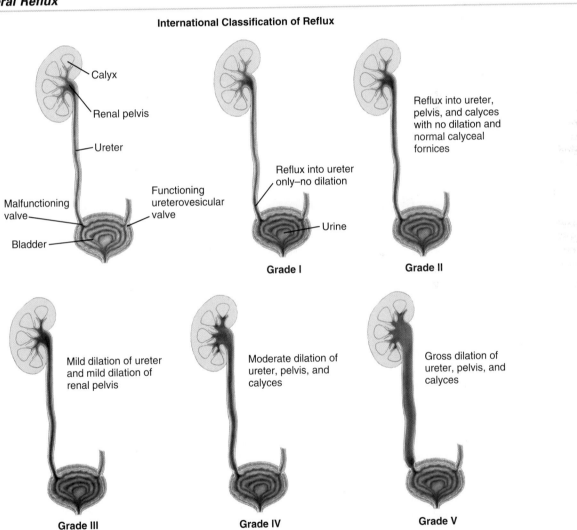

International Classification of Reflux

Calyx

Renal pelvis

Ureter

Malfunctioning valve

Functioning ureterovesicular valve

Bladder

Reflux into ureter only—no dilation

Urine

Grade I

Reflux into ureter, pelvis, and calyces with no dilation and normal calyceal fornices

Grade II

Mild dilation of ureter and mild dilation of renal pelvis

Grade III

Moderate dilation of ureter, pelvis, and calyces

Grade IV

Gross dilation of ureter, pelvis, and calyces

Grade V

A valvelike mechanism at the junction of the ureter and bladder prevents urine reflux into the ureters. As urine fills the bladder or as the bladder contracts during voiding, pressure in the bladder occludes the opening to the ureter. When a defect occurs at the vesicoureteral junction, vesicoureteral reflux (VUR) results. The defect at the vesicoureteral junction is considered a congenital abnormality, although transitory VUR associated with a lower UTI is also possible.

In VUR, two mechanisms contribute to the development of UTIs. Bacteria in the urine can be carried up to the kidney, causing pyelonephritis and renal damage with scarring. Also, when urine reflux into the lower ureter occurs, urine can return to the bladder, leaving urine residual that becomes a medium for bacterial growth.

The severity of VUR determines the potential risk for pyelonephritis and kidney damage. The International Classification of Reflux grades reflux on a scale of I through V. Grade I is described as reflux into the ureter only with no dilation. Grade V, the most severe, includes gross dilation of ureter, pelvis, and calyces and reflux involving the kidney.

BOX 20-1 MANIFESTATIONS OF URINARY TRACT INFECTION IN INFANTS AND CHILDREN

Infants
- Nonspecific
- Fever or hypothermia in neonate
- Irritability
- Dysuria as evidenced by crying when voiding
- Change in urine odor or color
- Poor weight gain
- Feeding difficulties

Children
- Abdominal or suprapubic pain
- Voiding frequency
- Voiding urgency
- Dysuria
- New or increased incidence of enuresis
- Fever

Children with Pyelonephritis
Same symptoms as for children with uncomplicated UTI plus:
- High fever, chills
- Back pain
- Costovertebral angle tenderness
- Nausea and vomiting
- Appears very ill

PATHOPHYSIOLOGY

Hydronephrosis

Obstruction at the ureteropelvic junction or other parts of the ureter causes dilation of the kidney. As the renal dilation increases, the risk of renal parenchymal damage and decreased renal function increases as well. In some instances, the obstruction is only partial, causing an initial dilation but no progressive renal function loss. Hydronephrosis can be associated with VUR.

Ultrasonography has facilitated prenatal diagnosis of hydronephrosis.* Since urinary tract obstruction is often silent, following birth, these infants need a complete evaluation including imaging studies.*

*Elder, J. (2011). Obstructions of the urinary tract. In R. Kliegman, B. Stanton, J. St. Geme, et al. (Eds.), *Nelson textbook of pediatrics* (19th ed., pp. 1838-1847). Philadelphia: Elsevier Saunders.

children, especially children who are not yet toilet trained. A child who can void on demand can provide a midstream clean-catch urine specimen. In infants and children who are not toilet trained, a sterile pediatric urine collection bag attached to the perineum can collect a urine specimen (see Chapter 13). Collecting urine by this method is less invasive but is clearly not as accurate for obtaining a culture as by other methods, and the urine specimen must be plated as quickly as possible. If the urine cannot be plated within 10 minutes of collection, it should be refrigerated.

When accurate determination of bacteria is the goal, more intrusive methods of bladder catheterization (see Chapter 13) or suprapubic aspiration are the collection methods of choice. If suprapubic aspiration is necessary, the area above the pubis is cleaned with an antiseptic solution, a needle attached to a syringe is inserted by the physician at a 90-degree angle into the bladder, and urine is aspirated. If

catheterization or suprapubic aspiration is used to obtain a urine culture, the growth of any bacteria indicates infection.

More intensive evaluation for underlying structural abnormalities is necessary for certain infants and children with UTIs. Evaluative studies include ultrasonography to detect kidney dilation resulting from obstruction and a voiding cystourethrography or radionuclide cystography to detect VUR.

Therapeutic Management

A 3- to 5-day course of oral antibiotics is the treatment of choice for an uncomplicated UTI without systemic symptoms (Elder, 2011d). The antibiotic should be one to which the specific bacterium (identified by culture) is sensitive, should be easily administered, and should have minimal adverse effects. Oral trimethoprim-sulfamethoxazole, nitrofurantoin, and cephalosporins are frequently used.

Children with pyelonephritis often require initial treatment with parenteral antibiotics followed by oral antibiotic treatment. The older child who does not need hospitalization can receive daily intramuscular ceftriaxone for 1 to 2 days, followed by 10 to 14 days of oral antibiotics. Infants and children hospitalized for treatment usually receive IV ampicillin and a cephalosporin or an aminoglycoside (e.g., gentamicin). Some children are treated with a cephalosporin alone. Oral antibiotics may follow this initial treatment with parenteral antibiotics.

When anatomic abnormalities are detected or UTIs recur, prophylactic antibiotic therapy might be initiated, although recent studies suggest that the risk for antibiotic resistance may be higher than the therapeutic value of prophylaxis (Agency for Healthcare Research and Quality, 2008). Prophylactic antibiotics are sometimes given to children after their initial course of treatment while they are waiting for imaging studies to confirm an underlying structural abnormality.

Because the majority of children with grades I through III VUR have a spontaneous resolution of the reflux, most physicians choose nonsurgical management of this condition (Elder, 2011e). Children are often given prophylactic antibiotics, although this has become controversial (Montini, Rigon, Zucchetta et al., 2008), and screened for UTI every 2 to 4 months and when febrile. A voiding cystourethrogram (VCUG) is performed every 12 to 18 months to monitor resolution of reflux (Elder, 2011e).

First-line surgical treatment for children with persistent grade I through III VUR is the endoscopic injection of bulking material into the submucosa of the affected ureter. The material, Deflux injectable gel, builds a protective wall inside the ureter to prevent the backflow of urine. Open surgical repair, reimplantation of the ureter into the bladder, is indicated for children who continue to have reflux and breakthrough UTIs despite antibiotic therapy, severe grade IV or V reflux, or two or three failed Deflux treatments (Elder, 2011e).

NURSING CARE OF THE CHILD WITH A URINARY TRACT INFECTION

▪ Assessment

The nurse obtains a history from the child and family inquiring about age-specific signs and symptoms of UTI. Determining bowel elimination patterns is important as well, because constipation can increase the risk for UTI in certain children.

Physical assessment includes temperature, blood pressure, abdominal examination for masses, examination for costovertebral angle tenderness, and examination for genital abnormalities. It is important to obtain a urinalysis and urine culture before initiating antibiotics.

■ Nursing Diagnosis and Planning

The nursing diagnoses and expected outcomes that apply to the child with a UTI and the child's family are as follows:

- Risk for Injury to the kidney related to complications from the infectious process.

Expected Outcome. The child will be free of recurrent UTIs, as evidenced by the absence of voiding frequency and urgency, dysuria, and fever and the presence of a negative urine culture.

- Deficient Fluid Volume related to decreased intake and increased fluid loss from fever.

Expected Outcome. The child will maintain adequate intake of fluids and electrolytes for age, as evidenced by an output normal for age (see Chapter 16).

- Deficient Knowledge related to incomplete understanding of the disease process, diagnostic tests, antibiotic administration, and preventive measures for UTI.

Expected Outcomes. The parent or child will explain the disease process, diagnostic tests, and preventive measures for UTIs. The family will follow through with appropriate follow-up care, including antibiotic administration and imaging studies, if recommended.

■ Interventions

Infants admitted to the hospital with fever of unknown source often are evaluated to rule out a focal infection or septicemia, as well as UTI, which is one of the most frequent causes of fever in infants. The evaluation includes blood studies and cultures, lumbar puncture, and urinary catheterization or suprapubic aspiration for urine culture. The parent already is anxious about the infant, so it is imperative that the nurse inform the parent about why procedures are being done. An IV line is established at the time of the workup because parenteral antibiotics are given while waiting for laboratory results and for several days thereafter if the child has a UTI.

The nurse encourages the parents to express concerns, and provides reassurance about the infant's condition. Every effort should be made to maintain the infant's routine; the mother continues to breastfeed, ensuring that the IV site is protected as she holds the infant. If the breastfeeding mother is unable to remain with the infant, she will need to pump her breasts. Allowing parents to participate in the infant's care provides them a measure of control in an uncertain situation. The infant with a documented UTI will require renal ultrasonography at the earliest convenient time.

Nursing care of the child who is not hospitalized includes ensuring administration of antibiotics, promoting comfort, maintaining good hydration, preparing the child and parent for diagnostic procedures, and monitoring for responses to treatment and possible complications.

The child and family are educated about the prevention of UTIs (see the Patient-Centered Teaching: How to Manage and Prevent Urinary Tract Infections box). The nurse emphasizes the importance of adhering to the treatment regimen and obtaining follow-up studies. Because repeated UTIs can contribute to renal damage, prevention is critically important. For older children, once-daily antibiotics are best administered at bedtime because of urinary stasis during the night.

Good hydration is essential for the child with a UTI, especially if the child has been febrile, nauseated, vomiting, or feeding poorly. The nurse encourages oral fluid intake, if possible. IV hydration may be required, especially for young infants. The child must be observed for signs of dehydration: poor skin turgor, dry mucous membranes, a sunken fontanel, decreased output, and decreased peripheral perfusion. Daily weights, intake and output measurements, and urine specific gravity are indicators of the child's hydration status.

PATIENT-CENTERED TEACHING

How to Manage and Prevent Urinary Tract Infections

If your child has been diagnosed with a urinary tract infection, it is most important for you to do the following:

- Give your child the prescribed medication for the full number of days your physician or nurse practitioner recommends. Some children need to continue on a lower dose of the antibiotic after the initial treatment is finished.
- Take a follow-up urine culture to the laboratory if your physician or nurse practitioner has requested one. Use a sterile container to collect the urine. If the laboratory has not given you a sterile plastic container, you can use a glass container and a cover that have been sterilized. Make sure the urine stays refrigerated or in a cooler while you take it to the laboratory.
- Keep the appointment for follow-up studies of your child's urinary system, if ordered by the physician or nurse practitioner. These studies can help diagnose a structural problem with your child's urinary system or monitor the kidneys for any problems.
- Call your physician or nurse practitioner if your child has a fever or symptoms that make you think the infection has returned.

Preventing a urinary tract infection from recurring is important because repeated infections can cause kidney damage. Some suggestions that can help prevent a urinary tract infection are as follows:

- Wipe babies and teach young girls to wipe from front to back after going to the bathroom. This takes any germs away from the opening that leads into the urinary system. Be sure to keep the foreskin on uncircumcised baby boys as clean as possible without forcible retraction.
- Encourage your toilet-trained child to avoid "holding" urine and to urinate at least four times per day, emptying the bladder completely.
- Give your child lots of fluids throughout the day to help flush out the bladder.
- Avoid dressing your child in tight clothing or diapers. Use cotton underwear, rather than synthetic fabric.
- Avoid bubble baths, which can irritate your child's urinary system.
- Emphasize proper hygiene if your daughter is sexually active and encourage her to urinate immediately after having sexual intercourse.

For children with VUR, the nurse explains the treatment plan, including medical or surgical management, to the parent and child in a simple, age-appropriate manner. If medical management with antibiotic therapy is elected, both parents and the child should understand that treatment may last for years and that adherence is imperative. Follow-up includes urine cultures, renal function tests (blood urea nitrogen [BUN], serum creatinine), blood pressure monitoring, and imaging studies.

If surgical treatment is required, the parents and child are given information regarding the procedure and preoperative and postoperative care. They need to understand that inpatient hospitalization is required. Medications are given for pain and bladder spasms, which frequently occur after surgery. Postsurgical care involves administering prophylactic antibiotics until a cystogram is performed and indicates that the VUR has been corrected.

■ Evaluation

- Is the child free of frequency, urgency, and dysuria?
- Is the urine culture negative?
- Is the child taking fluids in amounts expected for age?
- Is the child's urine output adequate (see Chapter 16)?

- Has the child continued on the prescribed antibiotic therapy regimen?
- Has the child received follow-up diagnostic testing and antibiotic therapy?
- Can the parent or child describe symptoms of recurrence and measures to take if infection occurs?

⚠ NURSING QUALITY ALERT

Evaluation after a Documented Urinary Tract Infection

Radiologic studies are indicated for infants and children who are likely to have renal damage associated with structural abnormalities. Studies can diagnose underlying abnormalities and monitor the extent of potential renal scarring. The following are recommended follow-up studies and evaluations:

- Radiographic imaging studies for at-risk infants and children (all boys with UTIs and all girls younger than 5 years) after the first UTI. Evaluation of older girls with recurrent UTIs.
- Renal ultrasonography before discharge in all infants and children hospitalized for treatment of a febrile UTI or suspected pyelonephritis.
- VCUG or isotope cystogram for at-risk children when symptoms have disappeared and the urine culture is negative. Some practitioners prefer to wait 4 to 6 weeks after the resolution of the UTI to allow transitory VUR to resolve.
- Renal scan for children diagnosed with VUR and children with suspected pyelonephritis.
- Comprehensive evaluation of children after the first UTI who have hypertension, who have a family history of urinary tract abnormalities, or who exhibit delayed growth.

CRYPTORCHIDISM

Cryptorchidism (undescended or hidden testes) occurs when one or both testes fail to descend through the inguinal canal into the scrotal sac.

Incidence

Congenital cryptorchidism is a common urologic problem, with approximately 4.5% of normal, healthy boys having at least one undescended testis discovered at birth (Elder, 2011b). Premature male infants have a significantly higher incidence at 30% (Elder, 2011b). Cryptorchidism is also seen more frequently in low-birth-weight or smaller-than-average-length newborns (Acerini, Miles, Dunger et al., 2009). Most infants have spontaneous descent of their testes during the first 6 months of life. An increased incidence of acquired (ascending) undescended testes (testes descended at birth no longer remain in the scrotal sac) is being seen in boys ages 4 to 10 years (Acerini et al., 2009; Elder, 2011b).

Manifestations

Testes that are not palpable or not easily guided into the scrotum and a previously descended testis that ascends into an extrascrotal position are manifestations of cryptorchidism. Children with undescended testes are at increased risk for testicular malignancy and infertility (Elder, 2011b).

Diagnostic Evaluation

One or both testes may be undescended. If the testis is not palpable, in some instances ultrasonography, computed tomography scan, or magnetic resonance imaging can determine its location. The missing

---

PATHOPHYSIOLOGY

Cryptorchidism

In normal fetal development, the testes begin their descent from the abdomen between 32 and 36 weeks of gestation. The exact reason for failure of the testes to descend is not known. Factors including maternal hormones, genetics, prematurity, and low-birth-weight or length influence the prevalence of undescended testicles.*† Sperm production is decreased in the undescended testis, and there is increased risk for development of a malignancy when the child reaches adulthood. Inguinal hernias are commonly associated with cryptorchidism.

*Ashley, R., Barthold, J., & Kolon, T. (2010). Cryptorchidism: Pathogenesis, diagnosis, treatment, and prognosis. *Urologic Clinics of North America, 37*(2), 183-193.
†Elder, J. (2011). Disorders and anomalies of the scrotal contents. In R. Kliegman, B. Stanton, J. St. Geme, et al. (Eds.), *Nelson textbook of pediatrics* (19th ed., pp. 1858-1864). Philadelphia: Elsevier Saunders.

testis may be found at any point along the process vaginalis, may be located in the abdomen, or may follow an aberrant course and come to lie in the inguinal area, base of the penis, or perineum.

Location of an intraabdominal testis may require surgical exploration by laparoscopy; an orchiopexy can be performed at the same time, if appropriate (Elder, 2011b). When neither testis can be palpated, the child may be evaluated for their presence by hormonal stimulation and measurement of testosterone response. Elevated follicle-stimulating hormone and luteinizing hormone levels accompanied by absent testosterone indicate testicular absence. True absence of both testes is rare.

Therapeutic Management

Initially, the infant with cryptorchidism is managed by observation because spontaneous descent of the testes during the first 6 months of life is common. If the condition persists, an orchiopexy is performed to bring the testis down into the scrotal sac and suture it in place. This surgery is typically done on an outpatient basis using a laparoscopic approach (Ashley et al., 2010). The most common complications are bleeding and infection. The optimal time for surgery is controversial; it is performed with increased frequency at age 6 months, and no later than age 9 to 15 months (Elder, 2011b). The purpose is to reduce the risk of infertility and malignancy (Ashley et al., 2010) as well as provide a normal-appearing scrotum. It is important for the adolescent male to perform testicular self-examinations throughout his life to screen for malignancy.

▌ NURSING CARE OF THE CHILD WITH CRYPTORCHIDISM

■ Assessment

Absence of the testis in the scrotal sac can be discovered through routine physical examination of the newborn. The nurse also must assess the parents' knowledge of undescended testes and the importance of treatment.

■ Nursing Diagnosis and Planning

The nursing diagnoses and expected outcomes that apply to the child with cryptorchidism and the child's family are as follows:

- Deficient Knowledge (parental) related to cause and management of cryptorchidism.

! NURSING QUALITY ALERT

Assessing for Cryptorchidism

Testes can retract into the inguinal canal if the infant is upset or cold. The cremasteric reflex, testicular retraction in response to tactile stimulation to the front inner thigh, can lead to a false diagnosis of cryptorchidism.

- Examine the infant in a warm environment. Be sure the infant is calm before the examination.
- Warm your hands before touching the infant.
- Milk each testis downward from the groin and document its distal point.
- Examine the older child in both a sitting and a frog-leg position (see Chapter 13).
- Most testes descend by the time the infant is 1 year old.

Expected Outcome. The parents will be able to explain cryptorchidism, its management, and possible sequelae.

- Risk for Ineffective Health Maintenance related to possible decreased fertility and increased risk of testicular malignancy.

Expected Outcomes. The parents will help the child learn to perform regular testicular self-examination during adolescence, and the individual will seek referral for fertility testing as warranted.

■ Interventions

Nursing care should be directed at educating parents and providing them with information and resources. If the child has bilateral undescended testes or absence of testes, referrals to a counselor, psychologist, or specialist may be appropriate. The nurse provides routine postoperative care after orchiopexy, monitoring the child's voiding patterns, pain level, and swelling, and observing for signs of bleeding or infection.

■ Evaluation

- Are the parents able to explain cryptorchidism and its management?
- Do the parents state their responsibilities to guide their child when he is an adolescent to perform regular testicular self-examination and to seek fertility testing if appropriate?

HYPOSPADIAS AND EPISPADIAS

Hypospadias is a congenital anomaly in which the actual opening of the urethral meatus is below the normal placement on the glans of the penis (Figure 20-1). The degree of misplacement of the urethral opening can vary. The urethra may open only slightly ventral to the glans or as far back as the penoscrotal junction. *Chordee,* or downward curvature of the penile shaft, is usually seen in more severe forms of hypospadias. Associated anomalies may include undescended testes and inguinal hernias. Dorsal placement of the urethral opening, or epispadias, also may occur but is less common.

Etiology and Incidence

Hypospadias is one of the most common congenital anomalies, occurring in 1 of every 250 male children (Elder, 2011a). Risk is increased if either the father or a sibling has the anomaly. Other contributing factors include maternal age over 35 years, intrauterine exposure to environmental chemicals, and possible genetic mutation (Elder, 2011a). Testes are undescended in 10% of affected children, and risk for inguinal hernias is increased. Epispadias is extremely rare and is often associated with bladder exstrophy.

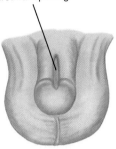
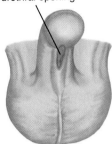

Dorsal placement of urethral opening

Ventral placement of urethral opening

Epispadias   **Hypospadias**

FIG 20-1 Epispadias and hypospadias are congenital anomalies in which the urethral opening is above or below its normal location on the glans of the penis. Stenosis of the opening could occur, leading to possible UTIs or hydronephrosis. Hypospadias might interfere with fertility if it is left uncorrected.

PATHOPHYSIOLOGY

Hypospadias

Hypospadias occurs from incomplete development of the urethra in utero. The exact cause of the defect is not known, but it is thought to be related to genetic, environmental, and hormonal influences.*

The displacement of the urethral meatus does not usually interfere with urinary continence. Stenosis of the opening, however, would give rise to partial obstruction of outflowing urine. Further, ventral placement of the urethral opening might interfere with fertility in the mature man if it is left uncorrected.

*Elder, J. (2011). Anomalies of the penis and urethra. In R. Kliegman, B. Stanton, J. St. Geme, et al. (Eds.), *Nelson textbook of pediatrics* (19th ed., pp. 1852-1858). Philadelphia: Elsevier Saunders.

Manifestations and Diagnostic Evaluation

Ventral placement of the urethral opening, altered urinary stream, and chordee are physical manifestations of hypospadias. A defect on the topside of the penis is indicative of epispadias and the appearance of lower urinary tract structures outside the abdominal wall is seen with bladder exstrophy. Diagnosis is based on physical examination.

Therapeutic Management

Correction of hypospadias is accomplished by surgical intervention, which is usually done in one stage and on an outpatient basis. The surgeon releases the chordee, lengthens the urethra, positions the meatus at the penile tip, and reconstructs the penis. The surgical procedure should be done before the age of toilet training because the location of the meatus may make it difficult for the child to urinate standing up. Surgery is ideally done when the child is between 6 and 12 months of age (Elder, 2011a). Infants with hypospadias should not be circumcised because the foreskin may be used in the surgical reconstruction. After surgery, the child may have some type of temporary urinary diversion to allow for healing of the meatus. Indwelling urinary catheters or urethral stents are commonly used. In addition, the child's activity must be restricted for several days. These treatments are tolerated better by the younger child. The goal of surgery is to make urinary and sexual function as normal as possible and to improve the cosmetic appearance of the penis.

Surgical correction of epispadias can include bladder neck reconstruction and lengthening of the penis and urethra. If bladder exstrophy is present, surgical correction is more complex and may be performed in multiple stages; ongoing management of the urinary drainage system is required.

NURSING CARE OF THE CHILD WITH HYPOSPADIAS

■ Assessment

Hypospadias is usually discovered during the newborn examination. In the infant with hypospadias, the abdomen is palpated for a distended bladder or enlarged kidneys. The urinary stream should be observed, if possible. For the older infant with hypospadias, the parents are asked about UTIs, quality of urinary stream (whether it is steady or intermittent), dribbling, or family history of genitourinary problems. The nurse assesses the parents' understanding of hypospadias and the surgical procedure and follow-up care necessary for correction.

■ Nursing Diagnosis and Planning

The nursing diagnoses and expected outcomes that apply to the child with hypospadias and the child's family are as follows:

- Deficient Knowledge (parental) related to diagnosis of hypospadias, surgical procedure, and postoperative care.

Expected Outcomes. The parents will describe hypospadias and the reason for surgical correction. The parents will actively participate in the postoperative care.

- Risk for Infection related to indwelling catheter.

Expected Outcome. The child will remain free of UTI, as evidenced by normal urinalysis and culture and absence of fever.

- Acute Pain related to surgery.

Expected Outcomes. The child will exhibit infrequent episodes of crying and demonstrate normal sleep patterns.

- Impaired Physical Mobility related to surgical procedure on the penis.

Expected Outcome. The child will tolerate activity restriction, as evidenced by participating in developmentally appropriate bedside play.

■ Interventions

The nurse should provide parents with detailed preoperative teaching and encourage them to participate in the postoperative care of their child. The child has a pressure dressing to decrease edema, which is removed by the physician after approximately 4 days. Some infants have a stent that drains directly into the diaper, whereas others require a closed drainage bag system. The parents should be able to demonstrate proper care of the catheter or stent before discharge.

The nurse advises the parents to encourage the child to drink frequently. High fluid intake is necessary to maintain hydration and a free flow of urine. The parents are taught to monitor the child's temperature and observe urine for cloudiness or foul smell. Any signs of a UTI should be reported immediately. Postoperative prophylactic antibiotics are usually prescribed.

The parents should provide the child with a variety of quiet diversional activities, being careful not to traumatize the site. The child is given medication as ordered for pain. The parents can provide environmental stimulation and a feeling of mobility by transporting the child in a carriage, wagon, or cart. Parents are encouraged to bring favorite toys or music to help the child feel less anxious.

■ Evaluation

- Can the parents explain the surgical procedure and postoperative care of their child?

- Are the parents participating in the care of their child?
- Is the child afebrile, and are the child's urinalysis and culture within normal limits?
- Is the child happy, comfortable, and able to sleep?
- Is the child participating in age-appropriate play within restrictions?

MISCELLANEOUS DISORDERS AND ANOMALIES OF THE GENITOURINARY TRACT

Other disorders and anomalies associated with the genitourinary tract are described in Table 20-1. Most require surgical correction. For both psychological and mechanical reasons, these defects are usually corrected at a young age; some may require more than one surgery.

ACUTE POSTSTREPTOCOCCAL GLOMERULONEPHRITIS

The term *glomerulonephritis* refers to a group of kidney disorders characterized by inflammatory injury in the glomerulus. Infection or a systemic disease process, such as lupus erythematosus (see Chapter 17) or Schönlein-Henoch purpura (an autoimmune vasculitis), can cause glomerular inflammation. Acute glomerulonephritis refers to disorders that occur suddenly, are self-limiting, and resolve completely. Acute poststreptococcal glomerulonephritis, the most common type, is characterized by sudden onset of hematuria, proteinuria, hypertension, edema, and renal insufficiency (Pan & Avner, 2011).

Etiology and Incidence

Acute poststreptococcal glomerulonephritis occurs as an immune reaction to a group A beta-hemolytic streptococcal infection of the throat or skin.

This disorder occurs most frequently in young children with ages ranging from 5 to 12 years and is rarely seen before age 3 years. Clinical symptoms usually develop 1 to 2 weeks after a streptococcal pharyngitis or 3 to 6 weeks after a streptococcal skin infection (pyoderma) (Pan & Avner, 2011).

Manifestations

Hematuria, which is a cardinal sign of poststreptococcal glomerulonephritis, ranges in severity from microscopic to gross, as evidenced by smoky or tea-colored urine. Edema, which is worse in the morning, affects primarily the eyelids and ankles. This can be accompanied by decreased urinary output. Hypertension can be severe. The child may be febrile. Many children experience fatigue. Pulmonary edema is a life-threatening complication.

Diagnostic Evaluation

History, presenting symptoms, and laboratory results can establish the diagnosis of acute poststreptococcal glomerulonephritis. A urinalysis reveals macroscopic or microscopic hematuria with red blood cell (RBC) casts, which indicates glomerular injury. Proteinuria is also present but not severe. Blood chemistry values are usually within the normal range. If renal insufficiency is severe, however, BUN and creatinine levels are elevated. Electrolyte disturbances, such as high serum potassium and low serum bicarbonate levels, can result from inadequate glomerular filtration.

The complete blood cell count usually demonstrates normal WBCs and mild anemia. The lower hemoglobin and hematocrit values reflect the dilutional effect of extra fluid in the blood as a result of decreased glomerular filtration.

TABLE 20-1 MISCELLANEOUS DISORDERS AND ANOMALIES OF THE GENITOURINARY TRACT

DISORDER OR ANOMALY	THERAPEUTIC MANAGEMENT
Hydrocele: Painless swelling of the scrotum caused by a collection of fluid.	In the majority of infants, hydroceles resolve by 12 months of age. A large, tense hydrocele or one that persists beyond 12 to 18 months should be surgically repaired.*
Phimosis: Inability to retract the prepuce (foreskin) at an age when it should be retractable (usually 3 yr).	Accumulation of sebaceous gland secretions. Mild cases can be corrected through cleaning and gentle manual retraction. More severe cases require surgical enlargement of the phimotic ring or circumcision.
Testicular torsion: Rotation of the testicle that interrupts its blood supply, causing irreparable testicular damage if not corrected quickly. Manifests by sudden onset of severe, progressive scrotal pain, erythema, and edema. More common in adolescents and infants.	This is a surgical emergency. Surgery straightens and fixates the affected testicle and the other testicle to prevent torsion. If the affected testicle is necrotic, it is removed.
Bladder exstrophy: The extrusion of the urinary bladder to the outside of the body through a developmental defect in the lower abdominal wall. Associated with epispadias and other anomalies.	The exposed bladder tissue is covered with nonadhering plastic wrap until surgery. Surgical management is done in one or several stages and includes closing the abdominal defect and reconstructing the bladder and genitalia to allow the child to achieve urinary continence. It is important to address attachment issues with parents, who might be overwhelmed by their infant's appearance. Preventing UTI is essential.
Disorders of sex development† *46,XX DSD:* Normal internal female structures with virilized external genitalia. The most common cause is congenital adrenal hyperplasia (CAH) (see Chapter 27). *46,XY DSD:* Internal structures are testes; external genitalia are female, ambiguous, or demonstrate incomplete virilization. *Ovotesticular DSD:* Both ovarian and testicular tissues are present, with ambiguous external genitalia; most are genetically female.	Most infants are identified at birth because of ambiguous external genitalia or by signs of CAH. Because gender identity is influenced more by a combination of genetic, neurologic, family, and social factors, rather than external appearance, gender assignment is a complex process. It begins with karyotyping for sex chromosomes, and is followed by imaging studies to identify gonadal and reproductive structures, and a variety of hormonal studies. Decisions about surgical and other treatment approaches are based on potential fertility, external appearance, and the complexity of the proposed surgical reconstruction; parents and a variety of specialists (e.g., endocrinologist, surgeon, urologist, psychiatrist) are consulted. In some instances surgery is postponed until the child is old enough to participate in the decision. Surgery can reconstruct external genitalia to match the gender assignment. Psychological support for the family should be provided on a regular basis throughout the child's life starting at birth.

UTI, urinary tract infection.

*Elder, J. (2011). Urologic disorders in infants and children. In R. Kliegman, B. Stanton, J. St. Geme, et al. (Eds.), *Nelson textbook of pediatrics* (19th ed., pp.1858-1864). Philadelphia: Elsevier Saunders.

†Data from Houk, C., Hughes, I., Ahmed, S., & Lee, P. (2006). Summary of consensus statement on intersex disorders and their management. *Pediatrics, 118*(2), 753-757; Donahoue, P. (2011). Disorders of sex development. In R. Kliegman, B. Stanton, J. St. Geme, et al. (Eds.), *Nelson textbook of pediatrics* (19th ed., pp. 1958-1968). Philadelphia: Elsevier Saunders.

Immunologic studies are important in diagnosing acute poststreptococcal glomerulonephritis. Serum complement (C3) may be low because of the fixation of complement in immune complexes. An antistreptolysin (ASO) titer, which indicates the presence of antibodies to streptococcal bacteria, or a Streptozyme test can be elevated. The ASO titer might not be elevated in a streptococcal skin infection. Culture of the throat or skin lesion (if present) may be helpful for isolating the bacterium, however, this is useful only if the infection is recent and the child has not received antibiotics. A renal biopsy may be indicated for those children whose signs and symptoms are not characteristic of acute poststreptococcal glomerulonephritis or for those children whose symptoms do not improve as expected.

Therapeutic Management

There is no specific therapy for acute poststreptococcal glomerulonephritis. Supportive care and medical management are directed to the associated signs and symptoms and guided by the degree of renal dysfunction. A 10-day course of antibiotic therapy may be required. Children with acute renal failure should be hospitalized to allow for fluid and electrolyte management until their renal function has stabilized.

Antihypertensive therapy may be necessary. This can be accomplished by limiting sodium and water intake and by administering diuretics and antihypertensive medication. The prognosis for children with acute poststreptococcal glomerulonephritis is excellent. The acute clinical episode is usually self-limiting, with diuresis signaling the beginning of resolution. Most children have a complete recovery; laboratory values usually return to baseline in 6 to 12 weeks.

NURSING CARE OF THE CHILD WITH ACUTE POSTSTREPTOCOCCAL GLOMERULONEPHRITIS

■ Assessment

The nurse assesses the child for presence of periorbital or lower extremity edema. Obtaining vital signs and monitoring daily weight are important for determining the degree of fluid retention and hypertension. An appropriate-size blood pressure cuff must be used to obtain accurate blood pressure measurements (see Chapter 13). The child's levels of fatigue and anxiety are monitored as well.

The child is evaluated for the presence of any respiratory difficulty, such as cough, increased respiratory rate, or increased work of

PATHOPHYSIOLOGY

Acute Poststreptococcal Glomerulonephritis

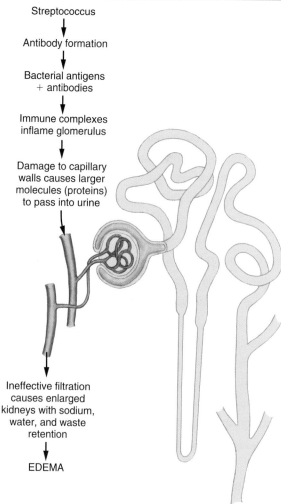

Streptococcus

↓

Antibody formation

↓

Bacterial antigens + antibodies

↓

Immune complexes inflame glomerulus

↓

Damage to capillary walls causes larger molecules (proteins) to pass into urine

↓

Ineffective filtration causes enlarged kidneys with sodium, water, and waste retention

↓

EDEMA

Acute glomerulonephritis after a streptococcal infection is thought to occur as a result of an immunologic response. The body responds to the *Streptococcus* bacteria by forming antibodies, which combine with the bacterial antigens to form immune complexes. As these antigen-antibody complexes travel through the circulation, they become trapped in the glomerulus and activate an inflammatory response in the glomerular basement membrane. Products of the inflammatory response damage the glomerular capillaries and reduce the size of the capillary lumen. This process can cause a decrease in the glomerular filtration rate, leading to renal insufficiency. Sodium and fluid are retained, and the child exhibits edema and oliguria. In addition, injury to the capillary walls interferes with their permeability so that larger molecules and structures such as RBCs, casts, and proteins can pass through into the urine.

---

breathing. Breath sounds are auscultated for crackles. Laboratory values, especially urinalysis and serum electrolytes, are monitored.

The nurse determines what the child and family understand about the illness and the reasons for hospitalization. The parents may be anxious about permanent damage to the child's kidneys as a result of this condition.

■ Nursing Diagnosis and Planning

The nursing diagnoses and expected outcomes that apply to the child with acute poststreptococcal glomerulonephritis and the child's family are as follows:

- Risk for Imbalanced Fluid Volume related to retention of sodium and fluid and dietary fluid restriction.

Expected Outcome. The child will maintain a normal fluid balance, as evidenced by urine output appropriate for age-group (see Chapter 16), moist mucous membranes, adequate skin turgor, normal blood pressure, no increase in weight, and no symptoms of respiratory distress.

- Risk for Activity Intolerance related to fatigue.

Expected Outcome. The child will be rested, as evidenced by the ability to tolerate daily care and play activities.

- Risk for Impaired Skin Integrity related to edema and decreased activity.

Expected Outcome. The child will exhibit no signs of skin breakdown, as evidenced by skin that is intact, normal color for race, and nontender to touch.

- Imbalanced Nutrition: Less Than Body Requirements related to diet restrictions.

Expected Outcome. The child will have adequate nutrition, as evidenced by maintenance of weight at the preillness level.

- Anxiety related to insufficient knowledge about disease process or hospitalization.

Expected Outcomes. The child and parents will demonstrate decreased anxiety, as evidenced by cooperation with daily care and interest in developmentally appropriate play. Parents or caregiver will describe the disease process and its usual resolution.

■ Interventions

■ **Preventing the Consequences of Fluid Excess.** Frequent, accurate assessment of intake and output is essential for evaluating fluid volume status. Children with severe renal impairment might require measurement of intake and output every 1 to 2 hours. Fluid intake includes oral intake and IV fluids. If urine output is less than 1 mL/kg/hr, this must be reported to the physician (see Chapter 16), because oliguria suggests impending renal failure or inadequate fluid intake.

Comparing the child's weight each day is important for determining fluctuation in fluid balance. The nurse must obtain accurate daily weights, using the same scale at approximately the same time every day for maximum consistency. Infants and young children should be weighed without diapers, and older children should wear only a gown.

Because hypertension from fluid overload and glomerular damage is a severe consequence of this condition, the nurse measures blood pressure with an appropriate-size cuff every 4 to 8 hours and documents the results. Increased values are reported immediately to the physician. More frequent readings might be required if the child has significant hypertension or is receiving antihypertensive medication.

Breath sounds are auscultated every 4 to 8 hours noting adventitious sounds and signs of increased work of breathing. Rapid respirations, retractions, nasal flaring, and crackles are signs of developing pulmonary edema, which can result from fluid overload.

Limits on fluid intake may be ordered. This may be difficult; some children may "sneak" drinks or obtain beverages from people unaware of restrictions. The nurse should inform parents, visitors, and hospital staff of the need to limit fluids. The child's favorite fluids are listed on the nursing care plan. The child is encouraged to consume fluids gradually, rather than drink large amounts all at once. The nurse provides the child with only the amount of fluids allowed for a given time period. Sodium intake can increase fluid retention. The nurse ensures that a low-sodium diet is followed if ordered and informs parents and visitors of any dietary restrictions.

■ **Providing Adequate Rest.** If fatigue is present, it is essential that the child is given ample opportunities to rest. Children with glomerulonephritis may tire easily when first hospitalized. Most children continue to participate in activities according to their level of fatigue. If needed, the nurse can limit play time to short periods and then extend the limits as the child's condition improves. The nurse needs to arrange daily care so that the child has some uninterrupted time for sleep and naps. Parents are asked to bring a favorite sleep toy or blanket for the child and to allow for nap time and bedtime to coincide with the child's home schedule as much as possible. Following home rituals can promote rest and sleep as well.

■ **Maintaining Skin Integrity.** Frequent position changes decrease pressure on bony prominences and help decrease edema in dependent areas. The nurse prompts the child to change position at least every 2 hours during the day. If the child has edema of the lower extremities, the extremities are elevated when the child is sitting or lying in bed. As the child's condition improves, engaging in activities that increase circulation and promote reabsorption of fluid from edematous areas is encouraged.

To prevent skin breakdown, the nurse maintains good hygiene by giving baths and cleaning the skin well after bowel movements and diaper changes. Using a small amount of lotion to massage the skin helps prevent dryness and promotes active circulation.

■ **Maintaining Nutritional Status.** Low-sodium foods taste different, and children may refuse to eat them. Offering a variety of low-sodium foods or treats may encourage the child to eat. The nurse consults with the dietary department about palatable low-sodium foods and drinks. Parents are allowed to bring favorite foods from home if they comply with the child's dietary restrictions.

A small fluctuation in weight can indicate fluid losses or gains as well as weight loss from decreased food intake. After obtaining the child's preillness weight, the nurse weighs the child daily to monitor for any fluid shifts or underlying weight loss. In addition, the nurse monitors the child for signs of dehydration (dry mucous membranes, listlessness, poor skin turgor, tachycardia) that would coincide with fluid restriction, diuretic administration, and diuresis.

■ **Relieving Anxiety.** Allowing the parents and the child to voice their concerns provides support and a basis for evaluating their understanding of the disease process and prognosis. The nurse reassures the family that most children recover from this condition with no residual effects. Parents are encouraged to participate in the child's care, helping to make the child comfortable and providing suitable play activities and emotional support.

Information enables the child and parents to understand the course of the condition and to anticipate procedures and events. Knowing what to expect helps decrease anxiety. It is especially important to provide information and prepare the family for the child's care at home. If the child has been hypertensive or is to be discharged on antihypertensive medications, the nurse instructs parents on how to measure the child's blood pressure and emphasizes that blood pressure should be taken before medication administration. A blood pressure cuff of appropriate size and a stethoscope or an automated blood pressure device is obtained before discharge so the parents can learn how to use it. The nurse explains the parameters for when to withhold medication or when to call the physician related to blood pressure readings.

■ Evaluation

- Does the child demonstrate adequate urine output for weight and normal blood pressure for age?
- Are the child's mucous membranes moist, and does the child appear to be well hydrated?
- Is the child's respiratory status stable?
- Has the child's weight changed from the preillness weight?
- Is the child able to tolerate usual activities for age?
- Is the child's skin intact, appropriate color, and nontender to touch?
- Is the child relaxed enough to cooperate with care activities and maintain interest in play?
- Do parents participate appropriately in the child's care, providing comfort to the child?
- Can the parents describe the disease process and care required?

NEPHROTIC SYNDROME

Nephrotic syndrome refers to a kidney disorder characterized by proteinuria, hypoalbuminemia, and edema. Nephrotic syndrome can be classified as primary or secondary. *Primary nephrotic syndrome,* or minimal change nephrotic syndrome (MCNS), results from a disorder within the glomerulus of the kidney and is the most common type seen in children. A child also can acquire nephrotic syndrome as the result of a systemic disease, such as hepatitis, systemic lupus erythematosus, heavy metal poisoning, or cancer.

Etiology

The cause of primary nephrotic syndrome is not fully understood, but it can arise from one of four types of renal lesions. Success

⚠ NURSING QUALITY ALERT

Differences between Children with Glomerulonephritis and Children with Nephrotic Syndrome

The signs and symptoms of glomerulonephritis and nephrotic syndrome in children can be confusing. It is important for nurses to be able to discriminate between the two.

POSTSTREPTOCOCCAL GLOMERULONEPHRITIS	NEPHROTIC SYNDROME
Manifestations	
• Hematuria: cola-colored urine	• Severe proteinuria: Frothy urine
• Edema: abrupt onset, mild periorbital or lower extremity	• Edema: Insidious onset, massive edema from shift of fluid into interstitial spaces, worsens during the day
• Hypertensive	
• Proteinuria	• Hypovolemia
• Usually young school-age child	• Normotensive
	• Pallor, fatigue
	• Toddler or preschool-age child
Laboratory Findings	
• RBCs, casts, small amount of protein in urine (0 to 3+)	• Protein in urine (3+ to 4+), possible microscopic hematuria
• Normal serum albumin, cholesterol, and triglyceride levels; decreased or normal hemoglobin and hematocrit values	• Hypoalbuminemia (less than 2.5 g/dL), elevated cholesterol and triglyceride, hemoglobin, hematocrit, and platelet levels
• Altered electrolytes, elevated blood urea nitrogen or creatinine levels	• Normal serum electrolytes, complement levels, ASO titer
• Elevated ASO titer or Streptozyme, decreased complement	
Management	
• Supportive	• Prednisone to initiate remission (0 to trace protein in urine for 5 to 7 days)
• Antihypertensives and diuretics; antibiotic treatment for active streptococcal infection	• Diuretics, possible albumin administration
• Low-salt diet	• Prevent infection and skin breakdown
• Possible fluid restrictions	• No-added-salt diet

in controlling the disease by the use of immunosuppressive drugs suggests the possibility of an immunologic component. In most children, minimal alterations of the glomerulus are seen on histologic examination. Accordingly, the most common disorder, MCNS, accounts for almost 85% of childhood nephrotic syndrome (Pais & Avner, 2011). Nephrosis can develop as a result of focal segmental glomerulosclerosis, membranoproliferative glomerulonephritis, or mesangial proliferation.

Incidence

Primary nephrotic syndrome occurs most frequently in children between ages 2 and 6 years. The incidence is slightly higher in boys. The prognosis for children with MCNS is very good. Manifestations of the disease usually decrease with age, so relapses are rare in adolescence. Focal segmental glomerulosclerosis carries a poorer prognosis; the disease is progressive and often results in end-stage renal disease.

Manifestations

Manifestations of primary nephrotic syndrome include edema, anorexia, fatigue, abdominal pain, respiratory infection, and increased weight. Unlike the child with glomerulonephritis, the child with nephrotic syndrome usually has normal blood pressure.

Edema is usually first noted in the periorbital spaces and dependent areas of the body; its onset is often insidious. Children awaken with facial edema and, as the day progresses, become edematous in the abdomen, genital area, and lower extremities. The pitting edema is most noticeable over the bony prominences of the lower extremities. Abdominal pain can occur from the presence of extra fluid in the peritoneal area. Edema of the bowel may cause diarrhea and decreased absorption of nutrients. Many children are misdiagnosed with allergies because of periorbital edema and respiratory symptoms.

Diagnostic Evaluation

Nephrotic syndrome can be diagnosed on the basis of clinical presentation, age of the child, and laboratory results. Urinalysis demonstrates protein (3+ to 4+), and the urine appears dark and frothy. Microscopic hematuria may be present. Serum cholesterol, triglycerides, hematocrit, and hemoglobin values are elevated. Serum albumin is markedly decreased (less than 2.5 g/dL). The child has normal electrolyte levels and a negative ASO titer or Streptozyme test. Serologic tests for hepatitis, human immunodeficiency virus, syphilis, and antinuclear antibody titers are done to rule out underlying systemic disease.

In the event of an atypical presentation (a child older than 10 years or having gross hematuria or hypertension), a kidney biopsy might be done if a lesion other than MCNS is suspected. A biopsy is also indicated for the child who does not respond as expected to pharmacologic treatment.

Therapeutic Management

It is not unusual for the child with primary nephrotic syndrome to be hospitalized briefly during the initial onset of the disease to provide palliative treatment for the edema, perform necessary diagnostic testing, and initiate therapy. Parents are educated about the disease process and necessary home care. Before treatment begins, the child is tested for exposure to tuberculosis and varicella because treatment suppresses the immune system.

PATHOPHYSIOLOGY

Nephrotic Syndrome

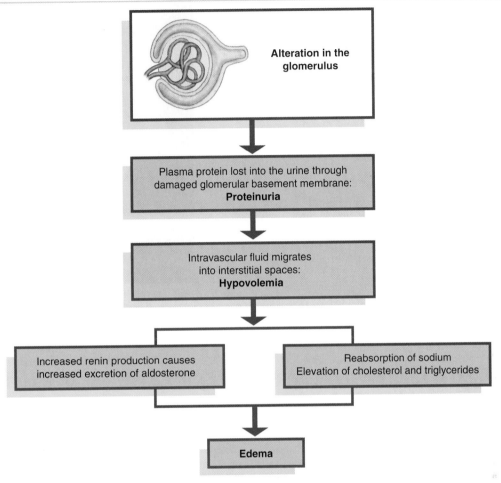

Alteration in the glomerulus

Plasma protein lost into the urine through damaged glomerular basement membrane:
Proteinuria

Intravascular fluid migrates into interstitial spaces:
Hypovolemia

Increased renin production causes increased excretion of aldosterone

Reabsorption of sodium
Elevation of cholesterol and triglycerides

Edema

Primary nephrotic syndrome occurs from an insult to the glomerular basement membrane. Damage to the membrane causes increased permeability and loss of substances that would normally prevent negatively charged proteins from crossing the membrane. Negatively charged proteins, particularly albumin, are cleared at an increased rate, resulting in loss of plasma proteins and in proteinuria. Proteinuria is essential for the diagnosis of nephrotic syndrome.

Blood albumin values are low (hypoalbuminemia) because of the loss of albumin through the defective glomerulus and the liver's inability to synthesize proteins to balance the loss. Decreased levels of albumin reduce the plasma oncotic pressure so that the intravascular fluid moves into the interstitial spaces. This shifting of fluid reduces the intravascular volume, causing hypovolemia and subsequent decreased renal blood flow. In an effort to increase blood volume, the kidney stimulates renin production. Renin causes increased excretion of aldosterone, resulting in renal tubular reabsorption of sodium, which in turn causes water retention. The net effect of this phenomenon is edema.

In addition, the serum values of cholesterol and triglycerides are elevated. This change is thought to result from increased stimulation of lipoprotein production because of the decrease in oncotic pressure. Loss of immunoglobulins into the urine is common in nephrotic syndrome. Most notably, levels of immunoglobulin G are decreased, which makes these children more susceptible to infection. Before the use of antibiotics, infection was a frequent cause of death in these children.

Children with nephrotic syndrome are in a hypercoagulable state, predisposing them to venous thrombosis. This tendency occurs as a result of several factors, including decreased intravascular volume (hypovolemia), which causes increased concentration of RBCs and platelets, and slowing of circulation. Urinary loss of proteins that inhibit coagulation also contributes to the risk of thrombus formation.

Remission Induction

Therapy for remission includes prednisone at a maximum daily amount of 60 to 80 mg divided into two or three doses. This regimen is continued until the child is in remission—defined as zero to trace urine protein for 3 to 7 consecutive days. Steroids usually are continued at the same daily dose for 4 to 6 weeks. After the initial treatment, the child's dose is decreased and changed to an alternate-day schedule and then slowly tapered.

In the event of a relapse, steroid therapy is less prolonged. Once remission is achieved, dosing decreases to alternate days and is tapered more quickly. This is done to minimize prednisone side effects (see Chapter 17).

Some children respond to steroids quickly and achieve remission in 5 to 7 days, whereas others may not respond for 4 weeks. If proteinuria continues beyond 8 weeks of daily steroid therapy, the child is said to be steroid resistant and a kidney biopsy is done to determine the exact nature of the disease.

Children who initially respond to steroid therapy but have relapses while on a tapering schedule or shortly after stopping steroids are said to be *steroid dependent* (Figure 20-2). These children may benefit from a course of an alkylating agent such as cyclophosphamide or chlorambucil. The risks and benefits of this therapy must be carefully considered, and the parents should be informed of all possible side effects. A kidney biopsy is usually done before therapy is started. The use of cyclosporine in children who remain steroid dependent despite a course of an alkylating agent, has proven to be effective in maintaining remission.

Additional Therapy

A no-added-salt diet is indicated. The parents should not use salt when cooking; the child should not be permitted to use the salt shaker; and the parents should avoid serving high-sodium foods such as pickles, salted chips, and cured meats. If edema is severe or if the child is hypertensive, sodium intake may be further restricted and the child may be placed on a fluid restriction.

Diuretic therapy may be initiated until urinary protein loss is controlled. If the edema is marked and causes the child to have decreased mobility, poor oral intake, or decreased urine output, salt-poor albumin may be given intravenously. Albumin helps restore normal plasma osmotic pressure and promotes the movement of interstitial fluid back into the intravascular compartments. Furosemide is given intravenously after the albumin infusion to enhance diuresis and decrease the chance of fluid overload.

Severe edema in the lower extremities can give rise to cellulitis because of fluid stasis and poor circulation. Peritonitis, a severe complication, can develop from stasis of ascitic fluid, which functions as a culture medium for organisms such as *Streptococcus pneumoniae.*

Live-virus vaccines are contraindicated in children receiving steroid therapy. In addition to routine killed-virus vaccines, the child

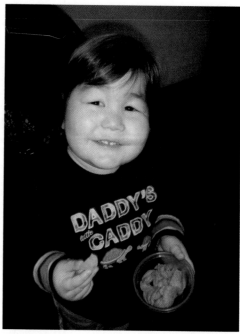

FIG 20-2 This child has nephrotic syndrome. He previously received steroid therapy and is now receiving CellCept immunosuppressant therapy to control the process. During the acute phase of the nephrotic syndrome, the child may have massive edema because blood proteins are lost in the urine. Skin pallor is also common. (Photo courtesy Cook Children's Pediatric Nephrology, Dialysis, and Transplant Services, Fort Worth, TX.)

should receive pneumococcal immunization to prevent pneumococcal infection in the event of a relapse. The child with nephrotic syndrome should receive an influenza vaccine each year because an exacerbation of the disease can occur after an infection. During remission and 1 month after steroids have been stopped, varicella and other live-virus vaccines may be given if needed (Pais & Avner, 2011).

◎ NURSING CARE PLAN

The Child with Nephrotic Syndrome

Focused Assessment
- Monitor child for early signs of infection every 4 to 8 hours.
  - Vital signs (temperature)
  - Laboratory data (WBCs)
- Assess fluid balance every 4 to 8 hours.
  - Monitor vital signs for indicators of hypovolemia (increased pulse rate, low BP) or fluid overload (elevated BP)
  - Check laboratory data (hemoglobin, hematocrit)
  - Accurate daily weights
  - Strict measurement and documentation of fluid intake and urine output
  - Auscultate breath sounds and observe for respiratory distress
- Assess the amount of edema present and condition of skin every 4 to 8 hours.
  - Check periorbital areas, abdomen, genitalia, and lower extremities
- Daily check laboratory data for amount of protein in the urine.
  - Indicates severity of disease if increased or effectiveness of treatment if decreased

- Obtain a nursing history.
  - Immunizations received
  - Recent exposure to communicable diseases
- Assess understanding of the child and family regarding the disease process and treatment.
  - Determine need for referrals to appropriate support services
  - Evaluate educational needs

Planning
Nursing Diagnosis
Risk for Impaired Skin Integrity related to edema and decreased circulation.

Expected Outcome
The child will remain free from skin breakdown, as evidenced by the absence of redness, tenderness to touch, and ulceration.

The Child with Nephrotic Syndrome—cont'd

Intervention/*Rationale*

1. Ensure that the child changes position every 2 hours.
   Frequent position change decreases pressure on body parts and helps relieve edema in dependent areas.
2. Maintain good hygiene by giving baths and changing linen daily. Use non–alcohol-based lotion for dry skin.
   Body secretions and debris on linens can irritate the skin. Gentle massage when bathing and applying lotion helps increase circulation.
3. Support or elevate edematous body parts while the child is in bed or sitting in a chair.
   Edema is gravity dependent. Elevation helps move fluid away from dependent body parts.
4. Promote physical activity as the child is able to tolerate by providing developmentally appropriate play activities.
   Increased activity helps promote circulation.

Evaluation

Is the child's skin intact without redness or tenderness?

Planning
Nursing Diagnosis

Risk for Infection related to urinary loss of gamma globulins and immunosuppressive therapy.

Expected Outcome

The child will be free of signs of an infection, as evidenced by normal WBC count, normal body temperature, and absence of abdominal pain and cough.

Intervention/*Rationale*

1. Screen visitors for signs of infection, such as upper respiratory symptoms, sore throats, or exposure to communicable diseases.
   Communicable diseases pose a serious threat because the child receiving immunosuppressive therapy is not able to respond appropriately to infection.
2. Administer antibiotics as ordered.
   Antibiotics are usually given for peritonitis prophylaxis during the edematous phase.
3. Use thorough hand hygiene techniques and instruct family members to do the same.
   Hand hygiene helps decrease transmission of organisms.
4. Monitor child for fever, cough, sore throat, and complaints of abdominal pain, and check laboratory values (CBC, differential) every 8 hours.
   Frequent monitoring ensures early detection of infectious processes. Abdominal pain can be an indication of peritonitis.

Evaluation

Does the child maintain normal body temperature and exhibit normal laboratory values?
Is the child free from cough, pain, or other signs of infection?

Planning
Nursing Diagnosis

Risk for Deficient Fluid Volume (intravascular) related to proteinuria, edema, and effects of diuretics.

Expected Outcome

The child will maintain adequate fluid volume, as evidenced by normal blood pressure measurement, urine output appropriate for age, and normal hematocrit and hemoglobin values.

Intervention/*Rationale*

1. Monitor vital signs, including blood pressure and pulse, every 4 to 8 hours. Report variance from baseline.
   Low blood pressure and increased heart rate are signs of hypovolemia. Blood pressure may be elevated because of renin release.
2. Monitor intake and output every 4-8 hr. Report if child has output of less than 1 to 2 mL/kg/hr of urine (see Chapter 16).
   Accurate intake and output measurement is essential for evaluating fluid status.
3. Monitor laboratory values, particularly hemoglobin and hematocrit.
   Increasing values of hemoglobin and hematocrit may indicate hemoconcentration or low intravascular volume.
4. Observe for signs of dehydration such as dry appearance of mucous membranes, poor skin turgor, increased capillary refill time, and decreased level of activity. (Capillary refill may be altered because of edema; assess in nonedematous area.) Report abnormal findings to the physician.
   The pathophysiologic mechanisms of nephrotic syndrome may predispose the child to decreased intravascular volume. This condition is compounded by the use of diuretics.

Evaluation

Are the child's vital signs and hematocrit and hemoglobin within normal limits?
Is the urine output normal for age-group (see Chapter 16)?
Does the child have moist mucous membranes and appropriate skin turgor?

Planning
Nursing Diagnosis

Excess Fluid Volume related to decreased excretion of sodium and fluid retention.

Expected Outcome

The child will not exhibit signs of fluid overload, as evidenced by stable daily weights and normal respiratory pattern.

Intervention/*Rationale*

1. Monitor intake and output every 4 to 8 hours.
   Accurate intake and output are essential for evaluating fluid balance.
2. Obtain accurate daily weights. Weigh child on the same scale, at same time each day in a gown only.
   Daily weights are necessary to detect changes in fluid volume status. Clothing or presence of wet diaper can alter weight. Readings of weight can vary from scale to scale and time of day.
3. Adhere to no-added-salt diet and fluid restriction if ordered.
   *Excessive sodium intake can increase amount of water retention. If the child is hyponatremic, fluid restriction may be indicated.**
4. Measure and record abdominal girth each day. Ensure accuracy by measuring in the same area each time.
   Edema commonly occurs in the abdomen. Ascites may increase during course of the disease.
5. Monitor blood pressure at least once every 8 hours.
   Increased total-body fluid volume and concurrent steroid therapy can result in increased blood pressure.
6. Administer diuretics as ordered. Ensure adequate potassium intake.
   Diuretics may aid in the elimination of excessive fluid. Diuretics can increase excretion of potassium.
7. Monitor respiratory status every 4 to 8 hours. Auscultate breath sounds checking for crackles. Observe for signs of increased work of breathing (retractions, nasal flaring, increased respiratory rate) and cough.
   Fluid overload can result in pulmonary edema.

---

*Pais, P., & Avner, E. (2011). Nephrotic syndrome. In R. Kliegman, B. Stanton, J. St. Geme, et al. (Eds.), *Nelson textbook of pediatrics* (19th ed., pp. 1801-1807). Philadelphia: Elsevier Saunders.

Continued

NURSING CARE PLAN

The Child with Nephrotic Syndrome—cont'd

Evaluation
Does the child maintain a stable weight?
Is the child free from respiratory distress?

Planning
Nursing Diagnoses
Anxiety (parental) related to hospitalization of child and caring for a child with a chronic disease.
Deficient Knowledge about home management related to incomplete understanding.

Expected Outcomes
The parents will demonstrate decreased anxiety, as evidenced by participating in the care of their child and explaining the normal course of the disease process.
The parents will be able to explain principles of home management.
The child will gain understanding of disease management per developmental level.

Intervention/Rationale
1. Allow parents to verbalize frustration and fears; encourage them to ask questions. Provide the parent and child with information about nephrotic syndrome and its treatment.
   Verbalization of fears is often therapeutic. Information helps decrease anxiety by reducing fear of the unknown.

2. Incorporate the parents into the child's daily care including urine protein testing with Albustix, taking blood pressures, and assessing edema. Involve the child in care activities that are developmentally appropriate.
   Nephrotic syndrome can be a chronic condition and it is usually managed at home. It is important for the parents to feel comfortable providing care for their child.

3. Arrange for a dietary consultation.
   Steroid therapy stimulates appetite. Children should be informed about low-calorie snacks and portion size. Encourage the parents to cook without salt and remove the salt shaker from the child's access.

4. Teach parents how to maintain a daily calendar of urine protein readings, obtain daily weights, administer approved medications only, and perform hand hygiene and other actions to prevent infection. Encourage parents to report any exposure to communicable disease.
   Education allows the family to manage the child's care. The child's urine protein results are monitored for signs of relapse. Parent must check with the nephrologist before giving any over-the-counter medications; some can aggravate hypertension. Children receiving steroids are immunosuppressed and may require prophylactic treatment if exposed to communicable diseases.

Evaluation
Can the parents describe their child's condition and required treatment?
Do the parents actively participate in the child's care?
Do the parents accurately demonstrate procedures they will be required to do at home?
Does the child participate in care activities?

ACUTE RENAL FAILURE

Acute renal failure (ARF) is defined as the sudden, severe loss of kidney function. In acute renal failure, the kidneys can no longer filter waste products, regulate fluid volume, or maintain chemical balance. Most children with acute renal failure regain renal function.

Etiology and Incidence

The three types of ARF are prerenal, intrinsic renal, and postrenal. Causes of prerenal failure are dehydration, perinatal asphyxia, hypotension, septic shock, hemorrhagic shock, and renal artery obstruction. Nephrotoxins (e.g., aminoglycosides, contrast dye), lupus erythematosus, hemolytic uremic syndrome (HUS), glomerulonephritis, and pyelonephritis all can cause intrinsic renal failure. Postrenal failure is associated with structural abnormalities such as ureteropelvic junction obstruction, ureterovesical obstruction, posterior urethral valves, neurogenic bladder, and outlet obstruction by stones, tumor, or edema (Sreedharan & Avner, 2011).

Acute renal failure occurs in 8% of neonates and 2% to 3% of children admitted to intensive care units and tertiary care centers (Sreedharan & Avner, 2011). HUS is one of the most frequent causes of acute renal failure in children (Sreedharan & Avner, 2011). It is an acute disorder characterized by anemia, thrombocytopenia, and ARF. HUS is often associated with *Escherichia coli (E. coli)* infection that results from improperly cooked meat or contaminated dairy products.

Manifestations

Manifestations of acute renal failure include electrolyte abnormalities, fluid volume shifts, increased BUN and serum creatinine levels, acid-base imbalances, and nonspecific symptoms such as poor feeding, decreased appetite, vomiting, lethargy, seizures, and pallor. In children

PATHOPHYSIOLOGY

Acute Renal Failure

Acute renal failure (ARF) is categorized as prerenal, intrinsic, or postrenal. *Prerenal ARF* is the result of decreased perfusion of the kidney. The kidney must have adequate blood flow for effective functioning. The decreased blood flow and subsequent ischemia cause cellular swelling and injury and possible cell death. *Intrinsic ARF* is the result of actual damage to kidney tissue from certain diseases including prolonged hypoperfusion. *Postrenal ARF* is the result of obstruction of urine outflow. The obstruction increases pressure within the kidney, which decreases renal function.

Impaired perfusion markedly decreases the glomerular filtration rate (GFR), triggering oliguria (decreased urine output), azotemia (elevated blood levels of urea, creatinine, and uric acid), and associated electrolyte imbalances. Tissue injury further magnifies the damage and the decreased perfusion.

As the underlying problem is treated, recovery of the renal endothelial and tubular cells begins and renal function gradually improves. Because the GFR returns to normal faster than the tubular transport mechanisms, diuresis occurs first with the child voiding large amounts of dilute urine. This puts the child at increased risk for dehydration related to the fluid loss. In most cases, renal function progressively returns to normal.

with HUS, gastrointestinal illness is characterized by abdominal pain, fever, vomiting, and bloody diarrhea.

Diagnostic Evaluation

Determining the underlying cause of acute renal failure is very important. If the cause can be reversed, renal function usually returns to normal.

History

The history often gives an indication of the underlying cause of the acute renal failure. Vomiting, diarrhea, and fever may indicate dehydration and prerenal acute renal failure. It is necessary to ascertain any recent history of bloody diarrhea that might suggest HUS.

Fluid Volume Status

Prerenal ARF is usually associated with dehydration whereas children with intrinsic ARF from glomerulonephritis often are fluid overloaded and have edema, crackles, and hypertension. Urine output can be normal, increased, or oliguric (less than 1 mL/kg/hr) (see Chapter 16).

Laboratory Data

Serum creatinine and BUN levels are increased. BUN, an end product of protein catabolism, may reflect the child's nutritional status. Metabolic acidosis can occur, as indicated by low serum bicarbonate. Serum potassium may be increased. Serum sodium may be increased or decreased, depending on fluid volume status. The child with HUS exhibits hemolytic anemia, thrombocytopenia, hematuria, proteinuria, and in some cases, a stool culture that is positive for *E. coli*.

PATHOPHYSIOLOGY

Hemolytic Uremic Syndrome

Most affected children have an associated prodrome of gastrointestinal symptoms, including bloody diarrhea, which suggests that an infectious agent may be the cause of HUS. Most cases are the result of an antecedent infection by Shiga toxin-producing strains of *E. coli*, especially the O157:H7 serotype.* Two important characteristics of *E. coli* O157:H7 contribute to the development of HUS. First, because this bacterium attaches itself to the intestinal mucosa, its clearance through normal intestinal peristalsis is decreased, allowing the bacteria to grow and multiply. Second, the bacteria produce a toxin that damages the endothelial cells of capillary walls, and the subsequent inflammatory response results in occlusion of capillaries. This is especially significant in the renal glomeruli. The occlusion of glomerular vessels decreases filtration which results in acute renal failure. However, it is important to understand that the vascular process seen in HUS can affect any organ. Anemia results from fragmentation of RBCs, which are damaged as they try to pass through the occluded vessels and are removed from circulation by the spleen. Thrombocytopenia occurs because the platelets get trapped within the small vessels.

*Thorpe, C. (2004). Shiga toxin-producing *Escherichia coli* infection. *Clinical Infectious Diseases, 38,* 1298-1303.

Physical Examination

The child may be hypertensive. Edema resulting from decreased urine output and fluid overload may be present. The child may be in respiratory distress because of fluid overload.

Imaging Studies

Renal ultrasonography may help with the diagnosis of obstruction and postrenal ARF. A renal scan can be helpful in determining the cause of all ARF types. It can assess blood flow, kidney function, and obstruction.

Therapeutic Management

Many children in acute renal failure are managed without dialysis. Therapeutic management focuses on correcting imbalances.

Fluid Imbalances

Maintaining a normal fluid volume status is critical for the child with ARF. If the child is dehydrated, precise fluid replacement is performed.

Fluid restriction is necessary for a child who has decreased or absent urine output and is adequately hydrated or fluid overloaded. Fluid intake is calculated to replace insensible fluid loss and urinary output. Maintaining fluid restrictions can be difficult for some children. It is helpful to give small amounts of fluids as often as possible. Older children can participate in decisions about the kind and frequency of fluids.

Electrolyte Imbalances

Potassium. Most children with acute renal failure have a high serum potassium level, requiring intervention when the level reaches 6 mEq/L. Potassium is restricted from the diet and IV fluids. Interventions to remove potassium include instituting gastric suction; administration of an exchange resin, such as Kayexalate; or administration of sodium bicarbonate, glucose, and insulin.

Sodium. The serum sodium level may be elevated or decreased. It is more common for the level to be decreased because of fluid overload, in which case fluid restrictions help improve the sodium level. Any replacement sodium is adjusted to maintain a normal serum sodium level.

Acid-Base Imbalances. Children with acute renal failure are unable to excrete hydrogen ions and ammonia through the kidney, so metabolic acidosis (low serum bicarbonate) develops. Additional sodium bicarbonate can be administered orally or intravenously.

Nutrition

Nutritional support of children with acute renal failure is critical. Foods should be low in sodium and potassium.

The underlying principle of nutritional therapy for these children is to provide maximum calories. If the child is critically ill, parenteral hyperalimentation with essential amino acids may be administered (Sreedharan & Avner, 2011).

❗ NURSING QUALITY ALERT

Indications for Dialysis in Acute Renal Failure

- Severe fluid overload
- Pulmonary edema or congestive heart failure caused by fluid overload
- Severe hypertension
- Metabolic acidosis not responsive to medications
- Hyperkalemia not responsive to medications
- Blood urea nitrogen level greater than 120 mg/dL

Dialysis

Dialysis is a process of removing waste products and excess body fluid and regulating electrolytes and minerals. The two principal types of dialysis are hemodialysis and peritoneal dialysis.

Nursing Considerations

Most children with acute renal failure are cared for in special-care units. Principles of nursing care include (1) monitoring and maintaining fluid, electrolyte, and acid-base balances, (2) preventing infection, (3) providing adequate nutrition, (4) reducing parent and child anxiety, and (5) teaching about the disease process, treatment, and dialysis (Box 20-2).

CHRONIC RENAL FAILURE AND END-STAGE RENAL DISEASE

Chronic renal failure is an irreversible loss of kidney function that usually occurs over months to years. It can be managed conservatively

BOX 20-2 DIALYSIS

Dialysis is a process of removing waste products and excess body fluids and regulating electrolytes and minerals. It is sometimes necessary in acute renal failure. When chronic renal failure progresses to end-stage renal disease (ESRD), dialysis or kidney transplantation is required. The two principal types of dialysis are hemodialysis and peritoneal dialysis.

Hemodialysis

Hemodialysis cleanses the blood by circulating it through a special filter called an *artificial kidney*. Blood is pumped through the artificial kidney and returned to the body. Hemodialysis occurs through a surgically placed, vascular access, such as a double-lumen central line or an **arteriovenous fistula** or shunt. Children who receive long-term dialysis usually receive treatments three times per week for 3 to 4 hours each time.

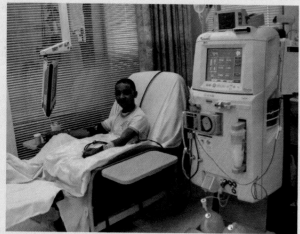

Teenager receiving hemodialysis. (Photo courtesy Cook Children's Pediatric Nephrology, Dialysis, and Transplant Services, Fort Worth, TX.)

 The major complications of hemodialysis include access infection and access obstruction. In addition, school, social, and family lives are disrupted because of the treatment schedule. However, children treated with hemodialysis in a specialized pediatric unit can thrive. Hemodialysis is technically more difficult for infants and small children, and fluid and electrolyte shifts are more pronounced.

 Hemodialysis is more efficient and requires less time than peritoneal dialysis. In addition, the family has less direct responsibility for the actual dialysis process since it is performed by personnel in a dialysis center.

Peritoneal Dialysis

In peritoneal dialysis, fluid enters the peritoneal cavity through a catheter that is placed in the child's abdomen, at the bedside or in the operating room. The dialysis fluid remains in the cavity for a prescribed time, during which waste products, chemicals, and fluid pass through the peritoneal membrane into the fluid. The fluid is then drained out of the body, and the process is repeated.

 In children receiving long-term dialysis, the exchanges are often performed at home every night with an automated cycler while the child is asleep.

 Peritoneal dialysis is technically easier than hemodialysis. Advantages over hemodialysis include more independence for the child and family and a more stable physiologic state because of more frequent dialysis. The disadvantages include the risk of infections (peritonitis, catheter exit site) and the stress often experienced by the family and child due to treatment demands.

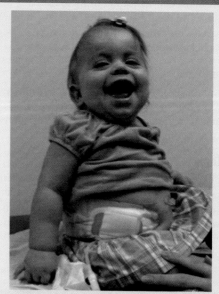

Peritoneal dialysis. Implanted line allows instillation of the dialyzing fluid into this child's peritoneal cavity. (Photo courtesy Cook Children's Pediatric Nephrology, Dialysis, and Transplant Services, Fort Worth, TX.)

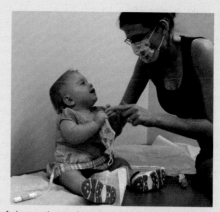

Infection of the peritoneal cavity is the chief hazard of peritoneal dialysis. When the lines are open to begin or end the dialyzing cycle, both adult and child wear masks. (Photo courtesy Cook Children's Pediatric Nephrology, Dialysis, and Transplant Services, Fort Worth, TX.)

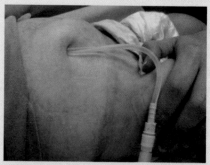

Peritoneal dialysis catheter exit site. (Photo courtesy Cook Children's Pediatric Nephrology, Dialysis, and Transplant Services, Fort Worth, TX.)

with medications and diet restrictions. Chronic renal failure progresses to end-stage renal disease (ESRD), which is the permanent, irreversible loss of kidney function such that conservative treatment alone can no longer sustain the child's health and life. ESRD usually is diagnosed when the glomerular filtration rate (GFR) decreases to 10%.

Etiology

The causes of chronic renal failure in children are different from those in adults. The most common causes, especially in younger children, are congenital anomalies such as obstruction, VUR, and renal dysplasia. Chronic renal failure can develop in children from diseases such as glomerulonephritis, pyelonephritis, and HUS. In general, secondary causes of ESRD such as diabetes and high blood pressure, are not seen in children.

Incidence

The incidence of chronic renal failure with ESRD among children younger than 19 years is approximately 18 in 1 million (Sreedharan & Avner, 2011). The incidence is higher in adolescents, in boys, and in whites.

Pathophysiology

Regardless of the initial cause of kidney damage, chronic renal failure progresses to ESRD. The exact mechanisms are unclear. Factors that contribute to the development of ESRD include continuing immunologic injury, hyperfiltration (the overwork of the remaining nephrons), high dietary phosphorus intake, persistent proteinuria, and hypertension.

Manifestations

Manifestations of chronic renal failure and ESRD include electrolyte abnormalities, fluid volume shifts (dehydration or fluid overload), acid-base imbalances, renal osteodystrophy (rickets), anemia, poor growth, hypertension, fatigue, decreased appetite, poor feeding, nausea and vomiting, and neurologic symptoms from accumulation of wastes in the blood.

Diagnostic Evaluation

Chronic renal failure may manifest nonspecifically. Physical examination may reveal short stature and failure to thrive. The child may be hypertensive. Blood work reveals electrolyte abnormalities (varying according to the underlying disease process), calcium and phosphorus abnormalities (decreased calcium and bone calcium resorption, elevated serum phosphorus), and anemia. Rising serum creatinine and BUN levels suggest ESRD. Creatinine clearance testing measures the ability of the renal system to excrete metabolic products; it gives an approximation of the GFR. As renal function deteriorates, the creatinine clearance decreases. Bone radiographs diagnose renal osteodystrophy. The child may have normal fluid volume, be dehydrated, or have fluid overload.

The history may or may not include known renal disease. Diagnostic tests may be performed to determine etiology and prognosis. These may include a voiding cystourethrogram (VCUG), renal ultrasonography, renal scan, and renal biopsy.

Therapeutic Management
Chronic Renal Failure

The diet of a child with chronic renal failure is modified because of the decreased ability of the kidneys to regulate fluids, electrolytes, minerals, and waste products. Reductions in sodium and fluid intake are necessary to prevent fluid overload and hypertension. Phosphorus is restricted to manage bone disease (renal osteodystrophy). Serum potassium levels are closely monitored and decreased intake may be required because of impaired excretion by the kidneys. Protein intake is carefully regulated to decrease the accumulation of waste products while providing the child with essential amino acids and other nutrients.

Diuretics may be indicated to control fluid overload, and antihypertensives are given for hypertension. Sodium bicarbonate tablets are taken to maintain acid-base balance. Synthetic, active vitamin D and phosphorus-binding medications are given to increase serum calcium, decrease phosphorus blood levels, control parathyroid gland activity, and treat renal osteodystrophy.

Children with chronic renal failure should receive all childhood immunizations and a yearly influenza vaccine, unless immunosuppressive treatment precludes live-virus vaccines. It is advantageous to administer live-virus vaccines as soon as possible within the normal childhood schedule so the child is fully immunized before undergoing kidney transplantation which requires lifelong immunosuppressant therapy (Sreedharan & Avner, 2011).

Advances in the treatment of infants and children with chronic renal failure, such as recombinant erythropoietin and recombinant growth hormone, have improved the quality of life of these children (Sreedharan & Avner, 2011). Recombinant erythropoietin is used to treat anemia, thus improving the energy level and avoiding repeated blood transfusions. The use of recombinant growth hormone has significantly improved the growth of children with chronic renal failure (Sreedharan & Avner, 2011).

End-Stage Renal Disease

The diagnosis of ESRD is made by monitoring serum creatinine levels, glomerular filtration rate, and the quality of the child's life. Dialysis or kidney transplantation is required once ESRD is diagnosed with only 5% to 10% of kidney function remaining.

Kidney Transplantation

Transplantation is the therapeutic goal for most children with ESRD; it offers the best opportunity for relatively normal lives and continued growth and development. Unfortunately, transplantation is not a cure. Children with kidney transplants must continue to take immunosuppressive medications daily, have frequent blood tests, and attend regular clinic appointments.

Kidneys come from either living donors or cadaveric donors. A living donor is often someone in the child's family, such as a parent, older sibling, or grandparent, although persons without a biologic relation may also donate a kidney. The donor must be in good health and have healthy kidneys. A cadaveric donor kidney is obtained from a person who has been declared brain dead and whose family has consented to the donation. The cadaveric donor kidney must have normal function. The blood and tissue types of the donor and recipient need to be compatible. Transplants with kidneys from living-related donors are generally more successful in children than transplants using cadaveric donor kidneys.

Rejection by the child's immunologic system of the transplanted kidney is the most common complication. Immunosuppressive medications are taken to prevent rejection; these include cyclosporine (Gengraf or Neoral), prednisone, tacrolimus (Prograf), and mycophenolate (CellCept or Myfortic).

As with all medications, immunosuppressive medications have side effects. When the immune system is suppressed, risk of infection is increased, related to the body's decreased ability to fight infection. Children with renal transplants should be monitored for infection and may take antiinfective medications routinely.

High blood pressure is also a complication of transplantation. Underlying renal disease, the transplanted kidney, or immunosuppressive medication side effects can cause high blood pressure.

NURSING CARE OF THE CHILD WITH CHRONIC RENAL FAILURE AND END-STAGE RENAL DISEASE

Assessment

The assessment of the child with chronic renal failure or ESRD is directed toward clinical manifestations of the renal failure and its possible complications. Blood is monitored for abnormalities and response to interventions. Monitoring hemoglobin and hematocrit assesses for potential anemia and assesses response to therapy in the child receiving recombinant erythropoietin. Serum calcium and phosphorus, alkaline phosphatase, and parathyroid hormone levels and bone radiographs are obtained to monitor for renal osteodystrophy.

The nurse assesses fluid volume status for fluid overload and dehydration by obtaining the child's weight, monitoring blood pressure and heart rate, and observing and documenting findings related to edema, skin turgor, mucous membranes, and fontanels.

Accurate weights and height measurements are obtained regularly and plotted on growth curves to assess the child's growth and development. Parents are asked to provide the child's dietary and caloric intake history. Information regarding attainment of developmental tasks, school performance, and peer relationships is important to include in the nurse's assessment.

Nursing Diagnosis and Planning

The nursing diagnoses and expected outcomes that apply to the child with chronic renal failure and the child's family are as follows:

- Imbalanced Nutrition: Less Than Body Requirements related to decreased appetite and dietary restrictions.

Expected Outcome. The child will receive adequate nutrition for growth and health as measured by appropriate growth for age.

- Deficient Knowledge about disease process, treatment, or diet restrictions related to anxiety or incomplete understanding of principles.

Expected Outcomes. The child and parents will be able to explain the disease process, its treatment, and dietary restrictions.

- Risk for Imbalanced Fluid Volume related to fluid and electrolyte shifts secondary to renal dysfunction.

Expected Outcome. The child will exhibit no signs of fluid overload or deficit, as measured by weight, blood pressure, and absence of edema or signs of dehydration.

- Delayed Growth and Development related to restricted diet, chronic illness, and anemia.

Expected Outcomes. The child will continue to grow and develop at acceptable rates according to standard measuring instruments.

- Interrupted Family Processes related to having a child with a chronic and potentially life-threatening disease.

Expected Outcome. The child and family will use successful coping strategies, as measured by their ability to care for the child, meet the needs of other family members, and access appropriate support.

- Risk for Impaired Skin Integrity related to edema and poor nutrition.

Expected Outcome. The child's skin will be intact without redness, irritation, or breaks.

Interventions

The care of the child with chronic renal failure is complex and requires a multidisciplinary team. Maintaining adequate nutritional intake within the dietary restriction parameters is a challenge. The nurse individualizes the diet of the child with chronic renal failure and includes foods the child likes. Small, frequent meals are helpful. Diet supplements may be necessary to meet caloric needs. Administration of recombinant growth hormone may allow the child to have adequate growth.

Children with chronic renal failure and their families have multi-faceted information requirements. The parents need information regarding diet, medications, potential adverse effects of the renal failure, and side effects from treatment. Most children with chronic renal failure will need dialysis. Children and their families will be most successful with dialysis if the method chosen fits their lifestyle (Gilman, Miller, & Rabetoy, 2006). The goal is to optimize physical, social, and emotional development while addressing complex physical requirements. Additionally, children and parents need to be informed about other treatment options including transplantation.

The nurse is diligent in providing the correct amount of fluid intake and ongoing assessment of fluid volume status. The child and family are educated about fluid restrictions and hydration assessment parameters such as weight, blood pressure, and appearance of edema.

The child is encouraged to participate in school and other age-appropriate activities. Parents may find it difficult to allow their child to be independent and may need assistance in this area.

Children with chronic renal failure and their families need support from a multidisplinary team of health care providers. They need opportunities to ask questions, verbalize feelings, and express concerns. Involving children in their own care and decisions regarding treatment is beneficial. It is important to determine the coping strategies used successfully by the family in the past and then encourage family members to use those same strategies again. The nurse considers making referrals to social workers, child life specialists, play therapists, psychologists, or psychiatrists when the need for additional support is indicated.

Evaluation

- Does the child maintain the age-appropriate growth percentile on a growth chart despite dietary restrictions?
- Can the parents and the child discuss the disease course and management?
- Is the child adapting to diet restrictions?
- Is the child free of edema?
- Has the integrity of the child's skin been maintained?
- Does the child have moist mucous membranes and adequate urine output (see Chapter 16)?
- Does the child continue to achieve age-appropriate developmental milestones?
- Is the family involved in the child's care?
- Has the family demonstrated appropriate coping strategies to meet the needs of all family members, and do they access appropriate support?

KEY CONCEPTS

- The kidneys reach near-adult function at 6 to 12 months of age.
- Infants cannot concentrate urine as efficiently as older children and adults.
- With therapeutic intervention, nocturnal enuresis can be resolved for most children.
- The clinical manifestations of UTI vary in relation to the child's age, gender, underlying anatomic or neurologic abnormalities, and frequency of recurrence.
- UTI is the most common clinical manifestation of vesicoureteral reflux (VUR).
- To prevent UTI, nurses educate the parents and child about perineal hygiene, increased fluid intake, emptying the bladder, and wearing cotton underwear.
- Cryptorchidism will spontaneously resolve in most infants during the first year of life.

- Goals for hypospadias corrective surgery are normal urinary and sexual function and improved cosmetic appearance of the penis.
- Children with glomerulonephritis should be assessed for signs and symptoms of hypertension and fluid overload.
- Children with edema should have their position changed at least every 2 hours and their lower extremities elevated when they are sitting or lying in bed.
- Edema related to nephrotic syndrome is first noted in the periorbital spaces and dependent areas of the body. Prednisone usually induces a remission in the child with nephrotic syndrome.
- Most children with acute renal failure regain renal function.
- Children with chronic renal failure (ESRD) and their families require multidisciplinary care.

REFERENCES

Acerini, C., Miles, H., Dunger, D., et al. (2009). The descriptive epidemiology of congenital and acquired cryptorchidism in a UK infant cohort. *Archives of Disease in Childhood, 94*(11), 868-872.

Agency for Healthcare Research and Quality. (2008). *Antibiotics to prevent children's recurrent urinary tract infections have unclear benefits and potential risks.* Retrieved from www.ahrq.gov/research/jan08/0108RA2.htm.

Ashley, R., Barthold, J., & Kolon, T. (2010). Cryptorchidism: Pathogenesis, diagnosis, treatment, and prognosis. *Urologic Clinics of North America, 37*(2), 183-193.

Elder, J. (2011a). Anomalies of the penis and urethra. In R. Kliegman, B. Stanton, J. St. Geme, et al. (Eds.), *Nelson textbook of pediatrics* (19th ed., pp. 1852-1858). Philadelphia: Elsevier Saunders.

Elder, J. (2011b). Disorders and anomalies of the scrotal contents. In R. Kliegman, B. Stanton, J. St. Geme, et al. (Eds.), *Nelson textbook of pediatrics* (19th ed., pp. 1858-1864). Philadelphia: Elsevier Saunders.

Elder, J. (2011c). Obstructions of the urinary tract. In R. Kliegman, B. Stanton, J. St. Geme, et al. (Eds.), *Nelson textbook of pediatrics* (19th ed., pp. 1838-1847). Philadelphia: Elsevier Saunders.

Elder, J. (2011d). Urinary tract infections. In R. Kliegman, B. Stanton, J. St. Geme, et al. (Eds.), *Nelson textbook of pediatrics* (19th ed., pp. 1829-1834). Philadelphia: Elsevier Saunders.

Elder, J. (2011e). Vesicoureteral reflux. In R. Kliegman, B. Stanton, J. St. Geme, et al. (Eds.), *Nelson textbook of pediatrics* (19th ed., pp. 1834-1838). Philadelphia: Elsevier Saunders.

Elder, J. (2011f). Voiding dysfunction. In R. Kliegman, B. Stanton, J. St. Geme, et al. (Eds.), *Nelson textbook of pediatrics* (19th ed., pp. 1847-1852). Philadelphia: Elsevier Saunders.

Gilman, C., Miller, D., & Rabetoy, C. (Ed.). (2006). Controversies in nephrology nursing: Peritoneal dialysis is the treatment choice for pediatric patients. *Nephrology Nursing Journal, 33*(2), 219-220.

Marild, S., Hansson, S., Jodal, U., et al. (2004). Protective effect of breastfeeding against urinary tract infection. *Acta Paediatrica, 93*(2), 164-168.

Montini, G., Rigon, L., Zucchetta, P., et al. (2008). Prophylaxis after first febrile urinary tract infection in children? A multicenter, randomized, controlled, noninferiority trial. *Pediatrics 122*(5), 1064-1071.

National Institute for Health and Clinical Excellence. (2007). *Urinary tract infection in children: Diagnosis, treatment and long-term management.* Retrieved from www.nice.org.uk/nicemedia/pdf/CG54fullguideline.pdf.

Pais, P. & Avner, E. (2011). Nephrotic syndrome. In R. Kliegman, B. Stanton, J. St. Geme, et al. (Eds.), *Nelson textbook of pediatrics* (19th ed., pp. 1801-1807). Philadelphia: Elsevier Saunders.

Pan, C. & Avner, E. (2011). Glomerulonephritis associated with infections. In R. Kliegman, B. Stanton, J. St. Geme, et al. (Eds.), *Nelson textbook of pediatrics* (19th ed., pp. 1783-1786). Philadelphia: Elsevier Saunders.

Shaikh, N., Morone, N., Lopez, J., et al. (2007). Does this child have a urinary tract infection? *Journal of the American Medical Association, 298*(24), 2895-2904.

Sreedharan, R. & Avner, E. (2011). Renal failure. In R. Kliegman, B. Stanton, J. St. Geme, et al. (Eds.), *Nelson textbook of pediatrics* (19th ed., pp. 1818-1826). Philadelphia: Elsevier Saunders.

The Child with a Respiratory Alteration

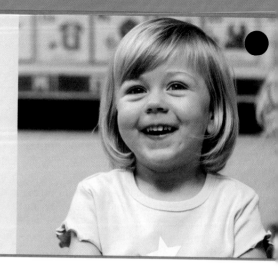

evolve WEBSITE

http://evolve.elsevier.com/James/ncoc

LEARNING OBJECTIVES

After studying this chapter, you should be able to:

- Describe the differences in the anatomy and physiology of the infant's or child's respiratory system that increase the risk for respiratory disease.
- Outline nursing care for a child with allergies to inhalants.
- Discuss the pathophysiology, clinical manifestations, and therapeutic management of common acute and chronic respiratory alterations.
- Identify the nursing care needs of infants and children with acute and chronic respiratory alterations.
- Develop guidelines for the home care of a child with an acute respiratory alteration.
- Identify common triggers of asthma symptoms.
- Apply measures that can be taken to prevent and treat asthma episodes.

- Identify teaching needs for children with asthma and their families.
- Describe the nursing care of the child with cystic fibrosis.
- Discuss measures to maintain adequate oxygenation and provide appropriate developmental stimulation for the child with bronchopulmonary dysplasia.
- Describe the correct method of administering and evaluating tuberculosis skin tests.
- Identify ways to prevent the transmission of tuberculosis and explain the importance of administering antituberculosis medications as prescribed.

CLINICAL REFERENCE

REVIEW OF THE RESPIRATORY SYSTEM

The respiratory system consists of the nose, pharynx, larynx, trachea, bronchi, and lungs. It is further divided into the *upper respiratory tract* (nose, pharynx, larynx) and the *lower respiratory tract* (trachea, bronchi, lungs).

The Upper Airway

Air enters the body through the *nares,* or nostrils, two nasal cavities lined with mucous membrane. In older infants and children, air can also enter through the mouth into the *pharynx,* or throat. The *nasopharynx* is located immediately behind the nasal cavity; the *oropharynx* is located behind the mouth. The *laryngeal pharynx* lies below the

oropharynx and opens into the larynx toward the front and into the esophagus toward the back.

The *larynx* is located between the pharynx and the trachea. The vocal cords are at the upper end of the larynx. The proximity of the upper esophagus to the upper respiratory system can put an individual at risk for inhaling food or liquids, but the *epiglottis* covers the larynx during swallowing and helps keep food out of the lower respiratory tract.

Cilia are hairlike processes that move mucus and fluid. Damage to cilia interferes with the removal of mucus from the respiratory tract. Ciliated mucous membranes line the larynx and filter dust and other particles from the air. The particles are then carried to the pharynx to be removed by sneezing, blowing, or coughing. After being filtered, the

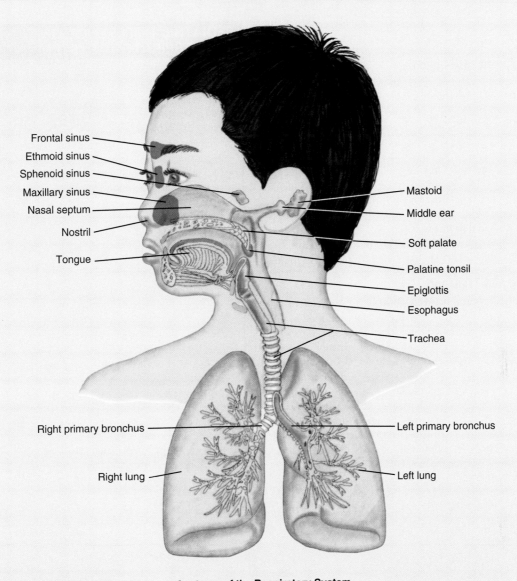

Anatomy of the Respiratory System

air that enters the respiratory system is humidified and warmed before proceeding into the lungs.

Tonsils are located in the posterior oropharynx. The three types of tonsils are the oval *palatine tonsils,* located on either side of the pharynx; the *lingual tonsil,* located below the palatine tonsils at the base of the tongue; and the *pharyngeal tonsils,* or *adenoids,* located at the nasopharyngeal border. The tonsils are composed mainly of lymphoid tissue. They help filter the circulating lymph of bacteria and other foreign material that enter the body, especially through the mouth and nose.

The Lower Airway

The *trachea* conducts air between the larynx and the lungs. It divides into right and left main *bronchi* at its lower end, the *carina.* The right main bronchus is shorter and wider than the left. The main bronchi divide into *lobar bronchi, segmental bronchi,* and *bronchioles* and terminate in *alveoli.* Mucus-secreting goblet cells line the bronchi and protect the lungs from dust and bacteria.

The *lungs* are two cone-shaped structures within the thoracic cavity. The right lung has three *lobes* (upper, middle, and lower); the left has two lobes (upper and lower). The *pleura* consists of two layers, the *parietal pleura* and the *visceral pleura.* The parietal pleura lines the entire thoracic cavity; the visceral pleura encases each lung. The pleura help maintain lung stability. Negative pressure within the intrapleural space prevents the lungs from separating from the thorax. *Diffusion* of gases takes place in the lungs. Terminal bronchioles lack mucus-secreting goblet cells and cilia, and gas exchange does not take place here.

Distal to the terminal bronchioles are the alveoli, where most gas exchange occurs. Thinness of the alveolar walls aids in gas exchange. An almost solid sheet of capillaries is within the alveolar walls, so the alveolar gases are proximate to the capillary blood.

Prenatal Respiratory Development

The respiratory system must mature before birth for the neonate to survive. The placenta performs oxygenation in utero, but to adapt to extrauterine life the neonate must be able to inflate the lungs, establish

Animation—Bronchi and Bronchioles

481

continuous breathing, and transfer the gases needed to meet metabolic needs.

Postnatal Respiratory Changes

Postnatal changes in the respiratory system occur as follows:

1. Compression of the thorax during vaginal delivery forces out some fetal lung fluid.
2. Respirations are stimulated by hypoxemia; hypercarbia; cold, tactile stimulation; and a possible decrease in the concentration of prostaglandin E$_2$.
3. Inflation of the normal lung is complete within a few breaths, and most alveoli have expanded within the first hour of life.
4. Surfactant in the lung liquid lowers surface tension and facilitates lung expansion.
5. Pulmonary blood flow increases.
6. Closure of the foramen ovale and the ductus arteriosus (see Chapter 22) establishes the pulmonary and circulatory systems.

Gas Exchange and Transport

Two-way diffusion takes place between the walls of the alveoli. In *diffusion,* molecules move from an area of greater concentration to one of lesser concentration. Blood entering the lung capillaries is somewhat low in oxygen. Oxygen will diffuse from the alveoli, where its concentration is higher, into the blood. Similarly, carbon dioxide moves out of the blood and into the alveoli. Most oxygen that diffuses into the capillary blood in the lungs is bound to the hemoglobin of red blood cells. A small percentage is dissolved in plasma. For oxygen to enter the cells, it must separate from hemoglobin. Carbon dioxide diffuses into the blood from the tissues and is transported to the lungs by the blood. In this activity, hemoglobin is a buffer that enables blood to take up carbon dioxide without altering the blood pH significantly. The uptake and delivery of gases by the blood is a continuous process.

Ventilation occurs through *inspiration* and *expiration.* In inspiration, the diaphragm contracts and flattens, expanding the vertical dimension of the chest; the lung volume increases. In expiration, the

PEDIATRIC DIFFERENCES IN THE RESPIRATORY SYSTEM

- Surfactant is lacking in premature infants. Infants born before 34 weeks of gestation have a higher risk for respiratory distress syndrome (RDS).
- Smaller lower airways and undeveloped supporting cartilage predispose the child to an increased risk for obstruction by mucus, edema, and foreign bodies. The neonate's airway is 50% smaller than that of adults. A premature infant has a more compliant chest wall and weaker respiratory muscles than a term infant.
- Lung size is proportional to body height. Therefore, lung volumes and capacities do not vary from age to age.
- Infants are obligatory nose breathers; they have difficulty breathing through the mouth. If the infant has nasal congestion, breathing becomes more difficult.
- The diaphragm is the neonate's major respiratory muscle. Intercostal muscles are not well developed. Retractions are more common in the infant than in older children and adults.
- Brief periods of apnea (10 to 15 seconds) are common in the neonate. The respiratory pattern may be irregular.
- Children's normal respiratory rate is higher than that of adults.
- An increased metabolic rate increases oxygen needs.
- Alveoli develop from approximately 20 million to 200 million by age 3 years. Alveolar development gradually decreases after age 3 years; few develop after age 8 years.
- The lung surface increases until age 5 to 8 years. Actual lung growth continues into the adolescent years.
- Eustachian tubes are relatively horizontal, which increases the risk for bacteria entering the middle ear.
- Tracheal size approximately triples by adulthood.
- Tonsillar tissue is normally enlarged in early school-age children.
- Infants and children use abdominal muscles to inhale until about age 5 to 6 years.
- The child's flexible larynx is more susceptible to spasm.

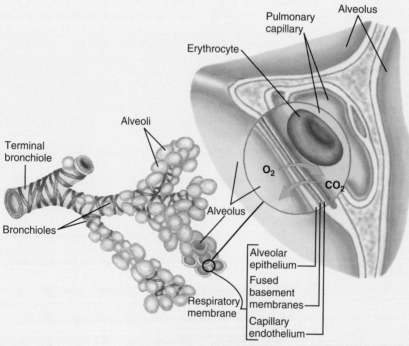

Mechanisms of Gas Exchange

diaphragm and chest wall relax, decreasing thoracic volume. Intrathoracic pressure increases, and gas flows out of the lungs, taking with it the carbon dioxide that was delivered to the lungs by the blood. Ventilation of the lungs is intermittent. Inspired air is 21% oxygen; end-expired air is 16% oxygen and 35% carbon dioxide.

DIAGNOSTIC TESTS

In most instances, respiratory tract disorders are diagnosed from the findings on physical examination and the clinical manifestations. Sometimes, however, specific diagnostic tests are needed.

COMMON LABORATORY AND DIAGNOSTIC TESTS FOR RESPIRATORY DISORDERS

TEST	DESCRIPTION	NORMAL FINDINGS	INDICATIONS	NURSING CONSIDERATIONS
Chest radiography, posterior, anterior and lateral views	Shows airways, lungs, heart, great vessels	Normal appearance of internal structures of chest	To detect respiratory disease of lungs	Assist in holding child.
Computed tomography	Shows lesions in chest wall, pleural space, mediastinum, and lung parenchyma	Normal cross section of lung tissue	To image tumors or masses; to evaluate response to therapy aimed at defined lesions	Assist with sedation and immobilization of child. Withhold feedings 3-4 hr before the test because of frequent use of contrast medium.
Bronchoscopy	Provides viewing of tracheobronchial tree through a scope	Normal appearance of tracheobronchial tree or successful removal of foreign body or mucous plugs	To view a lesion and obtain biopsy material for culture; to remove foreign body or mucous plugs	Rigid bronchoscopy is usually performed with child under general anesthesia. Fiberoptic flexible bronchoscopy can be performed while child is awake or sedated. Observe child closely for signs of airway obstruction. Mist may be given to decrease swelling and edema.
Laryngoscopy	Provides direct viewing of larynx with a scope	Normal appearance of larynx	To identify cause of stridor and local abnormalities	Mirror (indirect) laryngoscopy can be performed on children age 4 yr or older. In infants and younger children, direct laryngoscopy or transnasal laryngoscopy with flexible bronchoscope will give much better results. General anesthesia is usually required; topical anesthesia and mild sedation may be provided for fiberoptic examination. Fluids and foods are withheld until effects of local anesthetic have worn off and gag reflex has returned.
Cultures	Throat, blood, nasopharyngeal, sputum, induced sputum	No culture growth or normal flora only	To isolate and identify pathogens	See Chapter 13 for procedures.
RAST for IgE	Measures quantity of IgE antibodies in serum after exposure to specific antigens	If the child is not allergic to the antigen, IgE antibody is not detected. A test result is positive in relation to a specific antigen if the value is above 400% of control	To identify specific allergens; systemic reactions to insect venom, drugs, and chemicals; to monitor response to desensitization procedures; also performed at the onset of asthma, hay fever, or dermatitis	Prepare child for peripheral blood sample to be drawn. Determine whether child has undergone any radioisotope tests within past week because such tests may alter the results.

IgE, immunoglobulin E; *RAST*, radioallergosorbent test.

Continued

COMMON LABORATORY AND DIAGNOSTIC TESTS FOR RESPIRATORY DISORDERS—cont'd

TEST	DESCRIPTION	NORMAL FINDINGS	INDICATIONS	NURSING CONSIDERATIONS
Pilocarpine iontophoresis (sweat test)	Measures sweat electrolyte concentration for diagnosis of CF Sweating is stimulated on the child's forearm with a small electrical current and pilocarpine; a sweat sample is then collected on preweighed, dry, sterile gauze or filter paper and the amounts of sweat sodium and chloride are measured	Normal chloride: <40 mEq/L Suggestive of CF: 40 to 60 mEq/L Positive for CF: >60 mEq/L	To diagnose cystic fibrosis	No physical preparation is needed. Offer parents and child support as they face the implications of a positive diagnosis. Inform child and parents that the test is painless and that it is usually performed twice to ensure accurate results. Because an adequate amount of sweat is difficult to obtain from infants, the sweat test is usually unreliable in infants younger than 2 wk.
Mantoux test	Skin test for TB PPD, 5 TB units (0.1 mL) is injected intradermally into volar surface of forearm with short, 26- to 27-gauge needle, beveled side up A wheal 6-10 mm in diameter should appear during injection The site is checked in 48-72 hr by a health care professional Results are recorded in millimeters (not simply as positive or negative). The reading is based on induration (hardness), not redness	Positive result: area of induration ≥15 mm (in children 4 yr of age and older); area of induration ≥10 mm in children younger than 4 yr or at high risk for exposure; area of induration ≥5 mm in highest risk group Negative result: Mantoux test cannot rule out the presence of TB, particularly in young infants	To screen and test individuals suspected of having TB or of having been exposed to TB	Test is fairly difficult to administer. After PPD is injected, withdrawal of needle should be delayed 2-3 sec to minimize leakage of PPD at the puncture site. In most children, skin testing will elicit positive reaction 3-6 wk after initial infection. Steroids and immunosuppressants given within 4-6 wk can cause false-negative skin test results. Positive tuberculin reactivity usually continues for person's lifetime, even with treatment.

CF, Cystic fibrosis; *PPD*, purified protein derivative; *TB*, tuberculosis.

Blood Gas Analysis

Arterial blood gas analysis plays an important role in the investigation of pulmonary function. Arterial blood gas values most frequently determined include the partial arterial oxygen tension (PaO_2), the partial pressure of carbon dioxide in arterial blood ($PaCO_2$), the acid-base balance (pH), and bicarbonate (HCO_3^-). Arterial blood is more reliable than capillary or venous blood for these tests, especially in children with poor peripheral perfusion. Arterial blood gas values are used primarily to determine acid-base balance, not oxygen saturation (see Chapter 16).

Pulmonary Function Tests

Probably the most useful measures of ventilatory function are the *vital capacity* and the *expiratory flow rate*, both measured by spirometry. Spirometry can be performed at an acceptable level by most preschool-aged children (Gaffin, Shotola, Martin, & Phipatanakul, 2010). Accurate measurements are difficult to obtain in younger children because they are unable to follow commands. Infant pulmonary function testing is now being performed at many institutions with the use of conscious sedation. Pulmonary function tests assess the degree of pulmonary disease, the response to therapy, and the presence of restrictive or obstructive disease. They are also done to test the child's response to bronchodilators should pulmonary function be affected.

The child must be given instruction and practice in blowing, pushing, and holding respirations. The child should become familiar with the mouthpiece and the nose clip to feel comfortable with their use.

Pulse Oximetry

Pulse oximetry is a simple, noninvasive, intermittent or continuous method for measuring oxygen saturation for the purpose of determining the need for or response to oxygen therapy (see Chapter 13). The goal of treatment for most respiratory conditions is an oxygen saturation value greater than 95%. For children with chronic respiratory disease, however, a realistic goal may be slightly lower.

Transcutaneous Monitoring

Transcutaneous monitoring continuously checks oxygen and carbon dioxide concentrations in the body through an electrode placed on the child's skin. Electrode sites must be changed every 3 to 4 hours to prevent burning the skin, and the machine must be recalibrated each time electrodes are changed. The readings may not be accurate if tissue perfusion is poor.

End-Tidal Carbon Dioxide Monitoring

End-tidal carbon dioxide monitoring, often used in conjunction with pulse oximetry, measures carbon dioxide in the exhaled breath noninvasively. It is useful in verifying endotracheal tube position, in evaluating asthma, and during procedural sedation. It can also be a primary indicator of worsening respiratory distress or impending respiratory failure because results are thought to mimic $PaCO_2$ measurement (Burton, Harrah, Germann, & Dillon, 2006).

RESPIRATORY ILLNESS IN CHILDREN

Respiratory alterations are the most common causes of illness in the infant and child. Upper respiratory disorders affect the ears, nose, pharynx, and larynx; lower respiratory disorders include those disorders that involve the trachea, bronchi, and lungs.

Infants and children younger than 3 years of age are at greater risk than older children and adults for development of respiratory infections because of their immature immune systems, smaller upper and lower airways, and underdeveloped supporting cartilage. Although most respiratory infections are self-limiting, in infants and young children respiratory distress can occur quickly as mucus and edema obstruct their small airways.

Parents should be taught preventive measures, including adequate rest, optimal nutrition, and good hygiene, with an emphasis on hand hygiene. Even with the most careful hygiene and preventive practices, however, most children will have some type of respiratory infection each year. School nurses often see children with respiratory problems in the school health office and may be the primary health care providers for these children.

Most children can be cared for at home by their parents and do not need hospitalization. Those children who are hospitalized are being discharged from the hospital earlier in their recovery than in the past. The current health care environment underlies the need for nurses to teach parents appropriate home care techniques, including careful observation and recognition of signs that indicate the need to contact health care providers. Parents, especially first-time parents, often are frightened by the sudden onset of respiratory symptoms, which may indicate a severe problem. Teaching them the signs and symptoms of serious illness will help them develop appropriate decision-making skills.

Children with chronic conditions have many special needs, and the child with a chronic respiratory disease is no different. Medications and treatments become a way of life for many of these children. Their activity level is often altered, and some may have a shortened life span.

Children with chronic respiratory conditions are now becoming adults with those same conditions. As advances in treatment modalities are made and children with these conditions are living longer, the transition to adult care becomes a necessity.

The nurse plays an important role in the care of the child with a chronic respiratory disease. Beyond giving acute care to the hospitalized child, the nurse must coordinate and facilitate the child's long-term care. Because of advances being made in the treatment of chronic pediatric respiratory conditions, the treatment and care of children affected by these disorders are constantly changing and improving, requiring the nurse to stay current in these areas.

ALLERGIC RHINITIS

Allergic rhinitis is an inflammatory disorder of the nasal mucosa. It is usually seasonal, recurrent, and triggered by specific allergens (see Chapter 18). It is sometimes referred to as *seasonal allergic rhinitis* or *hay fever*. Some children have symptoms year round (*perennial allergic rhinitis*).

Etiology and Incidence

Agents that commonly cause allergic rhinitis include dust mites, feathers, animal dander, mold spores, and pollens of trees, grasses, and weeds. There is usually a family history, similar to that seen in individuals with atopic dermatitis and asthma. Unlike atopic dermatitis, however, allergic rhinitis does not predispose to the development of asthma.

The onset of allergic rhinitis usually occurs during childhood but rarely before age 2 years. It is estimated that 20% to 40% of children have this type of allergic response (Milgrom & Leung, 2011).

PATHOPHYSIOLOGY

Allergic Rhinitis

Allergens (pollens, molds, spores, dust mites, animal dander) are deposited on the nasal mucosa, causing local inflammation and increased capillary permeability. Local immunoglobulin E (IgE) is produced, and sensitization of the respiratory tissues occurs. Mast cell mediators are released, producing vasodilation, mucosal edema, mucus secretions, stimulation of itch receptors, and a reduced threshold for sneezing.

Manifestations

The classic symptoms of allergic rhinitis are clear rhinorrhea, associated with itching of nose, eyes, ears, and palate, and paroxysmal sneezing. Additional signs and symptoms include the "allergic salute"—an upward rubbing of the nose with the palm of the hand, which can leave a crease below the bridge (Figure 21-1); allergic shiners—dark circles under the eyes from congestion and edema; dry lips from mouth breathing; pale, boggy nasal mucous membranes; and nasal

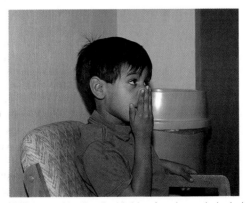

FIG 21-1 Children with allergic rhinitis often have dark circles under their eyes, called *allergic shiners*, and may be seen rubbing their noses upward with the palm—the "allergic salute." (Courtesy Parkland Health and Hospital System Community Oriented Primary Care Clinic, Dallas, TX.)

obstruction. Children with allergic rhinitis have symptoms as long as they are exposed to the allergen.

It is important to distinguish allergic rhinitis from viral *nasopharyngitis* (the common cold), which is usually caused by a rhinovirus and is spread by droplet or by contact with contaminated items. Usually children with nasopharyngitis have the associated symptoms of sore throat, fever, cough, and fatigue. The condition is self-limiting and usually resolves within 2 weeks. The quality of the nasal discharge in children with nasopharyngitis often changes from clear to cloudy or yellow. Management is supportive. Because young infants are obligatory nose breathers, the infant's blocked nasal passages can be relieved with instillation of normal saline solution drops followed by gentle bulb suction.

Diagnostic Evaluation

A thorough personal and family history usually elicits a description that suggests an allergic rather than infectious pattern. The nasal smear may demonstrate eosinophils. Allergy skin testing is done if signs and symptoms continue after treatment with medication. The radioallergo-sorbent test (RAST) is used only when skin testing is difficult because of generalized dermatitis, the child is very young, or the child is too ill for skin testing. A complete blood cell count might reveal elevated eosinophils, a finding associated with allergic manifestations.

Therapeutic Management

The treatment of choice is to eliminate the allergen from the child's environment; however, complete elimination may be difficult in children (Turner & Kemp, 2010). When this is impossible, as in the case of pollen in the air, medication can control symptoms.

Antihistamines or intranasal corticosteroids may be effective in treating allergic rhinitis. Antihistamines are most effective when given before or very early in an allergic episode. Because they can cause drowsiness, they should be given at night. Some of the newer antihistamines (e.g., loratadine, cetirizine, fexofenadine) are long acting, have fewer side effects and require only one or two doses daily. They are prescribed according to the child's age. Decongestants may be effective in relieving nasal congestion, but are not recommended in children. Decongestants have side-effect profiles that include insomnia, behavior problems and even cardiac events; therefore, their use is no longer recommended (Turner & Kemp, 2010).

Short-term topical intranasal corticosteroids (e.g., fluticasone, mometasone, and budesonide) are highly effective and may be used as first-line therapy for children with allergic rhinitis (Milgrom & Leung, 2011; Turner & Kemp, 2010). It usually takes several days of treatment before the child feels the effects of topical corticosteroids.

Leukotriene inhibitors (e.g., Singulair) may be used in the treatment of allergic rhinitis, although results may be suboptimal. These medications have a good safety profile and seem to work well for children with both allergic rhinitis and asthma (Turner & Kemp, 2010).

Finally, immunotherapy (allergy shots) may be considered for children whose condition is not responsive to either environmental modification or medication. Immunotherapy involves injecting the child with progressively larger doses of the allergen in an effort to reduce the magnitude of the body's allergic response. Injections are given once or twice a week until a maintenance dose is reached; monthly maintenance injections can continue for several years.

Nursing Considerations

Nursing care focuses on early identification of clinical signs and symptoms of allergic rhinitis and the therapeutic management of the condition. The nurse assesses and records the applicable history and helps the family identify allergens to which the child is sensitive. Once the allergens are known, the nurse counsels parents regarding administration of medications, environmental control, and immunotherapy as appropriate (see Patient-Centered Teaching: How to Implement Environmental Modifications box). Allergic rhinitis can negatively affect quality of life and school performance—not only does allergic rhinitis impair cognitive function, but allergies are also one of the most common reasons for missed school days, topping 2 million annually (Nathan, 2007).

PATIENT-CENTERED TEACHING

How to Implement Environmental Modifications

To reduce your child's exposure to allergens, take the following measures.

Pollen and Dust
- Wash your child's sheets and blankets weekly in hot water.
- Avoid using wool and down blankets.
- Encase pillows and mattresses in dust-proof covers.
- Replace carpet with wood, tile, slate, or vinyl.
- Replace drapes and blinds with curtains and shades.
- Replace upholstered furniture with wood or plastic.
- Keep closet doors shut.
- Cover hot air vents with filters.
- Install air cleaners.
- Use multilayer vacuum bags.
- Clean with a towel treated to attract dust.
- Run an air conditioner.
- Keep household humidity at 40% to 50%.

Mold
- Clean with a mold inhibitor.
- Dry everyone's shoes thoroughly.
- Use a moisture remover in closets.
- Encourage your child to stay out of the basement.
- Replace foam rubber mattresses with inner spring mattresses.
- Run an air conditioner.
- Keep the humidity below 35%.
- Run a dehumidifier.
- Ventilate the house.
- Store firewood outside.
- Limit the number of indoor plants.

Dander
- Keep pets outside if possible.
- Ventilate the house.
- Install air cleaners.
- Encase mattresses and pillows in dust-proof covers.

For further information, contact: Allergy & Asthma Network/Mothers of Asthmatics, Inc. website: www.aanma.org, a family site that provides information on asthma, products, kits, and books.

Side effects of medications used to treat allergic rhinitis can further impair functioning. Drowsiness, the most common side effect of antihistamines, can usually be alleviated if the child takes the medication at night. Some children may have dry mucous membranes or excitability. Warm water or saline solution irrigations of the nasal passages can be used to moisten mucous membranes, soften crusted secretions, and wash out irritants. Saline solution can be mixed by adding ¼ teaspoon of salt to a cup of warm water. Saline solution nose drops are also available without prescription.

When specific allergens have been identified, they should be eliminated or controlled. During the pollen season, the child should stay indoors as much as possible and the windows should be kept closed if the house is air conditioned. After being outdoors, the child should shower and wash his or her hair to remove pollens from the body. Animals that have been outside may also be a source of contamination.

Receiving immunotherapy can be a traumatic experience for the child. It is often difficult for children to understand how an injection will help them. Allergy injections must be given in a physician's office because the risk of an anaphylactic reaction to the allergy serum exists. Monitor the child closely (vital sign changes, difficulty breathing) for 20 to 30 minutes after the injection in case anaphylaxis develops. Keep emergency epinephrine ready.

SINUSITIS

Sinusitis, although not itself a serious disorder, can lead to life-threatening complications. Inflammation and infection of the sinuses can be acute or chronic.

Etiology and Incidence

Acute sinusitis often follows an upper respiratory tract viral infection. Children with chronic sinusitis often have allergic rhinitis or otitis media with effusion (OME) as well. Hypertrophied adenoids, immune deficiencies, and foreign body obstruction in the nose also predispose one to sinusitis. Children with cystic fibrosis have a high incidence of sinusitis because of highly viscous mucus secretions and nasal polyps. The most common causative organisms are *Streptococcus pneumoniae, Haemophilus influenzae, Moraxella catarrhalis,* and *Staphylococcus aureus* (Pappas & Hendley, 2011).

Sinus infections can occur in infancy as well as in childhood but are most common in the 2- to 6-year-old (Revai, Dobbs, Nair, et al., 2007).

PATHOPHYSIOLOGY

Sinusitis

Acute sinusitis occurs when the sinus cavity is invaded by bacteria, causing mucosal inflammation and edema that block narrow sinus channels. The volume of secretions increases, and the affected sinuses fill with purulent material. Inflammation and infection interfere with the protective cleansing action of the cilia covering the sinus mucous membranes. Impaired mucociliary transport leads to stagnation of secretions within the sinuses; the stagnant secretions provide a medium for bacterial growth.

Chronic sinusitis is usually a complication of acute sinusitis. Prolonged or repeated infections result in irreversible changes in the mucosal lining of the sinus. Nasal polyps, a deviated septum, and enlarged adenoids inhibit sinus drainage, which can lead to infections. The frontal and sphenoid sinuses are most often involved in children.

Infection from sinusitis can spread to the middle ear, causing otitis media. Serious complications occur when infection spreads either directly through the bone or along the venous channels of the skull into adjacent structures, such as the orbit or the central nervous system.

Manifestations

Sinusitis is characterized by signs and symptoms of a cold that do not improve after 14 days, low-grade fever, nasal congestion with purulent nasal discharge, halitosis, cough (which usually increases when the child is lying down), and headache, tenderness, and a feeling of fullness over the affected sinuses. Young children may become irritable. Occasionally, children have facial edema. Children with chronic sinusitis have many of the same symptoms except that the cough is chronic and the headache is recurrent. The child's sense of taste or smell may be impaired, and the child may be fatigued.

Diagnostic Evaluation

Sinus radiographs show mucosal thickening, opacification, and air-fluid levels in children older than 1 year. Sinus radiographs are of no value in younger children because of their small sinuses. Computed tomography is the diagnostic tool chosen most often for evaluation of sinus disease because it provides detailed anatomic information (Leo, Mori, Incorvaia et al., 2009). Because of the thick bone of the maxilla in the anterior part of the face and the small size of the sinus, transillumination of the sinuses is not useful.

Therapeutic Management

Most cases of acute sinusitis are self-resolving and do not require antibiotics (Suhaili, Goh, & Gendeh, 2010). When a prescription is required, amoxicillin or amoxicillin–potassium clavulanate (Augmentin) is used most frequently (DeMuri & Wald, 2010). In addition to antibiotics, treatment includes analgesics, hydration, and the application of moist heat. The use of decongestants or antihistamines in the treatment of sinusitis should be avoided in children secondary to inefficacy and potential risks posed to children (DeMuri & Wald, 2010). Antihistamines may be used to treat allergy symptoms associated with chronic sinusitis, but they tend to impair sinus drainage by thickening secretions. Steroid nasal sprays may be used to reduce inflammation while avoiding the rebound effect of decongestant nose drops. Saline nasal washes may also be helpful (DeMuri & Wald, 2010). Obstructive deformities, such as enlarged adenoids or polyps, are sometimes surgically corrected (Novembre, Mori, Pucci, et al., 2007).

If orbital cellulitis develops, the child should be hospitalized immediately and parenteral antibiotic therapy begun (Pappas & Hendley, 2011).

Nursing Considerations

The nurse assesses the location of pain or fullness. Pain can occur in the forehead or over the cheek bones or upper teeth, or it may radiate to the top of the head. Inspect and palpate the face for edema, document any fever, and inspect the nose and throat for purulent discharge. The nasal mucous membranes are inspected for erythema and edema.

Nursing care focuses on teaching the parents antibiotic administration, comfort measures, how to monitor for response to treatment, and how to identify complications. Emphasize the importance of the child taking the antibiotics as prescribed. Sinus drainage is facilitated by increasing the child's intake of clear fluids and by using a bedside humidifier.

Warm, moist compresses applied two or three times daily help decrease swelling and pain. Acetaminophen is given for fever and discomfort. Breathing warm mist in a hot shower or through hot, moist towels can help liquefy and mobilize nasal mucus, as can saline solution nose drops. The nurse teaches the parent to administer nose drops after the nasal passages have been gently cleaned. The amount, color, and consistency of nasal drainage should be noted and evaluated to determine whether the child is responding to treatment.

Carefully evaluate the child's response to treatment and the development of complications. Advise parents to contact the physician promptly if symptoms become worse, if the child has any periorbital redness or edema, or if the child does not seem to be feeling better after 3 to 4 days.

OTITIS MEDIA

Otitis media is one of the most common illnesses of infancy and childhood. The term *otitis media* refers to *effusion* (fluid) and infection or blockage of the middle ear. *Acute otitis media* (AOM) is effusion and inflammation in the middle ear that occurs suddenly and is associated with other signs of illness. *Otitis media with effusion* (OME) refers to the presence of fluid behind the tympanic membrane without signs of infection. Otitis media with effusion often follows an episode of AOM and usually resolves in 1 to 3 months.

Etiology

The bacterial pathogens that usually cause AOM are *S. pneumoniae*, *H. influenzae*, and *M. catarrhalis* (Coates, Thornton, Langlands et al., 2008). Although viruses do not cause otitis media, they are thought to predispose the child to ear infection by altering host defenses and contributing to eustachian tube dysfunction. Allergies are also thought to precipitate otitis media.

Attendance at daycare centers may predispose children to otitis media. Infants younger than 1 year who attend daycare have a significant risk for acquiring AOM. Other risk factors include age (highest in 6- to 24-month-olds), ethnicity (higher in Native Americans, Alaskan Inuit, and Canadian Inuit), exposure to household cigarette smoke, and pacifier use (Ramakrishnan, Sparks, & Berryhill, 2007).

Bottle feeding can contribute to ear infection because of the position of the infant during feeding. Reflux of formula into the eustachian tube from the nasopharynx occurs when the infant swallows while supine. Breastfeeding offers some protection from ear infection by providing maternal antibodies and by decreasing the incidence of allergy; also, the more upright position of the infant while nursing is protective against ear infection (Abdullah, Hassan, & Sidek, 2007).

Incidence

The incidence of otitis media peaks between ages 6 months and 6 years, with most episodes occurring in children younger than 3 years. Most initial episodes occur at about age 6 months, when maternal antibody levels decline. Early onset of AOM (during infancy) increases the risk for recurrent episodes (Lasisi, Olayemi, & Irabor, 2008).

By the end of the third year of life, more than 80% of all children have had at least one episode of AOM (Kerschner, 2011). Most children younger than 5 years have two or three episodes of otitis media each year. Boys have a slightly higher incidence of otitis media than girls. The incidence of otitis media is highest in winter and spring and lowest in the summer months.

Manifestations

AOM is characterized by the following:
- Otalgia (earache); infants may pull their ears or roll their heads.
- A bulging, opaque tympanic membrane that usually looks red, with decreased mobility; diffuse light reflex; and obscured landmarks (Figure 21-2).
- Drainage, usually yellowish green, purulent, and foul smelling (indicates perforation of the tympanic membrane).

These signs and symptoms might also be accompanied by irritability, sleep disturbances, persistent crying in infants, fever, vomiting, anorexia, or diarrhea (especially in infants).

OME differs from AOM in that there are no signs of acute infection. The tympanic membrane appears retracted and either dull gray or yellow, and an air-fluid level or air bubbles may be visible through the tympanic membrane. The mobility of the tympanic membrane is decreased, and landmarks are distorted. Associated signs and symptoms can be subtle and can include the following:
- Tinnitus, popping sounds
- Hearing loss (usually conductive) below 35 decibels, with delays in speech development possible from prolonged hearing loss; in the older child, hearing loss may manifest as behavior problems, poor school performance, disturbed sleep, irritability, and decreased responsiveness
- Mild balance disturbances that may result in delays in motor skills
- A flattened tracing and negative pressure on the tympanogram (a graphic representation of tympanic mobility and middle ear pressure)

AOM is considered to be persistent if the child experiences symptoms while being treated or within 1 month after treatment is complete. AOM is viewed as recurrent if the child experiences more than three episodes over a 6-month period or four episodes in a year (Kotsis, Nikolopoulos, Yiotakis et al., 2009).

Diagnostic Evaluation

The diagnosis of otitis media is based on the history of signs and symptoms and pneumatic otoscopy. In pneumatic otoscopy, a small puff of air is blown into the ear canal through the otoscope; the examiner can discern the appearance and mobility of the tympanic membrane. In addition to pneumatic otoscopy, tympanometry or tympanography can be used to confirm what was seen with the eye.

Therapeutic Management

The emergence of resistant organisms has created much discussion around the use of antibiotics to treat AOM because spontaneous resolution of the infection occurs in about 80% of children. In 2004, the American Academy of Pediatrics (AAP) issued two policy recommendations regarding identification and management of AOM and OME in healthy children ages 2 months to 12 years (AAP, 2004; American Academy of Pediatrics Subcommittee on Otitis Media with Effusion, American Academy of Family Physicians, & American Academy of Otolaryngology—Head and Neck Surgery, 2004). Recommendations include the following:
- Accurate discrimination between AOM and OME before treatment decisions are made
- Adequate pain relief for children with AOM
- Symptomatic treatment and observation for 48 to 72 hours after diagnosis as an alternative to initiating antibiotic therapy for selected children older than age 6 months with AOM
- Reassessment and treatment initiation for children with positive AOM after the 48- to 72-hour observation period
- Use of amoxicillin at a dose of 80 to 90 mg/kg/day for 5 to 10 days when treatment is indicated
- Encouraging reduction of risk factors as a method for preventing AOM episodes
- Treating children with OME who are not at risk for hearing, language, or learning problems with 3 months of "watchful waiting"

Alternative antibiotics such as azithromycin or a second- or third-generation cephalosporin may be prescribed for penicillin-resistant organisms or in cases of penicillin allergy (Kerschner, 2011). The pneumococcal conjugate vaccine was approved in 2001 for use in

PATHOPHYSIOLOGY

Otitis Media

Older child

The eustachian tube normally ventilates the middle ear by opening and closing regularly. This equalizes pressure and permits middle-ear drainage. It also protects the middle ear from nasopharyngeal secretions and sound pressure.

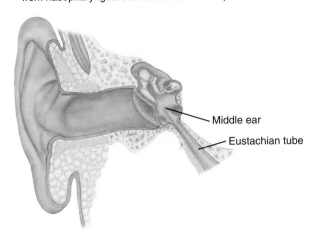

Middle ear

Eustachian tube

Infant/toddler

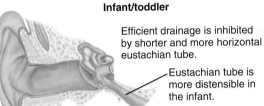

Efficient drainage is inhibited by shorter and more horizontal eustachian tube.

Eustachian tube is more distensible in the infant.

Lack of cartilage support causes eustachian tube to collapse easily, restricting drainage.

The immature anatomy of the child's middle ear and eustachian tube predisposes infants and toddlers to otitis media. When the eustachian tube is obstructed, as frequently occurs with enlarged adenoids or mucosal edema from an upper respiratory tract infection, effective drainage and ventilation of the middle ear cannot occur. Air that is normally present in the middle ear is absorbed by the blood, causing a vacuum or negative pressure in the middle ear. Effusion accumulates within the middle ear space, creating a medium for bacterial growth. After an upper respiratory tract infection, pathogens travel from the nasopharynx to the eustachian tube. In the presence of effusion, negative pressure in the middle ear draws mucus through the eustachian tube whenever the child cries, yawns, or sucks forcefully on a nipple. Purulent fluid accumulates in the middle ear space, causing the pressure and pain of acute otitis media.

If the eustachian tube remains nonfunctional for a prolonged period, the fluid within the middle ear becomes thick and dark (glue ear). Mild temporary conductive hearing loss (see Chapter 31) often occurs in otitis media with effusion because of the decreased mobility of the ossicles and the tympanic membrane. Permanent conductive hearing loss can result from repeated episodes of otitis media and may interfere with the development of language and cognitive skills. Chronic otitis media with effusion is the most common cause of hearing loss in children.

Complications of otitis media include conductive hearing loss and sensorineural hearing loss. The infection of acute otitis media can spread to surrounding tissues, causing mastoiditis or intracranial complications such as meningitis or brain abscess. Inflammation and pressure from otitis media may result in *tympanosclerosis* (scarring of the tympanic membrane), perforation of the tympanic membrane, and *cholesteatoma* (a cyst formed from pus and debris in the middle ear).

children and should be administered to all children younger than 2 years according to the recommended schedule (see Evolve website). After the approval of this vaccine in 2001, episodes of AOM caused by *S. pneumoniae* decreased substantially (Zhou, Shefer, Kong, & Nuorti, 2008).

A recent Level I meta-analysis of the usefulness of decongestants and antihistamines in the treatment or prevention of otitis media in children concluded that these medications provide minimal relief and have the risk for adverse side effects; therefore, they are not recommended (Coleman & Moore, 2008). Acetaminophen is given to help relieve the pain and fever of AOM.

In children with recurrent and persistent ear infection despite multiple courses of antibiotic therapy or with OME that persists for more than 3 months and is associated with hearing loss, *myringotomy* with insertion of *tympanostomy tubes* (pressure-equalizing tubes) may be performed (Kerschner, 2011). During this operation, mucoid material is removed from the middle ear and a tympanostomy tube is inserted through the tympanic membrane. A tympanostomy tube is a small polyethylene tube that is inserted into the middle ear to equalize the pressure on both sides of the tympanic membrane and to keep the ear aerated. Negative pressure in the middle ear is relieved, allowing the middle ear mucosa to return to normal and growth of the eustachian

tube to occur. The tube usually falls out spontaneously in 6 to 12 months. This period may provide enough time for the effusion process to resolve, but some children need repeated insertions of tympanostomy tubes because of persistent eustachian tube dysfunction. Tympanostomy tubes are inserted with the child under general anesthesia, usually in an outpatient surgery setting.

NURSING CARE OF THE CHILD WITH OTITIS MEDIA

■ Assessment

Ask the parent whether the child has had a recent upper respiratory tract infection or previous ear infections. Assess the child for fever and pain. Because signs of ear infection may be subtle in infants, the nurse should assess not only for obvious signs of ear pain, such as head rolling and pulling at the ear, but also for nonspecific findings, such as irritability, diarrhea, or decreased appetite. Older children may complain of pain or a feeling of fullness in the affected ear. The nurse may examine the ear with a pneumatic otoscope, noting the color, mobility, and translucency of the tympanic membrane and the appearance of the external canal. The tympanic membrane should be inspected

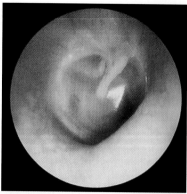

Normal right tympanic membrane and middle ear.

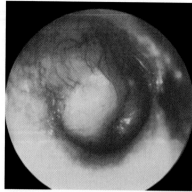

Acute otitis media: bulging right tympanic membrane.

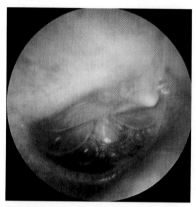

Otitis media with effusion: air-fluid level and bubbles visible through right retracted, translucent tympanic membrane.

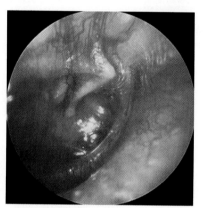

Otitis media with effusion: severely re-tracted, opaque right tympanic membrane.

FIG 21-2 Appearance of tympanic membrane in otitis media compared with normal tympanic membrane. (From Bluestone, C. D., & Klein, J. O. [1995]. *Otitis media in infants and children* [2nd ed.]. Philadelphia: Saunders.)

carefully for signs of perforation. The nurse may obtain a culture of any drainage and notes the color, consistency, and odor. Hearing and language development should be assessed.

▪ Nursing Diagnosis and Planning

The nursing diagnoses and expected outcomes that may be appropriate for the family and infant or child with otitis media are as follows:

- Acute Pain related to inflammation and pressure in the middle ear.

Expected Outcomes. The child will be free of pain, as evidenced by sleeping through the night, not pulling at the ears, and decreased crying. The child's tympanic membranes will appear shiny and pearl-gray, with normal landmarks, a visible light reflex, and normal mobility on tympanography.

- Deficient Knowledge related to incomplete understanding of the disease process and treatment regimen.

Expected Outcomes. The parents will demonstrate (1) methods of feeding the infant that decrease the risk for otitis media, (2) how to keep the child's ears dry if tympanostomy tubes are in place, and (3) ways to follow the treatment regimen, including administering the entire course of antibiotics.

- Risk for Imbalanced Body Temperature related to inflammation.

Expected Outcome. The child will display a normal body temperature.

- Risk for Deficient Fluid Volume related to elevated temperature and decreased intake.

Expected Outcome. The child will have moist mucous membranes, good skin turgor, and appropriate intake and output for age.

▪ Interventions

Teach the parents the importance of giving prescribed antibiotics on time and for the prescribed number of days. Because the child usually feels much better after a few days of medication, parents may believe that the antibiotics are no longer necessary and stop giving them. Increase adherence by giving written and oral instructions for administering medications. Providing a medication record form on which to record doses taken and a calibrated measuring device for liquid medications is also helpful.

The nurse also advises the parents to discard any unused antibiotic rather than save it and not to give the child an antibiotic without consulting the physician first.

Acetaminophen can be given to relieve discomfort. The child's fluid intake should be increased if fever is present. Advise the parents to notify the physician if the child's condition has not improved after 48 hours of observation without antibiotics, after 48 hours of antibiotic treatment without improvement in symptoms, or if there is drainage from the affected ear. If a follow-up visit is recommended, emphasize the importance of keeping the appointment.

The nurse can enhance medication adherence through specific teaching about administration of antibiotics. For example, the nurse might say, "After a few days, your child may seem to be well and show no signs of the ear infection. If you stop giving the antibiotic at that time, some of the germs that caused the otitis media might still be alive and your child can have a relapse."

If the child is undergoing myringotomy with insertion of tympanostomy tubes, the nurse prepares the child and parents as for any outpatient surgical procedure. Explain the procedure in clear terms and answer questions simply and honestly.

Postoperatively, the child is monitored for ear drainage. A small amount of reddish drainage is normal for the first few days after surgery, but the parents should report any heavier bleeding or bleeding that occurs after 3 days. The parents should also be instructed to report any fever or increased pain. The child should avoid blowing the nose for 7 to 10 days.

Most physicians prefer that the child's ears be kept dry if tubes are in place, but some believe that a small amount of water in the ears is not harmful. Bath and lake water are potential sources of bacterial contamination, however, and chlorinated swimming pool water can be irritating to tympanic membranes with tubes. The usual recommendation is to place ear plugs or cotton balls covered with petroleum jelly in the ears during baths and shampoos. Swimming is allowed only with ear plugs and the physician's approval. Diving and swimming deep under water are prohibited. The size and appearance of the tympanostomy tubes should be described to the parents, and they should be reassured that if the tubes fall out it is not an emergency but that the physician should be notified.

Otitis media is usually a chronic problem, with frequent recurrences of infection and effusion. The nurse teaches the parents the early signs of ear infection and the importance of seeking care if these signs should occur. Because hearing impairment from middle ear effusion can be very difficult for parents to detect, the child with chronic otitis media should undergo periodic hearing evaluations.

The nurse should teach parents methods to decrease the risk for recurrent otitis media, such as breastfeeding during infancy, discontinuing bottle feeding as soon as possible, feeding the infant in an upright position, and refraining from giving a bottle to the infant in bed. Parents should be told not to smoke in the child's presence because passive smoking increases the incidence of otitis media.

■ Evaluation

- Is the child sleeping an appropriate amount of time for age with decreased episodes of crying or pulling at ears?
- Have otoscopic findings returned to normal?
- Did the parents complete the treatment regimen by giving the entire dose of the prescribed antibiotic, and are they able to demonstrate appropriate feeding methods?
- Were follow-up appointments kept to determine the resolution of the otitis media?
- Is the child afebrile?
- Does the child appear well hydrated with moist mucous membranes and good skin turgor?

PHARYNGITIS AND TONSILLITIS

Pharyngitis, inflammation of the pharynx and surrounding lymphoid tissue, can be viral or bacterial in origin. Although pharyngitis is a self-limiting and relatively minor disorder, streptococcal infections can have serious complications—among them, rheumatic fever and acute glomerulonephritis.

Tonsillitis is the term commonly used to describe inflammation and infection of the two palatine tonsils. *Adenoiditis* refers to infection and inflammation of the pharyngeal tonsils, or adenoids, which are located above the palatine tonsils on the posterior wall of the nasopharynx. The purpose of these lymphoid tissues is to filter and protect the respiratory and digestive tracts from invasion by pathogens, but often the tonsils become a site for infection.

Etiology

A variety of viruses play a role in pharyngitis, most notably adenoviruses, coronaviruses, enteroviruses (e.g., coxsackievirus), and respiratory syncytial virus. Group A beta-hemolytic streptococcal (GABHS) bacteria are an important bacterial cause of pharyngitis (Hayden & Turner, 2011). Streptococcal pharyngitis is rare before age 3 years. Streptococcal infection is spread by close droplet transmission. Tonsillitis, like pharyngitis, may be bacterial or viral in origin. The most common bacterial agent is group A beta-hemolytic *Streptococcus*.

Incidence

The incidence of pharyngitis and tonsillitis peaks between ages 4 and 7 years, when most children begin preschool and elementary school and have increased exposure to microorganisms. Group A beta-hemolytic streptococcal infection occurs most frequently in the winter and is spread more readily in crowded living situations. The incidence of tonsillitis decreases during middle childhood as the lymphoid tissue undergoes normal shrinkage.

Manifestations

Signs and symptoms differ between viral and bacterial pharyngitis (Table 21-1). The only reliable means of determining whether a case of pharyngitis is viral or bacterial in origin is with a throat culture. Not all children with pharyngitis complain of a sore throat, particularly if they are of preschool age. Instead, the child may complain of a stomachache or simply refuse to eat. The child with tonsillitis demonstrates the following:

TABLE 21-1	COMPARISON OF VIRAL AND BACTERIAL PHARYNGITIS
VIRAL PHARYNGITIS	**BACTERIAL PHARYNGITIS**
Gradual onset	Abrupt onset (may be gradual in children <2 yr old)
Sore throat (reaches a peak on the second or third day)	Sore throat (usually severe)
Erythema and inflammation of the pharynx and tonsils (may be slight), vesicles or ulcers on tonsils	Erythema and inflammation of the pharynx and tonsils
Fever (usually low grade but may be high)	Fever (usually high, 103° to 104° F [39.4° to 40° C], but may be moderate), begins early in illness and usually lasts 1-4 days
Hoarseness, cough, rhinitis, conjunctivitis, malaise, anorexia (early)	Abdominal pain, vomiting, headache
Cervical lymph nodes may be enlarged and tender	Cervical lymph nodes may be enlarged and tender
Usually lasts 3-4 days	Usually lasts 3-5 days

EVIDENCE-BASED PRACTICE

Otitis Media: Treatment versus Watchful Waiting

Acute otitis media (AOM) is the most common condition in children for which antibiotics are prescribed (Siegal, 2010). AOM accounts for as many as 2.6 million emergency department visits and almost 17 million practitioner's office visits a year (Johnson & Holger, 2007). In the United States, many caregivers expect the practitioner to write a prescription when AOM is diagnosed. The practice of watchful waiting, or observation, has come to the forefront. Watchful waiting involves controlling pain and observing symptoms, while refraining from prescribing antibiotics for the first 48 to 72 hours after definitive diagnosis.

In 2004, the American Academy of Pediatrics developed clinical management guidelines for AOM. The first component of the guidelines is a definitive diagnosis of AOM. This includes a rapid onset of ear pain, the presence of a middle ear effusion, and middle ear inflammation. The next component involves relief of pain. The third component offers two options: Observation or treatment with antimicrobials. If treatment is initiated, amoxicillin is recommended. If observation is chosen, the child is observed for 48 to 72 hours, with proper pain relief provided. If improvement is noted, the observation continues. If the symptoms worsen or fail to improve, then antimicrobial agents are prescribed (American Academy of Pediatrics, American Academy of Family Physicians, & Subcommittee on Management of Acute Otitis Media, 2004).

There are several reasons noted in the literature for initiation of the observation period. Research has shown that up to 30% of AOM may have a viral cause; therefore, antibiotics may not be beneficial. Resistance to antibiotics from overprescribing is a concern as well (Siegal, 2010).

Patient and caregiver teaching is an integral part of the observation process. Caregivers must be informed of signs and symptoms that may indicate worsening of the child's condition. Some serious complications of untreated otitis media are meningitis and mastoiditis, both of which could require hospitalization. The incidence of these conditions after otitis media is very low. Caregivers must be informed of the signs to look for in both disease processes. They must be instructed to have their child reevaluated immediately if any of those symptoms are observed.

Pain control is another teaching point in the observation process. Caregivers are much more likely to be adherent to the observation intervention if their child is not in pain (Johnson & Holger, 2007). A proper assessment of pain must be done and appropriate analgesic treatment initiated.

Of course, realize that watchful waiting is presented as an option. Good communication between the caregiver and the practitioner must be in place for this option to be successful. The caregiver must understand the procedure and must be aware of the need for reevaluation if complications should occur. Often times, a "safety-net" prescription for antibiotics is written and sent home with the parent, with the instructions to fill and begin the medication at the end of the 72-hour waiting period if there is no improvement.

The goal behind the watchful waiting option is multifaceted. It could reduce the cost of health care, reduce antibiotic resistance, and increase parental satisfaction (Johnson & Holger, 2007).

As a nurse, what are some of the teaching points you will be sure to relay to caregivers? What are some of the signs and symptoms that the child's condition is worsening? What might you say to the caregiver who is resistant to the idea of watchful waiting?

References

American Academy of Pediatrics, American Academy of Family Physicians, & Subcommittee on Management of Acute Otitis Media. (2004). Clinical practice guideline: Diagnosis and management of acute otitis media. *Pediatrics, 113*, 1451-1465.

Johnson, N. C., & Holger, J. S. (2007). Pediatric acute otitis media: The case for delayed antibiotic treatment. *The Journal of Emergency Medicine, 32*(3), 279-284.

Siegal, R. M. (2010). Acute otitis media guidelines, antibiotic use, and shared medical decision-making. *Pediatrics, 125*(2), 384-385. Retrieved from www.pediatrics.org/cgi/doi/10.1542/peds.2009-3208.

- Sore throat, which may be persistent or recurrent
- Tonsils enlarged and bright red; may be covered with white exudate or cryptic plugs
- Difficulty swallowing
- Mouth breathing and an unpleasant mouth odor
- Enlarged adenoids, which may cause a nasal quality of speech, mouth breathing, hearing difficulty, otitis media, snoring, or obstructive sleep apnea

Older children and adolescents can have a *peritonsillar abscess* associated with pharyngitis or tonsillitis. A peritonsillar abscess usually is unilateral, with the enlarged tonsil displacing the uvula to the opposite side. The child might refuse to talk or swallow because of severe pain that often radiates to the ear. There is a risk for airway obstruction and dehydration with this condition.

Diagnostic Evaluation

Rapid streptococcal antigen tests ("rapid strep test") can accurately screen for group A beta-hemolytic streptococcal infection, but because rapid strep tests have an approximately 20% incidence of false-negative results, if the child's symptoms suggest a streptococcal infection, culture of a throat specimen obtained by swab should be done simultaneously. Because a small percentage of children carry group A

PATHOPHYSIOLOGY

Pharyngitis

Pharyngitis often accompanies the common cold. Tonsillitis is usually present with pharyngitis. Infection and inflammation of the tonsils cause them to enlarge. The palatine tonsils may meet in the midline ("kissing tonsils") and cause difficulty swallowing and breathing. If adenoids enlarge, they can obstruct the eustachian tubes, resulting in otitis media and hearing impairment. Hypertrophy of the adenoids can also block the passageway between the nose and the throat, causing mouth breathing or obstructive sleep apnea.

beta-hemolytic streptococci in their throats, a positive throat culture is not proof of active infection.

Therapeutic Management

During the acute phase of pharyngitis or tonsillitis, treatment is symptomatic, focusing on pain relief and rest. Acetaminophen or ibuprofen is used for pain; older children may find gargling with warm saline solution comforting. Cool, bland liquids are tolerated best because of the discomfort caused by swallowing solids or irritating liquids.

Antibiotics should be restricted to those children who test positive on antigen detection tests or cultures. Streptococcal pharyngitis is most commonly treated orally with penicillin given two or three times daily for 10 days. Recent studies have shown that a shorter course of amoxicillin is as effective as or more effective than the traditional 10-day penicillin therapy because of superior adherence, lower incidence of side effects, improved patient/parent satisfaction, and lower drug costs (Hayden & Turner, 2011). Erythromycin or a cephalosporin may be used in children who are allergic to penicillin (Casey & Pichichero, 2007). A single intramuscular dose of procaine penicillin and benzathine penicillin G might be considered in children for whom adherence is expected to be a problem. Children given penicillin therapy are noninfectious to others 24 hours after therapy is initiated.

Surgical removal of the tonsils, or tonsillectomy, is controversial. Although some physicians think that a tonsillectomy is warranted in cases of recurrent tonsillitis, the prevailing attitude is more conservative, and the procedure is generally reserved for cases of upper airway obstruction, peritonsillar abscess, obstructive sleep apnea, or other serious problems. Tonsillectomy is generally not performed in children younger than 3 years because of the tendency for remaining tonsillar tissues to hypertrophy. Contraindications to tonsillectomy include active infection and cleft palate (see Chapter 19). Surgical removal of the tonsils while they are infected can result in spread of the infecting organism and sepsis. In children with cleft palate, the tonsils help prevent air escape during speech. Adenoidectomy alone may be performed in cases of recurrent otitis media caused by eustachian tube obstruction or for persistent nasal or airway obstruction.

Many parents believe that a tonsillectomy will solve their child's problems of frequent sore throats, mouth breathing, and poor weight gain. There is no evidence that a tonsillectomy reduces the incidence of recurrent pharyngitis. The nurse should be prepared to discuss the current treatment philosophy with parents and address their concerns. If tonsillectomy is chosen as the method of treatment, the procedure is often done in a day-surgery setting.

Nursing Considerations

Assessment of the child with pharyngitis or tonsillitis includes inspecting the pharynx for erythema, exudate, or petechiae. The skin should be inspected for rash and color changes. Some children with streptococcal pharyngitis have a pink, sandpaper-like rash on the trunk (see Chapter 17). The child is questioned about the onset and location of throat, ear, or abdominal pain. The parent of a preverbal child may report that the child refuses to eat or begins to cry during feedings. The nurse also assesses the child's temperature and respiratory status and asks the older child or parent about the onset of symptoms and any known contact with streptococcal infection in the school or family. Also ask whether the child has been taking any antibiotics at home, because antibiotics will interfere with the results of the throat culture.

Measures to relieve throat discomfort include administering acetaminophen, warm salt water gargles ($\frac{1}{4}$ teaspoon of salt per 8-oz glass of water), and warm or cool compresses applied to the neck. Recent studies demonstrate pain relief with the use of oral steroids; however, steroids are not recommended as a primary pain reliever (Wing, Villa-Roel, Yeh, et al., 2010). The child should not be forced to eat. Offer cool, bland liquids to prevent dehydration. Soft foods such as gelatin, soup, mashed potatoes, puddings, Cream of Wheat, and flavored ice pops appeal to children the best. Bed rest is advisable while the child

has a fever. The nurse should advise the parents to call the health care provider if the child has difficulty breathing or increased difficulty swallowing or if the fever has lasted more than 3 days. If a fever, sore throat, or headache develops in any family members, they should have a throat culture. Instruct the parents that leftover antibiotics from siblings or friends should never be used.

Moist mucous membranes and adequate urine output are signs of proper fluid balance. At the end of treatment, the child should be free of signs of infection and show no signs of complications of the disease.

NURSING CARE OF THE CHILD UNDERGOING A TONSILLECTOMY

■ Assessment: Preoperative Period

A complete history is taken, with special attention given to allergy symptoms, difficulty swallowing, or airway obstruction. The child is assessed for signs of active infection (fever, elevated white blood cell [WBC] count) and redness and presence of exudate in the throat. The child should be questioned about the presence of pain in the throat or ears. Because the tonsillar area is so vascular, any bleeding history must be recorded and communicated to the primary physician.

Laboratory results (prothrombin time, partial thromboplastin time, platelet count, hemoglobin, hematocrit, urinalysis) are reviewed, and the child should be checked for loose teeth to decrease the risk for aspiration during surgery. A complete current medication list should be reviewed as well.

■ Nursing Diagnosis and Planning: Preoperative Period

The nursing diagnoses and expected outcomes that may be appropriate for the child undergoing a tonsillectomy and the child's family are as follows:
• Anxiety related to surgery.
Expected Outcome. The child and parents will exhibit a decreased level of anxiety, as evidenced by relaxed body posture and involvement in play activities.
• Deficient Knowledge related to surgery and procedures.
Expected Outcome. The child and parents will restate preoperative teaching.

■ Interventions: Preoperative Period

The nurse reassures the child that talking will not be a problem after surgery. Providing the child a way to communicate will reduce postoperative anxiety. Emphasize to the child that it is important to drink liquids after surgery, although the child's throat will be sore (see also Chapter 16). It is important to maintain hydration postoperatively to promote healing. Teach the child's family about postoperative pain assessment and appropriate analgesia administration because many parents undermedicate their children. Undermedication can interfere with optimal postoperative recovery.

■ Evaluation: Preoperative Period

• Does the child demonstrate relaxed body posture and the ability to engage in play while waiting for surgery?
• Can the parents describe what to expect during the postoperative period?

■ Assessment: Postoperative Period

Immediately after surgery, the child should be assessed for bleeding and ability to swallow secretions. Postoperative hemorrhage is the most serious and life-threatening complication of tonsillectomy (Leonard, Fenton, & Hone, 2010). If bleeding occurs, the child is returned to surgery for recauterization. The rate and quality of respirations and breath sounds should be assessed. Vital signs, including blood pressure, should be monitored frequently until discharge. Suction equipment should be available, but do not suction unless there is airway obstruction. The child is assessed for bleeding (frequent swallowing; restlessness; a fast, thready pulse; or vomiting bright red blood). When visually assessing the site for clots or bleeding, use a flashlight for illumination and avoid using a tongue depressor if at all possible. If a tongue depressor is necessary, use a sterile tongue depressor and keep it as far forward in the mouth as possible.

■ Nursing Diagnosis and Planning: Postoperative Period

The nursing diagnoses and expected outcomes that may be appropriate for the child who has undergone a tonsillectomy and the child's family are as follows:

- Risk for Injury (hemorrhage) related to surgery.

Expected Outcome. The child will experience minimal postoperative bleeding, as evidenced by vital signs within normal limits and absence of excessive swallowing, bright-red vomitus, or restlessness.

- Ineffective Airway Clearance related to throat discomfort.

Expected Outcome. The child will maintain a clear airway without jeopardizing the operative site.

- Acute Pain related to surgical removal of tonsils.

Expected Outcome. The child will describe relief from pain and will be able to rest.

- Risk for Deficient Fluid Volume related to difficulty swallowing and nothing-by-mouth (NPO) status before surgery.

Expected Outcome. The child will have adequate fluid intake for age and minimal fluid loss.

- Deficient Knowledge related to home care.

Expected Outcome. The parents will describe how to care for their child at home.

■ Interventions: Postoperative Period

The child should be placed in a prone or side-lying position to facilitate drainage. Although not all clinicians are in agreement, straws and forks may be withheld to prevent trauma to the surgical site. If bleeding occurs, the child is turned to the side and the physician notified.

Vomiting of old blood ("coffee-grounds" emesis) is common. Antiemetics are given as ordered to decrease throat pain caused by retching. If vomiting occurs, keep the child on NPO status for 30 minutes and then resume clear liquids.

Nonaspirin analgesics (e.g., acetaminophen) are given as ordered. In some instances, the surgeon prescribes acetaminophen with codeine liquid to provide adequate analgesia (avoid administering oral medications in suspension that are colored red because they can be confused with blood in vomitus). Adequate analgesia increases fluid intake. It is common to prescribe the analgesic every 4 hours for the first 24 hours because throat discomfort is expected. An ice collar can be applied for comfort.

Provide clear, cool liquids when the child is fully awake. Avoid citrus drinks, carbonated drinks, and extremely hot or cold liquids because they may irritate the throat. Milk and milk products (puddings, ice cream) can coat the throat, causing a need to clear the throat and thus increasing the risk for bleeding. Adequate fluid intake promotes healing and maintains hydration. The nurse teaches the parents the principles of home management and ensures that the child is retaining fluids before discharging the child from the surgical unit. Be sure to tell the

---

⚡ SAFETY ALERT

Caring for the Child Who Has Had a Tonsillectomy

Assessing the child for postoperative bleeding is most important. Because the operative site is not as readily visible as other sites, the nurse needs to look for the following:

- Excessive swallowing
- Elevated pulse; decreasing blood pressure
- Signs of fresh bleeding in the back of the throat
- Vomiting bright-red blood
- Restlessness that does not seem to be associated with pain

---

parent to monitor the child for postoperative bleeding both within the first 24 hours and again 7 to 10 days after surgery (see Patient-Centered Teaching: Caring for a Child after a Tonsillectomy box).

PATIENT-CENTERED TEACHING

Caring for a Child after a Tonsillectomy

- Encourage your child to participate only in quiet activities for 1 week after surgery.
- Encourage abundant liquid intake. Avoid citrus juices, which irritate the throat, for 10 days.
- Avoid red liquids, which will give the appearance of blood if your child vomits.
- Add full liquids (cream soups, gelatin, puddings, and other soups) on the second day and soft foods (mashed potatoes, soft cereals, eggs) as your child tolerates them. Avoid rough or scratchy foods (bacon, chips, popcorn), citrus foods, or spicy foods for 3 weeks.
- Encourage your child to chew and swallow because this exercises pharyngeal muscles and promotes healing.
- Do not give your child any straws, forks, or sharp pointed toys that could be put in the mouth.
- Use acetaminophen for pain relief; your child may have a prescription for acetaminophen with codeine for sore throat. Do not use aspirin or any medicine containing aspirin because it might affect the clotting time of the blood.
- Pain should not persist past the first week. Notify your physician if pain persists.
- Discourage your child from coughing, clearing the throat, or gargling.
- Bad mouth odor is normal and may be relieved by drinking more liquids.
- Earache and slight fever are common.
- Call your physician for any bleeding, persistent earache, or fever greater than 101° F (38.3° C).
- Bleeding caused by tissue sloughing during the healing process can occur 7 to 10 days after surgery. Such bleeding requires immediate medical attention.
- To protect your child from catching a cold, keep the child away from crowds for 2 weeks.
- Your child may return to school when directed by the physician, usually in about 10 days.
- Bring your child for a follow-up appointment in 1 to 2 weeks.

■ Evaluation: Postoperative

- Does the child have minimal bleeding, nausea, and vomiting, and are vital signs within normal limits?
- Is the child taking clear liquids and avoiding liquids that irritate the throat?

- Are the child's complaints of pain and irritability minimal?
- Can the parents describe home care measures?

LARYNGOMALACIA (CONGENITAL LARYNGEAL STRIDOR)

Flaccidity of the epiglottis and supraglottic aperture and weakness of the airway walls contribute to laryngomalacia, the most common cause of inspiratory stridor in the neonatal period (Breysem, Goosens, Vander Poorten, et al., 2009). Laryngomalacia may be caused by immature neuromuscular development in the airway.

Manifestations

Noisy, crowing inspiratory respiratory sounds (stridor) are present, with or without retractions. The infant usually remains acyanotic despite the stridor. Stridor is usually present at birth but may begin as late as age 2 months. Symptoms increase when the infant is supine or when the infant is crying. The diagnosis is based on a thorough history and on findings on direct laryngoscopy.

Therapeutic Management

Symptoms usually resolve without treatment by age 18 to 24 months. In rare instances, endotracheal intubation or tracheostomy may be required.

Nursing Considerations

The nurse observes the neonate for stridor, retractions, and dyspnea, noting any signs of acute respiratory distress. Because some infants have feeding problems, the infant should be observed for feeding difficulties and appropriate growth and development patterns. The infant's respiratory status is assessed, and findings are recorded every 2 hours and as needed. Obstruction may increase during crying or when the child has a respiratory infection. Stridor may increase when the child is supine with the neck flexed. Positioning with the neck hyperextended improves the child's breathing by reducing the obstruction and therefore improves the stridor.

As part of discharge teaching, parents are taught the signs of respiratory distress so that they can monitor for changes that might indicate respiratory tract infection. If the bottle-fed infant has feeding difficulties, the parents can try using a smaller nipple. Smaller, more frequent feedings are sometimes better tolerated by infants with respiratory difficulties. Reassure the parents that the condition usually resolves by the time the child is 2 years old. The ability of parents to comfortably care for their child indicates the effectiveness of the discharge teaching.

CROUP

Croup refers to a group of conditions characterized by inspiratory stridor, a harsh (brassy or croupy) cough, hoarseness, and varying degrees of respiratory distress (Table 21-2). The major types of croup are acute spasmodic croup, laryngotracheobronchitis, bacterial tracheitis, and epiglottitis. Although epiglottitis is a type of croup, it is discussed separately because it is a bacterial infection with unique symptoms and treatment.

Etiology and Incidence

Parainfluenza viruses cause most cases of viral croup. The cause of acute spasmodic croup is unknown.

Laryngotracheobronchitis, the most common form of croup, usually affects infants and toddlers, and it is one cause of airway obstruction in children ages 6 months to 6 years. The incidence of croup is higher in boys than in girls, and the disease occurs more often during the winter than in other seasons.

Acute spasmodic croup occurs most often in children ages 1 to 3 years. Spasmodic croup occurs more often in anxious and excitable children. There seems to be hereditary predisposition to spasmodic croup.

Bacterial tracheitis is less common than laryngotracheobronchitis and acute spasmodic croup. It progresses from an upper respiratory tract infection and may be confused with laryngotracheobronchitis because of similar manifestations. Treatment for laryngotracheobronchitis is not effective if the child has bacterial tracheitis.

The following discussion focuses on acute spasmodic croup and laryngotracheobronchitis, the most common types of croup leading to hospitalization.

Manifestations

Croup often begins at night and may be preceded by several days of symptoms of upper respiratory tract infection. The child with laryngotracheobronchitis may have a gradual onset and a fever along with other signs and symptoms; occasionally the fever is as high as 104° F (40° C). Children with spasmodic croup do not have a fever. Other manifestations include the following:

- The sudden onset of a harsh, metallic barky cough; sore throat; inspiratory stridor; and hoarseness
- The use of accessory muscles (substernal, intercostal, suprasternal retractions) to breathe
- Frightened appearance
- Agitation
- Cyanosis

Diagnostic Evaluation

The diagnosis is made mainly from observation of clinical symptoms. Differentiation between viral croup and bacterial epiglottitis is very important because treatment differs. However, the use of the *H. influenzae* type B (Hib) vaccine has reduced the incidence of epiglottitis. A croup score is often used to describe the severity of respiratory distress. Arterial blood gas values or pulse oximetry readings may be monitored to detect decreased PaO_2 levels.

Therapeutic Management

The goal of treatment is to maintain a patent airway. Children with acute spasmodic croup can usually be cared for at home. Treatment for acute spasmodic croup includes a calm approach and increased oral fluid intake if the child is not in respiratory distress. Taking the child out into the cool, humid night air may relieve mucosal swelling. Evidence suggests that using mist, either cool or warm, does not alter the course of the child's illness (Roosevelt, 2011).

Crying aggravates the airway obstruction. Children who develop stridor at rest, cyanosis, severe agitation or fatigue, or moderate to severe retractions or who are unable to take oral fluids should be seen in the emergency department.

PATHOPHYSIOLOGY

Croup

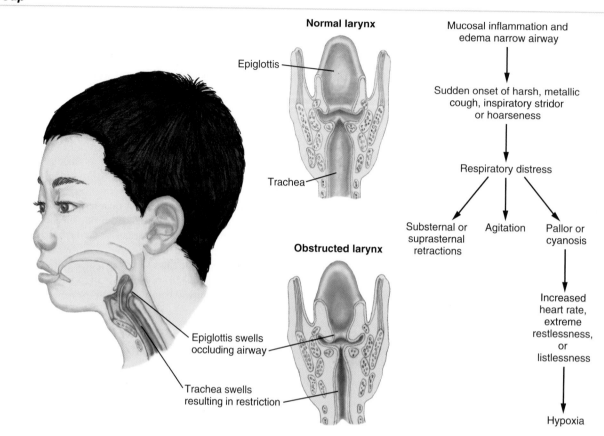

Normal larynx

Epiglottis

Trachea

Obstructed larynx

Epiglottis swells
occluding airway

Trachea swells
resulting in restriction

Mucosal inflammation and
edema narrow airway

Sudden onset of harsh, metallic
cough, inspiratory stridor
or hoarseness

Respiratory distress

Substernal or
suprasternal
retractions   Agitation   Pallor or
cyanosis

Increased
heart rate,
extreme
restlessness,
or
listlessness

Hypoxia

Croup is a viral infection of the upper airway. Although the entire upper, or nonreactive, airway is involved to some extent in all forms of croup, each type is named according to the anatomic area most severely involved. For example, laryngotracheobronchitis affects the larynx, trachea, and bronchi. In acute spasmodic croup, the larynx is the area of most severe inflammation.

In all forms of croup, mucosal inflammation and edema cause narrowing of the airway. This narrowing is more dangerous in infants and young children than in adults because of their small airway diameter and flexible larynx, which is more susceptible to spasm.

Symptoms are usually worse at night and better in the day; they may recur for several nights. Croup usually lasts 3 to 4 days.

Children with laryngotracheobronchitis, usually a more severe type of croup, are more often hospitalized than are those with acute spasmodic croup. Racemic epinephrine nebulized with oxygen may be given to decrease the laryngeal edema and bronchospasm. The child must be observed closely for changes in respiratory status and should not be treated with epinephrine on an outpatient basis because the effects of epinephrine are temporary. Rebound stridor may occur. Children who receive epinephrine should be observed in the emergency department for at least 3 hours after treatment and should not be discharged if stridor or retractions are present.

Oral dexamethasone in a single dose of 0.15 to 0.6 mg/kg decreases airway inflammation and reduces the necessity for hospitalization for many children (Roosevelt, 2011). Antibiotics are not indicated unless a bacterial infection is present. Acetaminophen is given to reduce fever.

For children with more severe symptoms (progressively worsening stridor, cyanosis, decreased oxygen saturation, retractions), hospitalization is necessary. Humidified oxygen and IV fluids are given

until respiratory distress subsides and the child can take adequate fluids by mouth. Sedatives are contraindicated because they depress respirations and could mask restlessness, an early sign of hypoxia.

If signs of moderate or severe hypoxia develop, the child is intubated immediately and is transferred to an intensive care unit. Usually the tube remains in place for 3 to 5 days and is removed when the child can breathe around the tube and the inflammation subsides.

NURSING CARE OF THE CHILD WITH CROUP

Assessment

A nursing history typically reveals a recent upper respiratory tract infection. Assess the child for inspiratory stridor, barking cough, hoarseness, and increased heart rate and respiratory rate. Record any signs of respiratory distress, such as the use of accessory muscles; substernal, intercostal, and suprasternal retractions; nasal flaring; restlessness and irritability; and pallor or cyanosis. Cyanosis, increased

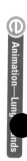

TABLE 21-2   COMPARISON OF TYPES OF CROUP

	ACUTE SPASMODIC LARYNGITIS (SPASMODIC CROUP)	ACUTE LARYNGOTRACHEOBRONCHITIS (LTB)	ACUTE EPIGLOTTITIS	ACUTE TRACHEITIS
Age usually affected	1-3 yr	3 mo-3 yr	3-7 yr	1 mo-6 yr
Location of swelling and inflammation	Subglottic (below vocal cords)	Vocal cords, subglottic, and tissue below vocal cords, including bronchi	Supraglottic (above vocal cords)	Mucosa of upper trachea
Cause	Viral, emotional, or genetic predisposition	Usually viral but may be bacterial	Bacterial (usually *Haemophilus influenzae* type B [Hib])	*Staphylococcus* (most common)
Assessment	Sudden onset, usually at night Child awakens with harsh cough, inspiratory stridor, dyspnea, and hoarseness	Gradual onset, usually at night Child awakens with harsh cough and inspiratory stridor	Sudden onset, which may rapidly progress to complete airway obstruction and death Sore throat, dyspnea, high fever	Progresses from upper respiratory infection (1-2 days) High fever Stridor Croupy cough Purulent secretions
Treatment	Humidity Increased fluids May treat at home	Humidity Racemic epinephrine IV fluids during respiratory distress Hospitalization may be necessary	IV antibiotics Artificial airway IV fluids Emergency hospitalization	Humidified oxygen Antipyretics IV antibiotics May require intubation

heart rate and respiratory rate, extreme restlessness, or evidence of fatigue or listlessness may be signs of hypoxia and should be reported to the physician immediately. The lungs should be auscultated for adventitious breath sounds or areas of decreased breath sounds. Temperature and hydration status should also be assessed.

Nursing Diagnosis and Planning

The diagnoses and expected outcomes that may be appropriate for the child with croup and the child's family are as follows:
- Ineffective Airway Clearance related to mucosal swelling and obstruction of the upper respiratory tract.

Expected Outcomes. The child will breathe without difficulty and have a heart rate and respiratory rate within normal limits for age.
- Risk for Deficient Fluid Volume related to inadequate oral intake and tachypnea.

Expected Outcome. The child will have adequate fluid intake for age and weight.
- Fear related to dyspnea and hospitalization.

Expected Outcomes. The child will appear less fearful, as evidenced by resting quietly, decreased crying, and cooperating with nursing care as appropriate for age. The parents will demonstrate decreased fear, as evidenced by their ability to assist the child to deal with stressors of hospitalization and illness.
- Deficient Knowledge related to the course of croup and home care.

Expected Outcomes. The parents will have accurate knowledge of croup symptoms, state that they are comfortable in home management of croup, and seek assistance appropriately if symptoms become severe.

Interventions

Facilitating Airway Clearance. The nurse monitors the child's breathing continuously for signs and symptoms of increased respiratory distress (increased respiratory rate, stridor at rest, nasal flaring, retractions, cyanosis, changes in level of consciousness or increased

irritability, decreased or adventitious breath sounds, tachypnea). A child with respiratory distress should never be left alone, and the physician should be notified immediately. If epiglottitis is suspected, the physician should be contacted and the throat should not be inspected because this may result in laryngospasm and airway obstruction. The nurse should administer humidified oxygen at the ordered flow rate and mist only if ordered. Monitor vital signs and pulse oximetry readings frequently. There should be emergency intubation equipment (e.g., intubation tray, oxygen, suction, manual resuscitation bag-valve-mask) closely available should the child's condition change rapidly. Aerosolized racemic epinephrine is often administered to decrease laryngeal edema, and dexamethasone is given as an antiinflammatory agent. The child should be observed for recurrence of obstruction, which may occur within a few hours after administration of racemic epinephrine.

The child should be kept as quiet as possible because crying may aggravate laryngospasm and increase hypoxia. Encourage parents to stay nearby. Maintain a calm, quiet environment. Observe the child closely but disturb as little as possible. Support the child in an upright position with the head of the bed elevated to facilitate respiration.

Maintaining Fluid Balance. Tachypnea causes insensible water loss, and difficulty swallowing leads to decreased intake. Therefore, the nurse monitors the child's hydration status with intake and output and urine specific gravity measurements. Check mucous membranes, skin turgor, and presence of tears. Weigh the child daily on the same scale and at the same time of day. Offer the child clear, room temperature liquids as tolerated when the child no longer exhibits signs of respiratory distress. Observe the child's ability to swallow because tachypnea and laryngospasm often cause dysphagia. IV fluids are administered in the acute phase of croup because oral fluids are contraindicated in the setting of severe respiratory distress that heightens the risk for aspiration. The child's temperature is monitored every 4 hours, and acetaminophen is administered as ordered.

Decreasing Fear. Maintain a calm, restful environment for the child and organize nursing care so as to disturb the child as little as possible and allow for periods of uninterrupted rest. Encourage parents to touch and cuddle the child, because a parent's presence is important in reducing fear in infants and young children. Also, encourage parents' participation in care and explain ways that they can make their child more comfortable. Caring for a child in the hospital is exhausting to parents, and fatigue magnifies feelings of anxiety and helplessness. Therefore, provide parents with breaks as needed and assure them that their child will be cared for in their absence. Allow the child to keep a favorite toy or blanket and use developmentally appropriate communication techniques (e.g., play, puppets) when explaining treatments and procedures. Allow the child and parents to ask questions and to discuss fears and concerns, because croup symptoms can be frightening and parents sometimes feel guilty for not having brought the child in for treatment sooner.

■ **Providing Teaching.** The nurse determines the parents' level of understanding of croup and previous experiences in coping with the illness. Teach the parents that once a child has had an attack, croup may recur. Teach the parents that maintaining a stable environmental temperature and humidity and keeping the child well hydrated may help decrease the severity of attacks. Teach that croup is a viral infection and that avoiding large groups of people and practicing good health habits to prevent infection may decrease the risk for recurrence of croup. Teach parents the signs and symptoms of respiratory distress and symptoms that should prompt a call to the physician:

- Increased difficulty breathing or worsening of symptoms
- Retractions (tugging in of the skin between, above, or below the ribs with inspiration)
- Lips turn bluish or dusky
- Breathing cool or warm mist does not improve symptoms in 20 minutes
- Inability to drink much over the past 24 hours
- Drooling or difficulty swallowing
- Fever (higher than 103° F [39.4° C])
- Lethargy, listlessness, or severe agitation

The nurse emphasizes the importance of adequate hydration and nutrition. Parents are taught that acetaminophen or ibuprofen is effective in reducing fever and will help the child feel more comfortable. A humidified environment may also help increase the child's comfort. Cough syrups and cold medicines are avoided because they can dry and thicken secretions.

■ Evaluation

- Are the child's respiratory rate and heart rate within normal limits for age, and is the oxygen saturation greater than 95%?
- Does the infant have moist mucous membranes, good skin turgor, and urine output appropriate for age (see Chapter 16)?
- Does the child exhibit decreased signs of agitation or being upset (less crying), and is the parent able to comfort the child?
- Can the parents explain the appropriate treatment of croup and when medical help is needed?

EPIGLOTTITIS (SUPRAGLOTTITIS)

Epiglottitis, the acute inflammation and swelling of the epiglottis and surrounding tissue, is a life-threatening, rapidly progressive condition that may cause complete airway obstruction within a few hours of onset.

Etiology and Incidence

Epiglottitis is almost always caused by *H. influenzae*. Other organisms, such as *Staphylococcus aureus*, *Haemophilus parainfluenzae*, *S.*

pneumoniae, and group A beta-hemolytic streptococci, cause the infection less frequently. Viral epiglottitis is rare.

Epiglottitis occurs most often in children ages 3 to 7 years. The incidence is about equal in boys and girls. The incidence decreased markedly after the introduction of the Hib vaccine; however, vaccine failure and the emergence of epiglottitis caused by atypical organisms make it a relevant topic for discussion.

Manifestations

Unlike croup, epiglottitis has an abrupt onset with rapid progression of symptoms. Often parents report that the child was put to bed well and awakened with a severe sore throat and difficulty swallowing. The child demonstrates a high fever (102.2° to 104° F [39° to 40° C]) and appears to be in a toxic condition and very ill. The accompanying sore throat can progress to acute respiratory distress in a few hours. The child appears anxious and frightened and may be irritable or lethargic. One of the classic signs of epiglottitis is that the child insists on sitting upright, often in a tripod position (leaning forward supported on the arms), with the chin thrust out and the mouth open. Respiratory symptoms include nasal flaring; suprasternal, substernal, and intercostal retractions; pale skin color to cyanosis (depending on the degree of airway obstruction); and tachycardia. The epiglottis appears edematous and cherry red.

Diagnostic Evaluation

The most reliable diagnostic sign of epiglottitis is an edematous, cherry-red epiglottis. However, examination and visual observation of the epiglottis *are contraindicated* until emergency intubation equipment and qualified personnel are available to support the child in case of sudden airway obstruction. The child's WBC count is usually elevated (20,000 to 30,000/mm^3).

⚡ **SAFETY ALERT**

Cardinal Signs and Symptoms of Epiglottitis

Drooling
Dysphagia (difficulty swallowing)
Dysphonia (difficulty talking)
Distressed inspiratory efforts

Do not examine or obtain material for culture from a child's throat if epiglottitis is suspected because any stimulation with a tongue depressor or culture swab could trigger complete airway obstruction.

Do not leave a child with epiglottitis unattended.

Therapeutic Management

Treatment for epiglottitis should achieve a patent airway as quickly as possible. The child with epiglottitis has an edematous epiglottis, which can completely obstruct the airway at any time. Radiographs are best obtained at the bedside, where the child can be constantly monitored and emergency equipment is readily available. The danger of airway obstruction is so great that usually all invasive procedures, such as venipuncture, are postponed until the child is intubated. Once the airway is secured, the child is transferred to the intensive care unit. Oxygenation status is closely monitored with arterial blood gas values or pulse oximetry, and humidified oxygen is administered. Mechanical ventilation is sometimes instituted.

Throat and blood specimens are obtained for culture after the child is intubated. Antipyretics are given for fever. Antibiotics are

PATHOPHYSIOLOGY

Epiglottitis

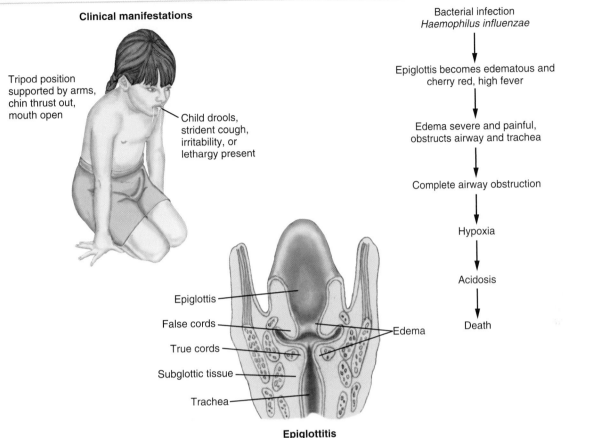

Clinical manifestations

Tripod position supported by arms, chin thrust out, mouth open

Child drools, strident cough, irritability, or lethargy present

Bacterial infection
Haemophilus influenzae

Epiglottis becomes edematous and cherry red, high fever

Edema severe and painful, obstructs airway and trachea

Complete airway obstruction

Hypoxia

Acidosis

Death

Epiglottis
False cords
True cords
Subglottic tissue
Trachea
Edema

Epiglottitis

Epiglottitis is a bacterial form of croup. The epiglottis and surrounding structures become inflamed as bacterial infection invades the soft tissue. The epiglottis becomes edematous and cherry red and may become so swollen that it completely covers the glottis and obstructs the airway. Secretions pool in the hypopharynx and larynx. As the disease rapidly progresses, swelling becomes so severe that the child is unable to swallow and begins to drool. The child's voice is muffled, and the throat is very sore. Inspiratory stridor, cough, and irritability are present. Complete airway obstruction can occur rapidly, resulting in hypoxia, acidosis, and death.

The onset of epiglottitis is usually sudden. The child may have had symptoms of a mild upper respiratory tract infection for a few days before symptoms began. Children with epiglottitis can progress from wellness to complete airway obstruction within 2 to 6 hours.

administered IV until the child is extubated. Usually the child improves dramatically after 48 hours of antibiotic therapy and can be extubated at this time. The usual course of treatment is 7 to 10 days. Discharge occurs in about 3 to 7 days, and the child is sent home on a regimen of oral antibiotics.

Nursing Considerations

The nurse should continuously assess for signs of respiratory distress (stridor, nasal flaring, tachypnea, tachycardia, retractions, drooling, changes in level of consciousness, cyanosis). A sudden decrease in respiratory effort may be a sign of exhaustion and impending respiratory arrest. Arterial blood gas values and pulse oximetry findings are monitored. On pulse oximetry, the oxygen saturation should remain above 95%, with the PaO_2 between 80 and 100 mm Hg.

Maintenance of a patent airway is essential. The nurse should also keep the child as calm and quiet as possible. If temperature is taken, it should be by the axillary or tympanic route rather than the oral route. The child should be supported in a position of comfort, usually sitting straight up (orthopneic); never force the child to lie down. Children who are anxious and in respiratory distress are often less fearful sitting on their parents' laps. Parents should be encouraged to hug and comfort their child. The parents' anxiety level must be assessed and controlled because their anxiety is easily transferred to the child.

Humidified oxygen is delivered in high concentrations. Oxygen therapy is usually less upsetting if the parent holds the oxygen tubing in front of the child's face. All procedures are explained to the parent and child clearly, calmly, and according to the child's level of understanding.

Emergency intubation equipment (i.e., oxygen, laryngoscope, endotracheal tube, suction equipment) should be immediately available in case of complete airway obstruction. Worsening of the child's condition should be reported to the physician immediately.

Antipyretics are given rectally for fever. Because of the risk for aspiration, the child is kept on NPO status and fluids are given IV. The nurse must closely monitor the ordered IV rate and the urine specific gravity and other indicators of hydration. IV antibiotics are administered as ordered.

If the child has an artificial airway, with either an endotracheal tube or a tracheostomy, the nurse must observe the child closely for respiratory distress and suction the airway as needed. The endotracheal tube must be securely taped to decrease movement of the tube and to minimize the chance of accidental extubation. Once intubated, the child needs to be restrained and sedated to prevent accidental extubation. It may be impossible to reintubate the child because of the severe swelling of the epiglottis. The endotracheal tube is usually kept in place for approximately 24 to 48 hours. After extubation, the child must be watched carefully and is usually placed in a mist tent for 24 hours before being transferred to a pediatric unit. Normal respiratory rate and rhythm and normal color serve as evaluation criteria.

Because epiglottitis progresses rapidly and acute respiratory distress is frightening, both parents and child have high anxiety levels. The nurse cares for the child calmly and efficiently and offers the family much-needed support during hospitalization. On discharge, the parents need to be taught how to administer the child's oral antibiotics. Reassure them that epiglottitis rarely recurs. The child should be free of respiratory difficulty, resting well, and without other distress. The nurse encourages parents of young children to have their children immunized against *H. influenzae* (see Chapter 4) to decrease the risk for contracting epiglottitis. Prophylaxis with rifampin is given to underimmunized contacts or family members younger than 4 years old and to any child contact who is immune depressed (Roosevelt, 2011).

BRONCHITIS

Bronchitis is a disease that rarely exists by itself but occurs together with other conditions of the upper and lower respiratory tracts. It can be confused with asthma. A cough is the major sign; it usually resolves without therapy in approximately 2 weeks.

Etiology and Incidence

Acute bronchitis is usually viral in origin. Rhinoviruses are the most common causative organisms. Other viruses thought to cause bronchitis include respiratory syncytial virus, influenza virus, parainfluenza virus, and adenovirus. Most bacterial infections occur secondary to a primary viral infection or some other airway problem. They may also occur as a result of foreign body aspiration. Air pollution has also been implicated in the disease.

The disorder is more common in young children and boys. It can occur anytime but is more common during the winter months than in other seasons.

PATHOPHYSIOLOGY

Bronchitis

Inflammation of the trachea and major bronchi is present in bronchitis. Mucus production is increased, and the mucosa is congested. Because of nonspecific leukocytic migration, purulent secretions can occur even in the absence of a bacterial infection.

Acute bronchitis is a self-limiting disease. Chronic bronchitis in children may indicate an underlying chronic respiratory dysfunction.

Manifestations and Diagnostic Evaluation

Bronchitis is characterized by the gradual onset of rhinitis and a cough that is initially nonproductive but may change to a loose cough with increased mucus production. Auscultation may reveal coarse and fine, moist crackles and high-pitched rhonchi (resembling the wheezing of asthma). Associated symptoms include malaise, low-grade fever, and increased mucus, which may be purulent.

Chest radiographs are usually normal. The diagnosis is based on the clinical findings.

Therapeutic Management

Treatment is mainly symptomatic and includes rest, humidification, and increased fluid intake. Exposure to cigarette smoke should be avoided. Cough suppressants are not recommended unless the cough interferes with the child's ability to rest. Antihistamines should be avoided because of their drying effect on secretions. Antibiotics should be given only if a bacterial infection is confirmed by culture or if the clinical findings support the diagnosis.

Nursing Considerations

The nurse should assess temperature, appearance of secretions, and respiratory effort every 2 to 4 hours. The child's intake should be monitored, and the nurse should observe for signs of sleep deprivation related to the persistent cough.

Advise the parents to encourage fluids by frequently offering small amounts of the child's favorite liquids and to humidify the child's room. The child should be monitored for signs of dehydration; this includes taking daily weights if the child is hospitalized. Acetaminophen is administered for an elevated temperature (usually above 101° F [38.3° C]). Quiet activities should be provided for diversion.

BRONCHIOLITIS

Bronchiolitis, or inflammation of the bronchioles, is a significant cause of hospitalization in infants younger than 1 year. Respiratory syncytial virus (RSV) is the causative agent in more than half of cases (Garcia, Bhore, Soriano-Fallas, et al., 2010).

Etiology and Incidence

Infants usually acquire the disease from an older child or adult, particularly a family member or daycare contact, who has a minor respiratory illness. RSV infection is easily communicable and is acquired mainly through contact with contaminated surfaces and hand-to-hand transmission. Nosocomial outbreaks in pediatric hospitals are common. RSV can live on skin or paper for up to 1 hour and on cribs and other nonporous surfaces for up to 6 hours. Although it is not airborne, it is highly communicable. It is usually transferred by inadequately washed hands. Meticulous hand hygiene decreases the spread of organisms.

In addition to RSV, other causative organisms include *Mycoplasma*, parainfluenza virus, and some adenoviruses. RSV infection occurs in annual epidemics during the winter and early spring, mainly from November to March in northern climates. The incidence peaks at age 6 months. By age 2 years, nearly 100% of children will have had RSV. Immunity does not occur, but the incidence and severity decrease with age.

Manifestations

A mild upper respiratory tract infection usually precedes the development of bronchiolitis. Serous nasal drainage, sneezing, low-grade fever, and anorexia are present for several days, followed by the onset

PATHOPHYSIOLOGY

Bronchiolitis

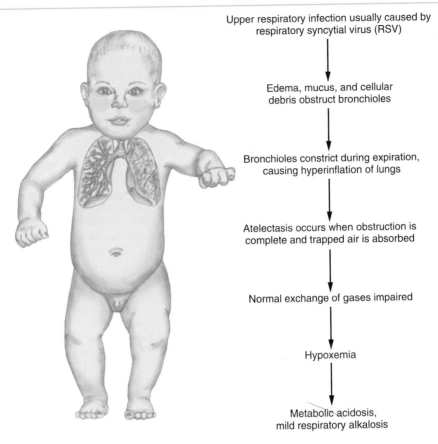

Upper respiratory infection usually caused by respiratory syncytial virus (RSV)

↓

Edema, mucus, and cellular debris obstruct bronchioles

↓

Bronchioles constrict during expiration, causing hyperinflation of lungs

↓

Atelectasis occurs when obstruction is complete and trapped air is absorbed

↓

Normal exchange of gases impaired

↓

Hypoxemia

↓

Metabolic acidosis, mild respiratory alkalosis

In bronchiolitis, edema and the accumulation of mucus and cellular debris cause obstruction of the bronchioles. Infants' bronchioles are very small and can become obstructed quickly. Airway resistance is increased during the inspiratory and expiratory phases of respiration because of the small air passages. Hyperinflation of the lungs results from air trapping because the bronchioles constrict during expiration. Atelectasis can occur if obstruction becomes complete and trapped air is absorbed. Normal gas exchange is impaired, and the infant becomes hypoxic. Some infants have mild respiratory alkalosis; more frequently, metabolic acidosis is observed.

The child with bronchiolitis is most acutely ill during the first 48 to 72 hours after the onset of the disease. Improvement usually occurs in a few days. Symptoms may last for 10 to 14 days. Mortality rate is less than 1%. There have been studies that show a predisposition for asthma later in life when an infant in hospitalized for severe bronchiolitis.*

*Carroll, K., Wu, P., Gebretsadik, T., et al. (2009). The severity-dependent relationship of infant bronchiolitis on the risk and morbidity of early childhood asthma. *Journal of Allergy and Clinical Immunology, 123*(5), 1055-1061.

of acute respiratory distress, manifested by the following signs and symptoms:
- Tachypnea: Respiratory rates of 60 to 80 breaths/min
- Tachycardia: Heart rate more than 140 beats/min
- Wheezing, crackles, or rhonchi
- Intercostal and subcostal retractions with or without nasal flaring
- Cyanosis

Feeding may be difficult because of increased respirations, which interfere with sucking and swallowing. The body temperature varies from hypothermic to as high as 105.8° F (41° C).

Diagnostic Evaluation

The clinical presentation and the age of the child suggest the diagnosis. Chest radiographs, if performed, may show hyperinflation of the lungs and an increased anteroposterior chest diameter on lateral views. There are scattered areas of consolidation in some infants, a finding attributable to atelectasis caused by obstruction or inflammation of the alveoli. In some infants, the chest radiographs appear normal. If, based on clinical symptoms and epidemiologic factors, the diagnosis is not definitively determined a rapid virus identification can be performed on respiratory secretions obtained by nasal or nasopharyngeal washing (Watts & Goodman, 2011).

Therapeutic Management

Infants with mild bronchiolitis can be treated at home with fluids, humidification, and rest. Infants with respiratory distress are hospitalized for supportive treatment. Cool, humidified oxygen is delivered if the oxygen saturation decreases to less than 90% on room air to relieve dyspnea, hypoxemia, and insensible water loss from tachypnea (Watts & Goodman, 2011). Zhang, Mendoza-Sassi, Wainwright, & Klassen (2008) conducted an integrative literature review that suggests that inhalation of hypertonic (3%) normal saline solution improves respiratory status and decreases the hospital stay of infants with bronchiolitis.

Parenteral administration of fluids may be necessary for acutely ill infants who are dehydrated from tachypnea or poor intake. The infant should be positioned with the head and chest at a 30- to 40-degree angle and the neck slightly extended to maintain an open airway and decrease pressure on the diaphragm.

Antibiotics are not given unless there is a secondary bacterial infection. Although some health care providers routinely prescribe bronchodilators, epinephrine, or corticosteroids, randomized clinical trials have failed to demonstrate clinical efficacy in the use of these medications (Da Dalt, Callegaro, Carraro et al., 2007).

RSV prevention is of the utmost importance to reduce hospitalizations for young, at-risk infants and children. Intramuscular palivizumab (Synagis) administered monthly throughout the RSV season has significantly reduced the hospitalization risk for premature infants (less than 35 weeks of gestation) younger than 6 months and children younger than 24 months with chronic lung disease or congenital cardiac disease (Morris, Dzolganovski, Beyene, & Sung, 2009). Prophylaxis is done on an outpatient basis.

NURSING CARE OF THE CHILD WITH BRONCHIOLITIS

■ Assessment

The nurse assesses the infant for signs and symptoms of respiratory distress (tachypnea, dyspnea, retractions, cyanosis, nasal flaring) every 1 to 2 hours during the acute phase and as needed if changes occur. Auscultate the lungs for breath sounds. Apnea monitoring and cardiorespiratory monitoring are indicated for the infant with acute disease. Make sure that the alarms on the cardiorespiratory monitor are appropriately set, and document any periods of apnea.

Assess the infant for signs of dehydration (dry mucous membranes, decreased urine output, sunken fontanel, weight loss) and monitor body temperature. The infant should be placed in a room near the nurses' station for easy observation. Assess the family's understanding of the disease and family members' level of anxiety. Observe the infant for signs of anxiety, restlessness, or irritability.

■ Nursing Diagnosis and Planning

The diagnoses and expected outcomes that may be appropriate for the infant with bronchiolitis and the infant's family are as follows:

- Impaired Gas Exchange related to airway edema and increased mucus.

Expected Outcome. The infant will have adequate gas exchange, as evidenced by oxygen saturation above 95% on room air.

- Ineffective Airway Clearance related to increased secretions.

Expected Outcome. The infant will exhibit clear breath sounds and normal respiratory rate, depth, and rhythm.

- Deficient Fluid Volume related to decreased intake and insensible loss.

Expected Outcome. The infant will maintain adequate hydration, as evidenced by moist mucous membranes, a flat fontanel, urine output normal for age, and stable weight.

- Ineffective Thermoregulation related to illness.

Expected Outcome. The infant will demonstrate a body temperature within normal limits.

- Anxiety related to hospitalization and the child's dyspnea.

Expected Outcomes. The infant will demonstrate decreased anxiety, as evidenced by adequate sleep and stable vital signs. The parents will verbalize understanding of the infant's condition and be able to participate appropriately in the infant's care.

■ Interventions

Many hospitals are now using clinical pathways for children with respiratory disease. Even when using a clinical pathway, the nurse needs to focus on appropriate nursing interventions.

■ **Facilitating Gas Exchange.** The nurse documents the infant's vital signs and respiratory status every 1 to 2 hours or more often as needed. Particularly note the rate, quality, and depth of respirations along with any adventitious breath sounds and the presence of retractions. Close monitoring with a cardiorespiratory monitor or continuous pulse oximetry will ensure early identification of impending respiratory distress.

Oxygen administration is indicated for infants who are hypoxic or in respiratory distress. Administer humidified oxygen (at 35% to 40% concentration) in the manner most comfortable for the infant (by hood, mask, or nasal prongs) to decrease hypoxia and bronchial edema. Positioning the infant's head at a 30- to 40-degree upright angle with the neck slightly extended will maintain an open airway and ease respirations by decreasing pressure on the diaphragm. Scheduling periods of uninterrupted rest between care episodes decreases oxygen demand.

■ **Preventing Transmission.** Isolate the infant with RSV infection in a single room or place the infant in a room with other RSV-infected infants. Meticulous hand hygiene is imperative. Nurses caring for these infants should not care for other high-risk children. Maintaining Contact Precautions (i.e., wearing a gown and gloves) reduces nosocomial transmission of RSV.

Emphasize to parents and other visitors that touching the infant or surfaces within 3 feet of the infant can transmit the organism to the hands and clothes. It is essential to stress the importance for parents and visitors to use protective gloves and gown and practice meticulous hand hygiene before entering the infant's room and after removal of the gown and gloves to avoid transmitting the infection to others.

■ **Maintaining Fluid Balance.** Most infants with bronchiolitis can take fluids orally; IV fluids are administered if respiratory distress is severe enough to risk aspiration. If the infant's nasal passages are blocked with mucus, instill saline solution nose drops (one or two drops in each nostril, followed by gentle suctioning with a bulb syringe) before feeding. Offer the infant frequent, varied clear liquids (juices, Pedialyte, Ricelyte). Older infants may enjoy frozen electrolyte pops. The infant's hydration status (skin turgor, fontanel, mucous membranes) and electrolyte values are monitored, and daily weights and intake and output are documented.

■ **Reducing Fever.** The nurse monitors the infant's temperature every 2 to 4 hours and as needed. Control environmental temperature by maintaining the room temperature between 72° and 75° F (22° and 24° C) and dress the infant in light clothing. Fluid intake is encouraged, if respiratory rate is within normal limits, and liquid acetaminophen or ibuprofen is administered as ordered to reduce fever.

■ **Decreasing Anxiety.** Encourage the parent to stay with the infant when possible and to participate as much as possible in the infant's care. Hospital routines and all procedures and treatments should be explained to reduce fear of the unknown. Because adult anxiety can be transferred to the infant, maintain a calm environment and

Animation—Pneumonia

encourage parents to do the same. Parents need to be allowed to express concerns.

■ Evaluation

- Does the infant demonstrate adequate oxygenation (oxygen saturation greater than 95%), clear breath sounds, and stable respiratory status?
- Does the infant have moist mucous membranes, good skin turgor, stable weight, a flat fontanel, and urine output of at least 2 to 3 mL/kg/hr? (For appropriate urine output in older children, see Chapter 16.)
- Is the infant's body temperature within normal limits?
- Does the infant demonstrate reduced crying or irritability and increased rest?
- Do the parents verbalize understanding of the disease, have a relaxed appearance, and demonstrate comforting behaviors toward the infant?

PNEUMONIA

Pneumonia is an inflammation of the lung parenchyma. It can occur as a primary or a secondary disease. Pneumonias can be classified by anatomic distribution or by the agents that cause them. Environment, immune system status, and the child's age are factors in the pathogenesis of the disease.

The two most common types of infectious pneumonia are *viral* and *bacterial* (Table 21-3). Viruses are the most common causative agents in infants and children younger than 5 years old, particularly influenza and RSV (Sandora & Sectish, 2011). Community-acquired pneumonia is a significant problem worldwide. In the United States the prevalence of pneumonia in children has decreased markedly with the institution of routine vaccination with pneumococcal conjugate vaccine during infancy (Sandora & Sectish, 2011). Children with chronic and acute conditions, such as acquired immunodeficiency syndrome, cystic fibrosis (CF), congenital defects, and foreign body aspiration, are at increased risk for development of pneumonia. Opportunistic infections (*Pneumocystis jiroveci* [formerly *carinii*] pneumonia) may be associated with acquired immunodeficiency syndrome (see Chapter 18). Secondary pneumonia can result from aspiration of hydrocarbons contained in household products or lipids (e.g., mineral oil given to treat severe constipation).

NURSING CARE OF THE CHILD WITH PNEUMONIA

■ Assessment

Every 2 hours, or more frequently depending on the severity of respiratory distress, assess the child's breath sounds, respiratory rate and rhythm, color, vital signs, and degree of restlessness. Immediately

TABLE 21-3 COMPARISON OF TYPES OF PNEUMONIA

ETIOLOGY AND INCIDENCE	PATHOPHYSIOLOGY	MANIFESTATIONS	THERAPEUTIC MANAGEMENT
Viral Most often caused by influenza viruses, parainfluenza virus, and RSV. Viruses cause 80%-85% of all pneumonias. Most common in children younger than 3 yr.	Cell destruction with sloughing of cellular debris into lumen of terminal airways and alveoli causes patchy infiltrate that affects multiple lobes.	Low to high fever, cough, crackles, wheezing (more common with RSV), headache, malaise, myalgia, abdominal pain. Infiltrates seen on chest radiography. WBC count <20,000/mm³. Usually lasts 5-7 days.	Supportive. No antibiotics are prescribed unless coexisting bacterial infection is suspected. Severely ill infants and children may be hospitalized for oxygen and fluid therapy.
Bacterial and Bacterial-like Caused primarily by *S. pneumoniae* in infants and children younger than 5 yr. *M. pneumoniae* and *C. pneumoniae* are more commonly seen in children older than 5 yr. Also may be caused by *H. influenzae* and group A streptococci. *Chlamydia trachomatis* is seen mainly in infants.	Alveoli fill with fluid and cells in small segment or entire lung. Bacteria enter bloodstream through pulmonary lymphatics. Vital capacity and lung compliance decrease as consolidation increases.	Preceded by upper respiratory infection. Abrupt onset of high fever, chills, cough, chest pain, decreased breath sounds, signs of respiratory distress (retractions, nasal flaring, tachypnea), restlessness, and apprehension. Symptoms may be vague in infants; older children can have gastrointestinal symptoms, chest pain, and abnormal breath sounds. Onset of the bacterial-like pneumonias may be more insidious. Radiography reveals consolidation; WBC count is elevated.	Oral antibiotic therapy, usually with amoxicillin, cefuroxime, or amoxicillin-clavulanate for mild episodes; erythromycin for penicillin-allergic children; azithromycin or fluoroquinolone for older children or adolescents. IV cefotaxime or parenteral ceftriaxone for children needing hospitalization. Hospitalization for severely ill infants and children who will need oxygen and fluid therapy. Chest tube drainage of fluid or purulence from pleural cavity may be necessary (particularly for children with staphylococcal pneumonia).

IV, Intravenous; *RSV,* respiratory syncytial virus; *WBC,* white blood cell.

report any signs of increased respiratory distress, including dyspnea, tachypnea, cyanosis, use of accessory muscles of breathing, diminished breath sounds, and crackles. Also note any fever, tachycardia, malaise, anorexia, discomfort, and changes in condition.

Nursing Diagnosis and Planning

The nursing diagnoses and expected outcomes that may be appropriate for the child with pneumonia and the child's family are as follows:

- Ineffective Airway Clearance related to bronchial obstruction.

Expected Outcome. The child will have clear airways, as evidenced by the absence of abnormal breath sounds and dyspnea.

- Ineffective Breathing Pattern related to increased mucus production and pain with inspiration.

Expected Outcome. The child will demonstrate effective breathing, as evidenced by respiratory rate and rhythm within normal limits for age and absence of retractions.

- Impaired Gas Exchange related to increased mucus and accumulation of exudate.

Expected Outcome. The child will maintain adequate gas exchange, as evidenced by decreased restlessness, appropriate oxygen saturation, and improved mucous membrane and nail bed color.

- Deficient Fluid Volume related to fever, decreased intake, and tachypnea.

Expected Outcome. The child will maintain fluid balance, as evidenced by moist mucous membranes, good skin turgor, urine output appropriate for age, and maintenance of age-appropriate weight.

- Deficient Knowledge related to the disease process and home care.

Expected Outcome. The parents will explain the disease process and describe the child's care.

- Anxiety (parental) related to infant's dyspnea and hospitalization.

Expected Outcome. The parents will show a decrease in anxiety, as evidenced by decreased irritability and increased periods of rest. The parents will verbalize and demonstrate comfort and ease when caring for the child.

- Acute Pain related to coughing and difficulty breathing secondary to disease process.

Expected Outcome. The child will have decreased pain, as evidenced by less irritability, verbalization of increased comfort (if age appropriate), and a relaxed body posture.

Interventions

The severity of the illness and the cause of the disease direct the nursing care of the child with pneumonia. Many children will be cared for at home, whereas others will be hospitalized on a general pediatric unit or special care area.

For the hospitalized child, elevating the head of the bed and changing the child's position every 2 hours assist respiratory effort and promote pulmonary drainage. Older children may assume a position of comfort but still must change their position every 2 hours. The use of infant seats should be avoided because pressure may be placed on the diaphragm, thus actually decreasing lung expansion.

The older child should be assisted with coughing and deep breathing and splinting as necessary to ease discomfort. Oxygen should be humidified and monitored. Pulse oximetry aids in monitoring oxygen saturation and the adequacy of air exchange. A cardiorespiratory monitor is used when available.

Oral or IV fluids are given as ordered. IV fluids may be indicated when oral intake increases the stress put on an already compromised

body. The nurse monitors intake and output and observes for signs of dehydration (oliguria, poor skin turgor, dry mucous membranes, sunken fontanels, weight loss). Weight should be measured daily. The specific gravity of urine also is checked to monitor hydration status.

Because conserving energy aids oxygenation, nursing care is planned to provide for periods of rest. Quiet diversional activities, such as reading, puzzles, videos, and board games, are suggested. The nurse maintains a quiet and cool environment and limits visitors to allow the child maximum rest. Visits by anyone with an infection should be restricted.

Administer antipyretics, antibiotics, and analgesics as ordered. Normal breathing may cause discomfort. If an analgesic is not ordered, the physician should be notified of any discomfort the child has. Splinting of the affected side by lying on that side may decrease discomfort. Diversional activities and manipulation of the environment are often effective for pain relief.

The family and child (if of appropriate age) need to receive information about the disease and its treatment. The nurse explains all procedures and treatments and encourages the parents to stay with their child and participate in the child's care. The nurse conveys empathy for the family's feelings and concerns. The nurse also teaches the family about home management of the infant or child (see Patient-Centered Teaching: Home Management of the Child with Pneumonia box).

PATIENT-CENTERED TEACHING

Home Management of the Child with Pneumonia

- Provide rest.
- Increase your child's fluid intake. Offer favorite fluids more frequently than usual, and be sure your child is urinating appropriate amounts. Warm liquids (lemonade, apple juice, Pedialyte, Ricelyte) help loosen secretions. Call your health care provider if the child's mucous membranes appear dry or if urination decreases.
- Administer acetaminophen for fever and discomfort.
- Use a cool-mist humidifier and follow the manufacturer's instructions for cleaning.
- Administer antibiotics as ordered; give the correct dose and the entire prescribed amount.
- Avoid exposing your child to cigarette smoke.

Evaluation

- Are the child's vital signs and respiratory status within normal limits?
- Is the child's oxygen saturation greater than 95%?
- Does the child appear hydrated, with moist mucous membranes, good skin turgor, and adequate urinary output for age?
- Can the parents describe home care techniques?
- Do the parents appear relaxed, and are they able to fully participate in the child's care?
- Can the child comfortably participate in quiet activities and rest quietly when appropriate?
- Is the child in pain?

FOREIGN BODY ASPIRATION

Foreign body aspiration is seen most frequently in children ages 6 months to 5 years. Children who play, run, or laugh with objects in

BOX 21-1 COMMON ITEMS OF ASPIRATION

- Nuts
- Pins
- Screws
- Coins
- Seeds
- Grapes
- Bones
- Earrings
- Small toys
- Chunks of food
- Parts of toys
- Hard candy
- Latex balloons
- Popcorn
- Hot dogs
- Carrots

their mouths are at risk. Certain items have an increased incidence of aspiration by infants and children (Box 21-1).

Etiology and Incidence

Children's curiosity, oral needs, and occasionally lack of supervision contribute to the occurrence of foreign body aspiration. Infants and children love to explore and investigate objects. Exploration often includes putting objects into their mouths. Children also have the uncanny ability to remove small parts from toys and to find other objects that parents thought were out of their reach (e.g., pins, screws, nuts, coins, earrings). Adults may give infants and small children foods they are not developmentally prepared to ingest (hard candy, popcorn, uncooked carrots, hot dogs, peanuts). Latex balloons account for a significant number of deaths from aspiration per year. Childhood aspiration can occur at any age, but it occurs most frequently in children under 2 years of age (Shlizerman, Mazzawi, Rakover, & Ashkenazi, 2010).

Pathophysiology

Most foreign bodies become lodged in the bronchi. The right main bronchus is a more common site than the left main bronchus because of its anatomic development. Objects lodged in the larynx cause edema and inflammation. Bronchial obstruction manifests as obstructive emphysema, pneumonia, or atelectasis. Failure to remove obstructing foreign objects is almost always fatal. Most can be removed mechanically without complications; a delay in treatment can lead to aspiration pneumonia and airway trauma.

Manifestations

Immediate signs and symptoms include sudden, violent coughing; gagging; wheezing; vomiting; brief episodes of apnea; and possibly cyanosis.

After aspirating a foreign object, the child may remain asymptomatic for hours or weeks. If the object is not found and removed, signs and symptoms related to edema and increased irritation and obstruction may develop. Signs and symptoms of laryngeal and tracheal obstruction include choking, dysphagia, hoarseness, croupy cough, stridor, and possibly dyspnea with cyanosis. Coughing, wheezing, unilaterally decreased breath sounds, pneumonitis, and possibly respiratory arrest can indicate bronchial inflammation and obstruction.

Diagnostic Evaluation

The diagnosis is based on an accurate history and the clinical manifestations. Fluoroscopy, magnetic resonance imaging (MRI), computed tomography (CT) scan, or chest radiography may be used to reveal the presence of a foreign object in the respiratory tract. Radiographs may

not be particularly helpful, because a nonmetallic object may not be visible. Rigid bronchoscopy confirms the diagnosis and may provide an avenue for removing the object.

Therapeutic Management

Foreign bodies are removed from the respiratory tract by direct laryngoscopy or bronchoscopy. After the procedure, the child should remain hospitalized for observation for laryngeal edema and respiratory distress. Antibiotics are unnecessary unless respiratory signs and symptoms suggest an infection. Cool mist and administration of bronchodilators or corticosteroids 24 to 48 hours after the removal of the foreign body may be indicated.

Nursing Considerations

The degree of obstruction should be assessed to determine the appropriate action to take. If the child is aphonic (not speaking) and not breathing, the nurse should follow the current guidelines for managing an obstructed airway (see Chapter 10). Children with a partially obstructed airway are observed for signs of increasing obstruction.

After the object has been removed, the child is observed for signs of obstruction caused by laryngeal edema and soft tissue swelling (restlessness, dyspnea). The child should be placed on a cardiorespiratory monitor.

Liquids are withheld until the child's gag reflex returns after anesthesia. Oral fluids should be started slowly and increased as the child tolerates the intake. Intake and output should be recorded. If the child refuses to drink because of a sore throat or is unable to take fluids orally, the physician should be notified so that IV fluids may be started. The parents' knowledge of respiratory distress is also evaluated before discharge.

Parental anxiety and guilt are common after an episode of aspiration. In addition to supporting the parents, the nurse assesses their knowledge of safety. Prevention is the key to reducing the incidence of aspiration. Safety is discussed at every well-child visit (see Chapters 5 through 8).

PULMONARY NONINFECTIOUS IRRITATION

Although we think of foreign body aspiration as the most common type of pulmonary noninfectious irritation in children, other forms of irritation may cause respiratory difficulties. These include acute respiratory distress syndrome (ARDS), passive smoking, and smoke inhalation.

Acute Respiratory Distress Syndrome

Although there is not uniform agreement as to what constitutes acute respiratory distress syndrome, it is generally agreed that ARDS represents severe diffuse lung injury precipitated by a variety of illnesses. The mechanism of lung injury in children is similar to that of adults and usually occurs from 8 to 48 hours after the initial illness, which may be, but is not limited to, aspiration, trauma, drug ingestion, shock, and massive transfusions.

Pathophysiology

The mechanism that initiates and perpetuates the lung injury is not understood. There is a breakdown in the alveolar-capillary barrier with fluid accumulation in the interstitium and alveoli. ARDS has acute and chronic stages. Initially there is capillary congestion and pulmonary edema. Fibrosis of the lungs develops in children who do not recover from the acute stage.

TABLE 21-4   PULMONARY NONINFECTIOUS IRRITANTS

ACUTE RESPIRATORY DISTRESS SYNDROME (ARDS)	PASSIVE SMOKING	SMOKE INHALATION
Clinical Manifestations		
Acute, subacute, and chronic phases	Increased respiratory infections	Singed nasal hair
Pulmonary manifestations may be minimal during acute phase but will move toward respiratory distress (dyspnea, tachypnea, retractions, grunting, cyanosis)	An effect on respiratory function and growth in infants and small but significant reduction in airway function in older children	Cough
		Hoarseness
	Possible negative effect on linear growth of children with cystic fibrosis	Hemoptysis
Severe hypoxemia and, occasionally, hypercapnia may develop		Soot in sputum
		Cyanosis
Note that there is a primary disease, and manifestations of that disease process will also be present		Wheezing
		Carbon monoxide effects:
		Mild: Headaches, mild dyspnea, visual changes, confusion
		Moderate: Irritability, diminished judgment, dim vision, nausea
		Severe: Hallucinations, confusion, ataxia, collapse, coma
Therapeutic Management		
Need to be treated in ICU	Awareness of problem and preventive teaching	100% oxygen by mask
Treat underlying cause	Effective programs to prevent smoking in parents and minors	Close monitoring of carboxyhemoglobin levels
Oxygen/mechanical ventilation		Arterial blood gases
Pulse oximetry		Intubation and tracheostomy equipment available
Maintain cardiac function		Aerosolized bronchodilators
Stabilize hematocrit		Balance fluid therapy between need for large volume of fluid and need to limit fluid to decrease pulmonary edema
Prevent infection		Prophylactic antimicrobial therapy is controversial
Nursing Care		
Monitor respiratory status	Involvement in community projects to designate "no smoking" ordinances in public places	Respiratory assessment
Monitor blood gas analysis		Support of pulmonary therapy
Psychological support of child and parents	School-based prevention programs	Psychological support of child and family as a result of the fear of the trauma of the fire or insult that caused the injury
Monitor urine output, capillary filling, perfusion	Education of parents as part of anticipatory guidance of dangers of smoking, both active and passive	
	Role modeling no smoking	Children who have lost a family member will need long-term psychological support
Prognosis		
High mortality rate, usually more than 50%	Increased numbers of studies have shown correlation between smoking and respiratory disease; more studies needed to show long-term effects	Most will return to near-normal pulmonary function, and few will have long-term problems associated with the injury
Those who survive have a good chance of full recovery		

ICU, Intensive care unit.

Table 21-4 discusses clinical manifestations, therapeutic management, nursing care, and prognosis.

Passive Smoking

Increased attention has been paid to the role of passive smoking in the development of respiratory disease in children. Children with a history of exposure to cigarette smoke, both prenatally and postnatally, have more frequent upper and lower respiratory complications, more hospitalizations for those complications, and a greater tendency to develop wheezing than do nonexposed children. *Prenatal* exposure can be associated with impaired lung growth as well (Håberg, Stigum, Nystad, & Nafstad, 2007).

Pathophysiology

Smoke is an irritant that can cause increased airway reactivity and inflammation.

See Table 21-4 for a discussion of clinical manifestations, therapeutic management, nursing care, and prognosis.

Smoke Inhalation

As many as 50% of all fire-related deaths are caused by smoke injuries. The severity of lung injury is related to the nature of the material inhaled, the products of incomplete combustion that are generated, and the child's confinement in a closed space. Besides the noxious gases, fine particles of soot may also be inhaled, which may have toxic gases adsorbed on them or which may cause thermal burns.

Pathophysiology

Because the upper airway has a built-in cooling system, most thermal airway injury is limited to the areas above the larynx. Steam inhalation injury is an exception. Combustion of the materials involved causes a wide variety of noxious gases. These include but are not limited to oxides of sulfur and nitrogen, corrosive alkalis, and carbon monoxide. Exposure to and inhalation of these gases can cause mucosal edema, airway obstruction, atelectasis, necrosis of the pulmonary mucosa, and pulmonary edema (Antoon & Donovan, 2011).

Carbon monoxide poisoning is a complication of smoke inhalation caused when carbon monoxide combines with hemoglobin to form carboxyhemoglobin, causing severe hypoxia.

See Table 21-4 for a discussion of clinical manifestations, therapeutic management, nursing care, and prognosis.

RESPIRATORY DISTRESS SYNDROME

Respiratory distress syndrome (RDS), not to be confused with acute respiratory distress syndrome as discussed earlier, is also known as *hyaline membrane disease*. It occurs when there is immature development of the respiratory system or an inadequate amount of surfactant in the lungs. Infants with RDS are unable to keep their lungs expanded and the alveoli open. RDS is the leading cause of respiratory failure in the preterm infant.

RDS occurs in infants with immature lung development or insufficient amounts of surfactant. Predisposing factors include prematurity, asphyxia at birth, cesarean delivery, a diabetic mother (especially <38 weeks' gestation), acute antepartum hemorrhage, multiple gestation, and a sibling who had RDS. Affected boys outnumber affected girls 2 to 1.

Incidence

The incidence of RDS increases as gestational age decreases. The degree of prematurity is directly related to the risk for RDS. Maternal diabetes is another risk factor, as is perinatal asphyxia and birth by cesarean delivery (Hallman & Haataja, 2007). On the other hand, factors that tend to cause chronic fetal stress, such as maternal hypertension, drug abuse, and prolonged rupture of membranes, decrease the incidence of RDS.

Pathophysiology

In the preterm infant, anatomic immaturity of the chest wall, lung parenchyma, and capillary endothelium contributes to the development of RDS. The immature chest wall anatomy increases the chances of lung collapse at the end of expiration. Immaturity of the lung parenchyma and capillary endothelium results in less surface area for gas exchange. In the preterm as well as the term infant, RDS may be caused by a decreased total amount of pulmonary surfactant or a qualitative alteration of the surfactant present. The resulting inability to keep the lungs expanded causes the lung to be relatively noncompliant with changes in intrathoracic and extrathoracic pressure, decreasing air exchange. Lung repair begins after 24 to 48 hours, even as

further cell damage takes place. Hyaline membranes, consisting of debris from necrotic cells enmeshed in a proteinaceous filtrate of serum, are destroyed by macrophages. Cuboidal cells replace the damaged alveolar and airway epithelium and eventually flatten. New capillaries develop and make contact with the regenerating cells of the alveoli. Surfactant synthesis begins and helps the repaired alveoli remain expanded. Diuresis is usually a sign that the acute phase of RDS has ended and recovery is taking place. The differential diagnosis of RDS should include transient tachypnea of the newborn, pulmonary insufficiency of prematurity, group B streptococcal pneumonia, and anatomic malformations. An immature chest wall, decreased surfactant, and immature lung tissue may contribute to RDS.

Manifestations

Symptoms of RDS usually appear at or shortly after birth, worsen over the first 24 to 48 hours, and gradually improve over the next 3 to 5 days. Signs and symptoms include tachypnea, inspiratory retractions (e.g., suprasternal, substernal, intercostal), paradoxic seesaw respirations, inspiratory nasal flaring, and an audible expiratory grunt. Radiographs of the chest may show overall hypoventilation and a reticular granular pattern (i.e., ground-glass appearance). Apnea occurs as lung function worsens. Central cyanosis (a late, ominous sign) indicates increased hypoxemia and an advanced stage of deterioration. Blood gases initially show a decrease in the concentration of oxygen in the blood. Carbon dioxide levels in the blood rise as respiratory failure occurs from repeated apnea or poor air exchange. As respiratory failure progresses, metabolic acidosis slowly develops, and, as the concentration of carbon dioxide in the blood increases, a mixed metabolic and respiratory acidosis develops. Some complications of RDS may include pneumothorax, patent ductus arteriosus, necrotizing enterocolitis, intraventricular hemorrhage, retinopathy of prematurity, and death (Soll & Özek, 2009). Respiratory failure may result in death if supportive management is not timely and appropriate.

Therapeutic Management

Supportive Care

The goals of supportive care are to keep oxygen consumption as low as possible and to maintain adequate nutrition and hydration. Every effort should be made to maintain the infant in a neutral thermal environment. Oxygen consumption increases rapidly above or below the neutral thermal environment. Evaporation is a significant contributor to fluid loss in premature infants. Measures should be taken to minimize fluid loss by evaporation and loss of heat. Because handling stimulates movement and oxygen consumption, the infant should be handled as little as possible. A minimum of 60 kcal/kg/day should be provided with sufficient amino acids to prevent catabolism of endogenous proteins and ketoacidosis.

Respiratory Care

Oxygen should be given to maintain partial pressure of oxygen (PO_2) within the normal range. Interrupting oxygen administration, even briefly, may cause hypoxemia, pulmonary vasoconstriction, and reduced cardiac output. Mechanical ventilation should be started when the infant's respiratory system requires additional assistance. Apnea with bradycardia that is unresponsive to stimulation, regardless of the blood gas values, is also an indication that mechanical ventilation is needed. With intubation and continuous positive airway pressure or positive-pressure ventilation, radiographic changes usually appear less severe.

⊖ Prenatal steroids, surfactant replacement, continuous positive airway pressure (CPAP) ventilation, and, if necessary, mechanical ventilation are all integral parts of the therapeutic management of RDS (Verder, 2007).

NURSING CARE OF THE CHILD WITH RDS

▪ Assessment

The nurse identifies infants at risk for RDS by reviewing the perinatal history for risk factors. The respiratory system is assessed for signs of respiratory distress, including tachypnea, apnea, retractions, nasal flaring, and grunting. During auscultation of the chest, the nurse assesses the infant's breath sounds, comparing and contrasting the left and right sides and noting the equality of breath sounds, the quality of air entry, and the presence of rhonchi, crackles, and wheezes.

Assessment of the cardiovascular system includes determining the heart rate and noting any murmurs that may indicate a cardiac malformation or patent ductus arteriosus. A shift in the location of the point of maximal impulse may indicate a shift in heart position from a pulmonary air leak.

Peripheral cyanosis may progress to central cyanosis, which in the neonate usually indicates severe hypoxia. Peripheral cyanosis may become obscured as the infant's color further deteriorates to pale gray. Initially, extremely ill infants may have a blood pressure that is slightly higher than normal, progressing to hypotension as the infant's condition deteriorates.

The nurse discusses the results of laboratory tests for abnormal findings. Blood gas abnormalities, acid-base imbalances, disturbances in electrolyte and glucose homeostasis, and early signs of complications, such as sepsis, require immediate intervention.

▪ Nursing Diagnosis and Planning

The nursing diagnoses and expected outcomes that may be appropriate for the neonate with RDS and the family are as follows:

- Impaired Gas Exchange related to immaturity of the lungs and chest wall or insufficient amounts of surfactant.

Expected Outcome. The infant will be able to maintain adequate gas exchange, as evidenced by blood gas values and oxygen saturations within normal ranges.

- Ineffective Airway Clearance related to obstruction or inappropriate positioning of an endotracheal tube.

Expected Outcome. The infant's artificial airway will be correctly positioned and patent, as evidenced by equal and adequate breath sounds and chest wall movement.

- Ineffective Breathing Pattern related to asynchronous breathing between the infant and the ventilator, ventilator malfunction, or inappropriate ventilatory support.

Expected Outcome. Ventilatory support will appropriately complement the infant's respiratory efforts, as evidenced by blood gas parameters within normal ranges.

- Risk for Injury related to extremes in acid-base balance, oxygen levels, carbon dioxide levels, or barotrauma from mechanical ventilation.

Expected Outcome. The respiratory assistance provided will prevent or promptly treat extremes in blood gas parameters and will minimize potential barotrauma.

- Risk for Impaired Parenting secondary to situational crisis (sick newborn infant).

Expected Outcomes. The parent will exhibit signs of parent-child attachment and develop role identity as a parent.

▪ Interventions

Infants with RDS are cared for in the special care nursery. The nurse monitors the infant's vital signs and respiratory status for evidence of respiratory distress. Blood gas monitoring and pulse oximetry are also done, and results are reported to the physician. Continuous cardiorespiratory monitoring will provide for early recognition of respiratory distress.

Proper positioning of the infant to maximize lung expansion is achieved in the supine position with the neck slightly extended and the nose pointed toward the ceiling. Positioning the infant this way prevents narrowing of the airway. Suctioning of the endotracheal tube as needed optimizes ventilation. The nurse works closely with the respiratory therapist to administer and monitor respiratory support.

If ventilatory support is indicated, settings are checked hourly and the nurse observes the infant to ensure synchronous breathing between the ventilator and infant. Ventilatory changes are made as ordered if blood gas results fall outside established parameters. The nurse encourages the parents to verbalize fears and concerns and to participate in caring for the infant as appropriate. The nurse may also consider directing the parents to contact outside resources for further support.

▪ Evaluation

- Does the infant maintain normal oxygen saturations on pulse oximetry?
- Does the infant maintain a normal respiratory rate?
- Are the infant's breath sounds and chest wall movements adequate and equal bilaterally?
- Are the infant's blood gases within normal limits?
- Are ventilatory settings adjusted in a timely manner whenever blood gas results fall outside established parameters?
- Does the family assume appropriate caregiving responsibilities?
- Are the parents able to hold, feed, and interact with the infant?

APNEA

Manifestations

Apnea is the cessation of breathing for a period of 20 seconds or longer, or for a shorter period but accompanied by bradycardia or cyanosis. True apnea differs from periodic breathing, which might be seen in premature infants. In periodic breathing, there is a shift from regular rhythmic breathing to brief episodes of apnea. This type of breathing pattern consists of three or more respiratory pauses of longer than 3 seconds, with less than 20 seconds of respiration between pauses. Rarely, periodic breathing is associated with changes in heart rate or color. Periodic breathing is common in premature infants and decreases as the infant's gestational age increases. The cause is unknown; periodic breathing may be a normal event.

Apparent life-threatening events (ALTEs) are sudden episodes characterized by apnea, a color change, a change in muscle tone, choking, or gagging in an infant who otherwise appears healthy. The observer of the event relates the belief that the infant would have died if not for intervention. Apparent life-threatening events most often occur in infants of 37 weeks of gestational age or older while they are sleeping, feeding, or awake. Infants who have had such an event are usually hospitalized for observation and testing (Scollan-Koliopoulos & Koliopoulos, 2010).

Two categories of true apnea events are apnea of prematurity and infant apnea (Table 21-5).

TABLE 21-5   APNEA OF PREMATURITY COMPARED WITH INFANT APNEA

ETIOLOGY AND INCIDENCE	PATHOPHYSIOLOGY	THERAPEUTIC MANAGEMENT
Apnea of Prematurity		
Most common type of apnea; occurs in neonates of 24-32 wk gestational age, with onset usually within first week of life. It usually resolves by 38 wk. Although neonate's age may be similar to the age at greatest risk for sudden infant death syndrome (SIDS), apnea of prematurity is not considered to predict risk for SIDS.*	Varies among neonates but may be caused by upper airway obstruction, immaturity of central control mechanisms, compliant chest wall, or abnormal response during REM sleep. Apnea often occurs during feeding because of immaturity of breathing, sucking, and swallowing coordination.	Gentle cutaneous stimulation is used to stimulate breathing in neonates with mild apnea (<10 episodes/day with little desaturation). For persistent apnea, use oxygen administration, cardiorespiratory monitor; consider CPAP for neonates with severe apnea. Drug therapy may include caffeine, oral theophylline, or IV aminophylline to increase central respiratory drive and improve carbon dioxide sensitivity.
Infant Apnea		
Most infant apnea has no known cause. Underlying conditions such as gastroesophageal reflux, seizures, or hypoglycemia should be ruled out.	Three types: • *Central:* Absence of respiratory effort and air movement. • *Obstructive:* Apparent respiratory efforts without air movement or sound. • *Mixed:* Absence of respiratory effort and nasal air movement followed by resumption of respiratory effort without air movement. Short episodes of apnea are usually central apnea; apnea episodes that last 15 sec or more are usually mixed.	If no underlying disorder is identified, home monitoring with a respiratory stimulant (e.g., caffeine).

*Scollan-Koliopoulos, M., & Koliopoulos, J. (2010). Evaluation and management of apparent life-threatening events in infants. *Pediatric Nursing, 36*(2), 77-83.
CPAP, Continuous positive airway pressure; *REM*, rapid eye movement.

Diagnostic Evaluation

Tests are selected for the clinical indications and to rule out any underlying condition. Cardiorespiratory and neurophysiologic studies are commonly ordered. These studies include chest radiography, blood chemistry studies, electrocardiography, and electroencephalography. Pneumocardiography specifically tests for apnea by recording the heart rate and chest wall movements; however, the reliability of the test in predicting apnea has not been well established. Sleep studies also are useful in determining which infants might benefit most from home apnea monitoring (Scollan-Koliopoulos & Koliopoulos, 2010).

NURSING CARE OF THE INFANT WITH APNEA

▪ Assessment

The infant's heart rate and respirations are monitored continuously. The nurse should ascertain that the alarms on the cardiorespiratory monitor are set. Resuscitative equipment should be available.

If an apneic episode is observed, the nurse should record the time and duration of the episode, the skin color change, heart rate, and oxygen saturation. The nurse should also describe what the infant was doing before the episode and any actions the nurse took to stimulate breathing.

▪ Nursing Diagnosis and Planning

The nursing diagnoses and expected outcomes that may be appropriate for the infant with apnea and the family are as follows:

• Ineffective Breathing Pattern related to apnea secondary to prematurity of respiratory control mechanisms (premature infant) and related to apnea of known or unknown etiology (term infant).
Expected Outcome. The infant will have regular breathing patterns, as evidenced by respiratory rate and rhythm within normal limits for age.

• Anxiety (parental) related to the possibility of the infant's death.
Expected Outcome. The parents will verbalize feelings concerning the infant's periods of apnea.

• Deficient Knowledge (parental) related to unfamiliarity with apnea monitoring equipment and cardiopulmonary resuscitation (CPR).
Expected Outcome. The parents will learn how to perform infant CPR and how to operate the apnea monitor.

▪ Interventions

The nurse sets the heart rate parameters of the cardiorespiratory monitor according to the infant's age and the respiratory pause at greater than 15 seconds. Resuscitative equipment should be available, and the nurse should be proficient in using it.

The apneic infant can be stimulated by gently tapping the infant's foot or trunk or turning the infant over. The infant should not be shaken vigorously. If breathing does not resume, institute bag-and-mask ventilation.

Maintain a neutral thermal environment while the infant is hospitalized and avoid suctioning if possible. Several studies have shown that

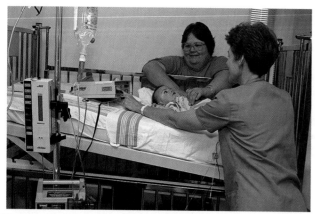

FIG 21-3 Teaching the family about using an apnea monitor and how to respond to alarms is an important element in caring for the child with infant apnea. The nurse must assess the parents' ability to tolerate the stressors of living with a child who is prone to apnea and support them as they deal with these stressors.

<table>
<tr><td>

BOX 21-2   HOME APNEA MONITORING

- Home apnea monitors track respiratory movements and, usually, cardiac rate; recordings of events are downloaded into a computer for evaluation.
- The parent or caregiver should record in a diary conditions leading up to an event, time of the event, how long it lasts, and the condition of the infant afterward. These results are compared with the computer record.
- Parents should routinely check manufacturer instructions, the ordered alarm settings, leads, wires, and belt to be sure they are in the correct position.
- Parents should be taught to stimulate the child when an event is observed and not wait for the monitor to alarm.
- The parents must be trained to do CPR and understand conditions for calling the health care provider.
- Twenty-four-hour medical, police/fire, electrical and technical (equipment troubleshooting) coverage is mandatory; there should be a backup plan for power outages.
- Although apnea is not directly correlated with SIDS, parents should follow the recommendations that apply for SIDS prevention in any infant.

</td></tr>
</table>

Data from Scollan-Koliopoulos, M., & Koliopoulos, J. (2010). Evaluation and management of apparent life-threatening events in infants. *Pediatric Nursing, 36*(2), 77-83.

feeding affects ventilation. Therefore, infants should be monitored closely when being fed.

Home apnea monitoring remains controversial, and there are few clear guidelines related to which infants would benefit most from home monitoring. In general, infants who appear to be at risk for recurrent events should be monitored at home (Silvestri, 2009). If home apnea monitoring is ordered, the family should be instructed in the use of the monitor and in CPR (Figure 21-3) (Scollan-Koliopoulos & Koliopoulos, 2010). Stimulating action should be taken if the infant becomes bradycardic, even if the apnea monitor does not alarm. Home pulse oximetry assists the parent with assessment of the infant's respiratory status (Scollan-Koliopoulos & Koliopoulos, 2010). Emphasize to the parents that when the monitor alarm is triggered, they should immediately assess the infant rather than focus on the machine (Box 21-2).

Parents of infants who are monitored at home may have emotional needs that need to be met. Witnessing their infant during an apneic episode can be frightening and traumatic for parents. Some parents experience a type of posttraumatic stress disorder and need to be referred for appropriate mental health evaluation (Scollan-Koliopoulos & Koliopoulos, 2010).

■ Evaluation

- Does the infant demonstrate normal respiratory rate and rhythm?
- Have the parents verbalized their fears associated with the infant's apnea?
- Have the parents demonstrated the ability to operate monitoring equipment and to perform CPR?

SUDDEN INFANT DEATH SYNDROME

Sudden infant death syndrome (SIDS) is defined as the sudden and unexplained death of an infant younger than 1 year. The exact cause is unknown despite a thorough investigation that includes a complete autopsy, examination of the death scene, and review of the clinical history. It is sometimes referred to by the public as *crib death.* SIDS usually occurs during sleep.

Etiology and Incidence

Although numerous theories have been proposed, the cause of SIDS is unknown. Proposed contributing factors include prematurity, brainstem defects, infections, and genetic predisposition. Some studies have suggested a connection with lower socioeconomic status, substance use during pregnancy, cultural influences, lack of prenatal care, smoking during pregnancy and exposing the infant to smoke, having a sibling with SIDS, and season (winter). It is generally accepted that SIDS is the result of an interaction among nonmodifiable and modifiable factors that include underlying susceptibility (genetic predisposition, brain abnormalities), developmental stage (rapid growth leading to physiologic instability during early infancy), and environmental stress (prone positioning, upper respiratory infection, exposure to smoke, and overheating) (National Institute of Child Health and Human Development [NICHHD], 2007, p. 9).

Numerous reports from countries outside the United States have found a significant association between a prone sleeping position and the incidence of SIDS. On the basis of this information, the AAP (2005/2009) updated its recommendations that healthy infants be placed on their backs to sleep, rather than prone or side-lying. Since the AAP issued its initial recommendations in 1992, SIDS has declined nearly 70% in the United States (Hunt & Hauck, 2011).

Risk factors are also associated with the use of soft bedding. Infants may suffocate by rebreathing carbon dioxide–laden expired air when sleeping face down on soft bedding (NICHHD, 2007). To reduce the risk of SIDS, the AAP (2005/2009) recommends using mattresses with a firm sleeping surface, avoiding exposing the infant to secondhand smoke, and offering a pacifier for sleep. The AAP does not recommend bed sharing and advises parents to put the infant in a safe bassinet or crib in the parent's room for sleeping (AAP, 2005/2009).

SIDS occurs most frequently between the second and fourth months of life, with 95% of cases occurring before age 6 months. It is more common in boys, low-birth-weight infants, and infants from lower socioeconomic groups. It occurs more often during the winter months. American Indians have the highest incidence, followed by African-Americans.

PATHOPHYSIOLOGY

Sudden Infant Death Syndrome

Autopsy findings in infants who have died of SIDS have varied widely. Non-specific findings such as mild pulmonary edema, vascular congestion, or pulmonary inflammation are common. Other consistent findings include retarded postnatal growth, increased pulmonary arterial smooth muscle, retention of brown fat, brainstem gliosis, and intrathoracic petechiae. Partial upper airway obstruction in association with rebreathing may be an explanation for many deaths from SIDS.* No single cause has been identified.

Prevention is of the utmost importance. Nurses must be role models and teachers about infant sleep positioning and other risk factors associated with SIDS. Teaching begins at the earliest contact the nurse may have with the infant and parents and as soon as possible after delivery.

*National Institute of Child Health and Human Development (2007). *Curriculum for nurses: Continuing education program on SIDS risk reduction.* Washington, DC: U.S. Government Printing Office. Retrieved from www.nichd.nih.gov.

Manifestations

The principal manifestation of SIDS is silent death. The child may be found in any position and may be clutching bedding.

Diagnostic Evaluation

Diagnosis is confirmed through autopsy. A medical history of the infant and family should be taken. The infant is examined for signs of illness or trauma. The death scene is also investigated.

NURSING CARE OF THE FAMILY OF THE INFANT WHO HAS DIED OF SUDDEN INFANT DEATH SYNDROME

■ Assessment

The nursing care involved in a SIDS case is family centered, not patient centered. When an infant is brought into the emergency department with suspected SIDS, the family is often confused. If resuscitation was begun at home, they may assume that it was effective and that their infant is alive. Assessment of the family's understanding of the situation is necessary to plan for teaching and support. The nurse should assess the family's emotional status and coping strategies.

The nurse interviews the family in a calm, slow, and nonthreatening manner. Questions should not imply negligence or any involvement in the death. Parents need to be given time to think before they answer questions. Because the parents will be overwhelmed, questions may need to be repeated for clarity.

■ Nursing Diagnosis and Planning

The nursing diagnoses and expected outcomes that may be appropriate for the family of the infant victim of SIDS are as follows:
- Interrupted Family Processes related to death of a child.
Expected Outcome. The parents and family will verbalize feelings related to the death of the infant.
- Compromised Family Coping related to death of a child.
Expected Outcome. The parents and family will identify strengths and accept support of other family members, friends, professionals, and support groups.
- Deficient Knowledge related to not understanding the cause of death.

Expected Outcome. The parents will verbalize an understanding of the cause of their child's death.

■ Interventions

The nurse working with a family whose child has died of SIDS should provide calm and compassionate support. The parents are confused about the death and are trying to cope with many emotions. Most parents will experience a combination of guilt, anger, and emotional pain.

A quiet room with dim lighting and a rocking chair should be provided for the family, and someone should remain with them. Assist the family to call family, friends, or clergy. The nurse should accompany the physician when the parents are told their infant is dead. At this time the parents should also be told that the apparent cause of death is SIDS and that nothing could have been done to prevent the death. This information may help minimize feelings of guilt.

Parents should be given the opportunity to say good-bye to their child. Because the parents may not think to ask to see their infant, the nurse should provide this opportunity.

The nurse might say, "Would you like to have some time alone with your baby? We will bring him to you, and you can take as long as you would like to hold him."

The infant should be cleaned and wrapped in a blanket and brought to the parents. Parents who are not given the opportunity to hold their child and say good-bye often regret it later, but parents who do not want time alone with their baby should have their decision respected. The nurse should accept the parents' decision in this matter. Each parent will cope in an individualized way.

The need for an autopsy should be explained. The autopsy will verify the cause of death and confirm for the parents that they did not cause the death.

Before the parents leave the hospital, arrangements for follow-up care should be made. Many hospitals have a team consisting of a social worker, chaplain, and nurse that is called when a suspected SIDS death occurs.

The nurse may refer the family to a local SIDS program for information, support, and counseling (American SIDS Institute, 509 Augusta Dr., Marietta, GA 30067; website: www.sids.org). Nurses who are involved in home visiting can encourage the family to communicate their feelings. Siblings should not be overlooked; parents may be so overwhelmed with their own grief that they forget their other children. The nurse may suggest local grief counseling resources that target siblings specifically. Another reaction might be to overprotect their other children. The nurse should guide the family in identifying the members' various responses and in treating them at the appropriate developmental level. Children in the family who perhaps resented the new baby may have tremendous guilt feelings. The loss of a sibling may be especially traumatic to a toddler, who does not understand the changes that are taking place in the family. Routines and rituals that are important to the toddler may be disrupted.

■ Evaluation

- Is the family able to verbalize feelings associated with the death of the child?
- Has the family joined a support group or identified a support system?
- Has the extended family mobilized to support the family?
- Is the family using effective coping skills to work toward an understanding of the child's death?

ASTHMA

Asthma is a leading cause of acute and chronic illness in children and the most frequent admitting diagnosis in children's hospitals. Despite advances in medical treatment, the incidence and death rate from asthma have continued to increase, and the prevalence of asthma in children is 9.6% (Akinbami, Moorman, & Liu, 2011).

Etiology

It is unclear why some children's airways are more reactive than others. It is known, however, that asthma is caused by an interaction between genetic and environmental factors and that the underlying physiologic alteration is inflammatory (National Heart, Lung, and Blood Institute [NHLBI] & National Asthma Education and Prevention Program [NAEPP], 2007). Asthma occurs more frequently in African-American children and those children living in crowded urban areas where they are exposed to a variety of adverse environmental and psychosocial triggers (Liu, Covar, Spahn, & Leung, 2011). Onset usually occurs before age 6 years, and persistence is related to underlying allergy in most cases (Liu et al., 2011).

An asthma episode can be triggered by a variety of stimuli, among them cold air, smoke, allergens, viral infection, stress, exercise, odors, and medications (particularly aspirin and nonsteroidal antiinflammatory drugs) (Ritz, Kullowatz, Kanniess, et al., 2008; Wills-Karp, 2007). Foods are occasionally the trigger in infants but less commonly in older children.

The immature anatomy of infants and small children predisposes them to increased distress from asthma. Children's smaller, narrower airways and decreased elastic lung recoil make them more prone to airway obstruction. The child's flexible rib cage and underdeveloped chest muscles and diaphragm lead to exhaustion when respiratory effort increases. Although asthma is not actually outgrown, the severity of asthma attacks often decreases as the child gets older because of increased airway size, improved diaphragmatic support, and better clearing of mucus. Asthma is considered a lifelong condition and may become increasingly severe after a period of remission.

Incidence

Since the early 1980s, the incidence of asthma has risen in the United States and other parts of the world. Asthma affects an estimated 7.1 million American children younger than age 17 years (Akinbami et al., 2011).

Manifestations

The manifestations of asthma may vary. A child with an asthma episode may have only a dry cough. Wheezing is a classic sign of asthma, but other signs may be present, including shortness of breath, cough, or dyspnea on exertion. Other manifestations may have a sudden or an insidious onset:

- Retractions, nasal flaring, or stridor
- Nonproductive cough (with or without wheezing) that later becomes productive
- Tachypnea, orthopnea
- Restlessness, apprehension, diaphoresis
- Abdominal pain resulting from the strain placed on the abdominal muscles during labored breathing
- A hunched-over sitting position with arms braced (tripod position)
- Fatigue and difficulty performing simple tasks, such as eating, walking, or even talking, because of shortness of breath

PATHOPHYSIOLOGY

Asthma

Asthma is a reversible obstructive airway disease characterized by the following:

- Increased airway responsiveness to a variety of stimuli
- Bronchospasm resulting from constriction of bronchial smooth muscle
- Inflammation and edema of the mucous membranes that line the small airways and the subsequent accumulation of thick secretions in the airways

Immediate Reaction (Early-Phase Response)

Allergens or other trigger substances activate immunoglobulin E (IgE) receptors on sensitized airway mast cells, causing mast cell degranulation and release of chemical mediators (histamine, leukotrienes, prostaglandins). These mediators cause bronchoconstriction shortly after exposure to the trigger; the bronchoconstriction resolves within 1 to 2 hours.

Delayed Reaction (Late-Phase Response)

Chemical mediators attract immune system cells (eosinophils, neutrophils, basophils) to the respiratory tract. Infiltration by these cells and their release of additional inflammatory substances damage the epithelial and smooth muscle cells, causing airway edema, mucous plugging of small airways, and additional inflammation. Bronchoconstriction recurs and can persist for several hours. The airway hyperresponsiveness resulting from this inflammatory process can last several weeks or months.

Late asthmatic responses can occur without a previous early (immediate) response. When asthma is precipitated by nonallergenic stimuli (exercise, cold air), bronchospasm usually lasts less than 1 hour and is not followed by a late response.

During an asthma episode, the mucous membranes lining the bronchioles become edematous and secrete large amounts of thick mucus. As a result, the airways narrow, leading to increased airway resistance and respiratory distress. Because small airways are normally wider on inspiration than expiration, the child is able to inhale but has difficulty exhaling through the narrowed bronchioles. Wheezing can be heard as air is forced through the narrow passages during expiration. Air becomes trapped, causing hyperinflation of the alveoli.

Airway obstruction is more severe in some parts of the lungs than in others, and air flows more easily into areas with the least resistance. The blood that flows to the less-ventilated portions of the lungs is inadequately saturated with oxygen. Thus a mismatch between ventilation and perfusion in poorly ventilated areas of the lung occurs, resulting in incompletely saturated blood entering the systemic circulation and in decreased PO_2 levels (hypoxia).

As the child struggles to get enough air, the respiratory rate increases (tachypnea). Tachypnea lowers carbon dioxide levels in the blood (hypocapnia). As the child tires from the increased work of breathing, hypoventilation occurs and carbon dioxide levels increase. Increased levels of carbon dioxide in the blood (hypercapnia) during an asthma episode may be a sign of severe airway obstruction and impending respiratory failure.

- A feeling of chest tightness followed by a dry cough, wheezing, and dyspnea
- Worsening of symptoms after the child goes to bed at night because of increased narrowing of the airways at night and pooling of secretions

At the beginning of the asthma episode, wheezing may be heard only with a stethoscope. As the severity of the episode increases, wheezing may be audible to the unaided ear. Children in severe respiratory distress may not demonstrate wheezing because of decreased air movement; decreased wheezing in a child who is not improving clinically may signal an inability to move air. This is referred to as a *silent chest* and is an ominous sign during an asthma episode. With treatment, increased wheezing may actually signal that the child's condition is improving.

Diagnostic Evaluation

For children older than 5 years, an objective measure of airflow by spirometry is necessary for diagnosis. Improvement of symptoms in response to nebulized bronchodilators is strongly suggestive of asthma as opposed to other pulmonary disease (NHLBI & NAEPP, 2007). History of associated allergic manifestations or family history of asthma supports the diagnosis. Other conditions that cause a chronic cough in young children, such as gastroesophageal reflux disease (GERD) (see Chapter 19) and sinusitis, need to be ruled out. However, both of these conditions can coexist with asthma in children and need to be managed (Liu et al., 2011).

Chest radiographs are usually normal except in cases of severe asthma, in which hyperinflation of the airways can be seen. Pulmonary function tests reveal a decreased forced expiratory volume in 1 second, increased residual volume from air trapping, and decreased vital capacity (the maximum amount of air exhaled after a maximum inhalation). Other pulmonary function test results might be altered as well. The peak expiratory flow rate (PEFR) is used to monitor children with chronic asthma.

Rhinitis, sinusitis, and nasal polyps are often present in children with asthma. Eosinophilia is present in both the blood and the sputum. Skin tests are often performed to identify specific allergens. The RAST may be used to identify specific antigens. Arterial blood gas measurements may be ordered in children having a severe asthma episode because of initial respiratory alkalosis and subsequent metabolic acidosis. Pulse oximetry values provide information about oxygenation.

Therapeutic Management

The NHLBI and NAEPP periodically update guidelines for asthma management. Management is based on four interacting components: (1) accurate assessment of severity and regular monitoring for control of symptoms; (2) creating and maintaining a partnership for care that includes the child, parent, health provider, and school nurse; (3) management or elimination of environmental triggers and coexisting conditions; and (4) pharmacologic therapy (NHLBI & NAEPP, 2007).

Acute Asthma Episode

A child who is having an episode of wheezing along with other symptoms of asthma is usually seen at a physician's office or an emergency department. First, a bronchodilator, usually a short-acting beta$_2$-adrenergic agonist (SABA) such as albuterol, is administered by a powered nebulizer or metered-dose inhaler (MDI) as often as every 20 minutes for 1 hour or continuously. Oxygen is administered as well. Close monitoring of the child's respiratory status after each course of medication assesses resolution of the episode.

If the child improves (PEFR greater than 70% of baseline, sustained oxygen saturation greater than 92% on room air for 4 hours), the child can return home with a SABA prescription and instructions for assessing respiratory status or with instructions for administering the SABA more frequently along with routine asthma medications. A short course of an oral corticosteroid (liquid preparations are available for infants) and an inhaled corticosteroid, if not part of the child's usual therapy, are prescribed (Liu et al., 2011). If symptoms continue to worsen, administration of the bronchodilator every 20 minutes for an additional hour is warranted. Indicators for hospital admission include the following (Gorelick, Scribano, Stevens et al., 2008):

- PEFR less than 50% of baseline
- Inspiratory and expiratory wheezing
- Tachycardia and tachypnea
- Dyspnea, retractions, use of accessory muscles
- Oxygen saturation 91% or lower after aggressive treatment
- Child's mental status depressed
- Prolongation of expiration

Once the child is hospitalized, humidified oxygen is administered at 30%, either by nasal prongs or by facemask, to keep the oxygen saturation at 95% or greater. An IV line delivers fluids and provides venous access for parenteral medications (e.g., methylprednisolone) as ordered, although most children, if not in severe respiratory distress, can manage oral steroids. Chest radiography, arterial blood gas determinations, or pulse oximetry may be performed to further evaluate the child's oxygenation status. The child receives a bronchodilator by nebulizer every 20 minutes to 1 hour initially, with the interval between doses increased as the child's condition improves. Some providers choose to deliver the nebulized bronchodilator continuously at a dose of 5 to 15 mg/hr (Liu et al., 2011). Ipratropium bromide (Atrovent), an anticholinergic agent, has been found to be an effective bronchodilator when administered along with albuterol in some children with severe exacerbations.

Increasingly severe asthma that is unresponsive to vigorous treatment measures is termed *status asthmaticus*. Status asthmaticus is a medical emergency that can cause respiratory failure and death. Hospitalization, usually in an intensive care unit, is indicated. The child is placed on a continuous cardiorespiratory monitor and continuous pulse oximeter. Blood gas and serum electrolyte values are monitored, as is fluid status. In addition to the previously discussed measures, the child may receive continuous nebulized albuterol and ipratropium bromide every 6 hours. If the child's condition does not respond to these medications, oral or intravenous steroids are then administered. Levalbuterol is a relatively new treatment for acute asthma; it is delivered by a nebulizer. Endotracheal intubation with mechanical ventilation may be necessary, along with other adjunctive approaches (Liu et al., 2011). Antibiotics may also be administered to treat concurrent infection (e.g., pneumonia).

Long-Term Management

Long-term asthma treatment should minimize and control symptoms, prevent acute asthma episodes, avoid the side effects of therapy, and help the child maintain a normal lifestyle. The NHLBI and NAEPP (2007) recommend an in-depth and regular education process that facilitates self-management of asthma. Beginning with the first and second follow-up visits after diagnosis, the provider teaches about the etiology of asthma, the goals of management and control, environmental assessment, triggers, self-assessment of symptoms, and medications. These are reviewed at every follow-up visit thereafter (NHLBI & NAEPP, 2007). A resource for parents is the Asthma and Allergy Foundation of America, 1233 20th St. NW, Washington, DC 20036; website: www.aafa.org.

Environmental Control

Irritants and allergens. Children with asthma and their parents can decrease the frequency and severity of asthma episodes by recognizing and controlling the triggers that precipitate symptoms. Common environmental irritants include cigarette smoke, smoke from wood-burning stoves and fireplaces, fumes, deodorants, overhumidified air, and perfume. Allergenic triggers, such as animal dander, cockroaches, dust mites, seasonal pollens, and molds, often cause problems (Liu et al., 2011).

The extent of environmental control needed depends on the severity of the asthma. If the asthma is mild, prohibiting smoking in the house and controlling dust with frequent house cleaning may be adequate. If the child continues to have problems after these interventions, additional steps should be taken to minimize environmental triggers.

Immunotherapy (allergy shots) can be helpful in decreasing asthma symptoms caused by specific allergens the child cannot avoid. Immunotherapy is used in conjunction with, not in place of, other asthma therapies.

Exercise. Exercise can be a trigger of asthma in asthmatic children. Exercise-induced bronchospasm may be triggered by rapid breathing of large volumes of cool, dry air (e.g., with mouth breathing during exercise). The symptoms of exercise-induced asthma usually begin after 5 to 10 minutes of exercise and often last from 30 to 60 minutes. Measures to prevent exercise-induced asthma include the following:

- Warming the air by breathing through the nose or covering the mouth and nose with a scarf when exercising in cold weather
- Using an inhaled beta$_2$-agonist 30 minutes before exercise
- Practicing techniques to decrease hyperventilation (e.g., progressive muscle relaxation, diaphragmatic breathing)

Because athletics and active play are important parts of a child's life, children with asthma should not be restricted from physical activity. Exercise not only increases physical fitness but also enhances self-esteem and offers valuable opportunities for socialization. Swimming is frequently recommended as an ideal sport for children with asthma because the air is humidified and exhaling underwater prolongs exhalation and increases end-expiratory pressure. Other sports that do not require sustained exertion, such as gymnastics, baseball, and weight lifting, are also well tolerated, and if asthma is well controlled, the child can usually participate in any type of sport.

Infection. Viral respiratory infections are the most frequent triggers of pediatric asthma. It is advisable for children with frequent or severe asthma to avoid exposure to individuals with a viral respiratory infection. Children with asthma also benefit from influenza vaccine.

Emotions. Asthma is not caused by psychosocial problems. Emotional upset, however, can exacerbate asthma symptoms. Laughing, crying, or shouting can act as mechanical triggers of bronchoconstriction. Also, a child with asthma may become angry or frustrated and refuse to take medication or adhere to a treatment regimen. Moreover, anxiety during an episode may cause the child to hyperventilate, aggravating asthma symptoms.

Monitoring Symptoms. Asthma symptoms can best be treated if they are detected early. Children and their parents should be taught the subtle early symptoms of an asthma episode (itchy chest or chin, cough, irritability or tired feeling, increased breathing rate, dry mouth, unusually dark circles under the eyes).

A useful device for monitoring breathing capacity is the peak flow meter, which measures the flow of air in a forced exhalation in liters per minute. Peak flow monitoring can help identify the start of an asthma episode, often before the child is aware of symptoms. It can also help determine the need for treatment modification. Home monitoring of PEFR may be performed several times a day. The results can be compared with the child's normal predicted level and with results obtained over the preceding several days, providing an objective assessment of respiratory status (Box 21-3). Children with moderate to severe persistent asthma should do daily PEFR monitoring. Ideally, PEFR results should be compared with the child's "personal best" value.

BOX 21-3   MONITORING BREATHING CAPACITY WITH A PEAK FLOW METER

The peak flow meter is a device to help children monitor their asthma on a daily basis. Results gained from daily monitoring are related to an overall action plan (see Figure 21-4) prescribed by the child's health care provider.

Procedure

1. Remove gum or food from the mouth and stand up.
2. Move the pointer on the meter to 0, its lowest point.
3. Hold the meter horizontally, being sure to keep your fingers away from vent holes and the marker.
4. Relax and take a few slow, deep breaths. Then, slowly take the deepest breath you possibly can with your mouth wide open.
5. While holding your breath, place the mouthpiece of the meter on your tongue and close your lips tightly around the mouthpiece.
6. Blow out as hard and fast as possible. Give a short, sharp blast, like blowing a loud whistle, not a slow blow. (The meter records the fastest blow, not the longest.) Look at the number by the marker on the numbered scale. Write it down.
7. Repeat two more times. Wait at least 10 seconds between attempts. (Be sure to move the pointer to 0 after each try.)
8. Record the highest of the three readings in your daily asthma diary.
9. It is best to take peak flow readings every day, preferably in the morning and before and after you take a bronchodilator.

⚡ SAFETY ALERT

Emergency Asthma Management

The following symptoms indicate the need for emergency treatment of asthma:

- Worsening wheeze, cough, or shortness of breath
- *No* improvement after bronchodilator use
- A peak flow rate that decreases or does not change (even after use of an inhaled beta$_2$-adrenergic agonist) or that is less than 60% of the child's predicted baseline level or personal best
- Difficulty breathing (the child's chest and neck are pulled in with each breath, or the child hunches over or struggles to breathe)
- Trouble with walking or talking
- Discontinuation of play without the ability to resume activity
- Listlessness and weak cry in an infant; refusal to suck bottle or breast
- Gray or blue lips or fingernails (in which case the child needs emergency treatment *immediately!*)

This value is the number on the meter reached most often over a 2-week period, when the child is feeling well.

Even with teaching, parents and children sometimes do not appropriately recognize or provide appropriate treatment for worsening asthma signs and symptoms. This observation underscores the need for thorough teaching guidelines for home asthma management, including the following (NHLBI & NAEPP, 2007):

- A written asthma action plan (Figure 21-4) that includes details of home management and lists indications for seeking physician or emergency department care
- Daily use of a peak flow meter (in children older than 5 years) to monitor pulmonary status and response to treatment

Asthma Action Plan

For: _____ Doctor: _____ Date: _____

Doctor's Phone Number _____ Hospital/Emergency Department Phone Number _____

GREEN ZONE

Doing Well

- No cough, wheeze, chest tightness, or shortness of breath during the day or night
- Can do usual activities

And, if a peak flow meter is used,

Peak flow: more than _____
(80 percent or more of my best peak flow)

My best peak flow is: _____

Take these long-term control medicines each day (include an anti-inflammatory).

Medicine	How much to take	When to take it
_____	_____	_____
_____	_____	_____
_____	_____	_____

Before exercise   □ _____   □ 2 or □ 4 puffs   5 to 60 minutes before exercise

YELLOW ZONE

Asthma Is Getting Worse

- Cough, wheeze, chest tightness, or shortness of breath, or
- Waking at night due to asthma, or
- Can do some, but not all, usual activities

-Or-

Peak flow: _____ to _____
(50 to 79 percent of my best best peak flow)

First Add: quick-relief medicine—and keep taking your **GREEN ZONE** medicine.

_____ (short-acting beta₂-agonist)   □ 2 or □ 4 puffs, every 20 minutes for up to 1 hour   □ Nebulizer, once

If your symptoms (and peak flow, if used) return to GREEN ZONE after 1 hour of above treatment:
□ Continue monitoring to be sure you stay in the green zone.

-Or-

If your symptoms (and peak flow, if used) do not return to GREEN ZONE after 1 hour of above treatment:

Second □ Take: _____ (short-acting beta₂-agonist)   □ 2 puffs or □ Nebulizer

□ Add: _____ (oral steroid) _____ mg per day For _____ (3–10) days

□ Call the doctor □ before/ □ within _____ hours after taking the oral steroid.

RED ZONE

Medical Alert!

- Very short of breath, or
- Quick-relief medicines have not helped, or
- Cannot do usual activities, or
- Symptoms are same or get worse after 24 hours in Yellow Zone

-Or-

Peak flow: less than _____
(50 percent of my best peak flow)

Take this medicine:

□ _____ (short-acting beta₂-agonist)   □ 4 or □ 6 puffs or □ Nebulizer

□ _____ (oral steroid) _____ mg

Then call your doctor NOW. Go to the hospital or call an ambulance if:
- You are still in the red zone after 15 minutes AND
- You have not reached your doctor.

DANGER SIGNS
- **Trouble walking and talking due to shortness of breath**
- **Lips or fingernails are blue**

→ **Take □ 4 or □ 6 puffs of your quick-relief medicine AND**
- **Go to the hospital or call for an ambulance (_____ phone) NOW!**

FIG 21-4 Asthma action plan. (From National Heart, Lung, and Blood Institute. [2007, April]. *Asthma action plan,* NIH Publication No. 07-5251. Washington, DC: U.S. Department of Health and Human Services.)

- Home initiation of inhaled beta$_2$-adrenergic agonists, and oral steroids when daily control medications are ineffective for resolving symptoms
- Prompt communication with the health care provider for deteriorating respiratory status or reduced response to medication

Medications. Initiating daily pharmacologic treatment is based on classification of severity and usually begins when the child exhibits symptoms of mild and persistent asthma. In general, for children, the decision to initiate long-term therapy is based on the following (NHLBI & NAEPP, 2007, pp. 72 and 73):

- Presence of symptoms or need for SABA more than 2 days per week but not as often as daily
- Wakes at night because of symptoms one to four times per month (depending on age)
- Experiences minor limitations in usual activity
- Frequent exacerbations (more than two every 6 to 12 months, depending on age) that require short bursts of oral steroids or, in children younger than 5 years, more than four episodes of wheezing a year lasting longer than 24 hours and presence of asthma risk factors

Generally, asthma is treated with a combination of medications from two categories: bronchodilators and antiinflammatory agents. The first-line treatment recommended to all children for long-term control of persistent asthma, regardless of severity, is an inhaled corticosteroid in a dose that reflects the severity of the asthma. Other control medications are determined using a "stepwise" system, which is a flexible approach to asthma control in which approaches and pharmacologic intervention increase or decrease based on severity of symptoms (NHLBI & NAEPP, 2007). The medication regimen depends on the classification of the child's asthma and can be changed at home according to symptoms and peak flowmeter readings (Box 21-4). It is important to differentiate rescue medications (those used for immediate relief of an exacerbation) and routine medications.

Rescue medications. Some medications used to relieve an asthma episode are described here:

- *Short-acting beta$_2$-adrenergic agonists (SABAs):* Albuterol (Ventolin, Proventil), levalbuterol (Xopenex), and terbutaline (Brethine, Brethaire) relax bronchial smooth muscle and inhibit the release of mediators from mast cells. They are delivered by MDIs or by nebulizer three or four times daily if the child is symptomatic or before exercise.
- *Anticholinergic:* Ipratropium bromide (Atrovent) is used in combination with beta$_2$-adrenergic agonists in older children (older than 12 years) with severe asthma.
- *Mast cell inhibitors:* Cromolyn sodium (Intal), an inhaled nonsteroidal antiinflammatory drug, prevents asthma symptoms by blocking the release of mast cell mediators. It can be given 30 minutes before exposure to triggers. Another antiinflammatory asthma medication, nedrocromil sodium (Tilade), is available for use in children age 12 years or older.
- *Systemic corticosteroids:* Prednisone or prednisolone decreases airway inflammation. They are preferably given in short-burst courses of 5 to 7 days.

Routine medications. Additional medications are recommended for long-term asthma control:

- *Inhaled corticosteroids:* Beclomethasone, budesonide, fluticasone, flunisolide, and triamcinolone acetonide deliver topical antiinflammatory action directly to the airway.
- *Long-acting beta$_2$-adrenergic agonists (LABAs):* Salmeterol (Serevent) and formoterol (Foradil).

BOX 21-4   CLASSIFICATION OF ASTHMA SEVERITY

Intermittent
- Symptoms less than or equal to twice per week or only with exercise
- Asymptomatic with normal peak expiratory flow rate (PEFR) between episodes; PEFR 80% of predicted rate during exacerbation
- Brief episodes
- Infrequent use of bronchodilator (<2 days a week)
- Few missed school days
- Rare activity limitation
- Symptoms rarely disturb sleep (less often than twice monthly)

Mild Persistent
- Symptoms more often than twice per week but less than once per day
- Exacerbations may begin to affect activity
- Exacerbations that require a burst of oral corticosteroids experienced more frequently (twice or more yearly; more often in children younger than 4 years)
- Nighttime symptoms 1 to 4 times per month depending on age
- PEFR >80% predicted

Moderate Persistent
- Daily symptoms occur and bronchodilator used daily; exacerbations requiring a corticosteroid burst twice or more yearly
- More than 9 school days missed per year
- Some activity limitation
- Sleep disturbed by symptoms more than once per week
- PEFR 60% to 80% of predicted

Severe Persistent
- Throughout the day on a daily basis
- Use of bronchodilator several times per day
- Severely limited physical activity
- Frequent sleep disturbance
- Exacerbations requiring corticosteroid bursts occur frequently (twice or more yearly)
- PEFR less than or equal to 60% of predicted

Modified from National Heart, Lung, and Blood Institute & National Asthma Education and Prevention Program. (2007). *Expert panel report 3: Guidelines for the diagnosis and management of asthma.* Retrieved from www.nhlbi.nih.gov.

- *Combination medications:* Budesonide and formoterol (Symbicort, a combination inhaled corticosteroid and LABA), fluticasone and salmeterol (Advair, a combination inhaled corticosteroid and LABA)
- *Leukotriene blockers:* Montelukast diminishes the mediator action of leukotrienes. Montelukast is available in sprinkles and chewable tablets and can be given to children as young as 1 year old.
- *Anti-immunoglobulin E (anti-IgE) antibody:* Omalizumab (Xolair) for allergic-type moderate to persistent asthma is approved for use in children older than 12 years. It is administered subcutaneously every 2 to 4 weeks.

Children with intermittent asthma use a SABA as needed for symptom relief. Children and families need to be cautioned not to overuse these medications and to notify the health care provider if the medications are needed more than twice per week or more frequently than every 3 to 4 hours during a 12-hour period.

Children with mild to moderate persistent asthma should take daily antiinflammatory medications. Beclomethasone by MDI (children older than 5 years) or nebulized budesonide for younger children is preferred. It can take up to 3 weeks of daily dosing to realize a therapeutic effect. In addition, SABAs are used to relieve symptoms. For moderate persistent asthma in children older than 5 years, an LABA is added to keep the inhaled corticosteroid (ICS) dosage lower. A leukotriene modifier may be given as an alternative to the LABA (NHLBI & NAEPP, 2007).

PEFR monitoring helps the child with mild to moderate asthma monitor symptoms and pulmonary function. The family is given a written management plan.

Children with persistent severe asthma take daily inhaled corticosteroids and LABAs or leukotriene blockers. Oral corticosteroids are considered for management of exacerbations.

Medication delivery. Inhaled medications are delivered either by nebulizer (see Patient-Centered Teaching: Tips on Using a Nebulizer box) or by MDI (see Chapter 14). Both can be used for older and younger children. A spacer attached to an MDI may make it easier for younger children to use the MDI. It also provides a more even distribution of medication. If using a spacer, the child attaches the spacer to the outlet of the MDI, closes the lips around the spacer mouthpiece, activates the canister, and then inhales. Earlier types of MDIs contained a chemical that was damaging to the ozone layer. In 2008, these inhalers were reformulated. Newer inhalers contain hydrofluoroalkane (HFA), a chemical that is less damaging to the ozone (Mangan, Bailey, & Gerald, 2009).

Dry-powder inhalers (DPIs) are now available as well. They are easier to use and do not contain the ozone-damaging chlorofluorocarbons that some MDIs still use. In addition to the single-dose DPI, a multidose tubular inhaler (for budesonide) and a multidose disk-shaped inhaler (for fluticasone and salmeterol) are now available (Mangan et al., 2009).

PATIENT-CENTERED TEACHING

Tips on Using a Nebulizer

- Wash your hands before setting up the nebulizer equipment. You should have available the nebulizer machine, clean tubing (attached to the nebulizer), and the reservoir for medication with dome cover attached to the T-shaped mouthpiece, or mask, if preferred.
- Unscrew the reservoir from the dome and place the ordered amount of liquid medication in the reservoir; most medications will have additional normal saline solution added.
- Reattach the dome cap tightly, attach to the tubing and turn on the machine. You will see mist begin to come out of the mouthpiece.
- Ask the child to put the mouthpiece in the mouth with the lips forming a seal around the mouthpiece. The child should be sitting upright, if possible, or on your lap.
- Your child should breathe at a normal rate, but deeply. As the treatment progresses, condensation may build up on the sides of the reservoir. It is all right to gently tap the reservoir so the liquid will drop to the bottom.
- Most nebulizer treatments take approximately 15 to 20 minutes.
- When the treatment is complete, be sure to clean the equipment carefully according to manufacturer recommendations and store it in a clean, dry place.

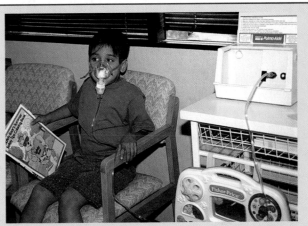

The powered nebulizer delivers a bronchodilator to the child who is having an acute asthma episode. This boy has a viral respiratory infection, which is a common trigger of acute asthma episodes in the pediatric population. (Photo courtesy Parkland Health and Hospital System Community Oriented Primary Care Clinic, Dallas, TX.)

◎ NURSING CARE PLAN

The Child Hospitalized with Asthma

Focused Assessment
- Obtain a thorough history, including family history of asthma or allergy, past asthma or allergy episodes.
- Document treatments used and their effectiveness.
- Assess vital signs, oxygenation, level of consciousness, and respiratory status.
- Assess for signs of impending respiratory distress (retractions, nasal flaring, tachypnea, dyspnea, and fatigue).
- Auscultate breath sounds and document adventitious or diminished breath sounds.
- Assess fluid status (urine output, status of mucous membranes, presence of tears, skin turgor, and weight).

- Document the child's usual routines, previous hospitalizations, and child's and family's emotional state.
- Determine any child or family teaching needs.

Planning
Nursing Diagnoses
Ineffective Airway Clearance related to bronchospasm and mucosal edema.
Impaired Gas Exchange related to air trapping in the bronchioles.

Expected Outcomes
The child will be able to clear the airway, as evidenced by a respiratory rate and rhythm appropriate for the child's age, the ability to expectorate mucus, and normal vital signs for age.

Continued

◎ NURSING CARE PLAN

The Child Hospitalized with Asthma—cont'd

Expected Outcomes—cont'd

The child will have improved gas exchange, as evidenced by clear breath sounds, a pulse oximetry value of greater than 95% on room air, no use of accessory muscles, pink mucous membranes and nail beds, and a capillary refill time of less than 2 seconds.

Intervention/*Rationale*

1. Monitor respiratory rate and effort, color, heart rate, and blood pressure every 15 to 30 minutes, with the interval lengthened as the child improves. Auscultate the chest for breath sounds. Monitor arterial blood gas values, pulse oximetry values, and pulmonary function test results. Notify the physician of any significant change (increased respiratory rate and effort, changes in wheezing, retractions, nasal flaring, severe cough, decreased alertness, cyanosis, increased dyspnea, apprehension).
   Subtle changes in the child's condition may serve as an early warning of increased airway obstruction.
2. Administer humidified oxygen at the ordered flow rate. If the child has chronic carbon dioxide retention, do not exceed 2 L/min.
   Supplemental oxygen decreases hypoxia caused by airway edema, mucus, and bronchospasm. Administration of oxygen to a child with chronic carbon dioxide retention may lead to respiratory depression by decreasing the stimulus to breathe.
3. Help the child assume an upright position or position of comfort. The older child may be most comfortable leaning forward on a pillow or an overbed table.
   An upright position aids in expansion of the lungs and decreases pressure on the diaphragm.
4. Administer medications as ordered and monitor for effectiveness. Assess whether medications are effectively relieving the child's symptoms. Monitor the child for side effects.
   Short-acting bronchodilators provide relief fairly quickly. Oral or IV prednisolone begins to reduce airway inflammation.
5. Keep the child on nothing-by-mouth (NPO) status during periods of severe respiratory distress, as ordered by the physician.
   Oral intake is contraindicated for the child in severe respiratory distress because of the risk for aspiration.
6. Obtain and maintain IV access. *IV access is necessary for administering medications and fluids.*
7. Ensure that respiratory treatments are given as ordered. Listen to and document the child's breath sounds before and after treatments. Encourage the child to cough and deep breathe, especially after treatments. Suction as needed.
   Breathing treatments help loosen or eliminate secretions and re-expand lung tissue. Mucous plugs can cause atelectasis and alveolar collapse.
8. Ensure that emergency equipment is available (e.g., appropriate-size ventilation bag, endotracheal tubes, laryngoscope, emergency medication).
   The child's condition can deteriorate rapidly. Immediate resuscitation may be necessary in the event of severe respiratory distress.
9. Keep the child as calm as possible. Offer support during periods of respiratory distress.
   Anxiety increases bronchospasms.

Evaluation

Does the child have clear breath sounds with free movement of air?
Does the child expend minimal respiratory effort?
Does the child maintain a patent airway?
Is the respiratory rate within normal limits for age, and is the oxygen saturation greater than 95%?

Planning
Nursing Diagnosis

Fatigue related to hypoxia and increased work of breathing.

Expected Outcome

The child will exhibit decreased fatigue, as evidenced by less irritability and restlessness, uninterrupted sleep periods, and ability to perform usual activities.

Intervention/*Rationale*

1. Observe the child for signs and symptoms of hypoxia, including restlessness, fatigue, irritability, increased heart rate, and increased respiratory rate.
   Irritability and agitation may be early signs of hypoxia. Prompt treatment of hypoxia decreases fatigue.
2. Organize nursing care to provide periods of uninterrupted rest and sleep.
   Periods of quiet decrease stress and promote rest.
3. Encourage the parents' presence, particularly if the child is young.
   The parents' presence decreases fear and anxiety.
4. Provide for the child's physical comfort. Encourage quiet, age-appropriate play activities as the child's condition improves.
   Physical and emotional comfort confers a sense of well-being and promotes rest.
5. Implement measures to relieve respiratory distress. Monitor the frequency of nebulized medications.
   Restlessness, agitation, and inability to sleep are side effects of some asthma medications.

Evaluation

Is the child able to play or perform usual activities without undue fatigue?

Planning
Nursing Diagnosis

Risk for Deficient Fluid Volume related to increased respiratory rate, diaphoresis, and decreased oral intake.

Expected Outcomes

The child will drink adequate fluid for age and weight.
The child will not become dehydrated.

Intervention/*Rationale*

1. Monitor intake and output, status of mucous membranes, body weight, tearing, and urine specific gravity. Maintain urine specific gravity at 1.002 to 1.030. Monitor electrolyte levels. Observe the child's sputum for color, tenacity, and amount.
   Rapid respiratory rate, diaphoresis, and increased pulmonary secretions may cause dehydration and increased viscosity of excretions.
2. Maintain IV infusion at the ordered flow rate. Avoid excessive amounts of fluid.
   Adequate hydration enhances liquefaction of secretions, and thinner secretions are more easily expectorated. Excessive fluids may lead to pulmonary edema.
3. Encourage oral fluids when the respiratory distress has decreased, with the amount consumed being determined by the child's calculated needs. Offer favorite fluids. Provide liquids at the bedside.
   Oral fluids are contraindicated during acute respiratory distress to minimize the risk for aspiration. Children are most likely to drink fluids if they are offered fluids they like.

◉ NURSING CARE PLAN

The Child Hospitalized with Asthma—cont'd

Intervention/*Rationale*—cont'd

4. Offer liquids at room temperature. Avoid milk and milk products.
   Cold liquids may aggravate bronchospasm. Milk sometimes causes increased coughing and production of mucus.
5. Provide a humidified atmosphere.
   Humidification helps liquefy secretions and helps maintain hydration.

Evaluation

Does the child ingest adequate fluid for age and weight?
Does the child maintain a urine specific gravity of 1.002 to 1.030?
Does the child maintain preillness weight?
Are moist mucous membranes and good skin turgor present?
Does the child have urinary output appropriate for age (see Chapter 16)?

Planning
Nursing Diagnosis

Anxiety related to hospitalization and respiratory distress.

Expected Outcomes

The child will exhibit reduced anxiety, as evidenced by a relaxed body position and a decrease in negative behaviors.
The parents will demonstrate reduced anxiety by verbalizing an accurate knowledge of asthma and participating in the child's care in a calm manner.

Intervention/*Rationale*

1. Teach the child techniques to control panic and anxiety and to slow the breathing rate (e.g., visually imagining staying calm, breathing exercises, pursed-lip breathing, belly breathing).
   Concentration on such activities during an asthma episode calms the child and decreases the fear of suffocation.
2. Maintain a calm, quiet environment and a reassuring manner. Stay with the child. Provide care efficiently and calmly.
   The ability to remain calm decreases the child's oxygen demand and work of breathing.
3. Reassure the child that there is someone nearby to assist if breathing difficulties develop. To allay any fears about going to sleep, tell the child that someone will be watching at night. Make the call light available for older children.
   Calm reassurance by the nurse can decrease the child's fear of suffocation and facilitate rest.
4. Use play therapy.
   Therapeutic play allows the child to work through fears in a nonthreatening manner.
5. Encourage the parents to stay with the child. Praise the parents for rooming-in and supporting the child.
   The presence of a familiar person can decrease fear and anxiety.
6. Keep parents informed of treatments, routines, and the child's condition.
   Reassuring the parents can help calm the child because parental anxiety is quickly transferred to the child. Frequent and accurate updating of the child's condition reassures parents and decreases fear of the unknown.
7. Encourage expression of feelings by child and parents.
   Expressing feelings can help relieve stress and guilt.
8. Avoid the use of sedatives.
   Sedatives may depress respirations.
9. Explain all procedures in an age-appropriate manner.
   Procedures and an unfamiliar hospital setting may produce anxiety. Explanations decrease fear of the unknown.

10. Facilitate trust by being truthful and acknowledging the discomfort of procedures.
    Honesty fosters trust.

Evaluation

Does the child cooperate with and participate in treatment and appear relaxed?
Does the child obtain adequate rest and sleep?
Do the parents verbalize decreased anxiety about the hospitalization and the child's condition?

Planning
Nursing Diagnosis

Interrupted Family Processes related to the possibility of a chronic illness.

Expected Outcome

The family will demonstrate the ability to cope with the child's illness and adhere to management in a way that promotes the child's normal growth and development.

Intervention/*Rationale*

1. Provide opportunities for the family to express feelings. Recognize and accept negative feelings about the child and the illness.
   This nonjudgmental approach helps the family work through fear, guilt, anxiety, and economic problems.
2. Explore previous coping mechanisms used in times of stress.
   Identification and review of previously successful coping skills can assist the family in dealing with the current crisis.
3. Explain all procedures and treatments.
   A thorough explanation decreases fear of the unknown and anxiety.
4. Keep parents informed of the child's condition.
   Knowledge gives parents a sense of control.
5. ⊖ Arrange for the family to meet with others affected by asthma. Identify available community resources (see Evolve website).
   Meeting others with asthma can assist with problem solving and provide support.

Evaluation

Is the family able to provide necessary care?
Can the family describe how to access helpful resources?

Planning
Nursing Diagnosis

Deficient Knowledge about the disease process and home management related to inexperience with asthma.

Expected Outcomes

The family will identify asthma triggers.
The family will describe home management principles.

Intervention/*Rationale*

1. Determine the child's and parents' understanding of asthma. Explain unfamiliar procedures and equipment at the child's level of understanding. Teach the family about the disease, its triggers, and prescribed medications and treatments.
   Understanding increases adherence to treatment.
2. Help the family identify precipitating factors (e.g., exercise, infections, allergens, weather changes).
   An awareness of triggers may decrease future asthma episodes.

Continued

Additional Resources—Resources for Health Care Providers and Families

NURSING CARE PLAN

The Child Hospitalized with Asthma—cont'd

Intervention/Rationale—cont'd

3. Explain the role of emotions and stress in the development of asthma symptoms.

   Stress and emotional upset can trigger bronchospasm.

4. Teach the child and family about the importance of taking medications as prescribed. Assess ability to afford medications. Provide written information and instructions about medications (names, side effects, dosages, times of administration). Teach the family to recognize signs and symptoms that warrant notification of the physician. Reinforce the need to keep follow-up appointments.

   Knowledge of medications increases adherence to the therapeutic regimen; adherence helps maintain serum drug levels within a therapeutic range.

5. Assist in developing an exercise program for the child. Medication may be needed before exercise. Teach the importance of a healthy lifestyle (regular exercise, adequate fluids and nutrition, rest, prevention of infection).

   Exercise promotes pulmonary and cardiovascular health and assists the child in leading a normal life.

6. Refer the family to a support group.

   Meeting with other children and families affected by asthma provides an avenue for expressing feelings and sharing information.

7. Teach self-management of asthma. Teach the necessary skills for home care. Encourage the child to take charge of asthma. The child should know what triggers to avoid, early warning signs of an episode, the correct use of treatment aids (MDI, DPI, nebulizer, peak flow meter), and proper administration of medications and techniques for stress reduction and relaxation. Encourage the child and family to participate in programs designed to develop effective self-management and decision-making skills.

   Knowledge of asthma decreases anxiety during acute episodes. The frequency and severity of episodes will be minimized if the child knows the appropriate actions for controlling symptoms. Learning about the condition can help decrease anxiety during episodes and increase the child's ability to take appropriate action to control symptoms. The frequency and severity of asthma episodes will be minimized if the child knows what triggers to avoid, the early warning signs of an episode, and the correct treatment of symptoms.

8. Teach the importance of follow-up care and routine health maintenance, such as keeping immunizations up to date.

   Preventing infection and practicing healthy living habits help decrease asthma triggers.

Evaluation

Do the child and family verbalize an accurate knowledge of asthma and its treatment?

Do the child and family keep follow-up appointments?

Does the child resume normal daily activities?

BRONCHOPULMONARY DYSPLASIA

Bronchopulmonary dysplasia (BPD) is a chronic obstructive pulmonary disease that occurs as a result of acute lung injury in some infants who have received supplemental oxygen and mechanical ventilation. BPD is now commonly referred to as *chronic lung disease of infancy.*

Etiology

Lung immaturity seems to be a key factor in the development of BPD, but many other factors affect its development as well. Some major risk factors for BPD are premature birth, respiratory infection, oxygen supplementation, and mechanical ventilation (Bhandari & Bhandari, 2009). Infants with BPD often also have patent ductus arteriosus (see Chapter 22). Because lung development varies among infants, gestational age alone does not always predict the development of BPD.

PATHOPHYSIOLOGY

Bronchopulmonary Dysplasia

The pressures of mechanical ventilation damage bronchial epithelium. Macrophages and polymorphonuclear inflammatory cells invade the airways, causing airway edema. Alveolar walls become thickened, and fibrotic changes occur in the airways and alveoli. The continued use of oxygen affects the growth and development of lung structures, significantly reducing the number of developing alveoli.

Cystic and atelectatic areas develop in the lungs, predisposing the infant to pulmonary hypertension. Loss of ciliated cells also may occur, which decreases the lungs' ability to remove mucus and leads to mucous plugs, atelectasis, and pneumonia.

Incidence

BPD is a significant cause of morbidity and death among very low-birth-weight infants (less than 1000 g) and infants who have survived RDS. It is the most frequently seen chronic lung condition in infants.

The rates of severe BPD in infants with gestational age less than 33 weeks have increased from 3.6% in 1999 to 9.5% in 2006 (Yoder, Harrison, & Clark, 2009).

Manifestations

Manifestations of BPD include tachycardia and tachypnea related to decreased oxygenation; an increased work of breathing, retractions, and prolonged exhalation with the increased use of abdominal and accessory muscles; pallor associated with chronic hypoxia; and cyanosis and activity intolerance (feeding, handling). Affected infants also exhibit weight loss or poor weight gain related to the increased metabolic workload, hypoxia, and poor feeding; restlessness and irritability related to hypoxia; wheezing (intermittent or chronic) associated with a hyperresponsive airway; and puckering or pursing of the mouth with flaring of the nares (early signs of impending respiratory distress).

Diagnostic Evaluation

The diagnosis is based on clinical manifestations and radiographic abnormalities. Infants with respiratory symptoms that persist beyond 28 days of life, who need supplemental oxygen by 1 to 2 weeks of age and are still oxygen dependent after 28 days, or who need mechanical ventilation during the first week of life are suspected of having BPD. Chest radiographs may show infiltrates.

Therapeutic Management

Treatment goals for the infant with BPD include maintaining adequate oxygenation to promote growth and development, preventing further lung disease, and promoting healing of the damaged lungs. Treatment consists of oxygen therapy, drug therapy, and nutritional support.

Positive-pressure ventilation should be discontinued as soon as possible. If mechanical ventilation is necessary to maintain life, the lowest possible inflation pressures should be used, together with expiratory times that allow the lung to empty completely. Weaning from the ventilator may be a slow process, requiring constant attention to subtle changes in the infant; however, earlier weaning strategies may lead to more positive outcomes (Greenough & Sharma, 2007).

Oxygen Therapy

Oxygen can be administered through a hood, facemask, or nasal cannula. Oxygen saturation rates should be monitored closely and are usually maintained between 88% and 95%, although there is no consensus on an acceptable saturation for infants with BPD (Bhandari & Bhandari, 2007). Many infants are discharged from the hospital while still oxygen dependent.

Medications

Diuretics and fluid restriction are initiated to treat pulmonary interstitial edema. Furosemide is the most common diuretic used, with some physicians attempting to change the medication to chlorothiazide and spironolactone once enteral feeding is tolerated. Because infants with BPD often have fluid overload and edema, fluid and electrolyte status should be monitored closely. Supplemental calcium, potassium, and chloride may be indicated for the infant receiving diuretics.

Inhaled bronchodilators, especially albuterol, when given in the early stages of BPD, can lessen airway resistance and decrease the possibility of lung damage. Theophylline or caffeine may be used to enhance lung compliance and improve respiratory status by relaxing the smooth muscles. Administration of dexamethasone is no longer recommended, but an inhaled corticosteroid may be helpful to hasten extubation (Dudell & Stoll, 2007).

Infants with BPD have frequent infections related to increased susceptibility and exposure to invasive treatments and procedures. After the initial stages of BPD, the risk for infection is probably the greatest risk to survival for these infants. Antibiotics are often needed. Palivizumab is highly recommended for the prevention of RSV in infants with BPD (Wang, Cummins, Bayliss et al., 2008).

Nutrition

The infant needs increased nutritional intake for lung growth and repair beyond that required for normal infant growth. Other factors, such as frequent respiratory exacerbations and feeding problems, also increase caloric needs. A calorie intake of about 150 kcal/kg/day to produce a weight gain of 20 to 30 g/day is an appropriate goal. High-calorie formulas (24 or 27 cal/oz) assist with meeting this requirement, especially in infants in whom fluids are restricted. Medium-chain triglyceride oil or glucose polymers, if added to the formula, increase the calories per ounce.

Prognosis

Most infants with BPD do improve. The mortality rate ranges from 10% to 25%; death usually is a result of pulmonary complications. Most infants with BPD will require continuing therapy at home, and in some chronic airway hyperreactivity will develop, which may progress to bronchial asthma. Many infants with BPD are rehospitalized during the first year of life because of acute respiratory tract infections. Infants may have growth retardation and developmental delay as well.

Nursing Considerations

Because of their low birth weight and possible RDS, most neonates with BPD are initially cared for in a special-care nursery. Nursing intervention before discharge includes meticulous planning for home care, coordinating referrals, and teaching home management.

Home care of the infant with BPD decreases the risk for hospital-acquired infection and reduces health care costs. Care at home also improves social development by encouraging interaction between the child and family.

Preparation for discharge and home care requires a great deal of education and reassurance. Educating the family with a chronically ill or technology-dependent child must begin early with basic care—feeding, bathing, holding, and playing. This care progresses to medical, nursing, and respiratory procedures. The infant may continue to receive supplemental oxygen at home or may have a tracheostomy. Some infants are discharged while they are still ventilator dependent. Families must be taught the necessary precautions for safe use of oxygen in the home (Patient-Centered Teaching: Safe Use of Oxygen at Home). Before hospital discharge, the nurse contacts emergency services, utility companies, and the telephone company to notify them that a technology-dependent child will be living in their area (Figure 21-5). Required actions for contacting these services in case of emergency should be reviewed with the family.

PATIENT-CENTERED TEACHING
Safe Use of Oxygen at Home

SAFETY GUIDELINES	RATIONALE
Secure the oxygen tank in an upright position.	Oxygen tanks are highly explosive. If a horizontally positioned tank explodes, the rapid release of oxygen can catapult it through both animate (human bodies) and inanimate (walls) objects.
Keep oxygen tanks at least 5 feet from heat sources and electrical devices (e.g., space heaters, heating vents, fireplaces, radios, vaporizers).	
Ensure that no one smokes in the room or in the area of the oxygen tank.	Smoking increases the risk for fire, which could cause the tank to explode; escaped oxygen would feed the fire.
Avoid using alcohol-based substances or oil to relieve dryness around your child's mouth (e.g., petroleum jelly, vitamin A & D ointment, baby oil).	Both alcohol and oil are flammable and increase the risk for fire.
Keep a fire extinguisher readily available.	A fire extinguisher may be needed to put out a fire immediately.
Turn off both the volume regulator and the flow regulator when oxygen is not in use.	If the volume regulator is on when the oxygen is turned on, the child might receive a rapid, forceful flow of oxygen in the face that could be frightening and uncomfortable. Oxygen leakage, which might not be detected because oxygen is odorless, can cause a fire.

Evaluating the family's response to the infant's illness and their coping strategies is critical for optimal home management of the infant with a chronic condition. The nurse should help the family identify physical and psychological strengths and weaknesses. Because the care of an infant with BPD can be extraordinarily expensive, the nurse should consider referring the family to social services for access to potential financial assistance.

CYSTIC FIBROSIS

Cystic fibrosis (CF), the most common lethal genetic disease in whites, is a chronic multisystem disorder affecting the exocrine glands. The mucus produced by the exocrine glands (particularly those of the bronchioles, small intestine, and pancreatic and bile ducts) is

---

ELECTRIC COMPANY
REQUEST FOR SPECIAL CONSIDERATION

Date: _____

Name: _____

Address: _____

_____

Phone: _____

Account Number: _____

Attention: Customer Service

Our infant/child, _____, is under the care of

Dr. _____ at _____ for

_____

This condition(s) requires the use of a cardiorespiratory monitor and/or other life support equipment, specifically:

_____

The necessary equipment selected for home care is equipped with a battery back-up system that will power the equipment in the event of a power failure for a **limited period of time.** If a power failure occurs, it is imperative to restore service to this home as soon as possible. Please place this home on a priority list for restoration of electric service. If you have advance warning of a temporary interruption in electric service, please notify the parents so alternative arrangements can be made. If you have questions regarding the specifications of the equipment provided, please contact our equipment provider, Pediatric Home Care Associates.

Thank you for your cooperation.

Sincerely yours,

OUR EQUIPMENT PROVIDER IS:

FIG 21-5 Example of a letter that can be used to notify the local public service company that a technology-dependent child is living in the service area. (Courtesy Pediatric Home Care Associates, Garfield, NJ. From Barnhart, S. L., & Czervinske, M. P. [1995]. *Perinatal and pediatric respiratory care* [p. 662]. Philadelphia: Saunders.)

---

abnormally thick, causing obstruction of the small passageways of these organs. Although CF is incurable, the life expectancy of affected children has increased dramatically. The median survival age is 37 years, making CF a disease not only of children but also of young adults (Cystic Fibrosis Foundation, 2008). The discovery of the mutated gene encoding a defective chloride channel in epithelial cells (named *cystic fibrosis transmembrane conductance regulator*) has improved clinicians' understanding of the disorder's pathophysiologic features and has significantly aided diagnosis.

Etiology

CF is transmitted as an autosomal recessive trait, which means that both parents must carry the gene for the child to be affected. If both parents carry the CF gene, each pregnancy has a 25% chance of producing an affected child. The CF gene has been localized to the long arm of chromosome 7.

Incidence

The incidence of CF in white children is approximately 1 in 3500 live births (Egan, 2011). The prevalence in African-Americans, Hispanics, and Asians is lower than that in the white population (Egan, 2011). Of all patients with CF in the United States, 70% are diagnosed by 2 years of age (Cystic Fibrosis Foundation, 2008).

Manifestations

Signs and symptoms of CF, the extent of specific organ system involvement, and the age at which symptoms begin vary widely among affected children. Symptoms gradually worsen as the disease progresses, and the outcome is eventually fatal.

Respiratory System

Signs and symptoms of respiratory involvement include wheezing and a dry, nonproductive cough (earliest pulmonary manifestations), repeated bouts of pneumonia and bronchitis, and purulent and copious sputum accompanying chronic bacterial infections. The cough at this stage is wet and paroxysmal and may be followed by vomiting. Crackles, wheezes, and diminished breath sounds; accessory muscle use, retractions, hypoxia, and cyanosis; and increased cough, dyspnea, tachypnea, and cyanosis occur as the disease progresses. Emphysema and atelectasis may develop as the airways become increasingly obstructed with secretions; cor pulmonale and congestive heart failure resulting from fibrotic lung changes can be seen in later stages of the disease. Spontaneous pneumothorax or hemoptysis (blood-stained sputum) is seen in later stages as well. Nasal polyps (10% to 25% of patients), sinusitis (evident on radiography in nearly 90% of patients), digital clubbing (Figure 21-6), and a barrel chest (increased anteroposterior chest diameter) are also noted.

Digestive System

Digestive system involvement is marked by steatorrhea (frothy, foul-smelling stools two to three times bulkier than normal) and flatus. Malnutrition and growth failure may be evident despite normal caloric intake; deficiencies in the fat-soluble vitamins A, D, E, and K are caused by an inability to absorb fats. Vitamin A deficiency may lead to xerophthalmia (abnormal thickening of eye tissue), and vitamin K deficiency may result in bleeding, especially in infants. Children with CF are usually thin and underweight, but with adequate treatment most attain normal height. A protuberant abdomen, barrel chest, wasted buttocks, and thin extremities are common.

PATHOPHYSIOLOGY

Cystic Fibrosis

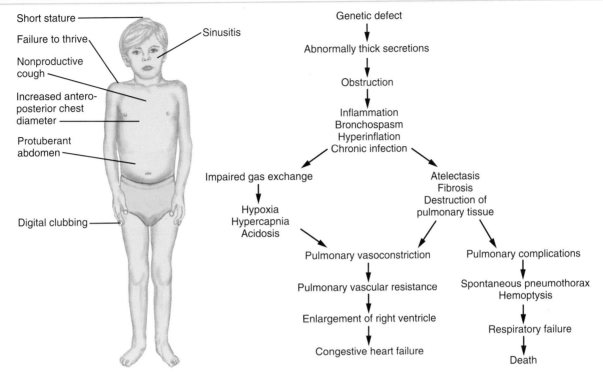

Short stature
Failure to thrive
Nonproductive cough
Increased antero-posterior chest diameter
Protuberant abdomen
Digital clubbing
Sinusitis

Genetic defect
↓
Abnormally thick secretions
↓
Obstruction
↓
Inflammation
Bronchospasm
Hyperinflation
Chronic infection

Impaired gas exchange
↓
Hypoxia
Hypercapnia
Acidosis
↓
Pulmonary vasoconstriction
↓
Pulmonary vascular resistance
↓
Enlargement of right ventricle
↓
Congestive heart failure

Atelectasis
Fibrosis
Destruction of pulmonary tissue
↓
Pulmonary complications
↓
Spontaneous pneumothorax
Hemoptysis
↓
Respiratory failure
↓
Death

Cystic fibrosis (CF) affects the exocrine glands throughout the body and causes respiratory, digestive, integumentary, and reproductive dysfunction and damage.

Respiratory System

Abnormally thick, sticky secretions cause obstruction of both the small and large airways. Stasis of secretions from bronchial obstruction provides a medium for bacterial growth. Chronic infection causes the release of toxic chemicals that damage lung tissues and alter host defenses within the airways, thus exacerbating the infection and inflammation. Inflammation may also cause bronchospasm, worsening airway blockage. Because airways dilate on inspiration and constrict on exhalation, air trapping occurs in the peripheral airways narrowed by mucus secretions. Hyperinflation is one of the first findings on chest radiographs of a child with CF. Chronic infection leads to atelectasis and eventual fibrosis and destruction of pulmonary tissue.

As the disease progresses, the lungs of almost all children with CF eventually become colonized with *Pseudomonas aeruginosa*, an organism that most clinicians believe can never be completely eradicated from the respiratory tract but can be controlled with vigorous antibiotic therapy. Chronic respiratory tract infection and impaired oxygen and carbon dioxide exchange cause varying degrees of hypoxia, hypercapnia, and acidosis. Fibrotic lung changes occur as the disease worsens and hypoxia increases. Alveolar hypoxia leads to pulmonary vasoconstriction, increasing pulmonary vascular resistance. Increased pulmonary vascular resistance causes the right side of the heart to work harder to pump blood into the lungs. Enlargement of the right ventricle in response to

increased pulmonary resistance (cor pulmonale) results. Heart failure may develop. Pulmonary complications include sinusitis, spontaneous pneumothorax, and hemoptysis. Death in individuals with CF is almost always the result of respiratory failure.

Digestive System

The pancreatic ducts, blocked by thick mucus, are unable to secrete trypsin, amylase, and lipase into the small intestine. Without these digestive enzymes, proteins, carbohydrates, and fats are poorly absorbed. Bowel obstruction from thickened intestinal mucus and pancreatic insufficiency may be present at birth (meconium ileus). The islets of Langerhans in the pancreas are normal in patients with CF, but they may decrease in number as the disease progresses and the pancreas undergoes fibrotic changes. Type 1 diabetes sometimes develops in older children with CF. Abnormalities of the gallbladder are common.

Integumentary System

The sweat glands of children with CF secrete normal amounts of sweat. The levels of sodium and chloride in the sweat, however, are two to five times the normal range.

Reproductive System

Ninety-five percent of males with CF are sterile because of obstruction of the deferent ducts and seminal vesicles. Females have reduced fertility because of abnormally thick cervical mucus, which impedes sperm penetration of the cervical canal.

Meconium ileus in the neonate is the earliest clinical manifestation of CF. Intestinal obstruction later in life, called *meconium ileus equivalent,* may occur and is the result of impacted feces at the ileocecal junction. Rectal prolapse and intussusception may also occur. Liver disease, as manifested by biliary cirrhosis, portal hypertension, and esophageal varices, resulting from obstruction of the bile ducts, is com-

monly seen in the first decade of life, with a prevalence of 26% to 45% (Witters, De Boeck, Dupont et al., 2009). Diabetes mellitus has evolved as a complication because of increased longevity. The prevalence of diabetes has been reported upward of 20%, but it is unusual in patients younger than age 10 years (Cystic Fibrosis Foundation, 2008).

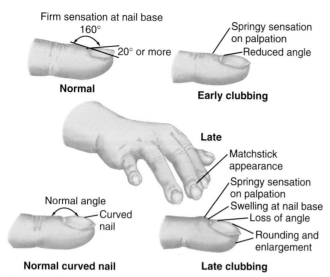

FIG 21-6 Digital clubbing may be an indication of hypoxia, which often occurs in cystic fibrosis and other respiratory disorders.

Exocrine Glands

Abnormally high concentrations of sodium and chloride in sweat are an early sign of CF (mothers often report that their infants taste salty when kissed). The risk for electrolyte imbalance during hot weather is high; infants are especially prone to development of hyponatremia and hypochloremia, as well as dehydration. Many children complain of dry mouth and have an increased susceptibility to infection.

Reproductive System

Reproductive system involvement is marked by an average of 2 years' delay in the development of secondary sex characteristics. Females with CF may have difficulty becoming pregnant because of the thick cervical mucus, which acts as a barrier to sperm. This impairment of fertility should not be relied on as a birth control method. Women with mild CF can carry a pregnancy to term with conscientious prenatal care (Egan, 2011). Sterility caused by lack of sperm is noted in approximately 95% of male patients with CF; otherwise, sexual function is normal (Egan, 2011).

Diagnostic Evaluation

CF has been called the great imitator because failure to thrive and chronic respiratory infection are signs of many other childhood conditions. In some infants, CF is evident at birth because of symptoms of severe bowel obstruction (meconium ileus) caused by intestinal plugging by thick, tenacious secretions. Nearly all U.S. states now test for CF with the routine newborn screening. The current test uses the immunoreactive trypsinogen assay, which has a high number of false-positive results, so follow-up of a positive screen with definitive testing is necessary. The early diagnosis and treatment of CF make a difference in the quality and length of life for these children.

The diagnosis of CF requires a positive sweat test result (obtained on two separate occasions) or deoxyribonucleic acid (DNA) testing that identifies two CF mutations and a positive newborn screening test, or a family history of CF or clinical signs consistent with CF (Egan, 2011). The sweat test, *pilocarpine iontophoresis*, measures the amount of sodium and chloride in sweat and is simple, painless, and reliable. A chloride level greater than 60 mEq/L is considered to be diagnostic for CF; a level of 40 to 60 mEq/L is suggestive of CF and requires repeating the test. A sample of at least 50 mg of sweat is required for

accurate results. Because this amount is difficult to obtain from small infants, the sweat test is usually not reliable in infants younger than 2 weeks.

In addition to the sweat test, the following studies may also be performed: 72-hour fecal fat determination; liver function tests (alanine aminotransferase aspartate aminotransferase); fasting blood glucose test; chest radiography; sputum culture (for identification of infective organisms); and pulmonary function tests.

DNA analysis of chorionic villi samples or amniotic fluid testing can establish a diagnosis prenatally. DNA analysis (by buccal smear or blood sample) can also determine whether siblings of the affected child are carriers.

Therapeutic Management

Therapy is individualized for each child and is aimed at preventing and treating pulmonary infections, maintaining optimal nutritional status, and promoting psychological adjustment. Children with CF are cared for at home most of the time. They are hospitalized during acute pulmonary infections, periodically for IV antibiotic treatment and vigorous chest physical therapy (CPT), and for end-stage disease.

Respiratory Problems

Because chronic respiratory infection is a major cause of lung damage in patients with CF, treatment goals are to relieve airway obstruction by mobilizing secretions, to decrease the number of bacteria by removing secretions, and to treat infections by administering antibiotics.

Segmental percussion and postural drainage (see Chapter 13) with inhalation therapy are performed several times a day to loosen secretions and move them from the peripheral airways into the central airways where they can be expectorated. Newer airway management techniques, such as forced exhalation and positive expiratory pressure (PEP) devices (PEP valve, Flutter device, Acapella device), have been successful in mobilizing mucus. Mucolytic agents (inhaled recombinant DNase or Pulmozyme), inhaled bronchodilators, and antiinflammatory agents (ibuprofen, steroids, macrolides) are often used with postural drainage to decrease the viscosity of secretions or clear the airways (Borowitz, Robinson, Rosenfeld et al., 2009).

Exercise is an important part of pulmonary treatment. Regular aerobic exercise, such as jogging or swimming, and/or weight training can improve or maintain lung function (Egan, 2011). Children with CF who exercise regularly have fewer pulmonary exacerbations and generally feel better than those who do not.

Antibiotics have played a major role in increasing the life expectancy of children with CF. Depending on the course of the child's condition, the symptoms and history, and the underlying organism involved, organism-sensitive oral antibiotics may be prescribed intermittently or continuously (Egan, 2011). Children with CF frequently need higher-than-usual doses of antibiotics because of their rapid metabolism of these drugs. Aerosolized antibiotics, tobramycin and aztreonam, the latter of which was approved by the U.S. Food and Drug Administration in 2010, are used to control organisms that are resistant to oral antibiotics, most specifically *Pseudomonas aeruginosa* (Cystic Fibrosis Foundation, 2010).

IV antibiotics are the usual treatment of choice during acute pulmonary exacerbations. IV antibiotics are usually administered during hospitalization, but home IV therapy is becoming more widely accepted, offering substantial savings and minimizing disruption of daily activities. Aerosolized antibiotics may be used as an adjunct to IV therapy (Egan, 2011).

Because they decrease inflammation in the lung, steroids are sometimes prescribed when pulmonary symptoms are unresponsive to antibiotics and increased CPT; however, adverse side effects, including growth retardation and altered glucose tolerance, are problematic with long-term steroid treatment. Long-term ibuprofen administration has demonstrated positive benefits in delaying disease progression. Azithromycin has been found to decrease length of hospital stay (Cystic Fibrosis Foundation, 2010). Oxygen therapy is used with caution because many children with CF have chronic carbon dioxide retention and are at risk for oxygen-induced carbon dioxide narcosis.

Digestive Problems

Early in the course of CF, the child may exhibit a huge appetite but not gain weight. Chronic pulmonary infections, increased work of breathing, and malabsorption place an increased caloric and protein demand on the child with CF. The child's calorie requirements are approximately 150% of the normal recommended daily allowance. Children with CF are managed with a high-calorie, high-protein diet, pancreatic enzyme replacement therapy, fat-soluble vitamin supplements, and, if nutritional problems are severe, nighttime gastrostomy feedings or total parenteral nutrition. Fats are not restricted unless steatorrhea cannot be controlled by increased pancreatic enzymes.

Infants are sometimes given a predigested formula (Pregestimil, Nutramigen), which is more easily absorbed than regular formula. Formulas may also be concentrated to provide increased calories. For the older child, caloric intake may be increased with food supplements or enteral tube feedings. The administration of growth hormone has shown significant improvement in both height velocity and weight gain in children with CF (Egan, 2011).

Enteric-coated microencapsulated pancreatic enzyme preparations (Creon, Pancreaze) are administered with every meal and snack. Enzyme dosage is adjusted according to stool formation: fewer enzymes with constipation; more enzymes with loose, fatty stools. Still, the enzyme dosage should be individualized for each child and kept as low as possible while still maintaining the child's nutritional status. Often, histamine (H_2)-receptor blockers (ranitidine) or proton-pump inhibitors are prescribed to decrease the overly acidic intestines because enzymes will only work in an alkaline environment. Extra salt is added to the diet in extremely hot weather or when the child exercises vigorously.

NURSING CARE OF THE CHILD WITH CYSTIC FIBROSIS

■ Assessment

The child with CF should be assessed for signs and symptoms in each of the systems usually affected by the disease and for psychosocial adaptation to this chronic condition.

■ **Respiratory Assessment.** The child may have had frequent episodes of pneumonia or bronchitis. Auscultate the chest to detect any crackles, wheezes, areas of diminished breath sounds, or a prolonged expiratory phase of respiration. Note signs of long-standing respiratory difficulty, such as barrel chest or digital clubbing. The respiratory status is assessed by noting the rate, depth, and ease of respirations; the color of the nail beds and mucous membranes; and pulse oximetry. The characteristics of the child's cough and the color, amount, and quality of sputum should be documented, along with any fever. Exercise tolerance and the child's ability to sleep lying down at night should also be assessed.

■ **Digestive Assessment.** The nurse weighs and measures the child, plotting the results on a standardized growth chart. Signs of malabsorption (e.g., steatorrhea; loose, bulky stools; protuberant abdomen

with thin extremities) should be noted. A diet history is useful in assessing the child's caloric intake. The use of vitamins and dietary supplements should be recorded. Determining the number and consistency of stools assesses the adequacy of intestinal enzyme replacement. Because ulcers and intestinal obstruction often accompany CF, complaints of abdominal pain, blood in the stools, and constipation should be noted. Use of antacids, H_2-receptor blockers, or antireflux medications should also be assessed.

■ **Reproductive Assessment.** Girls should be assessed for vaginal itching or drainage, which may indicate a vaginal infection. Contraception should be discussed with adolescents.

■ Nursing Diagnosis and Planning

The nursing diagnoses and expected outcomes that often apply to children with CF are as follows:

- Ineffective Airway Clearance related to increased pulmonary secretions.

Expected Outcome. The child will be able to remove secretions from the airway.

- Impaired Gas Exchange related to air trapping within the alveoli secondary to obstruction of the airways by thick mucus.

Expected Outcome. The child will maintain an oxygen saturation level of greater than 95%.

- Risk for Infection related to tenacious secretions and altered body defenses.

Expected Outcome. The child will remain free of infection.

- Imbalanced Nutrition: Less Than Body Requirements related to poor intestinal absorption of nutrients.

Expected Outcomes. The child's nutritional status will improve, and the child will exhibit normal growth; the child's stools will be of normal consistency, frequency, and color.

- Activity Intolerance related to pulmonary congestion and poor absorption of nutrients.

Expected Outcomes. The child will rest comfortably and will engage in age-appropriate activities.

- Situational Low Self-Esteem related to physical changes from chronic illness.

Expected Outcome. The child will demonstrate a positive self-concept and feelings of independence, as demonstrated by participating in self-care and in age-appropriate activities.

- Ineffective Coping (individual) and Compromised Family Coping related to chronic illness.

Expected Outcomes. The child and family will adhere to the treatment regimen, will verbalize feelings about the impact of the illness on their lives, and will use available support systems and community resources.

- Grieving related to a potentially fatal diagnosis.

Expected Outcomes. The child and family will make realistic plans for the future and will be able to discuss feelings about the child's prognosis.

■ Interventions

■ **Facilitating Airway Clearance and Gas Exchange.** Perform CPT two or three times a day and as needed; perform treatments at least 1 hour before or 2 hours after meals to reduce gastrointestinal upset. The child's respiratory status should be determined before and after CPT. Note the child's tolerance of the procedure. Teach "huffing" (forced expiration) to mobilize secretions. The child should take a deep breath and then exhale rapidly while whispering the word "huff." Administer ordered bronchodilators or Mucolytic in conjunction with CPT or as ordered. There are now many techniques from which to choose to facilitate airway clearance. These include positive expiratory pressure devices, autogenic drainage, active cycle of breathing, high frequency vibratory vest, and even exercise (Flume, Robinson, O'Sullivan et al., 2009).

To facilitate gas exchange, administer humidified, low-flow (2 L/min or less) oxygen as ordered. The recommended amount of oxygen should not be exceeded because too much oxygen administered to children who are chronically hypoxic can depress respirations. Elevate the head of the bed, or support the child in an upright position, if the child is dyspneic. Be sure to stay with the child during coughing episodes.

■ **Preventing Infection.** Children with CF are prone to respiratory infection, especially airway colonization with *Pseudomonas aeruginosa*, and oral or inhaled antibiotic therapy may be routine. IV antibiotics may be required during acute exacerbations. Pay meticulous attention to hygiene measures, especially hand hygiene, and teach the child and family to do the same. Monitor the child for signs of respiratory infection (fever, chills, increased respirations, dyspnea, cough, purulent secretions, increased WBC count). Advise the family to avoid exposing the child to others who are ill. Children with CF should receive all routine childhood immunizations at ages recommended by the AAP (see Evolve website). An annual influenza vaccine also is appropriate, on the basis of the recommendations by the Centers for Disease Control and Prevention.

■ **Providing Optimal Nutrition for Growth.** Provide a well-balanced diet that is high in calories, protein, and carbohydrates and that includes the child's favorite foods. Oral or enteral high-calorie supplements can increase the child's calorie intake.

The child needs to take pancreatic enzymes (which come as enteric-coated capsules containing the enzyme beads) as ordered within 30 minutes of eating all meals and snacks. The child should not mix the enzymes with hot foods because enzymes are inactivated by heat. Older children can swallow the enteric-coated pancreatic enzyme capsules. For children who cannot swallow capsules, the capsules may be opened to display the beads, which can then be mixed with a small amount of a nonprotein food. Because prolonged contact with enzyme beads may cause excoriation of oral mucosa, wipe off any beads that remain on the child's lips. Advise the family to note the color, consistency, and frequency of the child's stools because enzyme replacement is correlated with the child's bowel elimination pattern (e.g., an acceptable pattern is one or two stools daily in older children and more often in infancy). The enzyme dosage should be increased when high-fat foods are eaten. Administer multivitamins; water-miscible, fat-soluble vitamins; and iron supplements as ordered. Monitor the child's appetite and food intake. Extra salt and fluid are required when the weather is hot.

■ **Promoting Increased Exercise Tolerance.** For the child in acute exacerbation, provide rest periods between treatments and organize nursing care to ensure periods of uninterrupted rest. The child's activity level is increased as tolerated. Arrange age-appropriate activities geared to the child's energy level. When the child is feeling well, encourage active play and activities, such as swimming and gymnastics.

■ **Meeting the Child's and Family's Emotional Needs.** Encourage the child to express feelings about the chronic illness and its effect on feelings of self-worth. Identifying a support system is especially important for adolescents as they begin to take responsibility for their health. Helping the child identify personal strengths and areas of accomplishment will increase the child's self-esteem. Teach parents the importance of fostering their child's independence. As the child grows, encourage discussion about areas of concern, such as dating, sexuality, and peer acceptance. Assist families with the child's transition from pediatric to adult health care providers.

Introducing the family to other families affected by CF can increase problem-solving strategies and facilitate support. Provide information about available community resources, such as the Cystic Fibrosis Foundation and the American Lung Association (see Evolve website). The family also should be encouraged to communicate with personnel at the child's school to ensure coordination of care between home and school.

Although tremendous progress has been made in treating CF, it remains a chronic disease with no cure. Provide the family with honest information about the disease and its prognosis. Refer the family for counseling and listen if they wish to discuss feelings about the disease, the future, and possible death.

■ **Home Care.** Preparation for home care involves teaching family members how to carry out CPT, how to provide breathing treatments, and how to give medications at home. Written instructions should describe the specifics of all aspects of the child's care. Families may need assistance in obtaining home care equipment.

■ Evaluation

- Does the child exhibit improved breath sounds, oxygen saturation greater than 95% on room air, and stable respiratory status?
- Are the child's body temperature and WBC count within normal limits? Has the sputum amount decreased?
- Is the child growing in height and weight along the normal growth curve?
- Are the child's stools of normal consistency, frequency, and color?
- Is the child able to engage in appropriate physical activity?
- Does the child appear to be developing age-appropriate cognitive, emotional, and social skills and an appropriate level of self-care?
- Does the child demonstrate an attitude of acceptance of self and of the illness?
- Does the family demonstrate appropriate coping strategies, adherence to the child's treatment plan, and the ability to access needed resources?
- Can the parents demonstrate CPT, inhalation therapy, and other treatments to be performed at home?
- Are the child and family able to appropriately express feelings of anger, sadness, and fear without guilt?

TUBERCULOSIS

Tuberculosis (TB) is a reportable contagious disease with high morbidity and mortality rates throughout the world. Between 1985 and 1992, cases of TB in the United States increased by 20%. Since then, the incidence of TB has decreased 53%, with the decrease slowing in the past 10 years (Wallace, Kammerer, Iademarco et al., 2009). The Centers for Disease Control and Prevention (2010) estimates that worldwide more than 9 million people are newly infected with TB per year. Left untreated, each person with active TB will infect between 10 and 15 people each year.

Etiology

Mycobacterium tuberculosis, an acid-fast bacillus, causes TB. Contamination occurs chiefly through inhalation of droplets from a person with active TB. Droplets produced by coughing and sneezing remain suspended in the air. When they are inhaled, they can reach the bronchioles and alveoli.

The risk for infection by the organism is thought to depend on several physiologic and socioeconomic factors. Most children are infected by a family member, babysitter, or other person with whom they have frequent contact (Box 21-5).

BOX 21-5 RISK FACTORS FOR THE DEVELOPMENT OF TUBERCULOSIS

- Contact with adults with infectious TB
- Chronic illness, immunosuppression, human immunodeficiency virus (HIV) infection
- Malnutrition
- Age (infancy, adolescence)
- Nonwhite racial and ethnic groups; immigration from areas with a high incidence of TB
- Urban, low-income living conditions
- Incarcerated adolescents
- Children in close contact with any of the following groups of adults: HIV-infected persons, users of IV or other street drugs, poor or medically indigent city dwellers, residents of nursing homes, migrant farm workers

BOX 21-6 DEFINITION OF A POSITIVE MANTOUX SKIN TEST

Area of Induration ≥5 mm Considered Positive in
- HIV-infected persons
- Recent contact with a person who has TB disease
- Persons with fibrotic changes on chest radiograph consistent with prior TB
- Persons who are immunosuppressed for other reasons (e.g., taking the equivalent of >15 mg/day of prednisone for 1 month or longer, taking tumor necrosis factor-α antagonists)

Area of Induration ≥10 mm Considered Positive in
- Recent immigrants (<5 years) from high-prevalence countries
- Injection drug users
- Residents and employees of high-risk congregate settings
- Mycobacteriology laboratory personnel
- Persons with clinical conditions that place them at high risk
- Children <4 years of age
- Infants, children, and adolescents exposed to adults in high-risk categories

Induration ≥15 mm Considered Positive in
- Any person, including persons with no known risk factors for TB.

From Centers for Disease Control and Prevention Division of Tuberculosis Elimination. (2010). Retrieved from www.cdc.gov.

Incidence

In 2008, there were 1.3 million deaths worldwide from TB. In the Americas, there were 282,000 new cases diagnosed. That constitutes 3% of the world's infected population (World Health Organization, 2010). In the pediatric population, TB occurs most commonly in infants and adolescents and in children with immunosuppressive conditions. Of particular concern is the increase in multidrug-resistant TB. Because this is most often caused by poor adherence to drug therapy, directly observed therapy is indicated for anyone being treated for tuberculosis disease (Volmink & Garner, 2007).

PATHOPHYSIOLOGY

Tuberculosis

The bacillus multiplies in lung tissue, alveoli, and regional lymph nodes. After an incubation period of 2 to 12 weeks, hypersensitivity develops; at that time, skin tests of the infected child will test positive. Most infected children are asymptomatic at the time of the initial positive skin test result.

The *disease* of TB is differentiated from TB *infection* by the presence of clinical manifestations. The risk for development of TB disease is highest in the first 2 years after infection, but many infected children never progress to clinical disease.

The immunologic response of most people is usually strong enough to keep the bacteria from multiplying and spreading. If the host response is adequate, the organism is walled off and the tubercle becomes a healed calcified mass. TB bacilli can remain dormant and cause active disease at a later time if the child's resistance is lowered. If the lesion does not heal and is not walled off, it may continue to enlarge and spread into nearby tissues or it may enter the blood and spread to other sites (middle ear, brain, kidney, bones, joints, skin).

TB disease destroys host tissue. When tubercle bacilli multiply, they may damage tissue so badly that the center of the infected area turns to liquid pus. When this liquid escapes through an airway, it is coughed up as sputum, leaving a tiny hole (cavitation) in the lung. The bacteria-laden sputum is infectious. Children rarely have active TB with cavitation, in which case they can be infectious to others. Because children with primary pulmonary TB have small lesions and minimal cough, they are not contagious (AAP, Committee on Infectious Diseases, 2009). The duration of infectivity of treated adults and adolescents depends on the drug susceptibility of the infecting organism and cough frequency. Although infectivity usually lasts only a few weeks after treatment is begun, it may last longer if the person fails to take the prescribed medication or is infected with a resistant strain.

Manifestations

Children ages 3 to 15 years are usually asymptomatic, have normal chest radiographs, and can be identified only through a positive skin test. Some children have malaise, fever, night sweats, a slight cough, weight loss, anorexia, lymphadenopathy, or more specific symptoms related to the site of extrapulmonary infection (e.g., kidneys, brain, bone).

Diagnostic Evaluation

Skin testing is the initial method of screening and testing for TB. In most children, skin testing will become positive 2 to 12 weeks after the initial infection, and once positive, tuberculin reactivity usually continues throughout life, even with treatment.

Skin testing with 5 tuberculin units of purified protein derivative (PPD) (Mantoux test) is the preferred method of screening. The PPD is administered by intradermal injection on the forearm. The skin reaction is read by an experienced professional 48 to 72 hours after placement. A 15-mm induration in any child older than 4 years is considered a positive sign of TB. Induration of more than 5 mm suggests TB in children younger than 4 years and in certain populations of children. A negative tuberculin skin test does not rule out TB, particularly in infants (Box 21-6).

Children with positive skin test results undergo follow-up examinations, which include periodic chest radiography and sputum cultures and smears for the presence of acid-fast bacilli. Because children often swallow sputum rather than expectorate it, gastric washings to obtain swallowed sputum are sometimes done. A thorough history should be obtained, and all contacts of the affected child should be tested for the disease.

Therapeutic Management and Nursing Considerations

It is important to understand the differences between TB exposure, infection, and disease. *Exposure* is recent and significant contact with an individual diagnosed with contagious TB. The skin test is often negative at this point, and the child is asymptomatic. TB *infection* is defined by a positive skin test. The child continues to lack signs and symptoms of TB, and there may be no chest radiograph changes at this time. Prophylactic treatment is instituted to prevent the progression to disease. TB *disease* is defined by chest radiograph changes along with signs and symptoms of disease and a positive skin test.

Tuberculosis Infection

After a chest radiograph is obtained, asymptomatic children with positive tuberculin tests and no previous history of TB receive daily isoniazid (INH) for 9 months. Children with drug-resistant TB need an individualized treatment regimen; the most commonly used alternative drug is a 6-month course of rifampin. Rifampin may be teratogenic and can alter the efficacy of oral contraceptives, so alternative methods of birth control must be used if an adolescent girl requires treatment with this medication (AAP, Committee on Infectious Diseases, 2009). Household contacts (especially children younger than 4 years) and immunosuppressed contacts should undergo skin testing and chest radiography. Even if the skin test is negative, asymptomatic contacts should receive INH for at least 8 to 10 weeks after contact has been broken or until a negative skin test can be confirmed (second test taken at least 10 weeks after last exposure) (AAP, Committee on Infectious Diseases, 2009). Reporting cases of TB is required by law in all states in the United States. Nurses should assist in searching for the source case and others infected by the source case.

Bacillus Calmette-Guérin vaccine is the only anti-TB vaccine available. Unfortunately, the vaccine varies in the immunity it provides and has resulted in serious reactions. In the United States, it is used mainly for children who test negative for tuberculosis but who are continuously exposed to (1) contacts who are not treated or undertreated for contagious pulmonary TB, and the child cannot take antituberculosis

medications, or (2) contacts who have INH and rifampin-resistant pulmonary TB (AAP, Committee on Infectious Diseases, 2009).

Tuberculosis Disease

A 6-month course of combination antituberculosis medications (INH, rifampin, ethambutol, and pyrazinamide for the first 2 months; INH and rifampin for the next 4 months), optimal nutrition, and preventing exposure to infection, which could further compromise the child's already challenged immune system, are the mainstays of treatment (AAP, Committee on Infectious Diseases, 2009). Most children are treated at home. The nurse needs to emphasize to the family the importance of following the prescribed medication regimen meticulously and for the appropriate length of time because inappropriate medication dosing contributes to the growth of drug-resistant organisms. The AAP Committee on Infectious Diseases (2009) recommends directly observed therapy (DOT) for children taking medication for tuberculosis. In most cases, supervision of medication administration is done by a visiting nurse or public health nurse.

Children with TB may be hospitalized, depending on the severity of the disease, the age of the child, the need for more extensive testing, or the child's family and social environment. Unless the child is acutely ill, bed rest is not required. Isolation usually is not required because children with TB are rarely contagious.

Prevention and Screening

Promptly identifying cases and treating appropriately are the focus of disease prevention. Because most children are infected by a family member, the best way to stop transmission of the disease is to identify those who are infected and to provide TB therapy.

Early detection of the disease is accomplished by screening. Children at high risk for TB should be tested annually with the Mantoux test. Annual skin testing of children in low-prevalence areas who have no risk factors is not indicated.

▌KEY CONCEPTS

- Infants and children younger than 3 years are at increased risk for development of respiratory tract infections because of their immature immune system, smaller airways, and underdeveloped supporting cartilage. Infants should be placed on their backs to sleep to prevent sudden infant death syndrome.
- Nursing care for children with respiratory conditions may include symptomatic relief, encouraging fluids, assessing for increased respiratory effort or airway obstruction, oxygen therapy, pain relief and, in some instances, antibiotic administration and teaching.
- Inflammatory conditions affecting the upper respiratory tract include rhinitis, sinusitis, otitis, pharyngitis, and the various forms of croup. Epiglottitis is a rare manifestation of bacterial infection.
- Any child in respiratory distress needs to be seen immediately for emergent care; scheduling nursing care to maximize rest is essential.
- Bronchiolitis, an inflammation of the lower airways, is most often caused by RSV infection, which is highly communicable. For infants hospitalized with bronchiolitis, Contact Precautions and meticulous hand hygiene will assist with preventing spread of infection to others.
- During an apneic episode, the time and duration of the episode, color change, bradycardia, oxygen saturation, what the infant was doing before the apneic period, and any actions that stimulated breathing should be recorded.

- Asthma is the most common chronic disease of childhood. Asthma is characterized by bronchospasm, edema of the bronchiolar mucous membranes, and increased secretion of mucus in the airways, which can be triggered by a variety of stimuli that include allergens, cold air, weather changes, infection, exercise, fatigue, and emotional distress.
- Status asthmaticus, or continued severe respiratory distress despite medical treatment, places the child in imminent danger of respiratory arrest and requires immediate hospitalization.
- In addition to general care for a child with a respiratory condition, nursing care for the child with acute and chronic asthma involves administration of inhaled antiinflammatory medications and bronchodilators and teaching the child and parent about daily monitoring with a peak flow meter.
- BPD is a chronic obstructive pulmonary disease characterized by thickening of the alveolar walls and bronchiolar epithelium, usually seen in premature and low-birth-weight infants who have been mechanically ventilated with high concentrations of oxygen for prolonged periods.
- Nursing care of the infant with BPD includes supportive interventions to maintain adequate oxygenation and the provision of appropriate stimulation to promote normal growth and development.
- CF is an inherited (autosomal recessive), multisystem disorder characterized by widespread dysfunction of the exocrine glands.

Abnormal secretion of thick, tenacious mucus causes obstruction and dysfunction of the pancreas, lungs, salivary glands, sweat glands, and reproductive organs.

- Nursing care of the child with CF includes maintaining a patent airway by administering bronchodilators and performing or supervising respiratory treatments, administering antibiotics and pancreatic enzymes, and teaching the child and family about CF and its treatment.

- Nursing care of the child with TB includes administering and evaluating TB skin tests and administering anti-TB medications as ordered. The nurse also instructs the child and family about the importance of adequate rest, a nutritionally adequate diet, adherence to the medication regimen, and ways to prevent the transmission of TB infection.

REFERENCES

Abdullah, B., Hassan, S., & Sidek, D. (2007). Clinical and audiological profiles in children with chronic otitis media with effusion requiring surgical intervention. *Malaysian Journal of Medical Sciences, 14*(2), 22-27.

Akinbami, L., Moorman, J. & Liu, X. (2011). Asthma prevalence, health care use, and mortality: United States 2005-2009. *National Health Statistics Reports, 32*, 1-14.

American Academy of Pediatrics. (2004). Clinical practice guideline: Diagnosis and management of acute otitis media. *Pediatrics, 113*, 1451-1465.

American Academy of Pediatrics. (2005, reaffirmed 2009). The changing concept of sudden infant death syndrome: Diagnostic coding shifts, controversies regarding the sleeping environment, and new variables to consider in reducing risk. *Pediatrics, 116*, 1245-1255.

American Academy of Pediatrics Subcommittee on Otitis Media with Effusion, American Academy of Family Physicians, & American Academy of Otolaryngology—Head and Neck Surgery. (2004). Otitis media with effusion. *Pediatrics, 113*, 1412-1429.

American Academy of Pediatrics, Committee on Infectious Diseases. (2009). *Report of the Committee on Infectious Diseases, 2009 Red Book* (28th ed.). Elk Grove Village, IL: American Academy of Pediatrics.

Antoon, A., & Donovan, M. (2011). Burn injuries. In R. Kliegman, B. Stanton, J. St. Geme, et al. (Eds.), *Nelson textbook of pediatrics* (19th ed., pp. 354-355). Philadelphia: Elsevier Saunders.

Bhandari, A., & Bhandari, V. (2007). Bronchopulmonary dysplasia: An update. *Indian Journal of Pediatrics, 74*(1), 73-77.

Bhandari, A., & Bhandari, V. (2009). Pitfalls, problems, and progress in bronchopulmonary dysplasia. *Pediatrics, 123*(6), 1562-1573.

Borowitz, D., Robinson, K., Rosenfeld, M., et al. (2009). Cystic fibrosis foundation evidence-based guidelines for management of infants with cystic fibrosis. *Journal of Pediatrics, 155*(6, Suppl. 1), S73-S93.

Breysem, L., Goosens, V., Vander Poorten, V., et al. (2009). Vallecular cyst as a cause of congenital stridor: Report of five patients. *Pediatric Radiology, 39*(8), 828-831.

Burton, J. H., Harrah, J. D., Germann, C. A., & Dillon, D. C. (2006). Does end-tidal carbon dioxide monitoring detect respiratory events prior to current sedation monitoring practices? *Academic Emergency Medicine, 13*(5): 500-504.

Carroll, K., Wu, P., Gebretsadik, T., et al. (2009). The severity-dependent relationship of infant bronchiolitis on the risk and morbidity of early childhood asthma. *The Journal of Allergy and Clinical Immunology, 123*(5), 1055-1061.

Casey, J. R., & Pichichero, M. E. (2007). The evidence base for cephalosporin superiority over penicillin in streptococcal pharyngitis. *Diagnostic Microbiology and Infectious Disease, 57*(3, Suppl. 1), S39-S45.

Centers for Disease Control and Prevention. (2010). *Tuberculosis.* Retrieved from www.cdc.gov.

Coates, H., Thornton, R., Langlands, J., et al. (2008). The role of chronic infection in children with otitis media with effusion: Evidence for intracellular persistence of bacteria. *Otolaryngology—Head and Neck Surgery, 138*(6), 778-781.

Coleman, C. & Moore, M. (2008). Decongestants and antihistamines for acute otitis media in children. *Cochrane Database of Systematic Reviews. Issue 3.* CD001727.

Cystic Fibrosis Foundation. (2008). *Patient registry 2008 annual data report.* Bethesda, MD: Cystic Fibrosis Foundation.

Cystic Fibrosis Foundation. (2010). *Therapies for cystic fibrosis.* Bethesda, MD: Cystic Fibrosis Foundation.

Da Dalt, L., Callegaro, S., Carraro, S., et al. (2007). Nasal lavage leukotrienes in infants with RSV bronchiolitis. *Pediatric Allergy and Immunology, 18*(2), 100-104.

DeMuri, G. P., & Wald, E. R. (2010). Update on acute sinusitis in children. *Pediatric Health, 4*(1), 99-105.

Dudell, G., & Stoll, B. (2007). Respiratory distress syndrome (hyaline membrane disease). In R. Kliegman, R. Behrman, H. Jenson, & B. Stanton (Eds.), *Nelson textbook of pediatrics* (18th ed.), Philadelphia: Elsevier Saunders.

Egan, M. (2011). Cystic fibrosis. In R. Kliegman, B. Stanton, J. St. Geme, et al. (Eds.), *Nelson textbook of pediatrics* (19th ed., pp. 1481-1497). Philadelphia: Elsevier Saunders.

Flume, P., Robinson, K., O'Sullivan, B., et al. (2009). Cystic fibrosis pulmonary guidelines: Airway clearance therapies. *Respiratory Care, 54*(4), 522-537.

Gaffin, J., Shotola, N., Martin, T., & Phipatanakul, M. (2010). Clinically useful spirometry in preschool-aged children: Evaluation of the 2007 American thoracic society guidelines. *Journal of Asthma, 47*(7), 762-767.

Garcia, C., Bhore, R., Soriano-Fallas, A., et al. (2010). Risk factors in children hospitalized with RSV bronchiolitis versus non-RSV bronchiolitis. *Pediatrics, 126*, e1453-e1460.

Gorelick, M., Scribano, P., Stevens, M. W., et al. (2008). Predicting need for hospitalization in acute pediatric asthma. *Pediatric Emergency Care, 24*(11), 735-744.

Greenough, A., & Sharma, A. (2007). What is new in ventilation strategies for the neonate? *European Journal of Pediatrics, 166*, 991-996.

Håberg, S. E., Stigum, H., Nystad, W., & Nafstad, P. (2007). Effects of pre- and postnatal exposure to parental smoking on early childhood respiratory health. *American Journal of Epidemiology, 166*(6), 679-686.

Hallman, M., & Haataja, R. (2007). Genetic basis of respiratory distress syndrome. *Frontiers in Bioscience, 12*, 2670-2682.

Hardin, D. S., Adams-Huet, B., Brown, D., et al. (2006). Growth hormone treatment improves growth and clinical status in prepubertal children with cystic fibrosis: Results of a multicenter randomized controlled trial. *Journal of Clinical Endocrinology & Metabolism, 91*(12), 4925-4929.

Hayden, G., & Turner, R. (2011). Acute pharyngitis. In R. Kliegman, B. Stanton, J. St. Geme, et al. (Eds.), *Nelson textbook of pediatrics* (19th ed., pp. 1439-1440). Philadelphia: Elsevier Saunders.

Hunt, C., & Hauck, F. (2011). Sudden infant death syndrome. In R. Kliegman, B. Stanton, J. St. Geme, et al. (Eds.), *Nelson textbook of pediatrics* (19th ed., pp. 1421-1429). Philadelphia: Elsevier Saunders.

Kerschner, J. (2011). Otitis media. In R. Kliegman, B. Stanton, J. St. Geme, et al. (Eds.), *Nelson textbook of pediatrics* (19th ed., pp. 2199-2213). Philadelphia: Elsevier Saunders.

Kotsis, G. P., Nikolopoulos, T. P., Yiotakis, I. E., et al. (2009). Recurrent acute otitis media and gastroesophageal reflux disease in children: Is there an association? *International Journal of Pediatric Otorhinolaryngology, 73*(10), 1373-1380.

Lasisi, A. O., Olayemi, O., & Irabor, A. E. (2008). Early onset otitis media: Risk factors and effects on the outcome of chronic suppurative otitis media. *European Archives of Oto-Rhino-Laryngology, 265*(7), 765-768.

Leo, G., Mori, F., Incorvaia, C., et al. (2009). Diagnosis and management of acute rhinosinusitis in children. *Current Allergy and Asthma Reports, 9*(3), 232-237.

Leonard, D. S., Fenton, J. E., & Hone, S. (2010). ABO blood type as a risk factor for secondary post-tonsillectomy hemorrhage. *International Journal of Pediatric Otorhinolaryngology, 74*(7), 729-732.

Liu, A., Covar, R., Spahn, J., & Leung, D. (2011). Childhood asthma. In R. Kliegman, B. Stanton, J. St. Geme et al. (Eds.), *Nelson textbook of pediatrics* (19th ed., pp. 780-801). Philadelphia: Elsevier Saunders.

Mangan, J. M., Bailey, W., & Gerald, L. B. (2009). *Patient information: Asthma inhaler techniques in adults.* Up to Date. Version 17.3.

Milgrom, H., & Leung, D. (2011). Allergic rhinitis. In R. Kliegman, B. Stanton, J. St. Geme, et al. (Eds.), *Nelson textbook of pediatrics* (19th ed., pp.775-780). Philadelphia: Elsevier Saunders.

Morris, S., Dzolganovski, B., Beyene, J., & Sung, L. (2009). A meta-analysis of the effect of antibody therapy for the prevention of severe respiratory syncytial virus infection. *BMC Infectious Diseases, 9*(1), 106. Retrieved from www.biomedcentral.com/1471-2334/9/106.

Nathan, R. A. (2007). The burden of allergic rhinitis. *Allergy and Asthma Proceedings, 28*(1), 3-9.

National Heart, Lung, and Blood Institute & National Asthma Education and Prevention Program. (2007). *Expert panel report 3: Guidelines for the diagnosis and management of asthma.* Retrieved from www.nhlbi.nih.gov.

National Institute of Child Health and Human Development. (2007). *Curriculum for nurses: continuing education program on SIDS risk reduction.* Washington, DC: U.S. Government Printing Office. Retrieved from www.nichd.nih.gov.

Novembre, E., Mori, F., Pucci, N., et al. (2007). Systemic treatment of rhinosinusitis in children. *Pediatric Allergy and Immunology, 18*(Suppl. 18), 56-61.

Pappas, D., & Hendley, O. (2011). Sinusitis. In R. Kliegman, B. Stanton, J. St. Geme, et al. (Eds.), *Nelson textbook of pediatrics* (19th ed., pp. 1436-1438). Philadelphia: Elsevier Saunders.

Ramakrishnan, K., Sparks, R., & Berryhill, W. (2007). Diagnosis and treatment of otitis media. *American Family Physician, 26*(11), 1650-1658.

Revai, K., Dobbs, L. A., Nair, S., et al. (2007). Incidence of acute otitis media and sinusitis complicating upper respiratory tract infection: The effect of age. *Pediatrics, 119*(6), e1408-e1412.

Ritz, T., Kullowatz, A., Kanniess, F., et al. (2008). Perceived triggers of asthma: Evaluation of a German version of the asthma trigger inventory. *Respiratory Medicine, 102*(3), 390-398.

Roosevelt, G. (2011). Infectious upper airway obstruction. In R. Kliegman, B. Stanton, J. St. Geme, et al. (Eds.), *Nelson textbook of pediatrics* (19th ed., pp. 1445-1448). Philadelphia: Elsevier Saunders.

Sandora, T., & Sectish, T. (2011). Community acquired pneumonia. In R. Kliegman, B. Stanton, J. St. Geme, et al. (Eds.), *Nelson textbook of pediatrics* (19th ed., pp. 1474-1479). Philadelphia: Elsevier Saunders.

Scollan-Koliopoulos, M., & Koliopoulos, J. (2010). Evaluation and management of apparent life-threatening events in infants. *Pediatric Nursing, 36*(2), 77-83.

Sectish, T., & Prober, C. (2007). Pneumonia. In R. Kliegman, R. Behrman, H. Jenson, & B. Stanton (Eds.), *Nelson textbook of pediatrics* (18th ed., pp. 1795-1799). Philadelphia: Elsevier Saunders.

Shlizerman, L., Mazzawi, S., Rakover, Y., & Ashkenazi, D. (2010). Foreign body aspiration in children: The effects of delayed diagnosis. *American Journal of Otolaryngology, 31*(5), 320-324.

Silvestri, J. (2009). Indications for home apnea monitoring (or not). *Clinical Perinatology, 36*(1), 87-99.

Soll, R., & Özek, E. (2009). Multiple versus single doses of exogenous surfactant for the prevention or treatment of neonatal respiratory distress syndrome. *Cochrane Database of Systematic Reviews*, Issue 1. CD000141.

Suhaili, D. N., Goh, B. S., & Gendeh, B. S. (2010). A ten year retrospective review of orbital complications secondary to acute sinusitis in children. *Medical Journal Malaysia, 65*(1), 49-52.

Turner, P. J., & Kemp, A. S. (2010). Allergic rhinitis in children. *Journal of Paediatrics and Child Health*, 1-9.

Verder, H. (2007). Nasal CPAP has become an indispensable part of the primary treatment of newborns with respiratory distress syndrome. *Acta Paediatrica, 96*, 482-484.

Volmink, J., & Garner, P. (2007). Directly observed therapy for treating tuberculosis (review). *Cochrane Database of Systematic Reviews*, Issue 4. CD003343.

Wallace, R. M., Kammerer, J. S., Iademarco, M. F., et al. (2009). Increasing proportions of advanced pulmonary tuberculosis reported in the United States: Are delays in diagnosis on the rise? *American Journal of Respiratory and Critical Care Medicine, 180*(10), 1016-1022.

Wang, D., Cummins, C., Bayliss, S., et al. (2008). Immunoprophylaxis against respiratory syncytial virus (RSV) with palivizumab in children: A systematic review and economic evaluation. *Health Technology Assessment, 12*(36), iii, ix-x, 1-86.

Watts, K., & Goodman, D. (2011). Wheezing in infants: Bronchiolitis. In R. Kliegman, B. Stanton, J. St. Geme, et al. (Eds.), *Nelson textbook of pediatrics* (19th ed., pp. 1456-1459). Philadelphia: Elsevier Saunders.

Wills-Karp, M. (2007). Complement activation pathways: A bridge between innate and adaptive immune responses in asthma. *Proceedings of the American Thoracic Society, 4*(3), 247-251.

Wing, A., Villa-Roel, C., Yeh, B., et al. (2010). Effectiveness of corticosteroid treatment in acute pharyngitis: A systematic review of the literature. *Academic Emergency Medicine, 17*(5), 476-483.

Witters, P., De Boeck, K., Dupont, L., et al. (2009). Noninvasive liver elastography (fibroscan) for detection of cystic fibrosis-associated liver disease. *Journal of Cystic Fibrosis, 8*(6), 392-399.

World Health Organization. (2010, November). *Tuberculosis fact sheet.* Retrieved from www.who.int/mediacentre/factsheets/fs104/en.

Yoder, B. A., Harrison, M., & Clark, R. H. (2009). Time-related changes in steroid use and bronchopulmonary dysplasia in preterm infants. *Pediatrics, 124*(2), 673-679.

Zhang, L., Mendoza-Sassi, R., Wainwright, C., & Klassen, T. (2008). Nebulized hypertonic saline solution for acute bronchiolitis in infants. *Cochrane Database of Systematic Reviews*, Issue 4. CD0006458.

Zhou, F., Shefer, A., Kong, Y., & Nuorti, J. P. (2008). Trends in acute otitis media-related health care utilization by privately insured young children in the United States, 1997-2004. *Pediatrics, 121*(2), 253-260.

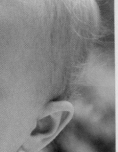

The Child with a Cardiovascular Alteration

WEBSITE

http://evolve.elsevier.com/James/ncoc

- Describe the anatomy and physiology of the normally functioning heart.
- Describe the major circulatory changes that occur in the fetus during the transition from intrauterine to extrauterine life.
- Discuss specific techniques used in a comprehensive cardiac assessment.
- Explain the various classifications of congenital heart disease, describe their underlying mechanisms, and list the associated congenital cardiac defects.
- Discuss the nursing process used for an infant or child with congestive heart failure.
- Discuss the major physiologic features and the therapeutic management of a child with a heart defect, including left-to-right shunting lesions, right-to-left shunting lesions, and obstructive or stenotic lesions.
- Discuss the importance of early recognition and treatment of infective endocarditis.
- Describe nursing care of a child with rheumatic fever, Kawasaki disease, or hypertension.
- Explain why high cholesterol is an important health issue for children and adolescents, and describe the assessment and nursing management of this problem in children in the community.
- Explain the effects of childhood obesity on future cardiovascular health.

CLINICAL REFERENCE

REVIEW OF THE HEART AND CIRCULATION

Normal Cardiac Anatomy and Physiology

The heart is a muscular pump divided into four chambers. The two upper chambers are the atria, and the two lower chambers are the ventricles. The atria are referred to as the filling chambers and the ventricles as the pumping chambers. There are two atrioventricular (AV) valves, the tricuspid valve and the mitral valve, and two semilunar valves, the pulmonary valve and the aortic valve. In normal blood flow, desaturated venous blood returning from the body flows from the superior vena cava and inferior vena cava into the right atrium. It then moves through the tricuspid valve into the right ventricle and is pumped into the main pulmonary artery and branch pulmonary arteries to the pulmonary circulation. In the lungs, carbon dioxide is removed and oxygen is added to the blood. This richly oxygen-saturated blood returns from the pulmonary circulation to the left side of the heart through the pulmonary veins and into the left atrium. From the left atrium, it flows through the mitral valve into the left ventricle and is pumped into the aorta and systemic circulation.

Mechanical contraction of the heart muscle starts with electrical stimulation. This electrical stimulation is normally initiated by a group of cells called the *sinus node,* located at the superior vena cava and right atrial junction. The electrical impulse spreads through the atrium to the relay station, the AV node, and is then transmitted to the ventricles through the bundle of His, the bundle branch system, and finally the Purkinje fibers. The result is rhythmic atrial electrical stimulation and then contraction, followed by ventricular stimulation and contraction.

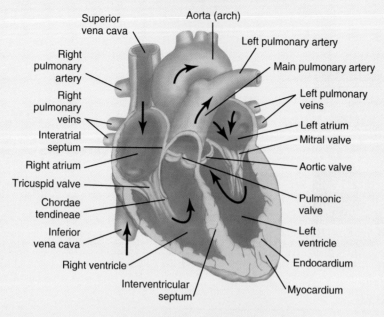

Anatomy of the Heart

The electrocardiogram records this electrical activity. The P wave reflects atrial depolarization; the QRS complex reflects ventricular depolarization; the T wave reflects ventricular repolarization. Each cardiac cycle consists of this electrical activity, which produces depolarization and subsequent repolarization of the cardiac muscle—more simply, a heartbeat.

The venous (or right) side of the heart is normally a lower-pressure system compared with the higher arterial (or left) side of the heart. The right ventricle has a range of normal pressure of 18-30/0-5 mm Hg and pulmonary artery pressure of 20-30/8-12 mm Hg. The left ventricle has a range of normal pressure of 90-140/5 mm Hg (age dependent), and the aorta has a normal pressure of about 100/60 mm Hg (age dependent). On average, the left-sided pressures are four to five times higher than those on the right side. In addition, the venous circulation normally has lower oxygen saturations, in the range of 65% to 80%. This compares with the arterial circulation, which has a normal range of 95% to 100%. Congenital or acquired malformations or anomalies in any of the cardiac structures can affect blood flow, pressures, and oxygen saturations, thereby altering hemodynamic stability.

Fetal Circulation

Fetal circulation differs from neonatal circulation in three areas: the process of gas exchange, the pressures within the systemic and pulmonary circulations, and the existence of anatomic structures that assist in the delivery of oxygen-rich blood to vital organ systems. In the fetus, oxygenation (gas exchange) takes place at the placenta. Oxygen and nutrients are carried by blood in the umbilical vein, which travels through the fetal liver to the inferior vena cava. A small amount of blood travels into the hepatic circulation to provide oxygen and nutrients to the hepatic tissue. Liver function is minimal in the fetus, so very little blood supply is required. The remainder of the blood

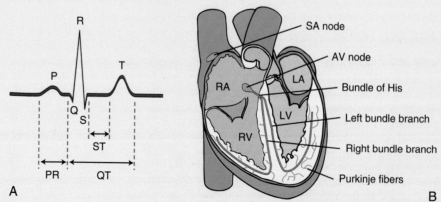

A, Normal heart cycle, represented as an electrocardiographic configuration. **B,** Cardiac electrical conduction system. (Modified from Park, M. K., & Guntheroth, W. G. [2006]. *How to read pediatric ECGs* [4th ed., p. 11]. St. Louis: Mosby.)

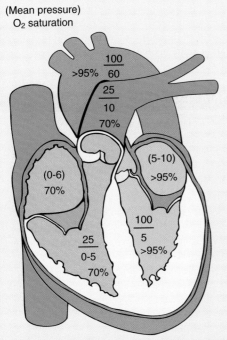

(Mean pressure)
O₂ saturation

Normal pressures (in millimeters of mercury) and saturations (percents). (Modified from Ko Chiang, L., & Ensor Dunn, A. [2000]. Cardiology. In G. K. Siberry & R. Iannone [Eds.], *The Johns Hopkins Hospital Harriet Lane handbook* [15th ed., p. 154]. St. Louis: Mosby.)

flows into the inferior vena cava through a fetal structure, the *ductus venosus.*

The inferior vena cava empties blood into the right atrium. The trajectory (direction) of the blood flow, as well as the pressure in the right atrium, propels most of this blood through a second fetal structure, the *foramen ovale,* into the left atrium. This richly oxygenated blood travels through the left ventricle into the aorta, feeding the coronary arteries and the brain—the two most oxygen-needy organ systems.

Blood returning from the upper body enters the right atrium through the superior vena cava. This blood is directed primarily through the tricuspid valve and the right ventricle into the pulmonary artery. Resistance in the pulmonary circulation is very high because the lungs are collapsed and filled with fluid. A very small amount of blood flows through the branch pulmonary arteries to provide oxygen and nutrients to the pulmonary tissue. Most of the blood flows through a third fetal structure, the *ductus arteriosus,* to the descending aorta. This blood is then distributed to the organ systems and tissues in the lower portion of the body and returns to the placenta for gas exchange through two umbilical arteries.

Transitional and Neonatal Circulation

Major changes in the circulatory system occur at birth. With the neonate's first breath, gas exchange is transferred from the placenta to the lungs. The fetal shunts (ductus venosus, ductus arteriosus, foramen ovale) functionally close in response to pressure changes in the

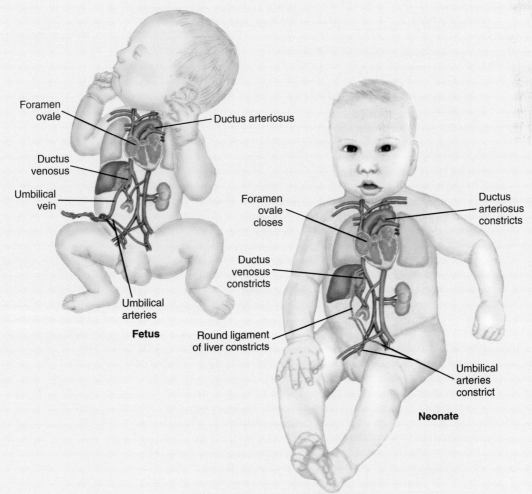

Changes in Circulation after Birth

533

systemic and pulmonary circulations and to increased blood oxygen content. Pulmonary vascular resistance begins to decrease, and pulmonary blood flow markedly increases. Closure of the ductus arteriosus, along with the increased pulmonary blood flow, enhances left ventricular filling. The increase in systemic arterial pressure as a result of clamping the umbilical cord at delivery and placental separation from the fetus increases the workload of the left ventricle, and the neonatal heart now functions on its own. The neonatal circulation is now normal. In some neonates, it may take several days for the fetal shunts to close.

DIFFERENCES IN THE HEART AND CIRCULATION OF NEONATES AND INFANTS

- The heart and the great vessels develop during the first 3 to 8 weeks of gestation. The fetus is most vulnerable to cardiac malformations during this period.
- Heart sounds in the neonate are higher pitched and of greater intensity than in the adult, and the pulse rate is higher. Many variations in these parameters are both possible and normal.
- The chest wall of infants and young children is thin because of the relative lack of subcutaneous fat and muscle tissue. Innocuous murmurs can be auscultated in structurally normal hearts because of the wall thinness.
- The neonate and infant's myocardial muscle is less efficient. The myocardial cells are smaller and contain fewer contractile elements; therefore, neonatal and infant hearts have decreased myocardial contractility. This makes neonates and infants particularly dependent on adequate heart rate and rhythm to maintain their cardiac output because they cannot increase their stroke volume as effectively as the older child or adult (Cardiac output = Stroke volume × Heart rate).

- The neonatal heart is highly dependent on calcium, glucose, and volume for optimal cardiac function.
- In a very sick child, the cardiac output should be evaluated as either adequate or inadequate to meet metabolic demands. Shock may be present even when the cardiac output is normal or high.
- Blood pressure is not a reliable indicator of clinical decompensation. Hypotension may indicate decompensated shock.
- Increased pulmonary vascular resistance in the neonate increases pressure on the right side of the heart. This may delay detection of left-to-right shunts in the newborn period because increased right-sided pressure decreases the left-to-right shunting and the intensity of cardiac murmurs. Normally, pulmonary vascular resistance decreases to the adult range over the first 4 to 6 weeks of life. Obvious signs and symptoms of left-to-right shunting may not be present until that time.

COMMON DIAGNOSTIC TESTS FOR CARDIAC DISORDERS

TEST	DESCRIPTION	PREPARATION AND NURSING CONSIDERATIONS	COMMENTS
Electrocardiogram (ECG)	Provides recording of heart's electrical activity from outside surface of body. Electrodes are placed over precordium and on the four extremities; electrodes are attached to lead wires. Lead wires are attached to an electrocardiograph that records and prints electrical activity.	Best done when the child is quiet and cooperative. Skin should be free of lotions and oils.	Displays heart rate and rhythm. Detects chamber enlargement and deviations in axis that may be caused by congenital or acquired heart defects or disease.
Holter monitor	Continuously records heart rate and rhythm for 24 hr. Electrodes and leads are attached to the child, who wears a compact recorder.	Same as for ECG.	Child or parent records times of activities, symptoms, or other events in a diary to be returned with the monitor. Important that diary be accurately completed.
Chest radiography	Provides x-ray picture of heart and associated organs and structures in the chest cavity.	Remove electrodes and lead wires if attached. Encourage the parent or family member to accompany the child to x-ray department.	Provides information about heart size, blood flow to lungs, sidedness of the stomach, liver, and heart.
Echocardiography	Uses high-frequency sound waves (ultrasound) to generate an image of the heart and associated structures. The study assesses location and relationship of intracardiac and extracardiac structures, cardiac function; measures size of cardiac chambers, valve function, size of septal or other defects; estimates gradients across structures and blood flow direction.	Must be done when the child is quiet and cooperative. If not cooperative, sedation may become necessary.	Methods of echocardiograms: • M-mode • Two-dimensional • Doppler Types of echocardiograms: • Transthoracic • Transesophageal • Directly on cardiac muscle • Fetal
Magnetic resonance imaging	A strong magnetic field surrounds the child; the field promotes rotation of nuclei (that normally spin) at predictable speed, allowing visualization of soft tissue, tumors, shunts, myocardial thickness, structure, and valve function.	Teaching about the procedure. Nothing-by-mouth status for at least 4 hr before procedure if requiring sedation. Assessment for allergy if contrast medium is to be used. All metallic items must be removed.	The child must be able to lie still for up to 1 hr or will require sedation.

COMMON DIAGNOSTIC TESTS FOR CARDIAC DISORDERS—cont'd

TEST	DESCRIPTION	PREPARATION AND NURSING CONSIDERATIONS	COMMENTS
Ventilation-perfusion scan	IV injection of isotope, which reveals distribution of pulmonary blood flow and ventilation; assists in quantifying percentage and pattern of pulmonary blood flow.	Requires an IV line for radioisotope injection.	The child must be able to lie still for a short time for the scan.
Pulse oximetry	A bandage probe is attached to a digit; measures oxygen saturation of blood noninvasively.	No specific preparation. The extremity needs to be relatively motion free for accurate reading. All nail polish must be removed.	If alarms (high or low), validate the child's heart rate corresponds to the monitor. Know the expected saturation range for the child's cardiac defect.

Cardiovascular alterations in children are either congenital or acquired. Congenital heart disease (CHD) denotes one or more structural abnormalities that develop before birth, although the clinical symptoms may not be present in the newborn period. Acquired heart disease, such as the cardiomyopathies, Kawasaki disease, or acute rheumatic fever (RF), develops after birth and may be seen both in children with normal hearts and in those with congenital heart disease. Over the past three decades, there have been major advances in the diagnosis and management of CHD. Because of these advances, approximately 90% of infants born with CHD can be expected to live into adulthood. In order to appreciate each defect or combination of multiple defects and their impact on a child's life, an understanding of normal cardiac anatomy and physiology, including development of the heart, circulation (including fetal, transitional, and postnatal), normal structures, and function is required.

CONGENITAL HEART DISEASE

Congenital cardiac defects are some of the most frequently seen congenital defects in infants and children and have an overall incidence of 8 in every 1000 live births (American Heart Association [AHA], 2011). As interventional cardiology becomes more effective, more adults are living with congenital heart disease; the prevalence of congenital heart disease in adults is approximately 4 per 1000 (AHA, 2011).

Although the non-genetic etiology and risk factors for congenital heart disease are not fully known, maternal diabetes mellitus, maternal infection during pregnancy, maternal smoking, maternal obesity, and maternal exposure to some chemicals and pollutants have been implicated (AHA, 2011). Children with certain genetic conditions or defects have an extremely high incidence of cardiac disorders, including children with chromosome aberrations, most specifically trisomy 21 (Down syndrome), in which the incidence of congenital heart disease is approximately 50% (Park, 2008). Other congenital conditions that increase the risk for congenital heart disease include Turner syndrome in girls (single X chromosome), Klinefelter variant in boys (genetically having additional X chromosomes), and children with Marfan syndrome or with velocardiofacial syndrome (DiGeorge syndrome) (Park, 2008). A family history of congenital heart disease increases the risk.

Classification of Congenital Heart Disease

Congenital heart defects can be classified according to structural abnormalities, functional alterations, or both (Table 22-1). Historically, defects were simply classified according to whether they were cyanotic or acyanotic. Currently, these classifications are subdivided into groups that are defined by blood flow patterns. These include presence of increased pulmonary blood flow, normal to decreased pulmonary blood flow, obstructive lesions, and miscellaneous complex lesions.

Clinical signs of congenital cardiac defects can manifest any time during the newborn period, infancy, or early childhood. The degree of symptoms, indications for medical, surgical, or transcatheter interventions, and chronicity of the condition depend on the diagnosis.

Shunting: Saturation Considerations

Abnormal blood flow from one part of the circulatory system to another is called a shunt. A shunt occurs when (1) there is an abnormal opening or connection between the cardiac chambers or great arteries, (2) the pressure is higher on one side of the heart compared with the other (pressure gradient), and (3) the oxygen saturation is increased or decreased in the normally desaturated or fully saturated blood. It is important to remember that the venous or right side is usually a low-pressure, desaturated (average 70%) system and the arterial or left side is usually a high-pressure, fully saturated (95% to 100%) system. The combination of pressure differences and the size of the abnormal opening determine the extent of shunting.

Blood Flow Considerations

Generally, the amount of blood flow to the lungs through the pulmonary artery is the same as the amount of blood flow to the systemic circulation through the aorta. This ratio of pulmonary to systemic blood flow is described as the *pulmonary-to-systemic ratio* (QP/QS ratio) and is usually 1:1. Patients with CHD may have normal, increased, or decreased pulmonary-to-systemic blood flow ratios. Understanding the principles of shunting and normal saturations in each of the heart's chambers helps clarify the blood flow direction in CHD.

PHYSIOLOGIC CONSEQUENCES OF CONGENITAL HEART DISEASE IN CHILDREN

There are two primary physiologic consequences of CHD in children. These include heart failure and cyanosis.

Heart Failure

The definition of *heart failure* (HF) is the heart's inability to circulate blood to maintain sufficient cardiac output to meet the metabolic demands of the body. Despite the causes of HF, the heart initially

TABLE 22-1	CLASSIFICATION OF CONGENITAL HEART DISEASE	
DEFECT	**UNDERLYING MECHANISM**	**EXAMPLES**
Left-to-right shunting lesions (lesions that increase pulmonary blood flow)	A defect in the atrial septum or persistence of a patent ductus arteriosus (PDA) causes saturated blood to shunt through the opening. This left-to-right shunting of blood results in a volume overload in the right side of the heart and in the pulmonary artery; cardiac workload (including ventricular strain, dilation, and hypertrophy) increases to manage the additional volume (pressure overload). This abnormal increase in highly saturated blood combined with the increased fluid volume in the lungs, results in altered gas exchange. One of the major consequences of left-to-right shunting lesions is HF. Other consequences include pulmonary vascular disease, pulmonary hypertension, Eisenmenger syndrome, and frequent upper and lower respiratory infections that can progress to respiratory failure.	Atrial septal defect (ASD) Ventral septal defect (VSD) Patent ductus arteriosus (PDA) Endocardial cushion defect
Obstructive or stenotic lesions, or lesions that decrease cardiac outflow	*Stenosis*, the narrowing or constriction of an opening, can occur in a valve or vessel constricting or obstructing blood flow through the area. Pressure rises in the area behind the obstruction; blood flow distal to the obstruction may be decreased or absent. Stenotic lesions can occur in the right or left side of the heart; obstruction on the left side of the heart decreases the amount of available blood for systemic perfusion. Physiologic effects of stenotic lesions include increased cardiac workload and ventricular strain, with clinical consequences of HF, decreased cardiac output, and pump failure.	Pulmonary stenosis Aortic stenosis Coarctation of the aorta
Cyanotic lesions with decreased pulmonary blood flow	These lesions arise from an error in fetal development that results in *hypoplasia* (incomplete development), malalignment, or obstruction on the right side of the heart, and decreased amount of blood volume to the lungs. Pulmonary blood flow may rely on having a PDA. There is abnormally decreased oxygen saturation in the left side of the heart. Physiologically, the child manifests hypoxemia, increased cardiac workload, and ventricular strain. The hypoxemia results in cyanosis, and even with oxygen administration, saturations do not approximate normal. Other clinical findings may include upper respiratory infection, severely limited pulmonary blood flow, and marked exercise intolerance.	Tetralogy of Fallot Tricuspid valve abnormalities Pulmonary atresia with intact ventricular septum
Cyanotic lesions with increased pulmonary blood flow	When the fetal heart fails to develop into separate pulmonary and systemic circulations or when there is a reversal of circulation so that desaturated blood goes to the systemic circulation and saturated blood to the pulmonary circulation, cyanosis occurs. Sometimes classified as mixing lesions, these defects cause increased cardiac workload, ventricular strain, and decreased cardiac output. Lesions are usually discovered early in the neonatal period. The infant might appear ruddy or cyanotic, with increased respiratory effort, or, if systemic circulation is compromised, may be dusky or gray and in cardiogenic shock (see Chapter 10). To support life, these complex cardiac defects may require intervention that allows for mixing of arterial and venous blood.	Truncus arteriosus Hypoplastic left heart syndrome* Transposition of the great arteries

*Also classified as a lesion that decreases cardiac outflow.

responds to the need for increased cardiac output by increasing the heart rate. Over time the heart may become enlarged (cardiomegaly), causing the muscle walls of the heart to grow weak and inefficient. This can reduce blood volume in the body, which causes the body's arteries to constrict and force the heart to work even harder. This poor function causes congestion in the body and/or lung tissues (pulmonary edema).

Etiology

The etiology of HF in neonates, infants, and children differs from that for adults. In infants and children, heart failure is most often related to an underlying congenital cardiac defect that causes volume or pressure overload, but may also develop from many other etiologies, including acquired heart disease. Examples of acquired heart disease include cardiomyopathies, arrhythmias, infections (e.g., endocarditis, myocarditis), and tumors. Damage to the heart also can occur as a

result of inborn metabolic disorders and exposure to certain drugs, and toxins (Park, 2008). Many times the symptoms can be treated by drugs. If there is an anatomic defect, correction of the cause either by surgery or transcatheter intervention is often needed.

Defects that lead to volume overload and cause symptoms of HF in infants and children include left-to-right shunts (e.g., atrial septal defects [ASDs], ventricular septal defects [VSDs], common AV canal defect [CAVC], and patent ductus arteriosus [PDA]). These defects allow excess blood to pass from the left side of the heart to the right, causing the heart to work harder to pump this extra volume to the lungs.

Defects that lead to pressure overload and cause symptoms of HF mainly include left-side heart obstructive lesions (e.g., critical aortic stenosis, severe aortic coarctation, congenital mitral stenosis, and hypoplastic left heart syndrome) (Park, 2008). These defects cause the heart to pump harder against an obstruction in order to get blood to the body. This extra work, over time, will cause the heart muscle to enlarge (hypertrophy) and become inefficient.

Defects that are acquired and cause symptoms of HF include primary myocardial diseases that attack the heart muscle and cause it to weaken. Arrhythmias disrupt the delicate balance of the electrical or conduction system of the heart; cause the heart rate to be slow, fast, or erratic; and, over time, lead to poor cardiac output. The incidence of HF in infants and children is difficult to estimate because of improvements in surgical options.

PATHOPHYSIOLOGY

Heart Failure

When a child develops HF, hemodynamic and neurohormonal changes occur in response to decreased cardiac output. Cardiac output is a function of stroke volume and heart rate. Stroke volume (SV) is defined as the amount of blood ejected from the heart with each heartbeat. It is expressed in liters/minute (L/min). Cardiac output equals heart rate multiplied by stroke volume. Other factors affecting cardiac output include preload, afterload, and contractility.

Neurohormonal changes include the stimulation of both the sympathetic nervous system and the renin-angiotensin system. Maintaining blood pressure, blood flow, and oxygen delivery to vital organs is the goal of this compensatory system. With decreased cardiac output, there is stimulation of the sympathetic nervous system. Initially this leads to increased heart rate, contractility, and stroke volume; increased systemic vascular resistance (afterload); and selective peripheral vasoconstriction. Tachycardia, although beneficial to compensate for early HF, increases myocardial oxygen consumption, decreases the diastolic filling time and resting phase of the heart, and decreases coronary artery perfusion.*

Decreased cardiac output also causes the renal system to have decreased renal blood flow and a diminished glomerular filtration rate. This leads to increased stimulation of the renin-angiotensin-aldosterone system. Sodium and water are reabsorbed, leading to fluid retention and thereby increasing intravascular volume. Initially, this volume retention increases preload and cardiac output. Later, the myocardium becomes more edematous and ventricular function decreases from volume and pressure overload.

The pulmonary system is also affected by this increased volume and interstitial edema develops. In addition, myocardial oxygen consumption increases and may exceed the oxygen availability. Finally, myocardial muscle can undergo cellular and muscular mass changes, or hypertrophy. Without intervention, heart failure progresses until the compensatory mechanisms are no longer effective.

*Bernstein, D. (2011). The cardiovascular system. In R. Kliegman, B. Stanton, J. St. Geme, et al. (Eds.), *Nelson textbook of pediatrics* (19th ed., pp 1527-1604.). St. Louis: Elsevier Saunders.

Manifestations

The earliest clinical manifestations of HF are often subtle. The infant may have mild tachypnea (70 to 100 breaths per minute) at rest and sometimes difficulty feeding. Parents may report that feedings take longer and the child requires frequent rest periods. This type of history describes a scenario where less nutrition is consumed while more energy is expended, resulting in fewer calories being consumed although metabolic demands are increased. Feedings therefore provide little satisfaction, and the infant may appear hungry and irritable soon after a feeding. Over time, the infant fails to gain weight and eventually develops a condition known as failure to thrive (FTT).

Children with HF may also exhibit respiratory-related symptoms. They may complain of dyspnea (particularly on exertion) and tachypnea. They are often described as having less energy than their peers. They may exhibit diaphoresis and complain of decreased appetite. This is due to chronic abdominal pain, usually related to poor circulation and decreased perfusion to the abdominal organs. This can also lead to failure to gain weight. Other clinical manifestations of HF include an abnormal cardiac rhythm known as a gallop; periorbital and facial edema, neck vein distention (in older children), hepatomegaly, and splenomegaly; and decreased peripheral perfusion, decreased urine output, mottling, and cyanosis or pallor.

Diagnostic Evaluation

The diagnosis of HF is established on the basis of clinical history, physical examination, chest radiographic appearance, electrocardiography (ECG), and echocardiography (ECHO). Chest radiographs may reveal cardiomegaly with increased pulmonary vascular markings. These markings reflect increased interstitial pulmonary fluid. Laboratory studies that may be indicated to determine the presence of heart failure in children include determinations of arterial blood gas values, serum electrolyte levels, complete blood cell count, erythrocyte sedimentation rate (ESR), serum glucose and calcium levels, and urinalysis.

Therapeutic Management

Management of a child with HF involves correcting the underlying problem as soon as it is feasible to do so. The medical management of HF is directed toward decreasing cardiac workload and improving cardiac output through the manipulation of the hemodynamics and neurohormonal responses. Supplemental oxygen can be helpful for increasing oxygen saturation, but it should be used with caution in children with left-to-right shunts. Because oxygen is a vasodilator, it may increase pulmonary blood flow. Pharmacologic agents used include positive inotropes (e.g., digoxin), diuretics, and angiotensin-converting enzyme (ACE) inhibitors. In addition, optimizing nutritional intake to meet the metabolic demands and improve growth is of paramount importance. Inability to decrease symptoms and achieve weight gain is an indication for surgical intervention.

Digoxin is a cardiac glycoside that increases cardiac output and improves cardiac effectiveness by several mechanisms. It has a positive inotropic effect that strengthens the force of myocardial contractions. It has a negative chronotropic effect that slows the heart rate and, at higher doses, conduction of cardiac impulses through the AV node, allowing the ventricles more time to fill with blood. It also improves blood flow to the kidneys and enhances diuresis.

Obtain a baseline ECG before initiating digoxin. Digoxin may be administered intravenously (IV) or orally. The effectiveness of digoxin depends on achieving and maintaining a therapeutic serum drug level. A loading or digitalizing dose according to the child's age and weight is administered in divided doses over 12 to 18 hours, and maintenance doses are given daily, usually in two divided doses. The range between therapeutic and toxic digoxin levels is narrow, with the therapeutic range 0.5 to 2.0 ng/mL (Skidmore-Roth, 2011). To avoid a falsely elevated serum digoxin level, serum digoxin levels should be measured at a minimum of 6 hours from the previous dose of digoxin. Measurement in the first 3 to 5 days after digitalizing could also yield elevated results, and so ECG changes are a more accurate sign of an elevated serum digoxin level during this time (Park, 2008). Levels are generally obtained when assessing for toxicity or medication adherence. Digoxin levels may be difficult to measure and monitor in preterm infants (Park, 2008). If a child is receiving digoxin and is having arrhythmias, a digoxin level should be obtained.

◎ NURSING CARE PLAN

The Child with Heart Failure

Focused Assessment

- Closely assess vital signs, cardiovascular status, and pulmonary status
- Observe the child for the worsening signs and symptoms of tachycardia, tachypnea, poor feeding, diaphoresis during feeding, and increased irritability or fatigue
- Obtain a history of fluid and nutritional status, feeding patterns, and growth
- Strictly monitor intake and output
- Weigh daily and report any weight increases

Planning

Nursing Diagnosis

Decreased Cardiac Output related to HF or decreased myocardial function.

Expected Outcome

The child will have adequate cardiac output, as evidenced by pink or baseline cyanotic (in cyanotic heart disease) mucous membranes and nail beds, a capillary refill time of less than 2 seconds, warm extremities, easily palpable peripheral pulses, adequate urinary output, no edema, appropriate heart rate, and an activity level within the normal limits of the defect.

Intervention/Rationale

1. Monitor peripheral perfusion by palpating peripheral pulses, noting temperature, color changes, and capillary refill time.
   Poor peripheral perfusion is usually evidenced by decreased or absent pulses in the extremities. Color and temperature changes (e.g., cyanosis, coolness, mottling) may be present in all extremities. Prolonged capillary refill time is an additional sign of poor perfusion.
2. Determine whether heart rate is appropriate for level of activity.
   Tachycardia occurs in an attempt to maintain adequate cardiac output.
3. Monitor and document hourly urine output.
   Altered renal perfusion caused by decreased cardiac output results in decreased urinary output.
4. Maintain a neutral thermal environment; use a warmer bed or incubator for the neonate; treat fever promptly.
   Episodes of hypothermia or hyperthermia increase oxygen demands and increase the cardiac workload.
5. Time nursing interventions to allow the infant or child rest periods. Anticipate and respond quickly to stressful events, crying, or restlessness.
   Rest periods reduce cardiac workload. Organizing nursing activities to promote rest results in decreased stress and fatigue for the child.
6. Administer digoxin (Lanoxin) as prescribed. Ascertain that the dosage is within safe limits. Count the apical rate for 1 full minute. Check the dosage with a second nurse. Withhold the dose and notify the physician if the heart rate is less than 100 beats/min in infants; the heart rate at which the medication should be withheld varies in older children and adolescents. If the withholding pulse rate is not ordered, withhold the medication and call the physician if the pulse rate is progressively decreasing or markedly lower than previous rates. Observe for signs of toxicity, and monitor for hyperkalemia in the child taking potassium-sparing diuretics.
   Digoxin is effective within a narrow therapeutic range (0.5-2 ng/mL)* although the pediatric range is not well defined. Safety in dosing is achieved by double checking the dose and counting the apical heart rate for a full minute. Digoxin toxicity can manifest with slow pulse, vomiting, and arrhythmias.

Evaluation

Are mucous membranes and nail beds pink or baseline cyanotic?
Is the capillary refill time less than 2 seconds?
Are peripheral pulses easily palpated, and is the child alert and active?
Is the heart rate in the expected range for activity?

Planning

Nursing Diagnosis

Excess Fluid Volume related to volume overload and HF.

Expected Outcome

The infant or child will remain free of evidence of fluid overload (e.g., infrequent urination, inappropriate water weight gain, inadequate balance between intake and output, edema [periorbital, hepatomegaly], respiratory distress, poor feeding).

Intervention/Rationale

1. Administer diuretics as prescribed, ensuring correct dosage, route, and effectiveness.
   Diuretics help the body eliminate excess fluid. Their effectiveness is evaluated from the urine output (either by measuring the amount of urine or by weighing diapers), weight, decreasing edema, decreasing respiratory distress, and improved feeding.
2. Maintain accurate intake and output records. The fluid intake and output should be about the same.
   If intake grossly exceeds output, the diuretics may need to be altered, the child may need fluid restriction, or both.
3. Maintain fluid restriction, if ordered.
   Fluid restriction will decrease pulmonary and liver edema.
4. Using the same scales, weigh the child daily at approximately the same time. Notify the physician of excessive weight gain (>50 g/day in infants, >200 g/day in children).
   Excess fluid volume is not always overtly visible. Weight changes may indicate fluid retention. Weighing the infant or child on the same scales at the same time each day ensures consistency.
5. Provide skin care and change position frequently.
   Edematous areas are extremely prone to skin breakdown because of stretching and opacity. Frequent position changes will prevent undesirable pooling of fluid in certain areas.
6. Monitor for increased or decreased edema (in infants and young children, edema is usually periorbital) and hepatomegaly; generalized edema in the preoperative patient is extremely rare.
   Changes in the amount of edema can indicate the effectiveness or ineffectiveness of therapies and interventions.
7. Monitor serum electrolyte levels, especially potassium.
   Diuretics may stimulate potassium loss.

Evaluation

Is the child urinating frequently in comparison with age-related norms (see Chapter 16)?
Is the child edematous?
Has the child lost or gained weight?
Are intake and output balanced?

Planning

Nursing Diagnosis

Ineffective Breathing Pattern related to pulmonary congestion.

Expected Outcomes

The child will demonstrate a respiratory rate within normal limits for age and a normal respiratory effort.
The child will have satisfactory rest periods.
The child will have color that remains pink or baseline cyanotic.

---

*Skidmore-Roth, L. (2011). *Mosby's nursing drug reference* (24th ed.). St. Louis: Elsevier Mosby.

The Child with Heart Failure—cont'd

Intervention/Rationale

1. Monitor respiratory rate and rhythm, the presence or absence of retractions or nasal flaring, the use of accessory muscles, and the presence or absence of crackles or rhonchi.
   Infants and children with HF have changes in their breathing pattern because of increased fluid retention in the lungs, liver, and other areas of the body.

2. Position the infant or child with the head of the bed elevated 30 to 45 degrees. Avoid clothing that constricts the chest. *An elevated position lowers the diaphragm and maximizes chest expansion.*

3. Administer oxygen as needed.
   Supplemental oxygen administration improves oxygen saturation and delivery to tissues. Cautious use of oxygen is indicated in left-to-right shunting lesions because of the effect of oxygen on lowering pulmonary vascular resistance, which can increase pulmonary blood flow and increase the degree of pulmonary congestion and symptoms of HF.

4. Plan nursing interventions to allow maximum rest for the child. Feed the child when the child is rested. Avoid performing multiple interventions at any one time.
   Clustering nursing activities decreases the child's fatigue, promotes feeding effort, and conserves metabolic demands.

5. Prevent exposure to individuals with respiratory illnesses. Prevent nosocomial exposures and infections.
   Respiratory infections with associated CHD can have a severe adverse impact on respiratory stability. Children with CHD are at a higher risk for nosocomial infections.

Evaluation

Is the child's respiratory rate within normal limits for age?
Are the child's mucous membranes and nail beds pink or at baseline cyanosis?
Is the child breathing easily?
Is the child able to obtain an appropriate amount of rest?

Planning

Nursing Diagnosis

Imbalanced Nutrition: Less Than Body Requirements related to increased energy expenditure and increased feeding effort.

Expected Outcome

The infant or child will demonstrate appropriate weight gain and no significant loss of weight over a short period.

Intervention/Rationale

1. Weigh the infant or child daily or before and after each feeding for breastfed infants. Use the same scale.
   Using the same scale ensures consistency.

2. Breastfeed or feed smaller volumes of concentrated formula (24-27 cal/oz) every 3 hours.
   Increased caloric content of formula increases caloric consumption and enhances weight gain. May require 120 to 150 kcal/kg/day for adequate weight gain. Additives are available that increase the caloric content of breast milk.

3. Use a nipple that the infant can comfortably adjust for flow rate and energy to express milk. May need a soft, large-hole nipple.
   Infants with HF tire easily. An appropriate nipple for the infant minimizes the level of energy required to express milk at a rate of flow the baby can swallow comfortably. A soft nipple with a large hole may facilitate easy sucking and decrease energy expenditure during feeding.

4. Implement gavage feedings if the infant tires before the recommended amount of feeding is consumed, takes longer than 30 minutes to feed, displays increased fatigue during or after feeding, or demonstrates poor weight gain on adequate caloric intake.

Gavage feedings decrease energy expenditure and allow calories consumed to be used for growth. Can be used in conjunction with timed nipple periods to maintain feeding skills.

5. Time the feedings to allow for adequate rest. Every 3 hours is a frequently used interval.
   Frequent disturbances increase oxygen consumption. Too frequent feedings disturb rest, whereas less frequent feedings require increased intake, which tires the infant.

6. Monitor for feeding intolerance.
   May not tolerate concentrated formulas. Also, gastroesophageal reflux may be present.

Evaluation

Has the infant or child maintained a steady weight gain?
Is the feeding pattern stable or changing?
Is the infant or child tolerating feedings without vomiting or other signs of intolerance?

Planning

Nursing Diagnosis

Deficient Knowledge related to anxiety and unfamiliarity with the disease process, treatment, interventions, and home care.

Expected Outcomes

Parents will describe the cardiac defect and current and future interventions.
Parents will demonstrate an ability to perform treatments, including medication administration.

Intervention/Rationale

1. Determine the parents' readiness to learn, anxiety level, knowledge needed to care for their child, and specific concerns. A baseline assessment of prior knowledge should be considered before developing a teaching plan.
   Addressing special concerns initially can facilitate parents' comfort level and receptiveness to new knowledge. Decreasing anxiety assists with information processing.

2. Provide brief, factual explanations of the child's defect or any treatments and interventions. Do so frequently.
   Parents are most likely to retain consistent, repetitive explanations.

3. Allow the parents and child to verbalize feelings and concerns related to hospitalization and caring for the child at home.
   Hospitalization is a frightening experience. By allowing verbalization of feelings and concerns related to the experience, nurses can assist in allaying fears and addressing concerns. Discussing care at home can also assist in allaying fears and addressing concerns.

4. Teach the parents to administer all necessary cardiac medications and explain their associated actions and potential adverse effects. Provide demonstrations and obtain return demonstrations by parents. Explain the use of oral syringes for accurate measurement of drugs. Provide a daily medication chart (which can be color-coded for specific medications) for children receiving multiple medications. Provide parents with written information about home care and signs and symptoms of concern (see Patient-Centered Teaching: Giving Your Child Digoxin Elixir box).
   Successful return demonstrations increase parents' confidence. Written information provides a ready reference for questions in the home setting.

Evaluation

Have the parents verbalized adequate and correct knowledge of the diagnosis and interventions?
Have the parents demonstrated confidence and competence in caregiving activities, including medicine administration?
Are the parents able to describe conditions that necessitate a call for medical or nursing advice?

Hypokalemia and hypomagnesemia can increase the risk for digoxin toxicity. In a child with altered renal function, the dosage needs to be decreased.

Diuretics are administered to eliminate excess water and sodium through increased urine production, thereby reducing systemic and pulmonary congestion. Furosemide is a potent loop diuretic and is preferred for initial diuretic therapy. Another classification of diuretics, the thiazides, acts at the distal renal tubules. These can be less potent than loop diuretics. These drugs cause the kidneys to waste potassium, placing the child at risk for hypokalemia. Potassium-sparing diuretics, such as spironolactone, are weak diuretics. This class of diuretics is often given with loop diuretics or thiazides to decrease the potential for hypokalemia. Potassium supplements can also be given in tandem with diuretics to replace these losses.

Vasodilators, such as hydralazine, captopril, or enalapril, may be used to relax vascular smooth muscles and reduce afterload (Park,

---

EVIDENCE-BASED PRACTICE

Breastfeeding Infants with Congenital Heart Disease

Level VI

In 2005, the American Academy of Pediatrics (AAP) updated its policy on breastfeeding for infants. Asserting that the beneficial effects of breastfeeding include protection from infection and enhanced maternal infant bonding, among others, the AAP recommends exclusive breastfeeding, or provision of breast milk by bottle, for the first 4 to 6 months of life, preferably until the child reaches 1 year of age or beyond.* In its report, the AAP (2005) recommends that health professionals provide support and education for breastfeeding mothers, promote policies that facilitate breastfeeding, and change policies that discourage breastfeeding (e.g., formula packages, discount coupons for formula, separating mother and infant in acute care settings).

As an important part of its policy on breastfeeding, the AAP states that breastfeeding should not be precluded for most high-risk neonates and infants. This includes infants with CHD who can derive the full benefits of breastfeeding from direct feeding or expressed milk (fortified or unfortified) from a bottle.*

Little nursing research exists that specifically addresses the benefits or problems associated with breastfeeding infants who have CHD. In the review of literature section of a recent study looking at breastfeeding in this infant population, Barbas and Kelleher (2004) cite data suggesting benefits of breastfeeding that include higher and more stable oxygen saturation measurements, improved weight gain, and shorter hospital stays. The major impediment to breastfeeding infants with CHD appears to be health professional attitudes and in-hospital practices that are discouraging to mothers who wish to breastfeed their infants.

The purpose of Barbas and Kelleher's Level VI study was to explore and describe breastfeeding outcomes, which included (1) length of time infants continued to breastfeed or receive expressed breast milk, (2) mothers' satisfaction with breastfeeding, and (3) perception of the level of breastfeeding support.† Mothers of 68 infants with various types of CHD were surveyed by mail 6 months after their children's discharge from a large children's medical center that had initiated a lactation support program for mothers of high-risk infants. The study occurred over a 2-year time period. Included in the study were infants who had had cardiac surgery before 1 month of age, who breastfed during their hospitalization, and whose mothers received breastfeeding education and support. The objective questionnaire requested information about preoperative breastfeeding patterns, postoperative breastfeeding patterns, maternal breastfeeding goals, and breastfeeding satisfaction; qualitative comments also were collected.†

Results from this study demonstrated some important aspects about breastfeeding in the infant with CHD. Most mothers reported a prebirth breastfeeding goal compatible with the AAP policy recommendation of exclusive breastfeeding for 6 months followed by continued breastfeeding for as long as possible; approximately half revised and met their goal to include combined breastfeeding and bottle feeding, fortifying with additional sources of calories, or expressing milk for bottle feeding.† Significant factors that contributed to satisfaction included the ability to exclusively breastfeed and the ability to increase breastfeeding after the infant's discharge from the hospital. As the study progressed, qualitative comments indicated a more positive perception of the support provided by nurses and other professionals and a marked increase in the number of mothers who initiated and persisted with breastfeeding. The authors conclude that, despite a relatively small sample size, some self-selection and recall bias, and a sample drawn from a center committed to lactation support, breastfeeding rates in infants with congenital cardiac disease are positively related to accepting attitudes by nurses and other health professionals, improved knowledge and education about the benefits of breastfeeding in this population, and hospital facilities and policies that enhance and facilitate maternal breastfeeding goals.†

Think about the implication of this research on clinical practice. When a nurse cares for infants who have CHD in a hospital setting, what kinds of policies, procedures, and resources might need to be readily available to facilitate breastfeeding initiation or the provision of breast milk? What suggestions might a student nurse think about for continued research in this area?

*American Academy of Pediatrics. (2005). Policy statement: Breastfeeding and the use of human milk. *Pediatrics, 115*, 496-506.
†Barbas, K., & Kelleher, D. (2004). Breastfeeding success among infants with congenital heart disease. *Pediatric Nursing, 30*, 285-297.

? CRITICAL THINKING EXERCISE 22-1

Lin, a 2-month-old infant, is seen in the pediatrician's office. She has gained 1 pound since birth and has a murmur. She is admitted to the pediatric unit with a diagnosis of HF. You will obtain a health history and perform an admission assessment.

1. What specific questions should you ask Lin's parents about her feeding patterns and behavior?
2. What physical assessment findings would you expect in an infant with HF?

List nursing interventions that would address Lin's nutritional and comfort needs.

! NURSING QUALITY ALERT

Feeding the Infant or Child with Heart Failure

Feed the infant or child in a relaxed environment. Time the feedings before multiple other activities to preserve the infant's energy. The infant with HF tends to tire easily during feedings. Frequent, small feedings may be less tiring. Holding the infant in an upright position may provide less stomach compression and improve respiratory effort during the feeding. If the child is unable to consume an appropriate amount during a 30-minute feeding period every 3 hours, nasogastric (NG) or nasoduodenal (ND) feedings should be considered. Assess for increased tachypnea, diaphoresis, or feeding intolerance (vomiting). Concentrating formula from the basic level of 20 kcal/oz to 24-30 kcal/oz, depending on age, can increase caloric intake without increasing the infant's work.

2008). Captopril and enalapril are called ACE inhibitors because they block the conversion of angiotensin I to angiotensin II and reduce vasoconstriction and sodium retention. In addition, ACE inhibitors also decrease norepinephrine release from the sympathetic nervous system.

PATIENT-CENTERED TEACHING

Giving Your Child Digoxin Elixir

Medication: Digoxin (Lanoxin)

Your child's dosage: _____ mL twice a day. Your child will be taking this medicine twice a day for several months to years.

What it does: Digoxin (Lanoxin) helps the heart pump blood more effectively, thereby improving the circulation of the blood, and promoting the normal elimination of excess fluid.

What you need to know:

- Digoxin (Lanoxin) is usually given every morning and evening. You may adjust the times to fit your and your child's schedule.
- Give the digoxin 20 to 30 minutes before a feeding. Give it at the same time every day so that it becomes part of your routine.
- The amount of digoxin you give your child must be measured carefully with a syringe, not the dropper provided with the medicine.
- Put a few drops of digoxin in your child's mouth and let the child swallow it before giving more.
- If you forget to give your child a single dose of digoxin, give the dose when you remember it; then resume your original schedule.
- If your child vomits after taking the digoxin, do not repeat the dose. Resume the digoxin at the next dosage time.
- *If you miss or your child vomits two doses in a row, call the cardiology department.*
- Rarely, children have too much digoxin in their body and can have vomiting. If your child vomits, call your pediatrician or cardiologist. You will be instructed what to do about your child's dosage.
- Keep the digoxin in a place where children living or playing in your home will not be able to reach it.
- If someone accidentally takes the digoxin, call poison control or take the person and the digoxin bottle to the emergency department.
- Obtain refills at least 1 week before you are out of medicine. Ask for new prescriptions as needed.

Modified and used with permission from Children's Hospital Oakland, Department of Cardiology, Oakland, CA. Developed and revised by Lili Cook, RN, MS, and Sally Higgins, PhD, RN, FAAN.

Pulmonary Hypertension

Pulmonary hypertension (PAH) is elevated blood pressure in the blood vessels of the lungs. Pulmonary hypertension is diagnosed when the mean pulmonary arterial pressure exceeds 20 mm Hg at rest (normal is 15 mm Hg at rest) (Park, 2008). The most common cause of pulmonary hypertension in children is congenital heart disease (Adatia, Kothari, & Feinstein, 2010). Initially, in an infant with a significant left-to-right shunting defect there is reversible pulmonary vasoconstriction and increased pulmonary blood flow that causes elevated pulmonary artery pressure. Pulmonary hypertension occurs over time when vascular changes eventually lead to vessel wall thickening, severe irreversible vasoconstriction, and vascular obstruction. This severe condition leads to a reversal of the cardiac shunting, becoming right-to-left (called *Eisenmenger syndrome*), with less blood being pumped to the lungs, so that a previously acyanotic child becomes

cyanotic as oxygen-poor blood gets pumped to the body. It is critical to time any surgical intervention before the development of irreversible vascular changes. This information is assessed clinically and in the cardiac catheterization laboratory. Repair of lesions with large left-to-right shunts is generally recommended in the first 3 to 6 months of life.

A child with a large left-to-right shunting lesion, particularly at the ventricular level, will have high pulmonary artery pressures but low pulmonary vascular resistance. Initially HF develops. Management is directed toward treating the symptoms of HF, including digitalis, diuretics, warfarin, and supplemental oxygen. Additionally, the family is advised to have the child avoid strenuous exercise and high altitudes. Vasodilators may be helpful if the child demonstrates adequate response when these medications are given during cardiac catheterization (Park, 2008). Inhaled nitric oxide has been shown to be an effective pulmonary vasodilator and is used in the treatment of persistent pulmonary hypertension of the newborn.

Pulmonary hypertension can also have heritable (genetic mutations) or idiopathic etiologies. Idiopathic disease occurs when no underlying disease can be found. Conditions leading to pulmonary hypertension include alveolar hypoxia, such as pulmonary parenchymal disease or airway obstruction that leads to vasoconstriction. Pulmonary venous hypertension is seen in left heart outflow obstructive lesions and connective tissue disorders.

There are many research studies and ongoing trials for PAH-specific therapies in children, but with early surgical intervention, a child with reversible pulmonary hypertension can have a return of normal pulmonary pressures postoperatively. Early intervention is important because, as increasing pulmonary vascular resistance caused by pulmonary vascular changes develops, the child will have an increased risk for surgical morbidity and mortality and for development of irreversible pulmonary hypertension. Management of a child with idiopathic or advanced pulmonary hypertension remains challenging, because current pharmacologic therapies (e.g., IV epoprostenol or oral bosentan) have somewhat improved survival but have not adequately addressed disease progression (Dunbar Ivy, Rosenzweig, LeMarie et al., 2010).

Cyanosis

Cyanosis, a bluish discoloration of the skin, nail beds, and mucous membranes, appears when tissues are deprived of adequate amounts of oxygen. Cyanosis becomes visible when hemoglobin that is not bound to oxygen reaches a level of approximately 5 g/dL blood and the measured oxygen saturation drops below 85%. A cardiac lesion produces cyanosis when desaturated blood from the venous system enters the arterial system without passing through the lungs, commonly through an abnormal opening that allows for shunting of the desaturated blood.

The degree of cyanosis varies; some children will appear pale and mildly cyanotic, whereas others will be quite dusky. In an anemic infant or child, the level of desaturation will be higher before cyanosis becomes apparent, because the lower hemoglobin level in anemia means that a larger percentage of the hemoglobin must be desaturated before cyanosis becomes visible. Concurrently, a child with significant *polycythemia* (increased number of red blood cells with resulting elevated hemoglobin level) will appear cyanotic when a lesser amount of hemoglobin is desaturated, because the higher hemoglobin level in polycythemia means that a smaller percentage must be desaturated before cyanosis is seen.

Cyanosis can occur when blood flow to the lungs is decreased (e.g., in severe pulmonary artery stenosis, pulmonary atresia, tetralogy of Fallot, or tricuspid atresia) or when desaturated blood is pumped to the body (e.g., in total anomalous pulmonary venous return, truncus arteriosus, and hypoplastic left heart syndrome). Cyanosis intensifies with crying in a child with these defects and is not alleviated by the administration of 100% oxygen.

The clinical consequences of cyanosis include polycythemia, anemia, clotting abnormalities, hypercyanotic episodes, central nervous system (CNS) injury caused by abscess or embolic events, pulmonary hypertension, and endocarditis. Developmental delay can be related to CNS injury, severe hypoxic events, or chronic illness.

Polycythemia is a compensatory response of the body to chronic hypoxia. The body attempts to improve tissue oxygenation by increasing the oxygen-carrying capacity of the blood—in other words, by producing additional red blood cells. Accelerated red blood cell production increases the viscosity of the blood and crowds the vascular space so there is less room for plasma and clotting factors. A child who is polycythemic is at greater risk for bruising and prolonged bleeding because of decreased specific clotting factors.

Increased blood viscosity makes the peripheral circulation sluggish and places the child at risk for CNS injury from a brain abscess or cerebrovascular accident. Depletion of iron stores may also result, and anemia may develop if iron is not available to participate in hemoglobin formation.

Dehydration can occur rapidly in a child with cyanotic heart disease. Hyperthermia (fever or environmental), poor oral intake, vomiting, and diarrhea can cause acute dehydration. Dehydration can be life threatening for the child with cyanotic heart disease because the fluid loss can contribute to the relative viscosity of the blood. The increased viscosity can close a shunt that is necessary for pulmonary blood flow (shunt thrombosis). Once the shunt closes, there is no pulmonary blood flow, resulting in metabolic acidosis and severe hypoxemia that can lead to cardiopulmonary arrest.

Hypercyanotic Episode

A serious, clinically significant, and dramatic event seen in children with cyanotic heart disease is the hypercyanotic episode. These events are often called *tet spells* because they frequently occur in children with unrepaired tetralogy of Fallot. The exact cause is unknown, but it is thought that the child has acute spasm of the right ventricular outflow tract as a result of agitation or another adverse event that dramatically decreases pulmonary blood flow, causing hypoxia and metabolic acidosis (Bernstein, 2011). These episodes include rapid and deep respirations, irritability and crying, peripheral vasodilation, increased systemic venous return, increasing cyanosis that can be very severe, and a decrease in the systolic murmur, reflecting decreased pulmonary blood flow (Bernstein, 2011). As the child becomes more cyanotic, the child has increased tachypnea and hyperpnea, which increase the degree of right-to-left shunting. The incidence of hypercyanotic spells is not directly related to the degree of baseline desaturation and cyanosis.

Hypercyanotic episodes are seen most frequently in the first 2 years of life and seem to occur mainly in the morning. Often the episode is preceded by crying, feeding, or defecation. The infant becomes agitated and may eventually lose consciousness. Although usually self-limiting, the spells can progress to a vicious cycle that can be fatal if not recognized and treated. Frequent or prolonged episodes may lead to diminished cerebral oxygenation and ischemic brain injury.

Treatment of the episode includes calming the infant, placing the infant in the knee-chest position, and administering oxygen. Morphine sulfate is administered to suppress the respiratory center and decrease the degree of hyperpnea (which contributes to vasodilation) (Park, 2008). Potent medications that cause vasoconstriction (e.g., phenylephrine) may be needed to increase systemic vascular resistance, decrease the degree of right-to-left shunting, and force blood into the pulmonary system. Preventing or treating hypovolemia is also an important factor. Hypercyanotic episodes indicate the need to surgically repair or palliate the defect.

NURSING CARE OF THE CHILD WITH CYANOSIS

Assessment

The nurse must know the source of pulmonary blood flow when caring for a child with cyanotic heart disease. An infant or child who is dependent on a shunt for pulmonary blood flow is at risk for shunt thrombosis (as detailed earlier). An infant with a right-to-left shunt is at increased risk for an arterial air embolus from an IV line because a small embolus can cross directly from the venous circulation to the arterial circulation through the shunt.

Evaluation of the child with cyanotic heart disease includes an assessment of baseline cyanosis and general appearance. Assess the level of activity, including irritability. Visible cyanosis is most easily seen in natural light and is evaluated by observing the skin of the central mucous membranes of the mouth and conjunctiva and the nail beds. General skin color is also assessed. Cyanotic children may be smaller than their peers and may demonstrate clubbing, thickening, and flattening of the fingertips and toes as a result of polycythemia (see Figure 21-6). Oxygen saturations should be obtained and compared with the child's baselines. To prevent infective endocarditis, some children with unrepaired cardiac defects require antibiotic prophylaxis for certain dental and surgical procedures until the defect is repaired and for several months afterward. This includes children who have had infective endocarditis; therefore, the nurse needs to document this.

The child may become dyspneic during feeding, crying, and other activities that require exertion and may have difficulty keeping up with peers. Children with cyanosis may have frequent respiratory infections, may miss more school days, and may, as a result, academically lag behind their classmates, although they are often developmentally normal. If the child requires an IV line for hydration or another indication, it is imperative that the nurse assess IV line patency and inspect IV tubing for the presence of air in the line because even a small amount of air in the circulation increases the risk of systemic air emboli causing a stroke or heart attack.. The use of an air filter is recommended.

Nursing Diagnosis and Planning

Nursing diagnoses and expected outcomes typical for the child with cyanosis and the child's family include the following:

- Deficient Knowledge related to inexperience with the management of a child with a life-threatening illness.

Expected Outcomes. The parents, and child if age appropriate, will explain the disease process, treatment, and interventions and will demonstrate the ability to perform home care treatments, including medication administration.

- Interrupted Family Processes related to impact of an acute, chronic, or life-threatening disease.

Expected Outcomes. The parents will express positive feelings for their child and for each other and will demonstrate the ability to meet the needs of the child, each other, and other family members.

- Delayed Growth and Development related to altered oxygenation or inadequate cardiac output to meet metabolic needs.

Expected Outcomes. The child will demonstrate adequate growth according to an optimal growth curve for age and condition and will perform motor, social, and expressive skills typical of age-group within the scope of the child's present capabilities. The parents will describe any developmental delay or deviation and make plans for intervention.

- Ineffective Peripheral Tissue Perfusion related to hypercyanotic episodes.

Expected Outcomes. The child will remain free of decreased tissue perfusion, as evidenced by the absence of profound cyanosis and by the child's activity level, affect, respiratory status, and oxygenation all being normal. The parents will list signs and symptoms that would signal the onset of hypercyanotic episodes.

- Risk for Infection related to the presence of infection-promoting conditions created by the underlying defect.

Expected Outcomes. The child will remain free of endocardial infection. The parents will understand and carry out any ordered antibiotic prophylaxis; and the parents will list when to seek medical attention for fevers.

- Deficient Knowledge related to unfamiliarity with the systemic complications from increased risk of clotting.

Expected Outcome. The parents will describe the signs and symptoms to report immediately, including increasing cyanosis, vomiting, and fever (signs of clotting of the pulmonary shunt), and new-onset facial or extremity weakness, slurred speech, clumsiness, or breathing difficulty (signs of a CNS clot).

■ Interventions

Cyanotic heart disease is usually diagnosed in the newborn period. The initial nursing interventions are directed toward stabilizing and preparing the child for medical or surgical intervention. Pulmonary blood flow in cyanotic heart disease may depend on the persistence of the ductus arteriosus. Prostaglandin (PGE$_1$), a vasodilator, is often administered to maintain ductal patency and restore pulmonary or systemic blood flow. Continuous infusion of the drug may improve arterial oxygen saturation and tissue perfusion, allowing the infant to be stabilized in anticipation of further diagnostic and treatment interventions. PGE$_1$ is rapidly metabolized through the pulmonary circulation and excreted through the renal system. It must be infused by continuous IV administration. The major side effect is apnea, and infants frequently require intubation. The nurse is responsible for monitoring PGE$_1$ infusion flow and evaluating peripheral perfusion and respiratory status.

Parental teaching and support at the time of diagnosis are a priority. Parents receive complicated information and are often asked to make important decisions that may affect their child's current therapy and, perhaps, future interventions. Parents need simple yet thorough explanations to help them make informed choices. The nurse may need to repeat the information several times. Help parents identify sources of emotional support and encourage communication within the family.

Parents of children with a cardiovascular disorder respond with a variety of reactions. Knowing this, the nurse has a responsibility to educate parents about their child's disorder and to stress the importance of the child interacting with the environment as normally as possible. For effective planning and provision of care, the child's condition must be placed in the context of the family's life.

In the child with cyanosis, careful monitoring of fluid status is necessary to prevent hemoconcentration. Intake and output are closely monitored, and daily weights may be recorded during hospitalization. Teach parents to recognize illnesses that place their child at risk for dehydration and to seek medical attention when their child has fluid losses.

Parents have concerns about worsening cyanosis and fear hypercyanotic episodes. Teach parents to recognize events that may trigger an episode and to respond calmly and place the infant in a knee-chest position. Review indications to seek medical care. Because most children with cyanosis limit their own physical activities, parents do not need to strictly limit the child's activities.

Prevention of infective endocarditis (IE) may be necessary for select patients and is accomplished through antibiotic prophylaxis. Parents may be given a copy of the American Heart Associations (AHA) guidelines (2008). Compared with previous guidelines, fewer patients are candidates to receive prophylaxis.

Children with cyanosis are prone to frequent respiratory infections. Respiratory infections may increase cardiac workload and lead to increased cyanosis and desaturation. Careful hand hygiene is necessary to reduce the risk of infection. Teach parents to avoid crowded areas and contact between their child and other people with respiratory infections.

The nurse's role includes the astute and vigilant assessment, monitoring, and collaborative treatment of a child with known or potential cardiovascular alterations. Rapid changes in acuity and decompensation can occur in children with certain congenital and acquired heart diseases. Thus the skills required of the pediatric nurse must be focused and refined to identify clinically significant changes that may have an impact on this often-complex population.

■ Evaluation

- Can the parent, or child (if appropriate), describe the cardiac defect and its implications?
- Are the parents able to monitor their child's condition, provide home treatments, administer medications, and support the child's fluid and nutritional needs?
- Are family members appropriately expressing feelings and supporting each other and the child, and can the parents meet the needs of siblings and each other?
- Is the child showing a steady increase in physical growth and attaining age-appropriate developmental milestones?
- Is the child undergoing any change in the level of cyanosis, activity, or respiratory status and oxygenation?
- Can the parents describe signs, symptoms, and management of hypercyanotic episodes?
- Is the child afebrile and free of other signs and symptoms of infection, and can the parents explain the necessity for seeking medical attention for any fevers?
- Are the parents able to list complications related to possible pulmonary shunt or CNS clotting?

ASSESSMENT OF THE CHILD WITH A CARDIOVASCULAR ALTERATION

Serious congenital cardiac lesions usually become symptomatic early in infancy. Remarkable technologic advances in the understanding of the cardiovascular system's function and needs have led to refinements in the tools and techniques for detecting, diagnosing, and treating congenital heart defects. Invasive procedures are now required less for initial diagnosis but rather to obtain more detailed hemodynamic information and for interventional procedures. Nevertheless, no tool or technique replaces obtaining a comprehensive history from both the child and the parents and performing a thorough physical examination (Table 22-2).

The cardiac assessment should take place in a quiet and nonthreatening environment with a parent present if possible. Parents know their child best, and they can offer a time line of events and subtle clinical information that may not be evident on examination. The nurse needs to establish an atmosphere of trust and cooperation—cardiac assessment is best and most easily performed on a cooperative infant or child.

The room should be warm and well lit. Natural light from windows will allow the nurse to accurately assess skin color. The assessment should begin with the least threatening steps—the history and inspection. During the parent interview, the child has the opportunity to observe the interaction between nurse and parent and has time to become comfortable with the nurse's presence. The child should be allowed to participate in the assessment and encouraged to touch and inspect each piece of equipment to be used during the examination.

Assessment progression includes inspection, auscultation, and palpation; each step requires more touching. The nurse must remember to warm the stethoscope used for auscultation, as well as the hands before touching the child's skin. This is particularly important when assessing a resting infant, who may become startled by the cold touch of the hands and stethoscope.

CARDIOVASCULAR DIAGNOSIS

Tests used to diagnose cardiac problems in children have been described previously. Cardiac catheterization is still considered the gold standard by which all other therapeutic modalities are measured. It usually constitutes the final definitive diagnostic test for many patients.

TABLE 22-2   CARDIAC ASSESSMENT FOR THE CHILD WITH CHD*

ASSESSMENT GUIDELINES	FINDINGS AND COMMENTS
Health History	
Inquire about a family history of CHD, sudden death, or fetal/infant death.	There may be an increased incidence of CHD in some families.
Ask about prenatal care, maternal illnesses, infections, medications taken during pregnancy.	Chronic maternal illness such as diabetes, lupus, perinatal infections such as rubella, and certain medications such as lithium have been linked to CHD.
Discuss pregnancy, birth history, associated birth defects or genetic anomalies.	There is an increased incidence of CHD with certain genetic anomalies or birth defects. Cyanosis, murmur, or other cardiac event present at birth may indicate cardiac disease.
Discuss feeding difficulties (including decreased intake or increased rest periods during feeding), tachypnea or increased work of breathing, frequency of respiratory infections, poor weight gain, fatigue, exercise intolerance, color changes with crying or Valsalva maneuvers, diaphoresis.	Poor weight gain and failure to thrive are often associated with cardiac disease. Cyanosis may be more prominent with crying or Valsalva maneuvers.
Inspection	
Color:	
Assess skin color in natural light if possible.	Central cyanosis can reflect cardiac or pulmonary alterations. Differential cyanosis may indicate complex heart disease that is dependent on PDA blood flow for systemic or pulmonary blood flow. Pallor, mottling, or ruddiness may indicate cardiac disease. Acrocyanosis (a painless disorder caused by constriction or narrowing of small blood vessels in the skin) may be seen in the healthy newborn.
Pay special attention to oral mucous membranes, nail beds, and conjunctiva, which can reflect central cyanosis.	
Assess hands, feet, and face.	
Assess body for differential or demarcated cyanosis or color differences.	
	Clubbing of nail beds may indicate chronic hypoxia. Usually present after 6 mo of arterial desaturation (see Figure 21-6).
Activity level:	Lethargy, irritability, or restlessness may indicate poor cardiac function.
Assess child while sitting and lying down.	
Observe level of activity and position of comfort.	Squatting may indicate cyanotic heart disease and attempts to improve hypoxia.
Observe for color changes with activity, feeding, or crying.	
Observe for exercise tolerance, including any respiratory distress or frequent rest.	
Chest:	PMI (apical pulse) may be seen in thin children. It is found at fourth left ICS in young children and fifth ICS in children older than 7 years. In neonates, PMI does not correspond with apical pulse. It is found at fourth ICS and can be more midline toward xiphoid because of right ventricular dominance in the fetal and neonatal heart.
Assess precordial activity, chest movement (including symmetry), and chest shape (including convex or concave).	
Assess for sternotomy or thoracotomy incisions.	
	An active precordium may indicate cardiac disease.
	A convex chest cavity shape may indicate cardiac disease.
Respiratory pattern:	Increased work of breathing and respiratory difficulty may indicate HF.
Observe work of breathing at rest and with activity, including feeding.	
Look for signs of respiratory alteration or distress (tachypnea, retractions, nasal flaring, crackles, grunting, and head bobbing are late signs of distress and may indicate impending respiratory failure).	

*A thorough cardiac workup will often include chest radiography, ECG, and echocardiogram.

TABLE 22-2   CARDIAC ASSESSMENT FOR THE CHILD WITH CHD—cont'd

ASSESSMENT GUIDELINES	FINDINGS AND COMMENTS
Auscultation	
Heart sounds	Heart sounds should be synchronous with palpable central or peripheral pulse.
Auscultate with both bell (for low-pitched sounds) and diaphragm (for high-pitched sounds) of stethoscope.	Rhythm normally is regular. A normal variation is sinus arrhythmia when the rhythm can alter and rate can increase with inspiration and decrease with expiration.
	Ask the older child to briefly hold a breath to allow the nurse to hear more clearly.
Identify first and second heart sounds.	S_1 is heard best at apex of heart (fourth or fifth ICS at left midclavicular line) and reflects closure of mitral and tricuspid valves. Correlates with palpable pulse.
	S_2 is heard best at base (right and left of sternum at second ICS) and reflects closure of aortic and pulmonic valves.
Identify additional heart sounds (S_3, S_4). These can be assessed with the child lying supine or on the left side.	S_3 can be heard at the LLSB or apex and can be a normal finding or reflect CHF.
	S_4 can be heard at the LLSB or apex and reflects cardiac disease.
	A gallop is an extra heart sound (S_3 or S_4), common in HF.
Identify presence of murmurs, clicks, precordial friction rubs.	Murmurs are caused by turbulent blood flow.
	Murmurs are described according to location, timing within cardiac cycle, intensity, pitch, quality, and duration.
	Clicks reflect abnormal valve motion.
	Precordial friction rubs can reflect pericardial inflammation.
Palpation	
Temperature	
Compare temperature of trunk with temperature of extremities.	Cooler extremities may indicate poor perfusion because of decreased cardiac output.
	If room is cold, cool extremities may indicate vasoconstriction to conserve heat.
Pulses	
Compare central and distal pulses.	Peripheral pulses may be diminished if cardiac output is impaired. Causes include HF and dehydration.
Assess pulses in all four extremities.	Weak or absent pulses in the lower extremities may indicate coarctation of the aorta.
Blood pressure	
Assess in all four extremities during initial assessment.	Discrepancies between upper and lower extremity blood pressure may indicate cardiac disease, including coarctation of the aorta.
Capillary refill	
Assess capillary filling in extremities; use fingertips to compress skin.	Normal is less than 2-3 sec.
Chest	
With fingertips, locate the PMI.	PMI located farther down than normal may indicate cardiac enlargement.
Assess for presence of vibratory thrills, heaves or lifts, or friction rubs.	Thrills are vibratory in nature.
	Heaves or lifts are palpable chest wall movement, separate from the PMI, and reflect hyperactive precordium.
	Friction rubs, caused by the presence of fluid in the cardiac or pleural space, produce a grating sound.
Abdomen	
Locate the liver border. It should be at or slightly below the right costal margin in infants and young children. In the neonate the liver can be 2-3 cm below the right costal margin and still be normal.	Normally the border should be firm and smooth.
	Liver may be boggy with a poorly defined edge and palpable more than 1-2 cm below the right costal margin when HF is present.
Percussion	
Percussion of the chest provides little useful data in a cardiac assessment.	PMI is a better indicator of heart size.

ICS, Intercostal space; *LLSB,* left lower sternal border; *PMI,* point of maximal impulse.

! NURSING QUALITY ALERT

Assessing Murmurs

Develop a systematic approach to assessing heart sounds with every examination. Abnormal heart sounds will be easier to detect once you can recognize a normal heart sound. Consider other clinical findings, including fatigue associated with anemia and fever, which can intensify a murmur by altering cardiac output.

Organic murmurs reflect an abnormality in the heart structures. Innocent (functional) murmurs do not reflect heart abnormalities but are the sounds made as the blood flows through the structurally normal heart. They can be loud or soft and are often vibratory in quality. Innocent murmurs do not affect growth or well-being and are common in children.

Cardiac Catheterization

Cardiac catheterization began as an invasive diagnostic procedure. It is now used as a diagnostic, interventional, and a therapeutic procedure. During a cardiac catheterization, catheters are advanced, generally through the femoral vein or artery, through the venous or arterial system and directly into the heart. Data obtained and interventions performed during the procedure include the following:

- Measurement of oxygen saturations in cardiac chambers and great arteries
- Measurement of pressures in cardiac chambers and great arteries and determination of gradients
- Evaluation of cardiac output
- Angiography to identify detailed images of structures and blood flow patterns
- Electrophysiologic studies to map the cardiac conduction system and identify the locus of arrhythmia-producing cells; radiofrequency catheter ablation is used for destruction of these cells
- Corrective, palliative, or therapeutic interventional procedures that include angioplasty of the pulmonary artery and branches, pulmonary valvuloplasty, aortic valve balloon angioplasty, stent placement to maintain patency of vessels, balloon/blade septostomy for creation of an atrial septal defect (ASD) (indicated for certain complex congenital heart defects), percutaneous pulmonary valve replacements, device closure of septal defects, and coil embolization of a patent ductus arteriosus (PDA) or collateral vessels

Complications

Complications may result both during and after the procedure. Potential complications of which the nurse should be aware include arrhythmias, hemorrhage, vascular damage, vasospasm of the catheterized vessel, thrombus or embolus formation, infection, reaction to the dye, and catheter perforation. Arrhythmias can be hemodynamically compromising. Vasospasm of the vessel results in poor perfusion to the affected leg. Thrombus formation at the catheter insertion site may impair perfusion to the affected limb and may shed emboli that may travel anywhere in the vascular system depending on the cardiac anatomy, including the lung or brain. A thrombus in the venous system can be associated with swelling or inflammation of the affected limb. A thrombus in the arterial system may be associated with coolness or discoloration of the extremity and loss of pulses distal to the thrombus. Thrombus formation may occur in the systemic-to-pulmonary artery shunts that provide pulmonary blood flow. Reactions to the dye may

be rash, pruritus, vomiting or, very rarely, severe anaphylaxis. Perforation by the catheter of the heart or vessels during the procedure can result in cardiac tamponade and cardiac arrest. Additional minor reactions to the procedure include anesthesia- or sedation-related nausea and vomiting or pressure ulceration of pressure points related to prolonged immobility and decreased subcutaneous tissue.

Nursing Care

Because impaired peripheral perfusion is a possible consequence of a cardiac catheterization, it is important for the nurse to locate and mark distal pulses before the procedure. Marking the location of pulses will assist the nurse with rapid postprocedure assessment.

After the procedure, the child is positioned with the affected leg straight for 4 to 6 hours; infants may be held prone on a parent's lap. Older children remain in bed with the head of the bed raised at only a 20-degree incline. Intravenous (IV) fluid administration continues until the infant or child is taking and retaining adequate amounts of oral fluids. Vital signs should be obtained frequently (every 5 to 15 minutes) for the first hour, with continuous initial monitoring of heart rate, blood pressure, respiratory rate and oxygen saturation, and temperature.

The insertion site dressing should be observed frequently, at least every 5 to 15 minutes, during the early postprocedure hours. Assess for bleeding not only on the dressing but also on sheets. Look under the child to check for pooled blood. Pull back bed linens and remove the infant's diaper (if applicable) to check the perineal area for bleeding under the skin. If bleeding occurs, place a gloved heel of the hand firmly on the insertion site. Apply pressure for at least 10 to 15 minutes and assess distal perfusion of the extremity. Immediately notify the cardiologist. Assess blood loss and the child's hemodynamic status.

Peripheral perfusion is also monitored. The affected extremity will frequently be mottled in appearance and cooler to touch than the other extremities. Distal pulses should, however, be palpable, although they may be weaker than in the contralateral extremity. Nonpalpable distal pulses should be checked with Doppler technology. Notify the cardiologist if distal pulses are absent on the affected extremity or the temperature or degree of mottling has changed or the child complains of increasing pain. Heparin drip infusions are initiated under certain circumstances, which may be related to pulse loss or catheter route, or with placement of stents, coils, or closure devices.

Children who have undergone a diagnostic cardiac catheterization are often discharged the same day. Children undergoing some types of interventional procedures or electrophysiologic studies may remain hospitalized overnight. The following day, the pressure bandage is removed and is replaced with an adhesive bandage (Band-Aid). Discharge instructions vary according to the institution but may include the following:

- Inspecting the catheter insertion site to assess healing or the presence of local infection
- Bathing limited to a shower, sponge bath, or brief tub bath (no soaking) for the first 1 to 3 days after the procedure
- Avoiding strenuous exercise (climbing trees, swimming, contact sports) for up to 1 week after the procedure or 6 weeks after a device is placed
- Returning to school on the third day after the procedure
- Notifying the cardiologist if the child has a fever above 101° F (38.3° C); bleeding or drainage (pus) from the catheter insertion site; or pallor, coolness, or numbness of the affected extremity
- Resuming normal feeding patterns and medication therapy, if applicable

- Reviewing the need to continue antibiotic prophylaxis for dental or other specific medical procedures
- Follow-up with a cardiologist at a scheduled visit

Congenital Cardiac Defects

Table 22-3 presents the most frequently seen cardiac lesions in infants and children.

THE CHILD UNDERGOING CARDIAC SURGERY

Most cardiac lesions are amenable to palliative or corrective repair, and the child with significant CHD will undergo a surgical or interventional catheterization procedure at some point during infancy or childhood. The timing of surgery is dictated by the child's clinical condition, but the trend in recent years is to intervene at an early age. The ultimate goal of intervention is for a two-ventricle repair, with physiologic and anatomic correction to normal or near-normal circulation. Complex lesions may require multiple, palliated stages with the goal of separating the saturated and desaturated blood, correcting cyanosis, and optimizing pulmonary and cardiac function.

Families anticipate surgery as a means of achieving a more normal lifestyle, but they also feel anxiety about the child's postoperative course and ultimate outcome. The nurse can help both the child and the parents cope with this stressful and traumatic event through support and education.

Preoperative Preparation

Preoperative teaching and preparation expose the child and family to the hospital environment and expected perioperative and postoperative care. The family should receive verbal, written, and visual information that describes the course of events throughout the hospitalization. Interpreter services should be used when indicated. It is important to evaluate the family's understanding of the surgical procedure and its expected outcomes. A multidisciplinary team, including physicians, nurses, a child life specialist, and social services, provides a comprehensive approach in the assessment of and interventions for the child and family. Barriers to actual hospitalization (e.g., financial, social, transportation) and discharge can be identified and interventions begun before the actual hospitalization. In addition, identifying positive coping mechanisms and providing anticipatory guidance can help the child and parent be empowered in their understanding and participation in care while the child is hospitalized. In family-centered care, the health care team works with the family in caring for the child.

The parents and child should tour the intensive care unit (Figure 22-1) and other units where the child will be during the hospitalization. This preparation allows them to become familiar with the physical environment and the noise and activity level. The visit should allow time for the family to meet members of the nursing staff and see equipment that will be used in the child's postoperative care. In addition, seeing other families and children who have undergone similar procedures as they progress and recover from the surgical process can be an encouraging experience.

Monitors, ventilators, and tubes should be described and shown to the family. Parents and children are reminded that invasive monitoring lines, chest tubes, and an endotracheal tube are inserted during surgery while the child is anesthetized, and they should be reassured that these tubes and lines will be removed as soon as the child's condition permits.

The sequence of events surrounding the day of surgery—when and where to arrive and where to wait during the procedure—should be reviewed. Parents should be assured that they will receive updates

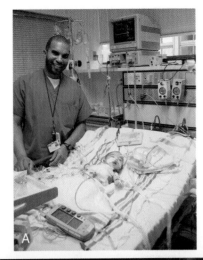

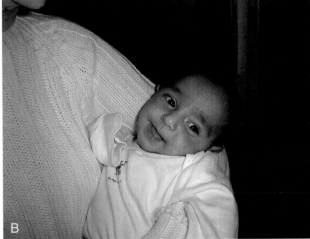

FIG 22-1 **A,** A preoperative visit to the intensive care unit and other units should be directed at an age-appropriate level for the child and the family before the child undergoes cardiac surgery. The experience prepares the family for the sights and sounds of the unit. **B,** Going home. (Courtesy Children's Hospital Oakland, Oakland, CA.)

about their child's condition throughout the procedure and will be permitted to visit soon after the surgery is completed.

Postoperative Management

Postoperative nursing management includes promoting hemodynamic and respiratory stability, preventing and identifying potential complications, providing comfort, ensuring pain assessment and interventions, and providing continuing educational and emotional support. Early postoperative care in the intensive care unit involves continuous monitoring of vital signs and cardiac output and frequent multisystem assessments. These assessments continue, with decreasing intensity, until discharge.

Cardiac surgical repair is either a closed heart procedure or an open heart procedure. The underlying cardiac defect and anticipated surgical intervention are the determining factors in the type of procedure performed.

In a closed heart surgery, the heart continues to pump and maintain cardiac function during the repair. Some examples of closed heart

Text continued on page 556

TABLE 22-3 CONGENITAL CARDIAC DEFECTS

INCIDENCE AND PATHOPHYSIOLOGY	ALTERED HEMODYNAMICS	MANIFESTATIONS	THERAPEUTIC MANAGEMENT
Left-to-Right Shunting Lesions *Patent Ductus Arteriosus (PDA)* 5%-10% of all congenital heart lesions* Often present with other lesions Caused by failure of the fetal ductus arteriosus to close completely after birth Normal closure within 24-72 hr after birth due to decreased prostaglandin (PG) levels and decrease in blood pressure in ductus lumen Eventual degeneration to the ductus ligamentum	Patent ductus arteriosus Due to a drop in pulmonary vascular resistance and failure of the ductus arteriosus to close, increased systemic pressure moves saturated blood from the aorta into the pulmonary arteries (left-to-right shunt), the lungs, and the left side of the heart causing both increased left-sided cardiac workload and increased pulmonary blood flow.	Signs of heart failure, which are related to the size of the lesion and amount of left-to-right shunting Continuous murmur (machinery-like sound) Widened pulse pressure (increased difference between systolic and diastolic readings) Bounding pulses Cardiac enlargement	*Medical Management* Interventions to address HF Administration of indomethacin (Indocin), a prostaglandin inhibitor, that constricts the ductus Monitor respiratory status, renal function, and growth *Interventional Cardiac Catheterization* A coil is placed to occlude the ductus. Tissue grows around the coil (endothelializes) forming permanent occlusion. *Surgical Management* Ligation of the ductus via left thoracotomy, usually within the first year of life
Atrial Septal Defect (ASD) 5%-10% of cardiac lesions; seen more often in girls Abnormal opening between the atria Three types predominate: (1) *Ostium secundum:* Located in the middle of the septum and is most commonly seen (2) *Ostium primum:* Lesion is low in the septum, associated with endocardial tissue formation defect, associated with cleft mitral valve (3) *Sinus venosus:* Located high in the septum near superior vena cava	Atrial septal defect Decreased right ventricular compliance (ease of ventricular filling during diastole) compared to left ventricular compliance leads to left-to-right shunting across the abnormal septal opening: right atrium is e[...]ed and pulmonary blood flow increased	May be asymptomatic depending on size of lesion Fatigue, dyspnea on exertion, palpitations, atrial arrhythmias Recurrent respiratory infections related to increased pulmonary blood flow Systolic murmur from increased blood flow across the pulmonary valve; diastolic murmur with large shunting Mitral valve regurgitation is possible HF may develop during young adulthood, if not repaired Risk for stroke	*Medical Management* Conservative, because spontaneous closure can occur Diuretics and digoxin for signs of HF; antiarrhythmics for atrial arrhythmias *Interventional Cardiac Catheterization* Occluder devices placed if criteria related to size of lesion, significance of shunting, and availability of septal tissue to anchor the device are met; usually done at age between 2-5 yr Daily low-dose aspirin for 6 mo following procedure (Park, 2008) *Surgical Management* Surgical placement of sutures or prosthetic patch through open heart procedure using cardiopulmonary bypass Surgical complications include arrhythmias and postpericardiotomy syndrome (inflammation[...] pericardial effusion)

Ventricular Septal Defect (VSD)

15%-20% of cardiac defects

Abnormal opening between the ventricles.

Three types according to location:
(1) conoventricular
(2) atrioventricular canal
(3) muscular

Depending on size, complete absence of the septum results in a common ventricle

Most common type of cardiac defect; may be accompanied by other defects

Decrease in pulmonary vascular resistance compared to systemic vascular resistance in the weeks after birth results in left-to-right shunting through the VSD. Increased pulmonary blood flow, pulmonary hypertension, and progressive pulmonary vascular disease can occur over time

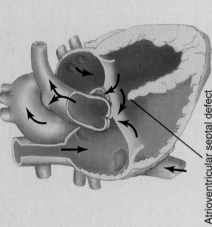

Ventricular septal defect

Signs and symptoms are related to the size of the defect—some children remain asymptomatic

Loud, harsh systolic murmur, varies in intensity and duration depending on degree of shunting and size of defect; palpable thrill, diastolic murmur and gallop rhythm may be present

HF may occur with moderate to large defects

Medical Management

Conservative: 30%-40% close spontaneously (Park, 2008)

Diuretics, digoxin, and medications for afterload reduction (e.g., angiotensin-converting enzyme [ACE] inhibitors)

Management of associated HF

Interventional Cardiac Catheterization

Insertion of an occluder device

May be done as a hybrid procedure using a surgical approach to visualize and directly access the ventricle and catheterization to place the device

Surgical Management

Suture or patch closure using open heart surgery with cardiopulmonary bypass

Consideration of pulmonary artery banding to reduce pulmonary blood flow for children with multiple defects and severe HF

Complications include residual VSDs, pulmonary hypertension, heart block that requires temporary or permanent pacemaker, abnormal rhythm (junctional ectopic tachycardia) that decreases cardiac output, and postpericardiotomy syndrome

Atrioventricular Septal Defect (Endocardial Cushion Defect)

2% of cardiac defects

Often associated with genetic syndromes (e.g., Down syndrome)

Abnormal endocardial tissue development affecting the atrial and ventricular septum and mitral and tricuspid valves (AV valves).

Three types:
(1) *Partial:* Ostium primum ASD and two separate AV valves but a mitral valve cleft
(2) *Intermediate or transitional:* ASD, beginning connection between the two AV valves, no VSD
(3) *Complete:* A single connected AV valve, ASD and VSD

Partial defect: Left-to-right shunting of blood with increased pulmonary blood flow related to differences in aortic and pulmonary pressure

Complete: Markedly increased pulmonary blood flow with associated pulmonary hypertension and risk for pulmonary vascular disease; mixture of saturated and desaturated blood as pressures change and right-to-left shunting occurs

Atrioventricular septal defect

Varying degrees of HF related to the size and number of defects and pressure differences

Systolic pulmonary flow murmur that develops over a few weeks after birth

Intermittent cyanosis

Medical Management

Symptomatic treatment of HF with diuretics, digoxin and ACE inhibitors

Surgical Management

Partial: If asymptomatic, ASD and mitral valve cleft are repaired in late infancy or early childhood

Complete: ASD and VSD are closed, construction of two separate AV valves from the common valve, possible mitral valve replacement; performed at 3-4 mo of age or later (but before pulmonary hypertension occurs) if child is asymptomatic

Children with small atria or ventricles may require palliative surgery (designed to relieve symptoms by directing venous blood return directly to the pulmonary artery)

Postoperative mortality is about 10% for complete repair; complications similar to VSD repair

Continued

*Prevalence statistics are from Park, M. K. (2008). *Pediatric cardiology for practitioners* (5th ed.). St. Louis: Elsevier Mosby.

TABLE 22-3   CONGENITAL CARDIAC DEFECTS—cont'd

INCIDENCE AND PATHOPHYSIOLOGY	ALTERED HEMODYNAMICS	MANIFESTATIONS	THERAPEUTIC MANAGEMENT
Obstructive or Stenotic Lesions			
Pulmonary Stenosis			
10% of cardiac defects	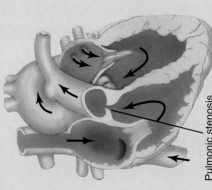 Pulmonic stenosis	Many asymptomatic; signs in symptomatic children include exercise intolerance, signs of right-sided HF	*Medical Management*
Narrowing at entrance to the pulmonary artery at the valve, below the valve, or above the valve	Obstruction causes resistance to blood flow at the right ventricular outflow tract; increased pressure in the right ventricle leads to right ventricular hypertrophy	Systolic ejection murmur, possible palpable thrill	Cardiac observation and antibiotic prophylaxis for children who are asymptomatic
The valve itself may be normal (tricuspid), bicuspid, or dysplastic	Critically severe pulmonary artery obstruction elevates right ventricular pressure severely, causing blood to regurgitate into the right atrium; rising right atrial pressure forces the foramen ovale open, allowing blood to flow from the right atrium to the right ventricle	Cardiomegaly on radiograph	Additional intervention related to increasing pulmonary pressure gradient across the pulmonary valve
		Cyanosis in severe cases	Interventional catheterization or surgical management for severe stenosis; PGE₁ (prostaglandin) infusion keeps the ductus arteriosus open so blood can return to lungs for oxygenation
			Interventional Cardiac Catheterization
			Balloon valvuloplasty with dilation of the valve to decrease the pressure; pulmonary regurgitation may be a complication; may have to be redone later
			Surgical Management
			Surgical valvulotomy for unsuccessful valvuloplasty or if stenosis is supravalvular
			Placement of a shunt from aorta to pulmonary artery (*systemic to pulmonary artery shunt*) for critical pulmonary stenosis with small right ventricle or for children who must remain on PGE₁ after interventional cardiac catheterization
Aortic Stenosis			
3%-6% of cardiac defects	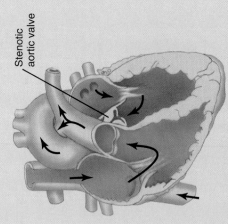 Stenotic aortic valve	*Mild/moderate:* Asymptomatic; exercise intolerance, ECG abnormalities with exercise, cardiomegaly, systolic ejection murmur with thrill or click; sudden death with strenuous exercise is a possibility	*Medical Management*
Narrowing of the entrance to the aorta; may be supravalvular, subvalvular, or at the valve level (most common); thickened, rigid, with some fusion of the leaflets; the valve may be bicuspid	Blood has difficulty flowing through the aortic valve, causing increased pressure and hypertrophy in the left ventricle, decreased cardiac output, decreased blood supply to the coronary arteries	*Severe:* Severe HF; decreased cardiac output with decreased peripheral perfusion (*critical aortic stenosis*); if uncorrected, chest pain, dizziness, and syncope	Mild/moderate—regular follow-up, especially for athletes; restriction from competitive athletics depending on degree of stenosis and severity of signs and symptoms
			Interventional Cardiac Catheterization
			Aortic balloon valvuloplasty decreases stenosis and improves cardiac output; may be performed to delay surgical intervention; aortic insufficiency, thrombosis, infection or artery damage may occur
			Surgical Management
			Surgical valvulotomy
			Aortic valve replacement for recurrent stenosis:
			(1) Mechanical valve replacement requires warfarin treatment; valve does not grow with the child
			(2) Use of child's pulmonary valve to replace the aortic valve; pulmonary valve homograft to replace the pulmonary valve; new aortic valve grows with the child; homograft will need later replacement

Coarctation of the Aorta

8%-... of cardiac defects

Aorta is constricted near the ductus arteriosus insertion location; associated with bicuspid aortic valve that can later become stenotic

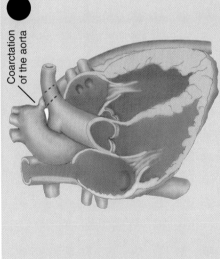

Coarctation of the aorta

Narrowing of the aortic structure obstructs the left ventricular output, increasing afterload to left ventricle; blood supply is decreased in the abdominal organs and the lower periphery; left ventricular pressure increases; aortic pressure is high proximal to the constriction and low distal; pulmonary edema can occur

If coarctation is mild, collateral blood supply can develop to channel blood past the constriction

Left-sided HF with low cardiac output, poor lower extremity peripheral perfusion, metabolic acidosis, shock

If PDA present: Right-to-left shunting with differential cyanosis (color and oxygenation differential between upper and lower extremities)

Asymptomatic children may show pulse and blood pressure differences between upper (systolic hypertension) and lower extremities; weakness, tingling, cramps in lower extremities

Systolic murmur accompanied by ejection click (with bicuspid aortic valve) or thrill

Medical Management

Diuretics and digoxin to improve cardiac output; PGE; infusion to open the ductus arteriosus and improve perfusion to the lower body

Interventional Cardiac Catheterization

Balloon dilation with placement of stent for recurrences; balloon angioplasty for the initial procedure can increase the incidence of recurrences (Park, 2008)

Surgical Management

Performed shortly after diagnosis in most cases

Several surgical procedures available—end-to-end anastomosis, use of prosthetic patch, left subclavian artery patch (results in postoperative absence of left palpable pulse)

Cyanotic Lesions with Decreased Pulmonary Blood Flow

Tetralogy of Fallot

5%-10% of congenital cardiac defects; most frequently seen cyanotic lesion

Constellation of lesions results from malalignment of the ventricular septum during fetal development

(1) Ventricular septal defect

(2) Right ventricular outflow tract obstruction (e.g., pulmonary stenosis)

(3) Overriding of the aorta (arises partially out of the right ventricle)

(4) Right ventricular hypertrophy

Equal right- and left-sided ventricular pressures related to the pulmonary artery obstruction and size of the VSD; desaturated blood enters the systemic system by shunting right to left across the VSD, or into the overriding aorta

Onset and severity of signs and symptoms are related to the extent of the obstructed pulmonary blood flow, which causes the right-to-left shunting; if lesions are mild, shunting is decreased and saturations are mildly low (pink tet)

Signs become worse in the neonate as the ductus arteriosus closes

Cyanosis, extreme fatigue, hypercyanotic episodes, chronic hypoxemia

Harsh systolic murmur with a palpable thrill; boot-shaped heart on radiography (related to poor development of the pulmonary artery)

Medical Management

PGE; infusion to maintain patency of the ductus arteriosus and blood flow to the lungs; management of hypercyanotic episodes; treatment of iron deficiency anemia

Surgical Management

Primary repair of defects during infancy is preferred; surgery occurs after 4 mo of age and is timed according to the degree of cyanosis and other symptoms

Surgery requires cardiopulmonary bypass

For infants who are poor candidates for early primary repair, palliative shunt procedures increase pulmonary blood flow; modified Blalock-Taussig procedure (creation of a systemic-to-pulmonary-artery shunt using a Gore-Tex tube) is used most frequently

Surgical complications: Rhythm disturbances, residual VSD, low cardiac output, residual right ventricular outflow obstruction, pulmonary valve regurgitation, residual right-sided HF; mortality is low

Continued

TABLE 22-3 CONGENITAL CARDIAC DEFECTS—cont'd

INCIDENCE AND PATHOPHYSIOLOGY	ALTERED HEMODYNAMICS	MANIFESTATIONS	THERAPEUTIC MANAGEMENT
Tricuspid Atresia 1%-3% of cardiac defects Nondevelopment of the tricuspid valve, patent foramen ovale or ASD, underdeveloped (hypoplastic) right ventricle. VSD of varying size, pulmonary artery may have normal position or may be transposed with the aorta, pulmonary stenosis of varying degrees	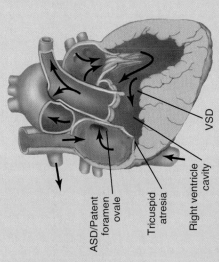 ASD/Patent foramen ovale Tricuspid atresia Right ventricle cavity VSD Desaturated blood enters the right atrium, shunts right to left through a patent foramen ovale into the left atrium; desaturated blood mixes with saturated blood in the left atrium, proceeds into the left ventricle and into the aorta; some blood shunts through the VSD to the right ventricle and into the pulmonary artery to the lungs; if the ductus arteriosus is open, some blood will flow from the aorta to the pulmonary artery; lesser pulmonary stenosis can contribute to pulmonary congestion	Profound cyanosis with decreased pulmonary blood flow Single second heart sound because of no closure of the tricuspid valve Systolic murmur from the VSD; PDA murmur if ductus remains open	*Medical Management* PGE₁ infusion to maintain patency of the ductus arteriosus *Interventional Cardiac Catheterization* Balloon atrial septostomy (creating an opening in the septum) if the foramen ovale begins to close; catheter is threaded through femoral vein, advanced into the right atrium, through the foramen ovale into the left atrium; balloon is inflated and pulled back into the right atrium through the foramen ovale and tearing the septum Catheter blade septostomy to cut the septum tissue, if balloon septostomy is not effective *Surgical Management* Goal is to separate desaturated and saturated blood and to optimize ventricular function by decreasing the workload on the heart Three-stage surgery: (1) Palliative systemic-to-pulmonary artery shunt (see Tetralogy of Fallot) (2) Creation of a connection between the superior vena cava and pulmonary arteries (bidirectional Glenn procedure); results in desaturated blood flow directly from the superior vena cava to the pulmonary artery and decreased volume in the left ventricle; performed at 4-6 mo of age; pulmonary hypertension may result (keep the child positioned with the head elevated postoperatively) (3) Modified Fontan procedure during early childhood; connection created from the inferior vena cava to the pulmonary arteries Surgical procedures result in a single ventricle and all desaturated blood going from the vena cavae directly into the pulmonary arteries Occasionally, a small connection (fenestration) between the venous and arterial circulation is kept to assist with adjustment to new flow and pressures; the fenestration is closed later

Pulmonary Atresia with Intact Ventricular Septum

<1% of cardiac defects

Failure of the pulmonary valve to develop; hypoplastic development of the pulmonary artery and right ventricle; extremely high right ventricular pressures; possible associated underdeveloped tricuspid valve

Profound cyanosis; survival depends on a PDA

Single second heart sound

PDA murmur

Medical Management

Continuous PGE₁ infusion

Interventional Cardiac Catheterization

Laser wire and radiofrequency valvulotomy with balloon dilation of the valve in some children (Park, 2008)

Surgical Management

Early management: Pulmonary valvulotomy or systemic-to-pulmonary artery shunt (Blalock-Taussig procedure) in children with adequate right ventricle size (Bernstein, 2011); as blood flow from the right ventricle to the pulmonary artery increases, the atrial right-to-left shunting decreases

Later management: ASD and systemic-to-pulmonary shunt may be closed

Bidirectional Glenn procedure or modified Fontan procedure if right ventricle remains small and cannot pump adequate blood to the pulmonary artery

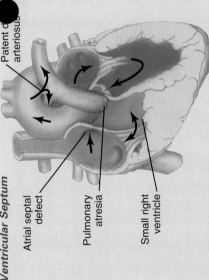

Patent ductus arteriosus

Atrial septal defect

Pulmonary atresia

Small right ventricle

Desaturated blood flows through the tricuspid valve to the right ventricle but cannot enter the pulmonary artery because there is no pulmonary valve; blood backs up through the tricuspid valve back into the right atrium, shunts right to left through the foramen ovale to left atrium; mixed desaturated and saturated blood flow into the left ventricle and out the aorta; blood is oxygenated through a left-to-right shunt from the aorta through a patent ductus arteriosus to the pulmonary artery and lungs

Total Anomalous Pulmonary Venous Return

1% of cardiac defects

Defect of fetal development during first 8 wk of pregnancy; pulmonary veins do not connect with the left atrium but connect somewhere else, such as to the superior vena cava (most frequently seen)

All four pulmonary veins connect to superior vena cava

Superior vena cava

Opening between atria

Tricuspid valve

Inferior vena cava

Pulmonary valve

Pulmonary vein

Mitral valve

Aortic valve

LA

PA

AO

RA

LV

RV

AO = Aorta
PA = Pulmonary artery
LA = Left atrium
RA = Right atrium
LV = Left ventricle
RV = Right ventricle

■ Oxygen-rich blood
■ Oxygen-poor blood
■ Mixed blood

Oxygen-rich blood that would normally return to the left side of the heart mixes with desaturated blood in the right side of the heart; associated heart defects (ASD, VSD, PDA) allow for communication between the right and left sides of the heart, delivering mixed blood to the systemic circulation

Cyanosis, severe respiratory distress, tachycardia, worsening pulmonary hypertension, progressive clinical deterioration with possible early death (first week to month after birth)

Murmur (systolic over the pulmonary area or tricuspid insufficiency murmur) may or may not be present

Decreasing peripheral pulses, increasing HF, enlargement of the liver, failure to thrive, frequent pulmonary infection in infants without pulmonary vein obstruction (Park, 2008)

Medical Management

HF and pulmonary edema treated with digoxin, diuretics, oxygen, mechanical ventilation

Treatment of metabolic acidosis

Enlargement of the septal defect through balloon or blade septostomy may facilitate right-to-left shunting

PGE, infusion to maintain patency of the ductus arteriosus

Surgical Management

Surgery between birth and 6 mo of age, depending on extent of obstruction

Goal of surgery is to reroute blood from the abnormally placed pulmonary veins to the left atrium

Surgical procedure varies according to the site of the abnormal circulation; all involve cardiopulmonary bypass, hypothermia, and total circulatory arrest; closure of the associated ASD occurs as well

Continued

TABLE 22-3   CONGENITAL CARDIAC DEFECTS—cont'd

INCIDENCE AND PATHOPHYSIOLOGY	ALTERED HEMODYNAMICS	MANIFESTATIONS	THERAPEUTIC MANAGEMENT
Cyanotic Lesions with Increased Pulmonary Blood Flow			
Truncus Arteriosus			
1% of cardiac defects		Signs of HF and cyanosis in neonate—determined by the volume of pulmonary blood flow (the higher the flow, the greater the symptoms of HF); pulmonary vascular disease can develop in early infancy; pulmonary stenosis limits the blood flow and increases cyanosis	*Medical Management*
Failure of the common great vessel, the truncus arteriosus, to divide into the pulmonary artery and aortic valve during fetal development; results in a single vessel and valve, which give rise to the pulmonary, systemic, and coronary circulations			Digoxin and diuretics for HF
			Preventing polycythemia is important
			Preventing frequent infections and assessing calcium and magnesium levels; this defect can be associated with DiGeorge syndrome, which is a syndrome that causes depressed immune system and hypocalcemia (Park, 2008)
Associated failure of septal development with VSD; the common vessel overrides the VSD and receives blood from both right and left ventricles	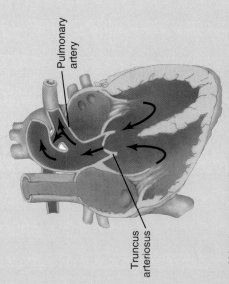	Harsh systolic murmur with thrill; diastolic murmur of truncal valve insufficiency may be heard; opening of the single truncal valve produces a click	*Surgical Management*
			Varies with the classification of truncus. In the more commonly seen type the VSD is closed and blood flow from the left ventricle is directed into the truncal vessel; a connection (conduit) is made between the right ventricle and the pulmonary artery, creating a pulmonary circulation; the conduit may need revision as the child grows
		Truncal valve insufficiency produces a bounding pulse and widened pulse pressure	Surgical mortality risk depends on the type of truncus and the extent of the required repair and is higher with truncal valve stenosis or insufficiency
Desaturated blood enters the right atrium, and through the tricuspid valve to the right ventricle; saturated blood from the left atrium flows through the mitral valve into the left ventricle; saturated and desaturated blood mix in the ventricles at the level of the VSD and common ventricular outflow tract; mixed blood flows into the common vessel and is circulated to the systemic, pulmonary, and coronary circulations			
Ventricles are under pressure and volume overload; oxygen saturation depends on the volume of pulmonary blood flow and determines the signs of HF, decreased cardiac output, and coronary artery ischemia			

Hypoplastic Left Heart Syndrome

1% of cardiac defects

Inadequate development of the left side of the heart results in one effective ventricle; associated with aortic valve atresia, hypoplasia of the left ventricle, hypoplasia of the ascending aorta, and mitral valve stenosis or atresia (Park, 2008)

Seen more often in males than females; if untreated, most infants die within the first few months of life

HF from increased pulmonary blood flow; tachypnea

Systemic hypoperfusion and shock as ductus arteriosus begins to close

Infant is grayish blue, has dyspnea and hypotension

Medical Management

Emergency management to correct acid-base and electrolyte imbalances

PGE₁ infusion to maintain ductus arteriosus patency until surgery

Surgical Management

Three options available:
(1) No intervention with supportive care
(2) Cardiac transplantation
(3) Three-stage palliative repair that will result in a single right ventricle, with different portions of the pulmonary artery acting to facilitate both systemic and pulmonary circulation

Surgical mortality from the initial stage of surgery can be as high as 35%, but approximately 50% of children who complete all stages of the surgery survive at least 4 yr (Park, 2008)

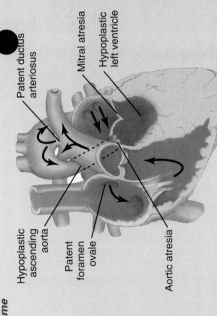

Patent ductus arteriosus
Mitral atresia
Hypoplastic left ventricle
Hypoplastic ascending aorta
Patent foramen ovale
Aortic atresia

Saturated blood returns to the left atrium but is unable to flow to the remainder of the left side of the heart; blood is shunted from left-to-right through a patent foramen ovale or ASD to the right atrium, where it mixes with desaturated blood; mixed blood enters the pulmonary circulation—some goes to the lungs, some to the ductus arteriosus, which remains open, and to the systemic circulation

Transposition of the Great Arteries

5%-7% of cardiac defects

Abnormal separation and rotation of the fetal common truncal vessel causes the aorta to arise from the right ventricle and the pulmonary artery to arise from the left ventricle

Associated VSD

Cyanosis at birth

Hypoxemia, despite oxygen administration

Progressive desaturation and acidosis; developing HF

Medical Management

Emergency PGE₁ infusion to maintain patency of the ductus arteriosus

Interventional Cardiac Catheterization

Balloon atrial septostomy to enhance mixing of blood in some infants

Surgical Management

Arterial switch procedure, which places the aorta and pulmonary artery in their anatomically correct positions and reimplants the coronary arteries in the new aorta

Long-term survival rates are positive (DeBord, Cherry, & Hickey, 2007)

Postoperative complications include low cardiac output, arrhythmias related to decreased coronary artery perfusion and myocardial ischemia

Patent ductus arteriosus
Pulmonary artery
LV
Aorta
ASD/PFD
RV

Desaturated blood returns to the right atrium, flows into the right ventricle and out the aorta to the systemic circulation; saturated blood returns to the left ventricle, out the pulmonary artery to the lungs

Survival depends on blood mixing through a patent foramen ovale/ASD and patent ductus arteriosus

Some infants have a VSD

procedures include repair of a PDA, coarctation of the aorta, and certain aorta-to-pulmonary artery shunts.

Potential complications include recurrent laryngeal nerve injury with associated vocal cord paralysis, pneumothorax, chylothorax, atelectasis, phrenic nerve injury and associated diaphragm paralysis, bleeding, infection, and, rarely, death.

Open heart surgery is done with the child on a cardiopulmonary bypass machine. The machine takes over the roles of the lungs and heart—oxygenation and the delivery of blood to the body. Special cannulas are placed in the venous side of the heart, and venous blood is diverted into the bypass circuit. In the circuit, the blood is oxygenated and filtered and returned to the aorta, where it is pumped to the brain and systemic circulation. The principles of hemodilution, hypothermia, and anticoagulation are critical to use of cardiopulmonary bypass. In addition, myocardial preservation is critical. The heart is generally not pumping during cardiopulmonary bypass, and all systems are supported. Potential complications from cardiopulmonary bypass include bleeding, stroke, myocardial infarction, arrhythmias, fluid and electrolyte imbalance, postpericardiotomy syndrome (an inflammatory process with the development of pericardial effusion), and death. Additional complications include those detailed for closed heart surgery (see previous paragraph). The majority of repairs are done with the child on cardiopulmonary bypass, including ASD, VSD, tetralogy of Fallot, and AVSD.

Monitoring Cardiac Output

The child's cardiac output is monitored through the assessment of vital signs and peripheral perfusion. Signs of low cardiac output include tachycardia, coolness and mottling of extremities, diminished peripheral pulses, delayed capillary refill time, hypotension, decreased urine output, metabolic acidosis, and changes in level of consciousness (difficult to assess in a sedated and intubated child). Intracardiac pressure monitoring is also used and assessed.

The components of cardiac output are heart rate, preload, contractility, and afterload. Problems with one or more of these components may develop during the early postoperative period. Changes in heart rate or rhythm affect cardiac function, and antiarrhythmic drugs or temporary cardiac pacing may be instituted to correct transient postoperative rhythm disturbances. Blood loss and leakage of fluid into the interstitial space may also influence preload. Transfusions of blood products, colloids, and crystalloids are frequently needed to maintain adequate circulating blood volume. Acid-base and electrolyte imbalances, as well as hypoxia, adversely affect contractility. Correction of these abnormalities may improve cardiac function, but most children will need some degree of continuous infusion of inotropic medications to support cardiac output. Changes in systemic and pulmonary vascular resistance influence afterload and the use of inodilators (medications with inotropic and vasodilator effects), such as milrinone, sometimes prove necessary.

Supporting Respiratory Function

During cardiopulmonary bypass, the lungs are not ventilated and expanded, placing the child at risk for postoperative atelectasis. Fluid may accumulate in the pleural and interstitial spaces during and after cardiopulmonary bypass. For surgery, the child will be intubated and mechanically ventilated and often returns to the intensive care unit intubated.

Airway patency is maintained, in part, through prudent suctioning of the endotracheal tube. The nurse must pay strict attention to oxygen saturation readings (and know the anticipated saturations for the specific cardiac defect and surgical intervention), including during suctioning, to avoid episodes of transient hypoxia. Frequently, the child receives bolus or continuous infusions of analgesia (sedative medications) to help maintain comfort during this time.

Once extubated, the child is encouraged to deep breathe and cough. Incentive spirometry or therapy is often used to enhance lung expansion. Supplemental oxygen is administered initially and then tapered off as the child's condition permits. Pain medication is given before treatments and pulmonary exercises to allow the child to participate with minimal discomfort. The child can be encouraged to splint the chest during coughing by hugging a favorite stuffed animal.

Chest tubes are placed during surgery to evacuate drainage and air and assist with lung reexpansion. These tubes are inserted in either the mediastinal or pleural space, depending on the surgical approach, and are removed when lung reexpansion is confirmed and drainage has ceased.

Initial chest tube drainage is bloody and changes to serosanguineous and then serous over time. Drainage is heaviest during the first 12 to 24 hours postoperatively, and it is measured and the color evaluated hourly. Increased chest tube drainage may indicate surgical bleeding or clotting abnormalities and must be strictly monitored and rapidly resolved.

Chest tubes are uncomfortable while in place; they restrict movement and cause discomfort when the child's position is changed. Chest tube removal is a painful experience, and the child should be premedicated with an opiate analgesic before the procedure.

Pulmonary hypertension presents a complicated and potentially life-threatening problem postoperatively. Intensive monitoring of pulmonary status (while intubated and extubated), saturations, and pulmonary artery pressures is indicated. In addition, special precautions before suctioning or other noxious stimuli are indicated while caring for these children.

Maintaining Fluid and Electrolyte Balance

Cardiac surgery and cardiopulmonary bypass affect fluid and electrolyte status. Blood loss and fluid shifts reduce circulating blood volume. Cardiopulmonary bypass stimulates secretion of aldosterone and antidiuretic hormone, resulting in water and sodium retention and potassium loss. Stress can increase calcium deposition in bone, placing the child at risk for hypocalcemia. In addition, administration of blood products can bind circulating calcium and lead to hypocalcemia.

Accurate recording of intake and output monitors fluid balance. Urine output is measured hourly, and weight is often measured daily. Fluid requirements are calculated on the basis of the 24-hour intake and output and child's weight. The child with fluid-volume deficit may require fluid boluses of crystalloid, colloid, or blood, whereas the child with fluid-volume excess may require fluid restriction and diuretic therapy.

Electrolyte imbalances adversely affect cardiac contractility. Serum electrolyte values are determined at regular intervals in the early postoperative period, and IV boluses of calcium or potassium are administered to correct abnormalities. Calcium chloride continuous infusions are often instituted in neonates who have undergone open heart surgery. These medications are delivered through a centrally placed venous line and given according to precise guidelines.

In addition, glucose is a critical factor in maintaining cardiac contractility, especially in the neonate and infant. Monitoring for and treating hypoglycemia are critical.

Promoting Comfort

Postoperative pain management is an important nursing function in the care of the child undergoing cardiac surgery. The experience is frightening to both the child and parents. Parents worry that their child will be in constant, severe pain after the procedure.

Optimal pain management in the initial postoperative period may require the use of a continuous IV infusion of an opiate analgesic, such as morphine sulfate or fentanyl. This infusion is often accompanied by the administration of sedatives and antianxiety agents. In addition, nonsteroidal antiinflammatory agents can be used. This combination of drugs controls pain, relieves anxiety, and allows the child to rest. Scheduled pain medication, along with as-needed doses, often provides better pain control than as-needed pain medication alone.

Once invasive monitoring lines and tubes have been removed, pain control can usually be achieved through the use of oral analgesics. Acetaminophen with or without an opiate additive or nonsteroidal antiinflammatory agents are frequently the drugs of choice. The incision site sometimes determines the amount of pain medication the child will need to remain comfortable. A thoracotomy incision usually divides muscle and necessitates spreading of the ribs for exposure; children who have undergone this surgical approach frequently have more postoperative discomfort than those who have had a midsternotomy incision.

Pain should be assessed frequently throughout the hospitalization. Preverbal children are unable to express their discomfort, and older children may not be able to accurately describe their pain. Pain assessment tools should be used to accurately assess the child's pain. The nurse also must be alert to nonverbal pain behavior, which includes restlessness and irritability, difficulty resting and sleeping, guarding, rigidity, resistance to movement, an increase in heart rate and blood pressure, and lack of interest in eating and other activities. Consulting the parents can help the nurse validate the assessment. Parents know their child best and are familiar with their child's response to stressful situations.

Promoting Healing and Recovery

A balance between rest and activity is necessary to promote healing. Children often feel fatigue during their postoperative recovery and may benefit from a planned schedule of progressive activity. Parents should be encouraged to allow their child to gradually resume the preoperative activity level. Regularly scheduled administration of pain medication provides comfort during activity, allows the child to rest, and reduces fatigue and anxiety.

Nutritional intake is monitored, and the child is encouraged to resume normal eating patterns. Infants and children who were in significant HF preoperatively from large left-to-right shunting lesions may demonstrate improved oral intake even before discharge home. Rarely, diet restrictions are implemented for the older child. These restrictions may be related to long-term anticoagulation with warfarin (Coumadin) or salt restrictions. Discharge teaching is important to ensure that parents feel comfortable managing their child at home (see the Patient-Centered Teaching: Care after Heart Surgery box).

ACQUIRED HEART DISEASE

Acquired heart disease encompasses all cardiac conditions that are not present at birth. Children with CHD may develop acquired cardiac problems, such as infective endocarditis and arrhythmias. Children with structurally normal hearts may be affected by these conditions and by other cardiac conditions such as rheumatic heart disease, Kawasaki disease, hypertension, and cardiomyopathies. Some factors that play a role in triggering these problems include genetic tendencies, autoimmune responses, and infection.

Infective Endocarditis

Infective endocarditis is an inflammation resulting from infection of the cardiac valves and endocardium by a bacterial or occasionally a fungal or viral agent. The infection can occur as the result of

---

PATIENT-CENTERED TEACHING
Care after Heart Surgery

Activity
- Resume regular nap and sleep schedules and play activities (infants).
- Omit contact play for several weeks; allow quiet inside and outside play as tolerated. Avoid wrestling, jumping, tugging on arms. Also, avoid sandbox play or swimming until the incision is healed.
- Avoid activities where the child could fall (e.g., riding tricycles or bicycles, swinging, playing on monkey bars or jungle gyms, sliding) for 4 to 6 weeks after hospital discharge.
- Avoid ill contacts.
- Resume regular bedtime (children).
- Avoid large crowds of people for up to 4 to 6 weeks after discharge (including daycare and places of public worship), especially during winter months.

Diet
- Resume regular or fortified formula (as instructed) and baby foods (infant).
- Do not give any new foods until after the first checkup (infant).
- Encourage adequate liquid intake.
- Appetite should improve at home.

Incision
- Do not bathe the infant or child until instructed to do so.
- When instructed, bathe the infant or child with soap and water in the usual way. Pat the incision; do not rub it while it is healing.
- If the infant drools saliva or formula, cover incision with gauze to prevent excessive moisture.
- Do not use creams, lotions, or powders on incision until it is completely healed and without scabs.
- Report any redness, drainage, or signs of infection at the incision or suture sites.

School
- The child may return to school the second to third week after hospital discharge.
- The child may return to school for half days for the first few days.
- The child should not participate in physical education until 2 months after the operation.

When to Call the Physician
- Faster, harder breathing than normal when child is at rest.
- Temperature above 100° F (37.7° C).
- New, frequent coughing.
- Turning blue or bluer than normal.
- Any swelling, redness, or drainage of the incision.
- Frequent vomiting or diarrhea.
- Pain worse instead of better.
- Appetite worse than at time of discharge.

Checkup
- An appointment should be made for a 1- to 2-week follow-up at the time of discharge.
- No immunizations should be given for 4 to 6 weeks postoperatively.

---

procedures such as dental work or invasive surgery to the respiratory tract; however, most cases are not attributable to an invasive procedure, and AHA-recommended IE prevention guidelines now suggest that the risk is greater from poor oral hygiene (Wilson, Taubert, Gewitz et al., 2007). Previously, distinction was made between acute bacterial endocarditis, with a rapid fulminant course of days to weeks, and infective endocarditis, with a slow, indolent course of several months' duration. The general term *infective endocarditis* is now more accepted, with further classification based on the organism responsible for the infection.

Etiology

IE in children occurs most commonly in the presence of CHD. Those with prosthetic heart valves, complex cyanotic heart disease, or surgically constructed systemic-to-pulmonary artery shunts, and those with a previous history of endocarditis are at greatest risk (Wilson et al., 2007). Acquired valvular disease with scarring (e.g., from rheumatic fever [RF]) may also present a risk for IE, but the incidence of this is decreasing as the incidence of RF has decreased (AHA, 2008). The bacterial organisms most commonly responsible for infective endocarditis are gram-positive organisms, including *Streptococcus viridans* and *Staphylococcus aureus*, and HACEK organisms *(Haemophilus, Actinobacillus, Cardiobacterium, Eikenella, Kingella)* (McDonald, 2009). Fungi are becoming more frequently implicated (Park, 2008).

Incidence

The incidence of IE is variable depending on the population. However, infective endocarditis is an important cause of hospitalization, with 0.5 to 1 in 1000 hospitalizations attributed to non-postoperative IE (Park, 2008).

PATHOPHYSIOLOGY

Infective Endocarditis

Children with congenital heart defects often have pressure gradients between the structures of their hearts. A pressure gradient causes turbulence, which may erode underlying tissue and result in damage to the endocardium or endothelium. A clot composed of fibrin and entrapped platelets may form at the site of the disruption. If bacteria are present (most commonly *Staphylococcus aureus* or *Streptococcus* organisms), they also may become entrapped in the clot and encircled by the fibrin and platelets. This is known as a vegetation. The vegetation increases in size as the microorganisms, fibrin, and platelets proliferate within a protective sheath of fibrin. The contained and protected bacteria can quickly destroy the surrounding tissue and valve structures. Because the vegetation is constantly exposed to pressure from blood flow, the vegetation may break off and migrate to other tissues. Particularly dangerous is a cerebral infarct.

Manifestations

The clinical manifestations of IE are highly variable depending on the organism and the host immune response. Manifestations include fever; nonspecific complaints of anorexia, nausea, fatigue, and malaise; arthralgias; chest pain; heart failure; petechiae; neurologic impairment as a result of embolic events; and presence of, or change in, a heart murmur (Bernstein, 2011; McDonald, 2009). Because murmurs are present in many children with underlying CHD, it is important to detect a change in the quality of the murmur.

Diagnostic Evaluation

The diagnosis of bacterial endocarditis is established on the basis of several blood cultures that yield the causative organism and on echocardiography findings. In 90% of cases, the first two blood cultures will be positive if the patient has not received antibiotics (Park, 2008). The visualization of a *vegetation* (an abnormal growth of infected tissue) on echocardiographic studies helps considerably in establishing the diagnosis, but a study that is negative for vegetations does not rule out IE. Echocardiography may help identify the subgroup of children who

may require early surgical intervention to prevent further hemodynamic compromise or neurologic complications, such as those with large, mobile, left-sided vegetations. Other laboratory tests that may help confirm the diagnosis include CBC, erythrocyte sedimentation rate, ECG, and rheumatoid factor (McDonald, 2009; Park, 2008). The development of AV block suggests extension of disease into the myocardium, which can be helpful in identifying another subgroup of children who may benefit from early surgery.

Therapeutic Management

Prevention is the most important therapeutic intervention for IE. Children at risk should establish and maintain an optimal oral hygiene routine to reduce the incidence of periodontal infections. Guidelines from the AHA (Wilson et al., 2007) have changed the recommendations for antibiotic prophylaxis in at-risk infants and children. Recognizing that the risk for IE is higher from poor oral hygiene than from periodic invasive dental procedures and that adverse effects from antibiotics (e.g., allergy, resistance) are increasing, the AHA recommends that antibiotic prophylaxis be given to the following patients only (Wilson et al., 2007, p. 1745):

- Those who undergo prosthetic valve replacement or repair
- Those who have unrepaired complex cyanotic heart disease or palliative shunts
- Those who are within a 6-month postprocedure period for repair of a cardiac defect with a prosthetic device or material
- Those who have residual defects near the site of a prosthetic repair
- Those who have had IE previously
- Those who have had a cardiac transplant with subsequent valve dysfunction

Additionally, prophylaxis is recommended only for dental procedures that involve "manipulation of gingival tissue or the periapical region of teeth or perforation of oral mucosa" (Wilson et al., 2007, p. 1746) and for invasive respiratory tract procedures such as tonsillectomy and adenoidectomy or biopsy. Prophylactic antibiotics are no longer recommended for gastrointestinal or genitourinary procedures. The standard general prophylactic agent is amoxicillin given orally 1 hour before the procedure. Clindamycin or azithromycin is the antibiotic of choice in children allergic to penicillin or amoxicillin (Wilson et al., 2007).

Treatment for IE caused by bacteria invariably includes parenteral administration of antibiotics for 2 to 8 weeks, depending on the pathogen and the clinical circumstances (McDonald, 2009). The prolonged course of antibiotics is necessary because total elimination of the bacteria is essential. Because the bacteria in vegetations are protected from host defense mechanisms by the deposition of platelets and fibrin, aggressive and prolonged treatment is necessary for bacterial eradication (Bernstein, 2011).

Surgical interventions such as excision of the vegetation or removal of an infected valve may be indicated, particularly in the acute forms of endocarditis. Indications for surgery include severe, unresponsive HF, abscess, and evidence of valve involvement (McDonald, 2009).

NURSING CARE OF THE CHILD WITH INFECTIVE ENDOCARDITIS

■ Assessment

Assessment of the child with IE requires close monitoring of temperature elevations and vital signs. Vital signs should be monitored every 2 to 4 hours, along with a thorough cardiovascular and neurologic assessment. If a heart murmur is present, any change in it should be reported to the physician.

■ Nursing Diagnosis and Planning

Nursing diagnoses and expected outcomes for the child with infective endocarditis include the following:

- Ineffective Cerebral and Peripheral Tissue Perfusion (peripheral and cerebral) related to hemodynamic instability as a result of impaired valvular or myocardial function and effects of a cerebral infarction.

Expected Outcome. The child will have adequate peripheral tissue perfusion, as evidenced by pink mucous membranes and nail beds, a capillary refill time of less than 2 seconds, strong peripheral pulses, vital signs within normal limits, and adequate cerebral perfusion, as evidenced by mental status and a level of consciousness within normal limits and no evidence of focal neurologic deficits.

- Hyperthermia related to bacterial infection.

Expected Outcome. The child will maintain a body temperature that is within normal limits.

- Acute Pain or Chronic Pain (headaches, arthralgias, myalgias) related to the body's immunologic response.

Expected Outcome. The pain associated with headaches, arthralgias, and myalgias will be reduced or eliminated.

- Deficient Knowledge about home care of the child with IE related to unfamiliarity of the information.

Expected Outcomes. The parents will be able to administer medications and monitor the child's condition. They will explain the need for antibiotic prophylaxis and when it is indicated.

■ Interventions

The child will need vigilant monitoring of vital signs, peripheral perfusion, and hemodynamic stability. Any change in the vital signs, neurologic status, heart murmur, or tissue perfusion should be immediately reported to the physician. The child's activity level may be diminished, necessitating assistance with activities of daily living. Opportunities for quiet activities, such as reading, watching videos, drawing, and doing puzzles, should be provided.

The child's temperature should be monitored every 2 to 4 hours and plotted on a graph. If the child is receiving an aminoglycoside antibiotic, serum peak and trough levels may be monitored. The nurse must administer the antibiotics at the appropriate time, with trough levels determined before and peak levels determined 1 hour after the dose is administered. Acetaminophen is administered as needed for fever, as ordered by the physician, once the initial blood samples have been drawn for culture. Acetaminophen may also be administered for persistent headaches, arthralgias, and myalgias. Reassure the child and parents that the aches and malaise will resolve.

The child may be discharged home receiving parenteral antibiotic therapy. It is imperative that the parents have access to adequate community resources. The nurse must confirm that they have undergone formal instruction in the use of the IV mode selected (e.g., heparin lock, implanted venous access device, Hickman catheter, percutaneous line) and the proper administration of antibiotics. Provide reassurance and support to the family and child regarding the extensive and lengthy therapy that will be needed.

■ Evaluation

- Have the child's vital signs improved?
- Does the child have a capillary refill of less than 2 seconds?
- Does the child have a negative neurologic examination?

- Is the child's body temperature within normal limits?
- Have symptoms of anorexia, malaise, arthralgia, and fever subsided?
- Can the parents demonstrate administration of medications and verbalize an understanding of the need and indications for antibiotic prophylaxis?
- Are the parents demonstrating the ability to manage their child's condition at home?

ARRHYTHMIAS

The identification of an arrhythmia, a cardiac rhythm disturbance, in childhood is an important finding. The most important aspect is to recognize that an arrhythmia is present and classify it quickly as life threatening or non–life threatening. Assessing the child hemodynamically is a critical factor in determining the interventions. Often, the nurse will note an abnormal rhythm during a child's or adolescent's well examination. After the assessment of an abnormal or irregular radial pulse measurement, the nurse should obtain an apical pulse, counting for a full minute.

Etiology

Cardiac rhythm disturbances have numerous causes. Arrhythmias may be associated with underlying CHD or may occur in structurally normal hearts. Either an abnormal impulse formation or abnormal conduction or a combination of these two factors causes an arrhythmia. Rhythm disturbances can be classified as tachyarrhythmic (rapid) or bradyarrhythmic (slow).

Arrhythmias may be seen in the postoperative period after repair or palliation of a cardiac lesion. Postsurgical arrhythmias result from injury to the conduction system, edema, ischemia, incision or suture placement, and acid-base or electrolyte imbalances.

Underlying acquired heart disease, such as myocarditis or cardiomyopathy, sometimes produces arrhythmias. Abnormal electrical pathways in the heart can cause certain arrhythmias. *Wolff-Parkinson-White syndrome* is the most common example. Abnormal electrical repolarization of the heart can cause disturbances such as prolonged QT syndrome, which can result in a life-threatening ventricular tachycardia. This can have a genetic cause. Noncardiac causes of rhythm disturbances include fever, temperature instability, hypoxia, electrolyte and metabolic disturbances, increased intracranial pressure, hypovolemia, cardiac tamponade, and drug therapy or reactions.

Incidence

Arrhythmias in children are not uncommon, most are not life threatening, and most appear in children whose hearts are structurally normal. Supraventricular tachycardia (SVT) is the most common primary symptomatic rhythm disturbance seen in infants and children (Park, 2008).

Manifestations

In tachyarrhythmias and bradyarrhythmias, cardiac output is diminished. The clinical presentation is of low cardiac output syndrome with poor end-organ perfusion. The earliest signs and symptoms may be subtle; later they can be quite dramatic. Clinical manifestations for the infant and toddler may include poor feeding, irritability, lethargy, pale or mottled color, poor peripheral perfusion (diminished pulses, mottling, cool extremities, delayed capillary refill time), decreased urine output, and HF.

In older children, palpitations, dizziness, syncope, and exercise intolerance may be demonstrated. Tolerance of rhythm disturbances

PATHOPHYSIOLOGY

Arrhythmias

Tachyarrhythmias

Primary tachyarrhythmias can originate in either the atria or the ventricles. The most common atrial tachyarrhythmia is supraventricular tachycardia (SVT). SVT is triggered by an atrial ectopic focus (a group of irritable cells somewhere in the atrium) or a re-entry circuit (accessory pathway permitting abnormal conduction within the heart). Ventricular tachycardia is uncommon; it is seen in prolonged QT syndrome or in the preoperative or postoperative period in children with underlying structural heart disease.

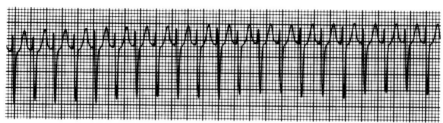

Supraventricular tachycardia. (Modified from Park, M. K., & Guntheroth, W. G. [2006]. *How to read pediatric ECGs* [4th ed., p. 224]. St. Louis: Mosby.)

Bradyarrhythmias

In children, primary cardiac bradyarrhythmias usually result from damage to the sinus node or the conduction pathway between the atria and the ventricles (AV block). Secondary bradyarrhythmias frequently result from surgery for congenital heart disease, especially surgery involving the atria. Children also can experience sinus bradyarrhythmia in which the pulse rate is markedly slower than expected for age.

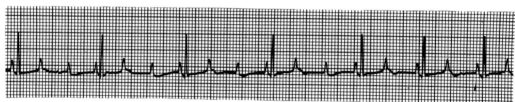

Heart block—two or three P waves for every QRS. Cardiac output is based on the rate of the QRS complexes—ventricular contraction. (Modified from Park, M. K., & Guntheroth, W. G. [2006]. *How to read pediatric ECGs* [4th ed., p. 232]. St. Louis: Mosby.)

Data from O'Connor, M., McDaniel, N., & Brady, W. (2008). The pediatric electrocardiogram part II: Dysrhythmias. *American Journal of Emergency Medicine, 26*(3), 348-358; Park, M. (2008). *Pediatric cardiology for practitioners* (5th ed.). St. Louis: Elsevier Mosby.

is based on the type of rhythm, underlying cardiac condition, and duration of rhythm and the effect on cardiac output.

In absent rhythms there is no cardiac output. This is a medical emergency. Cardiopulmonary resuscitation (CPR) and medical intervention must be initiated if the child is to survive.

Diagnostic Evaluation

The primary tool for diagnosing pediatric arrhythmias is the 12-lead ECG. Twenty-four-hour Holter monitoring and transtelephonic monitoring may be useful for documenting intermittent episodes of cardiac rhythm disturbances.

Therapeutic Management

Pediatric rhythm disturbances should be treated as emergencies if they compromise cardiac output or have the potential to degenerate into lethal (collapse) rhythms (e.g., ventricular fibrillation) (Van Hare, 2011). Management strategies include drug therapy, radiofrequency ablation, cardioversion, and pacemakers; the choice of treatment is guided by the origin of the arrhythmia and the clinical consequences.

Fast Pulse Rate

Supraventricular Tachycardia. SVT is a narrow QRS tachycardia. This narrow QRS configuration indicates that the impulse begins above the ventricles. Rates can be in the range of 220 to 300 beats/min. Children who are asymptomatic and hemodynamically stable can be treated conservatively. Vagal maneuvers may be used to terminate an episode of SVT by eliciting the diving reflex. Immersing the older child's face in ice water stimulates a vagal response that may stop the tachycardia; briefly placing an ice bag or bag of frozen vegetables over the infant's face accomplishes the same result. This should be done only while constantly monitoring the child and with emergency equipment available in case the child has a prolonged slow heart rate while converting to a normal rhythm.

If vagal maneuvers do not convert the child's heart to a normal rhythm, antiarrhythmics need to be considered. Antiarrhythmic drug therapy may also be successful in suppressing further episodes. Older children who continue to have episodes of SVT may benefit from radiofrequency ablation of the ectopic focus or accessory pathway.

Infants and children who are hemodynamically unstable require emergency intervention. If vascular access is present, the drug adenosine may be given. Adenosine is an effective antiarrhythmic because of its ability to slow conduction through the AV node and, in many cases, successfully terminate episodes of SVT rapidly and safely (Park, 2008). Synchronized cardioversion, however, remains the treatment of choice for the child with profound cardiovascular compromise.

Ventricular Tachycardia. Ventricular tachycardia is a wide complex tachycardia. This indicates that the impulse originates in the ventricle. The emergency management of ventricular tachycardia in unconscious children is synchronized cardioversion. Children with a wide complex tachycardia and no pulse (absent pulse) require CPR until defibrillation is available. Lidocaine, 1 mg/kg, may be administered before cardioversion, followed by a continuous infusion of the drug to prevent further episodes (Park, 2008). Once the tachycardia has been terminated, underlying causes should be explored.

Slow Pulse Rate

Bradyarrhythmias. Primary cardiac bradyarrhythmias include the varying degrees of heart block and junctional or ventricular "escape" rhythms caused by sinus node dysfunction. These arrhythmias are marked by dissociation between the P wave and the QRS complex, with the asynchrony between the atrial and ventricular contractions. They may be congenital, but are often seen in children who have undergone cardiac surgery, especially surgery of the atria (O'Connor, McDaniel, & Brady, 2008). Temporary or permanent cardiac pacing may be necessary to maintain adequate cardiac output.

Absent Rhythms. The classification of absent or collapse rhythms includes asystole, ventricular fibrillation, and pulseless electrical activity. In asystole, electrical cardiac activity is absent. Epinephrine is administered to stimulate cardiac activity. The heart is in electrical standstill, and there is no myocardial activity or cardiac output. The ECG rhythm strip is a "flat line." The emergency management of asystole is CPR and medical management. Epinephrine is administered to stimulate cardiac activity. The drug may be given IV, intraosseously, or through an endotracheal tube.

Ventricular fibrillation, rare in children, is frequently the result of underlying cardiac disease. The emergency management of episodes of ventricular fibrillation is defibrillation and CPR. Drugs administered during resuscitation efforts include epinephrine, lidocaine, and other antiarrhythmic agents.

Pulseless electrical activity indicates a hemodynamically compromised state in which cardiac electrical activity is unable to generate effective myocardial contraction and cardiac output. The ECG rhythm strip shows what looks like a normal rhythm. When the nurse palpates for a pulse or listens for a heartbeat, there will be none. CPR must be initiated. The underlying cause is usually noncardiac (e.g., respiratory arrest), and it must be identified and corrected for the child to survive the episode.

NURSING CARE OF THE CHILD WITH AN ARRHYTHMIA

▪ Assessment

Children with arrhythmias require a thorough cardiovascular assessment because they are at risk for development of cardiogenic shock. In a stable or compensated child with an arrhythmia, it is important to obtain a comprehensive and accurate history of activity tolerance. Older children may have unexplained episodes of dizziness, palpitations, or syncope. Irregular pulse may be noted. Nurses who have been trained to read pediatric ECG rhythm strips may observe signs of a particular arrhythmia.

▪ Nursing Diagnosis and Planning

Nursing diagnoses and expected outcomes for the child with an arrhythmia include the following:

⚡ SAFETY ALERT

Arrhythmias

If a child is having an arrhythmia, assess responsiveness and remember CAB*:

CIRCULATION assessment.
- Palpate and auscultate pulses for a maximum of 10 seconds.
- If no pulse, begin chest compressions.
- If slow pulse, assess the child's tolerance of slow pulse (including perfusion and pulses).

AIRWAY assessment.

BREATHING assessment.
- If no breathing, begin ventilation after first cycle of chest compressions.
- Obtain an ECG rhythm strip for assessment.
- Shock delivery if needed.

*Field, J. M. Hazinski, M. F., Sayre, M. R., , R., et al. (2010). American Heart Association guidelines for cardiopulmonary resuscitation and emergency cardiac care. *Circulation, 122,* S640-S656.

- Decreased Cardiac Output related to decreased ventricular filling or decreased rate of heart contractions.

Expected Outcome. The child will have pink or baseline cyanotic mucous membranes and nail beds, brisk capillary refill, good-quality pulses, and a normal level of consciousness.

- Risk for Injury related to episodes of syncope.

Expected Outcome. The child will remain free of injury during any episodes of syncope.

- Deficient Knowledge about care of a child with a potentially fatal condition related to unfamiliarity with the information.

Expected Outcomes. The family will describe medication administration, will demonstrate an ability to identify signs and symptoms indicative of arrhythmias, and will be able to perform CPR.

▪ Interventions

Nursing interventions involve immediate care of the child who has the arrhythmia and education of the child and family. The child and family will need information regarding monitoring for future signs and symptoms of arrhythmias, administering medications as ordered, and appropriate emergency measures to initiate, including CPR, once the child has been discharged from the hospital.

Educating the child and family is imperative for those children with life-threatening arrhythmias. Teach the child and family how to take a pulse or listen to the heart rate with a stethoscope. Teach the child and family to identify the signs and symptoms of arrhythmia, including poor feeding, color changes, palpitations, syncope/dizziness, respiratory distress, and fatigue. These signs and symptoms should be reported to the parent or teacher as soon as possible, and medical attention should be sought. Children who take antiarrhythmics at home need to adhere to the prescribed medication schedule closely and must be careful not to skip any doses. Medical alert bracelets should be worn by children who are in preschool or school. Parents and teachers also need to be aware of signs and symptoms that may indicate the early appearance of arrhythmias. All caretakers should complete a formal course in CPR and know how to activate the emergency medical services system.

▪ Evaluation

- Are the child's pulses of good quality and mucous membranes pink or baseline cyanosis, and does the child have a normal level of consciousness?

- Has the child remained free from injury related to falling as a result of syncope?
- Have the child, parents, and other caregivers demonstrated an understanding of medications, activity limitations, and the possibility of a life-threatening episode and how to activate the emergency medical services system?
- Have the child and parents demonstrated how to listen to the heart rate with a stethoscope or palpate a pulse?

RHEUMATIC FEVER

Rheumatic fever (RF) is a diffuse inflammatory condition, most probably of autoimmune origin (see Chapter 18), of the connective tissue, primarily of the heart, joints, subcutaneous tissues, brain, and blood vessels. The most serious complication is rheumatic heart disease, which can result in permanent damage to the cardiac valves, most commonly the mitral and aortic valves.

PATHOPHYSIOLOGY

Rheumatic Fever

Infection by group A beta-hemolytic streptococci located in the pharyngeal area triggers an abnormal humoral and cell-mediated immunologic response in children who have RF. Immune complexes cross-react with normal tissue in the heart, brain, skin, and joints, causing inflammation in these sites. Eventually, although the disease is self-limiting, permanent damage to cardiac valve tissue can occur. There may be a genetic predisposition to developing RF, although the evidence is unclear.*

*Steer, A., & Carapetis, J. (2009). Acute rheumatic fever and rheumatic heart disease in indigenous populations. *Pediatric Clinics of North America, 56*, 1401-1409.

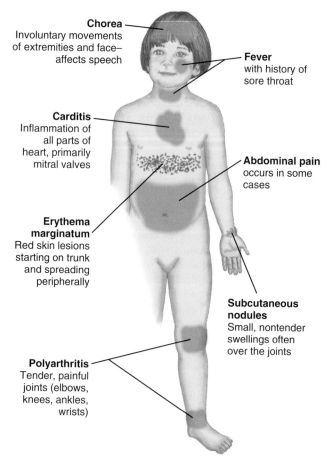

FIG 22-2 Clinical manifestations of rheumatic fever.

Chorea
Involuntary movements of extremities and face— affects speech

Fever
with history of sore throat

Carditis
Inflammation of all parts of heart, primarily mitral valves

Abdominal pain
occurs in some cases

Erythema marginatum
Red skin lesions starting on trunk and spreading peripherally

Subcutaneous nodules
Small, nontender swellings often over the joints

Polyarthritis
Tender, painful joints (elbows, knees, ankles, wrists)

Etiology

RF characteristically manifests 2 to 6 weeks after an untreated or partially treated group A beta-hemolytic streptococcal infection of the upper respiratory tract. The initial infection may or may not produce symptoms of pharyngitis. The major complication from rheumatic fever is rheumatic heart disease.

Incidence

Rheumatic fever has nearly disappeared from the United States and other developed countries. However, it is endemic worldwide in countries with overcrowding, poor access to health care, poor sanitation, and persistent exposure to streptococcal infections; it is also present in indigenous populations within developed countries (e.g., Alaskan natives and native Americans in the United States) (Steer & Carapetis, 2009).

Manifestations

Major manifestations of RF include the following (Figure 22-2):
- *Arthritis:* Tender, warm, erythematous joints, especially in the large joints, including the elbows, knees, ankles, and wrists; occurs in 75% of RF cases during the acute febrile period (first 1 to 2 weeks of illness). The typical presentation is a migratory polyarthritis, with inflammation moving rapidly from one joint to another and usually lasting less than 1 week for an individual joint before resolving.

- *Carditis:* Inflammation of the endocardium, including the valves, myocardium, and pericardium; may be subclinical and is usually diagnosed by the development of a cardiac murmur, cardiac enlargement or failure, or a pericardial friction rub. Mitral valve involvement is the most frequent manifestation of carditis.
- *Chorea:* Involuntary, purposeless, jerking movements of the legs, arms, and face, with speech impairment and emotional lability, caused by CNS involvement in RF. Also referred to as *Sydenham's chorea,* it is more common in girls and usually occurs in the absence of carditis or polyarthritis. Chorea has a longer latency period of up to 6 months after the initial streptococcal pharyngitis.
- *Erythema marginatum:* Red, painless skin lesions that start as flat or slightly raised macules, usually over the trunk. The erythema spreads at the margins of the lesion with central clearing.
- *Subcutaneous nodules:* Small, nontender lumps, attached to the tendon sheaths of joints and on bony prominences. They occur only rarely in RF and usually are associated with severe carditis.

Although arthritis is the most common manifestation, carditis is by far the most serious and the major cause of morbidity and mortality during both acute and chronic phases of the disease. Cardiac valvular disease is the major long-term consequence of RF (Gerber, 2011).

Minor criteria that assist in making a diagnosis of RF include a history of previous RF; arthralgias (joint pain) without arthritis; fever; elevated acute-phase reactants, including C-reactive protein and erythrocyte sedimentation rate; and first-degree AV block on the ECG.

Diagnostic Evaluation

A diagnosis of RF is made using the presence of the major and minor manifestations as previously described; these are referred to as the Jones criteria and are the gold standard for diagnosis of RF (American Heart Association, Council on Cardiovascular Diseases in the Young Special Writing Group of the Committee on Rheumatic Fever, Endocarditis, and Kawasaki Disease, 1992). According to the Jones criteria, a diagnosis of RF can be made if the patient manifests at least two of the major manifestations or one major and two minor manifestations. In addition, the patient must have evidence of a recent streptococcal infection diagnosed using at least one of the following diagnostic studies: positive throat culture, antistreptolysin O titer, Streptozyme, or anti-DNase-B assay; or by a history of scarlet fever.

Therapeutic Management

The management of RF includes eradication of the streptococcal bacteria and treatment of other symptoms, such as joint inflammation, HF, and chorea. Once RF has been confirmed, the child receives a 10-day course of oral penicillin or a single dose of benzathine penicillin intramuscularly. Cephalosporins or erythromycin may be used in penicillin-allergic children (Gerber, Baltimore, Eaton et al., 2009). Once the diagnosis is firmly established, antiinflammatory agents, including aspirin, or corticosteroids in the presence of significant carditis, are administered to speed resolution of the inflammatory process, although neither therapy has been proved to have an effect on the incidence or course of carditis. The duration of therapy is tailored according to the child's clinical course.

Children who have had RF are susceptible to recurrent attacks, risk further cardiac valve damage, and require secondary prophylaxis to prevent recurrence. The child without cardiac complications should receive antibiotic prophylaxis for 5 years or through age 21 years, whichever is longer. Those with rheumatic heart disease but no residual cardiac effects should continue prophylaxis for at least 10 years or until age 21 years (whichever is longer), and those with both rheumatic heart disease and residual cardiac issues continue prophylaxis for the longer of either 10 years or until 40 years of age (Gerber et al., 2009). The AHA recommends prophylaxis for life for those who have contact with children who may have group A streptococcal infection, such as teachers, health care workers, and parents of school-age children. Penicillin is the drug of choice, either by monthly intramuscular injection, which is more reliable in terms of adherence, or an oral dose of 250 mg twice daily (Gerber et al., 2009).

NURSING CARE OF THE CHILD WITH RHEUMATIC FEVER

Assessment

Children with RF often are admitted to the hospital on bed rest during the acute phase. Initially, the nurse determines whether the child or any family members have had a sore throat or unexplained fever within the past 2 months. The child should be monitored for cardiac symptoms throughout the course of hospitalization. Temperature, pulse, respiration, and blood pressure are assessed, and the child is observed for signs of carditis, including tachycardia; heart murmur; friction rub;

shortness of breath; or edema of the face, abdomen, or ankles. Examination of the joints may reveal very tender elbows, knees, ankles, and wrists, with subcutaneous nodules over extensor surfaces of the joints. Children with RF may have red skin lesions on the trunk or rapid, purposeless, involuntary movements (chorea), either on observation or by history.

Nursing Diagnosis and Planning

Nursing diagnoses and expected outcomes for the child with rheumatic fever include the following:

- Deficient Knowledge related to unfamiliarity with medications and activity restrictions.

Expected Outcome. The child will adhere to the medication regimen and activity restrictions.

- Ineffective Coping related to confinement.

Expected Outcomes. The child will participate in quiet activities and will maintain social contact.

- Acute Pain related to polyarthritis.

Expected Outcomes. The child will verbalize an increase in comfort and will indicate a decrease in pain using an age-appropriate pain tool.

- Risk for Injury related to subsequent streptococcal infection.

Expected Outcomes. The child will inform parents at the first sign of a sore throat, and the family will adhere to antibiotic prophylaxis.

Interventions

The nurse administers antibiotics, analgesics, and antipyretics as ordered and reports to the physician any fever or pain. Children with RF require bed rest during the acute febrile stage of the illness and should not return to school while there is clear evidence of rheumatic activity. While the child's activities are restricted, the nurse and family should talk about limiting visitors and arranging for quiet yet enjoyable activities. Family members and friends may provide board and computer games, movies, puzzles, and crafts for the school-age child. Such activities will help minimize activity and cardiac demand. The child may benefit from a daily schedule that includes rest periods interspersed with these diverse activities and some limited exercise (e.g., passive range-of-motion exercises). An art or play therapist can work with the child who is extremely anxious because of confinement.

Nursing comfort measures include alternating application of heat and cold to affected joints, repositioning, massage, and providing distraction by use of guided imagery and relaxation. Seizure precautions are warranted if the child has chorea. At home, parents must practice safety measures. For example, the child who cannot control movements may need to sleep on a mattress on the floor and may need assistance going up and down stairs. The child may be embarrassed by uncontrolled movements, especially in front of peers, and will need reassurance that these symptoms are temporary.

Emphasize to parents the importance of adherence to antibiotic prophylaxis. The family may be allowed to offer an adolescent the choice of monthly injections versus daily oral administration. If the child chooses the oral route, instruct the family about the required dose, frequency of administration, duration, effects, side effects, and potential cardiac complications if the regimen is not followed precisely.

Evaluation

- Is the child taking antibiotics as ordered?
- Is the child following modified bed rest guidelines?
- Is the child playing board games, reading, and visiting with friends as tolerated?

- Has the child verbalized a decrease in pain and indicated decreased pain on an appropriate assessment tool?
- Does the child take antibiotic prophylaxis as ordered and notify the parent if experiencing a sore throat?

KAWASAKI DISEASE

Kawasaki disease, also called *mucocutaneous lymph node syndrome,* is an acute, febrile, exanthematous illness of children with a generalized vasculitis of unknown etiology. Kawasaki disease is a major cause of acquired heart disease in children in the United States. Coronary artery aneurysms are seen in 20% to 25% of children with untreated Kawasaki disease (Son & Newburger, 2011).

Etiology

The cause of Kawasaki disease remains unknown. However, recent evidence suggests that it is an immune-mediated vasculitis triggered by an acute infection or by a bacterial toxin (see Chapter 18). Kawasaki disease may have a genetic component (Son & Newburger, 2011); it also has a seasonal component, being diagnosed most often in late winter and early spring.

Incidence

Kawasaki disease is seen most frequently in children younger than 5 years and is diagnosed less frequently in children older than 8 years. Affected boys outnumber affected girls (1.5 to 1), and there is an increased incidence in children of Asian ancestry (Park, 2008).

Manifestations

Kawasaki disease manifests in three phases. The acute stage lasts approximately 10 days and is characterized by a high fever that persists longer than 5 days. The fever is unresponsive to antibiotic treatment. Clinical signs include bilateral, nonpurulent conjunctivitis; changes in the mucous membranes (i.e., erythema, fissures, and cracking of the lips; strawberry tongue); changes in the peripheral extremities, such as swelling of the hands and feet and erythema of the palms and soles; a generalized erythematous rash (Figure 22-3); and enlarged cervical lymph nodes. Tachycardia and extreme irritability are also common.

The second or subacute phase lasts from approximately day 11 to day 25. The fever disappears, and most symptoms resolve. The phase is characterized by continued irritability, anorexia, desquamation of the fingers and toes, arthritis and arthralgia, and cardiovascular manifestations, including HF, arrhythmias, and the typical coronary aneurysms (Park, 2008).

Coronary aneurysm formation begins early in the second phase. A baseline echocardiogram at diagnosis with repeat studies at 2 weeks, 6

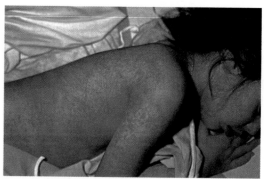

FIG 22-3 Erythematous rash of Kawasaki disease. (From Looking-bill, D. P., & Marks, J. G., Jr. [1992]. *Principles of dermatology* [2nd ed., p. 223]. Philadelphia: Saunders.)

PATHOPHYSIOLOGY

Kawasaki Disease

An infectious or possibly toxic trigger initiates an immune system response that affects medium-size arteries, especially the coronary arteries. A generalized immune response becomes more specific, with increasing numbers of T lymphocytes and B lymphocytes infiltrating the smooth muscle cells of the vascular walls. The infiltration causes edema and inflammation, which progressively weaken the vascular walls, leading to aneurysms. As the disease progresses, fibrous connective tissue forms at the inflammatory sites, eventually thickening and scarring the vascular walls. These vascular changes, along with the increased platelets that occur as part of the disease process, can cause thrombus formation, myocardial infarction, and death in some children.

to 8 weeks, and 6 to 12 months (optional) will help identify those with coronary artery involvement (Son & Newburger, 2011)). Severe thrombocytosis occurs during this period and marks the period of highest risk for coronary artery thrombosis in the areas of aneurysm, resulting in myocardial infarction.

The final or convalescent stage begins when most symptoms have disappeared and lasts until the erythrocyte sedimentation rate returns to normal. Deep transverse grooves, called *Beau's lines,* may appear on the child's nails.

Diagnostic Evaluation

Fever of 5 days duration in conjunction with at least four of the five following primary clinical findings for the acute phase establishes the diagnosis of Kawasaki disease (Son & Newburger, 2011):
- Bilateral nonpurulent conjunctivitis
- Oral mucosal alterations (e.g., strawberry tongue; pharyngeal erythema; dry, fissured lips)
- Redness of the hands and feet followed by desquamation
- Rash on the trunk
- Cervical lymphadenopathy with large nodes

and
- No other known disease process to explain the signs and symptoms

Laboratory data are nonspecific. The white blood cell count is elevated during the acute phase, as are the erythrocyte sedimentation rate and C-reactive protein level. There is sterile pyuria. The ECG in the acute phase may demonstrate first-degree heart block. Platelet levels dramatically rise during the subacute phase. Aneurysms are detected with echocardiography.

Therapeutic Management

Therapeutic management is directed toward preventing or reducing the coronary artery damage from Kawasaki disease. High-dose intravenous immune globulin (IVIG) in combination with aspirin has been shown to lower the prevalence of coronary artery abnormalities when given within 10 days of fever onset. At diagnosis, IVIG is given in a dosage of 2 g/kg over a 10- to 12-hour infusion (American Academy of Pediatrics [AAP], 2009). High-dose aspirin therapy is begun at the same time. Initially, the dosage is in the antiinflammatory range of 80 to 100 mg/kg/day in four evenly divided doses until fever resolves. The dosage is then reduced to an antiplatelet aggregation dose of 3 to 5 mg/kg/day once daily and continued through weeks 6 to 8 of the illness (AAP, 2009). If coronary artery abnormalities are identified, this dosage is continued indefinitely (Park, 2008). Corticosteroids may be considered if the child is unresponsive to standard therapy.

NURSING CARE OF THE CHILD WITH KAWASAKI DISEASE

■ Assessment

During the acute phase, the nurse must monitor the child's cardiac status closely, looking for clinical signs and symptoms of heart failure. Changes in pulse, respiration, blood pressure, and color, along with shortness of breath, chest pain, and decreased activity, may suggest cardiac complications. It is important to examine the child's eyes, mouth, and skin for signs of infection and the joints for redness, swelling, and tenderness.

The nurse should determine the parents' anxiety level. Parents are often frightened by how sick the child is and the threat of a possibly devastating outcome. Families appreciate talking about their fears; learning about the cause of the illness, the treatment plan, and the prognosis; and participating in the child's care.

■ Nursing Diagnosis and Planning

Nursing diagnoses and expected outcomes for the child with Kawasaki disease and the child's family include the following:
- Risk for Deficient Fluid Volume related to fever.

Expected Outcome. The child will maintain fluid and electrolyte balance, as evidenced by normal laboratory values and intake and output appropriate for age.
- Acute Pain related to fever, skin manifestations, and joint inflammation.

Expected Outcomes. The child will rest comfortably, as evidenced by periods of uninterrupted sleep, and will express decreased pain on an age-appropriate pain assessment tool.
- Fear related to changes in the child's behavior and uncertainty about the long-term prognosis.

Expected Outcome. The parents and child will discuss their fears related to having a serious disease with a long recuperative period.

■ Interventions

The nurse should administer aspirin with milk or food and infuse IVIG as ordered. During the infusion, it is important to monitor the child's vital signs and any adverse reactions to IVIG, including facial flushing, tightness in the chest, chills, dizziness, nausea, vomiting, diaphoresis, and hypotension. Blood pressure is checked every 15 minutes for the first hour and every 30 minutes thereafter until the infusion is complete. A precipitous fall in blood pressure may occur 30 to 60 minutes after the infusion has begun; this is often related to the rate of infusion. The physician will usually lower the prescribed rate of infusion if such a reaction occurs and may order diphenhydramine (Benadryl) and acetaminophen to control side effects. Epinephrine is given for anaphylactic reactions. IVIG may interfere with achieving immunity from live-virus vaccines, so some immunizations (e.g., measles, mumps, rubella, varicella) should be delayed for 11 months after IVIG therapy (AAP, 2009).

Nursing care focuses on comfort measures and adequate hydration. The nurse and parents must encourage fluid intake by offering ice pops or ice to numb affected mucous membranes; giving liquids that are high in calories and low in acid through a straw (avoiding citrus drinks and sodas); and offering favorite foods that are soft and bland. The nurse or family can apply salve to soothe cracked, dry lips.

Sponge baths with tepid water often decrease fever and relieve discomfort from skin manifestations. The child should be handled gently and only when necessary. If itching is severe, the physician should be notified.

Toddlers and preschool children fear hospitalization and body changes, often exhibiting regressive behavior and sleeping poorly. In addition, children with Kawasaki disease also manifest increased irritability during the acute phase. If possible, keep the environment calm by talking in gentle tones, playing soft music, and avoiding bright overhead lights. It may help to line the bed with soft blankets from home. Assure the family that the fever, pain, and irritability will eventually resolve and praise their hard work in keeping the child comfortable. Because the child's extreme irritability is an area of concern for parents, the nurse should provide support so the parent can take periodic breaks. Discharge instructions should include provisions for a cardiac follow-up. Parents' fears can be decreased through an understanding of the disease and treatment.

■ Evaluation

- Is the child taking adequate amounts of fluid and maintaining electrolyte balance?
- Is the child's urine output appropriate for age (see Chapter 16)?
- Is the child experiencing periods of uninterrupted rest?
- Does the child demonstrate decreased pain on an age-appropriate assessment tool?
- Are the parents able to verbalize their fears and discuss the course of the illness and their commitment to follow-up care?

HYPERTENSION

Hypertension is defined as an average systolic or average diastolic blood pressure that exceeds or is equal to the 95th percentile for age, height, and sex on the basis of measurements obtained on at least three occasions. Children with systolic blood pressure or diastolic blood pressure between the 90th and 95th percentiles are considered to be prehypertensive; prehypertension in adolescents is defined as blood pressure greater than or equal to 120/80 mm Hg (National High Blood Pressure Education Program Working Group on High Blood Pressure in Children and Adolescents [NHBPEP Working Group], 2007). Normal blood pressure is defined as a systolic or diastolic pressure that is less than the 90th percentile for age, height and sex (see Evolve website).

The two primary categories of hypertension are *primary* (idiopathic) and *secondary* (symptom of underlying disease). Primary hypertension predominates in the older adolescent, whereas secondary causes are overwhelmingly more common in the younger age-groups.

Etiology

Pediatric hypertension that is not the result of an underlying disease is referred to as essential hypertension, similar to that seen in adults. Pediatric hypertension has been increasing in the United States and is intimately related to the increasing prevalence of obesity (Lande, 2011). Essential hypertension is more prevalent among adolescents, teenagers, and those with moderately elevated blood pressure. The early development of essential hypertension is linked to childhood obesity, children with diabetes mellitus, and a strong family history of hypertension. Affected adults and children may exhibit exaggerated blood pressure responses to physical and emotional stresses compared with normotensive individuals. Some individuals with essential hypertension are negatively affected by increased levels of dietary sodium (Lande, 2011).

Height and weight are additional determinations of blood pressure in children. Children with elevated blood pressure are usually taller and heavier than their age-matched peers. The causes of secondary hypertension in children include various renal and renovascular diseases, coarctation of the aorta, endocrine and metabolic disorders, neurologic disease, and drug-related causes.

Of children with significant blood pressure elevations, the vast majority have renal or renovascular disease as the underlying cause. Renal arterial disease is a common etiology in the sick neonate and is usually caused by renal artery thrombosis resulting from the use of umbilical artery catheters or from polycythemia. Renal parenchymal disease, such as glomerulonephritis, obstructive uropathy, and hemolytic uremic syndrome are the most common causes of hypertension in children before adolescence.

Coarctation of the aorta is the primary cardiovascular cause of hypertension. Coarctation should be ruled out early in the course of the evaluation, because this is a treatable cause of hypertension, but one that may result in fixed vascular changes if not detected before adolescence. The heart itself is primarily an *end-organ,* in which hypertension can have long-term detrimental effects, as opposed to having any important etiologic role in hypertension. Endocrine causes include pheochromocytoma and congenital adrenal hyperplasia. Diabetes mellitus is frequently complicated by renal involvement and associated hypertension. Increased intracranial pressure from a tumor, trauma, or meningitis will produce acute, severe hypertension and is a medical emergency. Common causes of elevated blood pressure include use of corticosteroids, oral contraceptives, and sympathomimetic drugs (e.g., those found in over-the-counter cold preparations) and cocaine or amphetamine abuse.

Incidence

Hypertension is increasingly seen in children, with an overall prevalence of approximately 5 per 100 children (AAP, 2011). The majority of these children have only mild elevations of blood pressure, and those with significant blood pressure elevations often have secondary hypertension. Because adult hypertension is more prevalent in the African-American and Asian populations, adolescents from these racial groups should be monitored carefully. Children in families who have members with hypertension tend to have higher-than-normal blood pressures. Because of increasing prevalence of hypertension in young children, the NHBPEP Working Group (2007) recommends blood pressure measurement for all children beginning at 3 years of age, and earlier in children with underlying cardiac or renal disease or certain other underlying medical conditions.

PATHOPHYSIOLOGY

Hypertension

Systolic pressure reflects the stroke volume of the heart, the rate of blood ejected, and the elasticity of the aorta. Diastolic pressure reflects the resting pressure of the arterial system; it is affected by the peripheral vascular resistance or the diameter of the arteries and the heart rate. An increase in the heart rate decreases the diastolic or ventricular filling time. Together, these measurements form the arterial blood pressure and provide information about arterial function.

Hypertension, or increased arterial blood pressure over time, may produce cardiac enlargement and subsequent cardiac failure, cerebrovascular disease, renal disease and failure, retinal disease, and accelerated atherosclerosis and coronary heart disease. These effects are seen predominantly with primary or essential hypertension.

Manifestations

Children with primary hypertension rarely have clinical evidence of disease; the elevated blood pressure is usually detected on a routine physical examination. High elevations of blood pressure, however, can lead to the following manifestations:

- Essential or primary hypertension: Dizziness, headaches, epistaxis, and visual disturbances. Late signs of severe or acute hypertension include neurologic deficits, extremity weakness, and cerebrovascular accidents.
- Secondary hypertension—*renal:* Weight loss or failure to gain weight, facial or periorbital edema, pale mucous membranes, and unilateral or bilateral abdominal mass; *cardiovascular:* absent or decreased femoral pulses, decreased blood pressure in the lower extremities compared with the upper extremities, cardiomegaly, murmur, and signs and symptoms of HF.

Diagnostic Evaluation

Differentiating primary from secondary hypertension requires a comprehensive medical history and physical examination. Blood pressure measurements are done on all four extremities and repeated twice if elevated. Blood tests (complete blood cell count; blood urea nitrogen, creatinine, uric acid, and electrolyte levels), urinalysis, echocardiography, ultrasonography of the kidneys, and arteriography can rule out causes of secondary hypertension. Urinary catecholamines may be considered to rule out pheochromocytoma.

The diagnosis of primary, or essential, hypertension is established primarily by excluding an underlying disease. A hypertensive preadolescent or adolescent with a family history of hypertension is more likely to have primary hypertension as opposed to secondary hypertension. For younger age-groups, secondary causes of hypertension are much more prevalent.

Therapeutic Management
Primary Hypertension

Treatment of primary, or essential, hypertension during childhood emphasizes risk factor modification. Lifestyle counseling focuses on non-pharmacologic therapy that includes weight reduction, physical conditioning, dietary modifications, and stress modification. If the non-pharmacologic treatments are maximized, the need for pharmacologic therapy in children with hypertension should be reduced.

Weight Reduction

A direct relationship exists between obesity and hypertension. This relationship may be caused in part by increased sympathetic nervous system activity. Weight maintenance (children) or gradual weight reduction (adolescents) plays an important role in lowering blood pressure. Weight loss requires a program of diet, exercise, and lifestyle changes, and it is often very difficult to achieve significant results in asymptomatic young people. Even so, a modest 5- to 10-pound weight loss can have a positive effect on blood pressure reduction. Because of the long-term nature of primary hypertension, efforts should focus on education regarding a healthy lifestyle and the gradual incorporation of good dietary habits and activity into the child's everyday life. Success frequently depends on support from health care professionals, nutritionists, and family members.

Physical Conditioning An exercise program should be initiated in conjunction with a dietary weight reduction plan. Exercise not only facilitates weight loss, it also lowers blood pressure independent of weight loss. Thirty to 60 minutes of aerobic exercise several times per week may result in a consistently lower resting blood pressure. Recently, studies have also suggested that any increase in total physical activity during the day, such as climbing a flight of stairs several times per day instead of using an elevator, can show measurable benefit over months and years. The most successful approach in children and adolescents is to focus on activities that they enjoy and that provide a social outlet, such as organized sports or bike riding. Exercise in which the whole family can participate, such as walking or hiking, is also more likely to be successful in terms of maintaining a consistent lifestyle change.

Dietary Modification Avoidance of a high sodium intake is recommended in hypertensive and normotensive children and adolescents. Evidence suggests an association between alcohol and hypertension, believed to be related to alterations in the renin-angiotensin system and neurotransmitters. Smoking produces an aldosterone-like hypertension in young people. Therefore, avoidance of alcohol and tobacco is recommended.

Relaxation Techniques Relaxation techniques have resulted in modest reductions in blood pressure in the adult population. Information on efficacy in children is not yet available.

Pharmacologic Treatment Pharmacologic treatment of primary hypertension may be indicated if there is coexisting secondary hypertension, or if lifestyle modifications are ineffective. Diuretics, beta-adrenergic receptor blockers, and vasodilators are the mainstay of pharmacologic treatment. Pharmacologic therapy usually is begun with a diuretic and/or a beta-adrenergic receptor blocker; a vasodilator is added if these are not effective (Park, 2008).

Secondary Hypertension

Treatment of the underlying process is the focus of therapy in secondary hypertension. If the secondary disease is coarctation of the aorta or renal artery disease, surgery may be indicated. Therapy in patients with renal parenchymal or endocrine pathologic conditions focuses on the disease process. Effective treatment will often result in secondary control of blood pressure.

NURSING CARE OF THE CHILD WITH HYPERTENSION

■ Assessment

■ **Blood Pressure Screening.** Blood pressure screening should be initiated when a child is 3 years old and should continue through adolescence. Blood pressure should be checked at least yearly and more often

> ### ⚡ SAFETY ALERT
>
> #### *Infusing Intravenous Antihypertensive Medications*
>
> Intravenous antihypertensive medications must be infused very slowly, and an arterial line must be in place for monitoring. Sudden hypotension may result after initiation of antihypertensive drugs.

if the blood pressure reading is higher than recommended. The environment should be as quiet as possible, and the child's arm should be supported at the heart level. If an elevated blood pressure is found, measurement should be repeated two more times, allowing a 2- to 3-minute interval between blood pressure checks.

Cuff size is of critical importance. A too-small blood pressure cuff will result in an inappropriately high blood pressure reading. (See Chapter 13 for cuff measurement and selection.)

■ **Physical Assessment.** Assessment of a child with hypertension includes inspection of the skin to detect evidence of underlying disease, including edema (renal disease) and the presence of café-au-lait spots (neurofibromatosis) or moon facies (Cushing syndrome, steroid administration). The pulses should be palpated for symmetry and strength. A child with coarctation of the aorta is likely to have bounding upper extremity pulses and diminished or absent femoral and pedal pulses. The heart and chest are auscultated to determine the heart rate and to detect any heart murmur, gallop, or aortic bruit. The abdomen is auscultated for renal bruits. A neurologic examination is urgently indicated in children with acute, severe hypertension to rule out increased intracranial pressure.

■ Nursing Diagnosis and Planning

Nursing diagnoses and expected outcomes for the child with hypertension include the following:

- Ineffective Peripheral Tissue Perfusion, Ineffective Cerebral Tissue Perfusion, and Risk for Decreased Cardiac Tissue Perfusion related to elevation in systolic or diastolic arterial blood pressure.

Expected Outcome. The child will maintain normal tissue perfusion with blood pressure at a controlled level (below the 90th percentile for age).

- Ineffective Family Therapeutic Regimen Management related to excessive demands of dietary restrictions, physical conditioning, and a possible medication regimen.

Expected Outcomes. The child will describe and will engage in diet, physical conditioning, and medication therapy to lower blood pressure.

■ Interventions

Nursing interventions focus on education and family support and adherence to the treatment regimen. The nurse may consult a dietitian and collaboratively develop a teaching plan regarding a modified-sodium and weight-reduction diet if ordered. When the nurse counsels the family and child about dietary modifications, it is important to include the whole family in making dietary changes to increase motivation and adherence.

If a physical conditioning program is prescribed, physical activities the child enjoys are identified so that they can be incorporated into the plan. Family members and friends are encouraged to join the child in the exercise program. Praise the child for progress in weight loss and increased endurance. Encourage the child to express feelings about any possible problems related to home or school situations. Discuss methods for facilitating relaxation that may be helpful during periods of stress.

The child who is hospitalized with acute, severe hypertension may require medications. Once the child has been stabilized after an acute hypertensive crisis, oral antihypertensive medications will likely be prescribed. During discharge planning, reinforce the importance of adherence to the medication regimen and of periodic follow-up evaluations.

■ Evaluation

- Does the child maintain blood pressure below the 90th percentile for age?
- Has the child achieved weight loss?
- Is the child adhering to a modified-sodium diet?
- Is the child engaging in regular physical exercise according to the prescribed regimen?
- Is the child adhering to the medication regimen?

CARDIOMYOPATHIES

The cardiomyopathies are diseases of the heart muscle in which the cardiac pathologic condition is not the result of CHD, coronary artery disease, or other systemic disease. Cardiomyopathy is classified into three types on the basis of the size and function of the ventricles:

- *Dilated:* Decreased contractility and dilation of the ventricles without an increase in wall thickness (hypertrophy). There are congenital or genetic forms and acquired forms caused by infection or toxin exposure.
- *Hypertrophic:* Hypertrophy of the ventricles, generally with improved contractility but impaired ventricular filling because of increased "stiffness" of the ventricular walls. The interior chamber size of the ventricle may be decreased. Left ventricular outflow tract obstruction may occur and can be suddenly fatal. Hypertrophic cardiomyopathy is considered a genetic disorder.
- *Restrictive:* Impaired ventricular filling usually caused by infiltration of the muscle with abnormal material. The ventricular size and contractility are usually fairly normal. It may be congenital or acquired.

Hypertrophic cardiomyopathy (HCM), with a prevalence in children of less than 1%, is nevertheless one of the major causes of sudden cardiac death in adolescents (Movahed, Strootman, Bates, & Sattur, 2010). Approximately 50% of cases of sudden death in athletes are related to hypertrophic cardiomyopathy (Rowland, 2009). Through echocardiography screening, Movahed et al. (2010) demonstrated a significantly higher incidence in African-American adolescents than in adolescents of other races. Predicting sudden cardiac death from this cause is difficult because children with this disorder may have completely normal physical examination findings.

The assessment data that best predict whether a child or adolescent may be at risk are a family history of early or sudden cardiac death or a family history of HCM; the condition has a genetic predisposition (Park, 2008). If the adolescent is symptomatic, the most frequently seen signs and symptoms include dyspnea or chest pain with exertion, palpitations, presyncope, and syncope. Infants and children may fatigue easily. The thickened left ventricle is poorly compliant (stiff) and has impaired filling, causing pulmonary venous congestion and associated exertional dyspnea and orthopnea. On auscultation, the heart sounds are normal and there is often a systolic murmur at the left sternal border or apex. The murmur will characteristically vary in intensity depending on position or recent exertion.

The ECG may demonstrate left ventricular hypertrophy, deep Q waves, and ST-T abnormalities. Affected individuals should have a Holter monitor test to screen for asymptomatic ventricular arrhythmias. The chest radiograph may show mild cardiomegaly. The diagnosis is usually established by echocardiogram, often with concentric or localized ventricular hypertrophy, of the left and often the right ventricle.

All children with diagnosed HCM should be restricted from strenuous exertion and competitive sports. Beta blockade or calcium channel blockade (verapamil) is frequently used, especially in children with obstructive HCM, to decrease ventricular hypercontractility and outflow tract obstruction. Beta blockade is also used as prophylaxis against ventricular arrhythmias. Prophylactic therapy may be started in asymptomatic children with HCM, especially in the case of a family history of sudden death (Park, 2008).

Surgery is indicated in children who are symptomatic or who have severe outflow tract obstruction despite medical management. The most common procedure is a septal myomectomy, which is resection of a portion of the left ventricular septum to relieve obstruction. This often results in an improvement in symptoms with low surgical mortality risk but does not decrease the mortality rate of the disease itself.

A newer intervention is insertion of a pacemaker, which, by depolarizing the ventricle, causes dyssynchronous ventricular contraction and decreased outflow tract obstruction. In addition, children with life-threatening arrhythmias may be offered an implantable defibrillator pacemaker. The surgical risk of pacemaker or defibrillator insertion is much lower than that of myomectomy, and these options are likely to be used increasingly as long-term outcome data become available.

HIGH CHOLESTEROL LEVELS IN CHILDREN AND ADOLESCENTS

Preventive cardiology has become increasingly important during childhood and adolescence. Developing heart-healthy habits during these years reduces the risk for coronary artery disease and other cardiovascular problems during adulthood. Several major risk factors during childhood and adolescence appear routinely in the literature. They include the following (Daniels, Greer, & The Committee on Nutrition, 2008):

- Tobacco use
- High level of low-density lipoproteins (LDLs) and low level of high-density lipoproteins (HDLs)
- Hypertension (greater than the 90th percentile)
- Decreased physical activity
- Obesity
- Family history
- Type 1 or 2 diabetes mellitus

Recent statistics on overweight and obesity reveal that 10.7% of children age 2 to 5 years, 17.4% of middle-school children, and 17.9% of adolescents are obese (U.S. Department of Health and Human Services, 2010).

Assessment of Children at Risk

High cholesterol levels (dyslipidemia) can be the result of genetic or dietary factors or a combination. The AAP (Barlow & The Expert Committee, 2007) recommends that a child with a body mass index (BMI) at or above the 85th percentile be screened with a baseline lipid panel, regardless of age or risk factors. Acceptable cholesterol levels should be below 170 mg/dL. Borderline risk levels are 170 to 199 mg/dL; high risk level is over 200 mg/dL (Barlow & The Expert Committee, 2007). In addition, according to guidelines from the National Cholesterol Education Program (NCEP), the following children older than 2 years should be screened (McCrindle, Urbina, Dennison et al., 2007):

- Children whose parents or grandparents had vascular or cerebrovascular disease or have been diagnosed with coronary atherosclerosis before age 55 years should have fasting lipoprotein studies.
- Children who have at least one parent with a total cholesterol level greater than or equal to 240 mg/dL should have their total cholesterol measured, followed by two fasting lipoprotein levels if the average of two total cholesterol studies is 170 mg/dL or more or the initial total cholesterol level is greater than or equal to 200 mg/dL.

Other risk factors that may trigger cholesterol screening and treatment in healthy children include the presence of insulin resistance syndrome (metabolic syndrome), hypertension, tobacco use or exposure, and the presence of markers for cardiovascular risk (e.g., elevated level of homocysteine, presence of C-reactive protein). Children with any of these risk factors should be followed with periodic cholesterol level measurements. Recent discussions in the literature regarding targeted versus universal screening for high cholesterol levels suggest that targeted screening according to the NCEP screening guidelines may miss children with dyslipidemia and those who would be candidates for pharmacologic treatment for high cholesterol (Ritchie, Murphy, Ice et al., 2010).

Therapeutic Management

Children older than 2 years can follow a sensible low-fat dietary program. This includes using nonfat or low-fat dairy products, limiting red meat intake, and increasing intake of fish, vegetables, whole grains, and legumes. Children should avoid excessive intake of fruit juices and other sweetened drinks, sugars, and saturated fats. Adequate intake of dietary fiber and avoidance of processed foods also can contribute to lowering LDL levels (Daniels et al., 2008). Young children with elevated or borderline LDL levels will need to have their saturated fat and dietary intake monitored more closely. These children should limit their intake of saturated fat to less than 7% of total daily calories and reduce cholesterol intake to less than 200 mg/day (Daniels et al., 2008).

Other factors that contribute to a healthy lifestyle in children and adolescents include increased physical activity and avoidance of sedentary lifestyle (e.g., excessive television watching) and monitoring for coronary heart disease risk factors (Barlow & The Expert Committee, 2007).

Cholesterol-lowering medications generally are not used in the pediatric population. Medication therapy should be considered for children 8 to 10 years of age who have elevated LDLs or a strong history of individual and family risk factors; treating children younger than 8 years would require an LDL level that exceeds 500 mg/dL (Daniels et al., 2008). A variety of medications are used to treat high LDLs in children, and these include the statins, bile acid–binding resins (e.g., cholestyramine, colestipol), niacin, and cholesterol absorption inhibitors (Daniels et al., 2008).

Nursing Considerations

The most effective approach to decreasing risk factors during childhood and adolescence appears to be both population-based and individually targeted approaches, with continuing education about risk factors occurring in communities, schools, physicians' offices, and the media. Nurses play an important part in educating parents and children about healthy diets, the importance of regular exercise, and reduction of other risk factors.

■ KEY CONCEPTS

- With the neonate's first breath, gas exchange is transferred from the placenta to the lungs. The fetal shunts (ductus venosus, ductus arteriosus, foramen ovale) close, and resistance to flow in the pulmonary system decreases as systemic resistance increases. Pulmonary vascular resistance decreases, and a marked increase in pulmonary blood flow follows. Abnormalities during fetal development contribute to the incidence of congenital heart disease.
- Shunting is the movement of blood through an opening from one side of the heart to the other. In left-to-right shunts, blood is shunted to the right side of the heart because the pressure is lower on the right side and higher on the left; this can result in a volume overload in the right side of the heart and subsequent heart failure (HF).
- Right-to-left shunts can result in mixing of saturated and desaturated blood, with the physiologic consequence of hypoxemia.

- Assessment and management of the child and family of a child with a congenital cardiac defect should begin at diagnosis and supportively continue throughout the child's care continuum.
- Common nursing diagnoses associated with infants with congenital heart defects and their parents include Decreased Cardiac Output, Imbalanced Nutrition: Less than Body Requirements, Activity Intolerance, Deficient Knowledge, Anxiety, Interrupted Family Processes, Risk for Infection, and Ineffective Health Maintenance.
- Heart disease can be acquired through genetics, infection, or lifestyle-related causes. Examples of acquired heart disease and risk for heart disease include infective endocarditis, acute rheumatic fever, Kawasaki disease, cardiomyopathy, hypertension, and high cholesterol. Nursing care of children with these conditions is specific to the condition; however, prevention is the major focus of care.

REFERENCES

Adatia, I., Kothari, S., & Feinstein, J. (2010). Pulmonary hypertension associated with congenital heart disease: Pulmonary vascular disease: The global perspective. *Chest, 137*(6 Suppl.), 52s-61s.

American Academy of Pediatrics. (2009). *2009 Red book: Report of the Committee on Infectious Diseases* (28th ed.). Elk Grove Village, IL: American Academy of Pediatrics.

American Academy of Pediatrics. (2011). *High blood pressure in children*. Retrieved from www.aap.org.

American Heart Association. (2008). *Infective endocarditis (previously referred to as bacterial endocarditis)*. Retrieved from www.americanheart.org.

American Heart Association. (2011). American Heart Association statistical update: Heart disease and stroke statistics—2011 update. *Circulation, 123*, e18-e209.

Barlow, S., & The Expert Committee. (2007). Expert Committee recommendations regarding the prevention, assessment, and treatment of child and adolescent overweight and obesity: Summary report. *Pediatrics, 120*, S164-S192.

Bernstein, D. (2011). The cardiovascular system. In R. Kliegman, B. Stanton, J. St. Geme, et al. (Eds.), *Nelson textbook of pediatrics* (19th ed., pp. 1527-1604). St. Louis: Elsevier Saunders.

Daniels, S., Greer, F., & The Committee on Nutrition. (2008). *Lipid screening and cardiovascular health in childhood*. Retrieved from www.aap.org.

DeBord, S., Cherry, C., & Hickey, C. (2007). The arterial switch procedure for transposition of the great arteries. *AORN Journal*, 86(2), 211-226.

Dunbar Ivy, D., Rosenzweig, E., LeMarie, J., et al. (2010). Long term outcomes in children with pulmonary arterial hypertension treated with bosentan in real-world clinical settings. *American Journal of Cardiology*, 106(9), 1332-1338.

Field, J. M., Hazinski, M. F., Sayre, M. R., et al. (2010). American Heart Association guidelines for cardiopulmonary resuscitation and emergency cardiac care. *Circulation*, 122, S640-S656.

Gerber, M. (2011). Rheumatic fever. In R. Kliegman, B. Stanton, J. St. Geme, et al. (Eds.), *Nelson textbook of pediatrics* (19th ed., pp. 920-924). St. Louis: Elsevier Saunders.

Gerber, M., Baltimore, R. S., Eaton, C. B., et al. (2009). Prevention of rheumatic fever and diagnosis and treatment of acute streptococcal pharyngitis: A scientific statement from the American Heart Association Rheumatic Fever, Endocarditis and Kawasaki Disease Committee of the Council of Cardiovascular Disease in the Young, the Interdisciplinary Council on Functional Genomics and Translational Biology, and the Interdisciplinary Council on Quality of Care and Outcomes Research: Endorsed by the American Academy of Pediatrics. *Circulation*, 119, 1541-1551.

Lande, M. (2011). Systemic hypertension. In R. Kliegman, B. Stanton, J. St. Geme, et al. (Eds.), *Nelson textbook of pediatrics* (19th ed., pp. 1639-1647). St. Louis: Elsevier Saunders.

McCrindle, B., Urbina, E., Dennison, B., et al. (2007). Drug therapy of high-risk lipid abnormalities in children and adolescents: A scientific statement from the American Heart Association Atherosclerosis, Hypertension and Obesity in Youth Committee, Council of Cardiovascular Disease in the Young, with the Council on Cardiovascular Nursing. *Circulation*, 115, 1819-1846.

McDonald, J. (2009). Acute infective endocarditis. *Infectious Disease Clinics of North America*, 23(3), 643-664.

Movahed, M., Strootman, D., Bates, S., & Sattur, S. (2010). Prevalence of suspected hypertrophic cardiomyopathy or left ventricular hypertrophy based on race and gender in teenagers using screening echocardiography. *Cardiovascular Ultrasound*, 8, 54-59.

National High Blood Pressure Education Program Working Group on High Blood Pressure in Children and Adolescents. (2007). *A pocket guide to blood pressure measurement in children*. Retrieved from www.nhlbi.nih.gov/health/public/heart/hbp/bp_child_pocket/bp_child_pocket.pdf.

O'Connor, M., McDaniel, N., & Brady, W. (2008). The pediatric electrocardiogram part II: Dysrhythmias. *American Journal of Emergency Medicine*, 26(3), 348-358.

Park, M. K. (2008). *Pediatric cardiology for practitioners* (5th ed.). St. Louis: Elsevier Mosby.

Ritchie, S. K., Murphy, E. C., Ice, C., et al. (2010). Universal versus targeted blood cholesterol screening among youth: The CARDIAC project. *Pediatrics*, 12692, 260-265.

Rowland, T. (2009). Sudden unexpected death in young athletes: Reconsidering hypertrophic cardiomyopathy. *Pediatrics*, 123(4), 1217-1222.

Skidmore-Roth, L. (2011). *Mosby's nursing drug reference*. St. Louis: Elsevier Mosby.

Son, M.B., & Newburger, J. (2011). Kawasaki disease. In R. Kliegman, B. Stanton, J. St. Geme, et al. (Eds.), *Nelson textbook of pediatrics* (19th ed., pp. 862-867). St. Louis: Elsevier Saunders.

Steer, A., & Carapetis, J. (2009). Acute rheumatic fever and rheumatic heart disease in indigenous populations. *Pediatric Clinics of North America*, 56, 1401-1419.

U.S. Department of Health and Human Services. (2010). *Healthy People 2020*. Retrieved from www.healthypeople.gov.

Van Hare, G. (2011). Disturbances of rate and rhythm of the heart. In R. Kliegman, B. Stanton, J. St. Geme, et al. (Eds.), *Nelson textbook of pediatrics* (19th ed., pp. 1610-1619). St. Louis: Elsevier Saunders.

Wilson, M., Taubert, K., Gewitz, M., et al. (2007). Prevention of infective endocarditis: Guidelines from the American Heart Association: A guideline from the American Heart Association Rheumatic Fever, Endocarditis and Kawasaki Disease Committee, Council on Cardiovascular Disease in the Young and the Council on Clinical Cardiology, Council on Cardiovascular Surgery and Anesthesia, and the Quality of Care and Outcomes Research Interdisciplinary Working Group. *Circulation*, 116, 1736-1754.

The Child with a Hematologic Alteration

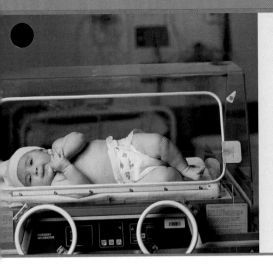

⊖volve WEBSITE

http://evolve.elsevier.com/James/ncoc

LEARNING OBJECTIVES

After studying this chapter, you should be able to:

- Describe the anatomy and physiology of the hematopoietic system.
- Discuss the pediatric differences related to blood and blood formation.
- Discuss the role of the nurse in the prevention of iron deficiency anemia.
- Describe common factors in the care of a child with anemia.

- Discuss the pathophysiology and therapeutic management of common hematologic alterations.
- List possible nursing diagnoses for children with hematologic alterations.
- Describe possible nursing care for children with hematologic alterations.

CLINICAL REFERENCE

REVIEW OF THE HEMATOLOGIC SYSTEM

Hematology is the study of the blood and blood-forming tissues. In fetal life, various tissues produce erythrocytes (red blood cells), but after birth, their production is controlled exclusively by the bone marrow, primarily in the long bones. With age, the more membranous bones of the vertebrae, sternum, and ribs assume red blood cell (RBC) production. Age, sex, and the altitude at which a person lives affect the number of RBCs.

Normally, RBCs are biconcave disks that are capable of changing shape as they flow through the microvasculature of the body. They have a fairly uniform size that is determined mainly by the amount of cellular content of substances, primarily hemoglobin. Their function is to transport oxygen to tissues. Essential to this ability to carry oxygen is an appropriate amount of hemoglobin, whose production depends on sufficient amounts of circulating iron. Iron is absorbed from dietary intake by the intestines and stored by the liver in both soluble and insoluble forms, to be used when necessary.

The stimulus for production of RBCs is a decrease in circulating oxygen, which in turn stimulates the kidneys to produce a hormone called *erythropoietin*. Erythropoietin stimulates the production of RBC precursors and causes them to mature rapidly. Disorders of the kidney can affect the individual's ability to produce this hormone and thus can affect RBC production by the bone marrow.

Anemia is a decrease in the number of RBCs, reduction in their hemoglobin content, or reduced volume of packed RBCs. Anemia results from one of two problems: either too rapid a loss of RBCs (by covert or overt bleeding or destruction) or too slow a production of RBCs. Anemias are categorized according to the size of the RBC (macrocytic, microcytic, normocytic) and the content of hemoglobin in the RBC (hypochromic, normochromic).

Polycythemia, which is an increase in the number of RBCs, is less frequently seen than anemia. *Polycythemia* can occur as a result of hypoxia, such as that experienced at high altitude or when oxygen is not sufficiently directed to the tissues, as in cyanotic heart disease.

⊖ White blood cells (WBCs), or leukocytes, are formed in the bone marrow and in lymphatic tissue. They assist in the body's ability to distinguish "self" from "nonself." WBCs destroy foreign cells through the processes of phagocytosis and antibody production.

PEDIATRIC HEMATOLOGIC SYSTEM

There are three important cells that are formed in the bone marrow. Those are red blood cells (RBCs), white blood cells (WBCs), and platelets.

Red blood cells are produced initially in the marrow of all bones. After 5 years of age, RBC production in the shafts of the long bones (tibia, femur) is reduced, and production ceases in these locations entirely at age 20 years. After 20 years of age, hematopoiesis takes place primarily in the marrow of the ribs, sternum, vertebrae, pelvis, skull, clavicles, and scapulas.

The number of erythrocytes (RBCs) varies according to age. The fetus has a higher oxygen-carrying capacity than an infant because of a considerably higher number of RBCs with proportionately elevated hemoglobin and hematocrit values.

The life span of RBCs in neonates is shorter than in older infants and children because of increased destruction during rapid growth.

By 2 months of age, erythropoiesis increases, leading to increased reticulocytes in the blood and a rise in hemoglobin.

Both phagocytes and antibodies destroy foreign cells and tissues perceived by the body as nonself (including, e.g., bacteria, fungi, viruses, parasites, and transplanted tissue) (see Chapter 18). WBC disorders result from an altered rate of production of WBCs (lymphocytosis or lymphopenia) or an alteration in function of the cells.

Platelets are the cells that promote hemostasis—the prevention of blood loss. They are formed in the bone marrow from megakaryocytes. Megakaryocytes later fragment into smaller cells known as *platelets*, either in the bone marrow or shortly after release into the systemic circulation. Platelets can circulate in the blood for about 10 days before they die; however, disease, fever, and infection can shorten a platelet's lifetime. Platelet disorders occur when the bone marrow cannot meet the production demands of the body.

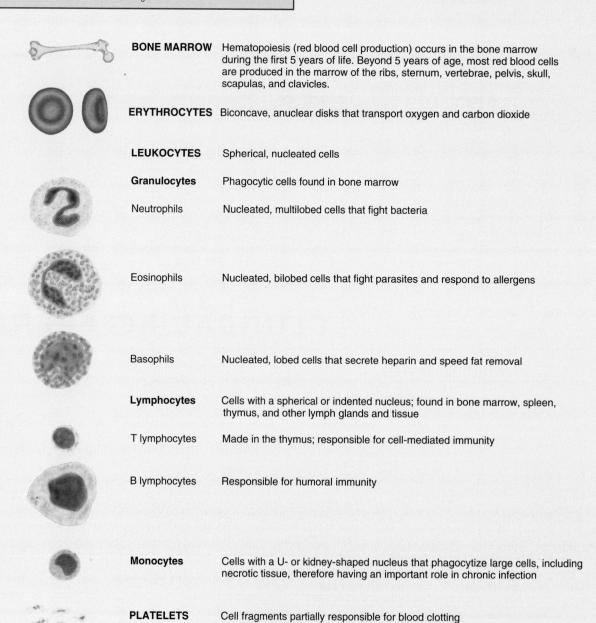

BONE MARROW	Hematopoiesis (red blood cell production) occurs in the bone marrow during the first 5 years of life. Beyond 5 years of age, most red blood cells are produced in the marrow of the ribs, sternum, vertebrae, pelvis, skull, scapulas, and clavicles.
ERYTHROCYTES	Biconcave, anuclear disks that transport oxygen and carbon dioxide
LEUKOCYTES	Spherical, nucleated cells
Granulocytes	Phagocytic cells found in bone marrow
Neutrophils	Nucleated, multilobed cells that fight bacteria
Eosinophils	Nucleated, bilobed cells that fight parasites and respond to allergens
Basophils	Nucleated, lobed cells that secrete heparin and speed fat removal
Lymphocytes	Cells with a spherical or indented nucleus; found in bone marrow, spleen, thymus, and other lymph glands and tissue
T lymphocytes	Made in the thymus; responsible for cell-mediated immunity
B lymphocytes	Responsible for humoral immunity
Monocytes	Cells with a U- or kidney-shaped nucleus that phagocytize large cells, including necrotic tissue, therefore having an important role in chronic infection
PLATELETS	Cell fragments partially responsible for blood clotting

Review of the Hematologic System

TYPES AND FUNCTIONS OF WHITE BLOOD CELLS

- Granulocytes: Phagocytic cells produced in the bone marrow and found in the circulation. These cells include:
  - Neutrophils: Primary defense in bacterial infection; capable of phagocytizing and killing bacteria.
  - Eosinophils: Influence the inflammatory process, fight parasites, and influence allergic hypersensitivity reactions.
  - Basophils: Activate the inflammatory response; contain histamine; other roles are unclear.
- Agranulocytes: Participate in inflammatory and immune reactions. These cells include:

- Monocytes/macrophages: Phagocytize large cells, including necrotic tissue; they are therefore important in fighting chronic infection.
- Lymphocytes: Found in bone marrow, spleen, thymus, lymph glands, tissues, and circulation.
- T cells: Made in the thymus and responsible for cell-mediated immunity.
- B cells: Responsible for humoral immunity (antibody production).
- Natural killer cells: Lymphocyte-like cells that can kill certain types of tumor cells and viruses directly.

When caring for infants and children with blood disorders, the nurse is challenged in the areas of preventive, acute, and chronic care. Depending on the disorder and the child's condition, care may be provided in the home, an outpatient setting, or the hospital. It is not unusual for a child to be seen in an outpatient setting (clinic, school), referred to a hospital for diagnosis and stabilization, and returned to the home for maintenance. Genetic counseling may be indicated for children or families with certain types of blood disorders.

Many medications for hematologic disorders can be given at home, including deferoxamine mesylate (Desferal), intravenous (IV) immune globulin (IVIG), IV antibiotics, coagulation factor products, and, in some instances, even blood transfusions. Parents are learning to manage infusion therapy in regard to initiating, monitoring, and discontinuing infusions when appropriate, with guidance from the collaborative efforts of the multidisciplinary health care team.

IRON DEFICIENCY ANEMIA

Iron deficiency is the most common cause of anemia during infancy, childhood, and adolescence. Iron deficiency anemia (IDA) may be characterized by mild or marked anemia.

Etiology and Incidence

Several factors can contribute to IDA, including decreased iron intake, increased iron or blood loss, and periods of increased growth rate.

IDA related to inadequate dietary iron intake is rare before age 4 to 6 months because of the presence of maternal iron stores; it occurs most often in children age 9 to 24 months as iron stores are depleted. Premature infants may develop iron deficiency early in life because they are born with insufficient maternal iron stores (Lerner & Sills, 2011). Decreased iron intake is often related to the intake of large amounts of cow's milk instead of breast milk or fortified formula and iron-fortified foods (Lerner & Sills, 2011). The incidence has dropped in recent years because of increased education about and availability of iron-fortified formula and cereals. Early transition from breast milk or infant formula to cow's milk can precipitate chronic diarrhea with occult intestinal bleeding in children younger than 2 years. This results from exposure to a protein found in cow's milk (Lerner & Sills, 2011). The rapid growth of infants and children younger than 2 years, if combined with decreased iron intake, further contributes to the increased incidence in this age-group.

Adolescents are also at risk for IDA because they too are undergoing increased growth and often have poor dietary habits. The situation is further complicated by the blood loss during menstruation in young women.

Manifestations

The clinical manifestations of IDA vary with the degree of anemia but may include extreme pallor with porcelain-like skin, pale mucous membranes and conjunctiva, tachycardia, tachypnea, lethargy, fatigue, and irritability. Children with lead poisoning often have associated IDA.

Diagnostic Evaluation

Any child with anemia should first have a complete history taken, with particular emphasis on assessment of nutritional intake. The results of a complete blood count (CBC) in individuals with IDA will show low hemoglobin levels (6 to 11 g/dL) and microcytic, hypochromic RBCs, reflected in a decreased mean cell volume (MCV) and decreased mean cell hemoglobin (MCH) (see Evolve website). The reticulocyte count is usually normal or slightly elevated. With these findings, serum ferritin levels and serum iron or iron-binding capacity should be assessed. Total iron-binding capacity (TIBC) is usually increased as a result of decreased serum iron levels. Serum ferritin and serum iron are low. Hemoglobin electrophoresis may be done to rule out causes other than IDA.

Therapeutic Management

Therapy is directed toward increasing the dietary intake of iron and iron supplementation. The absorption of dietary iron-rich foods can be unreliable and will not rapidly provide the body with enough iron to correct the iron deficiency. Therefore, affected children are given a daily oral iron preparation (often three times per day) of one of the available ferrous salts (ferrous sulfate, ferrous gluconate, or ferrous fumarate) on the basis of the content of elemental iron (dose should be 3 to 6 mg/kg/day [2 to 4 mg/kg/day for premature infants] in three divided doses).

Follow-up monitoring includes a CBC and reticulocyte count. The reticulocyte count should increase within days of the initiation of iron therapy. An increased hemoglobin level can be expected in 4 to 30 days. The response to iron therapy can often be positively predicted, so blood transfusions are rarely indicated to correct IDA. RBC transfusions are reserved for severe anemia and cardiovascular compromise. Oral iron therapy will be continued for 3 to 4 months after hemoglobin and hematocrit levels return to normal to replenish the child's iron stores. Administration of a daily multivitamin with iron can then be recommended.

PATHOPHYSIOLOGY

Iron Deficiency Anemia

Iron is one of the components necessary for the synthesis of hemoglobin. Without an adequate amount of iron, the bone marrow continues to manufacture RBCs, but their content of hemoglobin is decreased, rendering these RBCs inefficient at carrying oxygen to the tissues. The constellation of clinical signs evident with IDA results from compromised tissue oxygenation.

The full-term neonate is born with enough stored maternal iron to produce adequate amounts of hemoglobin for 4 to 6 months. The average life of an RBC is about 120 days. Thus IDA is usually not seen in children before age 9 months.

As RBCs undergo **hemolysis**, intracellular iron is released into the circulation for use by the body. Adults are able to use this breakdown of RBCs as a primary source of iron. Children, however, grow very rapidly and expand their circulating blood volume at the same time. Because children must produce additional RBCs to accommodate for their physical growth, their need for iron to synthesize new hemoglobin for RBC production is increased. Therefore, children must increase their dietary consumption of iron. The American Academy of Pediatrics (AAP) Committee on Nutrition* recommends routine iron supplementation with iron-fortified formula in nonbreastfeeding, full-term and preterm infants, as well as additional iron supplementation with elemental iron drops for all preterm infants. Neonates born before 32 weeks of gestation are at greater risk for anemia as a result of having less stored iron. Iron-fortified cereals are recommended when solids are introduced.

Iron deficiency can also result from inadequate iron absorption. Various factors can contribute to a lack of absorption of iron by the gastrointestinal tract. When cow's milk is introduced into the diet before age 1 year in place of breast milk or formula, infants do not ingest sufficient iron because cow's milk is a poor dietary source of iron. Often, the potentially large amount of cow's milk replaces iron-fortified cereals and iron-rich baby food. Although iron from breast milk is well absorbed, it is not a complete source of iron, and dietary iron supplements must be introduced to augment its nutrients when the infant is approximately 4 to 6 months old.

Iron deficiency can be the result of occult intestinal bleeding. Blood loss from an infant's intestine typically occurs very slowly and may have several causes. The immature intestine may be unable to tolerate the protein in cow's milk or milk-based infant formula. Irritation of the bowel results in hemorrhages of the microvasculature, resulting in blood loss in the stool. Although unusual, parasitic infections can also irritate the intestinal lining.

*American Academy of Pediatrics, Committee on Nutrition. (2009). *Pediatrics nutrition handbook* (6th ed.). Elk Grove Village, IL: American Academy of Pediatrics

---

❓ CRITICAL THINKING EXERCISE 23-1

Mrs. Anders has brought 18-month-old Jacob to the clinic because he is irritable, is running a low-grade fever, and has a cough. In the process of assessing Jacob, you note that he seems lethargic and his skin is very pale. You obtain a 24-hour diet history and suspect the child does not have adequate iron intake. A CBC confirms a diagnosis of iron deficiency anemia (IDA).

1. What do you think Mrs. Anders is most concerned about?
2. What is the nurse's role when a child enters the health care system with an acute illness?
3. What opportunities are present when a child is brought to an ambulatory care setting because of an acute illness?

PATIENT-CENTERED TEACHING

Home Care of the Child with Iron Deficiency Anemia

Dietary Changes
- Provide iron-fortified formula or breast milk with iron-fortified food supplements if the child is younger than 12 months.
- If the child is older than 12 months, limit intake of cow's milk to 24 oz/day or less.
- Increase the child's intake of age-appropriate iron-rich foods, with selections based on the age of the child: liver, dried beans, Cream of Wheat, iron-fortified cereal, apricots and prunes (and other dried fruits), egg yolks, and dark-green leafy vegetables.

Administration of Iron
- Administer iron in three divided doses between meals.
- Give with vitamin C–rich fluids such as orange juice.
- Administer iron through a straw or medicine dropper placed at the back of the mouth, away from the teeth. Brush or wipe off teeth because oral iron can stain the teeth.
- Recognize that iron supplementation causes black, tarry stools.
- Avoid administration of iron with milk or formula and cereal because iron binds with calcium, thus impeding absorption.

Follow-up Care
- Keep appointments for follow-up evaluations.
- Expect blood work to be done at follow-up visits.

❗ NURSING QUALITY ALERT

Obtaining a Dietary Intake History

Parents may not readily or accurately respond to questions about their child's dietary intake. Ask the parents to begin the dietary history at the time the child awoke yesterday, describing the child's activities and exactly what the child ate. Correlating activities with diet may enable the nurse to obtain a better history and may alert the nurse to feeding patterns for which counseling may be indicated. Determine the number of bottles of milk or juice that the child is taking each day and the size of the bottles. Parents often underestimate the ounces of milk or juice that the child is taking.

Children with iron deficiency anemia occasionally develop pica. Pica is an appetite for nonnutritive substances such as paper, cardboard, ice, or sometimes dirt. Ask about the intake of nonfood items, because parents may not openly share this information.

SICKLE CELL DISEASE

Sickle cell disease (SCD) is the generic term that refers to a group of genetic disorders characterized by the production of sickle hemoglobin (HbS), chronic hemolytic anemia, and ischemic tissue injury. The more common forms of SCD include homozygous HbSS disease (sickle cell anemia), HbSC disease (sickle hemoglobin C disease), and the sickle beta-zero thalassemia syndromes. SCD is an inherited, lifelong disease that affects primarily individuals of African, Mediterranean, Indian, and Middle Eastern descent. The morbidity and mortality rates from the severe forms of the disease have decreased as a result of newborn screening for the disease, routine prophylactic penicillin administration, and pneumococcal and *Haemophilus influenzae* vaccines.

Animation—Sickle Cell Anemia

◉ NURSING CARE PLAN

The Child with Iron Deficiency Anemia in the Community Setting

Focused Assessment

- Obtain history from parents addressing the following:
  - Decrease in child's activity level—more quiet than usual
  - Increased desire to be held
  - Infant given cow's milk before age 12 mo.
  - Increased milk consumption with exclusion of solid foods for infant and child
  - Child's heart "races" when at rest
- Conduct a physical examination and look for:
  - Pallor
  - Tired appearance
  - Mild to severe tachycardia
  - Heart murmur (due to severe anemia—is reversible)

Planning

Nursing Diagnosis

Imbalanced Nutrition: Less Than Body Requirements related to parents' lack of knowledge of age-appropriate nutritional needs.

Expected Outcome

The parents will have an understanding of the child's nutritional needs, as evidenced by verbal description of the child's dietary plan, including foods containing appropriate dietary iron.

Intervention/*Rationale*

1. Obtain the child's past and current nutritional history. Instruct the caregiver to continue to give the infant iron-fortified formula or breastfeed and give supplementary iron-fortified foods until age 12 mo. For a child older than 12 mo, instruct parents to limit cow's milk intake to a maximum of 24 oz/day and increase consumption of iron-rich foods.
   Cow's milk is poorly digested and is not rich in iron. The AAP recommends continuing breast milk or iron-fortified formula until age 12 mo. Decreasing milk intake will encourage the consumption of other iron-rich and iron-fortified foods (see Patient-Centered Teaching: Home Care of the Child with Iron Deficiency Anemia box).
2. Advise the parent to keep a dietary diary.
   Keeping a record of food and fluid intake assists with a dietary evaluation and identifies areas for additional teaching.
3. Explain to parents the need for iron in the manufacture of RBCs, how iron therapy affects laboratory test results, the potential outcome with no intervention, the lack of iron in cow's milk, and iron's effect on the body.
   Explaining the rationale for therapy can often help improve adherence.

4. Instruct the parents to administer oral iron supplements as ordered by the physician. Allow parents to practice medication administration, and then evaluate their technique, providing additional instruction as indicated (see Patient-Centered Teaching: Home Care of the Child with Iron Deficiency Anemia box).
   Iron supplements immediately increase iron intake beyond that absorbed from formula or food. Practice and additional instruction will build the parents' skills and confidence in giving their child medication.
5. Inform parents to give iron supplements with fruit juice and NOT with milk, formula, or cereal; when the child's stomach is empty.
   An acid stomach environment facilitates absorption. Calcium in milk products binds with iron to decrease iron absorption.
6. Instruct parents to administer vitamin C as ordered and encourage intake of foods rich in vitamin C.
   Vitamin C increases the absorption of iron by the body.
7. Instruct the parents to keep iron supplements (and all medications) out of reach of children and in a locked cabinet.
   Iron poisoning is possible with overdose. This can be serious and possibly fatal.
8. Instruct the parents to obtain follow-up laboratory tests when ordered, including reticulocyte count and hemoglobin and hematocrit levels.
   The reticulocyte count should peak in 5 to 7 days. It is an objective test that can determine the degree of adherence to iron therapy. The hemoglobin level should increase in 4 to 30 days.
9. Instruct the parents to monitor for and expect to see black, tarry stools. Verify that parents have observed this.
   Iron therapy causes black, tarry stools. If absent, this may indicate lack of adherence to therapy.
10. Refer to social services for enrollment in federal or state programs, if warranted.
    Poor nutritional practices may be attributable to a lack of resources to obtain appropriate foods.

Evaluation

Does the dietary diary reflect an increase in iron-rich and iron-fortified foods in the child's daily meal plan?

Does the child have normal iron, hemoglobin, and hematocrit levels?

Do the parents demonstrate adherence to the prescribed therapy and verbalize appropriate questions?

Has the child had a recurrence of IDA?

Etiology

SCD is a group of hemoglobinopathies in which normal hemoglobin, HbA, is partially or totally replaced by abnormal hemoglobin, HbS. SCD is an inherited, autosomal recessive condition. Each affected individual carries two copies of the gene that directs the production of hemoglobin. The normal hemoglobin gene is hemoglobin A (HbA). If one parent has the HbS trait (one copy of the HbA and one copy of HbS gene—HbAS) and the other parent does not (both copies HbA—HbAA), each pregnancy has a 50% risk of having the child inherit the trait. If each parent carries the trait (both parents with HbAS), there is a 25% chance that the child will be unaffected (HbAA), a 50% chance that the child will carry the trait (HbAS), and a 25% chance that the child will have the disease (HbSS). Although not a disease in and of itself, the carrier state of SCD—sickle cell trait (HbAS)—may produce clinical symptoms (e.g., hematuria, bacteriuria) in times of extreme stress, during extremely vigorous exercise, and at high altitudes.

Incidence

SCD affects approximately 1 in 500 African-Americans. Sickle cell trait is found in 8% of persons of African descent and is also prevalent in persons of Mediterranean, Middle Eastern, Indian, Caribbean, and Central and South American descent (Heeney & Dover, 2009).

Manifestations

All the clinical manifestations of SCD are a result of the obstructions caused by the sickled RBCs and the increased destruction of RBCs due

PATHOPHYSIOLOGY

Sickle Cell Disease

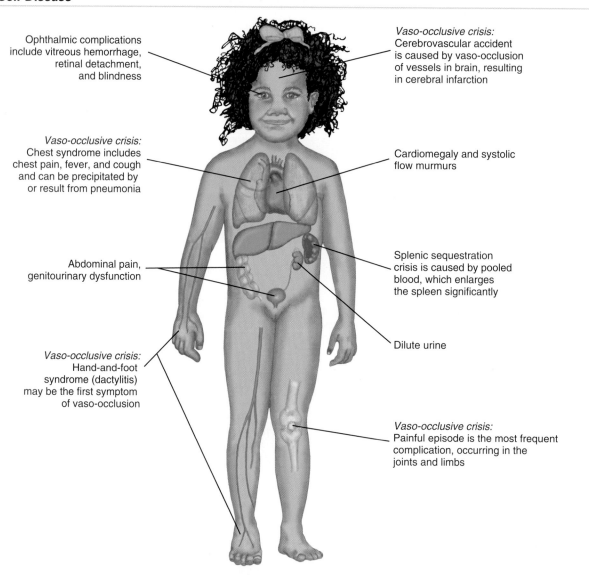

Ophthalmic complications include vitreous hemorrhage, retinal detachment, and blindness

Vaso-occlusive crisis: Cerebrovascular accident is caused by vaso-occlusion of vessels in brain, resulting in cerebral infarction

Vaso-occlusive crisis: Chest syndrome includes chest pain, fever, and cough and can be precipitated by or result from pneumonia

Cardiomegaly and systolic flow murmurs

Abdominal pain, genitourinary dysfunction

Splenic sequestration crisis is caused by pooled blood, which enlarges the spleen significantly

Dilute urine

Vaso-occlusive crisis: Hand-and-foot syndrome (dactylitis) may be the first symptom of vaso-occlusion

Vaso-occlusive crisis: Painful episode is the most frequent complication, occurring in the joints and limbs

The normal RBC is a smooth, biconcave disk that is capable of changing shape to enable it to flow easily through the microvasculature of the circulation. Under conditions of low oxygen concentration, acidosis, and dehydration, the RBCs in a child with SCD assume a sickle shape similar to a half moon, which prevents them from flowing easily through the smallest blood vessels. Sickled RBCs are stiff and nonpliable. These sickled cells clump together, causing occlusions in the small vessels. With reoxygenation, most of the sickled RBCs resume their normal shape. After repeated sickling (deoxygenation) and unsickling (reoxygenation), the cells become irreversibly sickled and their life span is reduced from 120 days to 12 days.

Sickled cells cause microvascular occlusion, leading to tissue ischemia, infarcts, and organ damage. The lungs, spleen, and brain are the organs most seriously affected by the complications of SCD. The normal spleen functions to filter bacteria in the blood. However, the spleen of a child with SCD does not function properly much beyond age 5 years because of this repeated microvascular occlusion and damage. The large vessels are also affected, leading to strokes and other vaso-occlusive events.

to their shortened life span in SCD. Large amounts of fetal hemoglobin (HbF) present in the first few months of life obscure the presence of HbS, so symptoms of the disease usually do not appear until age 4 to 6 months, when the infant begins to manufacture hemoglobin S.

The disease affects most organ systems. Delayed growth and puberty are common. The child usually has small stature throughout adolescence but may attain normal growth in the early 20s.

The general manifestations of SCD are chronic hemolytic anemia, pallor, jaundice, fatigue, cholelithiasis, delayed growth and puberty, avascular necrosis of the hips and shoulders, renal dysfunction, and retinopathy. Sickling events may also progress to acute episodic exacerbations known as *sickle cell crisis.* Infection, dehydration, hypoxia, trauma, or general stress may precipitate a crisis episode. The crisis may take one of three forms: vaso-occlusive, acute sequestration, or aplastic.

TABLE 23-1   CLINICAL MANIFESTATIONS AND THERAPEUTIC MANAGEMENT OF SICKLE CELL DISEASE COMPLICATIONS

COMPLICATION	CHARACTERISTICS	MANIFESTATIONS	TREATMENT
Vaso-Occlusive Crisis			
Painful episode	Most common type of crisis and reason for hospitalization Typically produces bone or joint pain, but pain can occur anywhere Pain may come and go Frequency of pain is individualized Pain is precipitated by infection, cold, stress, acidosis, local or generalized hypoxia	*Mild:* Joint or bone pain lasting a few hours *Severe:* Joint or bone pain lasting days	Oral analgesics initially and, if ineffective, IV opioids (usually morphine), which may be given by either intermittent or continuous infusion Oral or IV NSAIDs Oral and IV hydration Aggressive incentive spirometry use (10 breaths every 2 hr when awake) Consistent manner to assess subjective experience of pain is essential Use of nonpharmacologic pain management strategies in addition to medications
Acute chest syndrome	Common cause of hospitalization Sometimes confused with pneumonia Can recur	Chest pain, fever, cough, abdominal pain	IV hydration (1-1½ times maintenance), antibiotics, oxygen, RBC transfusion, analgesics
Dactylitis (hand-and-foot syndrome)	Occurs in children ages 6 mo to 4 yr Self-limiting complication	Swelling of hands or feet, pain, warmth in affected area	Oral analgesics, hydration (oral or IV), rest
Priapism (persistent erection of the penis)	Occurs if penile blood flow becomes obstructed	Persistent, painful erection	Analgesics; hydration Avoid hot and cold packs If prolonged, transfusion therapy
Cerebrovascular accident	Without treatment, mortality rate of 20%; 70% of patients have a recurrence	Hemiparesis or monoparesis, aphasia/dysphasia, seizures, alteration in level of consciousness, vomiting, vision changes, ataxia, headache	Long-term RBC transfusion therapy or erythrocytapheresis and possibly chelation therapy May require extensive rehabilitation
Acute Sequestration Crisis			
	Blood volume pooling in the spleen, causing splenic enlargement Life-threatening condition of hypovolemic shock Usually occurs in children ages 6 mo to 4 yr One episode increases the risk of future occurrences	Decreased hemoglobin level, acutely ill-looking child, pallor, irritability, tachycardia, impressively enlarged spleen, hypovolemic shock	Emergency treatment to restore circulating blood volume with crystalloid and colloid (blood) infusion Long-term transfusion therapy if recurrent Eventual splenectomy in cases of persistent recurrence
Aplastic Crisis			
	Profound anemia caused by diminished erythropoiesis Has been observed after parvovirus-like agent exposure	Pallor, lethargy, headache, fainting	RBC transfusions and treatment of symptoms

NSAIDs, nonsteroidal antiinflammatory drugs; *RBC,* red blood cell.

A vaso-occlusive crisis occurs when blood flow to tissues is obstructed by sickled RBCs, leading to hypoxemia and ischemia. This ischemic event causes the child to experience pain in the affected body part.

An acute sequestration event occurs when blood flow from an organ such as the liver, lungs, or spleen is obstructed by sickled RBCs. These organs then become engorged with blood, leading to acute anemia and, when in the lungs, acute chest syndrome with potential respiratory failure.

An aplastic event occurs when there is either an increased destruction or decreased production of RBCs. Increased destruction can be related to fever or infection. Decreased production is frequently associated with a viral infection such as parvovirus B19 (also known as Fifth disease).

Repeated vaso-occlusive crises and a virtually continual state of anemia produce long-term problems later in the life of the individual with SCD. Table 23-1 presents the clinical manifestations of SCD.

Diagnostic Evaluation

In the past, many infants died from complications of SCD before being diagnosed with the disorder. However, newborn screening for SCD has significantly decreased the mortality rate. A laboratory diagnosis of SCD is established on the basis of a CBC, isoelectric focusing, hemoglobin electrophoresis, and high-performance liquid chromatography.

Children with SCD have elevated reticulocyte counts because of the shortened life span and destruction of sickled RBCs. Prenatal diagnosis is an option and is made by chorionic villus sampling at 8 to 10 weeks of gestation or amniocentesis at 15 weeks of gestation.

Therapeutic Management

In SCD, the spleen often does not function properly or has been surgically removed because of complications. Functional or actual asplenia places children and adults with SCD in an immunocompromised state at high risk for infection. Splenic dysfunction can begin at 6 months of age, and those with HbSS may have total dysfunction by age 5 years. Bacterial septicemia poses a severe health risk to children with SCD (DeBaun, Frei-Jones, & Vichinsky, 2011a). The bacteria *Streptococcus pneumoniae* and *H. influenzae* are normally destroyed by the reticuloendothelial system of the spleen, but because the child with SCD does not have a properly functioning spleen, the child is considered to be more susceptible to infection with these bacteria.

The natural history of splenic dysfunction in children with HbSS places them at higher risk for fulminant septicemia and death during the first 3 years of life than children with HbSC. Prophylactic daily penicillin V therapy (given twice a day) is recommended for all children with suspected or actual diagnosis by age 2 months and is continued until at least age 5 years (American Academy of Pediatrics [AAP], Committee on Infectious Diseases, 2009). Although views regarding the use of penicillin differ, some experts will continue penicillin prophylaxis throughout childhood in high-risk patients with asplenia.

The possibility exists that pneumococcal infections will not be completely prevented by penicillin chemoprophylaxis because of the development of penicillin-resistant pneumococcal strains (AAP, Committee on Infectious Diseases, 2009). The pneumococcal polyvalent vaccine is routinely recommended for children at ages 2, 4, 6, and 12 to 15 months of age (AAP, Committee on Infectious Diseases, 2009). Routine vaccination against *H. influenzae* infections and routine immunization against hepatitis B are recommended as well. Moreover, children with SCD should receive the influenza vaccine annually and immunization against meningococcal disease after age 2 years (AAP, Committee on Infectious Diseases, 2009) because of their increased risk for related complications.

Stroke occurs in 7% to 13% of children with sickle cell anemia (HbSS). Stroke, caused by vaso-occlusion of blood vessels in the brain with sickled RBCs leading to ischemia, can result in significant motor and neuropsychological deficits. The goal of treatment is early identification of those at increased risk and intervention to prevent the occurrence of a stroke. The risk of stroke can be predicted by the performance of a transcranial Doppler ultrasound. Those with abnormal results are often managed to reduce their risk of stroke by either monthly transfusions or erythrocytapheresis. By maintaining the child's hemoglobin S at less than 30% with the transfusion of hemoglobin A–containing red blood cells, the marrow's production of additional hemoglobin S can be suppressed, therefore reducing the risk of stroke (Mazumdar, Heeney, Cox, & Lieu, 2007).

A child with SCD and a temperature of 101.3° F (38.5° C) or higher should receive prompt medical evaluation and treatment because of the overwhelming risk for infectious complications. Fever can be the first sign of bacteremia. Parenteral antibiotics, blood cultures, IV hydration, and general monitoring are the standard of care for children with SCD who have fever. Outpatient therapy with long-acting parenteral antibiotics may be provided in combination with rigorous evaluation and follow-up in those centers with the capabilities to do so. Children who are not eligible for outpatient therapy are those with the

---

PATIENT-CENTERED TEACHING
Home Care of the Child with Sickle Cell Disease

- Encourage fluid intake; increase fluid intake in hot weather or when there are other risks for dehydration.
- Expect frequent urination.
- Provide for adequate rest periods.
- Avoid cold, which can increase sickling, and extreme heat, which can cause dehydration.
- Avoid known sources of infection.
- Avoid prolonged exposure to the sun.
- Monitor the child's body temperature (know the proper use of a thermometer) and promptly notify the medical team in the event of a fever (avoid antipyretics until discussed with the medical team).
- Administer penicillin daily as ordered.
- Avoid use of aspirin; use acetaminophen or ibuprofen as an alternative.
- Be cautious when traveling with the child to avoid conditions or locations with decreased atmospheric oxygen.
- Call the primary caregiver if symptoms of infection are evident.
- Know the physician's telephone number.

---

following signs and symptoms (and thus they are considered at high risk for sequelae):

- Ill appearance
- Cardiovascular instability
- Age younger than 1 year
- Pulmonary infiltrate
- Prior splenectomy or history of pneumococcal sepsis
- Hemoglobin less than 5 g/dL
- Family's or child's lack of ability to adhere to outpatient therapy
- WBC count less than 500/mm^3 or more than 30,000/mm^3
- Dehydration

Opioids and nonsteroidal antiinflammatory drugs (NSAIDs) (i.e., ibuprofen, ketorolac) are the mainstays of analgesic treatment, particularly in combination for painful crises. Morphine is the current opioid of choice. Meperidine (Demerol) is not recommended for long-term pain management because of its side-effect profile. Opioids provide systemic relief, and the NSAIDs act locally to decrease inflammation at the site of vaso-occlusion and provide analgesia without the potential side effect of respiratory depression. Morphine has been very effective when administered IV, particularly when given using the patient-controlled analgesia method (see Chapter 15).

The treatment of SCD focuses on precise diagnosis, education about the disease, prevention of exacerbations, prompt identification of complications, and supportive care during crises (hydration, oxygenation, analgesia, RBC transfusion) (see Table 23-1). Additional therapies currently under investigation include erythrocytapheresis (removal of sickled erythrocytes by an exchange transfusion technique), phenotyping RBCs for transfusion ("tissue typing" blood products that can potentially reduce alloimmunization), and hydroxyurea administration (increases the production of fetal hemoglobin [HbF], which interferes with the RBC sickling process and is considered to be protective against exacerbations and severity of symptoms) (Heeney & Ware, 2008).

Research toward a cure continues; especially promising may be gene therapy. Another promising area of research is hematopoietic stem cell transplantation. It has been a successful treatment modality for a limited number of children. Logistic and ethical issues are related to candidate selection regarding this potentially curative strategy.

NURSING CARE PLAN

The Child with Sickle Cell Disease

Focused Assessment

- On initial diagnosis, obtain history related to parents' concern that their child is in pain. Ask if the child:
  - Has joint swelling
  - Refuses to move an extremity
  - Cries out when a joint is moved or touched
  - Has a fever
  - Is irritable
- Ask parents of a child with SCD for a more detailed history related to signs and symptoms of complications
- Assess for possible causes of pain other than SCD
- Assess the severity of the child's condition
- When assessing pain in adolescents with SCD, consider the following:
  - They want to fit in with their peer group, but they are different because of SCD.
  - They may verbalize continued symptoms in an attempt to gain attention from health care providers, avoid peers, and delay a return to normal activities.
  - Obtain objective data specific to the type of painful episode.
- Teach parents (and child) to closely monitor the child's condition, assess for complications, and check the size of the child's spleen, reporting enlargement to the physician

Planning

Nursing Diagnoses

Ineffective Peripheral Tissue Perfusion and Risk for Decreased Cardiac Tissue Perfusion related to red blood cell sickling.

Expected Outcomes

The child will demonstrate adequate tissue perfusion, as evidenced by palpable peripheral pulses; warm, dry skin; adequate urinary output for age; and oxygen saturation greater than 95%.

The child and family will describe the treatment regimen, including medications and their actions and possible side effects.

Intervention/*Rationale*

1. Monitor the child's vital signs and respiratory status every 4 hours and as needed.

   Vital signs and respiratory status are assessed frequently to detect changes in tissue perfusion and respiratory status. Signs of altered perfusion include increased respiratory rate, increased work of breathing, decreased SaO₂, poor color, mottled appearance, prolonged capillary refill time, decreased peripheral pulses, and altered level of consciousness. A change in the level of consciousness often indicates poor perfusion or oxygenation of the brain.

2. Monitor pulse oximetry and administer oxygen to keep SaO₂ greater than 95%.

   Oxygen saturation levels are monitored with pulse oximetry. Ensuring adequate oxygen can ease the child's work of breathing and facilitate tissue oxygenation. Oxygen does not reverse the sickling process but may prevent more sickling.

3. Ensure adequate hydration by measuring intake and output and administering crystalloids and colloids (RBCs) as ordered.

   Measuring intake and output monitors renal function and level of hydration. Transfusions of crystalloids and (nonsickled) RBCs will increase the oxygen-carrying capacity of the blood and decrease the relative number of sickled cells.

4. Determine the child's and family's understanding of SCD and the treatment regimen and provide information or clarification as necessary.

   Adequate understanding of SCD can increase adherence to preventive measures and prompt interventions during exacerbations and hospitalizations.

Evaluation

Are the child's vital signs and oxygen saturation within normal limits?

Does the child demonstrate palpable peripheral pulses, capillary refill time less than 2 seconds, and warmth of extremities?

Can the child and family demonstrate their ability to administer medication and describe possible side effects?

Have the child and family requested additional information or clarification related to treatment?

Planning

Nursing Diagnosis

Acute Pain related to vaso-occlusion.

Expected Outcome

The child will have decreased pain, as evidenced by a lowered score on the selected pain assessment tool.

Intervention/*Rationale*

1. Monitor and record pain level every 1 to 2 hours and more frequently if needed, using a pain assessment tool appropriate for the child's age.

   Pain can be severe in vaso-occlusive crisis and is relieved for only short periods. An assessment tool that measures the subjective experience of pain is helpful in determining the child's level of discomfort (see Chapter 15).

2. Administer analgesics as ordered.

   Analgesics may be administered intermittently, by a patient-controlled analgesic (PCA) pump (or PCA by proxy), and by continuous infusion through an IV line.

3. Increase oral fluids, if able to tolerate, or administer fluids IV at a rate that is 1 to 1½ times the maintenance rate.

   Increased fluid volume reduces the viscosity of the blood, thus alleviating sites of vascular occlusion and preventing further sickling caused by dehydration.

4. Administer RBCs as ordered.

   Maintaining an adequate hemoglobin level increases oxygen-carrying capacity to aid in further preventing sickling and microvascular ischemia.

5. Incorporate the use of age-appropriate nonpharmacologic pain relief measures.

   Comfort measures often help distract the child from discomfort (see Chapter 15).

6. Perform passive range-of-motion exercises and avoid exertion.

   Passive range-of-motion exercises promote circulation without exacerbating fatigue.

Evaluation

Does the child verbalize or demonstrate decreased pain?

Does review of the child's pain assessment tool rating show a decrease in discomfort?

Continued

◎ NURSING CARE PLAN

The Child with Sickle Cell Disease—cont'd

Planning
Nursing Diagnosis
Risk for Infection related to chronic immunocompromised state.

Expected Outcomes
The child will remain free from infection, as evidenced by normal vital signs and activity for age.
The child and family will verbalize signs and symptoms of infection and when to notify the medical team.

Intervention/Rationale
1. Monitor vital signs every 4 hours and more frequently as needed. Report any temperature elevations to the physician.
   Elevated temperature and increased respiratory rate may be signs of infection.
2. Administer antipyretics and antibiotics as ordered.
   Antibiotics may be given prophylactically because of the high risk for infection. Prompt intervention is critical in children with HbSS and sickle beta-zero thalassemia during febrile illness.
3. Administer penicillin daily as ordered. Administer preventive immunizations to decrease the risk of infection (pneumococcal, meningococcal, H. influenzae type b, influenza vaccines).
   Children are at a high risk for pneumococcal infections and should receive long-term penicillin therapy. The pneumococcal, meningococcal, and H. influenzae type b vaccines can prevent sepsis, and the influenza vaccine can prevent complications from influenza.
4. Teach the parents signs of infection to watch for and the proper way to obtain the child's temperature. Confirm that the parents have a thermometer. Instruct the parents when to notify the physician.
   A comprehensive teaching plan is essential. Do not assume that the parent has a thermometer or knows how to accurately obtain a temperature reading.

Evaluation
Is the child's body temperature within normal limits?
Can the child and family describe their plan to identify and respond to signs of infection?

Planning
Nursing Diagnosis
Ineffective Coping related to chronic illness.

Expected Outcomes
The child and family will adhere to the treatment plan and follow-up visits.
The child and family will verbalize feelings about the impact of the illness on their lives.
The child and family will use available support systems and community resources.

Intervention/Rationale
1. Teach the family the necessity of and rationale for following the treatment as outlined by the health care team (see Patient-Centered Teaching: Home Care of the Child with Sickle Cell Disease).
   Conscientious adherence to the treatment regimen decreases the frequency of hospitalizations and improves the child's health and longevity.
2. Provide written instructions on all aspects of the child's care, complications to watch for, when to contact the health care team, and names and phone numbers of who to contact.
   Education helps the family gain a sense of control and allows them to make informed decisions. Parents can refer to written instructions when less stressed and able to comprehend.
3. Listen and encourage the child and family to verbalize their feelings and express their concerns regarding SCD. Answer questions honestly and openly. Make a referral to the social work team to provide additional supports, as needed.
   Identifying concerns and clarifying misconceptions will help the family cope with the stress of chronic illness.
4. Introduce the family to other families of children with SCD.
   These families can offer support, suggestions, and strategies for dealing with problems.
5. ⊖ Encourage parents to contact health care team members when they have questions or concerns. Provide parents with the address and phone number of the local chapter of the Sickle Cell Foundation (see Evolve website).
   Knowing about available resources and how to access assistance decreases parents' feelings of frustration and helplessness.

Evaluation
Are the child and family demonstrating adherence to the treatment plan?
Do the child and family demonstrate positive coping mechanisms?
Do the child and family use available resources?
Is the family able to discuss problems related to caring for a child with a chronic disease?
Does the child share fears and frustrations related to having SCD?

THALASSEMIA

The thalassemias are a group of inherited disorders characterized by an abnormality in hemoglobin synthesis that results from a reduction in or absence of one of the chains found in normal hemoglobin. These disorders are categorized by the site of the aberrant globin synthesis (e.g., alpha-thalassemia, beta-thalassemia). The homozygous form of beta-thalassemia, also known as *thalassemia major* or *Cooley's anemia,* is the most common and severe form of thalassemia.

Etiology and Incidence

Inheritance is through an autosomal recessive pattern. The child who inherits only one gene for beta-thalassemia may have only a mild anemia, hence the term *thalassemia minor*. The child who inherits two genes for beta-thalassemia will have severe anemia, hence the term *thalassemia major*. Worldwide prevalence of genetic carriers of beta-thalassemia is 3% (DeBaun, Frei-Jones, & Vichinsky, 2011b). The thalassemias are found primarily in people of Mediterranean descent, although they have been reported in Asian and African populations. In the United States, the incidence of thalassemia is increasing in young Asian children (Cunningham, Sankaran, Nathan, & Orkin, 2009).

Manifestations

The clinical manifestations of beta-thalassemia include pallor, growth retardation, pubertal delay, severe anemia, characteristic facies (enlarged head, frontal and parietal bossing, severe maxillary hyperplasia, malocclusion), hepatosplenomegaly, and a bronze skin tone (Box 23-1).

EVIDENCE-BASED PRACTICE

Health-Related Quality of Life with SCD

Level IV

Children and adolescents with sickle cell disease (SCD), one of the most common genetic disorders, often experience acute complications such as painful episodes related to vaso-occlusive crises, chest syndrome, and infections. Chronic complications include stroke, avascular necrosis, delayed growth and development, and renal disease. These complications often result in high rates of hospitalization and school absenteeism (Dale, Cochran, Jernigan, et al., 2009).

Health-related quality of life (HRQOL) is often defined as not only the absence of disease but also the presence of physical, psychological, and social well-being. The closer a person's life is to the standard of normalcy, the better the HRQOL. Dale et al. (2009) hypothesized that hospitalizations and high school absentee rates result in a negative HRQOL.

Dale et al. (2009) conducted a study to assess the HRQOL in children and adolescents with SCD as compared to the HRQOL of healthy children and adolescents. The study team chose the PedsQL 4.0 Generic Scales because of its demonstrated validity and reliability for use in both healthy and chronically ill children and adolescents. A convenience sampling method was utilized to enroll 124 subjects who had either sickle cell anemia or sickle beta-zero thalassemia, the most severe form of SCD. The comparison group was from data published using the HRQOL tool in more than 10,000 healthy children and adolescents.

The results of the study showed that children and adolescents with SCD had significantly lower overall HRQOL than that reported for healthy children. A substantial portion of the study subjects with SCD were determined to have a significant risk for impaired overall HRQOL because their results were more than one standard deviation below that of healthy subjects (Dale et al., 2009).

This study indicated that the PedsQL 4.0 could be used to identify children and adolescents with SCD and with low HRQOL, who may benefit from additional treatments such as chronic transfusion, hydroxyurea therapy, or stem cell transplantation. More importantly, those children could be offered psychosocial interventions such as assistance with school work, counseling, or play therapy.

Consider what might be the next steps to further establish reliability and the usefulness of the PedsQL 4.0 to help children with SCD at high risk for low HRQOL.

Reference

Dale, J. C., Cochran, C. J., & Jernigan, E., et al. (2009). Health-related quality of life in children and adolescents with sickle cell disease. *The Journal of Pediatric Health Care*, doi:10.1016/j.pedhc.2009.12.006.

Diagnostic Evaluation

In addition to a CBC, laboratory testing should include quantification of reticulocyte count, serum iron level, total iron-binding capacity, hemoglobin electrophoresis, and hemoglobin A and HbF levels to confirm the diagnosis. The CBC will often reflect microcytic hypochromic erythrocytes. A detailed family history may also reveal a history of anemia and delayed growth and maturation.

Therapeutic Management

The management of beta-thalassemia centers on three techniques: (1) erythrocyte transfusions, (2) chelation therapy, and (3) splenectomy. To prevent the severe side effects and bony changes associated with the disease, the hemoglobin is maintained at approximately 11 g/dL, although this parameter is often individualized.

BOX 23-1 CHARACTERISTIC FEATURES OF A CHILD WITH BETA-THALASSEMIA

Features develop as a consequence of inadequate treatment:

- Frontal bossing (prominent and protruding forehead)
- Maxillary prominence
- Wide-set eyes with a flattened nose
- Hepatosplenomegaly
- Greenish yellow skin tone

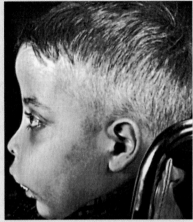

(Photo from Behrman, R.E., Kliegman, R.M., & Arvin, A.M. [Eds.]. [1996]. *Nelson textbook of pediatrics* [15th ed., p. 1402]. Philadelphia: Saunders.)

PATHOPHYSIOLOGY

Beta-Thalassemia

The abnormality of the beta-polypeptide chain in hemoglobin synthesis impairs the erythrocytes' ability to carry oxygen. Thalassemia is classified by the degree of imbalance in the globin chain and can be minor, intermediate, or severe.

Typically, during the second 6 months of life, a severe anemia develops. Erythrocytes are *hemolyzed* as they are produced. Because the body's natural response to a reduction in circulating hemoglobin is to try to produce more erythrocytes, the bone marrow begins massive production. Progressive disease constantly stimulates the bone marrow. The body perceives this as an inability to keep up with the need for erythrocytes. As a result, extramedullary (outside the bone marrow) sites of production of erythrocytes begin erythropoiesis. The result is a chronic state of production and destruction of erythrocytes, with a resulting inadequate amount of normal circulating hemoglobin.

Iron is necessary for the production of hemoglobin, and it is a byproduct of the hemolysis of RBCs. Normally the intestines absorb small amounts of iron. In this disorder, however, the body increases the absorption of iron. When increased iron absorption is combined with the increased iron introduced into the circulation by the transfusions necessary to treat thalassemia, *hemosiderosis* occurs, usually during the second decade of life. Hemosiderosis is the deposition of excess amounts of iron in tissue.

The results of excessive erythropoiesis and hemolysis are considerable. The bones become thin and fragile from excessive erythropoiesis. Hepatosplenomegaly occurs as a result of extramedullary erythropoiesis and hemosiderosis. Growth is impaired and puberty delayed. Without proper management, multisystem organ dysfunction ensues.

The major complication of long-term transfusion therapy is hemosiderosis. To prevent organ damage from excessive iron overload, these children must receive some form of chelation therapy.

The mainstay of chelation therapy has been with the drug deferoxamine (Desferal). It is most effective when given subcutaneously or IV. To avoid hospitalizing children who require deferoxamine therapy, the drug is often administered in the home by continuous subcutaneous infusion via a pump, over an 8- to 12-hour period at night. This approach can preserve some degree of normalcy in lifestyle for the family. Therapy is continued until the iron returns to an acceptable level. This goal can be accomplished within months of initiating chelation therapy. However, compliance with nightly subcutaneous infusions is often poor.

An oral chelation agent, deferasirox (Exjade), is now available in the United States for children older than 2 years. Compliance is improved with this orally administered medication. However, it is not without serious side effects, including gastrointestinal hemorrhage and kidney and liver damage (Hohneker, 2010).

Splenectomy may be indicated in children who are requiring 200 to 250 mL/kg of packed red blood cells each year to maintain their hemoglobin at 10 g/dL; the result is a moderate reduction in their transfusion requirements to 200 mL/kg per year (Cunningham et al., 2009). Splenectomy is a therapy that should not be considered casually because susceptibility to infection with *S. pneumoniae, H. influenzae,* and *Neisseria meningitidis* increases after splenectomy in children, particularly in those younger than 5 years. Standard therapy for asplenic individuals includes immunizations, prophylactic penicillin, and a high index of suspicion and aggressive antibiotic therapy for febrile illnesses as described previously for children with sickle cell disease (AAP, Committee on Infectious Diseases, 2009).

Bone marrow transplantation is the only available cure for thalassemia at this time. More than 1000 successful transplants have been performed. Only a small percentage of children (estimated at 30%) who have a matched donor and low risk factors, however, can undergo this procedure (Heeney & Dover, 2009).

PATIENT-CENTERED TEACHING

Home Chelation Therapy

Subcutaneous Route by Infusion Pump
- Know the technique for placing the subcutaneous needle, medication preparation, and infusion pump operation.
- Check needle security and placement.
- Check pump for proper infusion rate.
- Call the home care, clinic, or physician resource if the site becomes inflamed, red, or painful.
- Know indications for medication and side effects that require health care team notification; hearing loss or ringing in the ears, fever, diarrhea, visual disturbances, allergic reactions, and respiratory compromise.

Intravenous Route: Totally Implantable or Tunneled Access Device
- Know the technique for placing access needle or catheter connection, medication preparation, and infusion pump operation.
- Call the home care, clinic, or physician resource if the site becomes inflamed, red, or painful or the specific access device is obstructed.
- Have a list of home care resources for technique assistance, supplies, and problematic pump functioning.
- Know indications for medication and side effects that require health care team notification: hearing loss or ringing in the ears, fever, diarrhea, visual disturbances, allergic reactions, and respiratory compromise.

NURSING CARE OF THE CHILD WITH BETA-THALASSEMIA

■ Assessment

Subjective data may include the parents' observation that their child is not as active as other children of the same age. The child may sleep more than other children or want to be held often. The child appears pale, with laboratory values reflecting a microcytic, hypochromic anemia. Clinical symptoms are related to the degree of anemia, ranging from mild to severe.

An older child with the disease or a child who has not received adequate treatment will likely have characteristic facial deformities, including maxillary hyperplasia and malocclusion. These characteristics develop from extramedullary marrow expansion, a consequence of the marrow's effort to keep up with the demand for RBCs as a result of anemia. Hepatosplenomegaly is usually seen at this time in older children but not in infants.

■ Nursing Diagnosis and Planning

The nursing diagnoses and expected outcomes that may be appropriate after assessment of the child with thalassemia are as follows:
- Ineffective Peripheral Tissue Perfusion and Risk for Decreased Cardiac Tissue Perfusion related to anemia.

Expected Outcome. The child demonstrates adequate tissue perfusion, as evidenced by palpable peripheral pulses; warm, dry skin; urinary output appropriate for age; and the absence of cardiorespiratory distress (oxygen saturation >95%).
- Disturbed Body Image related to altered appearance and the perception of having a chronic disease.

Expected Outcome. The child and family will verbalize feelings related to changes in appearance and the limitations imposed by the disease process.
- Anxiety related to the diagnosis.

Expected Outcomes. The child and family will express feelings about the disorder, lifestyle disruptions as a result of treatment, and possible genetic transmission of the disease.
- Deficient Knowledge related to inadequate information about the disorder.

Expected Outcomes. The child and family will describe the disorder and its treatment regimen, including medications and their actions and possible side effects.

■ Interventions

Expect transfusions to begin immediately for an affected child while cardiovascular compromise from the anemia is being assessed. Preparing the child and family for diagnostic procedures will help alleviate fears. Once the diagnosis is made, education should begin. Parents need to understand the importance of proper and continuing follow-up. The family needs much support as they begin chelation therapy, which is very time consuming and interferes with family routines. The nurse must regularly monitor the family's adherence to therapy. If hematopoietic stem cell transplantation becomes an option, the parents will need referral to a specialty center and will need support from the entire health care team as they contemplate this course of treatment.

■ Evaluation

- Are the child's peripheral pulses palpable and oxygen saturation increased to 95%?
- Is the child's hemoglobin level improving?
- Is the child able to verbalize feelings associated with the treatment or the psychosocial implications of the disease?

- Is the child sharing feelings related to changes in appearance, limitations imposed by the disease, and having a chronic disease?
- Has the family sought genetic counseling?
- Does the family readily verbalize feelings about having a child with beta-thalassemia?
- Has the family demonstrated adherence to therapy?

HEMOPHILIA

Hemophilia is a lifelong hereditary blood disorder with no cure. Hemophilia A is associated with the deficiency of coagulation factor VIII. Hemophilia B, a deficiency in factor IX, has been associated with a constellation of symptoms similar to hemophilia A. Lack of factor XI, Hemophilia C, results in only mild bleeding tendencies (Bolton-Maggs, 2011). Congenital deficiencies in these three factors account for approximately 90% to 95% of the bleeding disorders referred to as *hemophilia*.

Etiology and Incidence

Hemophilia is an X-linked autosomal recessive disorder; carrier females pass on the defect to affected males. Women who never produce an affected male child may silently carry the gene for generations, but typically there is a history of hemophilia in the family. Rarely, female offspring are born with the disorder, but only if they inherit an affected gene from the mother and are the offspring of a father with hemophilia. The prevalence of factor VIII deficiency is 1 in 5000 males; factor IX deficiency prevalence is 1 in 35,000 males (National Hemophilia Foundation, 2010).

Manifestations

The disease severity is individual but tends to be familial. Bleeding occurs after surgery or serious trauma in all children with this disease. Bleeding occurs after tissue trauma in children with moderate and severe disease. Bleeding occurs spontaneously and for no apparent reason in children with severe disease. Affected children bruise easily, have episodes of epistaxis, and may have hematuria. They may also have bleeding with loss of deciduous teeth, from even minor lacerations, and from injections. Most commonly, bleeding develops in the muscles and joints (hemarthrosis), especially the knees, for those children with moderate and severe disease (Figure 23-1). Recurrent bleeding commonly occurs in the same joint in severely affected children, causing swelling, pain, bleeding, and stiffness.

PATHOPHYSIOLOGY

Hemophilia

More than 10 factors in the blood work in sequence to produce blood clotting. Factor VIII, or antihemophilic factor, and factor IX, or plasma thromboplastin component, are the two missing or defective constituents in the blood that cause hemophilia A, or classic hemophilia, and hemophilia B, or Christmas disease. When these factors are missing or defective, blood does not clot as it should. The two disorders are inherited in the same way and have similar manifestations. Normal factor activity is described as a percentage. The percentage of factor activity is closely related to the level of factor in the blood (e.g., 100 units/dL factor equals 100% factor activity). Normal levels of factor VIII are 50% to 150%. The severity of the disease is classified as follows:

Severe: Less than 1% factor activity
Moderate: 1% to 5% factor activity
Mild: 6% to 50% factor activity

Diagnostic Evaluation

Hemophilia is sometimes but not always diagnosed after circumcision, at which time prolonged bleeding may be observed. Because the most common sites of bleeding are in the muscles and joints, the diagnosis may be delayed until the toddler years, when the child becomes more active and the disease has an opportunity to manifest itself. By the preschool years, most affected children have had an episode of persistent bleeding from a minor traumatic laceration.

A diagnostic workup for the child with suspected hemophilia includes determining the prothrombin time (PT), partial thromboplastin time, bleeding time, fibrinogen level, and platelet count; quantitative immunoelectrophoretic assay; and factor VIII and factor IX assays.

Therapeutic Management

The management of hemophilia is highly individual and depends on the severity of the illness. Therapy aims to prevent excessive bleeding and tissue damage by supplying the body with additional factor, substituting for factor (VIII or IX) that is missing or ineffective.

Previously, treatment involved transfusions of blood products or administration of freeze-dried preparations manufactured from blood

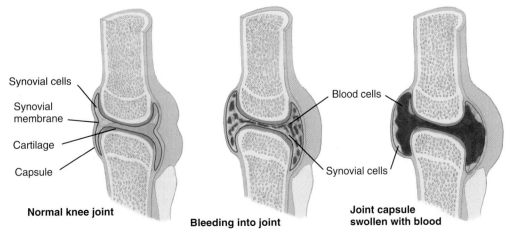

Synovial cells
Synovial membrane
Cartilage
Capsule

Normal knee joint

Blood cells
Synovial cells

Bleeding into joint

Joint capsule swollen with blood

FIG 23-1 Hemarthrosis and joint destruction are characteristic of hemophilia.

products. One of the major risks associated with this type of factor replacement therapy was contracting hepatitis or human immunodeficiency virus infection. Because of this risk, manufacturers began to heat-treat the blood factor to reduce the risk of viral transmission. Monoclonal products were then developed that were found to be even safer than the heat-treated products. The most recent development in the treatment of hemophilia is the availability of recombinant antihemophilic factor, which is not derived from human plasma but is produced synthetically from isolation of the gene. Recombinant factor eliminates the risk of virus transmission. Factor preparations must be reconstituted with sterile water before being given intravenously.

⚡ SAFETY ALERT

Acetylsalicylic Acid: Contraindication

Acetylsalicylic acid (e.g., aspirin, aspirin-containing products) should not be given to children with factor disorders because it inhibits platelet function. Because some over-the-counter medications may contain acetylsalicylic acid, it is important to read all labels carefully before giving the child the medication.

Prophylactic therapy is now being started in infants and young children with severe hemophilia to prevent joint problems (Rodriguez & Hoots, 2008). A regular schedule of factor replacement beginning in early childhood has been shown to delay the development of joint problems (Rodriguez & Hoots, 2008). Children with mild hemophilia A may be able to use desmopressin acetate (1-deamino-8-D-arginine vasopressin [DDAVP]) intranasal spray, because of its vasoconstrictor action, to stop bleeding. Children with hemophilias A and B can be given aminocaproic acid (Amicar) or tranexamic acid (Cyclokapron)—oral medications that stabilize oral clots and can also sometimes stop nosebleeds. In addition to factor prophylaxis, children with hemophilia must try to avoid activities that induce bleeding. Special precautions can be taken to protect joints, thereby allowing the child to lead a more normal life. Prophylactic factor replacement therapy should also be given before surgery and some dental procedures. Bleeding is treated with rest, ice, elevation of the affected part, and compression (also referred to as *RICE: rest, ice, compression, elevation*).

❗ NURSING QUALITY ALERT

Interviewing a Child with Hemophilia

Subjective data gathered from a child known to have hemophilia should include information about recent trauma and initial measures to stop bleeding. An important question is the length of time that pressure had to be applied before the bleeding subsided. Other questions to ask include whether the swelling increased after the surface bleeding stopped and whether swelling and stiffness occurred without apparent trauma.

◎ NURSING CARE PLAN

The Child with Hemophilia

Focused Assessment

- Consider these parameters when assessing children for signs and symptoms of hemophilia:
  - For male newborns, observe the circumcision site and injection sites for prolonged bleeding.
  - For children learning to crawl and walk, explore parental concerns about bruising easily after minor falls.
  - Ask parents about previous cuts and abrasions to determine if child needed more than the usual pressure application or time for the bleeding to subside
  - Inquire about a family history of bleeding disorders

Planning
Nursing Diagnosis
Risk for Injury related to prolonged bleeding.

Expected Outcomes
The child and family will recognize bleeding resulting from injury and promptly control it to prevent permanent tissue damage.

Intervention/Rationale

1. Monitor the area of injury hourly for bleeding over a 24-hour period.
   Bleeding may be prolonged and, especially in the case of head trauma, may not manifest immediately.
2. Measure the circumference of an injured joint.
   Joint measurement provides objective rather than subjective data for future comparisons.
3. In the case of head trauma, assess the child's level of consciousness at least hourly and note any behavioral changes.
   Decreased level of consciousness and unusual behaviors are early indicators of increased intracranial pressure resulting from hemorrhage.

4. Apply gentle pressure for 10-15 minutes to small superficial wounds and assess the area for subcutaneous bleeding.
   Small wounds may ooze blood into the subcutaneous tissue. Pressure facilitates clot formation.
5. Administer factor replacement as ordered.
   Factor must be reconstituted just before infusion. It may be given as a prophylactic measure even if no bleeding is apparent.
6. When a child is hospitalized, monitor factor blood levels, as ordered.
   With serious injuries, factor levels aid in prescribing dosages and establishing thresholds for the child.
7. If a muscle or joint injury occurs, immobilize, elevate, and apply ice to the affected part, as ordered by the physician.
   Initial immobilization will help prevent further injury until the bleeding resolves.
8. Offer suggestions for establishing a safe home environment for the child (see Patient-Centered Teaching: Home Care of the Child with Hemophilia box).
   A safe home environment will help prevent injuries.
9. Avoid rectal temperature measurement.
   Rectal temperatures may cause bleeding from tissue trauma.
10. Teach parents to provide for and expect behaviors consistent with normal growth and development per their child's age.
    Parents may tend to overprotect or provide special treatment for their child. This unnecessarily limits the child's opportunities for normal psychosocial development and decreases self-esteem.

Evaluation
Has the child had serious bleeding from injury?
Has the child adhered to the treatment regimen to control injuries?
Are there long-term complications from injury?

◎ NURSING CARE PLAN

The Child with Hemophilia—cont'd

Planning

Nursing Diagnosis

Deficient Knowledge related to the need for information about disease diagnosis and treatment.

Expected Outcomes

The child and family will explain the diagnosis.

The child and family will demonstrate adherence to the home care regimen.

Intervention/Rationale

1. Determine the child's and family's readiness for learning. Create an environment conducive to learning.
   The family may need time to adjust to the initial diagnosis before they are ready to be educated. Parents may need an educational setting away from the child so they can focus on learning.

2. On initial diagnosis and with subsequent follow-up visits, spend time with the child and parents explaining the diagnosis, sequelae, and treatment. Offer written literature and other educational materials.
   Education is ongoing and reinforcement is needed for stressed parents. Explaining the rationale for treatment and the disease's sequelae will help ensure adherence to therapy. Written or other forms of information (such as videotapes) can be reviewed later, improving parent comprehension.

3. Offer encouragement and praise for prompt recognition and response to bleeding.
   Praise will reinforce appropriate actions taken by the child and parents.

4. Teach techniques for reconstitution and infusion of factor at home. The infusion technique will depend on type of venous access (peripheral infusion, central venous line, implantable infusion device [port]) (see Patient-Centered Teaching: Home Care of the Child with Hemophilia box).
   Parents (and child per developmental level) are taught techniques for accessing the venous line or port, infusing the factor, and heparinizing the line or port.

5. Consider using a topical anesthetic, such as eutectic mixture of local anesthetics (EMLA), when accessing infusion ports or peripheral sites.
   The use of topical anesthetics decreases pain, thus causing the child less trauma and anxiety.

Evaluation

Are the child and family able to safely administer factor replacement at home?

Do the child and family promptly recognize and react to bleeding?

Planning

Nursing Diagnosis

Ineffective Coping related to chronic illness and guilt.

Expected Outcomes

The child and family will adhere to the treatment plan, as evidenced by safety alterations being made in the home and community.

The child and family will use available support systems and community resources.

Family members will verbalize concerns about the impact of the illness on the family.

Intervention/Rationale

1. Teach the family the need for safety precautions, correct response to injury, medication administration methods, and importance of following the treatment plan as outlined by health care providers (see Patient-Centered Teaching: Home Care of the Child with Hemophilia box).
   Conscientious adherence to the treatment regimen decreases the potential for long-term complications.

2. Listen to and encourage the child and family to verbalize their feelings and express their concerns regarding hemophilia. Answer questions honestly and openly. Be alert for feelings of guilt expressed by the mother.
   Identifying concerns and clarifying misconceptions help families cope with the stress of chronic illness. Mothers may experience guilt because of the genetic inheritance pattern of the disease.

3. Introduce the family to other families of children with hemophilia.
   Other families of children with hemophilia can offer support, suggestions, and strategies for coping.

4. ⊜ Provide referral to the National Hemophilia Foundation (see Evolve website).
   Access to information and assistance can help the family deal with the potentially overwhelming financial and emotional burdens of caring for a child with hemophilia.

5. Explore the child's feelings about restrictions in activities and participation in some sports due to having hemophilia. Assess the child's coping strategies and need for support.
   Discussing feelings related to a chronic disease provides an opportunity for the child to explore options and improve coping strategies.

Evaluation

Does the older child avoid contact sports and participate in other activities, such as swimming?

Has the family contacted the National Hemophilia Foundation?

Is the child able to balance limitations with normal childhood activities?

VON WILLEBRAND'S DISEASE

von Willebrand's disease (VWD) is the most commonly inherited bleeding disorder (Montgomery, Gill, & Paola, 2009) and has been estimated to occur in 1% to 2% of the general population, though that estimate is controversial.

Etiology

VWD is an autosomal inherited disorder with both dominant and recessive variants (Montgomery et al., 2009). At least 20 subtypes of VWD have been identified (e.g., type I, type IIA, type IIB). Type I is the most frequent subtype, occurring in approximately 75% of patients

with VWD. Almost all of the remaining 25% of patients with VWD have type IIA. The other subtypes are rare (Montgomery et al., 2009). VWD occurs equally in males and females, though the age of presentation differs, with females most commonly diagnosed after the onset of menstruation (National Hemophilia Foundation, 2010; Montgomery et al., 2009).

Pathophysiology

Children with VWD have either underproduction or dysfunction of von Willebrand's protein. The VWD protein occurs together with factor VIII in the circulation, making it a carrier protein for factor VIII. One of its most important functions is to bind and attract platelets to

PATIENT-CENTERED TEACHING

Home Care of the Child with Hemophilia

- Apply gentle, prolonged pressure to superficial wounds until the bleeding has stopped.
- Call the physician in the event of blunt trauma, especially trauma involving the joints.
- Establish an age-appropriate, safe environment:
  - Pad table corners.
  - Pad crib rails.
  - Provide extra joint padding on clothes.
  - Remove items that can tip over or be pulled down on the child.
  - Do not leave a crawling or toddling child unattended.
  - Use a toothbrush with soft bristles and a WaterPik for dental care.
  - Instruct older children to avoid contact sports and to take precautions with other sports.
  - Pad the knees and elbows for physical education class.
  - Use protective helmets for any sport in which head injury could occur (e.g., bicycling, skating).
  - Use an electric razor for shaving.
- Call the physician if any head injury occurs.
- Reconstitute and administer factor through an IV line or the child's central venous access device.
- If a child has an implantable infusion device, caregivers should understand the following:
  - Site preparation
  - Sterile technique for insertion of access needle
  - Technique for verification of needle placement
  - Administration of factor by IV push

- Saline solution and heparin flush
- Removal and proper disposal of needle
- Keep current with the schedule of immunizations, dental hygiene, and routine well-child care.
- Allow your child to set personal safety limits when possible.
- Provide for normal growth and development opportunities (safe activities, time with other children, limit setting, independence).

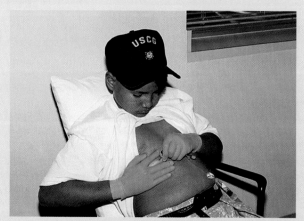

Control of deficient blood clotting in hemophilia requires injection of the missing clotting factors. This young man is injecting his factor into an implanted central venous access port. Sterile technique is essential. (Courtesy family of Jason Lee Davis.)

the site of endothelial tissue injury, thus facilitating the formation of a clot. Deficiency of von Willebrand's protein may result in a corresponding deficiency of factor VIII.

Manifestations

Clinical features and the need for treatment depend on the severity of the disorder. The clinical manifestations of VWD include a history of epistaxis, bleeding from the gums, prolonged bleeding from cuts, excessive bleeding after surgery or trauma, and menorrhagia (excessive menstrual bleeding) in females.

Diagnostic Evaluation

A thorough history will ascertain whether the episode of bruising is proportional to the degree of trauma. A family history of bleeding disorders is important. Recently researchers have developed scoring systems for identifying those at risk for von Willebrand's disease. Positive history of epistaxis, skin bleeding, oral/dental bleeding, gastrointestinal bleeding, muscle/joint bleeding, CNS bleeding, and significant bleeding after surgery are each evaluated and scored in these scoring systems. These scoring systems are not yet validated in children because of lack of specificity and sensitivity.

Laboratory evaluations are obtained once it has been identified, based on bleeding history, that a child potentially has von Willebrand's disease. Laboratory tests may include a bleeding time and a partial thromboplastin time, the results of which may be normal. Because both of these may be normal, children with a history of significant bleeding episodes must be further evaluated with more specific assays for von Willebrand's factor. The most clinically useful and widely used laboratory tests for diagnosing this disorder are the enzyme-linked

immunosorbent assay (ELISA) and the quantitative immunoelectrophoretic assay, which measure the quantity of von Willebrand's factor antigen in the plasma (Montgomery et al., 2009).

Therapeutic Management

Therapy is aimed at controlling bleeding episodes and replacing the missing or dysfunctional factor in the blood. A concentrate of antihemolytic factors that have undergone purification to inactivate viruses or possibly fresh frozen plasma is administered before surgery or after trauma with excessive bleeding (Robertson, Lillicrap, & James, 2008).

The treatment of choice is DDAVP, which is administered intravenously or intranasally. The DDAVP products are given for type I and type IIA VWD only (Montgomery et al., 2009). High-purity (not monoclonal or recombinant) factor VIII products that are specifically known to contain von Willebrand's factor can be used to treat type IIB disease. (Only a minority of currently available factor VIII concentrates actually contain von Willebrand's factor.)

NURSING CARE OF THE CHILD WITH VON WILLEBRAND'S DISEASE

▪ Assessment

A careful history detailing episodes of bruising and bleeding is essential. In addition, documenting a family history of bruising or bleeding assists with identifying the condition (Robertson et al., 2008). Possible causes of any previous episodes of bleeding, if any can be identified, should also be discussed. The nurse asks how many times the child has had a nosebleed, how long the child bleeds from minor injuries, and whether there is a history of prolonged bleeding associated with surgery or trauma.

Physical examination usually reveals a healthy child except for evidence of bruising greater than expected for the degree of trauma. If the child is being seen after a major bleeding episode, signs of hemorrhage or a decreased hemoglobin level (or both) will be seen.

■ Nursing Diagnosis and Planning

The nursing diagnoses and expected outcomes that may be appropriate after assessment of the child with von Willebrand's disease include the following:

- Ineffective Protection related to abnormal clotting.

Expected Outcome. The child will remain free of life-threatening episodes of hemorrhage.

- Deficient Knowledge related to the disorder.

Expected Outcomes. The child and family will explain the disorder, its management, and its chronic nature.

■ Interventions

Education of the family is aimed at producing an understanding of the precautions to take with the child and knowledge of when prophylactic therapy should be given before elective procedures. The child should wear a medical alert tag at all times. The degree of activity limitation will depend on the severity of the disorder. Limitations may include avoidance of contact sports, especially football. Avoidance of prescription and over-the-counter medications that affect platelet function, such as aspirin or NSAIDs, is also recommended. The nurse should advise the parents to check the labels of all over-the-counter medications for presence of aspirin or ibuprofen. If DDAVP is administered for a bleeding episode, the parents need to carefully monitor the child's fluid intake for 24 hours after administration to prevent hyponatremia, a complication seen in young children (Robertson et al., 2008). The family should be referred to the Hemophilia Foundation for support services.

■ Evaluation

- Are episodes of bleeding minimal and controlled?
- Does the family communicate an understanding of the importance of avoiding medications that affect platelet function and avoiding activities that increase the risk of bleeding?
- Does the family seek appropriate resources for information about the condition and its management?

IMMUNE THROMBOCYTOPENIC PURPURA

Immune thrombocytopenic purpura (ITP) is an acquired bleeding disorder characterized by thrombocytopenia (platelet count below 150,000/mm³), a purpuric rash, normal bone marrow, and the absence of signs of other identifiable causes of thrombocytopenia. It is classified as acute or chronic, with chronic being defined as the persistence of thrombocytopenia for more than 6 months.

Etiology and Incidence

ITP is estimated to be one of the most common acquired bleeding disorders in children. The incidence of symptomatic disease is approximately 3 to 8 per 100,000 children per year. Acute ITP is more prevalent among children younger than 10 years, affects males and females equally, and is more prevalent during the late winter and spring. Chronic ITP affects adolescents more than younger children, with females being affected more frequently than males (Wilson, 2009). The

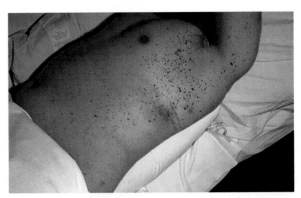

FIG 23-2 Multiple petechiae are characteristic of immune thrombocytopenic purpura. This disorder results in the destruction of circulating platelets and decreased bone marrow production of new platelets. (Courtesy Cook Children's Medical Center, Fort Worth, TX.)

etiology of ITP is unknown, although in the majority of children it follows a viral illness and is considered to be an autoimmune process.

Pathophysiology

In general, ITP is thought to occur as a result of the destruction of platelets by autoantibodies to glycoproteins normally expressed on platelet membranes. The spleen and other organs of the reticuloendothelial system subsequently destroy these antibody-coated platelets (Wilson, 2009).

Manifestations

Clinical manifestations of ITP include the sudden onset of bruising and petechiae, with bleeding involving the mucous membranes and gums, in a child who is in otherwise good health (Figure 23-2).

Diagnostic Evaluation

The initial diagnostic evaluation should include a thorough history and a CBC, including evaluation of a peripheral blood smear. A family history of ITP, information about any medications the child has taken that could cause thrombocytopenia, history of recent live virus vaccination, and any instances of illness, especially febrile illness, in the past month, are obtained. In an affected child, the initial CBC will reveal a low platelet count, often below 50,000/mm³, but the remainder of the CBC will otherwise be normal. The physical examination findings will be normal, aside from the signs of bleeding.

If any data in the history or CBC are suggestive of a diagnosis other than ITP, the physician may obtain a bone marrow aspirate to rule out an oncologic disorder and to determine whether megakaryocytes, the precursors of platelets, are present. Routine bone marrow examination is not warranted in a child with findings consistent with acute ITP.

Physical examination of the affected child reveals bruising and petechiae, the severity of which depends on how low the platelet count is and the child's tolerance of the low platelet count. The spleen and liver are generally normal in size. The greatest risk of a low platelet count is intracranial hemorrhage, so a neurologic assessment is important.

Therapeutic Management

The goal of treatment is to prevent rare, life-threatening bleeding events, such as intracranial bleeding. Additional goals include restoration of the platelet count to above 20,000/mm³ in children with mucocutaneous bleeding and a reduction in the duration of thrombocytopenia. Treatment is based on the child's presenting condition.

Treatment options have been an intense topic of discussion for years and have divided pediatric hematologists between what have been called *interventionists* and *noninterventionists* (Blanchette & Bolton-Maggs, 2008; Wilson, 2009). Because most cases of ITP are self-limiting, with a normal platelet count returning within 6 months, the noninterventionists recommend no therapy but frequent monitoring of platelet counts and bleeding status (Wilson, 2009). The mainstays of treatment are oral steroids and IVIG. Depending on whether the child is an inpatient or outpatient, IV or oral steroids may be administered over a 2- to 4-week period. Steroids block the autoimmune destruction of platelets. IVIG is administered once daily for 1 to 2 days. Often, the platelet count is dramatically increased after one dose of IVIG. In children with Rh-positive blood types (A+, B+, and O+), IV anti-D immune globulin may be used. However, an important side effect of anti-D immune globulin is intravascular hemolysis with a significant decrease in hemoglobin levels (Blanchette & Bolton-Maggs, 2008). Children treated with IV anti-D immune globulin must be monitored closely for signs and symptoms of hemolytic anemia.

ITP is considered to be acute if recovery of a normal platelet count occurs within 6 months. The condition becomes chronic if recovery takes longer than 6 months. Children with chronic ITP may initially respond to steroids with an increased platelet count, but it will not reach normal levels. These children may go for long periods without excessive bleeding or a low platelet count; the count will then begin to decline again, at which time steroid therapy should be resumed.

When steroids and IVIG do not control the thrombocytopenia in a child with chronic ITP, a splenectomy may be indicated. Splenectomy will cure most children with chronic ITP because the spleen synthesizes the antiplatelet antibody that results in the destruction of circulating platelets. The risk associated with removal of the spleen is sepsis from those organisms that the spleen's reticuloendothelial system fights, so ITP is managed without splenectomy, if possible, until age 5 years. Platelet transfusions are given in children only when active, uncontrolled bleeding occurs.

NURSING CARE OF THE CHILD WITH IMMUNE THROMBOCYTOPENIC PURPURA

■ Assessment

Parents usually bring their child to the physician because they have noticed excessive bruising or a "red rash" in the child's mouth or on the child's body. Although this "rash" (actually petechiae) may look remarkable to a nurse, it often evolves so gradually that it escapes the immediate notice of a parent who sees the child every day. As a result, health care may not be sought until very significant bruising and petechiae, even hematomas, are present.

Affected children usually demonstrate normal activity levels for their age because they do not "feel bad." Assessment should include observation for signs of any further bruising or bleeding, including epistaxis, hematuria, or blood in the stools, as well as for signs of a decreasing level of consciousness, which could indicate intracranial hemorrhage.

■ Nursing Diagnosis and Planning

The nursing diagnoses and expected outcomes that may be appropriate after assessment of the child with ITP are as follows:

• Ineffective Protection related to low platelet count.

PATIENT-CENTERED TEACHING

Home Care of the Child with Immune Thrombocytopenic Purpura

- Eliminate participation in high-risk activities, such as contact sports, bicycle riding, roller-skating, and diving, if the child's platelet count is low.
- Avoid medications that can affect platelet function (ibuprofen, aspirin). Be sure to read over-the-counter medication labels to check for these medications, which can be included in combination products, such as cold, flu, and upset stomach remedies.
- Use an extra-soft bristle toothbrush if the platelet count is less than 20,000/mm³.
- Establish an age-appropriate, safe home environment.
- Pad table corners.
- Pad crib rails.
- Offer extra joint padding on clothes.

For additional resources and information, contact national organizations (e.g., the ITP Society; see Evolve website, Additional Resources—Resources for Health Care Providers and Families).

Expected Outcome. The child will exhibit no signs of active bleeding or intracranial hemorrhage, as evidenced by pulse and blood pressure within normal limits and an alert and responsive child.

• Risk for Infection related to chronic use of steroids or splenectomy.

Expected Outcomes. The family will identify signs of infection and notify the health care team, and the child will respond rapidly to treatment for infection.

• Deficient Knowledge related to insufficient information about the disorder and its therapeutic management.

Expected Outcomes. The child and family will describe ITP and the treatment plan.

■ Interventions

The family is referred to a health care center to carry out medical treatments, and the family is educated about ITP and home care (see Patient-Centered Teaching: Home Care of the Child with Immune Thrombocytopenic Purpura box).

An IV access line may be established for the purpose of administering IV steroids or IVIG. It can be quite challenging to establish IV access in children with ITP because merely puncturing the skin may result in a hematoma, which may be confused with "blowing" the vein. Careful evaluation of blood return and flushing of the IV catheter with normal saline solution will confirm proper placement of the catheter.

Restricting the activity of toddlers and young children can be a challenge. Extra-soft bristle toothbrushes or Toothettes should be used for mouth care on all children whose platelet count is below 20,000/mm³. Until the platelet count returns to normal, activities such as bicycle riding, contact sports, and roller-skating should be curtailed.

Education includes teaching the family about the disease process of ITP; the side effects of steroids and IVIG, if used; the need to restrict the child's activity; and the importance of proper follow-up evaluations. Steroids can mask the presence of an infection. Parents should be instructed regarding the signs and symptoms of infection and what actions they should take if fever and other signs of infection are seen.

The nurse ensures that parents and the child's primary care physician are informed if the child receives IVIG. The AAP recommends delaying the administration of routine measles immunization for a

⚡ SAFETY ALERT

Actions to Avoid in Children with Low Platelet Counts

- Avoid administering intramuscular injections, aspirin, aspirin-containing products, and nonsteroidal antiinflammatory medications (e.g., ibuprofen) to children with low platelet counts.
- Avoid taking temperatures rectally, and perform invasive procedures with extreme caution.

minimum of 8 to 10 months after a child receives an immune globulin preparation because it may block the replication of live-virus vaccine immune response (AAP, Committee on Infectious Diseases, 2009).

If a splenectomy is planned, both the pneumococcal and Hib vaccines are given if not previously administered. After the splenectomy, the child must take prophylactic penicillin daily (Blanchette & Bolton-Maggs, 2008). Any signs and symptoms of infection should be reported immediately to the physician so that proper therapy can be initiated before the infection becomes life threatening.

■ Evaluation

- Are the child's vital signs within normal limits?
- Is the child responding in an age-appropriate manner?
- Have areas of ecchymosis and petechiae decreased?
- Does the family verbalize and implement a plan of care that decreases the risk of the child incurring an injury that is likely to cause hemorrhage?
- Does the family respond quickly to early signs of infection by notifying the primary health care provider?

DISSEMINATED INTRAVASCULAR COAGULATION

Disseminated intravascular coagulation (DIC) is an acquired hemorrhagic syndrome characterized by uncontrolled formation and deposition of fibrin thrombi, and by the resulting consumption of clotting factors, which leads to uncontrolled bleeding. In children, DIC does not have the high mortality rate seen in adults. The keys to recovery for children are identification and treatment of the underlying cause of the DIC.

Etiology

DIC is triggered by any factor that causes endothelial damage, liberation of tissue thromboplastin, circulating endotoxins, or immune complexes. In children, the most common causes are trauma, hypoxia, necrotizing enterocolitis, shock, liver disease, overwhelming viral or bacterial infections, and acute promyelocytic leukemia.

Manifestations

Manifestations of DIC involve an insidious onset, corresponding to changes in the platelet count and fibrinogen levels. Early indicators include excessive bruising and petechiae, oozing from puncture sites, oozing from sites of mild tissue trauma (e.g., site of insertion of a nasogastric tube), and mild gastrointestinal bleeding. As the disease progresses, manifestations of DIC include purpuric rash, worsening of bleeding, hemoptysis, hypoxemia, oliguria progressing to renal failure, progressive organ failure, and intracranial hemorrhage.

Diagnostic Evaluation

The diagnosis of DIC is confirmed by laboratory testing (Box 23-2).

PATHOPHYSIOLOGY

Disseminated Intravascular Coagulation

Disseminated intravascular coagulation (DIC) is a consumptive disorder caused by abnormal activation of the clotting mechanism, which causes rapid depletion of platelets, prothrombin, and fibrinogen. It is a pathologic syndrome resulting from the formation of thrombin, subsequent activation and consumption of certain coagulant proteins, and the production of fibrin thrombi. DIC manifests with diffuse microvascular coagulation caused by depletion of clotting factors, resulting in impaired hemostasis.

The pathophysiology of DIC is complicated and often not easily understood because both excessive bleeding and excessive clotting are occurring at the same time. The syndrome of DIC leads to deposition of platelet and fibrin plugs in the vasculature and the simultaneous depletion of platelets and clotting factor proteins.

The process of blood coagulation follows either an intrinsic or an extrinsic pathway.* Both pathways ultimately lead to the common pathway of prothrombin forming thrombin, which, in the presence of fibrinogen, forms fibrin. Alternately, fibrinolysis (clot destruction) requires the presence of thrombin. During this process, the enzyme *plasmin* lyses fibrin into fragments called *fibrin degradation products,* which interfere with the ability of platelets to adhere to one another. In DIC, initiation of the clotting process is stimulated by endothelial damage or some form of tissue injury. Platelets and clotting factors are subsequently depleted. As clotting is stimulated, the body perceives the need to produce substances to dissolve those clots, and there is an increase in the end result of clot lysis, fibrin degradation products. The overstimulation of both of these normal processes has four major effects on the body:

- Increased, uncontrolled bleeding resulting from the depletion of platelets and clotting factors and overstimulation of the fibrinolytic process
- Anemia caused by the excessive bleeding and the mechanical fragmentation of RBCs
- Organ damage resulting from the formation of emboli
- Tissue hypoxia leading to tissue necrosis

*Mann, K. G., & Brummel-Ziedens, K. (2009). Blood coagulation. In S. Orkin, D. Fisher, A. T. Look, et al. (Eds.), *Nathan and Oski's hematology of infancy and childhood* (7th ed., pp. 1399-1424). Philadelphia: Elsevier Saunders.

BOX 23-2   CONFIRMATORY LABORATORY FINDINGS IN DISSEMINATED INTRAVASCULAR COAGULATION

- Decreased RBC count
- Low platelet count noted on CBC
- RBC fragments on the smear
- Prolonged prothrombin time (PT)
- Decreased fibrinogen level
- Elevated levels of fibrin degradation products (e.g., D-dimer)

Therapeutic Management

To control DIC, the clinician must identify and then treat the underlying cause of the condition. Treatment then becomes symptomatic and directed at replenishing consumed coagulation factors. Depleted fibrinogen and other coagulation factors are replaced (e.g., fresh-frozen plasma) to normalize the PT. RBCs and platelet transfusions can aid in replacing cells lost with hemorrhage. Exchange transfusions may be used in neonates to minimize the excessive fluid volume required by replacing platelets, clotting factors, and RBCs. Vitamin K may also be administered to normalize the PT. The most frequent drug used to dissolve clots is heparin. However, heparin has a controversial role in the treatment of childhood DIC because it may increase the risk for bleeding.

Nursing Considerations

DIC typically develops in a child who is already hospitalized. The subjective and objective data assessed will depend entirely on the initial illness. The nurse must be cognizant of the child who is at risk for DIC. Evidence of bleeding at any site of integumentary interruption and at every orifice, must be assessed. The nurse also notes any changes in the pattern of vital signs. Adequate tissue perfusion should be confirmed because normal function of an organ is the end result of sufficient oxygenation of that organ. Children with full clinical manifestations of DIC are typically cared for in an intensive care setting owing to the multisystem sequelae and complex management of DIC.

Any areas of active bleeding should be located promptly and pressure applied, if possible. The nurse continues to monitor the child for overt and covert signs of bleeding. Care should be taken to avoid any unnecessary tissue trauma or injury. IV lines and indwelling tubes should be secured and protected to eliminate the additional trauma caused by reinsertion. Frequent monitoring of vital signs is necessary to identify changing patterns and ensure adequate cardiac output and end-organ perfusion. Laboratory results are also monitored carefully, with particular attention to the trending of values. Follow the physician's orders for administering medications, blood products, and treatments and closely monitor the child's tolerance and outcomes. Because hypoxemia and acidosis may actually cause DIC, adequate ventilation must be ensured to prevent or reduce compromised respiratory function.

Because DIC can be life threatening, the nurse helps parents deal with their anxiety about their child's condition. It is essential that the nurse be available to answer questions and update the parents on the child's progress.

The morbidity and mortality rates in children with DIC depend on the underlying causative condition. With prompt recognition of both the underlying cause and the diagnosis of DIC and with proper management, these children can have favorable outcomes.

APLASTIC ANEMIA

Aplastic anemia is a condition in which the bone marrow ceases production of the cells it normally manufactures. The result is peripheral pancytopenia, a condition in which all formed elements of the blood are simultaneously depressed.

Etiology and Incidence

Aplastic anemia can be congenital or acquired. Several rare, inheritable disorders are characterized by aplastic anemia. The most common of these is Fanconi anemia. Aplastic anemia can also be acquired, with a number of agents and conditions implicated as the probable cause. These most often include drugs or chemicals and less often radiation exposure, viruses (e.g., parvovirus B19), and immune diseases. Most cases (approximately 70%) of aplastic anemia in children are idiopathic—without an identifiable cause. Aplastic anemia results in a physiologic and anatomic failure of the bone marrow preventing the development of granulocytes, erythrocytes, and megakaryocytes. Annually, in the United States and Europe, the incidence of aplastic anemia is only 2 cases per million per year, as compared to leukemia

with an incidence of 50 cases per million per year (Shimamura & Nathan, 2009).

Manifestations

The clinical manifestations of aplastic anemia include petechiae, ecchymosis, pallor, epistaxis, fatigue, tachycardia, anorexia, and infection.

Diagnostic Evaluation

Although the diagnosis of aplastic anemia may be suspected from the child's history and the results of a CBC, bone marrow aspiration and biopsy must be performed for confirmation. Biopsy results should reveal the presence or absence of precursors of the mature cells found in a peripheral blood sample. In aplastic anemia, these precursors are notably absent from the marrow sample. This type of marrow is described as *hypocellular* and often contains a predominance of lymphocytes and yellowish fatty tissue.

PATHOPHYSIOLOGY

Aplastic Anemia

Aplastic anemia is characterized by cessation of hematopoiesis of granulocytes, erythrocytes, and megakaryocytes by the bone marrow. The disease may be classified as mild, moderate, or severe, depending on how low the values are for absolute neutrophil count, platelet count, and absolute reticulocyte count. The diagnosis of severe aplastic anemia requires two of the following anomalies: granulocyte count less than 500/mm^3, platelet count less than 20,000/mm^3, and reticulocyte count below 1% (after correction for hematocrit).* In addition, the bone marrow biopsy specimen must contain less than 25% of the normal cellularity.

*Hord, J. (2011). The acquired pancytopenias. In R. Kliegman, B. Stanton, J. St. Geme, et al. (Eds.), *Nelson textbook of pediatrics* (19th ed., pp. 1691-1692). Philadelphia: Elsevier Saunders.

Therapeutic Management

If the aplastic anemia is determined by history to be acquired, exposure to the causative agent is discontinued immediately. Treatment then is based on symptoms. Platelet and erythrocyte transfusions may be ordered. Granulocyte transfusions are not used routinely because of their short life span in the circulation. When signs and symptoms of infection are suspected or present, antibiotics are administered after appropriate cultures are obtained.

Bone marrow or allogeneic hematopoietic stem cell transplantation remains the treatment of choice for children with severe aplastic anemia for whom a suitable donor has been identified (Hord, 2011). (See Chapter 24 for a discussion of hematopoietic stem cell transplantation.) An immunosuppressant medication regimen of cyclosporine and antithymocyte globulin (ATG) effectively treats acquired aplastic anemia for many children for whom a suitable bone marrow or stem cell donor is not available (Hord, 2011).

NURSING CARE OF THE CHILD WITH APLASTIC ANEMIA

■ Assessment

The subjective assessment usually elicits parents' observations of bruising immediately after an event that would not normally result in a bruise. For example, an observant parent may have noted petechiae in the child's mouth while assisting the child in brushing the teeth.

The parent may also have observed extreme fatigue, headaches, and dizziness upon rising. Information should be elicited about medications recently taken or recent exposures to environmental substances outside the child's usual realm in an effort to determine possible drug- or chemical-related causes for the pancytopenia.

Petechiae, bruising, pallor, lethargy, and tachycardia are the usual abnormal findings and are directly related to the degree of pancytopenia. A history of fever is also commonly present in the child with aplastic anemia. Otherwise, the results of the physical assessment are usually normal.

■ Nursing Diagnosis and Planning

The nursing diagnoses and expected outcomes that may be appropriate for the child with aplastic anemia include the following:

- Risk for Infection related to inadequate secondary defenses or immunosuppression.

Expected Outcome. The child remains free from infection, as evidenced by being in the expected range for body temperature, neurologic assessment, cardiorespiratory assessment, gastrointestinal status, and genitourinary status.

- Ineffective Protection related to thrombocytopenia.

Expected Outcomes. The child will remain free of bleeding episodes and will demonstrate appropriate precautions to prevent or decrease bleeding.

- Ineffective Peripheral Tissue Perfusion and Risk for Decreased Cardiac Tissue Perfusion related to anemia.

Expected Outcome. The child's tissues will be perfused, as evidenced by palpable peripheral pulses, capillary refill less than 2 seconds, urine output appropriate for age, and absent respiratory distress.

- Deficient Knowledge related to incomplete information about the disease process.

Expected Outcomes. The child and family will describe the disease process and its potential complications.

■ Interventions

Nursing care initially focuses on providing supportive care and preventing any serious physiologic sequelae of pancytopenia. Because of the increased risk of bacterial and viral infection, affected children should be assigned to a private room, preferably a positive pressure room. All visitors as well as the child should be instructed in meticulous hand hygiene. Precautionary measures should be taken as for any individual with a low platelet count, including no injections; no rectal temperatures, examinations, or medications; use of an extra-soft bristle toothbrush or Toothette; abstinence from any contact sports or activity; and periodic assessment for increased bleeding.

Physician orders should be followed with regard to blood and platelet transfusions, acquisition of blood cultures, and antibiotic, antiviral, and antifungal medication administration. Usually, the platelet count will be maintained at a level greater than 20,000/mm^3 to prevent intracranial hemorrhage or active bleeding. The hemoglobin level is typically maintained above 7 g/dL. However, if a child is to receive a hematopoietic stem cell transplant, efforts are made to use blood transfusions only as necessary to avoid possible alloimmunization. If any symptoms of infection are present, blood should be drawn for culture. The decision to culture other body fluids or sites will be based on the child's clinical examination.

Antibiotics should be administered immediately to a febrile child with neutropenia, because of the risk for rapid onset of overwhelming sepsis. Children who are hospitalized, febrile, and neutropenic should be assessed frequently for signs of septic shock. Assessment includes the quality of peripheral pulses compared with central pulses, extremity temperature, capillary refill time, level of consciousness, vital signs, condition of cannulation sites, and presence of skin breakdown.

Education of the family and child should include information about the disease process and the complications that must be reported promptly to the health care provider. Often, referral is made to a transplant center. If so, intense pretransplant education is indicated. The Aplastic Anemia and MDS International Foundation, Inc. is a good source of information for children, parents, and health care providers. Follow-up studies should include frequent CBC and physical examinations.

■ Evaluation

- Is the child afebrile and do cannulation or other skin sites remain free of redness or swelling?
- Are assessment data related to other body systems within normal ranges?
- Has the child had any major bleeding?
- Is the child able to participate in age-appropriate activities without injury?
- Does the child demonstrate palpable peripheral pulses, capillary refill less than 2 seconds, urine output appropriate for age (see Chapter 16), and oxygen saturation more than 95%?
- Has the family received instruction regarding the disease and home care and verbalized an understanding of the information?

ABO INCOMPATIBILITY AND HEMOLYTIC DISEASE OF THE NEWBORN

The possibility of blood incompatibility exists whenever the fetal blood type is different from the maternal blood type. The most common difference is among the major blood groups of A, B, and O. Differences in Rh factor, although seen less often, are the most common cause of severe hemolytic disease of the fetus and newborn infant. Both types of incompatibility involve a maternal antibody response to antigens in fetal circulation. These maternal antibodies then cross the placenta into fetal circulation and destroy fetal erythrocytes, resulting in fetal anemia, referred to as *hemolytic disease of the newborn (HDN)*.

Three conditions must exist for HDN to develop: (1) maternal and fetal erythrocytes are antigenically incompatible, (2) maternal circulation contains or produces antibodies against fetal erythrocytes, and (3) immunoglobulin G (IgG) binds in sufficient amount to cause a widespread antigen-antibody–mediated hemolysis or splenic sequestration of erythrocytes.

Incidence

ABO incompatibility between the mother and fetus occurs in 15% to 25% of all pregnancies, with HDN (and subsequent hyperbilirubinemia) developing in approximately 1% of these neonates (Murray & Roberts, 2007). Rh incompatibility, the more serious cause of HDN, occurs in about 1 in 7 pregnancies with an Rh-negative mother and Rh-positive father (Liley, 2009). The prevalence of Rh hemolytic disease has decreased since the introduction of Rh$_o$(D) (RhoGAM) immune globulin (Liley, 2009).

Manifestations

Signs and symptoms of neonatal ABO and Rh incompatibility are the same and are listed in order of increasing severity of the hemolytic process:

- *Jaundice:* Resulting from an excess of unconjugated bilirubin formerly excreted by the maternal circulation

- *Anemia:* Resulting from an increased rate of RBC destruction caused by incompatibility
- *Hepatosplenomegaly:* Resulting from anemia and possibly sequestration of erythrocytes
- *Hydrops fetalis:* Constellation of symptoms resulting from the foregoing processes that results in overwhelming fetal edema and cardiovascular collapse

Diagnostic Evaluation

All women should have their blood typed before or during their initial pregnancies. The fetus affected by Rh incompatibility may be diagnosed with hydrops fetalis (a progressive condition with hemolysis that results in fetal hypoxia, generalized edema, and eventual circulatory collapse) during prenatal ultrasonographic testing. This condition may cause death in utero during the pregnancy. Routine screening of the neonate's blood type and direct Coombs test during the first hour after birth helps to identify neonates with blood group incompatibilities (the direct Coombs test evaluates for the presence of maternal antibody already bound to fetal erythrocytes). Assessment of the neonate's hematologic indices such as reticulocyte count, hematocrit level, and RBC morphologic features, helps to determine the extent of hemolysis. Neonatal bilirubin levels can also help to determine the severity of disease. The greater the increases in the bilirubin level from one time to the next, the more severe the hemolysis.

PATHOPHYSIOLOGY

ABO and Rh Incompatibility

The hemolytic process that occurs with hemolytic disease of the newborn begins in utero. In ABO incompatibility, the maternal blood type is usually O and the blood type of the fetus is either A or B, although it can also occur when the maternal type is either A or B and the fetal type is then B or A. The serum maternal type O contains antibodies against erythrocyte types A and B. These antibodies can cross the placenta and destroy the erythrocytes of the fetus. Most adults with type O erythrocytes also possess antibodies to types A and B, with ABO sensitization thereby occurring without fetal blood crossing into maternal circulation. Anti-ABO antibodies may in rare instances cross the placenta, but the potential for fetal harm is much less than what occurs with Rh factor incompatibility.

With Rh incompatibility, the maternal type is Rh negative and the fetal type is Rh positive. During placenta detachment (delivery or abortion), fetal and maternal circulation may mix. Unlike anti-ABO antibodies, Rh antibodies form only as the result of an actual exposure. When fetal blood cells enter the maternal circulation, the woman forms antibodies (IgG in nature) against the Rh factor that is perceived as foreign by the immune system. Once established, this anti-Rh antibody remains and recirculates through the reticuloendothelial system, crossing the placenta and causing an immune reaction during future pregnancies if the same Rh incompatibility exists between the maternal and fetal types. With this Rh incompatibility, serious consequences for the fetus may occur, such as hemolytic anemia, extramedullary erythropoiesis, hepatosplenomegaly, and the release of immature nucleated erythrocytes. Collectively, this is referred to as *erythroblastosis fetalis.* Without appropriate treatment, hydrops fetalis may occur, which can lead to fetal death as early as 17 weeks' gestation.

Therapeutic Management

Some neonates with mild ABO incompatibility may not require treatment. Most neonates requiring treatment respond well to aggressive hydration and phototherapy. Rarely does a neonate with ABO incompatibility have hemolysis severe enough to necessitate an exchange transfusion.

The best treatment for Rh incompatibility is prevention. $Rh_o(D)$ immune globulin (RhoGAM) suppresses the maternal immune response and antibody formation of Rh-negative individuals to Rh-positive erythrocytes. The specifics of dosing depend on the timing (prepartum, intrapartum, postpartum); however, the customary dose for postpartum prophylaxis is 300 micrograms administered intramuscularly to the mother (never the neonate) within 72 hours of delivery of *each* pregnancy. The widespread use of RhoGAM in women who are Rh negative and who give birth to Rh-positive neonates has significantly decreased the incidence of Rh incompatibility. Miscarriages or missed abortions of Rh-positive fetuses can sensitize an Rh-negative woman and account for Rh incompatibility in future pregnancies if RhoGAM was not appropriately administered.

When preventive measures for Rh incompatibility are not taken, the hemolytic process is almost always severe. Most neonates require a minimum of one exchange transfusion, and possibly more, to remove antibody-coated erythrocytes. The neonates may also require phototherapy to treat elevated levels of bilirubin, which may approach toxic levels shortly after birth. Additional erythrocyte transfusions for recurrent anemia may be necessary during the slow resolution phase of Rh incompatibility.

Nursing Considerations

Determination of the maternal blood type should be made prenatally or as soon after admission as possible to identify women at risk for giving birth to neonates with ABO or Rh incompatibilities. Blood typing and the direct Coombs test should be performed on cord blood soon after delivery whenever a neonate is identified as being at risk. Obtaining and assessing laboratory values in symptomatic neonates can help in the timely institution of appropriate treatment. Noting the rate of change in laboratory test results as well as the actual values can also help to determine the neonate's response to therapy.

If the neonate requires an exchange transfusion, the donor blood must be checked carefully to ensure that it is type O; Rh negative; low-titer anti-A, anti-B; and crossmatched with the maternal plasma and erythrocytes before transfusion. During the transfusion, the neonate should be monitored for changes in heart rate, blood pressure, oxygen saturation, body temperature, respiratory status, and integrity of indwelling IV catheter(s) used for the exchange. Both during and after the exchange transfusion, the neonate must be monitored for evidence of complications such as infection, thrombosis, air embolism, arteriospasms affecting the lower extremities, hypoglycemia, acid-base imbalance, hypernatremia, hypokalemia, hypocalcemia, coagulopathy, necrotizing enterocolitis, cardiac arrhythmias, volume overload, and hypothermia.

Adequate hydration of the neonate is ensured by administering appropriate fluids in adequate quantities. Phototherapy is provided according to established guidelines (see Nursing Care of the Neonate with Hyperbilirubinemia). The nurse monitors blood indices and bilirubin levels, and promptly reports deviations from normal or expected values. During an exchange transfusion, vital signs are checked according to the established routine and the neonate is monitored for evidence of complications (see Chapter 14).

HYPERBILIRUBINEMIA

Neonatal hyperbilirubinemia (also referred to as physiologic jaundice) is often a transient, benign disorder occurring during the first week of life. It is clinically significant, however, and does require follow-up to ensure that the disorder resolves. As bilirubin levels rise, the excess bilirubin is deposited in body tissues, resulting in a temporary yellow discoloration of the neonate's skin and sclerae. High bilirubin levels

TABLE 23-2   COMMON CAUSES OF HYPERBILIRUBINEMIA

MECHANISM	RELATED TO	CAUSED BY
Increased bilirubin availability	Overproduction of bilirubin	Polycythemia
		Decreased RBC life span
		Hemolysis (anemias, medication, infection)
		Extravascular blood (bruises, enclosed hemorrhages)
	Increased reabsorption of bilirubin from intestines	Delayed passage of meconium
		Increased enzyme activity
		Delayed enteral feedings
		Swallowed blood
Decreased bilirubin secretion	Altered liver metabolism of bilirubin	Prematurity; indicates immature liver
		Decreased uptake by liver
		Inadequate perfusion of liver
		Decreased enzyme activity (deficiency or inhibition)
	Liver obstruction	Biliary atresia
		Cystic fibrosis
		Hyperalimentation
		Tumor
Combined overproduction and undersecretion of bilirubin	Congenital infection: toxoplasmosis, rubella, herpes, syphilis, hepatitis	
	Asphyxia	
	Neonate of diabetic mother	
Uncertain mechanism	Breast milk jaundice	
	Neonates of Chinese, Japanese, Korean, African, or American Indian descent	

can penetrate and damage brain cells, a condition referred to as kernicterus.

Etiology

The most common causes of hyperbilirubinemia, including physiologic jaundice, are listed in Table 23-2. The discussion presented here will be limited to physiologic jaundice.

Incidence

Hyperbilirubinemia develops during the first few days of life in 45% to 60% of term neonates and in as many as 80% of preterm neonates (Bergeron & Gourley, 2009).

Manifestations

The yellow discoloration of the skin that is known as jaundice usually appears when the serum bilirubin level reaches 5 to 7 mg/dL. In the full-term neonate, peak levels are generally reached by the third to fifth day of life, followed by a gradual decrease in bilirubin levels until normal values are reached at about the 10th day of life. In the preterm neonate, peak levels are generally reached by the fifth day of life, followed by a slow decline in bilirubin levels until normal values are reached around the end of the first month of life.

Diagnostic Evaluation

Serum bilirubin levels should be obtained whenever clinical jaundice is present or in neonates with conditions known to cause hyperbilirubinemia. The direct bilirubin is a measurement of conjugated bilirubin, and the indirect bilirubin is a measurement of unconjugated bilirubin. The total bilirubin level is the direct level plus the indirect level. A total bilirubin level of 13 mg/dL or higher in premature neonates with clinical jaundice or in full-term neonates should be evaluated to determine the etiology of the jaundice. Total bilirubin levels are

PATHOPHYSIOLOGY

Hyperbilirubinemia

Physiologic jaundice in the neonate is caused by impaired bilirubin uptake and conjugation. The majority of the bilirubin produced in the neonate is derived from the normal breakdown of erythrocytes by enzymes in the liver and spleen. The hemoglobin in the erythrocytes is broken down into iron, protein, and bilirubin. The bilirubin then binds to albumin and is transported to the liver, where it undergoes conjugation, making it water soluble and able to be excreted from the body through the urinary and intestinal tracts. Conjugated bilirubin cannot be reabsorbed by the intestines; however, an enzyme present in the intestines of the neonate can convert the bilirubin back to the unconjugated form, which can be reabsorbed into the bloodstream. The process can contribute significantly to the amount of bilirubin the neonate must process. Unconjugated bilirubin is lipid soluble, not water soluble, and thus it is not as easily excreted from the body.

! NURSING QUALITY ALERT

Assessing Jaundice

Jaundice is often seen first in the face, especially the nose. It then descends to the torso and then to the extremities.

generally higher in breastfed neonates than in bottle-fed neonates and higher in neonates of Asian, African, or American Indian descent. Other diagnostic tests that may help to determine the etiology include a direct Coombs test, peripheral blood smear, and reticulocyte count, as well as the blood type and Rh type of both mother and neonate.

Therapeutic Management

The therapeutic management of physiologic jaundice is determined by the neonate's bilirubin level, gestational age, and feeding patterns, and by the caregiving capabilities of the mother or family. The treatment plan for other forms of neonatal jaundice is based on the underlying cause of hyperbilirubinemia; the neonate's gestational age, chronologic age, clinical status, weight, history, and risk factors; and the rate of rise in the bilirubin level.

Prevention of hyperbilirubinemia includes preventing the neonate from becoming dehydrated. Breastfeeding mothers should be encouraged to nurse at least 8 to 12 times a day (AAP, Committee on Nutrition, 2009), and bottle-fed babies should be fed the appropriate amount of formula. Newborn infants should be assessed routinely for the presence of jaundice, and follow-up laboratory studies should be conducted, if needed (AAP, Committee on Nutrition, 2009).

Treatment of hyperbilirubinemia usually begins with phototherapy, which consists of exposing the neonate to light from the blue part of the spectrum, ideally 420 to 470 nm. The light source can be a single quartz-halogen spotlight; a bank of fluorescent bulbs, either blue, cool white, or day bright; or a blanket of white light filaments with a fiber-optic light source. Phototherapy causes a chemical reaction in the skin that converts unconjugated bilirubin to a form that can be excreted by the body. Phototherapy also causes an oxidative reaction that allows unconjugated bilirubin removal by the liver and spleen. The therapeutic effect of phototherapy relies on the extent of hemolysis, amount of light energy used, distance from the neonate to the light source, amount of skin exposed, and the neonate's ability to excrete the bilirubin. Phototherapy is provided continuously with short breaks as dictated by other care needs, such as feeding, bathing, diapering, and stimulation (visual and tactile).

If phototherapy does not reduce the bilirubin level or if the bilirubin level is dangerously high, the neonate may require an exchange transfusion. A double-volume exchange, in which the neonate's blood volume is replaced twice, can lower the bilirubin level to approximately one half the original value. Exchange transfusions should always be performed in a setting familiar with the procedure and one capable of providing intensive care nursing support. Small amounts of the neonate's blood are removed, alternating with administration of small amounts of donor blood, of the appropriate type, through a venous access device, often an umbilical venous catheter. After exchange transfusion, phototherapy is often administered as an additional measure to lower the bilirubin level.

Some breastfed neonates may have elevated bilirubin levels that do not seem to decrease with the usual management. Breast-milk feedings are stopped and formula feedings are instituted for 24 to 48 hours; this can contribute to a decrease in the bilirubin level.

NURSING CARE OF THE NEONATE WITH HYPERBILIRUBINEMIA

■ Assessment

The nurse can assess the neonate for the presence of jaundice by pressing lightly on the skin with a fingertip, observing for a slight to moderate yellowish discoloration of the skin with blanching. The yellow color of jaundice will be easier to see over the fingerprint area than over the surrounding skin. Common assessment sites are the nose and upper chest. Assessment for jaundice should take place in natural light whenever possible. In neonates with dark skin, the first evidence of jaundice may be yellowing of the sclera. The nurse identifies neonates at risk for hyperbilirubinemia by assessing for evidence of bruising, petechiae, cephalohematoma, pallor, plethora, and enlarged liver or spleen, as well as prematurity and perinatal risk factors.

■ Nursing Diagnosis and Planning

The following nursing diagnoses and expected outcomes may be appropriate for the neonate with hyperbilirubinemia:

- Risk for Deficient Fluid Volume related to increased insensible losses from phototherapy.

Expected Outcomes. The neonate will have moist mucous membranes, flat fontanel, and urine output of 2 to 3 mL/kg/hr.

- Ineffective Thermoregulation related to heat from phototherapy lights or lack of clothing to expose skin to phototherapy.

Expected Outcome. The neonate will maintain body temperature within a normal range.

- Risk for Injury to neurologic system related to deposition of bilirubin in brain tissue.

Expected Outcomes. The neonate will demonstrate resolving jaundice and decreasing bilirubin levels.

- Deficient Knowledge related to unfamiliarity with phototherapy equipment.

Expected Outcomes. The parents will demonstrate proper use of home phototherapy equipment and describe when to contact appropriate support personnel.

■ Interventions

During hospitalization, to maximize the effectiveness of phototherapy, the neonate should be completely undressed or wearing only a diaper. While phototherapy is in use, the neonate's eyes MUST be covered with an opaque mask that is usually secured in place with a headband or cloth adhesive. Several types of eye shields are commercially available. Care must be taken to ensure that the eye shield does not slip down and cover the neonate's nares, compromising nasal breathing efforts. Eye shields can be removed when the light source is off to assess the eyes and allow the neonate visual stimulation. The neonate's position is changed frequently to ensure maximal skin exposure to the light source. Monitoring the neonate's bilirubin level is performed one to four times daily to assess the effectiveness of phototherapy.

The nurse monitors the neonate's temperature every 2 to 4 hours to ensure maintenance within normal limits. The additional heat generated by the phototherapy unit places the neonate at risk for hyperthermia. The lack of clothing on the neonate increases the possibility of heat loss through convection, conduction, radiation, and evaporation and may lead to hypothermia. Any signs of feeding intolerance, such as diarrhea or lactose intolerance, are recorded and reported so that appropriate feeding changes can be made. Because neonates receiving phototherapy have increased insensible water losses, their intake and output should be closely monitored to ensure adequate hydration. The neonates are removed from the light source briefly for feedings during which tactile stimulation is provided.

Full-term neonates who are otherwise healthy may be treated with phototherapy at home with the support of home health care. This practice not only reduces health care costs and saves resources but also allows the family to interact with the neonate in a more natural environment. The equipment and care are the same as for the hospitalized neonate. The nurse ensures that the parents know the precautions to take during home phototherapy treatments. Technicians should be available to service equipment. Home health nurses make visits once or twice each day during treatment to assess the neonate, obtain blood samples to measure bilirubin levels, and provide additional support to the parents as needed.

! NURSING QUALITY ALERT

Care during Phototherapy

- During phototherapy, special care should be taken to ensure that the neonate is well hydrated to offset the effects of increased insensible water loss brought on by the phototherapy.
- The neonate's eyes must be protected at all times during phototherapy to prevent retinal damage from the light source.
- To maximize the effect of phototherapy, expose as much skin surface as possible; leave the neonate clothed only in a diaper.

■ Evaluation

- Does the neonate have moist mucous membranes, a flat fontanel, and urine output of 2 to 3 mL/kg/hr?
- Has the neonate's body temperature remained within normal limits for age during phototherapy?
- Is the serum bilirubin level decreasing appropriately?
- Can the parent demonstrate proper home adaptations for phototherapy and describe situations that require notifying health care personnel?

■ KEY CONCEPTS

- For RBCs to carry oxygen, there must be an adequate amount of hemoglobin, which depends on sufficient circulating iron.
- Anemia results from blood loss, decreased production of RBCs or hemoglobin, or increased destruction of RBCs.
- Caring for children with blood disorders requires an understanding of the anatomy and physiology of blood and blood-forming tissues, genetics, and chronic illness.
- The number of RBCs in the blood varies according to age, sex, and the altitude at which a person lives.
- Iron deficiency anemia can be prevented by providing children from birth to 12 months with iron-fortified formula or breast milk with iron-fortified cereal and foods.
- Morphine is the drug of choice for children with a painful episode associated with SCD.
- Complications associated with sickle cell disease can be reduced through early screening, diagnosis, and treatment; routine and pneumococcal, meningococcal, and influenza immunizations; penicillin prophylaxis; and parent/child education.
- Children with decreased platelet counts and factor disorders should not receive aspirin or aspirin-containing products. To prevent hemorrhage, rectal temperatures must be avoided and invasive procedures done only when necessary, using extreme caution.
- Factor prophylaxis for infants and young children with hemophilia is warranted due to the risk of bleeding and joint damage.
- Bleeding associated with hemophilia is treated with rest, ice, compression, elevation, and factor replacement, as necessary.
- Family education about caring for a child with hemophilia at home should include management of bleeding episodes, environmental safety, administration of medications, health promotion, and normal growth and development.
- Educating the family of a child with ITP about activity restrictions and protection from injury is a major nursing challenge.
- Management of DIC is directed toward identifying and treating the underlying cause.
- Nursing care of the child with aplastic anemia focuses on the prevention of infection resulting from pancytopenia.
- Nursing care of the infant with hyperbilirubinemia, from any cause, is directed toward interventions that reduce serum bilirubin levels.

REFERENCES

American Academy of Pediatrics, Committee on Infectious Diseases. (2009). *2009 Red book* (28th ed.). Elk Grove Village, IL: American Academy of Pediatrics.

American Academy of Pediatrics, Committee on Nutrition. (2009). *Pediatrics nutrition handbook* (6th ed.). Elk Grove Village, IL: American Academy of Pediatrics.

Bergeron, M., & Gourley, G. (2009). Disorders of bilirubin metabolism. In S. Orkin, D. Fisher, & A. Look, et al. (Eds.), *Nathan and Oski's hematology of infancy and childhood* (7th ed., pp. 103-146). Philadelphia: Elsevier Saunders.

Bolton-Maggs, P. (2011). *Hemophilia C.* Retrieved from http://emedicine.medscape.com/article/955690-overview.

Blanchette, V., & Bolton-Maggs, P. (2008). Childhood immune thrombocytopenic purpura: Diagnosis and management. *Pediatric Clinics of North America, 55,* 393-420.

Cunningham, M., Sankaran, V., Nathan, D., & Orkin, S. (2009). The thalassemias. In S. Orkin, D. Fisher, & A. Look, et al. (Eds.), *Nathan and Oski's hematology of infancy and childhood* (7th ed., pp. 1015-1108). Philadelphia: Elsevier Saunders.

DeBaun, M., Frei-Jones, M., & Vichinsky, E. (2011a). Sickle cell disease. In R. Kliegman, B. Stanton, & St. J. Geme, et al. (Eds.), *Nelson textbook of pediatrics* (19th ed., pp. 1663-1670). Philadelphia: Elsevier Saunders.

DeBaun, M., Frei-Jones, M., & Vichinsky, E. (2011b). Thalassemia syndrome. In R. Kliegman, B. Stanton, & St. J.

Geme, et al. (Eds.), *Nelson textbook of pediatrics* (19th ed., pp. 1674-1677). Philadelphia: Elsevier Saunders.

Heeney, M., & Dover, G. (2009). Sickle cell disease. In S. Orkin, D. Fisher, & A. Look, et al. (Eds.), *Nathan and Oski's hematology of infancy and childhood* (7th ed., pp. 949-1014). Philadelphia: Elsevier Saunders.

Heeney, M., & Ware, R. (2008). Hydroxyurea for children with sickle cell disease. *Pediatric Clinics of North America, 55,* 483-501.

Hohneker, J. (2010). *Important information about Exjade (deferasirox) tablets for oral suspension.* Retrieved from www.fda.gov/downloads/Safety/MedWatch/SafetyInformation/SafetyAlertsforHumanMedicalProducts/UCM200858.pdf.

Hord, J. (2011). The acquired pancytopenias. In R. Kliegman, B. Stanton, & St. J. Geme, et al. (Eds.), *Nelson textbook of pediatrics* (19th ed., pp. 1691-1692). Philadelphia: Elsevier Saunders.

Lerner, N., & Sills, R. (2011). Iron-deficiency anemia. In R. Kliegman, B. Stanton, & St. J. Geme, et al. (Eds.), *Nelson textbook of pediatrics* (19th ed., pp. 1655-1658). Philadelphia: Elsevier Saunders.

Liley, H. G. (2009). Immune hemolytic disease of the newborn. In S. Orkin, D. Fisher, & A. Look, et al. (Eds.), *Nathan and Oski's hematology of infancy and childhood* (7th ed., pp. 67-102). Philadelphia: Elsevier Saunders.

Mazumdar, M., Heeney, M., Cox, C., & Lieu, T. (2007). Preventing stroke among children with sickle cell

anemia: an analysis of strategies that involve transcranial Doppler testing and chronic transfusion. *Pediatrics, 120*(4), 1107-1116.

Montgomery, R., Gill, J., & Paola, J. (2009). Hemophilia and von Willebrand disease. In S. Orkin, D. Fisher, & A. Look, et al. (Eds.), *Nathan and Oski's hematology of infancy and childhood* (7th ed. pp. 1487-1524). Philadelphia: Elsevier Saunders.

Murray, N., & Roberts, I. (2007). Haemolytic disease of the newborn. *Archives of Disease in Childhood Fetal and Neonatal Edition, 92,* F83-F88.

National Hemophilia Foundation. (2010). What are bleeding disorders? Retrieved from www.hemophilia.org.

Robertson, J., Lillicrap, D., & James, P. (2008). von Willebrand disease. *Pediatric Clinics of North America, 55,* 377-392.

Rodriguez, N., & Hoots, W. (2008). Advances in hemophilia: experimental aspects and therapy. *Pediatric Clinics of North America, 55,* 357-376.

Shimamura, A., & Nathan, D. G. (2009). Acquired aplastic anemia and pure red cell aplasia. In S. Orkin, D. Fisher, & A. Look, et al. (Eds.), *Nathan and Oski's hematology of infancy and childhood* (7th ed., pp. 275-306). Philadelphia: Elsevier Saunders.

Wilson, D. (2009). Acquired platelet defects. In S. Orkin, D. Fisher, & A. Look, et al. (Eds.), *Nathan and Oski's hematology of infancy and childhood* (7th ed., pp. 1553-1590). Philadelphia: Elsevier Saunders.

The Child with Cancer

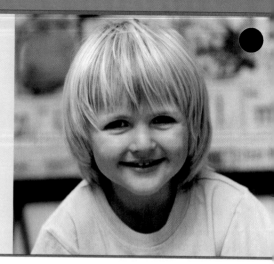

⊖volve WEBSITE

http://evolve.elsevier.com/James/ncoc

LEARNING OBJECTIVES

After studying this chapter, you should be able to:

- Identify the common clinical manifestations of childhood cancer.
- Discuss the treatment modalities used in the treatment of children with cancer

- Demonstrate an understanding of the nursing care associated with caring for a child with cancer.
- Discuss symptom management of the child with cancer.

CLINICAL REFERENCE

REVIEW OF CANCER

A *neoplasm* is any tumor that arises from new, abnormal cell growth. A tumor may be either benign or malignant. The distinguishing feature of cancer is its ability to invade surrounding tissue and spread to distant sites. Cancer cells spread in one of two ways: (1) by *invasion*, in which cells grow in an unrestricted, disorderly fashion at the site of origin; and (2) by *metastasis*, in which the cells grow in sites other than the site of the primary cancer. The cancerous cells grow progressively. The cells have lost the ability to perform their intended functions because changes in the cell's deoxyribonucleic acid (DNA) cause "wrong" information to be transmitted. As the cancerous cells continue to proliferate, they crowd out normal cells and compress vascular structures and vital organs, which results in symptoms.

Tumor staging is based on the results of diagnostic studies and, in some cases, surgical examination. Staging describes the extent of disease locally, regionally, and systemically and guides the therapy for most solid tumors. Each tumor has its own specific system of staging, which assists in determining treatment and prognosis.

The cause of most childhood cancers is unknown. One possible underlying cause of cancer is genetic. Alterations in normal DNA occur that predispose the child to the development of cancer. A small percentage of cancers are associated with an inherited predisposition related to chromosomal abnormalities (Asselin, 2011). A second, more controversial hypothesis contends that cancer develops as a result of failure of the immune system to distinguish between normal and abnormal cells. Inactivation of tumor suppressor genes is also thought to be implicated. Known carcinogens, such as radiation, physical irritation, and chemical irritants, contribute to the development of cancer.

The cardinal signs of cancer in children differ from those seen in adults. Most adult cancers are carcinomas, and more screening tools are available to assist with their early detection. The difficulty in diagnosing cancer in children is that symptoms resemble those of common childhood illnesses. Children are often not brought for medical care until obvious signs and symptoms are present. Primary care providers are understandably reluctant to think about cancer as the cause of the child's illness.

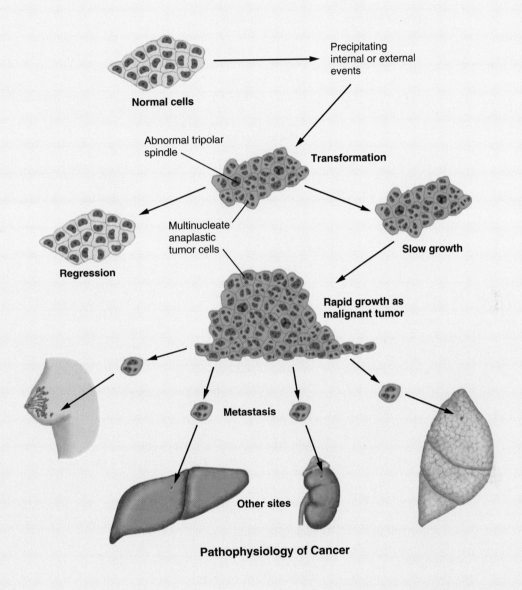

Normal cells

Precipitating internal or external events

Transformation

Abnormal tripolar spindle

Multinucleate anaplastic tumor cells

Regression

Slow growth

Rapid growth as malignant tumor

Metastasis

Other sites

Pathophysiology of Cancer

CARDINAL SIGNS AND SYMPTOMS OF CANCER IN CHILDREN

Overt Signs
- A mass
- Purpura
- Pallor
- Weight loss
- Whitish reflex in the eye
- Vomiting in early morning
- Recurrent or persistent fever

Signs and Symptoms that May Be Covert
- Bone pain
- Headache
- Persistent lymphadenopathy
- Change in balance, gait, or personality
- Fatigue, malaise

CLINICAL REFERENCE

DIAGNOSTIC TESTS AND PROCEDURES FOR CANCER

TEST	DESCRIPTION	PURPOSE	NURSING CONSIDERATIONS
Bone marrow aspiration	Bone marrow is aspirated from the anterior or posterior iliac crests (the tibia is sometimes used in infants).	Pathologic examination of the aspirated material shows the presence, absence, and ratio of cells that are specific to and diagnostic of certain diseases. Some conditions that can be diagnosed are leukemia, specific vitamin deficiencies, neoplastic diseases in which the marrow is invaded by tumor cells, and aplastic anemia.	1. Describe the procedure to the child and parents. Check the signed consent. Allow parents to stay with the child if they wish. 2. Depending on the protocol of the facility, the child may receive a wide range of sedative or anesthetic agents. Some centers use local anesthesia with no systemic sedation; others use a combination of a sedative and an analgesic. 3. The child should be positioned prone with a small pillow under the hips to facilitate access to the posterior iliac crest, the usual site. Tell the child that the physician will clean the site and that it will feel cold. Just before the needle insertion, the child should be told that some discomfort will be felt when the needle is inserted and the marrow aspirated but that the discomfort will last only a few seconds; it will help for the child to sing, count, or take slow, deep breaths. 4. Apply a dressing to the area. If the child's platelet count is less than 50,000/mm³, use a pressure dressing. Monitor vital signs until stable, and monitor the puncture site for bleeding and later for signs of infection.
Bone scintigraphy	A radiolabeled nucleotide is injected into the bloodstream. This tracer migrates to areas of the body in a predictable pattern.	Pattern of uptake in the axial skeleton is evaluated for variation from normal. Areas of increased uptake indicate increased cellular turnover related to growth, infection, trauma, or tumor activity.	Preparation similar to steps 1 and 2 for bone marrow aspiration. The child will be asked to lie still for 45-60 min to complete testing.
Gallium scan	Similar to bone scintigraphy.	In Hodgkin disease, 60%-70% of patients will have uptake of this isotope in active areas at diagnosis. Used as a marker for disease during and after therapy.	Preparation similar to steps 1 and 2 for bone marrow aspiration. The child will be asked to lie still for 45-60 min to complete testing.
Positron emission tomography (PET) scan	This study combines conventional nuclear medicine techniques with tomography and adds double-photon imaging, which displays metabolic activity.	PET scans reveal differences in metabolic processes. Tumor cells have accelerated glycolysis compared with the tissues of origin. PET scans can be useful for diagnosis, staging, and follow-up monitoring.	Be sure the patient is not pregnant. Younger children may need sedation.
Single-photon emission computed tomography (SPECT)	This study combines the techniques of conventional nuclear medicine imaging with that of computed tomography (CT) using gamma-emitting radioactive isotopes.	SPECT displays a normal organ in axial, parasagittal, and coronal sections.	Older children should be told about the scan and allowed to see the equipment.

See Chapter 28 for information about other diagnostics tests (CT, lumbar puncture, MRI). Refer to the Evolve website for laboratory tests (CBC, serum chemistry, urinalysis) used in the care of the child with cancer.

THE CHILD WITH CANCER

Cancer in children is often difficult to diagnose, and health care providers must be aware of the clinical manifestations that should raise the suspicion of cancer. The signs and symptoms depend on the type of tumor, the location of the tumor within the body, the extent of the disease, and the child's age. Testing, diagnosis, and initiation of therapy may occur within a very short period. The diagnosis of cancer can be devastating to both the child and the family. The nurse becomes the informational lifeline for the child and the family as they go through the treatment process.

Incidence

Cancer is uncommon in children; nevertheless, pediatric cancer is the second leading cause of death in childhood, after unintentional injuries, and is the leading cause of death from disease. Childhood cancer represents only approximately 1% of all new cancers diagnosed annually in both children and adults in the United States. The most common childhood cancers are leukemias, brain tumors, and lymphomas (Asselin, 2011) (Figure 24-1). Treatment challenges include minimizing treatment-related side effects while maintaining the child's normal growth and development.

Childhood Cancer and Its Treatment

Children with cancer are treated in a multidisciplinary setting. Pediatric oncology nurses play a prominent role in the care of children with cancer and their families. They support and educate the children and their families as they move through a stressful process. Pediatric oncology nurses are challenged to maintain a high level of technical

competence and an ability to provide the psychological support required by the child and family. Working with children with cancer can be an emotional experience. The nurse in this setting must have a support system and be aware of personal limitations and therapeutic relationship boundaries (Gerow, Conejo, Alonzo et al., 2010).

A great deal of research has been done over the past 30 years to improve the outcomes for children with cancer. Current survival rates are attributed to cooperative, systematic research through the Children's Oncology Group (COG) and the International Society for Pediatric Oncology. Each group meets twice a year to develop new research protocols and monitor the progress of current protocols; subgroups meet as needed throughout the year. Research protocols direct when drugs are to be given, how frequently, and in what dosages, and which diagnostic and follow-up studies are to be performed. Research has shown that children have better outcomes if they are treated by a scientifically derived protocol.

Because of the efforts of cooperative pediatric clinical trials, approximately 77% of children diagnosed with cancer will survive 5 years or longer after their diagnosis (American Cancer Society, 2009). The marked improvement in childhood cancer survival rates has placed renewed emphasis on the importance of identifying the long-term sequelae of cancer treatment in children and initiating timely intervention (American Cancer Society, 2009).

Even with apparently successful treatment of cancer in children, the disease may recur. A recurrence may occur during therapy, shortly after therapy has been completed, or years later. A second tumor may represent a new (or second) malignancy. Recurrence represents a resurgence of the initial disease, whereas a second cancer is a likely result of the initial treatment. For example, some children with acute lymphocytic leukemia (ALL) develop acute myelocytic leukemia (AML) after therapy is complete. Brain tumors may develop in a small number of children with ALL who were treated with radiation to their central nervous system (CNS).

Therapeutic Management

Chemotherapy, surgery, and radiation therapy are the primary treatment modalities for children with cancer. Hematopoietic stem cell transplantation (HSCT), steroid therapy, and biologic response modifiers are reserved for a specific subpopulation of children with cancer.

Chemotherapy

Chemotherapy is the use of drugs (antineoplastic agents) to kill cancer cells. Different drugs have different side effect profiles and modes of action. Combinations of drugs known individually to be active against the specific disease are used. Tumors possess the ability to develop resistance to chemotherapy agents, so a variety of active drugs are frequently used. Chemotherapy may be given orally, intravenously, intramuscularly, subcutaneously, or intrathecally (through the spinal canal). Depending on the protocol, a child may be hospitalized for chemotherapy, receive it on an outpatient basis, or be treated at home.

The side effects of chemotherapeutic agents represent challenges to caregivers. Chemotherapy nonselectively kills rapidly dividing cells. In addition to cancerous cells, the cells most often affected include cells of the hematopoietic system, gastrointestinal (GI) tract, and integumentary system (Box 24-1).

The bone marrow cells are one of the rapidly proliferating tissues adversely affected by many chemotherapy agents. Bone marrow production may become suppressed, resulting in neutropenia, anemia, and thrombocytopenia. The *nadir*—the time of the greatest bone marrow suppression when blood counts will be the lowest—generally occurs 7 to 14 days after chemotherapy administration, depending on

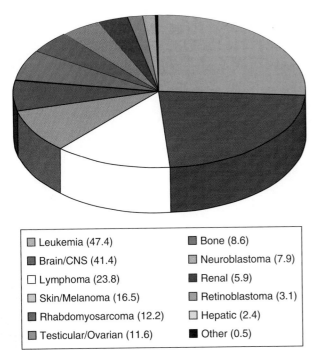

☐ Leukemia (47.4)	☐ Bone (8.6)
☐ Brain/CNS (41.4)	☐ Neuroblastoma (7.9)
☐ Lymphoma (23.8)	☐ Renal (5.9)
☐ Skin/Melanoma (16.5)	☐ Retinoblastoma (3.1)
☐ Rhabdomyosarcoma (12.2)	☐ Hepatic (2.4)
☐ Testicular/Ovarian (11.6)	☐ Other (0.5)

FIG 24-1 Incidence of cancers in children. Rate per million children under age 20 years, 2003–2007. (Data from U.S. National Institute of Health, National Cancer Institute, Surveillance Epidemiology and End Results. [2010]. *SEER cancer statistics review 1975–2007*.]. Retrieved from http://seer.cancer.gov/csr/1975_2007/browse_csr.php?section=29&page=sect_29_zfig.01.html)

BOX 24-1   COMMON SIDE EFFECTS OF CHEMOTHERAPY AND RADIATION THERAPY

Chemotherapeutic drugs and radiation therapy affect normal and abnormal cells, primarily cells that divide rapidly, such as cells of the GI tract, hair follicles, and bone marrow. As a result, children undergoing these therapies frequently have the following:

Chemotherapy Side Effects
- Bone marrow suppression
- Bruising
- Epistaxis and gingival bleeding
- Alopecia
- Malaise and fatigue
- Nausea
- Vomiting
- Anorexia
- Mucositis/Stomatitis

Radiation Side Effects
Acute (During and Shortly after Irradiation)
- Skin reactions
- Bruising
- Fatigue
- Bone marrow suppression
- Nausea
- Vomiting
- Anorexia
- Mucositis
- Brain edema
- Transient increase in neurologic symptoms

Subacute (1 to 6 Months after Irradiation)
- Somnolence syndrome: pronounced drowsiness, nausea, and malaise (typically 4 to 8 weeks after completing radiation therapy)
- Fever
- Irritability
- Ataxia
- Anorexia
- Dysphasia

Late Effects (More than 6 Months after Irradiation)
- Morphologic changes (e.g., cerebral atrophy, white matter degeneration, necrosis, calcification)
- Functional changes (e.g., encephalopathy, neuropsychological deterioration, focal neurologic deficits)
- Alopecia within the radiation field
- Mucositis of any mucous membrane and mouth ulcers

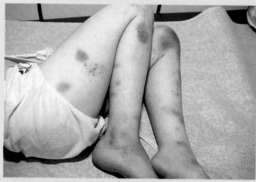

Suppression of the bone marrow because of chemotherapy or radiation therapy reduces the blood counts. Low platelet levels lead to spontaneous bruising, as shown. Nosebleeds and bleeding of the gums are other consequences. The nurse must make a special effort to observe for bruising in dark-skinned children because it will be more difficult to see.

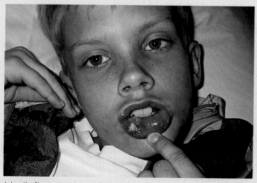

Mucositis (inflammation of the mucous membranes) and mouth ulcers are common side effects of chemotherapeutic drugs. Any mucous membrane can be affected.

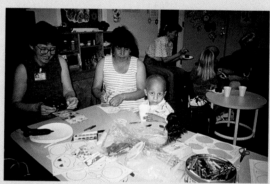

Hair loss is a distressing side effect of cancer treatment. School-age children and adolescents are most likely to feel this distress. Activities such as crafts or playgroups help children feel more normal and provide interaction with others in an accepting environment. (Photo courtesy Cook Children's Medical Center, Fort Worth, TX.)

the specific agent used. The greatest concern during the period of bone marrow suppression is infection.

Neutropenia places the child with cancer at risk for the development of opportunistic infections. Opportunistic infections are caused by nonpathogenic bacteria, viruses, and fungi that, because of compromised immunity, may invade and cause infection. Bacteria, generally present on the skin and within the intestinal tract, may invade the bloodstream through a break in the skin or mucous membranes, leading to a life-threatening infection. In the presence of markedly decreased white blood cells (WBCs), the usual inflammatory response (erythema, edema, swelling) indicative of an infection is not present. Fever is frequently the only indication of infection. Health care providers and families must remain acutely aware of elevated body temperature and breaks in the skin during periods of neutropenia.

The GI tract is affected in a number of ways. Chemotherapy represents a noxious stimulus that triggers nausea and vomiting. The treatment of nausea and vomiting was revolutionized in 1992 with the release of a class of nonsedating antiemetic drugs called *5-HT3 serotonin antagonists*. These drugs include ondansetron (Zofran), granisetron (Kytril), and dolasetron (Anzemet). 5-HT3 serotonin antagonists prevent serotonin from binding to vagus nerve receptors, consequently interrupting neurologic signals to the vomiting center of the brain. They have been more effective in combating chemotherapy-induced nausea and vomiting than earlier antiemetics.

Another nonsedating antiemetic drug has further improved the control of chemotherapy-induced nausea and vomiting. Aprepitant (Emend) belongs to a class of drugs known as substance P antagonists. Aprepitant works by binding to neurokinin-1 receptors in the central and peripheral nervous systems, thereby preventing activation of these receptors by substance P that would trigger vomiting. Aprepitant is used in conjunction with 5-HT3 serotonin antagonists and has proven to be very effective at preventing chemotherapy-induced nausea and vomiting.

Anorexia is associated with nausea and a change in taste experienced by some people in response to certain chemotherapeutic agents. Anorexia can lead to malnourishment resulting in weight loss and poor linear growth. Although antiemetics can be effective at preventing nausea and vomiting, they are not able to prevent alterations in taste that can occur with chemotherapy administration. This alteration in taste, often accompanied by an increased sensitivity to odors, contributes to anorexia.

Certain chemotherapeutic agents cause sloughing of the mucosal tissue of the GI tract, leading to the development of mucositis, both oral (stomatitis) and perianal, and esophagitis. These conditions can be painful and can contribute to poor nutrition. Bacteria and yeasts, present as part of the normal digestive process in the mouth and intestinal tract, may cross the open skin or mucous membrane and be absorbed into the bloodstream. The presence of breaks in the integument may lead to bacterial infections of the blood, particularly alpha-hemolytic streptococcus.

Decreased activity, pain medication, and poor oral intake may contribute to the development of constipation. Certain chemotherapeutic agents (such as vincristine) may also contribute to constipation. Passage of hard stool may cause abrasion of the delicate mucous membrane of the rectum. The stool is loaded with microorganisms as part of the digestive process. Again, the presence of breaks in the integument may lead to bacterial infections of the blood.

Hair loss (alopecia) has a tremendous psychological effect, especially on school-age children and adolescents. Some chemotherapeutic agents do not produce hair loss, but most do. Children should be reassured that their hair will grow back after the completion of therapy.

Accommodations should be made to ease the child's transition to alopecia, including the use of wigs, hats, or scarves. Although young children may respond casually to hair loss, teenagers, particularly girls, often struggle with this dramatic change in their body image.

Changes to the appearance of the skin and nails are common while receiving chemotherapy. These changes include hyperpigmentation of the skin, especially of the hands. Striae, or stretch marks, are also common with treatment regimens that include high-dose steroids. The nails may become brittle and appear either darkened or with whitish inclusions and/or scarring. These changes, with the exception of striae, typically resolve on completion of the chemotherapy regimen. In addition, many of the medications (e.g., methotrexate, trimethoprim-sulfamethoxazole) can lead to hypersensitivity to sunlight. The child should avoid excessive sun exposure by wearing long sleeves and hats and the application of sunscreen.

Treatment-related fatigue, common in adult cancer patients, is poorly reported in the child and adolescent populations, although an increasing body of research has identified and described fatigue in adolescents with cancer (Erickson, 2010). Other side effects are specific to the agent being used, as well as the dosage.

Nurses who administer chemotherapeutic agents should have evidence of special chemotherapy training by the institution in which they work. The Association of Pediatric Hematology/Oncology Nurses (APHON) (2011) has developed a Pediatric Chemotherapy and Biotherapy Provider Program to help standardize nursing education regarding administration of pediatric chemotherapy and biotherapy. The program consists of a provider course and an instructor course. Nursing responsibilities and precautions related to chemotherapy administration are detailed in Box 24-2.

BOX 24-2   NURSING RESPONSIBILITIES AND PRECAUTIONS FOR CHEMOTHERAPY

- Know Occupational Safety and Health Administration (OSHA) guidelines for administration of antineoplastic agents.
- Measure child's height and weight accurately.
- Confirm body surface area (BSA)—calculated in square meters and used to determine dosages.
- Always double-check the ordered dosage against protocol recommendations.
- Always double-check the medication against the original physician's order.
- A CBC count should be obtained within 48 hours preceding administration of chemotherapy.
- The WBC and platelet counts need to be at a predetermined level before chemotherapy is given.
- Know the potential side effects of the drugs being administered and appropriate actions to ameliorate those effects.
- Before giving any drugs, ensure the patency of IV tubing by checking for blood return.
- If using an implantable infusion device, ensure that needle placement is secure and blood returns.
- Vesicants (agents that produce blisters) should be given through a new IV site.
- Have appropriate emergency drugs available.
- Know and follow your agency's policies for administration of high-alert medications.

Surgery

Surgery is frequently part of cancer therapy for children. The surgery may be limited to a biopsy or may involve the removal of a solid tumor mass. The purpose of a biopsy is to obtain a small piece of the tumor for microscopic examination. Examination of the tissue by a pathologist confirms the tumor type and influences therapy decisions. Surgery may also be used for debulking or resecting a solid tumor mass. In some diseases, the tumor cannot be resected at the beginning of therapy. After the child has received a few rounds of chemotherapy, the mass may decrease in size and a less extensive surgical procedure can then be performed (see Chapter 13 for a discussion of preoperative care).

A central venous catheter (CVC) is frequently placed during an initial surgical procedure to facilitate chemotherapy administration. A central venous catheter is a central line that provides easy access to the venous system; the proximal tip of the catheter ends in the large vein just above the heart, the superior vena cava. Three types of central venous catheters are available. In an external catheter, the distal portion exits the skin and a tiny polyester cuff is "tunneled" under the exit site where the skin will adhere and hold the catheter in place. In an implanted venous access device (IVAD) or Port-a-Cath, the distal portion ends in a well or reservoir, which is placed in the subcutaneous tissue of the anterior chest wall. A percutaneously (peripherally) inserted central catheter (PICC) is usually placed by an interventional radiologist. The PICC is inserted in the brachial vein at or near the antecubital fossa using a technique that initially is similar to placement of a peripheral intravenous (IV) catheter. The PICC is then advanced up the veins of the arm until the tip ends in the superior vena cava.

The nurse should provide the child and family with information about the preparation for surgery (bowel preps, intake [NPO] restrictions) and what to expect in the postoperative period, such as pain control, wound healing, as well as signs and symptoms of bleeding. Because the risk of infection is higher for those receiving chemotherapy, the signs and symptoms of wound infection are important and may be subtle in an immunosuppressed child with a lower than usual WBC count. Those symptoms include warmth, redness, tenderness, and drainage. In addition, it is important for the nurse to check the most recent blood counts before surgery to ensure that the surgical timing is appropriate in relation to the last chemotherapy administration.

Radiation Therapy

Radiation may be given to cure or eradicate disease or given in low doses as a palliative therapy to control or prevent further growth of a tumor. To eradicate microscopic disease and promote bone marrow suppression, total body irradiation is given before some stem cell transplants. Radiation may be given in fractionated doses, in which the daily dose is split into smaller doses given more frequently to minimize side effects and increase tumor kill by decreasing the time for the tumor cells to repair between doses.

The nurse should prepare the child and family by teaching them about the process of radiation therapy as well as the side effects. Some institutions provide an introductory tour (often called a *simulation*) of the radiation facility so the child may experience the room and surroundings before therapy is started. During the tour, the child should be shown the window or monitor through which he or she will be observed while undergoing radiation alone in the room. Some children need to be sedated for radiation treatments; others can be coached to lie still with the help of child life specialists and parents. The child must lie still for what seems like long periods because the radiation

oncologist must carefully control the depth and peripheral margins of the radiation site.

During the simulation, computed tomography (CT) scans and radiographs are obtained to identify the site where the radiation therapy will be delivered. The child may receive skin markings with an indelible marker to help guide the radiation oncologists during each treatment. The markings are often covered with a transparent dressing. These markings (or tattoos) should be protected from inadvertent removal.

EVIDENCE-BASED PRACTICE

Fatigue in Adolescents with Cancer

Level IV

For many years nurses have assessed and provided interventions for fatigue, one of the most distressing symptoms in adult cancer victims. Fatigue and its effects on adolescents or children with cancer have only been recently studied. Erickson (2010) suggests that fatigue in adolescents with cancer is one of the most frequently reported and highest rated symptoms that is multifactorial in nature, requiring an integration of several different interventions at varying times.

In building on her early exploratory research, Erickson (2010) conducted a longitudinal, descriptive study of fatigue in adolescents. The objectives of her study were to describe patterns of fatigue in adolescents and the impact of fatigue during 1 month of chemotherapy, to explore variables that affect fatigue, and to explore the feasibility of collecting daily, self-report data in this population (Erickson, 2010). Erickson (2010) enrolled 25 subjects between the ages of 12 and 19 years receiving their second, third, fourth, or fifth month of chemotherapy. A longitudinal descriptive study design was used; data were collected from the same individuals at different points in time in order to describe the phenomenon of fatigue in adolescents on chemotherapy. Each study participant completed a daily fatigue report form and a weekly PedsQL Multidimensional Fatigue Scale (MFS). Participants' medical records were reviewed for treatment information such as the administration of chemotherapy agents and procedures performed (Erickson, 2010).

The study revealed that every adolescent experienced fatigue during the month of treatment, with great variability in severity and duration (Erickson, 2010). Fatigue was found to be a highly dynamic and variable state with two predominant patterns of fatigue. One pattern was that of a "declining rollercoaster" seen in those receiving chemotherapy once every 3 weeks, with fatigue gradually decreasing until the next scheduled chemotherapy. The other pattern was that of a "yo-yo" with fatigue seen in those who were receiving weekly chemotherapy that did not diminish over time. Treatment-related causes of increased fatigue included chemotherapy administration and cancer-related symptoms such as pain, nausea, and sleep disturbances.

The results from this study further expand the understanding of fatigue in adolescents on chemotherapy including interventions that alleviate fatigue symptoms and the effects of fatigue on activities of daily living. Of particular interest was the positive effect of exercise in alleviating fatigue symptoms. Erickson (2010) also suggests future areas for research including how nutrition, sleep patterns, cancer-related symptom control (such as pain and nausea), and exercise may influence fatigue in adolescents with cancer.

Consider what the experience of fatigue would mean to an adolescent who continues to attend school. What types of modifications to the adolescent's schedule could facilitate learning while conserving energy? How might a school nurse work with the school administrators to advocate for the adolescent with cancer?

Erickson, J. (2010). Patterns of fatigue in adolescents receiving chemotherapy. *Oncology Nursing Forum, 37*(4), 444-455.

The side effects of radiation are dose and treatment site specific. As with chemotherapy, the side effects result from the radiation's effect on healthy, rapidly dividing cells. The side effects usually appear 7 to 10 days after the initiation of therapy. Acute side effects usually dissipate a few days or weeks after the end of radiation therapy. Common side effects include fatigue, skin damage, hair loss, nausea and vomiting, and low blood cell counts. A child receiving cranial radiation is particularly affected by fatigue and an increased need for sleep during and shortly after completion of a course of radiation. Skin damage can include changes in pigmentation (darkening), redness, peeling, and increased sensitivity. Extra care must be taken to avoid excessive exposure of skin to heat, sunlight, friction (such as rubbing with a towel or washcloth), and creams or moisturizers. Only topical creams and moisturizers prescribed by the radiation oncologist should be applied to the irradiated skin.

The decision regarding irradiation dosage, frequency, and location depends on the purpose of the radiation and the disease process being treated. In general, radiotherapy is used more cautiously during childhood because a child's developing tissues and organs are more vulnerable to radiation's adverse and long-term effects (Bleyer & Ritchey, 2011).

Radiation therapy slows the growth of tumors and kills rapidly dividing cells nonselectively. Unfortunately, in a developing child, normal cell development may not be complete when radiation exposure occurs. Radiation therapy to developing brain tissue may alter cognitive potential. In children younger than 3 years, the effect of radiation therapy can be cognitively devastating. Bone growth is altered if radiation therapy is delivered to areas of growth potential, such as facial bones, spine, or growth plates in long bones. The result many years later may be skeletal malformations and failure to achieve anticipated growth.

Radiation exposure also has been linked to the development of certain types of cancer, and radiation exposure to treat cancer may lead to the development of a second malignancy. Between 3% and 10% of children treated for cancer will develop a second malignancy. Some of these secondary malignancies will be linked to the exposure to radiation as a primary treatment (National Cancer Institute, 2010).

Hematopoietic Stem Cell Transplantation

In recent years, the use of hematopoietic stem cell transplantation (HSCT) has become accepted therapy for the treatment of several hematologic and oncologic disorders. Transplantation allows extremely high doses of chemotherapy (with or without radiation) to be given without regard for bone marrow recovery because hematopoiesis will be restored through transplantation. Stem cells are harvested from bone marrow, peripheral blood, and umbilical cord blood. HSCT is often used interchangeably with the term bone marrow transplant (BMT) in the clinical setting even when referring to stem cells from cord or peripheral blood.

BMT uses bone marrow to reconstitute the immunologic function of the child after treatment with high-dose chemotherapy. Stem cell transplantation uses a unique immature cell present in the peripheral circulation to restore immunologic function in a similar manner. Stem cells are able to differentiate into any type of hematologic cell.

The healthy bone marrow cells or stem cells are infused into the bloodstream and migrate to the marrow space to replenish the child's immunologic function. The decision regarding the source of marrow or stem cells depends on the disease process being treated and the availability of an appropriate donor source.

Recent advances in the understanding of histocompatibility and in supportive care have improved outcomes in allogeneic (matched related or unrelated donor) transplants. The child's own harvested stem cells (an autologous transplant) using peripheral blood can be the source of stem cells in certain instances. This allows for aggressive chemotherapy that leads to almost total bone marrow ablation. Peripheral blood stem cells (PBSCs) are then given back to "rescue" and restore hematopoietic function of the child's bone marrow.

Umbilical cord blood is another source of transplanted stem cells. Because of the ability to "bank" or store umbilical cord blood, this source is becoming more significant. Cord blood from infants is easily harvested and banked. The donor undergoes no risk during harvesting of the cord blood, and the graft is thought to be more immunologically "tolerant" than stem cells from older donors. A national or international search for a matched, unrelated donor can be done through the National Marrow Donor Program (NMDP).

In preparation for a transplant, the child begins a regimen of chemotherapy with or without radiation (called *conditioning*). The goal of conditioning is to eradicate any disease from the body with high-dose chemotherapy and radiation therapy. WBC, red blood cell (RBC), and platelet counts begin to drop as the chemotherapy and radiation exert their effects on the bone marrow. When the conditioning phase is over, the child receives the donor marrow or stem cells by IV infusion.

Once the marrow is infused, nursing care focuses on (1) preventing profoundly immunosuppressed children from developing life-threatening infections and (2) minimizing treatment-related side effects. Parents and the child anxiously wait for the day when the CBC count begins to show signs of marrow engraftment. The production of WBCs, RBCs, and platelets from the transplantation of normal cells is evidence that the marrow has engrafted, or been accepted by the body.

Common complications in the days and weeks after HSCT include mucositis, diarrhea, fever, and nosebleed. The child should receive aggressive nutritional support since most will have substantial difficulty taking foods and fluids orally because of severe mucositis, GI discomfort, and diarrhea.

The major problem associated with allogeneic transplants is graft-versus-host disease (GVHD). GVHD results when the infused immunocompetent donor bone marrow recognizes the recipient's tissue as foreign and attacks the child's body, affecting numerous organ systems. Symptoms associated with GVHD include mild to severely elevated liver enzyme levels, mild to copious diarrhea, and maculopapular skin reactions ranging from rashes to full skin desquamation. Antirejection drugs such as prednisone, cyclosporine, and tacrolimus are given to prevent GVHD from occurring or to lessen its severity.

Transplantation is currently the standard therapy for children in first remission with Philadelphia chromosome–positive ALL (a genetically specific type of ALL with a 90% relapse rate), AML, stage IV neuroblastoma, severe aplastic anemia, severe combined immunodeficiency syndrome, as well as certain other hematologic disorders (see Chapter 23). Transplantation is also used to treat children with certain solid tumors, Hodgkin disease, and non-Hodgkin lymphoma that are resistant to conventional chemotherapy and radiation, and in children who experience relapses (Velardi & Locatelli, 2011).

Steroid Therapy

High-dose and/or long-term steroid therapy is a mainstay of treatment for children with leukemia, as an adjunct for control of nausea and vomiting, and for children with brain tumors complicated by increased intracranial pressure. High doses of steroids (e.g., dexamethasone, prednisone) cause many various side effects, including increased appetite, fluid retention, weight gain, hypertension, insulin-dependent diabetes (usually reversible once steroid therapy is stopped), emotional lability (mood changes), sleep disturbances, changes in appearance (abdominal striae, cushingoid features), and immunosuppression (Hinds, Hockenberry, Gattuso et al., 2007; Taketomo, Hodding, & Kraus, 2010).

The nurse should inform the child and caregivers about the side effects of steroid therapy because they can be quite frightening (sleep disturbances such as vivid dreaming) and disruptive (mood shifts from angry to sad to happy in very short periods of time). In addition, the family should be prepared for changes in the child's diet, such as craving salty food, which can contribute to increased fluid retention, weight gain, and hypertension. The child's caregivers should know to alert the health care team if the child has increased thirst and/or voiding at night, which can indicate hyperglycemia. The physical changes associated with steroid use can create body image disturbances for the child. These changes (cushingoid features) include puffy cheeks, abdominal weight gain, striae (stretch marks), increased acne, and a flushed, shiny appearance of the skin.

The child and caregivers should be reassured that these symptoms typically resolve over a period of weeks once the steroid therapy has been discontinued.

Biologic Agents

Recent additions to cancer therapy are the biologic response modifiers. Biologic response modifiers are naturally occurring substances found in small quantities in the body that influence immune system functions (e.g., colony-stimulating factors [CSFs]).

Used to enhance cell recovery, different CSFs work on different types of blood cells to reduce the time and severity of bone marrow suppression. The granulocyte colony–stimulating factors (GCSFs) stimulate WBC recovery. GCSFs may reduce the length of time a child has neutropenia by stimulating production of neutrophils, a type of granulocyte. Other CSFs promote recovery of platelets or RBCs and subsequently reduce the need for blood products.

Recently, clinical trials using immune-modulating agents have resulted in the approval of some as beneficial treatment modalities. Certain "targeted" monoclonal antibodies are used for very specific types of neoplasms and often are used in conjunction with other modalities, such as radiation and chemotherapy. They provide the advantage of effective treatment with less toxicity to normal tissue than other cancer modalities (Bleyer & Ritchey, 2011).

Complementary and Alternative Medical (CAM) Therapies

Complementary therapies include adjuncts to treatment that have been researched and proven to be helpful or therapies that are not yet scientifically proven but are deemed not to be harmful. Alternative therapies are those designed to replace conventional therapy in the treatment of individuals with cancer. The use of some CAM therapies, though often harmless and potentially beneficial for the child and family, can negatively affect the efficacy of therapy. Therefore, it is important to determine if the child is receiving any CAM therapies. One approach is to build a supportive, open rapport with the child and the family. However, not all families will disclose their use of CAM therapies without direct, but supportive, questioning. Most pediatric oncology centers provide an informational booklet to the family at the time of diagnosis. One technique for eliciting discussion regarding the use of CAM therapies is to include a description of their use and to emphasize the importance of discussing this issue with the child's health care providers.

When assisting families in their thinking about complementary and alternative therapies, health professionals should ask them to consider the following questions (National Center for Complementary and Alternative Medicine, 2010):

- What are the benefits and risks associated with the therapy?
- Do the benefits outweigh the risks?
- What side effects can be expected?
- What are the costs, and will the therapy be covered by insurance?
- What training and other qualifications does the practitioner have?
- Are there scientific articles or references about using the treatment?
- Could the therapy interfere with or delay conventional treatments?
- How long will the treatment last, and how often will it be assessed?
- Will it be necessary to buy equipment or supplies?
- Are there any conditions for which this treatment should not be used?

Family-centered care has the intent of developing mutually beneficial partnerships among health care providers, families, and patients. The first goal of the family-centered care approach regarding the use of CAM therapies includes preserving the dignity of the patient and the family. The nurse can achieve this goal by validating the feelings of the child and family regarding their desire to achieve a cure for the child's cancer. The nurse first seeks to understand what CAM therapy the family has chosen and why the family has made the choice. The next goal in the family-centered care approach is information sharing. The nurse provides the family with factual information and useful resources regarding CAM therapies and cancer. The ultimate decision regarding the use of CAM therapies rests with the family in consultation with the health care team. Nurses collaborate with the family in care planning that includes physician-approved CAM therapies.

❓ CRITICAL THINKING EXERCISE 24-1

When caring for children with cancer, nurses often encounter families who want to try (or are trying) a method of complementary or alternative medical (CAM) therapy to treat the child's cancer. It is not uncommon for families to try CAM therapies without disclosing this practice to the health care team for fear of alienating their providers. Families should be asked about the use of CAM therapies through direct questioning in a supportive, nonthreatening manner. Some CAM therapies can potentially decrease the efficacy of chemotherapy (such as folate supplementation in the child receiving methotrexate, an antifolate drug). Others may be vitamin supplements that can be obtained inexpensively, but perhaps were marketed to the family as a cure and are being provided at a very high cost. Unfortunately, even families in crisis are sometimes exploited. Think about the issues involved with the use of complementary and alternative therapies.

1. What is the difference between complementary and alternative medicine?
2. How might the nurse learn more about what particular CAM therapies can be incorporated into a child's plan of care?
3. As the nurse working with a parent of a young child with recurrent cancer that is resistant to conventional forms of therapy, how might you best assist the family to make decisions regarding the use of CAM therapies?

LEUKEMIA

As the first disseminated cancer shown to be curable, the approaches to caring for children with childhood leukemia set the standard for principles of pediatric cancer diagnosis, prognosis, and treatment (Tubergen, Bleyer, & Ritchey, 2011). Leukemia is the most common form of cancer in children younger than 15 years. The cause of disease is an abnormal proliferation of immature WBCs (blasts), which compete with normal cells for space and nutrients. Bone marrow production of other cells is suppressed, so very low numbers of RBCs (anemia) and platelets (thrombocytopenia) may be seen at diagnosis. Considerable progress in treatment has been achieved through years of research. Leukemia was uniformly fatal in the 1960s. Today, children diagnosed with the most common form of leukemia, acute lymphoblastic leukemia (ALL), can almost always achieve remission, with a 5-year disease-free survival rate approaching 85% (Campana & Pui, 2008).

Etiology

The cause of childhood leukemia is unknown. Geographic distribution varies around the world, with leukemia being uncommon in developing countries but more common in industrialized countries. This variation may be correlated with underdiagnosis in developing countries or exposure to environmental agents may be implicated in the development of leukemia in industrialized countries.

Genetic factors appear to play a significant role in the development of leukemia. When karyotyped, the leukemic cells in most children with the disease reveal chromosomal abnormalities. Some of these chromosomal abnormalities have become prognostic factors for the disease (Tubergen et al., 2011). Because of the genetic basis of this disease, identical twins have a significantly greater chance of sharing chromosomal abnormalities that later lead to disease. Therefore, the risk of a second twin developing the disease after the first has been diagnosed in infancy is significantly higher than that of the general population (Tubergen et al., 2011). The fraternal twin of a child who has had ALL has a two to four times higher likelihood of developing the disease than other children. Children with Down syndrome have a 10% to 20% greater risk of developing leukemia than the general population (Campana & Pui, 2008). Other less common preexisting chromosomal abnormalities, such as Fanconi anemia and neurofibromatosis, also have been correlated with the development of leukemia.

Exposure to ionizing radiation and certain chemical toxins has been shown to increase the risk of leukemia development. Leukemia was well documented in both the child and adult survivors of the atomic bomb detonations in Japan during World War II. Chemical exposure to alkylating agents, a drug class used to treat cancer, has been shown to increase the risk of developing acute myelogenous leukemia (AML).

Large epidemiologic studies are ongoing to examine links to pesticide exposure, electromagnetic fields, parental smoking, parental alcohol use, and parental exposures to occupational chemicals. Thus far, relationships between these exposures and leukemia have not been demonstrated.

Incidence

Leukemias represent approximately 31% of all cancers in children younger than 14 years in the United States, with the highest percentage of children diagnosed with leukemia having acute lymphocytic leukemia (>75%) (Leukemia and Lymphoma Society, 2010). ALL is more common in boys, and the peak incidence occurs between ages 2 and 3 years of age (Tubergen et al., 2011). With improvements in treatment, mortality in children younger than 15 years old has decreased markedly, and nearly 90% survive beyond 5 years after diagnosis (Leukemia and Lymphoma Society, 2010).

Manifestations

Clinical manifestations of leukemia include fever, pallor, excessive bruising, bone or joint pain (usually leg/knee pain), lymphadenopathy, malaise, hepatosplenomegaly, abnormal WBC counts (either lower or higher than normal for age), and mild to profound anemia and thrombocytopenia. The severity of the clinical manifestations varies with the cell type of leukemia and the length of time before diagnosis.

Diagnostic Evaluation

The diagnosis can be strongly suspected from a history of the clinical manifestations and an initial CBC. The confirmatory test for leukemia is microscopic examination of bone marrow obtained by bone marrow aspiration and/or biopsy. A bone marrow aspirate usually provides sufficient material to establish the diagnosis of ALL. A lumbar puncture is also performed to look for leukemic blast cells in the spinal fluid, which are indicative of CNS involvement.

Flow cytometry, the analysis of the bone marrow cells using a laser beam, is another test that is commonly performed on the initial bone marrow sample. Flow cytometry provides a rapid diagnosis by characterizing the type of leukemia within hours. In addition, a portion of the initial bone marrow sample is sent for cytogenetic analysis to determine the chromosomal changes that may have occurred in the leukemic blast cells. These results are typically available in 2 to 3 weeks and therefore are not useful for making induction treatment decisions. However, this chromosomal information can be used to determine the intensity of the child's consolidation and maintenance therapy, based on known prognostic indicators.

PATIENT-CENTERED TEACHING

Caring for the Child with Cancer

- Reinforce teaching concerning diagnosis, treatment, and side effects of chemotherapy.
- Encourage parents to participate actively in the child's care.
- Provide written and verbal instructions concerning home care, and provide ample opportunity for parents to give return demonstrations of the following:
  - Central venous access dressing changes
  - Oral medication administration
  - Assessment of oral mucous membranes and rectal mucosa
  - Temperature measurement by axillary, oral, temporal, and tympanic routes
- Teach the signs and symptoms of infection and bleeding that require immediate treatment and how to access after-hours emergency treatment.
- Provide telephone numbers parents can call to obtain answers to questions concerning the diagnosis, treatment, and side effects of chemotherapy.
- Make appropriate referrals to social services, a chaplain or other religious figure, and a home health nursing agency.
- Encourage parents to use community resources.
- Stress the importance of preventing infection (see Figure 24-2) and bleeding and the need for follow-up visits.

PATHOPHYSIOLOGY
Leukemia

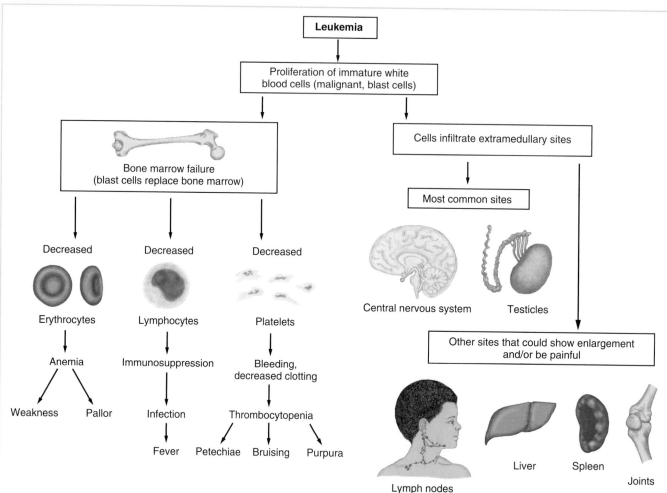

Leukemia most likely arises from a fundamental alteration in the genetic makeup of a WBC. Cells produced from the altered WBC have a defect that prevents maturation. These cells tend to replicate quickly, forming immature cells, or blast cells, in the bone marrow. The blast cells do not respond properly to the body's feedback mechanism and continue to replicate in great numbers. Blast cells are then released into the peripheral circulation and appear in a CBC blood test.

In leukemia, normal bone marrow is replaced by malignant blast cells. As the blast cells take over the bone marrow, eventually RBC and platelet production is impaired, and the child becomes anemic and thrombocytopenic. The symptoms of the disease reflect bone marrow failure and organ infiltration.

In addition to being present in the blood and bone marrow, leukemia cells infiltrate **extramedullary** sites, most commonly the CNS and the testicles.

Although extramedullary leukemia is not common at first diagnosis, these are common sites of relapse.

Leukemias are classified by the type of WBC affected. Broadly, acute lymphocytic leukemias are classified as ALL and acute nonlymphocytic leukemia (ANLL). ALL is an abnormality of the lymphocytes. ANLL is a broad term for leukemias not originating from abnormal lymphocytes. Acute myelocytic leukemia (AML) is an example of an ANLL. AML can be further classified as acute promyelocytic leukemia (APL), acute myelomonocytic leukemia (AMMoL), and acute monocytic leukemia (AMoL). ANLL tends to be less common in children, less responsive to therapy, more difficult to treat, and more likely to result in relapse than ALL.

Chronic leukemias are rare in children. The term *chronic* refers to the indolent nature of the disease. Whereas acute leukemias have a rapid onset to detectable disease, chronic leukemias have a slower onset of symptoms.

Therapeutic Management

Combination chemotherapy is the preferred treatment for leukemia. The particular drugs used and their dosage, route, and scheduling depend on the protocol customized for that specific type of leukemia. Children are placed into prognostic categories with specifically tailored therapies. Treatment of ALL is divided into phases: induction, consolidation, and maintenance. The aim of the first month of chemotherapy treatment, or induction, is to induce remission. Remission is the reduction of immature blast cells in the bone marrow to less than 5%. Approximately 98% of children with ALL achieve remission within 1 month (Tubergen et al., 2011).

Before induction, the child is treated for presenting signs, which may include sepsis, anemia, hemorrhage, and metabolic abnormalities. Serum electrolyte levels are determined to ensure metabolic stability before chemotherapy is initiated. An elevated level of uric acid, indicating rapid cell turnover, can be expected if the WBC count is very high.

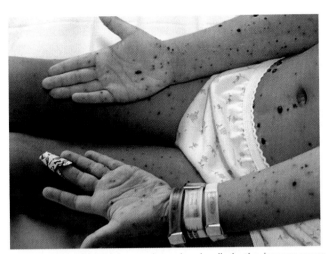

FIG 24-2 Varicella (chickenpox) can be deadly in the immunocompromised child. Thrombocytopenia (low platelet count) associated with chemotherapy can cause the varicella lesions to be hemorrhagic, like those shown here. Secondary infections of the lesions are also common because of low WBC counts. (Photo courtesy Cook Children's Medical Center, Hematology-Oncology Clinic, Fort Worth, TX.)

As WBCs break down in reaction to chemotherapy, they release uric acid. Uric acid has poor water solubility and can compromise kidney function (tumor lysis syndrome). When the WBC count is extremely high, allopurinol and IV fluids with sodium bicarbonate are given to decrease the serum uric acid level and alkalinize the urine before chemotherapy is initiated. Parenteral urate oxidase may be given in situations when lysing of the tumor by chemotherapy is expected to be significant. This recombinant enzyme oxidizes uric acid into a water-soluble product that can be excreted (Taketomo et al., 2010). During induction, the hospitalized child receives the first doses of chemotherapy while the response to the drugs is assessed. Remission can be verified within the first 28 days after the initiation of chemotherapy by sequential bone marrow aspirates and lumbar punctures. If a significant number of blast cells are still present, a new and stronger drug regimen is given. The presence of more than 5% blasts in the marrow at day 28 is an ominous sign indicating a poorer prognosis.

Once the child is medically stable, most chemotherapy treatment for ALL is given on an outpatient basis. The child is usually healthy and is able to return to school and engage in most age-appropriate activities.

Text continued on p. 611

◎ NURSING CARE PLAN

The Child with Leukemia

Focused Assessment

- Obtain history from parents of child's symptoms and the probably insidious onset of the disease
- Possible symptoms include decreased activity level, persistent or recurrent fever of unknown cause, more bruises than usual, intermittent stomachaches, and leg pains with refusal to walk (parents may interpret as child trying to avoid school, having growing pains, or being lazy)
- Conduct physical examination and comprehensive assessment
- Look for fever, fatigue, pallor, bruising on the extremities, petechiae in the mouth and sclera, hepatomegaly, very high WBC count, and bleeding
- Check mental and neurologic function due to risk of leukemic infiltration into the CNS
- Provide ongoing psychosocial assessment of the child and family to determine needs for intervention and support
- Parents may express guilt feelings that they delayed seeking treatment because they did not initially recognize their child's symptoms as signs of serious illness
- Observe the child's and parents' reactions to the disease. Assess how each person copes with the illness and treatment (Parents who are unable to cope may display a high level of anxiety that can be transferred to the child)
- Include these critical factors in the child's assessment: age, developmental level, and experiences with the health care system or providers (child may exhibit increased anxiety if he or she had a previous negative experience)

Planning

Nursing Diagnosis

Risk for Infection related to the immunosuppressed state.

Expected Outcomes

The child will be free of signs of infection, as evidenced by an afebrile state, no redness of the integument, no redness or swelling at the site of insertion of a central venous catheter, and negative culture results.

The parents and the child will recognize and verbalize early signs of infection.

Intervention/*Rationale*

1. Monitor vital signs every 4 hours and as necessary if the child is hospitalized. Instruct parents to measure the child's temperature as needed at home (by the oral, axillary, temporal, or tympanic routes only).

   In the presence of markedly decreased WBCs, an elevated temperature may be the only sign of infection. The risk of injury to the fragile mucous membranes is so great that only oral, tympanic, temporal, or axillary routes should be used to measure temperatures (NO rectal temperatures). Rectal abscesses can easily occur to friable rectal tissue. Report a single temperature of (101.3° F (38.5° C) or a temperature of 100.4° F (38.0° C) that continues for more than 1 hour.

2. Monitor CBC with differential as ordered. Report moderate to severe neutropenia.

Absolute Neutrophil Count (ANC) (cells/mm³)	Risk
1500–2000	Not significant
1000–1500	Minimal
500–1000	Moderate
<500	Severe

   The risk of infection increases significantly with moderate and severe neutropenia. The absolute neutrophil count can be easily calculated using the results from the child's CBC and this formula:
   (a) *Add the percent of neutrophils and the percent of bands*
   (b) *Convert the summed percentage into decimal form (e.g., 55% = 0.55)*
   (c) *Multiply that figure by the WBC (stated in thousands)*

3. Practice proper hand hygiene and teach this to the family.
   Proper hand hygiene is the best way to prevent the spread of infection.

4. Inspect the child's skin daily for breaks and redness.
   Some neutropenic children will not produce erythema or purulent drainage. Because pus is made of WBCs, drainage cannot be used as a sign of infection. Skin provides a barrier against infection.

Continued

◎ NURSING CARE PLAN

The Child with Leukemia—cont'd

Intervention/*Rationale*—cont'd

5. Inspect the child's mouth daily for oral ulcers, and inspect the perineum for fissures. Teach older children to do self-examination. No suppositories should be given.

   Mucous membranes are fragile and easily affected by chemotherapy and irradiation. Mouth ulcers and rectal fissures are common side effects of chemotherapy and radiation therapy and potential sites for bacteria entry because of the impaired mucosa.

6. Encourage and monitor regular bowel habits.

   Decreased activity, altered nutrition, and certain medications may predispose to constipation. The passage of hard stool may traumatize delicate rectal mucous membranes and create a potential site for entry of bacteria.

7. Teach the parents and child meticulous oral hygiene at diagnosis. The child should use a soft-bristled toothbrush or Toothettes when performing oral hygiene four times each day. If the platelet count is low, a cotton-tipped applicator, finger cot, or washcloth wrapped around a finger is used instead of a toothbrush.

   Prevention of dental caries and ulcerations on fragile oral mucosa will help prevent infections.

8. At the first signs of mouth ulcers, begin a mouth care regimen four times daily, which includes use of an antifungal drug as ordered by the physician. Do not use alcohol-containing mouthwashes.

   Fungal infections originating from the mouth or GI tract can quickly become disseminated in immunosuppressed children. Over-the-counter mouthwashes may have high alcohol content and may be drying to oral mucosa, thus increasing the risk of breaking down the protective barrier of the skin.

9. For the hospitalized neutropenic child, to decrease the risk of exposure to fungal spores, fresh flowers or plants are usually not permitted. Do not use humidifiers.

   Standing water and damp soil harbor Aspergillus and Pseudomonas organisms, to which these children are extremely susceptible.

10. Use sterile techniques to change any dressings and IV lines.

    A child with neutropenia is not able to fight infection normally; extra precautions must be taken.

11. In general, the child should not receive live-virus or live bacterial vaccines such as the measles-mumps-rubella (MMR) and the varicella vaccines. Special circumstances exist when risks of the disease outweigh risks of the vaccine. Siblings should receive inactivated polio vaccine and may also receive live (MMR) and varicella vaccines. Flu shots are recommended for the patient, family members, and close contacts.

    Live MMR vaccine could produce infection in the severely immunocompromised child, but no virus shedding occurs to create a threat if given to the sibling. Exposure to a rash produced by the varicella vaccine does have the potential of causing varicella disease in an immunocompromised child. If rash should occur in a vaccinated sibling, the immunocompromised child should be separated from the sibling until the rash resolves.

12. Keep any child with chickenpox or any child who has been exposed to the virus away from the child with cancer. Inform the teacher of the importance of notifying parents immediately if a case of chickenpox occurs in another child at school. Encourage vaccination of siblings who have not had varicella to create "herd" immunity.

    Immunocompromised children are unable to fight varicella adequately; chickenpox is life-threatening to them (Figure 24-2). If a child who has not had chickenpox is exposed to someone with varicella, the child should receive varicella zoster immune globulin within 96 hours of exposure.

13. Obtain specimens for culture as ordered and monitor the results.

    Physicians will order blood, urine, stool, and wound cultures as indicated when the neutropenic child has fever.

14. Administer acetaminophen for fever.

    Aspirin and ibuprofen given to a child who is thrombocytopenic can cause platelet dysfunction.

15. Administer antibiotics as ordered after cultures have been obtained. Cultures should be obtained and antibiotics should begin as soon as possible. Once the culture results are available, anticipate that antibiotic therapy will be tailored to treat any identified organisms. Organisms are not always identified, necessitating the continuation of broad-spectrum antibiotics until the child is afebrile, has continued negative cultures, and demonstrates recovering neutrophil counts.

    Cultures identify the specific organism so that the most effective antibiotic can be given. Appropriate antibiotic treatment should begin promptly.

Evaluation

Is the child afebrile and free of redness or swelling at insertion sites or other integumentary sites?

Have the child and parents promptly recognized and responded to warning signs of infection?

Planning

Nursing Diagnosis

Risk for Injury related to thrombocytopenia.

Expected Outcomes

The child will have no excessive, uncontrolled bleeding.

The parents and child will understand risk for hemorrhage, as evidenced by making the home environment safe and by their ability to respond appropriately to bleeding.

Intervention/*Rationale*

1. Apply gentle, firm pressure to any puncture sites. Apply a pressure dressing to sites of bone marrow aspiration.

   Additional pressure may be needed to stop bleeding if the platelet count is low.

2. For the child who is severely thrombocytopenic (platelet count <20,000/mm^3), monitor closely for signs of bleeding, including urine and stool checks for blood. Limit any activity that could result in injury and especially head injury; participation in contact sports is not allowed. Encourage the child to participate in quiet activities (e.g., reading books, watching videos, coloring). Provide a soft-bristled toothbrush or Toothettes for oral hygiene. Give stool softeners to prevent straining with constipation and do NOT use suppositories. Ensure the child avoid eating "sharp" foods such as chips that could cause injury to the oral mucosa.

   A decreased platelet count increases the risk for bleeding and intracranial hemorrhage is a potential risk.

3. Teach the child how to control nosebleeds and blow the nose gently.

   One of the most common sites of bleeding is the nose. Blood loss can be reduced through avoidance of nosebleeds.

4. Evaluate menstrual flow in adolescent girls.

   Menstrual bleeding can be severe when girls have low platelet counts. Occasionally, hormone therapy is required to inhibit menses.

Evaluation

Has the child had bleeding that could not be controlled?

Have the parents demonstrated what to do for a nosebleed?

Have the child and parents promptly recognized and responded to bleeding?

The Child with Leukemia—cont'd

Planning
Nursing Diagnosis

Imbalanced Nutrition: Less Than Body Requirements related to nausea and vomiting, mucositis, or taste changes.

Expected Outcomes

The child will experience no more than 5% weight loss and eat palatable foods that provide appropriate nutrients for growth.

Intervention/Rationale

1. Per physician orders, administer antiemetics prophylactically and as needed.
   Antiemetics help decrease or prevent vomiting.
2. When the child is nauseated, offer cool, clear liquids. Offer bland, soft foods at room temperature, served in small portions. Be creative with the liquids and foods offered to make them more interesting and inviting.
   Cool liquids and foods are soothing and better tolerated than hot ones, and the risk of burning fragile mucosa is eliminated.
3. Offer small, frequent meals of high protein and high calorie content. Fortify foods with nutritional supplements. Allow the family to bring favorite foods to the hospital.
   Small, frequent meals are better tolerated than large ones. Protein promotes tissue healing. A large number of calories are needed for growth. Children are more likely to eat their favorite foods.
4. Avoid offering favorite foods when the child is nauseated.
   Foods eaten within hours of nausea will be associated with feeling "sick."
5. Administer ordered mouth analgesics before oral intake.
   If mouth sores are present, analgesics will increase comfort and enable interest in eating.
6. Monitor daily weight. Keep strict intake and output records. Weigh the infant's diapers.
   Strict measurement ensures adequate intake and provides an objective assessment to alert the nurse that further interventions may be needed.
7. Involve the child in food selection.
   Allow the child as much control as possible over the foods to eat; this may increase interest and participation in eating.
8. Include a dietitian in the nutritional assessment and evaluation.
   A dietitian provides specialized input into developing a nutrition plan and evaluating the child's nutritional status.

Evaluation

Did the child have no more than 5% weight loss, as documented on a growth chart?
Does the child eat foods that provide appropriate nutrients for growth?

Planning
Nursing Diagnosis

Deficient Knowledge related to unfamiliarity with the disease process and treatment plan.

Expected Outcomes

The child and parents will explain the diagnosis and demonstrate adherence to treatment.

Intervention/Rationale

1. Determine the child's and parents' readiness for learning. Create an environment of learning.
   After the initial diagnosis, family members may need time to adjust before they are ready for education.
2. During each hospital and clinic visit, spend time with the family, explaining the diagnosis, its sequelae, and its treatment. Repeat key educational interventions for the child and family. Offer written information and video tapes of educational sessions (see Patient-Centered Teaching: Caring for the Child with Cancer box).

The diagnosis of cancer in a child is overwhelming. The family receives a flood of information and needs time to process. Educational interventions that are repeated over time as the family's stress decreases, reinforces learning and facilitates understanding.

3. During education sessions with the family, demonstrate procedures required for the child's care, discuss ways to approach nausea, explain the management of fatigue and other side effects, and address ways to encourage the child's normal development. Explain rationale for treatment and anticipated sequelae.
   Home care for the child is complex and the family needs comprehensive education. Understanding the rationale for treatment and expected outcomes encourages adherence to therapy.
4. Determine the family's preferred method of learning (demonstration, reading, listening, observing). Keep explanations at the family's level of understanding.
   Matching teaching techniques to preferred method of learning will facilitate the education process.
5. Offer encouragement for parents' recognition of danger signs and parents' appropriate use of medical care, to reinforce behavior.
   Parents want to know they are doing the right thing for their child.

Evaluation

Have the parents and child demonstrated an understanding of the treatment protocols by adhering to therapy and seeking appropriate medical care for danger signs?

Planning
Nursing Diagnosis

Disturbed Body Image related to hair loss.

Expected Outcomes

The child will adapt to alopecia, as evidenced by a return to socialization, and discuss concerns related to hair loss.

Intervention/Rationale

1. Instruct the child and parents on the progression of hair loss and potential changes in color and texture when the hair regrows. (Cranial irradiation can result in patches of permanent hair loss.) Suggest obtaining a wig before hair is lost or bringing a clipping of hair with a recent photograph.
   Knowing how hair loss occurs and that it is temporary for most children can be reassuring to the child and family. Matching a wig to original hair color, texture, and style is easier before hair is lost.
2. Encourage verbalization of feelings about hair loss. Enlist the help of a child life specialist to engage the child in play therapy.
   Allowing the child to verbalize concerns about returning to a social environment or school is important. Play therapy is a safe way for the child to express feelings and fears.
3. Discuss ways to minimize the reaction to alopecia by promoting creative solutions such as hats, wigs, or scarves.
   Allowing children to create their own head coverings may reduce the negative impact of hair loss.
4. Make visits to the child's classroom.
   Preparation of classmates for the child's school reentry will lessen classmates' negative reactions, fears, anxiety, and lack of understanding. It will also increase the support they can give the ill child.
5. Encourage a return to school as soon as possible.
   The sooner the child returns to school, the less likely it is that the child will begin a pattern of absenteeism. If the child returns to school before major body changes take place, the changes may not be so noticeable to the other children, thus decreasing undesirable reactions.

Continued

Evaluation

Is the child involved in prediagnosis social life?

Has the child discussed hair loss and feelings connected with body image?

Has the child experienced a successful reentry to school?

Planning

Nursing Diagnosis

Ineffective Coping (individual) or Compromised Family Coping related to chronic illness.

Expected Outcomes

The child will exhibit effective coping as evidenced by adherence to the treatment plan and identification of support systems (child life therapists, playroom activities, summer camps).

The parents will exhibit effective coping as evidenced by verbalization of their concerns about the impact of the child's illness on the family and utilization of support systems and community resources.

Intervention/Rationale

1. Teach the family the necessity of adhering to the protocol. Teach the warning signs of problems and how to access after-hours emergency care.

   Conscientious application of the treatment plan increases the chance of a positive outcome.

2. Listen and encourage the child and family to verbalize their feelings and express their concerns. Answer questions honestly and openly.

   Identification of concerns and clarification of misconceptions will help children and families cope with the stress of chronic illness.

3. Introduce the family to other families of children with cancer.

   Other families of children with cancer can offer suggestions and support.

4. Consult social services, child life specialists, and a chaplain or other appropriate religious figure.

   The financial and emotional burdens of caring for a child with cancer can be overwhelming.

5. Offer a list of local support groups appropriate to the child's age and the family's individual needs.

   Children and family members in similar situations can provide comfort and support to the child with cancer and the family.

Evaluation

Is the family adhering to the treatment plan?

Do the family and child verbalize appropriate concerns and questions?

Has the family contacted a local support group?

Planning

Nursing Diagnosis

Acute Pain and Chronic Pain related to the disease process and procedures.

Expected Outcome

The child will experience decreased discomfort, as evidenced by periods of uninterrupted rest, verbalization of increased comfort, a reduced pain score on an age-appropriate pain assessment tool, and participation in play activities.

Intervention/Rationale

1. Explain procedures to the child in an age-appropriate manner before performing them.

   Honest explanations build rapport and reduce fear.

2. Enlist a child life specialist's help before and during procedures.

   Child life specialists are trained to use distraction techniques with children and represent a "safe" person for the child to be with during repeated painful procedures.

3. Administer antianxiety drugs as ordered (see Chapter 15).

   Anticipation of a painful procedure may worsen the pain, especially in the adolescent. Giving an antianxiety drug may help calm the child so the procedure is better tolerated.

4. Monitor for signs and symptoms of pain such as inactivity for age, increased heart rate or blood pressure, grimacing, verbalization of discomfort, irritability, and crying. Use a developmentally-appropriate assessment tool and nonverbal cues to evaluate pain.

   Younger children will not be able to verbalize pain. Stoic children may not express discomfort. Nurses must watch for physiologic signs of pain.

5. Provide comfort measures as needed such as positioning, adjusting room temperature, and offering distractions appropriate for age.

   Comfort measures can decrease the perception of pain and even decrease the amount of analgesic needed.

6. Administer analgesics promptly as ordered. Use topical anesthetics for procedural pain. Ensure analgesia or nonpharmacologic strategies before painful procedures.

   Analgesics reduce the pain of procedures and of the disease. Delays in analgesic administration can increase anxiety and thus increase pain. Nonpharmacologic interventions can decrease anxiety and pain.

7. Explain the pain control regimen to the parents and child as age appropriate.

   Parents know their child and can help the nurse assess pain promptly.

8. Notify the physician if pain relief is not obtained with the ordered dose of analgesic.

   Pain tolerance varies greatly among children. Dosage increases may be needed, especially in the child with chronic pain or the dying child.

Evaluation

Does the child express decreased levels of discomfort, and have a reduced pain score on an appropriate pain assessment tool?

Is the child joining other children in play?

Planning

Nursing Diagnosis

Impaired Skin Integrity related to radiation therapy, chemotherapy, and immobility.

Expected Outcomes

The child's skin will remain free of skin breakdown.

The child and family will maintain the integrity of the child's skin.

Intervention/Rationale

1. Assess and document the child's skin condition each shift. (Skin erythema is common with radiation therapy but should not progress to skin breakdown.)

   Ongoing assessment and documentation will reveal early skin changes that require intervention to prevent skin breakdown.

2. Use only approved lotions and creams on the skin.

   Some commercial lotions can increase skin irritation and redness.

3. Avoid excessive scrubbing of skin, hot water, and abrasive soaps.

   Friction may increase skin breakdown. Hot water is uncomfortable to irritated tissue.

4. Offer loose clothing of soft materials.

   Tight clothing or abrasive fabrics may further irritate the skin.

5. Notify the physician if skin breakdown occurs.

   Additional orders for therapeutic creams may be needed.

6. If the child is immobile, gently turn and vary the position at least every 2 hours.

   Immobility may increase pressure on skin and promote breakdown.

◎ NURSING CARE PLAN

The Child with Leukemia—cont'd

Intervention/*Rationale*—cont'd

7. Teach the parents how to regularly assess the condition of the child's skin. Provide oral and written instructions to the family on the skin care techniques listed above.
   The family needs comprehensive education and detailed instructions in order to assess the child's skin and provide appropriate care.

Evaluation

Has the child's skin remained intact?
Can parents describe skin assessment and care techniques?

Planning

Nursing Diagnosis

Impaired Oral (and Anal/Rectal) Mucous Membranes related to chemotherapy and radiation therapy.

Expected Outcome

The child will not exhibit side effects from treatment, as evidenced by intact oral and anal/rectal mucous membranes.

Intervention/*Rationale*

1. Monitor the child's mouth and anus each shift for ulcers, erythema, or breakdown. Teach the parents and the child, if age-appropriate, how to perform this assessment. Report ulcerations to the physician.
   A breakdown in mucous membranes usually begins with erythema and progresses to ulcerations. Home care should include this assessment for the duration of therapy.

2. Begin meticulous mouth care, avoiding alcohol-based mouthwashes, several times a day with a soft-bristled toothbrush or Toothettes.
   Removing bacteria from the oral mucosa will decrease the risk of infection of irritated tissue.

3. Offer bland, nonirritating foods and cool liquids.
   Citrus products and spicy foods may be quite painful to an ulcerated mouth. Cool liquids are soothing. Ice pops and slushes are usually well tolerated.

4. If ulcerations occur, administer medications, mouth rinses and ointments per physician orders.
   Immediate treatment is essential to prevent infection and other complications.

5. Do not take a rectal temperature in a child undergoing chemotherapy or radiation therapy. Do not take oral temperatures if mouth ulcers are present. Teach parents how to take accurate axillary, temporal, or tympanic temperatures.
   The introduction of a thermometer into the rectum or mouth of a child with fragile mucous membranes, no matter how carefully done, can tear tissue.

6. If the anal/rectal mucosa becomes irritated, begin sitz baths several times a day and after bowel movements.
   Lukewarm sitz baths keep the perineum clean and soothe irritated tissue.

7. In diaper-wearing children, use only diaper wipes without alcohol or perfumes. If the perineum is very irritated, use only warm-water wipes on the area.
   Alcohol and perfumes will further irritate the skin and can cause great discomfort. Very few commercial diaper wipes are safe for these children.

Evaluation

Has the child exhibited signs of oral mucosal or anal/rectal ulceration?

Consolidation is the phase of therapy for ALL that follows induction and remission. The goal of consolidation therapy is to maintain remission and prevent disease in extramedullary "sanctuary sites" such as the testes and CNS where systemic therapy is not easily delivered. Intrathecal chemotherapy is given prophylactically to prevent relapse in the CNS. If the testes are involved, radiation therapy is administered.

Generally, after the initial induction and consolidation phases of chemotherapy are complete, a maintenance phase begins. Maintenance chemotherapy usually consists of lower dosage of chemotherapy given orally and possibly intravenously on a regular basis over a period of 2 to 3 years to "maintain" remission and prevent recurrence of the leukemia. Total treatment time for ALL is approximately $2\frac{1}{2}$ years for girls and $3\frac{1}{2}$ years for boys.

BRAIN TUMORS

Brain tumors are the most common solid tumor and the second most common childhood malignancy after leukemia. Brain tumors are a diverse group of tumors described by their tissue of origin, location within the brain, and rate of growth. Unlike other neoplasms, primary brain tumors are confined to the brain and spine and rarely metastasize to bone marrow or other organs. The mortality rate is significant (approaching 4.5%) (Kuttesch, Rush, & Ater, 2011).

Etiology

The cause of brain tumors remains unknown. Heredity and environment have both been associated with their development. Several inherited syndromes are associated with the development of brain tumors

in children, such as neurofibromatosis and tuberous sclerosis. Additional risk factors include immune system suppression and cranial irradiation. Although exposure to electromagnetic fields has been suggested to increase a child's risk of a brain tumor, no confirming evidence supports this theory (Maity, Pruitt, & Phillips, 2008).

Incidence

Approximately 3700 children younger than age 20 years are diagnosed with primary brain tumors annually in the United States (Kuttesch et al., 2011). CNS tumors represent 35% of solid tumor malignancies diagnosed in children (Santana, Rodriguez-Galindo, Dome, & Spunt, 2008) and 24% of all pediatric cancers (Maity et al., 2008). Nearly 50% of pediatric CNS tumors develop in the posterior fossa—the lower part of the brain that contains both the cerebellum and the brainstem (Kuttesch et al., 2011).

Manifestations

Manifestations of brain tumors vary with tumor location and the child's age and development. Symptoms produced by tumors in the posterior fossa include ataxia (unsteady gait), poor coordination of the upper extremities, visual changes (nystagmus, diplopia, strabismus) (see Chapter 28), and occasionally head tilt. Posterior fossa tumors are associated with increased intracranial pressure (ICP) caused by the tumor mass itself or, more commonly, by the tumor obstructing the normal flow of cerebrospinal fluid (CSF). Increased ICP often causes headaches, vomiting, and lethargy. These symptoms are usually most intense on arising in the morning.

Symptoms of increased ICP caused by a brain tumor are frequently subacute and nonspecific (see Chapter 28). Infants may be irritable, lethargic, and feed poorly, and have increased head circumference and bulging fontanels. Many younger children demonstrate loss of developmental milestones. School-age children may exhibit declining academic performance, fatigue, personality changes, and symptoms of vague, intermittent headache. Cranial nerve deficits and hemiparesis are usually associated with brainstem involvement.

Supratentorial tumors characteristically cause headaches, seizures, or focal neurologic deficits. Especially with slow-growing tumors, symptoms may be subtle and initially attributed to more common childhood illnesses.

Diagnostic Evaluation

Once a tumor is suspected, evaluation is considered to be an emergency. Imaging with magnetic resonance imaging (MRI), CT, or positron emission tomography (PET) may be performed. MRI is currently the imaging modality most commonly used to evaluate brain tumors. During MRI, the child must lie motionless inside a dark tunnel for approximately 1 hour. This is especially difficult for young children. In general, children younger than 6 years need sedation. A spinal MRI is

performed to look for metastatic disease in the spine. A CSF sample obtained from lumbar puncture is examined for the presence of tumor cells. In some cases, the tumor produces tumor markers such as alpha-fetoprotein that can be identified in the CSF or blood.

Usually the diagnosis is suspected from the child's signs and symptoms and the location of the tumor (Figure 24-3). Pathologic examination confirms the tissue type and tumor diagnosis. On the rare occasion when the tumor is not surgically accessible, the diagnosis must be made on the basis of location and radiologic evaluation alone.

! NURSING QUALITY ALERT
Signs of Brain Tumor in Children

The hallmark symptoms of children with brain tumors are headache and morning vomiting related to the child getting out of bed. The shift in intracranial pressure (ICP) with the change in position from lying flat (higher ICP) to standing up (lower ICP) causes the vomiting.

PATHOPHYSIOLOGY

Brain Tumors

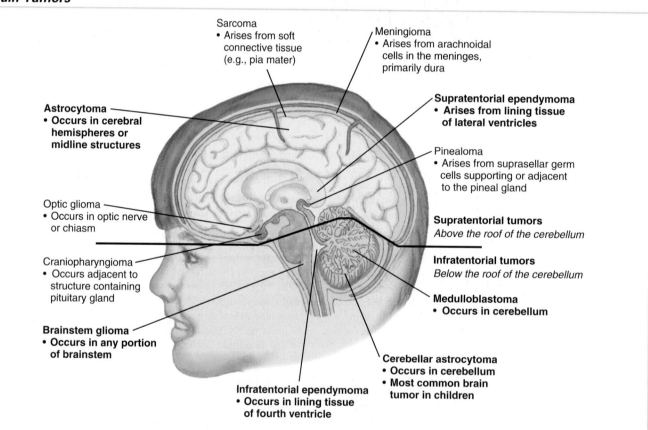

Brain tumors are classified according to cell histology and rate of tumor proliferation. Of the most commonly seen brain tumors, approximately 49% of pediatric brain tumors are astrocytomas, 15% are medulloblastomas, 15% are brainstem gliomas, 8% are craniopharyngiomas, 4% are ependymomas, and 9% other types.

The histology of brain tumors ranges from benign to highly malignant. The impact these tumors have on the brain and the clinical symptoms they produce often have more to do with the tumor size and location than with the aggressiveness of the tumor. Most astrocytomas are low grade or slow growing; however, if they persist after of treatment, they can produce significant neurologic deficits.

Kuttesch, J., Rush, S., & Ater, J. (2011). Brain tumors in childhood. In R. Kliegman, B. Stanton, J. St. Geme, et al. (Eds.), *Nelson textbook of pediatrics* (19th ed., pp. 1746-1753). Philadelphia: Elsevier Saunders.

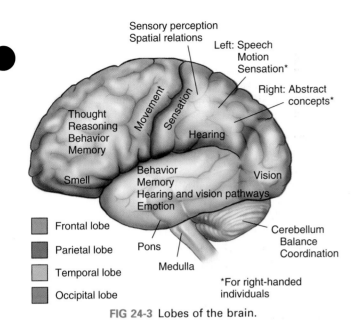

Sensory perception
Spatial relations

Left: Speech
Motion
Sensation*

Right: Abstract
concepts*

Thought
Reasoning
Behavior
Memory

Movement

Sensation

Hearing

Smell

Behavior
Memory
Hearing and vision pathways
Emotion

Vision

■ Frontal lobe

Pons

Cerebellum
Balance
Coordination

■ Parietal lobe

Medulla

■ Temporal lobe

*For right-handed
individuals

■ Occipital lobe

FIG 24-3 Lobes of the brain.

Therapeutic Management

Initial intervention for a child with a brain tumor is surgery. The goal is to remove as much of the tumor as possible while minimally disturbing the surrounding brain tissue so that the child's neurologic functioning is preserved to the highest degree possible. Complete removal of the tumor is associated with the best prognosis. In the case of a brainstem tumor or an optic pathway glioma, the risk to postoperative neurologic dysfunction outweighs the benefits of resection, so surgery is not performed.

Depending on the location of the tumor and the extent of surgical resection, a ventriculoperitoneal (VP) shunt may be inserted to relieve hydrocephalus, an excessive accumulation of CSF in the ventricles of the brain, and the symptoms associated with it (see Chapter 28). Children with tumors located above the roof of the cerebellum (supratentorial) are at risk for seizures from the tumor itself or from scar tissue formation after surgery. These children are prescribed anticonvulsants with monitoring of therapeutic levels.

The therapeutic regimen is based on the type of tumor, its location, the amount of residual tumor that remains after surgery, and the child's age. Some tumors, such as low-grade astrocytomas, require only surgery if the tumor can be completely resected. However, for malignant tumors, treatment is often multimodal involving complete surgical removal of the tumor and then radiation therapy and chemotherapy as indicated (Kuttesch et al., 2011). Radiation therapy in children younger than 5 years of age can have toxic effects on the developing brain. Use of chemotherapy has emerged in recent years as an alternative or adjunct to radiation treatment (Kuttesch et al., 2011). Imaging is performed at intervals to help determine the response to therapy. Prognostic percentages vary with the type of tumor, if all or only a portion of the tumor was resected, metastatic spread, child's age, physical status of the child, and individual responses to treatment.

Although more than 70% of children with brain tumors will be long-term survivors, most will have chronic neurologic problems as a result of the tumor and its treatment with surgery, radiation, and chemotherapy (Kuttesch et al., 2011). Problems include seizure disorders, focal motor and sensory abnormalities, learning disabilities, developmental delays, and neuroendocrine dysfunction causing growth failure and delays in the onset of puberty (Kuttesch et al., 2011). These children need ongoing medical management to control seizures and correct endocrine deficits. They will benefit from rehabilitation services and therapies as well as individualized educational programs.

NURSING CARE OF THE CHILD WITH A BRAIN TUMOR

■ Assessment

A thorough neurologic examination is paramount for any child diagnosed with a brain tumor. Knowing the location of the tumor heightens the nurse's understanding of neurologic deficits the child may have (see Figure 24-3). A psychosocial and developmental history is important to obtain, including information regarding the child's neurologic symptoms, achievement of developmental milestones in younger children, and school performance in older children. Children who have insidious loss of vision may have learned to compensate well; excellent nursing skills will be needed to identify vision loss. The nurse addresses impaired balance and coordination, brainstem dysfunction, and any loss of vision when evaluating the child's safety. The nurse should be especially vigilant when assessing for signs and symptoms of increased ICP in children who have just been diagnosed with a brain tumor, who are in the immediate postoperative period following tumor resection, and who have a VP shunt that can malfunction. Many children with brain tumors have seizures at some time during their illness, so seizure precautions should be considered even in the child with no previous history of seizures (see Chapter 28). It is essential to assess the child's nutritional status and watch for weight loss throughout treatment.

■ Nursing Diagnosis and Planning

The following nursing diagnoses and expected outcomes may be appropriate for the child with a brain tumor and the child's family:

- Acute Pain and Chronic Pain related to increased ICP.

Expected Outcome. The child will verbalize a decrease in the severity of headaches.

- Risk for Infection related to surgery or immunosuppression after chemotherapy.

Expected Outcomes. The child will remain free from signs of infection, as evidenced by body temperature within normal limits. The child and family demonstrate infection prevention measures.

- Anxiety (child and parent) related to the surgery and diagnosis.

Expected Outcome. The child and parents will exhibit decreased anxiety about the outcomes of surgery and therapy, as evidenced by verbalization of decreased stress and an increased ability to problem solve.

- Deficient Knowledge about the disease process related to unfamiliarity with the information.

Expected Outcomes. The child and parents will describe the disease process and its management.

- Disturbed Body Image related to a shaved head, hair loss, and/or neurologic deficits.

Expected Outcome. The child will demonstrate appropriate coping techniques for hair loss and changes in coordination or other abilities, as evidenced by maintaining social relationships and verbal statements indicating adaptation to the changed appearance.

Interventions

Nursing care focuses on controlling acute symptoms, preparation for surgery, and postoperative management. The family will also need education and support to cope with the significant anxiety caused by fear of the potential impact of surgery on the child's neurologic system, treatment failure, and the child's death. Preoperative teaching at the child's developmental level prepares the child and family for the potential outcomes of surgery. The child should be informed about anesthesia and should be prepared to be in the intensive care unit following surgery. (See Chapter 13 for a discussion of preoperative care.)

The child's head will be shaved before surgery. Although every effort is made to shave only as much hair as necessary, hair loss may still be traumatic for the child. The nurse should be aware of this and assist the child in verbalizing fears. Some children enjoy wearing a favorite cap or hat and make it a special event to buy a hat. The child must be prepared to wake up with a large dressing covering the head after surgery.

In addition to postoperative concerns of pain, hemorrhage, and infection, the nurse must also monitor the child for signs and symptoms of increased ICP. Increased ICP (see Chapter 28) is a risk in the postoperative period related to cerebral edema, hydrocephalus, or hemorrhage. The nurse performs and records vital signs measurements, mental status examinations, and neurologic function checks frequently after surgery. If indicators of increased ICP are noted, the nurse immediately notifies the physician and prepares the child for an evaluation, including an MRI or a CT scan. The child should not be placed in the Trendelenburg position because this may increase ICP and the risk of bleeding.

Many children return from the operating room with external ventricular shunts in place that temporarily remove CSF and reduce ICP. These external drains must be maintained at appropriate levels and CSF measured accurately. Normal CSF is colorless; bloody or discolored drainage can be a sign of contamination or bleeding and must be reported to the physician immediately (Bowden & Greenberg, 2007). Many children require placement of a permanent VP shunt because of secondary hydrocephalus.

After the child's condition has been stabilized, the child is assessed for functional deficits resulting from surgery or damage to normal brain tissue by the tumor. These deficits can be somewhat predictable if the involved area of the brain and the function of that area are known (Box 24-3). If radiation therapy is delivered, families need to be made aware of potential side effects and understand that acute side effects

will resolve over time. Chemotherapy may be delivered on an inpatient or outpatient basis; the nurse prepares the child and family for the side effects and how they are managed.

If neurologic deficits are significant and persist, rehabilitative therapy may be necessary to help the child regain function. Adequate academic support should always be considered for these children when they return to school.

Evaluation

- Are both verbal and nonverbal indications of a positive comfort level present?
- Does the child's rating on a pain assessment tool indicate decreased pain?
- Has the child remained afebrile, and do the child and family demonstrate infection prevention measures?
- Have the child and family expressed decreased levels of stress and the ability to rely on coping strategies?
- Is the family able to discuss the treatment plan and concerns related to the disease and treatment plan?
- Is the child relating with peers in the same manner as before the diagnosis and hospitalization, and is the child expressing adaptation to the changed appearance?

MALIGNANT LYMPHOMAS

Malignant lymphomas are neoplasms of lymphoid cells, a component of the immune system. Lymphomas represent 20% of childhood cancers in children younger than 20 years, making lymphomas the third most common childhood malignancy (Sandlund & Behm, 2008). Lymphomas are divided into two main types; non-Hodgkin lymphoma (NHL) and Hodgkin lymphoma.

In the United States, the average occurrence of NHL in children 19 years and younger is approximately 750 to 800 new cases per year (Waxman, Hochberg, & Cairo, 2011). NHL originates from a proliferation of either B or T lymphocytes. The three subtypes of pediatric NHL are: (1) small, noncleaved cell (Burkitt, Burkitt-like) lymphomas; (2) large-cell lymphomas; and (3) lymphoblastic lymphomas.

Hodgkin lymphoma in 15- to 19-year-olds comprises approximately 15% of all cancers seen in this age-group, accounts for 5% of all cancers seen in children 14 years and younger, and is rarely seen in children under age 10 years (Waxman et al., 2011). It represents approximately 40% of lymphomas. The presence of giant multinucleated cells (Reed-Sternberg cells) is the hallmark of Hodgkin disease.

The incidence of NHL increases gradually throughout life, unlike Hodgkin disease, which has a bimodal incidence curve (Sandlund & Behm, 2008). Because the incidence of Hodgkin disease peaks in children 15 years old and older, it accounts for a greater proportion of the lymphomas seen in older children. NHL in children younger than 5 years is uncommon.

Non-Hodgkin Lymphoma

NHL differs greatly from Hodgkin disease in its clinical behavior, pathology, mode of metastasis, and responsiveness to therapy. This disease has a rapid onset with widespread involvement at diagnosis.

Etiology

Viral, immunologic, and genetic factors may contribute to the development of NHL, although the exact cause is unknown (Waxman et al., 2011). Children with congenital immunodeficiency syndromes or acquired immunodeficiency syndrome (AIDS), as well as those who have undergone organ transplantation and have chronically

---

BOX 24-3	**POTENTIAL FUNCTIONAL DEFICITS RELATED TO A BRAIN TUMOR**

After surgery, the child should be assessed for functional deficits in the following areas:

- Gait: Look for ataxia, including head control and truncal stability
- Bilateral extremity strength and purposeful movement
- Speech
- Ability to swallow
- Vision and hearing
- Presurgical developmental task mastery
- Receptive and expressive language

If the deficits are significant, the child may need rehabilitative therapy to regain function.

suppressed immune systems, are at higher risk for developing NHL or other lymphoproliferative disorders (Sandlund & Behm, 2008).

Manifestations

Symptoms of abdominal disease include abdominal cramping, constipation, pain, anorexia, weight loss, ascites, and obstruction, with vomiting as a late sign. Painless, enlarged lymph nodes are found in the cervical or axillary region and less commonly in the inguinal area. If mediastinal disease is present, cough, respiratory distress, symptoms of bronchitis, and possibly significant tracheal deviation are seen. Bone marrow disease leads to a general decline in health and bone marrow suppression.

Diagnostic Evaluation

In addition to a physical examination looking for enlarged lymph nodes and hepatosplenomegaly, extensive laboratory work is necessary. Especially with Burkitt lymphoma, the uric acid level is often high, indicating a rapid turnover of cells.

A chest radiograph is obtained to look for mediastinal disease and tracheal deviation. The extent of disease is further evaluated with a CT scan of the neck, chest, abdomen, and pelvis; PET scans; and flow cytometry to identify the cell origin. Bone marrow aspirations and biopsies are performed to assess involvement of disease in the marrow. A lumbar puncture is performed to assess the CSF for disease. Pathologic findings are confirmed with a lymph node biopsy.

Therapeutic Management

Children with NHL, especially Burkitt lymphoma, often present in metabolic disarray because of the rapidity with which the disease progresses. These children are prone to tumor lysis syndrome from the large tumor burden and rapid tumor cell turnover, and cell death. Before chemotherapy can be started, the metabolic state must be stabilized.

In children susceptible to tumor lysis syndrome, intensive hydration with an IV fluid containing bicarbonate alkalinizes the urine to help prevent the formation of uric acid crystals, which damage the kidney. There should be no potassium in the IV fluid. Oral allopurinol is started to decrease the uric acid level. Parenteral urate oxidase (Rasburicase) may be indicated to further degrade uric acid (Taketomo et al., 2010). With the initiation of chemotherapy, serum electrolyte levels (electrolytes, calcium, magnesium, phosphorous, uric acid, and creatinine) may be checked several times a day to keep close surveillance on the child's metabolic state because these tumors respond rapidly to treatment. The urine may turn milky white as the tumor cells are filtered through the kidneys. Children who cannot be hemodynamically monitored on the general unit may be moved to the intensive care unit until metabolically stabilized.

! NURSING QUALITY ALERT

Tumor Lysis Syndrome

In tumor lysis syndrome, the intracellular contents are dumped into the extracellular fluid as the tumor cells are lysed, or killed. These intracellular contents have a different electrolyte concentration (higher potassium and phosphorus) compared with extracellular blood volume. The high concentrations of electrolytes overload the kidneys and, if the condition is not monitored and treated carefully, cause acute renal failure. Common electrolyte abnormalities in tumor lysis syndrome include hyperkalemia, hyperphosphatemia, and hypocalcemia. Tumor lysis syndrome is most common in children with leukemias who have very high WBC counts and in children with non-Hodgkin lymphomas, especially when extensive disease is present.

The primary treatment modality for all histologic classifications and stages of NHL involves multiagent chemotherapy. Surgery is used to obtain a diagnostic biopsy. In general, these lymphomas present as generalized disease, making them less amenable to treatment with radiation therapy; irradiation is reserved for emergent situations resulting from CNS disease or airway compromise. Chemotherapy is given over a 6- to 24-month period, depending on the type of lymphoma. Typically, a central venous catheter is placed to assist in delivering chemotherapy drugs. Frequent follow-up visits are made after the completion of treatment because the risk of recurrent disease is greatest immediately after therapy is stopped.

Survival rates of children with localized lymphomas approach 100%. Those children whose disease is advanced can achieve a survival rate of between 60% and 95% (Waxman et al., 2011).

NURSING CARE OF THE CHILD WITH NON-HODGKIN LYMPHOMA

■ Assessment

The parents of children with NHL will report an acute onset of symptoms that vary with the type of organ involved. Most parents will state that their child has become irritable and "just not himself." Children with metastatic disease often appear very ill. The nurse assesses lymph nodes and closely checks the respiratory system in a child with mediastinal disease, especially if the trachea is deviated. Signs of tumor lysis syndrome are considered and include subtle changes in behavior (restlessness and irritability) and changes in the sensorium. These are ominous signs indicative of electrolyte imbalances such as hyperuricemia, hyperkalemia, hyperphosphatemia, and hypocalcemia.

■ Nursing Diagnosis and Planning

The following nursing diagnoses and expected outcomes may apply to the child with NHL and the child's family:
- Ineffective Breathing Pattern related to mediastinal disease.

Expected Outcome. The child's respiratory status will remain stable, as evidenced by normal breath sounds for age and stable respiratory rate and rhythm.
- Risk for Injury related to electrolyte imbalances secondary to tumor lysis syndrome.

Expected Outcome. The child will maintain a normal fluid and electrolyte balance, as evidenced by a stable metabolic state and urine output appropriate for age.
- Risk for Infection related to the state of immunosuppression.

Expected Outcome. The child will exhibit no signs and symptoms of infection, as evidenced by normal body temperature.
- Deficient Knowledge related to unfamiliarity with the disease process.

Expected Outcomes. The child and parents will describe the disease process and its management.

■ Interventions

Initial nursing care focuses on following the physician's orders for maintaining a stable metabolic state before and during the induction phase of chemotherapy. The child undergoing induction chemotherapy should have intake and output and serum chemistry values strictly monitored. Occasionally, a child with Burkitt lymphoma will need a urinary catheter inserted for measurement of output. If a fever develops, urine and blood should be cultured to rule out an infection. The nutritional status of the child following chemotherapy induction needs careful evaluation and the child may require enteral feedings. If necessary, total parenteral nutrition may be given.

Parents will need support because the chemotherapy may initially make the child seem more ill. The nurse answers the family's questions directly and honestly. Once the child starts to recover from the initial chemotherapy, the nurse can provide more extensive education to the family about the disease and its treatment.

Consultations with child life specialists, chaplains or other religious figures, and social workers may enhance the psychosocial care of these families. Realistic expectations of therapy and of the child's response to therapy can help parents deal more effectively with their fears and anxiety (see Nursing Care Plan: The Child with Leukemia for other related nursing care).

▌Evaluation

- Has the child's respiratory status remained stable, with normal rate and rhythm and clear breath sounds?
- Is the child's urine output appropriate for age, and are electrolytes within normal range?
- Are the child's vital signs within normal limits?
- Are the parents asking questions about the disease process and the care of their child?

Hodgkin Disease

Hodgkin disease has a more indolent course than NHL. It frequently presents as localized disease. Systemic symptoms include unexplained fevers, weight loss, and night sweats. These systemic signs are used in diagnostic staging.

Etiology

The cause of Hodgkin disease is unknown. However, the possibility of an infectious agent is being investigated. Herpesvirus 6, cytomegalovirus, and Epstein-Barr virus (EBV) have been associated with Hodgkin disease, but the exact relation remains unknown. EBV readily infects Reed-Sternberg cells, and this infection can precede initiation of the malignant clone; however, this relation cannot be demonstrated in all cases (Horning, 2008). As with other cancers, no single environmental agent can be said to precipitate the disease process.

⚡ SAFETY ALERT

Prevention of Urinary Tract Infection in the Immunocompromised Child

Urinary catheters are used very infrequently in immunocompromised children because of the risk of introducing organisms into the urinary tract system.

Manifestations

Painless, firm, movable adenopathy in the cervical and supraclavicular regions is the most common presentation. Mediastinal involvement, with or without airway obstruction, occurs in two thirds of children. From 20% to 30% of children have constitutional symptoms that include fever, drenching night sweats, and weight loss. Other manifestations are hepatosplenomegaly and fatigue.

Diagnostic Evaluation

Biopsy of an involved lymph node and histologic classification of the tissue confirm the diagnosis. Laboratory tests include a CBC, renal and liver function tests, erythrocyte sedimentation rate (ESR), and serum copper and serum ferritin levels. Elevation of ESR or serum copper or ferritin level may be useful for follow-up evaluation if it correlates with disease activity at diagnosis. A gallium scan is performed to look for extent of disease. When a tumor demonstrates gallium uptake at diagnosis, a gallium scan can serve as a staging study as well as disease

response marker. PET scanning may be more sensitive and specific than CT or gallium scanning. Its use in diagnosis, staging, and follow-up surveillance imaging is being actively assessed (Horning, 2008). Chest radiography and CT of the chest, abdomen, and pelvis are performed to determine the extent of disease. Bilateral bone marrow aspirations and biopsies are done only if constitutional symptoms are present.

PATHOPHYSIOLOGY
Hodgkin Disease

Hodgkin disease originates in a single lymph node or a group of lymph nodes in the same anatomic region. Hodgkin disease is characterized by giant multinucleated cells called *Reed-Sternberg cells* that are thought to represent activated B and T lymphocytes. Hodgkin disease spreads predictably from lymph nodes to nonnodal sites such as the spleen, liver, bone, bone marrow, lungs, and mediastinum.

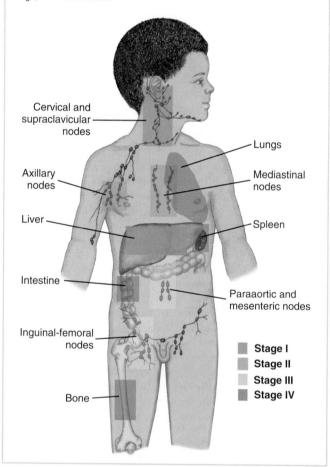

In the past, a surgical staging laparotomy was often performed. However, precise staging is less important now that most children receive systemic chemotherapy as part of their treatment. Universal staging laparotomy with splenectomy is no longer performed because of better diagnostic methods and better delivery of radiation therapy (Horning, 2008).

Some manifestations are of prognostic significance, and staging takes them into account. Children with unexplained weight loss of more than 10% of body weight in the preceding 3 months, unexplained fevers higher than 102.2° F (39° C), and night sweats are considered to have B disease as opposed to A (asymptomatic) disease. The presence of B symptoms is thought to affect prognosis negatively (Waxman et al., 2011). Four stages of the disease have been delineated, with stage I having limited disease and the most favorable prognosis.

Therapeutic Management

Therapy depends on the child's age at diagnosis, disease stage, and histologic type. If the mediastinal disease is expansive, it may compromise respiration. Radiation therapy may be used to shrink the tissue before any procedure requiring general anesthesia is performed.

Most children are treated with chemotherapy alone or chemotherapy and low-dose, involved-field radiation therapy. High-dose, extended-field radiation therapy alone may be used if the disease is detected in a single site or in older adolescents who are fully grown. Long-term survival rates of 95% or more can be expected in children with stage I or II disease and positive prognostic factors. For more advanced stages of disease, the long-term survival rate can approximate 90% (Waxman et al., 2011).

Nursing Considerations

The onset of Hodgkin disease is insidious. Frequently, when asked about activity level, children report not noticing any change until it was brought to their attention. Typically the child noticed lumps around the neck while bathing. Initial assessment of these children includes a thorough lymph node examination.

At least two thirds of children have some degree of mediastinal involvement. As with NHL, management of the airway is a concern if the child has any mediastinal disease. The nurse should assess the respiratory system for any changes in status with the child both sitting and lying down. If the airway is compromised, radiation therapy will be given locally to provide immediate relief.

Initially the nurse should prepare the child for diagnostic procedures and a surgical biopsy. A central venous catheter may be inserted at the time of diagnosis. Induction chemotherapy is begun as soon as the child is stable and staging of disease has been completed. In older children, a peripheral IV line may be placed at the time of each chemotherapy treatment to avoid a central venous catheter placement.

Education includes an explanation of the therapeutic protocol. Questions asked by the child and family should be answered honestly. Realistic expectations of response to therapy often help the child and family members cope more effectively. Hodgkin disease in first remission is treated on an outpatient basis at most centers. The nursing care is similar to that for a child with NHL.

NEUROBLASTOMA

Neuroblastoma is the most commonly diagnosed malignancy in infants and is only found in infants and children (Zage & Ater, 2011). It is an embryonal cancer of the sympathetic nervous system and presentation ranges from very aggressive tumors that are unresponsive to treatment to tumors that spontaneously regress (generally in children younger than age 12 months).

Etiology

The cause of neuroblastoma is unknown. Evidence exists that a familial form of neuroblastoma may occur; children in families with one or more affected members may be at increased risk for the development of neuroblastoma. It is also associated with certain congenital syndromes and possibly with maternal and paternal occupational exposure related to chemicals, farming items, and electronics, though no single environmental source is known to cause neuroblastoma (Zage & Ater, 2011).

Incidence

Neuroblastoma represents approximately 8% to 10% of all childhood cancers, with an annual incidence of 600 new cases in the United States (Zage & Ater, 2011). It is slightly more common in boys and in white children. The median age of presentation is 22 months, with 90% of cases diagnosed by 5 years of age (Zage & Ater, 2011).

Pathophysiology

Neuroblastoma arises from neural crest cells, which normally develop into the sympathetic nervous system and the adrenal medulla. Cells proliferate and begin to form a solid mass or tumor. These cells are immature and nonfunctional. Typically the tumor infringes and infiltrates into adjacent normal tissue and organs. Metastatic disease may be present in the lymph nodes, bone marrow, bone, liver and skin, and rarely in the lung or brain (Zage & Ater, 2011). Greater understanding of the cellular genetic makeup of this tumor has given researchers insight into prognostic indicators, which help with treatment planning.

Manifestations

The manifestations of neuroblastoma depend on the extent of disease and the location of the tumor. In most cases, a primary abdominal mass and a protuberant, firm abdomen are present. Other manifestations include impaired range of motion and mobility with pain and limping. Chest tumors may produce cough and decreased chest expansion, with respiratory compromise. Compression of the superior vena cava results in facial and periorbital edema. Spinal cord compression may cause inability to walk and impaired bowel and bladder function. Tumor infiltration may cause dark circles under the eyes, giving an appearance of "raccoon eyes." Bruising, drooping eyelids or small pupils may be evident, along with opsomyoclonus, or "dancing" eye movements and myoclonic jerks. These children act restless and uncomfortable.

Diagnostic Evaluation

The diagnostic workup includes chest radiography; CT of the chest, abdomen, and pelvis; and skeletal scintigraphy to determine the extent of disease. Bone marrow aspiration and biopsy, usually of both posterior iliac crests, are performed to evaluate marrow involvement. Tumor markers including urine catecholamine levels (homovanillic acid [HVA] and vanillylmandelic acid [VMA]) are elevated in 95% of children with neuroblastoma (Zage & Ater, 2011). In these children, serial monitoring of HVA and VMA are helpful as markers during treatment and for follow-up when treatment is complete.

Definitive diagnosis is made when tissue is obtained by biopsy. Tumor samples are sent to special reference laboratories to look at the genetic makeup of the tumor. The genetic information may reveal the aggressiveness of the tumor and help determine the prognosis and treatment plan.

Therapeutic Management

The treatment of neuroblastoma depends on the presence and extent of metastasis. The International Staging System for Neuroblastoma is used to compare patients. Staging is graded I through IV, with stage I representing localized disease and stage IV denoting distant spread. Staging criteria include the extent and location of metastases, lymph node involvement, and whether the tumor is unilateral or crosses the midline. Early-stage disease (stage I or II) without metastasis may require only surgical excision of the tumor and follow-up evaluations. Children with later-stage (stage IV) disease may undergo surgery to obtain tissue samples or to debulk a tumor for pain control.

Age at diagnosis is an important prognostic indicator. Children diagnosed before they are 1 year old have a better prognosis than children diagnosed at a later age. Approximately half of the infants diagnosed with neuroblastoma at younger than 1 year have a genetically less aggressive tumor type and may be watched carefully or treated with low-dose chemotherapy.

Treatment plans for children with advanced disease (stage III or IV) may include radiation therapy to tumor sites and systemic chemotherapy for several months. Another attempt may be made to resect the tumor after combination chemotherapy has been administered to reduce the tumor size. Autologous stem cell transplantation (ASCT) after high-dose chemotherapy has been shown to improve survival rates over chemotherapy alone (Zage & Ater, 2011). Administering the biologic modifier13-*cis*-retinoic acid orally after ASCT is used to eradicate any residual disease by decreasing proliferation and inducing differentiation in neuroblastoma cell lines (Freter & Perry, 2008). This treatment can further increase survival rates (Zage & Ater, 2011).

Children with stage I or II disease who are without poor prognostic factors have a long-term survival rate of more than 90%. The long-term survival rate for intermediate-risk children is approximately 70% to 80%. The long-term survival rate of high-risk children is approximately 25%, even with aggressive treatment (American Cancer Society, 2010a).

NURSING CARE OF THE CHILD WITH NEUROBLASTOMA

■ Assessment

Children with neuroblastoma typically appear pale, quite irritable, and uncomfortable. Parents may state that their child has wanted to be held more often than usual. Activity level and appetite are usually decreased. Because of large abdominal tumors, many have protuberant abdomens in which hard masses crossing the midline can be palpated. Range of motion and mobility are often impaired, so much so that the child cannot bear weight. If the tumor is compressing a nerve, neurologic changes may be noted. If the tumor is causing compression within the abdomen, vascular drainage may be compromised and GI obstruction may be present. Periorbital infiltration can cause characteristic ecchymosis or "raccoon eyes" (Zage & Ater, 2011).

■ Nursing Diagnosis and Planning

The following nursing diagnoses and expected outcomes may be appropriate for the child with a neuroblastoma and the child's family:

• Acute Pain related to tumor pressure.

Expected Outcome. The infant will exhibit pain relief, as evidenced by decreased crying and a relaxed body position.

• Anxiety (parents) related to a diagnosis of cancer, surgery, and the treatment plan.

Expected Outcome. The parents will express decreased anxiety about the outcomes of therapy.

• Deficient Knowledge related to unfamiliarity with the disease process and its management.

Expected Outcome. The parents will describe the disease process and its implications.

■ Interventions

Nursing care initially focuses on support of family members as they react and adjust to the diagnosis of cancer. The nurse facilitates the educational process to allay fears of the unknown. The child's initial care includes pain management, both preoperatively and postoperatively. The child with an abdominal tumor will return from surgery with a nasogastric (NG) tube in place. The nurses assesses the wound carefully for bleeding and signs of infection (see Chapter 13). In the case of tumors that are responsive to treatment, the child's condition and disposition will improve quickly.

Bowel habits may be altered because of pain, immobility, medication, surgery, and alteration in nutritional patterns. Children with large abdominal tumors may become obstructed because of tumor compression. The nurse should obtain a history of bowel habits and notify the physician if bowel habits are dramatically altered.

Management of the airway is of concern if the child has any mediastinal disease. It is critically important that the nurse monitor the child's respiratory effort, color, and pulses and place the child in a position that facilitates effective respirations.

■ Evaluation

• Has the child exhibited decreased crying and irritability?
• Does the child rest quietly and comfortably in the parent's arms and have uninterrupted periods of rest?
• Are the parents verbalizing their fears and expressing decreased anxiety?
• Are the parents asking questions related to the child's disease and treatment and seeking the support of family and friends?

OSTEOSARCOMA

Osteosarcoma (also called *osteogenic sarcoma*) is the most common primary bone malignancy in children. The symptoms of this disease in its earliest stage are almost always attributed to extremity injury or normal growing pains. Typically, unresolved pain attributed to trauma (often a sports-related injury) brings the tumor to the attention of medical personnel.

Etiology

The cause of osteosarcoma is unknown, although associations have been made between radiation therapy for other diseases and osteosarcoma. Familial tendencies have been seen, suggesting that genetic factors are involved (Arndt, 2011a).

Incidence

In the United States, the annual incidence of osteosarcoma is 5.6 new cases per 1 million children under the age of 15 years (Arndt, 2011a). The incidence of osteosarcoma peaks in the teenage years and is more common in males than in females. Osteosarcoma occurs at an earlier age in girls than in boys, which corresponds to the earlier maturation of girls (American Cancer Society, 2010b). Before adolescence, osteosarcoma is rare. If metastases are present, the lungs are the primary organ involved. Bone metastases, with "skip lesions" (tumor nodules growing outside the reactive rim but within the same bone or across a neighboring joint) are the second most common. Approximately 20% of affected individuals have metastatic disease at diagnosis (American Cancer Society, 2010b).

Pathophysiology

Osteosarcoma originates from bone-producing cells that invade the medullary canal of the bone and form a solid tumor. Incidence is higher in the most rapidly growing bones in adolescents—that is, the distal femur, proximal tibia, and proximal humerus. Since the highest risk period for osteosarcoma is during the adolescent growth spurt, there is a possible association between rapid bone growth and malignant transformation (Arndt, 2011a).

Manifestations

Manifestations of osteosarcoma include progressive, insidious, or intermittent pain at the tumor site; a palpable mass; limping, if a weight-bearing limb is affected; progressive, limited range of motion; and eventually pathologic fractures at the tumor site.

Diagnostic Evaluation

Initially radiographs of the primary site and chest are taken, and then CT or MRI and skeletal scintigraphy are performed. The CT scan includes the chest to search for pulmonary metastases, which helps stage the disease. A biopsy of the tumor must be performed with great care so that no local contamination of tissue by tumor occurs. Laboratory tests include a CBC count, chemistry levels, and serum alkaline phosphatase and lactate dehydrogenase (LDH) determinations. Surveillance alkaline phosphatase levels seem to correlate with osteoblastic activity and are therefore useful in monitoring response to therapy (Santana et al., 2008).

Therapeutic Management

The goals of therapy are to remove the tumor and prevent the spread of disease. Osteogenic sarcoma is treated with a combination of surgery and chemotherapy. After biopsy of the tumor by an orthopedic oncology surgeon, chemotherapy is administered for approximately 3 months before surgical resection of the tumor. To address the presence of microscopic disease, chemotherapy then resumes after recovery from the surgical resection and continues for an additional 9 months. Continuing chemotherapy is aimed at preventing the spread of disease by killing any microscopic tumor cells present anywhere in the body (American Cancer Society, 2010b). After resection, the tumor is sent to pathology for the determination of the percentage of tumor necrosis (how well the tumor responded to chemotherapy). Optimal response would be 100% tumor necrosis. Radiation therapy is used only for palliative pain control in advanced-stage disease, because osteosarcoma is generally unresponsive to irradiation.

Amputation was once the standard surgical intervention and is still necessary in some cases. Favorable tumor location allows specially trained orthopedic surgeons to perform a complex limb salvage operation. The affected tissue is removed with the certainty of clean margins, and limb function is preserved. The diseased bone is removed, and either bone grafts or surgically placed orthopedic devices are implanted.

The extent of disease at diagnosis, elevated LDH and alkaline phosphatase levels, and tumor necrosis found on surgical resection are the three most significant prognostic indicators. The cure rate is approximately 50% to 75% for children who respond well to chemotherapy treatment. The 20% of children with metastatic disease at diagnosis have a substantially poorer outcome (Santana et al., 2008).

NURSING CARE OF THE CHILD WITH OSTEOSARCOMA

■ Assessment

Subjective data to be gathered include a history of any injury to the affected limb and a history of discomfort. By the time children with osteosarcomas come to medical attention, they may be in considerable pain from the tumor. Warmth, erythema, and tenderness at the site of tumor are not uncommon. If the swelling is great, the skin may appear shiny and taut, with dilated blood vessels. Lung involvement is usually asymptomatic. As soon as a bone mass is identified, the child must become non–weight bearing on the affected limb (preferably using crutches). The bone surrounding the tumor is weakened by the tumor and is susceptible to a pathologic fracture, which can cause a spread of the cancer, necessitating an amputation of the affected limb.

To prepare the child for outcomes of surgery, an assessment of physical activity and sports involvement is essential, as is a psychosocial history. As for any child with cancer, body image changes, especially if the affected limb must be amputated, are of paramount importance. Preoperatively, the nurse should assess the child's values and fears and begin the process of preparing the child for postoperative lifestyle modifications.

■ Nursing Diagnosis and Planning

The following nursing diagnoses and expected outcomes may be appropriate for the child with an osteosarcoma and the child's family:

- Acute Pain related to disease process and procedures.

Expected Outcome. The child will have decreased pain, as evidenced by verbalization of adequate pain control and decreased pain rating on an age-appropriate pain assessment tool.

- Fear and Anxiety related to the potential loss or impairment of a limb and a diagnosis of cancer.

Expected Outcomes. The child and parents will express decreased fears and anxiety related to the surgery and diagnosis.

- Risk for Infection related to chemotherapy or surgery.

Expected Outcome. The child will remain free from signs and symptoms of infection, as evidenced by normal body temperature and no redness or purulent drainage from the surgical site.

- Disturbed Body Image related to loss or impairment of a limb.

Expected Outcome. The child will have a positive body image, as evidenced by a return to appropriate social situations and statements that indicate adaptation to the altered appearance and function.

- Impaired Physical Mobility related to loss or impairment of limb function.

Expected Outcome. The child will regain maximal mobility, as evidenced by ability to perform activities of daily living.

- Deficient Knowledge related to unfamiliarity with the disease process and anxiety.

Expected Outcomes. The child and parents will describe the disease process and potential postoperative adaptations.

■ Interventions

Initial care is focused on making the child comfortable. Preoperative teaching is extensive and procedure specific. If limb salvage is the procedure of choice, the surgeon and nurse will spend considerable time with the family explaining the planned procedure. The nurse reinforces preoperative and postoperative teaching.

In addition to the usual postoperative care, pain, infection, and potential hemorrhage are nursing concerns. The potential for postoperative pneumonia is increased in the child with pulmonary metastases.

If amputation occurs, phantom limb pain is a temporary condition that a child may experience. This sensation of burning, aching, or cramping in the missing limb is most distressing to the child. The child needs to be reassured that the condition is normal. Numerous pharmacologic agents are available to address postoperative neurogenic pain.

The child who undergoes amputation will be fitted with a permanent prosthesis once the surgical site has thoroughly healed. To begin to mold the stump for that, a temporary prosthesis may be used. A temporary prosthesis enables the child to maintain use and strength of surrounding muscles in preparation for the permanent device. A prosthesis can positively impact the issue of body image disturbance and enable the child to become independent in activities of daily living.

The nurse prepares the child for extensive work with physical therapists to achieve mobility with the prosthesis. Teenagers especially may become discouraged if they expect the prosthesis to enable them to immediately be fully mobile; some children may continue to have a limp or other awkward movements with the prosthesis.

The nurse must help the child verbalize feelings about changes in body image and function. The child is encouraged to participate in age-appropriate decision making concerning care. Promoting interaction with other children of the same age who have the same disease (support groups) can facilitate adaptation. It is of key importance that the nurse provide opportunities for the family to participate in the child's care as well as provide support and encouragement.

Follow-up outpatient visits need to include a careful assessment of psychosocial adjustment. Questions should include the topics of social interactions, school attendance and performance, and behavioral changes.

■ Evaluation

- Does the child have discomfort related to the surgical procedures?
- Does the child's pain rating on the pain assessment tool show decreased pain?
- Are the family and child discussing fears related to the disease and treatment?
- Is the child afebrile, and is the surgical site free of redness and purulence?
- Is the child relating with peers?
- Has the child made positive statements indicating beginning adaptation to the physical impairment?
- Is the child readily participating in physical therapy and returning to performing activities of daily living?
- Are the child and family asking questions related to the disease process?
- Do the family and child accurately describe the treatment regimen?

EWING SARCOMA

Ewing sarcoma is the second most common bone tumor seen in children. The diagnosis is often challenging to make because this disease mimics infection and may be difficult to differentiate from other malignancies. Ewing sarcoma may also manifest as a soft tissue mass. This tumor may also be referred to as a peripheral primitive neuroectodermal tumor (PPNET).

Etiology

It has been suggested that Ewing sarcoma may be caused by random factors because it has not been associated with other preexisting congenital chromosomal abnormalities. However, the cause remains unknown.

Incidence

The annual incidence of Ewing sarcoma in the United States is 2.1 per 1 million white children (Arndt, 2011a). The disease is very uncommon in African-Americans. Ewing sarcoma is rare in children younger than 5 years and yet is more common than osteosarcoma in children under age 10 years. Both Ewing sarcoma and osteosarcoma are more likely to occur in the second decade of life (Arndt, 2011a).

Pathophysiology

The diagnosis of Ewing sarcoma is made after all other solid tumors have been ruled out. Ewing sarcoma has no defining characteristics. As with osteosarcoma, this tumor invades the bone and is found most often in the flat bones of the axial skeleton such as the vertebrae, ribs, scapula, and pelvic bones. Gross metastasis is uncommon at diagnosis but does occur, most often to the lungs, bones, or bone marrow. As with osteosarcoma, microscopic disease is thought to be present early in the disease process.

Manifestations

Manifestations of Ewing sarcoma include pain, soft tissue swelling around the affected bone, and fever. If metastatic disease occurs, anorexia, fever, malaise, fatigue, and weight loss are seen. If a vertebral tumor is present, neurologic symptoms will be seen. If a rib tumor is present, respiratory symptoms may be seen.

Diagnostic Evaluation

The diagnostic workup is the same as for osteosarcoma and a biopsy is necessary to differentiate Ewing sarcoma from other neoplastic processes.

Therapeutic Management

A multidisciplinary approach with chemotherapy, surgery, and radiation is the basis of management. Treatment begins with chemotherapy to decrease the tumor bulk, followed by surgical resection of the primary tumor. Local control of the primary tumor site can be achieved with surgery or radiation therapy because this tumor is sensitive to radiation. Consideration is given to the expendability of the bone involved when surgery is a treatment option versus the potential late effects of radiation. Ribs and the proximal fibula are considered expendable and may be removed to excise the tumor without affecting function. Cure rates exceed 75% to 80% in children with small extremity tumors and no metastases (Santana et al., 2008). With gross metastasis, the cure rate is dramatically decreased.

Nursing Considerations

Nursing care is similar to that for children with osteosarcomas, with the addition of care for the child receiving radiation therapy.

RHABDOMYOSARCOMA

Rhabdomyosarcoma is a malignancy of muscle or striated tissue that most often occurs periorbitally, in the head and neck in younger children, or in the trunk and extremities in older children. Long-term survival rates vary with the child's age, the histologic subtype, and the location of the tumor.

Etiology

Although the exact cause is unknown, rhabdomyosarcoma has been associated with familial cancer syndromes.

Incidence

Rhabdomyosarcoma is the most common soft tissue malignancy in children and comprises approximately 3.5% of all pediatric cancers (Arndt, 2011b). The annual incidence in the United States is estimated at 4.3 cases per 1 million white children and 3.3 cases per 1 million African-American children. Two age-groups are predominant: children younger than 10 years and adolescents (American Cancer Society, 2010c).

Pathophysiology

There are two main histologic subtypes of rhabdomyosarcoma that occur in children. Approximately 60% of tumors are of the embryonal type and have an intermediate prognosis. Approximately 25% to 40%

of cases are of the alveolar type, which is found most often in the trunk and extremities and has the poorest prognosis. Lesions in the extremities (alveolar type) are most often found in the adolescent age-group (Arndt, 2011b).

The prognosis depends on several factors other than histologic type. If the tumor is in a location where manifestations appear early, rather than deeply buried in a body cavity, the prognosis is better because the tumor is usually found before it has metastasized. Abnormalities in the DNA content of the tumor cells have prognostic significance. Staging of the tumor is based on whether the tumor was resected completely, was resected with residual microscopic disease, was incompletely resected, or had metastasized to distant sites. Local failure is more common if the tumor cannot be completely resected.

Manifestations

The manifestations of rhabdomyosarcoma depend on the tumor location. Soft to hard, nontender, relatively immobile masses may be mistaken for a traumatic hematoma. If the lesion is periorbital, visual changes are present; the child may have ptosis, exophthalmos, or proptosis (bulging). Cranial nerve involvement may occur. If the lesion affects an extremity, range of motion will be limited. In the case of pelvic tumors, the function of organs around the tumor is disrupted.

Diagnostic Evaluation

CT, skeletal scintigraphy, and bone marrow aspiration and biopsy are performed to determine the extent of disease. The diagnosis is made after biopsy or attempted surgical resection of the tumor. A decision about treatment is made depending on the location of the tumor, histologic subtype, and the presence of distant metastases. Laboratory studies include a CBC, urinalysis, and renal and liver function tests.

Therapeutic Management

Rhabdomyosarcoma is treated with chemotherapy, surgery, and radiation therapy. Chemotherapy is used to decrease the tumor bulk and reduce the extent and morbidity of surgery. After surgical removal of the tumor, additional chemotherapy is provided. As with Ewing sarcoma, microscopic rhabdomyosarcoma is often present at the time of diagnosis. Discontinuation of chemotherapy after removal of the tumor generally results in recurrent disease. Tumor cells not removed by surgery are referred to as *residual disease*. Radiation therapy is used for children who have residual disease or whose tumor was not resectable. Only about 50% of children with metastatic disease at the time of diagnosis achieve initial remission, and of these, less than 50% are cured (Arndt, 2011b).

Follow-up care involves periodic CT or MRI studies to assess tumor response to therapy and monitor any development of disease progression. Most relapses occur within 2 years of diagnosis and during therapy, although late relapse (more than 5 years from therapy) is occasionally reported.

Nursing Considerations

Parents may relate that their first indication that something was wrong was a decreased activity level in a young child unable to verbalize pain. If the tumor is more superficially located, parents may have discovered a lump or swelling.

The physical examination findings will depend on the location of the tumor, but typically a soft to hard, nontender mass will be palpated. The surrounding lymph nodes should be palpated for enlargement, which may indicate tumor involvement. The CBC is usually normal unless the tumor has extended into bone marrow, causing a decrease in hemoglobin and platelet values.

Nursing care initially focuses on support of family members as they react and adjust to the diagnosis of cancer. Second, the nurse facilitates the educational process to allay fears of the unknown.

Postoperative care of the biopsy or surgical site involves careful observation for signs of infection, hemorrhage, and edema. If surgery involves excision of an abdominal or a pelvic tumor, the child will return from the operating room with an NG tube and possibly drains in place.

WILMS TUMOR

Wilms tumor is the most common renal tumor in children. Much research has been done on this disease, and the subsequent changes in therapy have resulted in improved outcomes. Prognosis is related to stage of disease at diagnosis, histopathologic features of the tumor, and child's age.

Etiology

Most Wilms tumors occur in children with no unusual physical features and no family history of the disease. These are considered "sporadic" cases. In approximately 1% to 2% of children with this disease, there is a genetic predisposition and familial occurrence. Certain genes for Wilms tumor have been identified (Anderson, Dhamne, & Huff, 2011). Wilms tumor can occur in one or both kidneys; bilateral disease is more common in familial cases than in sporadic cases. Though the cause of Wilms tumor is unknown, it has been associated with a variety of childhood syndromes and congenital anomalies including aniridia (absence of the irises), hemihypertrophy, cryptorchidism, and hypospadias (see Chapter 20).

Incidence

Approximately 8 new cases per 1 million children under age 15 years are diagnosed annually, representing 6% of childhood cancers (Anderson et al., 2011). Most children are diagnosed between the ages of 2 to 5 years; however, Wilms tumor is seen in neonates, adolescents, and adults. Bilateral Wilms tumors are seen in 7% of pediatric cases (Anderson et al., 2011).

Pathophysiology

Wilms tumor arises from the renal parenchyma of the kidney. Categories of Wilms tumor are based on favorable and unfavorable histologic findings; children with favorable histologic findings (the majority of children with Wilms tumor) have a better prognosis (Anderson et al., 2011). At the initial diagnosis, the disease is usually local, but metastasis to other organs occasionally occurs. The lungs are the most common site of metastasis. As with other tumors, a staging system directs treatment.

Manifestations

The most common clinical presentation of Wilms tumor is an asymptomatic, mobile, abdominal mass discovered by the parent or other caregiver while bathing the child or by a primary care provider during a routine physical examination. Additional manifestations include microscopic or gross hematuria, hypertension, abdominal pain, fatigue, anemia, and fever.

Diagnostic Evaluation

The diagnosis can be suspected from data in the child's history. Abdominal ultrasonography is the initial study done to detect a solid intrarenal mass. Abdominal CT or MRI, chest radiography, and chest CT are performed to further evaluate extent of disease. Laboratory tests include a CBC, electrolyte levels, liver and kidney function tests, and urinalysis. A definitive diagnosis is made at the time of surgery on the basis of pathologic findings. Palpation or any pressure on the tumor before surgery must be avoided to prevent possible rupture and spillage of tumor cells into the peritoneum.

Therapeutic Management

Treatment for Wilms tumor consists of surgery and chemotherapy alone or in combination with radiation therapy. In most cases the tumor can be completely removed by surgical resection at the time of diagnosis. During surgery, the surgeon is careful to prevent rupture of the tumor and spillage, which might necessitate more aggressive treatment (Anderson et al., 2011). In a few cases, complete surgical resection is considered too great a risk at the time of diagnosis and only a biopsy is performed to determine pathology. The goal of the initial chemotherapy treatments in these children is to reduce the tumor size before definitive surgery. All children receive chemotherapy after the tumor is surgically removed. Radiation therapy is added to the treatment of larger, more extensive tumors or those with an unfavorable histologic classification.

Survival rates for children with Wilms tumors are higher than rates for children with many other forms of cancer. Histologic features remain the most important determinant of prognosis. Five-year survival rates approach 90% for children with favorable tumor histology (Santana et al., 2008).

❗ NURSING QUALITY ALERT
Assessing the Child with a Wilms Tumor

The tumor mass should not be palpated during the assessment because of the risk of rupturing the protective capsule. Excessive manipulation can cause seeding of the tumor and spread of cancerous cells.

NURSING CARE OF THE CHILD WITH WILMS TUMOR

▪ Assessment

Parents often report that when bathing or dressing their child they noticed the child's stomach seemed swollen. Some parents state that the diapers no longer fit easily around the child's abdomen. More often than not, the child's activity level and appetite have not changed. Except for a palpable abdominal mass that usually does not cross the midline, the child's physical examination is normal.

▪ Nursing Diagnosis and Planning

The following nursing diagnoses and expected outcomes apply to the child with Wilms tumor and the child's family:
- Anxiety related to surgery with nephrectomy.

Expected Outcome. The child and parents will express decreased anxiety about the outcome of surgery.
- Risk for Infection related to surgical interventions.

Expected Outcome. The child will exhibit no signs and symptoms of infection, as evidenced by normal body temperature, intact incision site without redness and swelling, and absence of purulent drainage.
- Deficient Knowledge related to unfamiliarity with the disease process and treatment plan.

Expected Outcomes. The child and parents will describe the disease process and treatment plan.
- Risk for Deficient Fluid Volume related to having only one kidney postoperatively.

Expected Outcome. The child will demonstrate fluid balance, as evidenced by moist mucous membranes, normal electrolyte and urine values, and hourly urine output appropriate for age.

▪ Interventions

Because the child usually feels well, nursing care initially focuses on preoperative teaching for the parents and child. The nurse places a sign on the child's bed warning against palpating the abdomen. A nephrectomy is a serious surgical procedure, and family members will have anxiety about the child losing a kidney. Nurses must offer support and reassurance.

Postoperatively, monitor the child for GI activity, bowel sounds, stool production, abdominal distention, signs and symptoms of infection, hemorrhage, and changes in blood pressure. Careful assessment of urine output by the remaining kidney is essential. Intake and output are precisely measured and totaled at least every 4 hours. These children will probably return from surgery with an NG tube in place.

Once the tumor has been staged, the child is assigned to the appropriate therapeutic protocol. Teaching should center on the sequencing of tests and drugs on that protocol. The nurse provides support to the child and family and assesses their coping skills throughout the course of outpatient chemotherapy.

▪ Evaluation

- Are the parents and child using coping skills and mobilizing support systems?
- Has the child remained afebrile?
- Is the incision site dry and intact and free from redness, swelling, and purulent drainage?
- Is blood pressure within normal limits for age?
- Does the child have moist mucous membranes, are electrolytes and urinalysis within normal limits, and is hourly urine output appropriate for age?
- Is the family asking questions and sharing concerns and fears?

RETINOBLASTOMA

Retinoblastoma is a rare, malignant tumor of the embryonic neural retina. This tumor of the eye is found only in children. Observant parents may bring this disease to the attention of the physician when they look at a photograph and see a white reflection (leukocoria) in one of the child's eyes instead of the normal red color when the camera flash is reflected off the retina.

Etiology

Retinoblastoma is thought to result from a sequence of genetic mutations. The majority of these genetic mutations are sporadic, occurring within a single retinal cell that then multiplies to form the tumor. Hereditary, or familial, retinoblastoma occurs in individuals who have a germline mutation present. The mutation places the child at high risk of developing retinoblastoma, as well as other associated malignancies. A second mutation occurs in one or more of the retinal cells, which then multiply to form a tumor. Advances in genetic studies of this disease have led to genetic research on other forms of childhood cancer.

Incidence

Retinoblastoma represents 4% of all pediatric cancers. Forty percent of retinoblastomas are the hereditary form, and 60% are the non-hereditary form (Santana et al., 2008). The majority of children (60% to 75%) have unilateral involvement. Over 90% of cases are seen in children less than 5 years of age; the median age at diagnosis is about 2 years (Zage & Herzog, 2011).

Pathophysiology

The human retina does not reach maturation until approximately age 3 years. During this early, differentiating process, cells are at risk for abnormal division and neoplasia. The tumor develops on the retina, growing inward toward the vitreous humor or out toward the subretinal space. Retinoblastoma can develop at a single site or as multiple independent tumors that originate within the globe of the eye. The process of cells breaking off from the main mass and forming additional independent tumors is called *seeding*. If diagnosis is delayed these tumors can extend down the optic nerve and spread to CNS sites outside the eye (Zage & Herzog, 2011).

Manifestations

The most common findings of retinoblastoma are leukocoria and strabismus resulting from vision loss. In general, young children will not report vision loss limited to one eye. Manifestations may also include pain, redness, and inflammation of the eye.

Diagnostic Evaluation

Leukocoria or strabismus discovered by the parent or on a routine physical examination results in a referral to an ophthalmologist. A funduscopic examination with the child under general anesthesia is the best means of diagnosing and monitoring retinoblastoma. Ultrasound imaging confirms that the retinoblastoma tumors are present and determines their thickness and height. CT or MRI of the eyes, orbits, and brain is performed to evaluate the tumors within the eyes and search for extraocular spread. Skeletal scintigraphy, bone marrow aspiration and biopsy, and lumbar puncture generally are not necessary unless clinical evidence of metastasis is present (Santana et al., 2008).

Therapeutic Management

As with other cancers, a staging system has been developed to standardize descriptions of extent of disease confined to the eye and those tumors that have spread outside the eye and to other parts of the body. This system directs treatment and indicates prognosis.

The goals of treatment for retinoblastoma are to save the child's life and preserve the eye with useful vision. Treatment decisions are based on the size of the tumor and if it is confined to the eye or has spread to other parts of the body. Enucleation, removal of the eye, is becoming less frequent with the successful use of focal therapies (cryotherapy or laser photocoagulation) alone for small lesions or in combination with multiagent chemotherapy for larger tumors (Zage & Herzog, 2011). External-beam radiation therapy can be considered if chemotherapy plus focal therapy fails. Radiation can lead to orbital deformities and increased risk of secondary malignancies in children with familial retinoblastoma.

Enucleation is performed if there is no chance the child will have useful vision in the affected eye, if the tumor is unresponsive to nonsurgical treatment, or if the tumor recurs (Zage & Herzog, 2011). When enucleation is performed, the child does not require any further therapy and is monitored closely for tumor recurrence with serial examinations.

Since intraocular penetration of systemic chemotherapy agents is poor and the tumors can develop multidrug resistance, alternative treatment options are under investigation. These include use of new chemotherapy agents (topotecan) and infusing chemotherapy drugs directly into periocular and ophthalmic arteries (Zage & Herzog, 2011). The prognosis for children with retinoblastoma (confined in the orbit) is excellent, with a 5-year survival rate of 95% (Zage & Herzog, 2011). Retinoblastoma that extends to extraocular sites is associated with a poor prognosis. Routine eye examinations for children under age 7 years can result in early detection of a tumor before it spreads and successful treatment (Zage & Herzog, 2011).

NURSING CARE OF THE CHILD WITH RETINOBLASTOMA

■ Assessment

Except for leukocoria (a whitish reflex in the pupillary area), the findings on physical examination may be normal. The nurse assesses for strabismus, esotropia, exotropia, or decreased vision (See Chapter 31). The child may have compensated for loss of vision in one eye; therefore, the nurse must be very astute when assessing vision in these children.

■ Nursing Diagnosis and Planning

The following nursing diagnoses and expected outcomes apply to the child with retinoblastoma and the child's family:

- Anxiety (child and family) related to cancer, enucleation, and fear of blindness.

Expected Outcome. The child and family will express decreased anxiety about outcomes of therapy.

- Risk for Injury related to visual changes caused by the tumor or enucleation.

Expected Outcome. The child will develop compensatory mechanisms for vision, as evidenced by ability to safely perform activities of daily living.

- Deficient Knowledge related to unfamiliarity with the disease process and treatment.

Expected Outcomes. The child and parents will describe the disease process and the treatment plan and will demonstrate use of any prosthetic device, if required.

■ Interventions

Nursing care initially focuses on support of family members as they react and adjust to the diagnosis of cancer. Second, the nurse facilitates the educational process so families are informed of what to expect, decreasing fear and anxiety.

Postoperative care of the enucleated orbit entails careful observations for signs of infection, hemorrhage, and edema. The child will wear a patch over the socket for approximately 1 week postoperatively. To preserve the shape of the orbit for prosthesis, which will be fitted 5 to 6 weeks after surgery, a conformer is placed in the orbit. Nursing interventions include teaching the parents (and child if old enough) how to remove, clean, and reinsert first the conformer and then the prosthesis.

The nurse can reassure parents that children can generally accommodate to vision in only one eye. Protective eyewear must be worn when the child is participating in sports or other potentially hazardous activities, to protect the remaining eye.

Whatever the extent of involvement by tumor or the treatment modality used, careful follow-up with retinal examinations performed with the child under anesthesia and by CT, are indicated. Genetic counseling is recommended. If the retinoblastoma is found to be inherited, siblings should be periodically examined.

Children with familial retinoblastoma have a high incidence of developing second malignancies (primarily osteosarcoma) later in life because of the genetic origin of the disease. Although no specific screening is recommended, signs and symptoms should be carefully evaluated with a high index of suspicion.

■ Evaluation

• Are the child and family verbalizing fears and demonstrating a decrease in anxiety?
• Is the child able to compensate for loss of vision and safely continue daily activities?
• Is the child able to relate to peers and family?
• Are the child and family able to describe the disease and the treatment plan and demonstrate proper care of any prosthetic device?

RARE TUMORS OF CHILDHOOD

Several tumors not mentioned in this chapter occur infrequently in the pediatric population. These include soft tissue sarcomas other than rhabdomyosarcoma, primary tumors of the liver (e.g., hepatoblastoma and hepatocellular carcinoma), and gonadal (ovarian and testicular cancer) and extragonadal germ cell tumors. Carcinomas, melanomas, and primary cancer of the lungs are a few of the cancers seen in adults that are exceptionally rare in children. Many of the key principles of nursing care—pain management, nutrition, comfort, infection control, and emotional support—remain constant for all pediatric cancer diagnoses.

KEY CONCEPTS

• The signs and symptoms of childhood cancer vary according to the child's age, the type of tumor, and the extent of the disease.
• Childhood cancer is difficult to diagnose because most early symptoms may be attributed to common childhood illnesses.
• The decision to use allogeneic bone marrow, autologous peripheral blood stem cells, or umbilical cord blood stem cells is based on the disease process being treated and availability of hematopoietic cells.
• Nursing care of children with bone marrow transplants focuses on preventing infection until the marrow engrafts and WBCs are produced. All organ systems must be monitored for GVHD and toxicities from pretransplant chemotherapy and radiation.
• Biologic response modifiers are naturally occurring substances found in the body that influence the immune system.

• Chemotherapy is nonselective in its cytotoxic effect.
• Fatigue is a common side effect of radiation therapy; children may need longer or more frequent rest periods.
• Children receiving chemotherapy or radiation are at risk for breakdown of mouth and anal mucous membranes. Meticulous mouth and anal care should be provided. No rectal temperatures and limited use of oral thermometers are indicated.
• After surgical removal of a brain tumor, the child is at risk for increased intracranial pressure related to edema, hydrocephalus, or hemorrhage. The nurse should frequently check vital signs, mental status, and neurologic status.
• The abdomen of a child with Wilms tumor should not be palpated, as this may lead to rupture of the protective capsule and seeding of the tumor.

REFERENCES

American Cancer Society. (2009). *Childhood cancer: Late effects of cancer treatment.* Retrieved from www.cancer.org/Treatment/ChildrenandCancer/WhenYourChildHasCancer/childhood-cancer-late-effects-of-cancer-treatment.

American Cancer Society. (2010a). *Brain and spinal cord tumors in children.* Retrieved from www.cancer.org/acs/groups/cid/documents/webcontent/003089-pdf.pdf.

American Cancer Society. (2010b). *Osteosarcoma.* Retrieved from www.cancer.org/acs/groups/cid/documents/webcontent/003129-pdf.pdf.

American Cancer Society. (2010c). *Rhabdomyosarcoma.* Retrieved from www.cancer.org/acs/groups/cid/documents/webcontent/003136-pdf.pdf.

Anderson, P., Dhamne, C., & Huff, V. (2011). Wilms tumor. In R. Kliegman, B. Stanton, J. St. Geme, et al. (Eds.), *Nelson textbook of pediatrics* (19th ed., pp. 1757-1760). Philadelphia: Elsevier Saunders.

Arndt, C. (2011a). Malignant tumors of bone. In R. Kliegman, B. Stanton, J. St. Geme, et al. (Eds.), *Nelson textbook of pediatrics* (19th ed., pp. 1763-1766). Philadelphia: Elsevier Saunders.

Arndt, C. (2011b). Soft tissue sarcoma. In R. Kliegman, B. Stanton, J. St. Geme, et al. (Eds.), *Nelson textbook of pediatrics* (19th ed., pp. 1760-1762). Philadelphia: Elsevier Saunders.

Asselin, B. (2011). Epidemiology of childhood and adolescent cancer. In R. Kliegman, B. Stanton, J. St. Geme, et al. (Eds.), *Nelson textbook of pediatrics* (19th ed., pp. 1725-1728). Philadelphia: Elsevier Saunders.

Association of Pediatric Hematology/Oncology Nurses. (2011). *Pediatric chemotherapy and biotherapy provider program.* Retrieved from www.apon.org/education/ped.cfm.

Bleyer, A., & Ritchey, A. K. (2011). Principles of treatment. In R. Kliegman, B. Stanton, J. St. Geme, et al. (Eds.), *Nelson textbook of pediatrics* (19th ed., pp. 1731-1732). Philadelphia: Elsevier Saunders.

Bowden, V., & Greenberg, C. (2007). *Pediatric nursing procedures* (2nd ed.). Philadelphia: Lippincott Williams & Wilkins.

Campana, D., & Pui, C.-H. (2008). Childhood leukemia. In M. Abeloff, J. Armitage, J. Niederhuber, et al. (Eds.), *Abeloff's clinical oncology* (4th ed., pp. 2139-2170). Philadelphia: Elsevier.

Erickson, J. (2010). Patterns of fatigue in adolescents receiving chemotherapy. *Oncology Nursing Forum, 37*(4), 444-455.

Freter, C. E., & Perry, M. C. (2008). Systemic treatment. In M. Abeloff, J. Armitage, J. Niederhuber, et al. (Eds.), *Abeloff's clinical oncology* (4th ed., pp. 449-484). Philadelphia: Elsevier.

Gerow, L., Conejo, P., Alonzo, A., et al. (2010). Creating a curtain of protection: Nurses' experiences of grief following a patient death. *Journal of Nursing Scholarship, 42*(2), 122-129.

Hinds, P. S., Hockenberry, M. J., Gattuso, J. S., et al. (2007). Dexamethasone alters sleep and fatigue in pediatric patients with acute lymphoblastic leukemia. *American Cancer Society, 110*(10), 2321-2330.

Horning, S. J. (2008). Hodgkin's lymphoma. In M. Abeloff, J. Armitage, J. Niederhuber, et al. (Eds.), *Abeloff's clinical oncology* (4th ed., pp. 2353-2370). Philadelphia: Elsevier.

Kuttesch, J., Rush, S., & Ater, J. (2011). Brain tumors in childhood. In R. Kliegman, B. Stanton, J. St. Geme, et al. (Eds.), *Nelson textbook of pediatrics* (19th ed., pp. 1746-1753). Philadelphia: Elsevier Saunders.

Leukemia and Lymphoma Society. (2010). *Leukemia facts and statistics.* Retrieved from www.leukemia-lymphoma.org/attachments/National/br_1285360923.pdf.

Maity, A., Pruitt, A., & Phillips, P. (2008). Cancer of the central nervous system. In M. Abeloff, J. Armitage, J. Niederhuber, et al. (Eds.), *Abeloff's clinical oncology* (4th ed., pp. 1075-1136). Philadelphia: Elsevier.

National Cancer Institute. (2010). *PDQ® Late effects of treatment for childhood cancer.* Retrieved from http://cancer.gov/cancertopics/pdq/treatment/lateeffects/HealthProfessional.

National Center for Complementary and Alternative Medicine. (2010). *Selecting a complementary and alternative medical (CAM) practitioner.* Retrieved from http://nccam.nih.gov/health/decisions/D346.pdf.

Sandlund, J., & Behm, F. (2008). Childhood lymphoma. In M. Abeloff, J. Armitage, J. Niederhuber, et al. (Eds.), *Abeloff's clinical oncology* (4th ed., pp. 2171-2190). Philadelphia: Elsevier.

Santana, V., Rodriguez-Galindo, C., Dome, J., & Spunt, S. (2008). Pediatric solid tumors. In M. Abeloff, J. Armitage, J. Niederhuber, et al. (Eds.), *Abeloff's clinical oncology* (4th ed., pp. 2075-2130). Philadelphia: Elsevier Saunders.

Taketomo, C., Hodding, J., & Kraus, D. (2010). *Pediatric dosage handbook* (17th ed.). Hudson, OH: Lexi-Comp.

Tubergen, D., Bleyer, A., & Ritchey, K. (2011). The leukemias. In R. Kliegman, B. Stanton, J. St. Geme, et al. (Eds.), *Nelson textbook of pediatrics* (19th ed., pp. 1732-1739). Philadelphia: Elsevier Saunders.

Velardi, A., & Locatelli, F. (2011). Hematopoietic stem cell transplantation. In R. Kliegman, B. Stanton, J. St. Geme, et al. (Eds.), *Nelson textbook of pediatrics* (19th ed., pp. 757-763). Philadelphia: Elsevier Saunders.

Waxman, I., Hochberg, J., & Cairo, M. (2011). Lymphoma. In R. Kliegman, B. Stanton, J. St. Geme, et al. (Eds.), *Nelson textbook of pediatrics* (19th ed., pp. 1739-1746). Philadelphia: Elsevier Saunders.

Zage, P., & Ater, J. (2011). Neuroblastoma. In R. Kliegman, B. Stanton, J. St. Geme, et al. (Eds.), *Nelson textbook of pediatrics* (19th ed., pp. 1753-1757). Philadelphia: Elsevier Saunders.

Zage, P., & Herzog, C. (2011). Retinoblastoma. In R. Kliegman, B. Stanton, J. St. Geme, et al. (Eds.), *Nelson textbook of pediatrics* (19th ed., pp. 1768-1769). Philadelphia: Elsevier Saunders.

The Child with
Major Alterations in Tissue Integrity

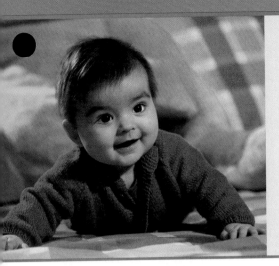

LEARNING OBJECTIVES

After studying this chapter, you should be able to:

- Describe the anatomy and physiology of normal skin.
- Contrast characteristics of the neonate's, child's, and adult's skin.
- Identify the manifestations of common skin disorders seen in infants and children.
- Discuss the management of skin disorders seen frequently in children, such as bacterial, fungal, and viral infections; infestations; inflammatory disorders; acne vulgaris; and insect bites and stings.

- Discuss common causes of burns in children and the prevention of burn injuries.
- Analyze the implications of burn injuries in children.
- Discuss the classifications of depth, extent, and severity of a burn injury.
- Describe the therapeutic management and nursing care of children with minor burns.
- Apply the nursing process to the care of infants and children with skin disorders.

CLINICAL REFERENCE

REVIEW OF THE INTEGUMENTARY SYSTEM

Knowledge of integumentary structure and function is necessary to understand the changes that occur with disease. There are a number of important differences between the skin of infants and young children and that of adults.

The skin has five major functions: (1) to protect the deeper tissues from injury, drying, and invasion by foreign matter; (2) to regulate temperature; (3) to aid in excretion of water; (4) to aid in production of vitamin D; and (5) to initiate the sensations of touch, pain, heat, and cold.

The skin is composed of two principal layers: the outer epidermis and the inner supportive dermis. Beneath these layers is the subcutaneous layer, which is composed largely of adipose tissue.

The epidermis is nonvascular stratified epithelium. It is divided into two major layers. The outermost layer, the stratum corneum, is a tough,

horny collection of dead keratinized cells that have migrated up from the underlying layers. Keratin, a fibrous protein, is also the principal component of nails and hair. Skin cells are constantly being shed and replaced with new cells from the layers below.

The stratum basale, or basal cell layer, anchors the epidermis to the dermis. It contains dividing, undifferentiated cells that migrate upward toward the stratum corneum, differentiating into keratinocytes on their way. Epidermal replacement is relatively rapid; the epidermis is completely replaced about every 4 weeks. The stratum basale also contains melanocytes—the source of melanin, the pigment that gives skin its color.

The dermis, composed of tough connective tissue, contains lymphatics and nerves. The highly vascular dermis nourishes the epidermis.

Appendages from the epidermis—sebaceous glands, sweat glands, and hair follicles—are embedded in the dermis. The sebaceous glands

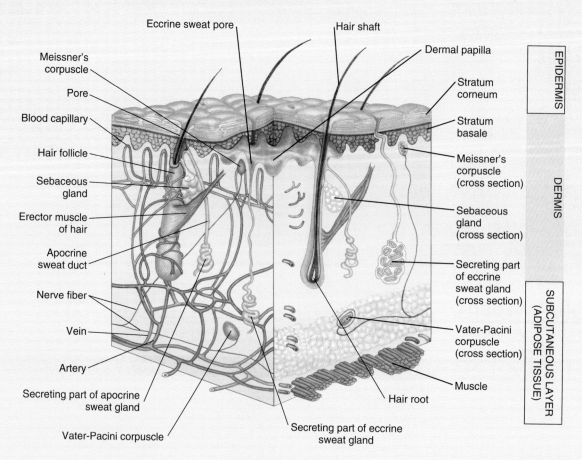

Eccrine sweat pore

Hair shaft

Dermal papilla

Meissner's corpuscle

Pore

Blood capillary

Hair follicle

Sebaceous gland

Erector muscle of hair

Apocrine sweat duct

Nerve fiber

Vein

Artery

Secreting part of apocrine sweat gland

Vater-Pacini corpuscle

Secreting part of eccrine sweat gland

Hair root

Muscle

Stratum corneum

Stratum basale

Meissner's corpuscle (cross section)

Sebaceous gland (cross section)

Secreting part of eccrine sweat gland (cross section)

Vater-Pacini corpuscle (cross section)

EPIDERMIS

DERMIS

SUBCUTANEOUS LAYER (ADIPOSE TISSUE)

Cross Section of the Skin

arise from the hair follicles and produce sebum, which lubricates the epidermis and is slightly bacteriostatic. Sebaceous glands are particularly abundant on the face and scalp. Hormones influence their activity, with testosterone increasing secretion and estrogen suppressing it.

There are two types of sweat glands. The eccrine sweat glands open directly onto the skin surface and produce sweat, which evaporates to reduce body temperature. Eccrine sweat glands are widely distributed over the body and are functionally mature by 2 months of age. The apocrine sweat glands produce a thick, milky secretion and open onto hair follicles. They are located mainly in the axillary and genital areas and become active during puberty.

Each hair is composed of a shaft and a root, which lie in a deep cavity of dermal cells called the hair follicle. There are several types of hair. Lanugo is the fine first hair that covers the body during fetal life and generally disappears before or shortly after birth. It is replaced by fine, nonpigmented vellus hair. Terminal hair covers all the ordinarily hairy parts of the body; it is coarse, long, and pigmented.

The subcutaneous layer, composed of fat cells, underlies the dermis. Adipose tissue helps cushion and insulate underlying structures.

PEDIATRIC DIFFERENCES IN THE SKIN

- The newborn's epidermis is thinner than that of adults. This results in increased permeability to topical agents and increased water loss through the skin.
- The ratio of skin surface area to body volume is greater in infants and small children than in adults, contributing to the risk of greater absorption through the skin. Topical medications should not be used without a physician's order.
- Premature infants have a proportionally greater body surface area than older infants and children, which increases evaporative fluid losses. Premature infants also have fewer cell attachments, which increases the tendency to blister.
- Eccrine glands do not reach mature function until age 2 or 3 years, making infants and young toddlers less able to regulate body temperature.
- Infants have fewer melanocytes than adults, which increases photosensitivity.
- IgA, secreted by the epithelial cells of the mucous membranes, does not reach adult levels until age 2 to 5 years. This makes the infant less resistant to organisms such as those occurring on the hands or other objects the infant might mouth.
- Hormonal changes during adolescence increase sebum production, which contributes to acne vulgaris.

Modified from Cohen, B. (2005). *Pediatric dermatology* (3rd ed., p. 15.). Baltimore: Elsevier Mosby.

The skin is a sensitive indicator of a child's general health. Skin disorders are among the most common health problems in children. They may cause pain, *pruritus*, or changes in local sensation. Because the skin is visible and its disorders are often disfiguring, skin disorders can cause emotional and psychological stress for the child and family. Whether it is the discomfort and stress produced by an infant's eczema or the emotional upset caused by an adolescent's acne, these disorders can influence the child's psychological and social development.

Nurses caring for children are in a unique position to assess the condition of children's skin and to help children and families cope with skin disorders. Nurses can play an important role by teaching parents and children strategies to maintain healthy skin and prevent future skin problems.

COMMON VARIATIONS IN THE SKIN OF NEWBORN INFANTS

Parents typically inspect every inch of their newborn infant's skin and continue to attend closely to variations in the skin of older infants. Regardless of whether the parent mentions it, the nurse may be sure the family is aware of spots, bumps, or rashes on the baby. Families frequently worry needlessly about skin lesions on infants, and the nurse can ease anxieties by pointing out and explaining the meaning and natural history of common skin variations.

COMMON BIRTHMARKS

Most birthmarks are composed of cells of one or more of the skin's normal elements. Any of the skin's components can produce a birthmark, including melanocytes, blood vessels, epidermal cells, connective tissue, and hair follicles. The great majority of birthmarks are benign, although some can signal congenital syndromes, some can be associated with an increased risk for malignancy, and others can interfere with function or be disfiguring.

Etiology

Port-wine stains are the result of capillary malformation, whereas hemangiomas result from the proliferation of dilated capillaries and endothelial cells of the capillary linings. Salmon patches (nevus simplex) represent distended dermal capillaries and are believed to result from persistent fetal circulation. Mongolian spots are not vascular but the result of collections of pigment deep in the dermis. They occur as a result of arrested migration of melanocytes from the neural crest to the skin during embryonic development. Café-au-lait spots, light-brown pigmented areas, can appear anywhere on an infant's body. Six or more of these lesions, if larger than 5 mm in diameter, suggest an underlying disorder, such as neurofibromatosis, Noonan syndrome, or McCune-Albright syndrome.

Incidence

Vascular birthmarks are extremely common, with most references estimating an incidence of occurrence in at least 20% to 40% of neonates. Port-wine stains occur in 3 in 1000 live births (Vascular Birthmarks Foundation, 2010), and about 1% to 2% of all newborn infants have hemangiomas (Morelli, 2011). The most common vascular lesion is the salmon patch, which some references estimate to occur in as many as 40% of neonates. The incidence of mongolian spots is proportional to the depth of the baby's pigmentation. As many as 80% of African-American, Asian, and American Indian infants are born with mongolian spots. Fewer than 10% of white infants have mongolian spots (Morelli, 2011).

Manifestations

The port-wine stain is present at birth. At first it is only faintly colored and flat, but it becomes darker as the child grows. In some cases, underlying bone and tissue may enlarge as well. The port-wine stain is permanent, and by middle age, the mark may be dark purple and rough or nodular. Hemangiomas, on the other hand, are not usually visible at birth but appear during the first few weeks of life and then grow during the first year. Generally, they begin to disappear spontaneously after 1 year of age and are gone by age 5 or 6 years. The salmon patch is a flat, pink, irregular-shaped spot on the nape of the neck, on the forehead, between the eyes, on the eyelids, or around the nasolabial folds. Commonly called "stork bites" or "angel kisses," these lesions are benign and usually fade during the first year of life. Salmon patches typically appear darker when the child is crying. Mongolian spots are present at birth and appear as flat, gray-green or blue lesions similar to bruises. They are most commonly distributed on the lumbosacral regions or buttocks, although they can appear on any part of the body. Mongolian spots generally fade completely by the time the child is 4 to 5 years old.

Diagnostic Evaluation

The appearance of most birthmarks is sufficient to make a diagnosis, although biopsy and histologic evaluation are definitive. Rarely, some hemangiomas are signs of more serious underlying disorders. Worrisome hemangiomas include those with large, segmented facial distributions, those with a beard distribution, and those that involve the gluteal cleft. Magnetic resonance imaging is typically performed to rule out underlying anomalies (Chan, Haggstrom, Drolet et al., 2008).

Therapeutic Management

Other than education, treatment for salmon patches and mongolian spots is not indicated. Treatment for port-wine stains is not indicated in the neonatal period, but their identification should prompt evaluation for associated congenital syndromes, such as Sturge-Weber, Beckwith-Wiedemann, and Klippel-Trénaunay syndromes. Conservative management of port-wine stains in older children includes instructions in concealing the lesions with makeup and psychotherapy if needed. Pulsed dye laser therapy is the treatment of choice for darker port-wine stains (Morelli, 2011).

The treatment for hemangiomas includes simple observation as the lesion involutes on its own, pharmacotherapy, surgical excision, radiation, and laser therapy. Active intervention is reserved for hemangiomas that interfere with function, such as those that obstruct the nose, mouth, or eyes or lesions that tend to ulcerate and bleed frequently. Pharmacologic approaches include injection of steroids into the lesion, oral steroids, and topical imiquimod. The argon laser tends to relieve the symptoms of ulcerated hemangiomas in a matter of days, and involution typically follows. A rapidly growing, deep hemangioma may be a sign of Kasabach-Merritt syndrome, a syndrome in which the child experiences a coagulation disorder that results in thrombocytopenia, severe anemia, and collecting of platelets within the hemangioma. This may be life threatening (Morelli, 2011).

Nursing Considerations

Assess the child's entire body for distribution, size, and shape of lesions. Assess hemangiomas for symptoms such as ulceration or bleeding and for potential to obstruct function. Assess the extent of the parents' knowledge regarding the infant's birthmarks.

Parents are frequently anxious about newborn infants' skin lesions, and it is not unusual to discover that parents already have acquired misinformation from friends and family members about the meaning and prognosis of birthmarks. Common anxiety-provoking beliefs include the ideas that prominent lesions are malignant or that the mother caused the lesions by careless behaviors during her pregnancy.

The parents should receive a simple, scientific explanation for the skin lesions and instructions regarding the usual skin care for neonates (see Patient-Centered Teaching: Care of Newborn and Infant Skin box). Parents should be made aware of the expected course of their child's lesion, and their expectations should be explored. Nurses can reassure parents when the lesions are benign and educate them thoroughly about what to expect when treatment is indicated.

PATIENT-CENTERED TEACHING

Care of Newborn and Infant Skin

Encourage parents to protect the infant's skin by teaching the following:

- Infants may be bathed and shampooed daily after the umbilical cord has fallen off. Use mild soap and warm water.
- Avoid overbathing, which dries the skin. Do not allow the infant to bathe longer than 10 minutes. Avoid bubble bath products; they dry and irritate the skin.
- Lotions, creams, and powders are not needed after the bath.
- Change diapers frequently and clean the diaper area with water at each change.
- Remove diapers for short periods during the day while the baby lies on a washable pad, to expose diaper area to air.
- Avoid hot environments and overbundling the baby. Infants do not sweat effectively, and heat results in rashes and problems with temperature regulation.
- Avoid direct exposure to the sun during the first 2 weeks of life and avoid sun exposure for more than 10 to 15 minutes daily thereafter during early infancy. Babies should wear hats or bonnets and shirts in the sun. Do not use sunscreen on infants younger than 6 months; keep them out of prolonged direct sunlight.

SKIN INFLAMMATION

Inflammatory conditions that affect the child's skin can be acute or chronic. A primary nursing goal when caring for a child with an inflammatory skin condition is to prevent secondary infection.

SEBORRHEIC DERMATITIS

Seborrheic dermatitis is a chronic inflammatory skin condition seen frequently in infants. It is referred to as "cradle cap" when located on the scalp. It often begins in the first 2 to 3 weeks of life and usually disappears by age 12 months. Seborrhea in older children might appear on the face, behind the ears, around the umbilicus, or in any other area with a large number of sebaceous glands. Although the precise cause is unknown, seborrhea appears to be related to sebaceous gland dysfunction and overgrowth of the fungi *Candida* and *Malassezia ovalis* (Poindexter, Burkhart, & Morrell, 2009).

Seborrheic dermatitis is characterized by nonpruritic, oily, yellow scales that block sweat and sebaceous glands, causing retained secretions and inflammation in affected areas (Figure 25-1). Confluent erythema might be present in the diaper and intertriginous areas and around the umbilicus (Figure 25-2). Often, there is overgrowth of normal skin bacteria and yeast, which increases inflammation and leads to secondary infection.

The nurse inspects the infant's scalp or other affected areas for lesions and inflammation and questions parents about the frequency and technique of washing the infant's scalp. Instruct the parents to remove the scales daily by shampooing with a mild baby shampoo or

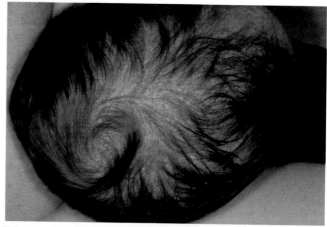

FIG 25-1 "Cradle cap," the most frequent form of seborrheic dermatitis in infants. The condition often begins in the first 2 to 3 weeks of life and usually disappears by age 12 months. (From Paller, S. A. [2012]. *Hurwitz clinical pediatric dermatology: A textbook of skin disorders of childhood and adolescence* [4th ed., p. 20]. Philadelphia: Saunders.)

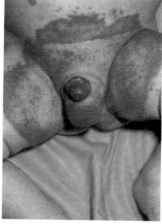

FIG 25-2 Seborrheic diaper dermatitis. (From Moschella, S. L., & Hurley, H. J. [1992]. *Dermatology* [3rd ed., p. 239]. Philadelphia: Saunders.)

an over-the-counter antiseborrheic shampoo containing sulfur and salicylic acid (Fostex Medicated Cleansing, P&S, Sebulex), selenium, or tar (Neutrogena T/Gel, Polytar). Ketoconazole 2% shampoo has been reported to be safe in infants less than 12 months of age (Poindexter et al., 2009). Massaging the scalp with warm mineral oil before shampooing helps loosen scales. Using a fine-tooth comb or a clean, soft-bristle toothbrush during the shampoo also helps loosen scales. Eyelid dermatitis (blepharitis) is treated with warm tap water compresses and cleansing with "no tears" baby shampoo. Care must be taken to keep topical medications out of the infant's eyes.

Teach the parents the importance of good hygiene of the infant's scalp and skin to prevent recurrence. Reassure them that the fontanel is not fragile and will not be damaged by gentle pressure and washing. Advise the parents to contact the physician if the sites become infected. Skin lesions that do not clear with frequent washing can be treated with hydrocortisone cream applied twice a day.

Seborrheic dermatitis of the diaper area is often secondarily infected with *C. albicans* and requires appropriate treatment. Lotions and creams tend to aggravate the condition and should not be used.

CONTACT DERMATITIS

Contact dermatitis is a skin inflammation that results from direct skin-to-irritant contact.

Etiology

Contact dermatitis can be caused by hundreds of substances. Among the most common causes of contact dermatitis are rubber products, clothing dyes, nickel (in jewelry, bra strap hooks, jeans fasteners), and plant oils. Scented or strongly alkaline soaps, skin lotions, cosmetics, and wool clothing also are irritating to many children.

Diaper dermatitis (diaper rash) is a contact dermatitis from irritants such as moisture, friction, and chemical substances. Urine ammonia, formed from the breakdown of urea by fecal bacteria, is extremely irritating to sensitive infant skin. Ammonia alone does not cause skin breakdown. Only skin damaged by infrequent diaper changes and constant urine and feces contact is prone to damage from ammonia in urine. Inadequate fluid intake, heat, and detergents in diapers aggravate the condition.

PATHOPHYSIOLOGY

Contact Dermatitis

Contact dermatitis is an inflammatory reaction of the skin either caused by direct exposure to an irritant *(irritant contact dermatitis)* or a delayed hypersensitivity response to an allergen *(allergic contact dermatitis).*

Irritant contact dermatitis can occur in any person who has repeated or prolonged contact with a primary irritant. Examples of primary irritants include citrus juices, detergents, bubble bath formulations, and urine. Diaper dermatitis is an example of irritant dermatitis that results from prolonged exposure to urine. Teething infants can have dermatitis on the face and neck folds from drooling.

Allergic contact dermatitis, a delayed hypersensitivity reaction, occurs in susceptible individuals who are sensitized to a substance by a previous exposure to the contact allergen. *Rhus dermatitis* (caused by poison ivy, oak, and sumac), the most common type of allergic contact dermatitis in children, is caused by oleoresins contained in all parts of the plant. Lesions appear several hours to several days after contact.

Incidence

Irritant contact dermatitis is more common in children than is allergic contact dermatitis. Many children have at least one episode of diaper dermatitis, usually occurring between ages 3 and 18 months, although it is most common between ages 8 and 10 months (American Academy of Pediatrics [AAP] Patient Education Online, 2010).

Manifestations

Manifestations of irritant contact dermatitis include dry, inflamed, and pruritic skin. The distribution of lesions correlates with the skin surface in contact with the offending agent (e.g., watchband, clothing). Diaper dermatitis begins with erythema in the perianal region and can progress to macules and papules, which form erosions and crusts (Figure 25-3). Manifestations of allergic contact dermatitis include blistering, weeping lesions over an area of inflamed skin, intense pruritus, and crusted, scaly lesions that heal in 10 to 14 days without treatment. Rhus dermatitis (e.g., poison ivy, oak, sumac) may cause severe systemic reactions.

Diagnostic Evaluation

The characteristic appearance of the lesions and a history of exposure to an irritating substance establish the diagnosis. Skin testing might be performed in children with persistent or recurrent dermatitis.

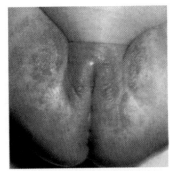

FIG 25-3 Contact diaper dermatitis. (From Moschella, S. L., & Hurley, H. J. [1992]. *Dermatology* [3rd ed., p. 239]. Philadelphia: Saunders.)

Therapeutic Management

Discontinuing exposure to the offending agent treats contact dermatitis. The skin should be washed thoroughly if any irritant remains on the skin. Cool compresses of tap water or Burow's solution or steroid cream (e.g., triamcinolone 0.1% or fluocinolone 0.025%) may be applied several times a day after application of compresses. Severe contact dermatitis might require treatment with oral steroids, which should be tapered gradually. Desensitization therapy is usually not effective in managing contact dermatitis.

NURSING CARE FOR THE CHILD WITH CONTACT DERMATITIS

■ Assessment

Investigate new or continuing exposure to any potentially irritating substances. Assessment of skin lesions includes noting their distribution and configuration and looking for evidence of pruritus.

For a child with diaper dermatitis, carefully inspect the diaper area, noting the type and extent of lesions. It is important to assess the infant's hygiene and the parents' knowledge of care related to the infant's skin integrity. Question parents about the type of diapers used, laundering practices, and frequency and method of cleaning the diaper area. Any recent changes in the infant's care, such as new foods, soaps, detergents, or lotions, should be investigated.

■ Nursing Diagnosis and Planning

The nursing diagnoses and expected outcomes that may be appropriate for the child with contact dermatitis and the child's family are as follows:

- Acute Pain related to skin inflammation.

Expected Outcomes. The child will have reduced skin irritation, as evidenced by decreased excoriation and increased healing. The child will exhibit decreased irritability, absence of scratching, and uninterrupted periods of sleep.

- Risk for Infection related to scratching of pruritic lesions.

Expected Outcome. The child will have no signs of secondary bacterial infection, as evidenced by clear intact skin.

- Deficient Knowledge of management and prevention of future skin inflammation related to incomplete understanding of therapeutic principles.

Expected Outcomes. The child and family will identify and avoid irritating substances and will carry out prescribed treatments correctly.

■ Interventions

Nursing care of the child with contact dermatitis is directed toward relieving itching, preventing infection, and identifying and removing offending substances. Cool compresses and tepid oatmeal (Aveeno) baths provide some relief from itching. Prescribed topical steroid creams should be applied in a thin layer. Antihistamines, such as diphenhydramine (Benadryl) or hydroxyzine (Atarax), also help the child rest. Because overheating increases itching, advise the parents to occupy the child with quiet activities and to keep the room temperature at a comfortable level.

Reassure the parents and child that the lesions are not contagious and cannot be spread to others or to other parts of the body by scratching. However, if oils from rhus plants remain on the skin, nails or on clothing, they may contact other parts of the child's body and cause new lesions at the point of contact. Keep the skin clean and help the child avoid scratching to prevent secondary infection. Instruct the parents to contact the health provider if the child has a fever or if the lesions produce purulent drainage.

Contact dermatitis is prevented by avoiding offending substances. Children should be taught to recognize plants of the rhus group. If the child is exposed to these plants, rinse the skin with cool water immediately (within 15 minutes) and wash clothing in hot, soapy water. Oleoresins in the plants can be spread not only by direct contact with the plant but also in the smoke of burning leaves or by touching pets that have contacted the plants.

Avoiding known irritants, such as cosmetics, jewelry, and canvas athletic shoes, can prevent other types of contact dermatitis. Nickel-sensitive children can usually tolerate 14-karat gold or sterling silver jewelry. Pierced earrings should have hypoallergenic or surgical stainless steel posts.

Diaper dermatitis is much easier to prevent than to treat. Successful treatment and prevention of diaper rash, regardless of the cause, depend on cleaning the diaper area thoroughly and keeping the skin dry. Prompt, gentle cleaning with water and mild soap (Dove, Neutrogena Baby Soap) after each voiding or defecation rids the skin of ammonia and other irritants and decreases the chance of skin breakdown and infection. Careful attention should be given to skin folds and creases. The parent should pat the skin dry with a soft cloth towel after washing. Air drying the skin and frequently exposing the skin to air and light promote healing of diaper rash. During bouts of diaper rash, the diaper may be left off during nap times.

A bland, protective ointment (A+D, Balmex, Desitin, zinc oxide) can be applied to clean, dry, intact skin to help prevent diaper rash. Ointments should not be applied to inflamed areas because they retain moisture. Occlusion increases the risk of systemic absorption of steroid; thus steroid creams are rarely used for diaper dermatitis because the diaper functions as an occlusive dressing. Frequent diaper changes decrease irritation from urine and feces. Encourage the parents to check the newborn infant's diaper every hour and the older infant's diaper every 2 hours. Using disposable diapers does not eliminate the need for frequent diaper changes. Although the "wicking" action of disposable diapers pulls moisture away from the skin toward the liner, ammonia and other byproducts are left behind on the infant's skin, causing irritation. Rubber or plastic pants increase skin breakdown by holding in moisture and should be used infrequently.

If cloth diapers are laundered at home, the parents should wash them in hot water, using a mild soap and double rinsing. Soaking diapers before washing in a quaternary ammonium compound (Diaperene) decreases ammonia in the diapers. Using $\frac{1}{4}$ cup of vinegar in the rinse is also helpful.

Advise parents to contact the health provider if the rash becomes solid and bright red, if it becomes raw or bleeds, if blisters or boils develop, if the rash does not improve in 3 days with treatment, or if the infant has a fever.

■ Evaluation

- Is the child's skin intact, with healed lesions and no evidence of pain or pruritus?
- Is the child's skin free from signs of secondary infection?
- Do the parents demonstrate understanding of proper skin and diaper area care?

ATOPIC DERMATITIS

Atopic dermatitis, or eczema, is a common chronic inflammatory disease of the skin characterized by severe pruritus. Atopic dermatitis can have distressing psychosocial effects on the child and family.

Etiology

The cause of atopic dermatitis (eczema) is unknown, but the disease is thought to be genetically determined and related to a malfunction in the body's immune system. Contributing factors include an inherited tendency for dry, sensitive skin; allergy; and emotional stress. Most children with atopic dermatitis have a family history of asthma, hay fever, or atopic dermatitis. Children with atopic dermatitis may present with asthma or allergic rhinitis. Although the role of allergy in the etiology of atopic dermatitis is controversial, immunoglobulin E (IgE)–mediated food allergy has been shown to be an exacerbating factor in some children (Leung, 2011).

Incidence

The prevalence of atopic diseases, including asthma, allergic rhinitis, and atopic dermatitis, has increased substantially in the past 30 years. Atopic dermatitis usually begins in infancy and clears by age 2 or 3 years, although it can persist through adolescence and adulthood. Data from the Prevention and Incidence of Asthma and Mite Allergy study show that high birth weight and daycare attendance increase the risk for atopic dermatitis in infancy, whereas exclusive breastfeeding decreases the risk (Scholtens, Gehring, Brunekreef et al., 2007). Atopic dermatitis affects all races. Symptoms tend to be worse during winter months.

PATHOPHYSIOLOGY
Atopic Dermatitis

Atopic dermatitis is an allergic skin condition. It has been suggested that infants who have atopic dermatitis have unusually slow maturation of T-cell function. The skin of affected children releases more histamine than that of normal children. The high levels of histamine trigger an inflammatory response, resulting in erythema, edema, and intense pruritus. Scratching increases itching, leading to an itch-scratch-itch cycle. Continual scratching and rubbing excoriate and damage the skin. Oozing, weeping, crusting, and cracking lesions develop. The skin of children with atopic dermatitis carries a higher-than-normal colonization of *S. aureus*, and secondary infection is common. Impetigo and viral infections (herpes, molluscum contagiosum) occur frequently in these children.

Scholtens, S., Gehring, U., Brunekreef, B., et al. (2007). Breastfeeding, weight gain in infancy, and overweight at seven years of age: The Prevention and Incidence of Asthma and Mite Allergy Birth Cohort Study. *American Journal of Epidemiology, 165*(8), 919-926.

Manifestations

During infancy, erythematous areas of oozing and crusting appear first on the cheeks and then on the forehead, scalp, and extensor surfaces of the arms and legs (Figure 25-4). Papulovesicular rash and scaly, red plaques become excoriated and lichenified. The affected scalp area resembles seborrheic dermatitis, but unlike seborrheic dermatitis, atopic dermatitis is intensely pruritic. Infants begin manifesting symptoms at approximately age 1 to 4 months.

Children who have atopic dermatitis after infancy have a rash pattern that differs from the rash seen during infancy. The flexor surfaces of the wrists, ankles, knees, and elbows are affected, as are the neck creases, the eyelids, and the dorsal surfaces of the hands and feet. There may be acute weeping areas, with or without secondary infection. Chronic lichenification results from persistent scratching.

Children and adolescents with atopic dermatitis readily experience intense itching, especially in response to sweating or contact with irritating fabrics, such as wool. Emotional upset increases sweating and precipitates itching and scratching. Dry skin is a hallmark of this condition.

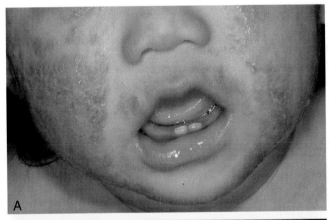

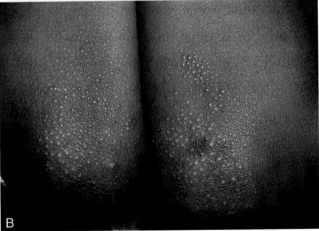

FIG 25-4 Atopic dermatitis, an allergic skin condition, usually begins in infancy and clears by age 2 to 3 years. However, it can continue into childhood. **A,** Lesions on cheeks often spread to the forehead, scalp, and extensor surfaces of arms and legs. **B,** Flexor surfaces of wrists, ankles, knees, and elbows may be affected in the childhood form of the disease. (From Paller, S. A. [2012]. *Hurwitz clinical pediatric dermatology: A textbook of skin disorders of childhood and adolescence* [4th ed., pp. 39-40]. Philadelphia: Saunders.)

Diagnostic Evaluation

The diagnosis is based on the clinical features of intense pruritus, the appearance of the lesions, the pattern of remissions and exacerbations, and a family history of allergy. IgE levels and eosinophils are often elevated. Skin testing for food allergies—usually milk, eggs, wheat, soy, peanuts, and fish—can help identify potential food triggers.

Therapeutic Management

The main goals of treatment are to control itching and scratching, moisturize the skin, prevent secondary infection, and remove irritants and allergens. Control of pruritus includes avoiding environmental triggers, such as overheating, soaps, wool clothing, and other skin irritants. Oral antihistamines, such as hydroxyzine (Atarax), diphenhydramine (Benadryl), and loratadine (Claritin), can be used to help break the "itch-scratch-itch" cycle. Nonsedating antihistamines, such as loratadine, may be preferred for school-age children. Itching is typically more severe at night; thus antihistamines should be given before bedtime. Secondary infection is treated with antibiotic therapy.

Proper skin hydration is essential. Either a "dry" or "wet" approach may be used. The dry approach depends on avoiding bathing and the liberal use of emollients on dry skin. The wet approach is currently more popular. It permits bathing for limited periods of time, and the use of wet compresses and occlusive creams and ointments are the mainstays of treatment. In humid climates bathing should be infrequent, and only lukewarm water and mild, nonperfumed soap (e.g., Purpose, white Dove, Basis) should be used. Emollients such as Eucerin cream or petroleum jelly applied immediately after bathing to damp skin help the skin retain moisture. Applying the moisturizer while the skin is still damp hydrates the skin. The child who lives in a dry climate should bathe frequently (several times a day), using a hydrophilic agent such as Cetaphil instead of soap, and should moisturize with a moisturizing ointment or cream immediately after bathing. The child should avoid lotions that contain alcohol because these can contribute to skin dryness. Regardless of the approach used, moisturizing the skin is maintenance therapy for atopic dermatitis and should become a daily routine for the child.

Antiinflammatory corticosteroid creams and ointments are prescribed for inflamed or lichenified areas. These creams are more effective when applied to damp skin. The lowest potency that controls signs should be used, and topical steroids are usually reserved for treatment of episodic flares.

Topical calcineurin inhibitors (TCIs), such as tacrolimus and pimecrolimus, have an antiinflammatory action and can be used in place of topical corticosteroids in children older than 2 years of age who do not respond well to other treatment approaches (Leung, 2011). Patients should avoid exposure to sunlight, tanning beds, sun lamps and any other sources of ultraviolet light while taking these medications.

These drugs are approved by the U.S. Food and Drug Administration (FDA) for children older than 2 years. They may be applied to 100% of the body surface if needed, and they may be used for longer periods of time than topical steroids may. Topical immunomodulators do not cause skin atrophy. Although they can penetrate the skin enough to suppress local inflammation, they are only minimally absorbed into the circulation.

Routine blood studies (to monitor for immunosuppression) in children using tacrolimus and pimecrolimus are not indicated. However, caution should be used in children whose skin integrity had widespread damage because immunosuppressives can be absorbed systemically in such cases.

Topical calcineurin inhibitors have become popular for use in children with atopic dermatitis; however, postmarketing surveillance

DRUG GUIDE

Topical Corticosteroids

Classification
Topical antiinflammatory.

Action
Reduce inflammation by causing vasoconstriction and inhibiting the movement of inflammatory cells from the bloodstream into local tissue.

Indications
Inflammatory skin diseases, such as atopic dermatitis.

Dosage and Route
Topical route; number of applications depends on the child's condition and the potency of the medication. Topical steroids are commonly divided into seven classes, with those of lowest potency assigned to the lowest (seventh) class.

Class I: Optimized betamethasone dipropionate 0.05% (Diprolene cream or ointment)

Class II: Triamcinolone acetonide ointment 0.5% (Kenalog); mometasone furoate ointment 0.1% (Elocon)

Class III: Triamcinolone acetonide ointment 0.1% (Aristocort A); triamcinolone acetonide cream (Aristocort-HP); fluticasone propionate ointment 0.005% (Cutivate)

Class IV: Hydrocortisone valerate ointment 0.2% (Westcort); mometasone furoate cream 0.1% (Elocon); desoximetasone cream 0.05% (Topicort-LP)

Class V: Fluticasone propionate cream 0.05% (Cutivate); hydrocortisone valerate cream 0.2% (Westcort); triamcinolone acetonide cream 0.025% (Aristocort)

Class VI: Desonide cream 0.05% (DesOwen); alclometasone dipropionate cream 0.05% (Aclovate)

Class VII: Hydrocortisone cream 0.5%, 1% (Cortizone, Hytone, generic)

Absorption
Better absorbed through the skin immediately after bathing.

Contraindications
Never apply to diaper rashes or chickenpox lesions. Superpotent topical steroids (class I) are rarely used for children. Only low-potency agents should be used on the face.

Precautions
Unless directed by the physician, do not bandage, wrap, or otherwise cover areas being treated with topical steroids. In general, the more potent the medication, the shorter the treatment time will be.

Adverse Reactions
Systemic side effects can occur with short-term use of high-potency topical steroids or with long-term use of lower-potency topicals. Systemic effects include suppression of the hypothalamic-pituitary-adrenal axis, resulting in growth suppression; suppression of immune response; osteoporosis; moon face; and obesity. Locally, thinning of the skin, striae, telangiectasia, atrophy, and purpura can occur.

Nursing Considerations
Advise the parent to apply to the child's skin within 5 minutes of bathing, to meticulously follow the physician's directions for use, and to immediately report any side effects.

reveals risks. An FDA advisory panel recommended adding a black box warning to labels informing consumers that calcineurin inhibitors are associated with increased risk for certain cancers, especially in children (American Academy of Dermatology [AAD], 2010).

Identifying and eliminating allergens can be helpful. Allergy-proofing the home might be recommended (see Chapter 18). Because allergy to certain foods is an exacerbating factor in some children, those foods should be eliminated from the diets of sensitive infants. Breastfeeding for the first year is recommended for infants at risk for allergy. Solid foods should not be introduced until the infant is at least 6 months old.

NURSING CARE FOR THE CHILD WITH ATOPIC DERMATITIS

■ Assessment

Obtain a thorough history that includes information about allergies in the family. Question parents about any environmental or dietary factors that seem to worsen the child's condition. Determine what treatments have been tried and their effectiveness. Examine skin lesions for type, distribution, and evidence of any secondary infection. Assess the child's comfort level and the family's feelings and coping methods.

■ Nursing Diagnosis and Planning

The nursing diagnoses and expected outcomes that may be appropriate for the child with atopic dermatitis and the child's family are as follows:

- Impaired Skin Integrity related to environmental and immunologic factors.

Expected Outcome. The child's skin will exhibit decreased evidence of dryness, irritation, and excoriation.

- Acute Pain related to dry skin, secondary infection, and external irritations.

Expected Outcomes. The child will have minimal pain and pruritus, as evidenced by decreased irritability, absence of scratching, and uninterrupted periods of sleep.

- Risk for Infection related to skin excoriation.

Expected Outcome. The child will have no signs of secondary bacterial infection, as evidenced by a normal body temperature and absence of purulent drainage.

- Deficient Knowledge about controlling itching, preventing secondary infection, and identifying aggravating factors related to anxiety or incomplete understanding of information.

Expected Outcomes. The child and family will identify and eliminate allergens and aggravating factors. The family will carry out prescribed treatments correctly. Family members will express any anxiety related to the child's condition.

- Interrupted Family Processes related to the child's pruritus and involved treatment.

Expected Outcome. The child and family will discuss their feelings and concerns.

- Disturbed Body Image related to perception of appearance.

Expected Outcomes. The child will engage in activities with other children. The child will verbalize positive ideas about self.

■ Interventions

Care of the child with atopic dermatitis is demanding, and the entire family routine may revolve around the affected child. Parents need support and reassurance as they care for an uncomfortable, often irritable child.

Keeping the child's skin hydrated will help relieve itching. Instruct parents to apply a moisturizing cream, such as Eucerin, several times a day and immediately after the child is bathed. Reassure parents that moisturizing creams contain no harmful drugs and should be applied whenever the child's skin looks dry. Soaks and cool, wet compresses are soothing and can be applied to remove crusts, reduce inflammation, and dry weeping areas. Provide parents with explicit instructions on the use of soaks and topical medications. Strips of old cotton sheets moistened in lukewarm or cool tap water work well for wet dressings. Wet compresses should not be used for more than 3 days.

Rough clothing can aggravate eczema, particularly wool or other fabrics that cause sweating. Soft cotton or cotton-polyester blends are tolerated best. Undergarments with irritating seams can be turned inside out so that the soft seam is against the skin. Heat and sweating increase pruritus, so instruct parents to be careful not to "bundle up" the child in heavy blankets or clothing. Because detergents and fabric softeners can also aggravate atopic dermatitis, clothes should be washed in mild detergent and rinsed twice.

Advise the parents to keep the child's fingernails clean and short. Cotton gloves or mittens might be needed to prevent excoriation from scratching but should be used with caution, preferably only at night, because overuse could interfere with fine motor development. Lightweight, long-sleeved tops and one-piece outfits discourage scratching.

The child's skin must be kept clean to minimize secondary infection. Avoid using soap. Bath oil or emulsifying ointment can be used as a soap substitute but must be used with caution because these cause both the child and the tub to become slippery. Tepid bath water helps prevent the child from becoming overheated and itchy. Instruct parents to contact the physician at the earliest signs of skin infection (weeping skin, pustules) and to administer topical and oral antibiotics as prescribed.

Children with atopic dermatitis who swim should apply moisturizer before swimming and immediately on exiting the pool. Prolonged immersion in water (more than 20 minutes) can have a drying effect. A humidifier in the child's room during winter months may decrease skin dryness. The child should avoid the drying effects of sun exposure.

Children and families of children with atopic dermatitis exhibit frustration when the condition does not resolve quickly. The parent or child might be concerned about the child's appearance, as well as the child's discomfort.

Help parents take control of the child's condition by empowering them with knowledge about therapeutic management. Allowing parents to verbalize frustrations and helping them learn management techniques that do not disrupt family routine are important interventions.

Although studies do not consistently support emotional upset as a direct cause of atopic dermatitis flares, it is helpful to teach an older child stress reduction techniques to help cope with the frustration and discomfort of the condition. A resource for families of a child with atopic dermatitis is the National Eczema Association for Science and Education.

■ Evaluation

- Is the child's skin intact and smooth?
- Have itching and pain been reduced?
- Is the child's skin free from redness or purulence that would indicate secondary infection?
- Do parents carry out prescribed treatments correctly?
- Are parents able to demonstrate appropriate coping techniques?
- Can the child demonstrate stress-relief measures to decrease itching?

SKIN INFECTIONS

Skin infections are common in childhood. Bacteria are normally present on healthy skin. The skin's susceptibility to bacterial infection depends on several factors, including the intactness of the skin, the virulence of the organisms, and the child's immune status. Children are susceptible to fungal and viral infections, as well. Unlike bacterial infections, which generally respond fairly quickly to treatment, fungal and viral infections can be more persistent and challenging to treat.

Although bacterial skin infections can be caused by a variety of microbes, *Staphylococcus* is a major pathogen, accounting for most of the skin infections of childhood. Skin infections predominantly caused by *Staphylococcus aureus* can range from minor, superficial lesions to severe generalized lesions with systemic effects. These skin infections include folliculitis, furuncles (boils), cellulitis, bullous impetigo, nonbullous impetigo, and staphylococcal scalded skin syndrome. Impetigo, a superficial, usually minor staphylococcal infection, is the most common bacterial skin infection of childhood. Folliculitis is inflammation of hair follicles. Furuncles, or boils, develop when the infection of an existing folliculitis progresses deeper. Cellulitis is infection of the subcutaneous tissues.

IMPETIGO

Impetigo often occurs as a secondary infection from another skin lesion, such as an insect bite. Close contact contributes to the spread of impetigo, which is highly contagious. Children in daycare facilities, schools, or camps and adolescent athletes are at increased risk. The incubation period for impetigo is 7 to 10 days, and it may spread to other parts of the child's skin or to others who touch the child, use the same towel, or drink from the same glass. Spread of the infection is fostered by poor hygiene, crowded living conditions, and a hot, humid environment. Lesions resolve in 12 to 14 days with treatment.

Etiology

Impetigo can be caused by *S. aureus*, group A beta-hemolytic streptococci, or a combination of these bacteria. *S. aureus* is the primary pathogen in most cases. Nonbullous impetigo, sometimes referred to as crusted impetigo, was formerly thought to be a result of streptococcal infection. Studies have shown that *S. aureus* is the primary cause of both bullous and nonbullous impetigo (Schor, 2010). Bullous impetigo is at the minor end of a spectrum of blistering disorders caused by the exfoliative toxins produced by some strains of *Staphylococcus*. Staphylococcal scalded skin syndrome is at the more severe end of that spectrum.

PATHOPHYSIOLOGY

Impetigo

Impetigo begins in an area of broken skin, such as an insect bite, scabies, or atopic dermatitis. The break in the skin allows for organism entry. The inflammatory process results in the formation of a pustular lesion. Honey-colored fluid from this lesion becomes crusted. In some children, nasal discharge containing the organism erodes healthy skin above the upper lip, allowing for organism entry.

Incidence

Impetigo occurs most often during hot, humid summer months. Toddlers and preschoolers are most commonly affected, often when recovering from an upper respiratory tract infection.

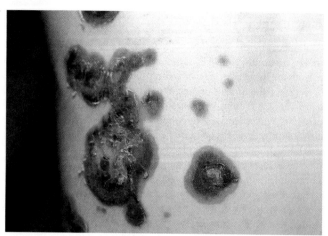

FIG 25-5 Impetigo lesions are usually located around the mouth and nose but may be located on the extremities. (From Paller, S. A. [2012]. *Hurwitz clinical pediatric dermatology: A textbook of skin disorders of childhood and adolescence* [4th ed., p. 322]. Philadelphia: Saunders.)

Manifestations

The primary lesions of impetigo occur in two forms. Bullous impetigo characteristically manifests as small vesicles that can progress to bullae. The lesions are initially filled with serous fluid and later become pustular. The bullae rapidly rupture, leaving a shiny, lacquered-appearing lesion surrounded by a scaly rim. Crusted impetigo appears initially as a vesicle or pustule that ruptures to become an erosion with an overlay of honey-colored crust. The erosions bleed easily when crusts are removed (Figure 25-5). Lesions are mildly pruritic. Scarring is uncommon but may occur if the child picks or scratches the lesions. Postinflammatory hyperpigmentation is a frequent sequel in dark-skinned children. The lesions are often located around the mouth and nose but can appear on any part of the body.

Diagnostic Evaluation

The characteristic appearance of the lesions usually confirms the diagnosis. Failure to respond to treatment may suggest community-acquired methicillin-resistant *Staphylococcus aureus* (CA-MRSA) (see Chapter 17), an increasing problem in children (Bar-Meir & Tan, 2010). If a culture is ordered, the specimen should be obtained from beneath the crust or from the fluid inside the lesions.

Therapeutic Management

Impetigo is treated with topical and oral antibiotics. The lesions should be gently washed three times a day with a warm, soapy washcloth and the crusts soaked and carefully removed. A topical ointment, such as mupirocin (Bactroban) or bacitracin (Baci-guent), is then applied to the lesions. Topical therapy lasts 7 to 10 days. Severe cases of impetigo or cases of impetigo around the mouth are treated with oral antibiotics that are effective against both staphylococcal and streptococcal organisms. Impetigo that is extensive is treated with intravenous (IV) antibiotics. Antibiotic treatment of streptococcal impetigo does not prevent glomerulonephritis, but it does hasten healing of the lesions.

Good handwashing and careful hygiene are imperative to prevent spread of the infection and should be emphasized to the child and parents. The child should not attend school or daycare for 24 hours after beginning treatment (AAP, 2009). The school should be notified of the diagnosis.

NURSING CARE FOR THE CHILD WITH IMPETIGO

■ Assessment

Assess the child's skin for the size, distribution, and spread of impetigo lesions. If the child is taking systemic antibiotics, monitor for signs of adverse effects, such as rashes or diarrhea. Observe for periorbital edema or blood in the urine, which may signal the development of acute glomerulonephritis if the impetigo is caused by group A beta-hemolytic streptococci.

■ Nursing Diagnosis and Planning

The nursing diagnoses and expected outcomes that may be appropriate for the child with impetigo and the child's family are as follows:
- Impaired Skin Integrity related to destruction of skin layers secondary to bacterial infection.

Expected Outcomes. The child will maintain skin integrity, as evidenced by confinement of the infection to the primary site. The area will heal without scarring or further infection.
- Deficient Knowledge related to unfamiliarity with measures to prevent spread of infection, care of impetigo lesions, and antibiotic administration.

Expected Outcomes. The child and family will adhere to measures to prevent the spread of infection. The parent will demonstrate care of the lesions and administration of medications.

■ Interventions

Teach parents to soak the crusts and then wash them off with a warm, soapy washcloth three times a day. Advise them to gently remove the crusts after soaking, taking care not to spread the infection to other parts of the body with the contaminated washcloth. Antibiotic ointment should then be applied to the lesions and the affected areas left open to air. A small amount of bleeding after crust removal is common.

The child should sleep alone and should be bathed daily, alone, with antibacterial soap. The caregiver should wear gloves when caring for the child. Emphasize the importance of administering the full course of topical or systemic antibiotics as prescribed.

■ Evaluation

- Are the lesions healing, and have they remained confined to the primary site?
- Do the child and family members practice handwashing and other techniques to prevent the spread of infection?
- Do the parents appropriately explain the necessity for administering the full course of treatment?

⚡ SAFETY ALERT
Caring for a Child with Impetigo

- The child can spread impetigo lesions merely by touching another part of the skin after scratching the infected area.
- Keep the child's fingernails short and wash the child's hands frequently with antibacterial soap.
- Emphasize good handwashing and careful hygiene for the child's entire household.
- Discourage family members from sharing towels, combs, or eating utensils with the infected child.

CHAPTER 25   The Child with Major Alterations in Tissue Integrity

CELLULITIS

Cellulitis is bacterial infection of the subcutaneous tissue and the dermis. It is usually associated with a break in the skin, although cellulitis of the head and neck can follow an upper respiratory tract infection, sinusitis, otitis media, or tooth abscess. Cellulitis occurs most commonly in the lower extremities and in the buccal (inside the cheek) and periorbital (around the eye) regions. Complications of cellulitis include septic arthritis, meningitis, and brain abscess. Periorbital cellulitis can lead to blindness.

Etiology and Incidence

Since the introduction of the *Haemophilus influenzae* type B vaccine, group A streptococci and *S. aureus* are the most common causes of cellulitis. Cellulitis is most common in children age 2 years and younger.

Pathophysiology

Bacteria overwhelm the defensive cells that normally contain inflammation to local areas. The result is more extensive invasion of the causative organism as the infection moves from superficial tissue to deeper subcutaneous tissue.

Manifestations

The affected area is red, hot, tender, and indurated. If *H. influenzae* is the suspected organism, the affected area might have a purplish tinge. Edema and purple discoloration of the eyelids and decreased eye movement are present in periorbital cellulitis. Lymphangitis may be seen, with red "streaking" of the surrounding area and enlarged regional lymph nodes (lymphadenitis). The child usually exhibits fever, malaise, and headache.

Diagnostic Evaluation

Usually a complete blood cell count, blood cultures, and culture of the affected area are done. If no drainage is present, the affected area can be aspirated. Orbital cellulitis can be diagnosed by computed tomography of the orbit.

Therapeutic Management

After an initial intramuscular or IV dose of an antibiotic, such as ceftriaxone, the child with cellulitis of an extremity is usually treated at home with a 10-day course of oral antibiotics (cephalosporin, cloxacillin, or dicloxacillin) and warm compresses. If the cellulitis involves a joint or the face, or if the child shows other signs of acute febrile illness, hospitalization and IV antibiotics are required. Incision and drainage of the affected area may be necessary. Community-acquired MRSA is increasingly becoming a problem in children and adolescents, particularly athletes (Hinckley & Allen, 2008). Lesions, especially abscesses, should be cultured for presence of methicillin-resistant staphylococcal organisms because treatment of CA-MRSA is tailored to sensitivity results. Effective antibiotics for CA-MRSA infection in children include sulfamethoxazole-trimethoprim, clindamycin, vancomycin, and linezolid (see Chapter 17).

NURSING CARE FOR THE CHILD WITH CELLULITIS

■ Assessment

Record the history and question the parent regarding recent ear infections, dental caries, or trauma to the skin surrounding the affected area. Other pertinent data include when the inflammation started and how rapidly it has progressed. Examine the skin, noting any temperature increase, swelling, redness, and drainage. Assess for fever, pain, guarding, and irritability.

■ Nursing Diagnosis and Planning

The nursing diagnoses and expected outcomes that may be appropriate for the child with cellulitis and the child's family are as follows:

• Impaired Skin Integrity related to bacterial invasion.

Expected Outcome. The child will exhibit signs of healing, such as decreases in redness, swelling, and fever.

• Acute Pain related to soft tissue swelling and inflammation.

Expected Outcome. The child will be able to sleep and will demonstrate decreased irritability.

• Deficient Knowledge related to unfamiliarity with the illness and treatment.

Expected Outcomes. The family will describe measures to prevent the spread of infection, will describe how to administer antibiotics as prescribed, and will demonstrate the ability to carry out treatment measures.

■ Interventions

The child should rest in bed with the affected extremity elevated and immobilized. Warm, moist soaks applied every 4 hours increase circulation to the infected area, relieve pain, and promote healing. Acetaminophen can be given to control fever and pain. Frequent hand hygiene is essential to prevent the spread of infection. If the child is hospitalized, IV antibiotics should be administered accurately and on time to maintain a therapeutic blood level. If the child is being treated at home, the parents must understand the importance of administering the entire course of antibiotics as ordered. The child should be carefully monitored for signs of sepsis (increased fever, chills, confusion) and spread of infection.

■ Evaluation

• Does the child's skin exhibit signs of healing?
• Is the child free from signs of infection and pain?
• Does the parent administer prescribed medications and carry out appropriate home care?

CANDIDIASIS

Thrush (oral candidiasis) (Figure 25-6) is a superficial fungal infection of the oral mucous membranes that is common in infants. Thrush occurs as a result of overgrowth of *Candida albicans*. In addition to oral lesions, the child may exhibit lesions in the diaper area, which are caused by *C. albicans* passing through the intestine. Moisture and heat in the diaper area create an environment favorable to the development of *Candida* dermatitis. Persistent candidiasis suggests that the child might be immunocompromised.

Etiology

A neonate can acquire candidiasis during delivery while passing through an infected vagina. An older infant may have a fungal overgrowth as a result of immunosuppression, during antibiotic therapy, from exposure to the mother's infected breasts, or from unclean bottles and pacifiers.

Incidence

Candidiasis occurs most often in infants. Predisposing factors in all age-groups include antibiotic therapy, diabetes, and altered immune status.

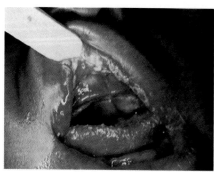

FIG 25-6 White, curdlike plaques of thrush (oral candidiasis, oral moniliasis), a common fungal infection in infants. (From Paller, S. A. [2012]. *Hurwitz clinical pediatric dermatology: A textbook of skin disorders of childhood and adolescence* [4th ed., p. 21]. Philadelphia: Saunders.)

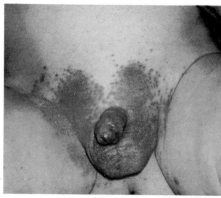

FIG 25-7 Diaper candidiasis. (From Feigin, R. D., & Cherry, J. D. [Eds.]. [2009]. *Textbook of pediatric infectious diseases* [6th ed., p. 774]. Philadelphia: Saunders.)

Manifestations

White, curdlike plaques are noted on the tongue, gums, and buccal mucosa in children with thrush. They can be distinguished from milk curds by the difficulty encountered in removing them and the bleeding of an erythematous base when plaques are removed. A child with severe infection may have difficulty eating. The lesions of diaper dermatitis are usually bright red and coalesced, with some satellite lesions spreading out to the child's abdomen and thighs (Figure 25-7).

Diagnostic Evaluation

The diagnosis of thrush and candidal diaper dermatitis is made from the clinical appearance of the lesions.

Therapeutic Management

Nystatin oral suspension (100,000 units/mL), swabbed onto the mucous membranes of the mouth, is effective in treating thrush. Because *Candida* is present in the gastrointestinal tract, oral nystatin also may be ordered to decrease the likelihood of recurrence. Oral fluconazole is an alternative therapy. Candidal diaper dermatitis is treated with a topical antifungal agent, such as nystatin or clotrimazole (Lotrimin).

NURSING CARE FOR THE CHILD WITH CANDIDIASIS

■ Assessment

Nursing assessment includes obtaining a history of maternal and infant *Candida* infections. Question the mother regarding vaginal itching or discharge or any nipple tenderness or redness. Also discuss methods used to clean bottles and pacifiers. Examine the infant's mouth and diaper area and assess nutrition and hydration status.

■ Nursing Diagnosis and Planning

The nursing diagnoses and expected outcomes that may be appropriate for the child with candidiasis and the child's family are as follows:
- Impaired Skin Integrity related to the effects of fungal infection.

Expected Outcome. The infant will exhibit signs of healing lesions, as evidenced by pink, intact mucous membranes or resolution of diaper rash.
- Acute Pain related to oral lesions or skin irritation.

Expected Outcome. The infant will have reduced discomfort, as evidenced by ability to take feedings without difficulty, decreased fussiness, and improved ability to sleep.
- Deficient Knowledge related to incomplete understanding of the cause of the infection and administration of medication.

Expected Outcomes. The family will demonstrate methods to prevent spread of infection and will administer the entire course of medication as prescribed.
- Imbalanced Nutrition: Less Than Body Requirements related to mouth irritation and altered taste.

Expected Outcomes. The infant will accept feedings and will consume appropriate amounts of nutrients.

■ Interventions

Teach the parent to swab 1 mL of oral nystatin suspension onto the infant's gums, tongue, and buccal mucosa every 6 hours until 3 to 4 days after symptoms have disappeared. Because cotton-tipped applicators tend to absorb the medication, a more effective method of administration is to rub the suspension onto the mucous membranes with a gloved finger. To increase the amount of time the medication is in contact with the mucous membranes, nystatin should be applied after feedings. Alternatively, oral fluconazole administered once a day may be used for treatment of thrush in infants.

Pacifiers, nipples, and bottles should be thoroughly cleaned to decrease the chance of reinfection. Teach the parents the technique and importance of good hand hygiene. If the infant is breastfed, the mother's breasts should also be treated with nystatin.

Suggest small, frequent feedings for the infant or child with thrush who is uncomfortable. Cool liquids are soothing to the older child.

For the infant with candidal diaper dermatitis, suggest that the parent apply nystatin or clotrimazole cream. Leaving the diaper area exposed to air reduces the moisture that facilitates fungal growth.

Advise the parent to contact the health care provider if the infant refuses to eat or fever develops or if the candidiasis does not clear with treatment.

■ Evaluation

- Have the lesions disappeared, leaving intact skin and oral mucous membranes?
- Does the child appear to be comfortable, sleeping well, and less irritable?
- Can the parents demonstrate proper medication administration?
- Is the child increasing the amount of oral intake?

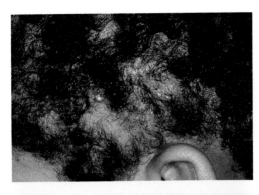

Tinea capitis
(scalp)

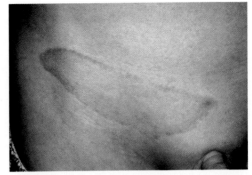

Tinea corporis
(trunk, face,
extremities)

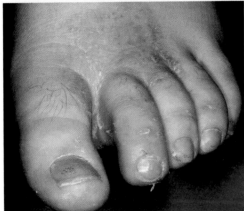

Tinea pedis (feet)

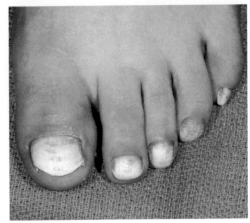

Tinea unguium
(nails, nail beds)

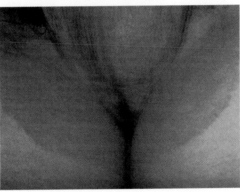

Tinea cruris
(groin, buttocks,
scrotum)

FIG 25-8 Tinea (ringworm) is an infection caused by dermatophytes, a group of fungi. Tinea is classified according to the part of the body affected. Five common types of tinea are shown here. (Tinea cruris from Hurwitz, S. [1993]. *Clinical pediatric dermatology: A textbook of skin disorders of childhood and adolescence* [2nd ed., p. 380]. Philadelphia: Saunders; remaining figures from Paller, S. A. [2012]. *Hurwitz clinical pediatric dermatology: A textbook of skin disorders of childhood and adolescence* [4th ed., pp. 392, 396, 400, 401]. Philadelphia: Saunders.)

TINEA INFECTION

Tinea is a superficial skin infection caused by a group of fungi known as dermatophytes. Tinea infections are designated by the word *tinea* followed by the Latin word for the affected part of the body. Figure 25-8 illustrates various types of tinea infections.

Etiology

Two types of dermatophytes, *Trichophyton* spp. and *Microsporum* spp., cause the majority of tinea infections. *Trichophyton* affects all keratinized tissue, including skin, nails, and hair. *Microsporum* invades the hair.

Incidence

Tinea capitis usually occurs in children ages 1 to 10 years, whereas tinea pedis and tinea cruris are most common in adolescent boys. Because a moist environment supports the growth of fungal infections, most tinea infections appear when the weather is hot and humid.

Manifestations

Common manifestations of tinea capitis include erythema and scaling of the scalp and one or more round patches of alopecia that slowly increase in size. Small papules at the base of hair follicles become crusting pustules and red scales. In some cases, thick, broken hairs close to

PATHOPHYSIOLOGY

Tinea Infection

Tinea infection occurs when the fungus causing tinea invades the hair, the stratum corneum of the skin, or the nails.

In *tinea capitis*, the fungus invades the hair shafts, causing the hairs to become brittle and to break off at the level of the scalp, leaving an area of stubby, black-dotted alopecia. An immune reaction to the fungus may develop in the form of a *kerion*, a boggy, red, tender scalp mass that may contain *S. aureus* and is often accompanied by fever and lymphadenopathy. Children with allergies seem to be more susceptible to tinea capitis.

Tinea corporis (ringworm) is a fungal infection of the face, trunk, or extremities. It can be transmitted by humans or by dogs and cats. Most lesions of tinea corporis clear without treatment in several months, but some may become chronic.

Tinea cruris (jock itch) is characterized by an intense inflammatory reaction with severe pruritus.

Tinea pedis (athlete's foot) may become chronic, particularly in adolescents who wear unventilated athletic shoes. Tinea lesions may become secondarily infected with bacteria or *Candida*.

Tinea infections are transmitted from person to person, by animal contact, or by contact with contaminated fomites (e.g., combs, hats, headrests, pillows). Tinea cruris (fungal infection affecting the groin and scrotal area) is not highly contagious. Poor hygiene, friction from tight clothing, and obesity are predisposing factors. Tinea pedis (athlete's foot) is a fungal infection of toes and feet. It is contagious but rarely develops on healthy, dry skin.

the scalp surface result in patches of black-dotted alopecia. *Kerion* formation may occur as a result of an inflammatory response to fungal antigens. A kerion is a boggy, fluctuant nodule, typically crusted and studded with pustules. Surrounding lymph nodes may be enlarged.

Tinea corporis, commonly seen on the trunk, face, and extremities, is characterized by ringlike plaques with clear centers and scaly, red margins. Lesions are usually ½ to 1 inch in diameter and mildly pruritic.

Manifestations of tinea cruris include pink papules and scales on the inner thighs, groin, scrotum, and buttocks (but not the penis). Pruritus is also present.

Tinea pedis, commonly referred to as "athlete's foot," produces fine vesiculopustular or scaly lesions on the soles of the feet, between the toes, and under the nails. The webs between the fourth and fifth toes are most commonly involved. Peeling, fissures, and maceration appear in severe cases, and pruritus and burning are typically present.

Diagnostic Evaluation

Most tinea infections can be diagnosed from the clinical appearance of the lesions. Fungal cultures or microscopic examination of skin scrapings prepared with potassium hydroxide confirms the diagnosis. *Microsporum* lesions fluoresce as a bright blue-green under a Wood light. However, the most common organism causing tinea today, *Trichophyton tonsurans*, does not fluoresce.

Therapeutic Management

Tinea Capitis

For treatment to be effective, medication must penetrate the hair follicles. Topical therapy alone is not effective for tinea capitis. Oral griseofulvin administered daily for at least 6 weeks is the treatment of choice; it is the only drug approved by the U.S. FDA for treating tinea capitis. Because griseofulvin is insoluble in water, its absorption is increased if it is taken with a high-fat meal or with milk. Other

antifungals, such as ketoconazole (Nizoral), terbinafine (Lamisil), or fluconazole (Diflucan), may be prescribed for older children who cannot tolerate griseofulvin or who fail to respond to it (Meadows-Oliver, 2009). Ketoconazole and other azole antifungals are used with caution in children because of the risk of hepatotoxicity during long-term therapy. Selenium sulfide shampoo should be used twice per week for 2 weeks to eliminate spores and to decrease transmission.

Tinea Corporis

Local treatment is usually effective for tinea corporis. Antifungal preparations, such as clotrimazole (Lotrimin) or miconazole (Monistat), can be used twice a day for approximately 4 weeks (AAP, 2009). Application of cream should extend 1 inch beyond the lesion borders to prevent spread. Infected pets should be treated as well, and the child should avoid close contact with infected pets.

Tinea Cruris

Management for tinea cruris is similar to that for tinea corporis. Topical antifungal preparations should be applied twice a day to the lesions and at least 1 inch beyond the borders. Care should be taken to apply the medication to all creases, and the adolescent should be advised to wear loose clothing.

Tinea Pedis

A prescribed topical antifungal agent, such as clotrimazole (Lotrimin), miconazole (Monistat), or oxiconazole (Oxistat), is applied twice a day until the lesions have been cleared for 1 week. If the lesions do not respond to topical therapy, oral griseofulvin may be given for 1 month or longer, to promote healing. Newer systemic antifungals, such as itraconazole (Sporanox), have demonstrated improved success over a shorter time than griseofulvin. If the affected area is inflamed and oozing, soaking the feet in Burow's solution can promote healing.

NURSING CARE OF THE CHILD WITH A TINEA INFECTION

■ Assessment

Obtain a history that includes a description of the skin lesions and possible contacts. Animals with which the child has played should be carefully inspected for ringworm. The child's siblings and playmates should also be examined.

■ Nursing Diagnosis and Planning

The nursing diagnoses and expected outcomes that may be appropriate for the child with a tinea infection and the child's family are as follows:

- Impaired Skin Integrity related to inflammation and excoriation.

Expected Outcomes. The child will exhibit intact skin over impaired areas. The skin lesions will exhibit progressive healing.

- Impaired Comfort related to pruritic lesions.

Expected Outcomes. The child will remain calm and will exhibit no evidence of discomfort or pruritus; scratching will decrease.

- Deficient Knowledge of the cause, treatment, and spread of the infection related to lack of information.

Expected Outcomes. The child and family will verbalize accurate information about the child's skin condition. The child and family will demonstrate behaviors that prevent spread of the fungus. Treatments will be performed correctly.

- Disturbed Body Image related to alopecia or unattractive lesions.

Expected Outcome. The child will return to or continue with social involvement.

■ Interventions

Adequate teaching is essential for successful treatment of tinea infection (see Patient-Centered Teaching: Home Care for a Child or Adolescent with a Tinea Infection box). In addition to teaching therapeutic management techniques specific for the child's particular type of tinea, emphasize to the parent that any prescribed oral medication regimen must be followed meticulously. Tinea infections are sometimes difficult to eradicate; discontinuing medication too soon risks recurrence. Treatment commonly continues for as long as 6 to 8 weeks and may continue for months for difficult infections of fingernails or toenails. It is important to advise the parent and the older child that the child taking griseofulvin must avoid sun exposure because griseofulvin makes the skin more susceptible to a photosensitivity reaction. If the child is taking itraconazole or longer courses of griseofulvin, the parent must ensure that the child undergoes any recommended liver-function studies.

PATIENT-CENTERED TEACHING

Home Care for a Child or Adolescent with a Tinea Infection

When providing information to the parent or older child with tinea, emphasize the following:

- Keep the infected areas as dry as possible.
- Do not share personal items, such as towels, washcloths, combs, hats, or hair ornaments.
- Athlete's foot: Wash the feet daily, and keep them dry. Nonventilated athletic shoes should dry thoroughly between wearing. Wear heavy cotton socks and change socks at least twice a day. Talcum powder or antifungal powder applied twice a day might help keep feet dry.
- Jock itch: Keep the groin area dry. Wear loose-fitting cotton underwear. Wash athletic supporters and underwear frequently. Wash the rash each day with plain water and dry carefully. Do not use soap on the affected area. Avoid scratching.
- Take oral medication as directed, even if the condition has improved. Discontinuing medication too soon can allow the infection to reappear.
- Call your physician if the infection has not improved in 4 weeks or if it continues to spread after 1 week of treatment.

Fungus thrives in a warm, moist environment, so it is important to keep infected areas as dry as possible. Teaching proper hygiene is essential for preventing and treating fungal infections. Teach children to avoid sharing personal items, such as combs, hats, and hair ornaments. Children with tinea infections should sleep alone and should not share towels and washcloths with others. Feet should be washed daily and kept dry. Advise children to allow their nonventilated athletic shoes to dry thoroughly between wearings. Heavy cotton socks absorb sweat and keep the feet dry. If tinea pedis is present, the child should change socks at least twice a day and go barefoot or wear sandals as much as possible. Talcum powder or antifungal powder applied twice a day might help keep feet dry. If the child showers at school or at a gym, shower shoes should be worn.

Tinea cruris heals much faster if the groin area is kept dry. Loose-fitting cotton underwear should be worn, and athletic supporters and underwear should be washed frequently. The rash should be washed each day with plain water and carefully dried. Soap should be avoided. Scratching delays healing, so instruct the child to avoid scratching the area. Reassure the young man and his parents that tinea cruris is not associated with sexually transmissible diseases.

Instruct parents to call the physician if the infection has not improved in 4 weeks or if it continues to spread after 1 week of treatment. Reassure parents that fungal infection is not an indication of poor hygiene or neglect. Avoid expressions of distaste or surprise when caring for children with severe alopecia or inflammation. Encourage parents to return the school-age child to school as soon as possible. Children with severe inflammatory tinea capitis may wish to wear a cap or scarf for a time until healing has progressed.

■ Evaluation

- Does the child have clean, intact skin?
- Is the child comfortable and without pruritus?
- Do the child and parents perform treatments correctly and verbalize ways to prevent the spread of infection?
- Does the child participate in usual social activities?

HERPES SIMPLEX VIRUS INFECTION

Herpes simplex types 1 and 2 (HSV 1, HSV 2) are responsible for a common, contagious, and often recurrent infection of the skin and mucous membranes. This infection can be asymptomatic or symptomatic and extremely painful. A wide spectrum of disease is caused by HSV: the common fever blister or cold sore (herpes labialis); corneal lesions; genital lesions (rare in children); and central nervous system infection.

Etiology

HSV is transmitted by infected body fluids and secretions coming in contact with breaks in the skin or mucous membranes. Delivery through an infected birth canal can cause infection in neonates. HSV can be transmitted by nurses who fail to practice careful hand hygiene. Children with burns, eczema, or diaper rash or those who are immunosuppressed are particularly susceptible to HSV infection.

Incidence

HSV is widespread. Infections in children are usually caused by HSV 1. Herpes labialis, commonly referred to as a "fever blister," is one of the most common manifestations of HSV 1. The primary infection with HSV 1 usually occurs before 20 years of age. Antibodies against this virus can be found in approximately 80% of adolescents (Opstelten, Neven, & Eekhof, 2008). Infection with HSV 2, which affects primarily the anal-genital area, is rare before age 14 years. Child sexual abuse should be considered in any child with a genital herpes infection.

Manifestations

Herpes Labialis ("Cold Sore," "Fever Blister")

Prodromal symptoms of herpes labialis are burning, itching, or tingling; these symptoms occur up to several days before lesions appear. Symptoms appear 2 days to 2 weeks after exposure. Lesions appear in clusters of fluid-filled vesicles that ulcerate, dry, and crust within 7 to 14 days (Figure 25-9). Usually one or two lesions are present on the lips, tongue, gingiva, or buccal mucosa. Pruritus and pain are present. Approximately 85% of active HSV 1 infections are asymptomatic.

Herpetic Gingivostomatitis

Herpes gingivostomatitis is a severe oral infection that affects children younger than 5 years. Vesicles and ulcerations, an edematous throat, and enlarged, painful cervical lymph nodes are seen. Associated signs and symptoms include chills, fever, malaise, bad breath, and drooling.

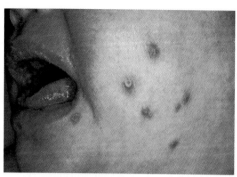

FIG 25-9 Herpes simplex infection in an infant. (From Feigin, R. D., & Cherry, J. D. [Eds.]. [2009]. *Textbook of pediatric infectious diseases* [6th ed., p. 760]. Philadelphia: Saunders.)

PATHOPHYSIOLOGY

Herpes Simplex Type 1 Infection

The four types of human herpesviruses are HSV types 1 and 2; cytomegalovirus; Epstein-Barr virus, which causes infectious mononucleosis; and varicella-zoster virus. HSV 1 causes the "oral" type of herpes and usually affects areas above the waist, producing cold sores, fever blisters, and corneal lesions. HSV 2 affects areas below the waist (anal-genital area). However, either type can affect any region of the body. After an initial HSV 1 infection, the virus remains dormant but alive within nerve cells innervating that portion of the skin originally infected. Fever, stress, trauma, sun exposure, menstruation, or immunosuppression can reactivate the virus. When reactivated, the virus migrates to the skin area innervated by the ganglia that harbor it, near the site of the initial infection. The recurrent infection can be symptomatic or asymptomatic, but it is just as contagious as the initial infection. Recurrent infections tend to be less severe than the initial infection.

The immune status of the host determines the severity of HSV infection. HSV 1 infection in the neonate or immunocompromised child can be fatal. HSV 1 is a common cause of viral encephalitis in children.

Herpetic whitlow, a painful HSV 1 infection of the fingers, can be transmitted to a nurse during oral or tracheal care of a child with herpes infection. Thumb-sucking children with oral HSV 1 infection can also develop this condition. Health care personnel with herpetic whitlow should not have patient contact until the infection has healed because the infection is highly contagious.

Herpetic Ocular Infection

Herpetic ocular infection (keratitis) is typically the result of rubbing the eyes with contaminated fingers. Herpetic keratitis causes irritation and inflammation of the conjunctiva or cornea with associated tearing and photophobia. Vesicles appear on the eyelid and mucous membranes of the eye. Children with HSV keratitis are at risk for recurrent episodes and vision loss (Potter, 2010).

Herpetic Whitlow

Symptoms of herpetic whitlow appear 3 to 7 days after exposure and include vesicles, swelling, pruritus, and severe pain of the affected fingers. Discomfort may continue for weeks after the vesicles have healed.

Diagnostic Evaluation

Clinical manifestations and the child's history suggest the diagnosis. A Tzanck smear can confirm a herpes infection, but a positive smear cannot differentiate between varicella-zoster virus and HSV 1, and a negative smear does not rule out HSV infection. Immunofluorescence assay to detect HSV-1 antigen and polymerase chain reaction to detect HSV 1 deoxyribonucleic acid can be performed on blood samples, but tissue culture is still considered the gold standard for diagnosis. Future diagnostic imaging studies may utilize high-resolution optical coherence tomography (OCT) (Wang & Ritterband, 2009).

Therapeutic Management

Treatment is symptomatic. The child with oral HSV 1 infection is usually cared for at home if able to take adequate fluids. If the child becomes dehydrated, IV fluids are needed.

Topical or oral acyclovir (Zovirax), if given early enough in the course of the infection, can reduce the time to recovery. Although there is no cure for HSV 1 infection, acyclovir given IV may be used in immunocompromised children, neonates, and children with encephalitis to decrease the severity of the infection (Stanberry, 2011). Treatment of ocular HSV 1 infection is determined in consultation with an ophthalmology specialist.

Antibiotic ointment may be used to treat secondary bacterial infection of lesions. Corticosteroids are contraindicated because they can worsen HSV 1 infection. Oral or rectal acetaminophen, with or without codeine, may be prescribed, and topical anesthetics may be dabbed on lesions to help relieve pain. A prescribed anesthetic mouth rinse of equal parts of diphenhydramine (Benadryl) elixir, Kaopectate, and 2% viscous lidocaine may decrease pain and help the child eat. Topical anesthetics, such as viscous lidocaine, must be used with caution. Overuse of topical anesthetics in small children can depress the gag reflex and increase the risk of aspiration.

NURSING CARE OF THE CHILD WITH A HERPES SIMPLEX INFECTION

▪ Assessment

Obtain a history, and ask the parent or child about previous HSV infections or contact with an infected person. Examine the skin carefully for lesions. Inspect the eyes for corneal ulcerations and edema and assess the child's vision for pain, blurring, and photophobia. Referral to an ophthalmologist is necessary for suspected ocular HSV infection. For the child with herpes gingivostomatitis, pay particular attention to assessing hydration status.

▪ Nursing Diagnosis and Planning

The nursing diagnoses and expected outcomes that may be appropriate for the child with a herpes simplex infection and the child's family are as follows:

- Impaired Skin Integrity related to inadequate secondary defenses.

Expected Outcomes. The child will demonstrate healing of lesions. The child will have no other signs of infection.

- Acute Pain related to inflammation and infection.

Expected Outcome. The child will have minimal pain, as evidenced by adequate fluid intake, decreased verbalization of pain, and decreased restlessness and irritability.

- Risk for Infection related to changes in skin integrity.

Expected Outcome. The child will have no signs of secondary bacterial infection, as evidenced by healing lesions and normal body temperature.

- Risk for Deficient Fluid Volume related to painful oral lesions.

Expected Outcomes. The child will maintain urine output appropriate for age and will exhibit moist mucous membranes and good skin turgor.

■ Interventions

Children with oral HSV infection may be extremely uncomfortable. Swallowing can cause severe pain, and dehydration is a real danger. Advise parents to contact the physician if the child has signs of dehydration. Fluid intake is very important, and the child must be encouraged to drink. Most children will accept ice pops, noncitrus juices, milk, and noncarbonated or "flattened" soft drinks. Frequent small feedings of bland, soft foods can be offered. Reassure parents that a few days without solid food will not harm the child as long as fluid intake is adequate.

To prevent secondary infection, the child's mouth should be rinsed often with normal saline solution, especially after eating. Hospitalized children infected with HSV should be placed on Contact Precautions. The child is considered contagious until the scabs from visible lesions have fallen off. Because scabs do not form on mucous membranes, these lesions are considered contagious until they are completely healed. All persons who have contact with the child should follow Contact Precautions meticulously and be particularly careful when touching the child near the lesions, when administering oral care or suctioning, and when handling bed linens or objects that might be contaminated with saliva or secretions from the lesions. Careful hand hygiene is essential.

Parents should take similar precautions when caring for the child at home to prevent spread of infection. Advise the parents to wash bottles, nipples, toys, eating utensils, and towels in hot, soapy water or in a dishwasher, if available. Family members should not share any of these items with the infected child.

Because the infection can be spread to other parts of the body, the child should not put his or her fingers near the mouth or infected area. Elbow restraints may be necessary for children too young to understand this. The child with HSV 1 infection is usually miserable and needs generous cuddling and comforting.

■ Evaluation

- Are lesions healed, with no sign of the infection spreading?
- Does the child demonstrate increased comfort?
- Does the skin remain free of signs of secondary infection (redness, swelling, drainage)?
- Is the child properly hydrated with adequate fluid intake and hourly urine output (see Chapter 16)?
- Can the parent or caregiver describe infection control measures?

SKIN INFESTATIONS

Children may become infested with a variety of parasitic insects that feed on human blood and cause intense itching with subsequent alterations in skin integrity. These include lice and mites that cause scabies. Infestations are extremely contagious and require a holistic management approach.

LICE INFESTATION

Lice are small, blood-sucking insects about 2 to 4 mm in length. *Pediculosis* refers to infestation of lice on the scalp or body. Although pediculosis is not a serious health problem, it can cause embarrassment and often elicits an emotional reaction among parents and school personnel who may mistakenly associate it with poor hygiene. Head lice are not responsible for the spread of any disease, although body lice are known to serve as vectors of several pathogenic bacteria (Centers for Disease Control and Prevention [CDC], 2008a).

Etiology

Lice live only on humans and are transmitted by direct contact with infected persons and indirect contact with infested objects (e.g., brushes, hats). Lice cannot jump like fleas, and clean hair is no deterrent to head lice.

Incidence

The prevalence of head lice is difficult to determine precisely because it is not a reportable condition. However, it is estimated that millions of children worldwide are infested each year (CDC, 2008a). Pediculosis rarely occurs in African-Americans. Girls are affected twice as often as boys. All socioeconomic groups are affected. The peak incidence is in preschool and young school-age children. Pubic lice are usually seen in adolescents or young adults and are generally transmitted by sexual contact.

PATHOPHYSIOLOGY

Pediculosis

Pediculosis may involve the scalp (pediculosis capitis), the body (pediculosis corporis), or the pubic area and eyelashes (pediculosis pubis). A specific type of louse, each of which has a similar life cycle, causes each of these infestations. All lice pierce the skin and suck blood. Severe itching caused by bites can predispose the child to secondary infection.

Head and pubic lice spend their life cycles on the skin of the human host; body lice live in clothing, coming to the skin only to feed. The female head louse lays eggs (nits) at the base of the hair shaft. The egg is covered with a gelatinous material, which hardens to semiopaque, tiny, pearly whitish masses that are stuck tight to the hair shaft (see Figure 25-10). Eggs incubate for about 1 week, and lice reach sexual maturity in about 2 weeks.

Pediculosis pubis is spread through sexual contact. Half of all patients with pediculosis pubis have another sexually transmissible disease, usually gonorrhea.

Lice can spread as long as the lice and nits remain alive on the infested person or belongings. Lice can live only 48 hours off the human host. Nits shed into the environment are capable of hatching for 10 days.

Manifestations

Pediculosis Capitis (Head Lice)

Nits are visible and are attached firmly to the hair shafts near the scalp. They are tiny, silvery or grayish white specks resembling dandruff, but they are more difficult to remove. They are commonly found behind the ears and at the nape of the neck. In active infestation, nits are found approximately $\frac{1}{4}$ to $\frac{1}{2}$ inch away from the scalp surface (Figure 25-10); nits found greater than $\frac{1}{2}$ inch from the scalp are considered to be nonviable (Bhatt, Curnutte, & Moore, 2008). Adult lice are difficult to see because of their small size and the fact that they crawl very fast to avoid light. Scattered lesions on the scalp, behind the ears, or on the back of the neck cause intense pruritus. These lesions are often associated with posterior cervical lymph adenopathy. Secondary scalp infection may develop from scratching.

Pediculosis Corporis (Body Lice)

Papular, rose-colored dermatitis, causing intense pruritus, appears on the skin in areas under tight clothing. Nits attach firmly to seams of the child's clothing or bedding.

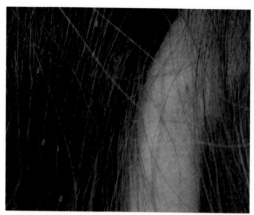

FIG 25-10 Head lice (pediculosis capitis). Note the nits attached to the hair shafts. (From Callen, J., Greer, K. E., Hood, A. F., & Swinyer, L. J. [1993]. *Color atlas of dermatology* [p. 373]. Philadelphia: Saunders.)

Pediculosis Pubis (Pubic Lice, Crab Lice)

Pediculosis pubis are lice that can be found in pubic hair and facial hair, in axillae, and on the body surface. The presence of pubic lice in the eyebrows or eyelashes of a prepubescent child suggests sexual abuse. Pubic lice also cause intense pruritus. Maculae ceruleae (blue spots) may be seen on the thighs and trunk in cases of heavy infestation. Dark-brown spots on underwear and sheets are insect waste materials.

Diagnostic Evaluation

The diagnosis of head lice is made by identification of nits or lice on the scalp. The examiner parts the hair with two tongue depressors and moves from side to side and front to back, paying particular attention to the crown, behind the ears, and the nape of the neck. The exposed scalp should be carefully examined under bright light or in a sunny area. A magnifying glass can assist in identification. Combing the hair with a fine-tooth nit comb can quickly aid in diagnosis (Bhatt et al., 2008). Unlike dandruff, nits are not easily removed from hair shafts. Pubic lice are diagnosed from a history of symptoms and visual inspection.

Therapeutic Management

Management of the child with pediculosis focuses primarily on killing active lice and nits, and preventing spread or recurrence by managing the environment.

Killing Active Lice and Nits

Approaches to treating pediculosis are changing as a result of the development of pediculicide-resistant strains of lice and because prescription lindane (Kwell) persists as a poison in the environment and can be neurotoxic if absorbed through the skin. Lindane, a hexachlorocyclohexane, has been nominated for elimination as a persistent organic pollutant under the provision of the Stockholm Convention on Persistent Organic Pollutants (United Nations Environmental Programme, 2009).

An over-the-counter pediculicide, permethrin 1% (Nix, Elimite, Acticin), kills head lice and pubic lice and eggs with one application and has residual activity (i.e., it stays in the hair after treatment) for 10 days. Nix crème rinse is applied to the hair after it is washed with a conditioner-free shampoo. It is applied as a lotion to pubic hair. Crème rinse or lotion should be rinsed out after 10 minutes. The hair should not be shampooed for 24 hours after the treatment. Even

though the kill rate is high and there is residual action, retreatment should occur after 7 to 10 days (AAP, 2010). Over-the-counter products containing pyrethrins (RID, Triple X, Tisit, R&C, Pronto) are safe and effective, but lice are becoming resistant to them. Because they lack residual activity, treatment with these products must be repeated on days 7 to 10 after the initial treatment. Ovicides should not be used routinely in children younger than 2 years (Bhatt et al., 2008); using a fine-tooth nit comb on wet, conditioned hair at least four times over a 2-week period is an evidence-based recommendation (Bhatt et al., 2008). Recent research that looked at a nonchemical treatment for lice suggested that an application of Cetaphil Gentle Cleanser followed by blow-drying may be effective as a suffocation-based therapy and is a safe alternative to chemical pesticides (Diamantis, Morrell, & Burkhart, 2009). Methods such as this show promise for future management of pediculosis.

Pubic lice are treated similarly to head lice, with the exception of areas around the eyes, which can be treated with two to four applications a day of petroleum jelly (AAP, 2010). Treatment and testing for other sexually transmissible diseases are required for sexual contacts of a person with pubic lice. For body lice, clothing and bedding should be washed in hot water and dried for 20 minutes at a hot dryer setting. Meticulous hygiene and regular laundering can eliminate body lice (AAP, 2010).

The pesticide malathion (Ovide) is approved for the treatment of lice in children older than 6 years, but it requires prolonged contact (i.e., 8 to 10 hours) to be effective. It is also flammable, and families should be cautioned not to use hair dryers or allow the child near fires or heaters while hair is being treated. The AAP recommendations for the treatment of head lice are revised every 3 years, and the interested reader is referred to that source for current guidelines (www.aap.org).

Addressing the Environment

Environmental objects, clothing, and bedding should be treated or washed. It is important to examine family members and others who might be in close contact with the infested child; only those with an observed infestation should be treated (Bhatt et al., 2008). The parent needs to notify the school if a child has an active case. Meticulous vacuuming of carpets in classrooms with affected children will help prevent transmission.

NURSING CARE OF THE CHILD WITH PEDICULOSIS

■ Assessment

Examine children for lice in an unobtrusive and private manner. In a school setting, classmates should be brought to the school nurse's office and admitted one at a time, rather than being seen together in a general check in a classroom setting. Use disposable tongue depressors or ice-pop sticks to part the hair, and discard these implements between children. Check all family members for the presence of nits or lice.

Assess adolescents with pubic lice for signs of other sexually transmissible diseases and ask about sexual contacts, because they will need treatment as well.

■ Nursing Diagnosis and Planning

The nursing diagnoses and expected outcomes that may be appropriate for the child with pediculosis and the child's family are as follows:

• Acute Pain related to inflammatory response and pruritus.
Expected Outcomes. The child will rest comfortably and will refrain from scratching.

• Risk for Infection related to scratching of scalp.

Expected Outcome. The child will have no signs of secondary bacterial infection, as evidenced by intact skin and normal-size cervical lymph nodes.

- Deficient Knowledge about treatment of lice infestation and the prevention of recurrence related to anxiety or incomplete information.

Expected Outcomes. The child or family will carry out the prescribed treatment. The parent will demonstrate measures taken to prevent reinfestation.

- Risk for Situational Low Self-Esteem related to social stigma associated with lice.

Expected Outcomes. The child or family will verbalize self-acceptance and will engage in usual social activities.

■ Interventions

Advise parents to carefully follow directions that come with over-the-counter pediculicides or to follow the physician's instructions for using prescription products. Caution parents against applying the medication more frequently than recommended.

Reassure parents that lice infestation does not reflect poor hygiene or low socioeconomic status. Advise them that it is necessary to notify the school nurse if the child is infested.

If the parent believes it is necessary to remove nits, teach the parent to remove them by back-combing with a fine-tooth comb. One hour before combing, nits can be loosened with a mixture of half vinegar and half water or a commercial product, such as Clear or Step 2. It is easier to comb the child's hair for nit removal when the hair is damp rather than wet or dry. Lice and nits can be removed from eyelashes by applying petrolatum to the eyelashes twice a day for 8 days. Many schools have a "no nit" policy, which requires that a child be free of all nits before re-entry, although such policies are strongly discouraged because of the missed school time and the low risk of transmitting the infestation to others (Rollins, 2010).

Advise parents to wash clothing (especially hats and jackets), bedding, and linens in hot water and dry at a hot dryer setting. Dress-up clothes, hair ornaments, bicycle helmets, batting helmets, headphones, and similar objects should be treated as well. Items that cannot be washed should be dry cleaned or sealed in plastic bags for 2 to 3 weeks.

Antilice sprays used for furniture and other environmental objects should never be used on a child. Thorough home cleaning is necessary to remove any remaining lice or nits. Parents should vacuum floors, play areas, and furniture to remove any hairs that might carry live nits. Combs and brushes should be boiled or soaked in antilice shampoo or hot water (greater than 140° F [60° C]) for at least 10 minutes. Routinely teach children not to share hats, combs, or hair ornaments with other children. At school, individually assigned lockers or separate hooks for coats can help inhibit spread of lice.

The child should be rechecked for infestation in 7 to 10 days. Advise parents to call the physician if itching interferes with the child's sleep, if the condition does not clear up after 1 week, or if scalp lesions look infected. The National Pediculosis Association provides information about this condition (see www.headlice.org). The Centers for Disease Control and Prevention is a resource that provides reliable, up-to-date information on the recommendations for combating head lice at www.cdc.gov/lice/head/treatment.html#supplement.

■ Evaluation

- Is the child free of infestation, pain, and pruritus?
- Is the skin intact, and does the child exhibit normal-size cervical lymph nodes?

- Do parents carry out the prescribed treatments?
- Can parents describe measures to prevent the spread of lice to others?
- Do the parents and child realistically describe the cause of pediculosis and continue to engage in usual social activities?

? CRITICAL THINKING EXERCISE 25-1

The pediatric clinic receives a phone call from an obviously upset mother about her 4-year-old daughter, who is in preschool. This is the third time in 1 month that the parent has been called at work to take her child out of school because the child was found to have lice. The mother states that she has properly treated her daughter and other family members, and she insists that the child is catching the condition from someone at school. The school maintains that no other child has this problem.

1. What should be the nurse's approach to this mother?
2. What kind of information will the nurse need to obtain to help this mother with her problem?

EVIDENCE-BASED PRACTICE

Pediculosis

Level V

Pediculosis is a worldwide problem, and its treatment is challenging for families. The cost associated with treating a family for a lice infestation can be high. In addition, resistance to pediculicide is increasing, potentially reducing the effectiveness of existing treatments. Treatment is effective only when 100% of adult lice are killed and eggs are prevented from hatching.

Bhatt, Curnutte, and Moore (2008) published a clinical practice guideline (Level V evidence) that addresses the diagnosis and treatment of pediculosis in children. Their recommendations for diagnosis and treatment of pediculosis have been described. This guideline provides good evidence that persistent infestation usually results from incomplete following of directions for using pediculicides, pediculicide resistance, or reinfestation. The guideline does not suggest, however, that complete removal of nits is necessary to prevent treatment failure.

The frustration felt by families whose members are repeatedly infested with lice has resulted in an upsurge in use of traditional home remedies or remedies obtained by searching the Internet. "No nit" policies in schools have contributed to interruptions in student education and achievement.

If you were doing a clinical placement in a school setting, where the school nurse was maintaining a "no nit" policy, what information might you want to give the nurse? How would you support your recommendation, and where might you refer the nurse for updated information? What kind of teaching might you do with families of children who have a problem with repeated infestations?

From Bhatt, V., Curnutte, E., & Moore, J. (2008). *Guidelines for the diagnosis and treatment of pediculosis capitis (head lice) in children and adults 2008.* Retrieved from www.guidelines.gov.

MITE INFESTATION (SCABIES)

Scabies is a contagious condition that has been recognized for many centuries. It results from infestation with *Sarcoptes scabiei*, the "itch mite."

Etiology

Scabies is transmitted by close personal contact with infected persons. Persons who share a bed or live in crowded conditions are likely to transmit scabies to each other. The scabies mite cannot survive for more than 3 days away from human skin. For that reason, transmission of scabies by bedding or clothing is infrequent.

Incidence

Scabies is widespread throughout the United States and it is prevalent in many schools. All socioeconomic groups are affected.

Pathophysiology

The female mite burrows into the epidermis, lays her eggs, and dies in the burrow after 4 to 5 weeks. The eggs hatch in 3 to 5 days, and larvae migrate to the skin surface to mature and complete the life cycle. The mites, eggs, and their excrement cause intense pruritus. One of the major complications of scabies is impetigo resulting from scratching.

Manifestations

Intense pruritus occurs, especially at night. Infants may be cranky, sleep fitfully, and rub their hands and feet together. Burrows (fine, grayish, threadlike lines) can be difficult to see because they are usually obscured by secondary changes of excoriation and inflammation. Papules, vesicles, and nodules are common (Figure 25-11) and are located mainly on the wrists, in the finger webs, on the elbows, in the umbilicus, in the axillae, in the groin, and on the buttocks. In infants, the head, palms, and soles may be affected.

Diagnostic Evaluation

The characteristic skin eruption and a history of intense pruritus, especially at night, are suggestive of scabies. The diagnosis is made by microscopic examination of scrapings of the lesions.

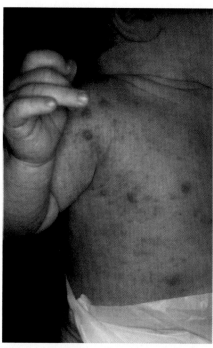

FIG 25-11 Scabies lesions on an infant. (From Callen, J. P., Greer, K. E., Paller, A. S., & Swinyer, L. J. [2000]. *Color atlas of dermatology* [3rd ed., p. 3283]. Philadelphia: Saunders.)

Therapeutic Management

Scabies can be treated with topical application of permethrin 5% (Elimite); lindane cream 1% (Kwell, Scabene) is used as an alternative if primary treatment with permethrin is not effective (AAP, 2009). Because of the risk of neurotoxicity, lindane should not be used in children younger than 2 years or in pregnant women. The medication is applied to the body and head (depending on age), avoiding the eyes and mouth. The medication must remain on the child for 8 to 14 hours (depending on the medication prescribed) to be effective, so applying it at bedtime is recommended. It is washed off in the morning. Retreatment in 1 week is usually recommended. Pruritus may last for several days to weeks after treatment and can be relieved with corticosteroid cream (e.g., hydrocortisone cream) and oral antihistamines.

Family members, even if asymptomatic, and daycare contacts (except for pregnant women) should also be treated. The child's bedding and clothing should be washed in hot water in a fashion similar to the environmental treatment for pediculosis.

Nursing Considerations

Nursing care of the child and family with scabies is similar to that for pediculosis. Inspect the child's hands, elbows, umbilicus, groin, and buttocks for burrows. Burrows may be difficult to see, however, and complaints of persistent itching may be the only symptom. Evaluate an adolescent with scabies for sexually transmitted disease.

Instruct parents to use the scabicide according to the manufacturer's instructions. The lotion is applied all over the child's body, including the soles of the feet, the scalp, behind the ears, in intertriginous areas, and under the toenails and fingernails. The lotion should be kept on for the recommended time (4 to 8 hours for lindane, 8 to 14 hours for Elimite), and then the child should be bathed. Infants should be clothed during treatment so they will not lick their skin. To minimize absorption and the risk of toxic effects from lindane, the lotion should not be applied for at least 30 minutes after bathing and should be applied only to cool, dry skin. Advise the parent that persistent itching after treatment is expected for about 2 weeks and is not a sign of reinfestation or an indication for repeated application.

Scabies is usually cured with one treatment; however, a repeat application in 1 week is recommended. Clothing and bed linen should be dry cleaned or washed in hot water and dried at a hot dryer setting.

ACNE VULGARIS

Acne is a disorder of the sebaceous hair follicles. Although acne is generally perceived as a minor disorder, it can cause significant anxiety and emotional pain for affected adolescents. The disfiguring lesions of acne can lead to physical and emotional scarring.

Etiology

Multiple factors play a role in the development of acne lesions, including abnormal sloughing of skin cells lining the sebaceous hair follicles, overgrowth of normal bacteria, and host factors, such as heredity, hormonal influences, and emotional stress. Acne of neonates may be triggered by infection with fungi, such as *Pityrosporum* species in some infants. Foods do not appear to cause or increase the severity of acne. Acne is unrelated to the general cleanliness of the skin.

Incidence

Acne affects approximately 85% of adolescents and up to 20% of neonates. Although acne may begin at any age, it usually develops during puberty and lasts into early adulthood. Acne is more common in boys than in girls. It tends to improve in summer and flare up in winter. Acne of newborn infants typically resolves spontaneously by 3 months of age.

PATHOPHYSIOLOGY

Acne Vulgaris

Acne begins when sebaceous glands, stimulated by androgens at the onset of puberty, enlarge and secrete increased amounts of sebum. The sebaceous glands become plugged and dilated with sebum. When the enlarged gland is open to the skin surface, an open comedo, or blackhead, is formed. The characteristic black color is not a result of poor hygiene but is produced as fatty acids are oxidized on the skin. If the gland does not have an opening, a closed comedo, or whitehead, is formed. Closed comedones are small, non-erythematous papules just beneath the skin surface. Because a closed comedo has only a microscopic opening on the skin surface, pressure from excess sebum and keratin causes the comedo walls to rupture. Fatty acids produced by bacterial action on sebum are released into the surrounding tissues, causing inflammation. If the rupture occurs close to the surface, a pustule is formed. Ruptures deep in the dermis result in cysts and abscesses, which can lead to significant scarring.

Bacteria, particularly *Propionibacterium acnes,* play a role in the development of acne lesions by increasing inflammation and disrupting the integrity of the follicle walls.

Manifestations and Diagnostic Evaluation

Acne consists of closed whiteheads, blackheads, papules, pustules, nodules, and cysts (Figure 25-12). Not all adolescents have all types of acne, and treatment is based on the type of acne. The areas most often affected are the face, neck, back, shoulders, and upper chest. The diagnosis is based on examination of the lesions and the child's history.

Therapeutic Management

The goal of treatment is to prevent scarring and to promote a positive self-image in the adolescent. Treatment must be individualized according to the severity of the condition, the types of lesion present, and the adolescent's gender. Improvement usually begins in 4 to 6 weeks, so the adolescent needs support to keep from feeling discouraged after treatment begins. Three to 5 months are needed for optimal results.

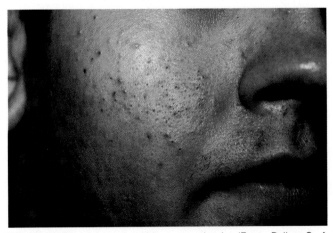

FIG 25-12 An adolescent with acne vulgaris. (From Paller, S. A. [2012]. *Hurwitz clinical pediatric dermatology: A textbook of skin disorders of childhood and adolescence* [4th ed., p. 168]. Philadelphia: Saunders.)

Topical therapy with a variety of agents is the primary treatment for acne. Commonly used agents include benzoyl peroxide, which reduces fatty acid production and is bactericidal for *Propionibacterium acnes,* and tretinoin (Retin-A), a vitamin A derivative. Tretinoin reduces comedo formation and eliminates the lesions already present. Benzoyl peroxide comes in a gel, cream, lotion, or soap in various strengths. Lower-potency formulas are available over the counter. Tretinoin is available in cream, gel, or liquid form by prescription. Sunscreen should be used with tretinoin to reduce photosensitivity. When applied together to the skin, benzoyl peroxide and tretinoin have a potentially offsetting effect that can reduce the overall effectiveness of each individual agent. For this reason, the health provider may order that the two medications be applied on alternate days or that benzoyl peroxide be applied in the morning and tretinoin at bedtime. In most instances it will take approximately 8 weeks for topical preparations to be effective (Morelli, 2011).

Topical antibiotics, such as clindamycin and erythromycin, decrease the number of *P. acnes* organisms in hair follicles and are often used for inflammatory acne. Topical antibiotics are preferred over systemic antibiotics.

Oral antibiotics (tetracycline, minocycline, erythromycin, clindamycin) might be prescribed for adolescents with severe inflammatory acne or those who are unresponsive to topical treatment. Exposure to sunlight should be avoided if tetracycline is used. Oral isotretinoin (Accutane) has dramatically improved the condition of adolescents with severe nodular/cystic acne. This drug suppresses sebum production and sebaceous gland activity. Because of the severity of side effects, isotretinoin is not indicated for all adolescents. Side effects include cataracts, cheilitis, dry skin, pruritus, conjunctivitis, nosebleeds, and depression. In some instances, depression associated with isotretinoin has possibly resulted in suicide (Morelli, 2011). Young women who anticipate becoming pregnant should not take isotretinoin because of its teratogenic effects. Sexually active female adolescents should use an effective form of contraception, or combination of contraceptive methods, from 1 month before treatment until 6 weeks after discontinuing treatment. A negative pregnancy test must be obtained before initiating therapy. Informed consent is recommended for treatment with isotretinoin.

Estrogen may be prescribed for young women who are unresponsive to antibiotic therapy or who cannot take isotretinoin. Some combination (progestin and estrogen) oral contraceptives may also be indicated for acne treatment. Although the dermatologist may mechanically express comedones, the adolescent should be cautioned not to pick or squeeze lesions. Although scars cannot be completely removed, techniques such as dermabrasion, plastic repair, and collagen implants may improve appearance.

NURSING CARE OF THE ADOLESCENT WITH ACNE VULGARIS

■ Assessment

Obtain a history that includes how long acne lesions have been present and the effect of menses, stress, and other aggravating factors on the severity and frequency of the lesions. Investigate acne treatments that have been tried and their effectiveness. Establish how often the adolescent washes the skin and hair and the type of cleansing agents used. Inquire about whether the adolescent uses cosmetics on a regular basis and what types of cosmetics are used. Try to assess the adolescent's understanding of the development and treatment of acne.

Examine the adolescent's face, chest, back, and neck for lesions. The depth of tissue involvement and the presence of pustules, papules, cysts, and scars should be noted. The adolescent's feelings about appearance and self-image and the effects acne may have had on social functioning should be explored.

■ Nursing Diagnosis and Planning

The nursing diagnoses and expected outcomes that may be appropriate for the adolescent with acne vulgaris are as follows:

- Impaired Skin Integrity related to increased sebaceous gland secretions, hormonal changes, and the action of bacteria on the contents of clogged follicles.

Expected Outcome. Affected areas will exhibit signs of healing.

- Risk for Infection related to inflammation of skin lesions.

Expected Outcome. The adolescent will have no signs of secondary bacterial infection, as evidenced by clear, intact skin.

- Disturbed Body Image related to appearance of skin lesions.

Expected Outcomes. The adolescent will verbalize feelings and concerns and will participate in desired social activities.

- Deficient Knowledge about skin care and treatment regimen related to being too embarrassed to ask questions.

Expected Outcome. The adolescent will carry out the prescribed treatment regimen to control excessive sebaceous gland activity.

■ Interventions

Because acne is a long-term condition, the affected adolescent needs support and encouragement if the treatment regimen is to be effective. Improvement may take as long as 12 weeks, and exacerbations are common. Although there is no cure for acne, much can be done to control inflammation and reduce scarring.

Explain the cause of acne and the rationale for treatment at the outset, so the adolescent can help plan the treatment regimen. Providing written instructions and involving the adolescent in care can help improve adherence. The treatment must be individualized, but all treatment regimens include measures to reduce oil on the skin. Gently cleaning the face twice a day with mild antibacterial soap and shampooing the hair daily are important facets of care. Warn the adolescent to avoid vigorous scrubbing and picking or squeezing of lesions, which can rupture pilosebaceous ducts and cause secondary infection. Teach the adolescent how to apply topical medications and caution against overusing these products to speed results. Because oily cosmetics and creams add to the plugging of follicles, only water-based cosmetics should be used.

A healthy lifestyle, including adequate rest, exercise, and a balanced diet, promotes healing of lesions. Explore the adolescent's feelings about appearance and coping mechanisms. Reinforce positive self-image and self-esteem. Concerns and fears should be openly discussed and myths about acne dispelled. Provide parents with needed information about acne to clear up misconceptions and to prevent needless nagging of the adolescent.

■ Evaluation

- Do the acne lesions exhibit signs of healing without signs of infection?
- Is the adolescent able to express feelings and concerns about possible change in body image?
- Does the adolescent appear confident and assured as the process of healing is occurring?
- Does the adolescent carry out the treatment regimen to control acne and prevent scarring?

MISCELLANEOUS SKIN DISORDERS

There are a large number of less common skin disorders of varied causes and manifestations. Several of these disorders, along with their manifestations, management, and special considerations, are listed in Table 25-1.

TABLE 25-1 **SKIN DISORDERS**			
DISORDER/ETIOLOGY	**MANIFESTATIONS**	**MANAGEMENT**	**COMMENTS**
Stevens-Johnson Syndrome			
Acute, sometimes recurrent autoimmune disease. May be triggered by infections or medications, such as sulfonamides or anticonvulsants. New lesions continue to erupt for 2-3 wk, followed by healing during the next 6 wk.	After a prodromal respiratory illness, bullae appear on the lips, mouth, eyes, and genitalia. Fever, chills, malaise, neutropenia, anemia, weakness. Purulent conjunctivitis is common. Skin lesions rupture and may lead to significant fluid loss.	Withdraw the triggering medication. Treatment of skin lesions similar to treatment of extensive burns: aseptic technique, IV fluids, air/fluid bedding, nutritional support, pain management. Give antibiotics for secondary infections. Obtain ophthalmology consultation for eye lesions.	Reassure the child that the skin lesions will disappear. Inform parents about the possibility of recurrence and encourage them to avoid any implicated medications.
Psoriasis			
Chronic, inflammatory rash caused by rapid proliferation of keratinocytes. Hereditary predisposition; onset in first two decades of life. Remissions and exacerbations; lasts throughout life. Exacerbations associated with stress. Arthritis is sometimes a complication.	Pruritus; erythematous, elevated plaques and silvery scales on the scalp, face, knees, elbows, and gluteal folds. Scales are attached at the center rather than edges and may bleed when removed.	Topical corticosteroids and tar preparations; keratolytic agents. Exposure to ultraviolet light and sunlight. Skin care to prevent secondary infection. Keratolytic agents enhance penetration of topical steroids. Sunlight may cause phototoxic reactions with tar preparations. To prevent tar folliculitis, tar should be applied down an extremity rather than up.	There is no cure for psoriasis. Cutaneous trauma and streptococcal infections (e.g., tonsillitis) are common aggravating factors. A resource for families of children with psoriasis is the National Psoriasis Foundation: www.psoriasis.org/home.

TABLE 25-1 SKIN DISORDERS—cont'd

DISORDER/ETIOLOGY	MANIFESTATIONS	MANAGEMENT	COMMENTS
Pityriasis Rosea Acute, inflammatory, self-limited skin disorder. Etiology unknown; may be viral.	Sudden eruption of salmon-pink, irregular patches on trunk and proximal portions of extremities. Symmetrical distribution of lesions, "Christmas tree" appearance on back. "Herald patch" precedes rash by 7-10 days.	No treatment required for asymptomatic children. Pruritus can be treated with antipruritic lotions, ultraviolet light, or sunlight.	Child generally feels well. Rash may last 6-12 wk.
Warts Skin infection caused by human papillomavirus. Incubation period is 1-6 mo. Can persist from a few months to 5+ yr.	Painless, hyperkeratotic papule. Begins as a round, flesh-colored papule; later becomes brown or tan with a rough surface. Most common sites: dorsum of hands, fingers, feet, face, genitalia.	Various methods of treatment: daily application of lactic acid and salicylic acid (e.g., Compound W); freezing with liquid nitrogen; topical application of cantharidin for plantar or periungual warts.	Most warts disappear without treatment in 2-3 yr. With treatment, they usually resolve in 2-3 mo. Picking at warts may cause them to spread to other areas of the body. Warts are not highly contagious to other people. Immunocompromised children are more susceptible to warts.
Molluscum Contagiosum Viral infection of the skin and mucous membranes. Transmitted by skin-to-skin and fomite-to-skin contact. May be transmitted by sexual contact.	Begin as pinpoint papules that increase in size to 2-3 mm or larger. Firm, solid, pink papules changing into soft, waxy, umbilicated papules. Curdlike core of the lesion can be expressed. Most common sites: face, trunk, extremities, oral mucous membranes, conjunctiva, genitalia.	Lesions may be treated with cantharidin, cryotherapy, tretinoin, or imiquimod. Condition usually responds well to treatment. Spontaneous disappearance is common.	Lesions may be spread to other parts of the body and may be transmitted to others. Lesions disappear spontaneously over time. Children with eczema or impaired immunity are at risk for generalized spread of lesions. (See Chapter 17 for additional discussion of genital warts [HPV].)
Frostbite Freezing of tissue resulting from exposure to extreme cold. Exposed areas (fingers, toes, nose, cheeks, ears) are most often affected. Cold causes arteriolar vasoconstriction, resulting in tissue anoxia and destruction.	Early signs: blanching of skin; stinging sensation followed by numbness and white, mottled appearance. Area feels cold, hard; may be without sensation. First-degree: redness and discomfort with return to normal in a few hours. Second-degree: redness; blisters and bullae 24-48 hr after rewarming. Pain during rewarming. Third-degree: cyanosis and mottling, followed by redness and swelling. Necrosis of epidermis, dermis, and subcutaneous tissue. Sensation is absent. Pain during rewarming. Fourth-degree: complete necrosis with gangrene, possible loss of body part.	Immediately cover affected areas with warm hands and warm clothing. Massaging areas causes further damage and should be avoided. Rapidly rewarm areas by immersion in a warm water bath (90°-106° F [32.2°-41.1° C]) until all frozen tissues are thawed and the skin appears flushed. Pain during thawing can be severe and should be treated with analgesics and sedatives. Severely damaged areas are treated as burns.	Children in cold climates should be taught to prevent frostbite by wearing adequate warm, layered clothing, hat, gloves, and two pairs of socks (one cotton, one wool). Children should be taught to warm themselves when hands or feet begin to sting. Young children should not be allowed to play outside in extremely cold temperatures.
Foreign Bodies Skin injury caused by penetration of splinters, gravel, cactus spines, bee stingers, glass, or other foreign objects.	Pain, erythema, possible secondary infection. Foreign body may or may not be visible.	Area surrounding foreign body should be washed with soap and water before removal. Superficial splinters can be removed with a needle and tweezers disinfected with alcohol or flame.	Deeply embedded foreign bodies, fishhooks, and other difficult-to-remove objects may require medical attention. Tetanus prophylaxis may be indicated.

INSECT BITES OR STINGS

Insects are found almost everywhere, and children often come in contact with them during play. The bites of most insects are not serious, usually causing only itching and mild pain; however, severe systemic reactions can occur in sensitized children. Systemic reactions to the venom of stinging insects, including wasps, honeybees, yellow jackets, hornets, and fire ants, is estimated to occur in nearly 1% of American children (Sicherer & Leung, 2011). Anaphylaxis from insect stings results in a number of deaths annually in the United States (Golden, Moffitt, & Nicklas, 2011). Children who are allergic to insect stings should wear a medical alert bracelet and be provided with an epinephrine autoinjector (EpiPen) and information on avoidance. Parents need to make sure the autoinjector is actually with the child or a responsible adult when the child is outdoors. The expiration date on the autoinjector must be checked regularly, and families must know how to obtain replacements when the autoinjector is outdated. Patients with a clear history of anaphylaxis after *Hymenoptera* stings should be referred to an allergist for immunotherapy (Golden et al., 2011). (See Chapter 18 for additional information about anaphylaxis.)

Arachnids (scorpions, spiders, ticks, mites) are found in areas where children play. Most arachnids are not dangerous or aggressive. In the United States, the bites from only one type of scorpion and two types of spiders (black widow, brown recluse) cause life-threatening reactions.

Topical insect repellents are an important measure in preventing insect bites. The CDC recommends the use of products that contain active ingredients registered with the Environmental Protection Agency. Repellents containing high concentrations of diethyltoluamide (DEET) should not be used on small children because of the risk of toxic encephalopathy. Likewise, products containing oil of eucalyptus are not indicated for children younger than 3 years. The AAP Committee on Environmental Health recommends that repellents with DEET should not be used on infants less than 2 months old. Such repellents should not be applied near the face, and children should be cautioned not to put their fingers in their mouths when wearing diethyltoluamide (CDC, 2008b).

The bites and stings of common insects and arachnids are discussed in Table 25-2. The table includes information on manifestations, treatment, and prevention.

TABLE 25-2 SKIN LESIONS CAUSED BY INSECTS AND ARACHNIDS

AGENT AND CHARACTERISTICS	MANIFESTATIONS	TREATMENT AND PREVENTION
Insects		
Mosquitoes, Fleas, Flies, Gnats Foreign protein in insect's saliva is injected as insect pierces skin to suck blood.	Itching, erythema, small wheal. Local reaction may occur that is difficult to distinguish from cellulitis.	Apply antipruritic lotions and cool compresses to relieve itching. Give antihistamines if needed for sleep. Prevention: Wear insect repellent when contact is anticipated. Treat potential breeding places (standing water for mosquitoes; pets, furniture, yard for fleas).
Hymenoptera (Bees, Wasps, Hornets, Yellow Jackets, Fire Ants) Venom is injected through a stinger.	Histamine and foreign proteins in venom cause local reaction of pain, swelling, redness, and itching. Systemic allergic reactions may be manifested by nausea, generalized edema, respiratory distress, and shock.	If visible, carefully remove stinger by scraping it out horizontally. Avoid squeezing stinger, because more venom will be released. Wash with soap and water. Paste made of powdered meat tenderizer and water is soothing. Apply ice and analgesics for discomfort, antihistamines for itching. For a systemic allergic reaction, give epinephrine and corticosteroids immediately; transport to emergency facility. Children allergic to *Hymenoptera* should wear medical identification. Prevention: Treat known hives or nests. Avoid wearing colorful clothing and perfumes when outside.
Arachnids		
Brown Recluse ("Fiddle Back") Spider Yellowish to reddish brown with a violin-shaped mark on its back. Venom injected by fangs. Bites only when threatened. Lives in dark, protected areas (woodpiles, basements, closets, trash heaps).	Mild stinging at time of bite. Within 2-8 hr, area around bite becomes painful and erythema develops, followed by a blister. Venom is necrotoxic. Edema, redness, and purpura may involve entire limb. Central portion of lesion develops an indurated wheal that progresses to deep, sloughing ulcer in 7-14 days. Ulcer often does not heal for several months. Usually results in a scar.	Immobilize and elevate affected extremity. Cool compresses, analgesics, tetanus prophylaxis. Observe for secondary infection. Skin graft may be necessary for large ulcers. No antivenin available. Prevention: Avoid areas inhabited by spiders.

Animation—Tick Paralysis

Animation—Pediatric Burns

TABLE 25-2 SKIN LESIONS CAUSED BY INSECTS AND ARACHNIDS—cont'd

AGENT AND CHARACTERISTICS	MANIFESTATIONS	TREATMENT AND PREVENTION
Arachnids—cont'd		
Black Widow Spider Shiny black with a red hourglass-shaped mark on abdomen. Female's venom is very poisonous to humans. Males do not bite. Female builds irregular web in dark, sheltered spots and aggressively defends eggs.	Bite may be painless initially. Within 1 hr pain develops at site. Severe muscle pains and numbness spread from bite, and puncture site becomes red, swollen, and pruritic. Neurotoxic venom enters the bloodstream within 1 hr, causing dizziness, headache, nausea, vomiting, cramps, tremors, and rapid, shallow respirations. Shock and renal failure may develop in young children.	Hospitalization for children. Antivenin if no allergy to horse serum. Supportive care, including IV calcium gluconate, morphine, muscle relaxants. Tetanus prophylaxis. Prevention: Avoid areas infested by spiders (woodpiles, outhouses). Carefully check packaged fruits and produce before reaching into bags or boxes.
Ticks Brown or gray; live in fields, pastures, woods. Feed on blood of humans, dogs, livestock, or deer. Larvae feed on rodents. Tick buries head and mouth parts in the skin to suck blood.	Bites may cause local reactions or, rarely, systemic reactions (tick fever, tick paralysis). Ticks can transmit Lyme disease, Rocky Mountain spotted fever, Q fever, and tularemia.	Methods to remove ticks: Remove with tweezers as close to the skin as possible, taking care to remove head. If mouth parts remain, remove with sterile needle. Wash site with soap and water. There is some evidence that prompt removal of ticks decreases chance of transmission of disease. Prevention: Wear long sleeves and pants and use insect repellent when walking in tick-infested areas. Inspect clothing and hair for ticks after walking through fields or woods. (See Chapter 17 for additional discussion.)
Scorpions Most scorpions are not dangerous. They rarely attack humans unless accidentally disturbed or stepped on. If disturbed, they inflict a painful sting. One type (found in Arizona), *Centruroides sculpturatus*, is extremely poisonous, and its sting can be fatal. Scorpions are found mainly in the southwestern United States. Scorpions hide by day in basements, garages, closets, crevices. Some varieties burrow and hide in gravel or children's sandboxes.	Sting is extremely painful. Local reaction of swelling at puncture site. Some species cause systemic reactions: tachycardia, hypertension, arrhythmias, irritability, seizures, pulmonary edema, coma. Fatal reactions most often occur in children younger than 3 yr.	Ice packs and tourniquet applied proximal to the site slow the spread of venom. Wound should not be excised. Topical steroids and antihistamines are used to relieve symptoms. For severe reactions, provide supportive care for pain, shock, seizures. Narcotic analgesics act synergistically with scorpion venom and are contraindicated. Antivenin is given for systemic reactions (available from the Antivenom Production Laboratory, Arizona State University). Prevention: Wear shoes to prevent stepping on scorpions. Inspect shoes and clothing before dressing. Apply creosote to garages, basements.
Chiggers (Harvest Mites) Live in tall grass and underbrush; burrow into hair follicles and skin pores to feed.	Tend to concentrate in warm areas where clothing is snug (underwear elastic). Cause erythematous papules and intense itching.	Antipruritic agents. Prevention of secondary infection. Prevention: Insect repellent on clothing, ankles, legs.

BURN INJURIES

Burn injury may involve a small, painful area that hurts until healing occurs, or it may involve most of a child's body, with resulting severe trauma or death. Infants and toddlers are at greatest risk for sustaining burns because they depend totally on others for safety.

Recovery from a major burn injury requires many months, and the child's appearance might be altered for life. Caring for a burned child entails a multidisciplinary approach with a focus on the child and the family. Nursing care involves treating the physical injury and its psychological effects on the child and family members. The challenges of burn nursing begin with acute burn care but continue through the rehabilitation phase until the child is restored to optimal function (Box 25-1).

Etiology

Burn injuries in children can be unintentional or intentional. In children younger than 5 years, unintentional burns are likely to occur as a result of environmental situations that are not controlled by caretakers. The young child's curiosity and increasing mobility contribute to the risk (Table 25-3). A child can start a fire by playing with matches (Figure 25-13) or flammable materials near open fires, or a child might be the victim of a house fire while sleeping or might be unintentionally scalded or electrocuted (Figure 25-14). (See Chapters 5 through 8 for a discussion of safety.) Either inattentive supervision or purposeful abuse can cause intentional burns (see Patient-Centered Teaching: Measures to Prevent and Initially Manage a Burn box).

BOX 25-1   PEDIATRIC DIFFERENCES IN THE EFFECTS OF BURN INJURY

- Very young children who have been severely burned have a higher mortality rate than older children and adults with comparable burns.
- Because a child's skin is thinner than that of an adult, lower burn temperatures and shorter exposure to heat or chemicals can cause a more severe burn.
- A larger body surface area compared with that of adults places severely burned children at increased risk for fluid and heat loss. Children are also at increased risk for dehydration and metabolic acidosis from diarrhea, evaporative water loss, and increased fluid requirements.
- The higher proportion of body fluid to mass in children increases the risk of cardiovascular problems because of their less effective cardiovascular response to changing intravascular volume.
- Burns involving more than 10% total body surface area (TBSA) require fluid resuscitation.
- Infants and children are at increased risk for protein and calorie deficiency because they have smaller muscle mass and lower body fat than adults. If they are not eating and their metabolism is increased, their protein and calorie needs will not be met.
- Hypertrophic scarring is more severe, and scar maturation is prolonged.
- An immature immune system means an increased risk of infection for infants and young children.
- A delay in growth may follow extensive burns.
- In children, Curling (gastroduodenal) ulcer occurs in the third or fourth week after a burn, which is later than in adults.

TABLE 25-3   AGE-RELATED RISKS FOR BURN INJURY

INJURY TYPE	RISK FACTORS
<5 Years of Age	
Flame	Playing with matches and cigarette lighters
	Playing with fires in fireplaces, barbecue pits, trash fires
Scald	Kitchen injury from tipping scalding liquids
	Bathtub scalds associated with lack of supervision or child abuse
	Most pediatric burn patients are infants and toddlers younger than 3 yr burned by scalding liquids
5-10 Years of Age	
Flame	Boys at increased risk
	Often associated with fire play and risk-taking behaviors
Scald	Girls at increased risk
	Likely to occur at home in kitchen or bathroom
Adolescent	
Flame	Injury associated with male peer-group activities involving gasoline or other flammable products
	Gasoline sniffing possibly involved
	Rarely occurs in female adolescents except in house fires or automobile accidents
Electrical	Occurs most often in male adolescents involved in dare-type behaviors, such as climbing utility poles or antennas
	In rural areas, may be associated with moving irrigation pipes that touch an electrical source

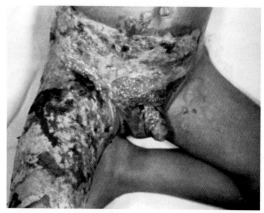

FIG 25-13 These burns were sustained when the child's pajamas caught fire while he was playing with matches. (From Cosman, B. [1973]. *Management of the burned patient.* New York: MEDCOM.)

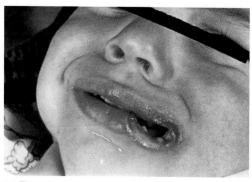

FIG 25-14 These burns were sustained when the child sucked on an electrical socket. (From Cosman, B. [1973]. *Management of the burned patient.* New York: MEDCOM.)

The extent of the injury determines whether burn-related problems are local or systemic. Other factors, such as the location of the burned area, whether the injury is an electrical injury, whether there is a concurrent inhalation injury or trauma, and whether there is a preexisting medical disease, contribute to morbidity and mortality rates. Morbidity and mortality rates are higher in children who have been burned than in adults.

Incidence

Fire and burn injuries are a leading cause of unintentional deaths in children ages 1 to 14 years in the United States (Antoon & Donovan, 2011). Scald burns are the most common burn injuries seen in pediatrics (Antoon & Donovan, 2011). Other burn injuries include those induced by flame, electrical, and chemical causes. It is estimated that as many as 10% of child abuse cases involve burn injuries (Goodis & Schraga, 2010).

Most children with severe burns are treated in burn centers. The American Burn Association has outlined criteria for referral to a burn center (Box 25-2).

Pathophysiology

In burn injury the injuring agent, whether flame, chemical, ultraviolet light, or electrical energy, denatures cellular protein, which destroys collagen linkages in connective tissue. As a result, osmotic and hydrostatic pressure gradients are disrupted, and intravascular fluid moves

BOX 25-2   BURN CENTER REFERRAL CRITERIA

The American Burn Association recommends that children with the following injuries be referred to a burn center after emergency assessment and stabilization:

- Second-degree burns greater than 10% body surface area
- Burns that involve major joints, face, hands, feet, genitalia, or perineum
- Third-degree burns
- Electrical burns, including lightning injury
- Chemical burns
- Inhalation injury with burns
- Preexisting medical disorders that might complicate recovery
- Coexisting trauma in which the burn injury poses the greatest risk to life or function
- Burned children in hospitals without qualified personnel to care for pediatric burn patients
- Children who will require specialized psychosocial or long-term rehabilitation

Modified from Committee on Trauma, American College of Surgeons. (2006). Guidelines for the operations of burn centers. *Resources for optimal care of the injured patient*, 2006, p. 79.

PATIENT-CENTERED TEACHING

Measures to Prevent and Initially Manage a Burn

Prevention

- Have periodic fire drills to teach your children how to evacuate the house in the event of a fire.
- Place child identification stickers, which can be obtained from most fire departments, on the outside of the bedroom door and in one window of each child's bedroom.
- Identify two or more exits from each room and a location to meet outside the house. Emphasize to your children that they should not return to the house under any circumstances, even if another family member or pet remains in the house.
- Be sure your child understands "stop, drop, and roll" as a measure to stop the burning process.
- Be sure to keep all matches and lighters out of reach. Check electrical cords regularly. Use outlet covers if children younger than 5 years are in the house.
- Check smoke and carbon monoxide detectors regularly and keep them clean. Replace the batteries regularly if they are battery operated.
- To reduce the number of scald burns, turn the hot water heater thermostat down to 120° F (48.8° C).
- Turn pot handles in and use back burners on the stove whenever possible.
- Do not sit a child on your lap while you are drinking a hot liquid.
- Keep your children away from outdoor grills and indoor wood- or coal-burning stoves. Keep older infants from crawling near floor heating grates.

Initial Emergency Burn Management

- Apply cool compresses or submerge minor burns in cool water, not ice.
- To prevent scalding, remove clothing soaked with hot water as quickly as possible.
- Contact the physician for any child with a burn that has blistered.
- Cover a child who has a major burn with a clean sheet while waiting for emergency personnel.
- Do not try to remove clothing that is adhering to burned skin.

into interstitial spaces. Inflammatory chemicals are released from injured cells, resulting in increased capillary permeability and adding to fluid shifts. Burn injuries are classified by depth and extent of tissue damage and by severity of injury. The combination of these factors determines referral and therapeutic management decisions.

Depth of Burn Injury

Depth of burn injury describes local tissue damage and is largely a factor of the duration of exposure and the temperature or destructive potential of the agent causing the damage. Depth of injury is classified as superficial, superficial partial thickness, deep partial thickness, or full thickness (Table 25-4).

Superficial burns, usually sunburns, affect only the epidermis. No blisters form in a true superficial burn, and the surface of the injury is dry. The pain of sunburns is usually delayed for several hours after sun exposure. Partial-thickness thermal, chemical, or electrical injury to the skin interferes with the skin's ability to carry out its normal physiologic functions of protection from infection or injury and preservation of fluid balance and temperature regulation. In addition, deep tissue injury damages sensory nerve endings and local circulatory patterns and adversely affects the skin's ability to regenerate or synthesize vitamin D.

Extent of Burn Injury

The extent of injury refers to the percent of total body surface area (TBSA) burned. The standard "rule of nines" used in adults gives an inaccurate estimate for children because of the differences in body proportion between children and adults. Many burn facilities use the Lund and Browder chart, which is a body surface chart corrected for age (Figure 25-15). Another method estimates burn percentage in smaller-area burns by calculating the complete palmar surface of the child's hand and assumes the area of the palmar surface equals 1% of the TBSA (Antoon & Donovan, 2011).

Severity of Burn Injury

Severity of burn injury is determined by the degree to which the skin's physiologic functions are disrupted beyond the body's normal ability to respond with compensatory mechanisms. Burn injuries are classified as minor, moderate uncomplicated, and major. The severity of burn injury is related to a combination of factors. These include age, medical history, extent and depth of burn, special care of the body area involved (e.g., face, hands), and the presence of associated trauma, such as fractures or head injury, sustained at the time of the burn. Burn severity relates to the child's eventual morbidity or mortality status.

Manifestations

Table 25-5 lists the clinical manifestations associated with burns of different severity. Assessment of the distribution of scald burns is of particular importance in infants and toddlers because of the possibility of child maltreatment. The classic forced immersion burn occurs when a child's extremity or buttocks are held under hot water. These burns have a "stocking" or "glove" appearance with a relatively sharp line dividing the burned from unburned skin. There are usually no smaller, scattered burns ("splash marks") that indicate attempts to remove the extremity.

Therapeutic Management
Superficial Burn Injuries

The most common cause of a superficial (epidermal layer only) burn is sunburn. Although uncomfortable, sunburn rarely requires intensive burn treatment. Cool compresses and application of soothing

TABLE 25-4 DEPTH OF BURN INJURY

	SUPERFICIAL	SUPERFICIAL PARTIAL THICKNESS	DEEP PARTIAL THICKNESS	FULL THICKNESS
Morphologic features	Destruction of epidermis; physiologic functions remain intact	Destruction of epidermis and some dermis	Destruction of epidermis and dermis	Destruction of epidermis, dermis, underlying tissue; may include fascia, muscle, tendon, bone
Blister formation	After 24 hr (e.g., from sunburn)	Within minutes; thin walled, fluid filled	May or may not appear as fluid-filled blisters; often are flat, dehydrated, and like tissue paper; body fluids lost through burn tissue must be replaced	Rare; may appear as a tissue paper–like layer that is flat and dehydrated
Appearance Healing time	Peels after 24-48 hr 3-7 days	Red to pale ivory, moist surface 7-21 days if no infection develops	Mottled, waxy white, dry surface 30 days to several months if no infection; if infected, this type of burn may convert to full-thickness burn	White, cherry red, or black Will not heal; skin grafting required; very small areas may heal from edges after a period of weeks
Patient reaction	Moderate discomfort, pain; chills; nausea; vomiting	May cause considerable pain	Severe pain on exposure to air or water because nerve endings are intact	No pain in area of full-thickness burn because nerve endings are destroyed; surrounding areas of lesser depth are painful
Scarring	None	Minimal; influenced by genetic predisposition	Greatest because the slow healing of these burns increases scar tissue; scar formation influenced by genetic predisposition	Autograft scarring is minimized by early excision and grafting; scar formation influenced by genetic predisposition

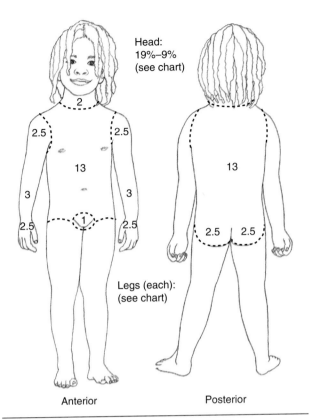

Head:
19%–9%
(see chart)

Legs (each):
(see chart)

Anterior   Posterior

Child Burn Size Estimation Table
(percent total body surface area)

Age in Years

	<1	1	5	10	15	Adult
Head	19	17	13	11	9	7
Neck	2	2	2	2	2	2
Anterior trunk	13	13	13	13	13	13
Posterior trunk	13	13	13	13	13	13
Buttock	2.5	2.5	2.5	2.5	2.5	2.5
Genitalia	1	1	1	1	1	1
Upper arm	2.5	2.5	2.5	2.5	2.5	2.5
Lower arm	3	3	3	3	3	3
Hand	2.5	2.5	2.5	2.5	2.5	2.5
Thigh	5.5	6.5	8	8.5	9	9.5
Leg	5	5	5.5	6	6.5	7
Foot	3.5	3.5	3.5	3.5	3.5	3.5

FIG 25-15 Calculating total body surface area (TBSA) burned in children. The standard "rule of nines" and standard body surface charts must be adapted because of the difference in body proportions between adults and children. (From Deitch, E., & Rutan, R. [2001]. *The challenges of children: The first 48 hours.* Chicago, IL: American Burn Association.)

topical lotions (especially those containing aloe) or mild topical corticosteroids provide symptomatic treatment. If the discomfort is disturbing the child's sleep, acetaminophen or ibuprofen can provide relief.

Preventing sunburn is especially important in children because frequent sunburn causes long-term damage to the skin. Children who are susceptible to sunburn are also susceptible to the later development of melanoma and nonmelanoma skin cancers (Skin Cancer Foundation, 2010). Children should avoid sun exposure, especially between the hours of 10 AM and 3 PM during the summer. During sun exposure, parents should apply to the child's skin an appropriate ultraviolet A and ultraviolet B protective sunscreen with a sun protection factor greater than 15. Hats and shirts are also desirable. Waterproof sunscreens are available for children who like to run in and out of the water, but frequent applications of sunscreen are still desirable. Recommend that parents check the date on the sunscreen to be sure it has not expired. Sunscreen is contraindicated for infants younger than 6 months. Parents should keep infants in the shade, away from reflecting sun rays.

Superficial Partial-Thickness Burn Injuries

In general, children with a minor burn injury are treated as outpatients in a physician's office, clinic, or hospital physical therapy department unless the extent of injury warrants hospital admission. Therapy is aimed at promoting wound healing, preventing infection, and providing pain relief. Burn wound care requires aseptic technique. Because anaerobic and aerobic bacteria can grow at the interface between burned and healthy tissue, tetanus toxoid is given to children who have not received tetanus immunization during the 5 years preceding the burn injury.

Wound Cleaning. Burn wounds receive care at least daily until closure is achieved. After old dressings are removed, the burned skin is cleaned with sterile saline solution or mild soap and water. If the child is hospitalized, hydrotherapy (Figure 25-16) can be used to remove old dressings and clean the wound and the child. During this cleaning process, the child can perform active range-of-motion exercises. Hydrotherapy can be done in a tank, tub, or shower. Some facilities use disposable plastic liners to prevent contamination between uses. Hydrotherapy should last no longer than 20 minutes to prevent electrolyte loss (through skin into water, as a result of osmosis). The room temperature is kept warm, and the child is covered and dried immediately after the procedure.

Débridement. Débridement is the removal of dead material within a wound to promote healing. In a burn injury, there is necrosis of skin and subcutaneous tissue. The burned tissue is called eschar. Eschar releases chemical mediators that stimulate leukocytes to digest debris, but this also damages capillaries and skin elements. Necrotic tissue within a wound prolongs inflammation and slows healing and epidermal coverage.

The initial débridement might be performed in the office, emergency department, or hydrotherapy treatment room. The burned area is débrided of loose debris and necrotic tissue. Blisters, particularly on palmar skin, are usually left intact in superficial partial-thickness burns. Subsequent to rupture, they are débrided (Antoon & Donovan, 2011). Old creams and ointments must be removed as part of the débridement, and loose tissue is trimmed around the burned area.

Application of Antimicrobial Agents and Dressings. Topical antibacterial agents (Table 25-6) are placed on burn wounds to penetrate the eschar and to control bacterial growth in and around the burn wound. Silver sulfadiazine (Silvadene) is the most commonly used topical agent, but it is not typically used on the face or on electrical burns. Facial burns are covered with a light layer of antimicrobial ointment. Mafenide (Sulfamylon) is the topical agent of choice for burns to the ear or electrical burns because of its deep penetration into the eschar. Mafenide should not be applied to the face. Acuzyme ointment, a topical enzyme, is an effective topical agent for débridement (Antoon & Donovan, 2011).

TABLE 25-5 CLASSIFICATION OF SEVERITY OF BURN INJURY IN CHILDREN

TYPE OF INJURY	CLINICAL MANIFESTATIONS
Minor Partial-thickness burn of <10% of TBSA Full-thickness burn of >2% of TBSA that does not involve special care areas (eyes, ears, face, hands, feet, perineum, joints) Excludes electrical injury, inhalation injury, concurrent trauma, all poor-risk children (e.g., those of extremely young age or with concurrent disease)	Localized pain and blister formation in the area of injury; white or black full-thickness injury No systemic effects Little or no scarring, except in areas of full-thickness injury
Moderate, Uncomplicated Partial-thickness burns of 10%-20% of TBSA Full-thickness burns of <10% of TBSA that do not involve special care areas Excludes electrical injury, inhalation injury, concurrent trauma, all poor-risk children (e.g., those of extremely young age or with concurrent disease)	Open wound that is a potential source of infection and a site for loss of fluids and electrolytes Pain that may interfere with routines of daily living Wound healing rate influenced by nutritional status Possible scarring in areas of partial- and full-thickness injuries
Major Partial-thickness burns of >20% of TBSA All full-thickness burns of ≥10% of TBSA All burns involving eyes, ears, face, hands, feet, perineum, or joints All inhalation injury, electrical injury, concurrent trauma, all poor-risk patients	Life-threatening injuries with risk for severe complications and death Volatile hospital course characterized by periods of relative physiologic stability followed, within hours, by life-threatening emergencies, such as shock Repeated operative procedures for skin grafting that are accompanied by major blood loss requiring multiple transfusions Potential risk for infection, either of the burn wound or related to pulmonary complications or systemic sepsis, until wound closure is achieved over 80% of the TBSA Much higher mortality rate associated with burn injury accompanied by inhalation injury than with burn injury alone

PATIENT-CENTERED TEACHING

Home Care for a Child with Burns

Often it is the parents' responsibility to care for the burn wound at home, supported by daily visits to the office or clinic for débridement and wound assessment.

Parents Will Need to Know the Following to Adequately Care for the Child:
- Type of cleaning method used to remove old antimicrobial ointment
- Where to obtain the topical ointment and dressing supplies
- How often to visit the office or clinic (the nurse provides the telephone number and a list of scheduled appointments)

Teach the Parents the Following:
- Use principles of aseptic technique. Use sterile gloves and applicators and know where to obtain these supplies. Know how to put on the gloves; give a return demonstration.
- Give the child medication for pain (if needed) 20 to 30 minutes before changing the dressing. Enlist other family members to provide distraction or to help hold the child.
- Wash the area with mild soap and tepid water or sterile saline solution. The old dressing can be soaked in tepid water to loosen it and decrease the discomfort of its removal.
- Apply the prescribed ointment and a light gauze dressing. Cover the area with a tubular net bandage, if possible, rather than wrapping with flexible gauze.
- Recognize signs and symptoms of infection, provide adequate fluids, and be sure the child's nutritional needs are met.
- Encourage the child in activities appropriate for age and development.
- Keep follow-up appointments.

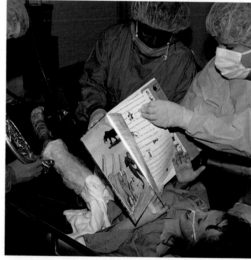

FIG 25-16 Burn dressings can be changed in the hydrotherapy room. The room is kept warm because children who have been burned have poor body temperature control. The child life therapist reads a book to the child to distract her from the discomfort associated with the procedure. (Courtesy Parkland Health and Hospital System, Dallas, TX.)

After application of the topical antibacterial agent, a dressing usually is applied. Depending on the burn care protocol, dressings are changed one to three times a day. Because exposed nerve endings can cause significant pain, wound assessment and care should be done as quickly as possible. Narcotic or nonnarcotic pain medications are administered 20 to 30 minutes before dressing changes to ensure maximum pain

TABLE 25-6   TOPICAL ANTIMICROBIAL AGENTS COMMONLY USED FOR BURNS

ADVANTAGES	SIDE EFFECTS AND DISADVANTAGES	NURSING CONSIDERATIONS
Silver Nitrate Solution Effective against most gram-positive and some gram-negative organisms	Hyponatremia, hypokalemia, hypochloremia Decreased penetration of eschar Not effective against established infection Requires large, bulky dressings that limit mobility	0.5% solution in distilled water applied to wet dressing every 2 hr Dressing changes twice daily Can cause staining of linens and clothing and interferes with accurate wound assessment
Mafenide Acetate Cream (Sulfamylon) Effective against a wide range of gram-positive and gram-negative organisms Rapid penetration through eschar (improved effectiveness in established infections) Permits open treatment of wound, thus increasing mobility	Painful on application May cause hypersensitivity reaction in 5%-7% of patients Associated with acid-base alteration (metabolic acidosis)	Applied to cleansed wound once or twice a day Treated area usually left open; a light dressing may be used Must be completely removed before reapplication Check sensitivity to sulfonamides
Silver Sulfadiazine Cream (Silvadene) Effective against a wide range of gram-positive and gram-negative organisms Soothing on application Moderate eschar penetration Absorbed slowly, reducing the possibility of nephrotoxicity	May cause hypersensitivity reaction in 5%-7% of patients Associated with initial decrease in leukocyte count (transient)	Applied to cleansed wound once or twice a day Wound may be left open or covered with light dressing Check sensitivity to sulfonamides Must remove all medication before reapplication

control at the time of the procedure. The child life specialist can assist with teaching the child how to use nonpharmacologic pain-relief techniques.

Besides pain control, measures to maintain the child's core body temperature, minimize shivering, and conserve energy also must be implemented as part of wound care activities. To the degree possible, the child's capacity for self-care should be optimized. Allowing the child to remove dressings provides a measure of control.

Aseptic technique is used during dressing changes. After dressings are applied to burn wounds, isolation is not necessary and the child does not need to be restricted to a room or to an area of the hospital.

Depending on the depth and extent of the burn, the physician might choose to cover the area with a biologic or synthetic dressing to reduce the chance of infection, provide pain relief, reduce evaporative fluid and heat loss, and promote healing. Such dressings are best used for partial-thickness burns. Commonly used biologic dressings include human skin, pig skin, and fresh human amniotic membrane (from the placenta). Synthetic dressings include plastic films, hydrocolloids, hydrogels, and collagen-impregnated dressings. The major risk associated with these dressings is infection; thus the wound must be clean and dry before dressing application.

CONDITIONS ASSOCIATED WITH MAJOR BURN INJURIES

For a child with a major burn injury, initial assessment and care focus on the primary survey (see Chapter 10) and particularly establishing and maintaining the child's airway, breathing, and circulation. After an airway and IV access have been established, a catheter is inserted into the bladder to begin hourly urine output measurements, and a nasogastric tube is inserted into the stomach to prevent aspiration.

Burn shock is a hypovolemic condition that develops after a burn injury affecting more than 15% to 20% of TBSA in children. Mechanisms of burn shock are not well understood, but the sequence of major burn injury followed by massive capillary leakage of circulating fluid into the surrounding tissues is well recognized.

Within minutes of a major burn injury, all the capillaries in the circulatory system, not just those in the area of the burn, lose their capillary seal, resulting in leakage of intravascular body fluid into the interstitial spaces. Erythrocytes and leukocytes remain in the circulation and produce an elevated hematocrit and leukocyte count. The process of burn shock continues for approximately 24 to 48 hours, at which time the capillary seal is restored.

Treatment for burn shock is aimed at supporting the child through the period of hypovolemic shock until capillary integrity is restored. To maintain adequate circulating volume, IV fluids are administered at a rate greater than the rate of fluid loss. Fluid resuscitation depends primarily on crystalloid solutions, particularly during the first 24 hours after injury, although recent studies show that colloid resuscitation (plasma) has the potential to decrease the amount of fluids needed to maintain adequate urine output and prevent complications, such as increased intraabdominal pressure (Zaletel, 2009). Various formulas are used to calculate the rate of fluid administration. The specific protocol for fluid resuscitation remains controversial. In the absence of clinical trials to identify best burn resuscitation practices, protocols are determined by the burn unit or health care facility. In general, the amount of fluid replacement in children is calculated according to body surface area. Typically, half the calculated fluid amount is given over the first 8 hours after the burn, and the remaining half is given over the next 16 hours.

Because urine output reflects end-organ tissue perfusion, IV fluids are administered at a rate sufficient to maintain the child's urine

Animation—Capillary Leak

The Child with a Minor Partial-Thickness Burn

Focused Assessment

- Rapidly assess for burn severity, considering the following:
  - Minor burn: Pain, wound condition, and potential for outpatient management
  - Moderate burn: Pain, wound condition, and possible need for fluid resuscitation
  - Severe burn: Multisystem assessment and possible transfer to a burn center
- Assess vital signs, particularly temperature, and determine risk for rapid heat loss leading to hypothermia
- Obtain neurologic signs: Child should be awake and alert
- Regular pain assessment both before and after intervention
- Assess extremity range of motion and child's ability to independently perform ADLs

Planning

Nursing Diagnosis

Risk for Infection related to thermal tissue injury.

Expected Outcome

The burn will heal without infection, as evidenced by normal temperature, lack of purulent drainage, normal granulating tissue, and restoration of the epithelial layer.

Intervention/Rationale

1. Clean and débride the wound daily and apply antimicrobial ointments and dressings as ordered. Document and record healing and any signs of wound infection, particularly fever and any change in wound appearance (drainage, odor). Obtain specimens for culture if ordered.
   Infection can be prevented by removing bacterial contamination, exudate, and previously applied medication. Early detection of infection will ensure proper treatment and prevention of complications.
2. Maintain aseptic technique for wound care.
   An open skin surface allows for organism entry.
3. Make sure that the child's tetanus toxoid immunizations are current.
   Anaerobic bacteria can cause infection at the interface between the burn wound and healthy tissue.

Evaluation

Is the tissue pink and free from exudate?
Is the child free of fever and other signs of infection?

Planning

Nursing Diagnosis

Impaired Skin Integrity related to thermal tissue injury and scratching of a healing wound.

Expected Outcome

The skin will exhibit progressively normal granulation, and restoration of the epithelial layer.

Intervention/Rationale

1. Administer antihistamines as ordered.
   Itching persists for several months after burns heal as new nerve endings and dermal elements reestablish themselves. Antihistamines such as diphenhydramine hydrochloride (Benadryl) reduce itching.
2. Apply soothing lotions, such as Nivea or Eucerin, to healing skin.
   These lotions reduce dryness, which is a factor contributing to itching.
3. Keep the child's hands clean at all times and the fingernails cut short. Encourage the child not to scratch or rub healing skin.
   These actions reduce the risk of impairing skin integrity.

4. Promote adequate fluid and nutritional intake. Offer, or encourage the parent to offer, high-calorie, high-protein meals and snacks. Provide foods that the child likes. Arrange the timing of meals so that they do not immediately precede or follow painful or distressing events.
   Healing occurs only in the presence of a positive nitrogen balance. The child's protein and calorie needs are elevated because of increased metabolism and catabolism.
5. Perform active and passive range-of-motion exercises of the affected parts of the child's body; this can be done at the time of dressing change and between dressing changes.
   Using the burned area promotes edema reabsorption and prevents contracture deformity.
6. Administer vitamins and minerals (vitamins A, B, and C and iron and zinc) as ordered, or encourage the parent to do so.
   Vitamin and mineral supplements facilitate wound healing and epithelialization.
7. Instruct the child and parents to keep the healed burn wound out of the sun for at least 1 year.
   Burned skin is more sensitive to sunlight, which increases the risk of sunburn.

Evaluation

Does the burn wound show signs of progressive healing?
Is the skin smooth and pink without excessive scar tissue?
Is the child's itching controlled in a way that reduces scratching?

Planning

Nursing Diagnosis

Acute Pain related to thermal injury and related procedures.

Expected Outcomes

The child will describe decreased pain on an age-appropriate pain assessment scale, except during procedures and physical therapy.
The child will exhibit age-appropriate behaviors, appropriate nutritional intake, and appropriate sleep patterns.

Intervention/Rationale

1. Determine the child's pain level with an age-appropriate assessment tool.
   The child's developmental stage affects response to pain, and the child's response to various pain assessment tools is related to developmental level.
2. Administer pain-relief measures and medication on a scheduled basis rather than on demand. Premedicate the child at least 20 to 30 minutes before painful procedures and advise the parent to do the same before the physician visit.
   Regular administration of pain-relief controls pain and prevents cyclic episodes of severe pain, which are more difficult to manage effectively.
3. Minimize the time spent on wound manipulation and exposure.
   Exposure of the burned area to air or water causes pain because the nerve endings are exposed. Dressing changes should be done as quickly as possible to minimize pain.
4. Use nonpharmacologic pain reduction measures.
   Distraction, relaxation techniques, therapeutic touch, and other measures may help alleviate pain.
5. Perform passive and active range-of-motion exercises. Be careful that dressings are applied so as to preserve function of body parts.
   Exercise, although painful in the acute stage, reduces the likelihood of contracture formation and increases functional ability.

⊚ NURSING CARE PLAN

The Child with a Minor Partial-Thickness Burn—cont'd

Evaluation

Except during times of direct wound care and physical therapy, is the child pain free, as evidenced by decreased pain assessment score and normal sleep, play, and eating patterns?

Is the child able to cooperate with dressing changes and range-of-motion exercises?

Planning

Nursing Diagnosis

Risk for Deficient Fluid Volume related to fluid shifts into burned tissue.

Expected Outcome

The child will maintain normal fluid and electrolyte balance, as evidenced by intake and output measurements and serum electrolyte values within normal ranges, moist mucous membranes, and good skin turgor on unaffected area.

Intervention/*Rationale*

1. Administer fluids orally or IV as ordered.
   Fluids help maintain capillary circulation to the viable skin appendages and general circulation to the vital organs. Fluid replacement continues until wound coverage is achieved.
2. Instruct the parents to monitor the child's intake and output frequently.
   Close monitoring is necessary to determine whether fluid resuscitation is adequate. Fluid intake sufficient to produce age-appropriate hourly urine output (see Chapter 16) ensures adequate tissue perfusion.
3. Weigh the hospitalized child daily.
   Weight is an accurate measurement of hydration status. Increasing weight may indicate fluid overload.
4. Monitor laboratory values for elevated electrolyte or hemoglobin levels.
   Early identification of abnormal laboratory values permits early treatment of fluid volume imbalances.

Evaluation

Is the child's urine output adequate for age (see Chapter 16)?

Are serum electrolyte values within normal ranges?

Does the child appear well hydrated with moist mucous membranes and appropriate skin turgor?

Does the child take fluids well?

Planning

Nursing Diagnosis

Disturbed Body Image related to altered appearance of the healing burn.

Expected Outcomes

The child will re-enter previous social settings and express a feeling of comfort in these areas.

The child will discuss feelings about others' reactions to the change in appearance.

The family will provide emotional support for the child.

Intervention/*Rationale*

1. Encourage the child to verbalize feelings about appearance and about returning to school.
   Identifying the child's concerns and anxieties is the first step in developing effective coping strategies.
2. Provide honest answers to the child's questions regarding appearance.
   Honesty builds trust and helps the child develop realistic expectations.
3. Encourage the family's involvement in the child's care (see Patient-Centered Teaching: Home Care for a Child with Burns box)
4. Encourage the child to provide age-appropriate self-care.
   Participating in self-care helps increase self-esteem.
5. Identify support systems and coping mechanisms used in previous times of stress or crisis.
   Strategies that were previously effective can be mobilized to aid the child and family through a stressful period.
6. Engage the assistance of a child life specialist to work with the child to identify feelings.
   Children can often best express feelings through play and art.
7. Discuss ways in which the child can "cover up" any disfigurement through clothing and makeup.
   Cosmetics can decrease or minimize the disfigurement.
8. Visit the child's school before the child's return or remain in contact with the school nurse.
   Prepare the child's classmates for the changes in the child's appearance and engage them in making the re-entry a positive experience through acceptance. If visiting is not possible, the school nurse can assist the child with the transition to school.

Evaluation

Does the child express a desire to reengage social contacts?

Is the child able to express fears related to the reactions of others?

Does the family support the child emotionally and encourage the child to express feelings?

---

output at a value appropriate for age (see Chapter 16). Inadequate urine output during burn shock is usually the result of insufficient administration of resuscitative fluids. Renal failure is not an expected component of burn shock if an adequate volume of IV fluids is being administered for burn shock resuscitation. It should be recognized that burn shock fluid resuscitation formulas are guidelines; individual children may need more fluids during the first 24 hours after the burn.

Table 25-7 lists additional physiologic effects caused by moderate to major burns. Once a child with a moderate or major burn has been stabilized, the child usually is transferred to a burn center for specialized care.

CONDITIONS ASSOCIATED WITH ELECTRICAL INJURY

Electrical injury is a major injury that often results in instant death because the electrical current disrupts the electrical rhythm of the heart. The child who does not die instantly is at risk for four major complications during the acute phase:

1. Cardiac arrest or arrhythmia
2. Tissue damage
3. Myoglobinuria (globulin from muscle serum appearing in the urine)
4. Metabolic acidosis

TABLE 25-7 BODY SYSTEM ALTERATIONS AFTER MODERATE TO SEVERE BURNS

SYSTEM/ALTERATION	CAUSE	MANAGEMENT
Respiratory		
Upper airway tissue injury with respiratory distress, possible obstruction	Edema from inhalation of superheated air	Establish adequate airway, provide moist mist with oxygen as needed
Lower airway tissue injury	Inhalation of smoke	Give oxygen as needed, place child in a head-elevated position, intubate with ventilatory support if necessary
Carbon monoxide inhalation, hypoxia	End products of combustion	Give 100% oxygen by mask; intubate and provide ventilatory support if necessary
Limited chest expansion	Circumferential burns	Escharotomy
Cardiovascular		
Fluid volume deficit with decreased cardiac output; tachycardia	Fluid shifts from vascular to interstitial compartment; massive leaking of fluid through the burn wound	Provide fluid and electrolyte replacement with or without colloids; goal is to achieve urinary output appropriate for age and good capillary refill
Initial vasodilation, then vasoconstriction	Compensatory mechanism to preserve fluid volume and prevent shock	
Edema, compartment syndrome	Increased fluid in interstitial spaces	
Elevated hemoglobin, hematocrit levels	Hemoconcentration caused by fluid loss	
Increase followed by decrease in serum potassium levels	Release of destroyed tissue cells into extracellular space	
Decreased serum sodium levels	Trapped in edema fluids	
Gastrointestinal		
Gastric dilation, paralytic ileus	Decreased perfusion to gastrointestinal tract as a result of hypovolemia	Restore fluid and electrolyte balance
Thirst	Hypovolemia	
Renal		
Oliguria, elevated blood urea nitrogen and creatinine values	Reduced circulation to kidneys	Adequate fluid resuscitation
Risk for acute tubular necrosis	Obstruction of renal tubules	
Metabolic		
Increased metabolic rate with elevated body temperature and massive evaporative heat loss	Insult of open wound	Provide caloric requirements two or three times basal requirements; provide high-protein diet or protein supplements; tube feed or use parenteral nutrition as necessary; provide vitamin C and vitamin A supplements
Catecholamine release	Burn stress; increased temperature and metabolic rate	
Hyperglycemia	Mobilization of glucagon and decreased insulin production	
Hematologic		
Decreased hematocrit level follows initial hematocrit increase (from hemoconcentration)	Increased red blood cell (RBC) hemolysis, decreased RBC production, blood loss from wound care	Packed RBC transfusion for low hematocrit
Coagulation disorders	Decreased platelet count and serum clotting factors	
Increased immature neutrophils to digest products of injury	Depletion of mature neutrophils	
High risk for infection, wound sepsis, septic shock (disorientation, fever, diminished bowel sounds are first signs, temperature falls below normal as body's resistance to infection decreases)	Open wound; altered protective mechanisms; decreased circulation to the skin	Burn excision and débridement followed by application of topical antimicrobial agents; may need biologic or synthetic skin coverings, graft
Pain		
	Tissue injury exposing nerve endings; edema; burn treatments	Meticulous pain management both around-the-clock and before treatments

Cardiac Arrest or Arrhythmia

The immediate risk is cardiac arrest or arrhythmia resulting from damage to the heart's electrical conduction system. If cardiac arrest occurs, standard cardiac life support measures are initiated (see Chapter 10).

Tissue Damage

The electrical current follows the path of least resistance through the body. Entering through the skin, electricity causes heat damage to the skin layers, bone, nerves, tendons, and blood vessels. The heat of the electrical current coagulates blood vessels and leaves the affected area without a blood supply. Gangrene develops in necrotic tissue unless it is removed. Amputation is necessary in more than 90% of children sustaining electrical injuries. The location of the damage depends on the child's position and exposure. Electricity may enter one hand and exit from the other, for example, or it may travel through the body and exit from one or both legs. The greatest damage occurs at the entrance and exit sites.

Myoglobinuria

Myoglobinuria develops from release into the blood of products found in normal muscle; the release can be occasioned by electrical injury. Myoglobin is a large molecule that can mechanically obstruct the renal tubules and lead to acute tubular necrosis unless large amounts of IV fluid are administered to flush the myoglobin out of the kidneys. Osmotic diuretics may be administered to promote increased urine volume. IV fluid is administered at a rate that maintains urine output at 2 mL/kg/hr until the myoglobinuria resolves.

Metabolic Acidosis

Metabolic acidosis follows electrical injury because of the associated cellular destruction and hypovolemic shock. Ringer's lactate solution,

the fluid used for fluid resuscitation, contains sufficient bicarbonate to manage the acidosis that accompanies burn shock but not enough to correct that associated with shock after electrical injury (i.e., pathophysiologic hypovolemic shock, not a "shock" from the electrical current).

Other Complications

The four complications just described usually resolve within 24 hours after injury. Other complications that follow electrical injury include loss of short-term memory and altered emotional states. Children can usually remember events up to the time of injury, including the names of family members and their own address, telephone number, and personal information, but they are unable to recall more recent events. This loss of memory can be distressing to the child and frustrating to the family. For example, the child may be unable to remember visits by the family and so may feel abandoned by them. It is difficult for the child to follow instructions because of the inability to retain instructions, and this may lead to difficulty in planning care. Altered emotional states may include an absence of affect and blank stares or the opposite type of emotional response—manic behavior, hyperactivity, swearing, physical violence, and feelings of paranoia. Emotional responses usually become normal after about 1 week but may persist longer in some children. The electrical injury need not be to the head for these altered states to occur.

The long-term sequelae of electrical injury may include neurologic deficits, amputations, and ocular cataracts. Ocular cataracts may occur in one or both eyes at varying times from 3 months to 18 months after injury. In the very young child, changes in visual acuity may not be noticed; therefore, regular eye examinations should be scheduled every 3 months for the first year after injury.

KEY CONCEPTS

- The functions of the skin include protection, thermoregulation, excretion, production of vitamin D, and sensation.
- The skin comprises two major layers—the outer epidermis and the inner supportive dermis. Beneath these layers is subcutaneous tissue, which attaches the dermis to the underlying structures.
- Developmental differences cause the skin of infants and children to be more susceptible to external irritants and infection than adults' skin.
- Neonates frequently exhibit a variety of birthmarks. Many of these resolve spontaneously, but some are associated with other congenital syndromes.
- Inflammatory skin conditions seen in children include contact or atopic dermatitis. Intervention is based on the cause of the inflammation.
- Impetigo, the most common skin infection of childhood, is highly contagious and nursing care addresses topical medication and infection prevention measures. Other skin infections seen in childhood include bacterial infection (cellulitis), fungal infections (tinea), and herpes simplex infection.

- Preventing reinfestation is a primary goal in the treatment of pediculosis and scabies.
- Nursing care of the adolescent with acne includes teaching about regular, gentle cleansing of the skin, applying topical medications, encouraging a healthy lifestyle and sensitivity to the adolescent's body image concerns.
- Insect bites and stings can cause severe systemic reactions in a sensitized child.
- Young children are at increased risk for burn injuries because they are curious, mobile, and totally dependent on their caretakers for safety.
- The depth, severity, and extent of a burn injury in a child determine the child's response and appropriate management.
- In comparison with adults, children who sustain burn injuries are at increased risk for fluid and heat loss, hypertrophic scarring, cardiovascular problems, infection, and protein and calorie deficiency.
- A child with a minor burn can be managed in the home; after stabilization, a child with a major burn is cared for in a burn treatment center because of multiple body system complications.

REFERENCES

American Academy of Dermatology. (2010). *Topical calcineurin inhibitors (TCIs)—ExzemaNet*. Retrieved from www.skincarephysicians.com/eczemanet/topical_calcineurin_inhibitors.html.

American Academy of Pediatrics. (2009). *Red book 2009: Report of the Committee on Infectious Diseases*. Elk Grove Village, IL: Author.

American Academy of Pediatrics. (2010). *Healthy children: Lice*. Retrieved from www.healthychildren.org

American Academy of Pediatrics Patient Education On-Line. (2010). *Diaper rash*. Retrieved from http://patiented.aap.org.

Antoon, A., & Donovan, M. (2011). Burn injuries. In R. Kliegman, B. Stanton, J. St. Geme, et al. (Eds.), *Nelson textbook of pediatrics* (19th ed., pp. 349-357). Philadelphia: Elsevier Saunders.

Bar-Meir, M., & Tan, T. Q. (2010). *Staphylococcus aureus* skin and soft tissue infections: Can we anticipate the culture result? *Clinical Pediatrics, 49*(5), 432-438.

Bhatt, V., Curnutte, E., & Moore, J. (2008). *Guidelines for the diagnosis and treatment of pediculosis capitis (head lice) in children and adults 2008*. Retrieved from www.guidelines.gov.

Centers for Disease Control and Prevention. (2008a). *Body lice fact sheet*. Retrieved from www.cdc.gov/lice/body/factsheet.html.

Centers for Disease Control and Prevention. (2008b). *Updated information regarding mosquito repellents*. Retrieved from www.cdc.gov/ncidod/dvbid/westnile/resources/uprepinfo.pdf.

Chan, L. C., Haggstrom, A. H., Drolet, B. A., et al. (2008). Growth characteristics of infantile hemangiomas: Implications for management. *Pediatrics, 122*(2), 360-367.

Diamantis, S., Morrell, D., & Burkhart, C. (2009). Treatment of head lice. *Dermatological Therapy, 22*(4), 273-278.

Golden, D., Moffitt, J., Nicklas, R. (2011). *Stinging insect hypersensitivity: A practice parameter update 2011*. Retrieved from www.aaaai.org.

Goodis, J., & Schraga, E. D. (2010). *Burns, thermal. Emergency medicine*. Retrieved from www.emedicine.medscape.com/article/769193.

Hinckley, J., & Allen, P. (2008). Community-associated MRSA in the pediatric primary care setting. *Pediatric Nursing, 34*(1), 64-71.

Leung, D. (2011). Atopic dermatitis (atopic eczema). In R. Kliegman, B. Stanton, J. St. Geme, et al. (Eds.), *Nelson textbook of pediatrics* (19th ed., pp. 801-806). Philadelphia: Elsevier Saunders.

Meadows-Oliver, M. (2009). Tinea capitis: Diagnostic criteria and treatment options. *Pediatric Nursing, 35*(1), 53-57.

Morelli, J. (2011). The skin. In R. Kliegman, B. Stanton, J. St. Geme, et al. (Eds.), *Nelson textbook of pediatrics* (19th ed., pp. 2215-2328). Philadelphia: Elsevier Saunders.

Opstelten, W., Neven, A., & Eekhof, J. (2008). Treatment and prevention of herpes labialis. *Canadian Family Physician, 54*(12), 1683-1687.

Poindexter, G. B., Burkhart, C. N., & Morrell, D. S. (2009). Therapies for pediatric seborrheic dermatitis. *Pediatric Annals, 38*(6), 333-338.

Potter, W. (2010). An overview of ocular herpetic disease. *Review of Optometry, 147*(5), 76-83.

Rollins, J. (2010). Back to school? The "no nit" policy. *Pediatric Nursing, 36*(5), 236-237.

Scholtens, S., Gehring, U., Brunekreef, B., et al. (2007). Breastfeeding, weight gain in infancy, and overweight at seven years of age: The Prevention and Incidence of Asthma and Mite Allergy Birth Cohort Study. *American Journal of Epidemiology, 165*(8), 919-926.

Schor, E. L. (2010). *Impetigo*. Retrieved from www.healthychildren.org/English/healthissues/conditions/skin/pages/Impetigo.aspx.

Sicherer, S., & Leung, D. (2011). Insect allergy. In R. Kliegman, B. Stanton, J. St. Geme, et al. (Eds.), *Nelson textbook of pediatrics* (19th ed., pp. 2215-2328). Philadelphia: Elsevier Saunders.

Skin Cancer Foundation. (2010). *Skin cancer*. Retrieved from www.skincancer.org.

Stanberry, L. (2011). Herpes simplex virus. In R. Kliegman, B. Stanton, J. St. Geme, et al. (Eds.), *Nelson textbook of pediatrics* (19th ed., pp.1097-1104). Philadelphia: Elsevier Saunders.

United Nations Environmental Programme. (2009). *Geneva hosts Stockholm Convention on Persistent Organic Pollutants from 4 to 8 May: Talks to spotlight nine new chemicals, alternatives to DDT and the challenges of a POPs-free future*. Retrieved from www.unep.org.

Vascular Birthmarks Foundation. (2010). *Port wine stain information*. Retrieved from www.birthmark.org/node/23.

Wang, J. C., & Ritterband, D. C. (2009). *Keratitis, herpes simplex differential diagnoses and workup*. Retrieved from http://emedicine.medscape.com/article/1194268-diagnosis.

Zaletel, C. L. (2009). Factors affecting fluid resuscitation in the burn patient: The collaborative role of the APN. *Advanced Emergency Nursing Journal, 31*(4), 309-320.

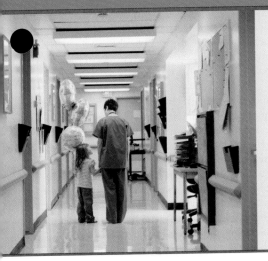

The Child with a Musculoskeletal Alteration

℮volve WEBSITE

http://evolve.elsevier.com/James/ncoc

LEARNING OBJECTIVES

After studying this chapter, you should be able to:

- Describe the implications of differences in the anatomy and physiology of the growing musculoskeletal systems of infants and young children in comparison to the mature musculoskeletal system
- Describe the pathology, etiology, manifestations, diagnostic evaluation, and therapeutic management of musculoskeletal alterations frequently seen in infants, children, and adolescents.
- Identify characteristic assessments that indicate alterations in musculoskeletal function.

- State appropriate nursing diagnoses for children with an alteration in musculoskeletal function.
- Summarize the treatment modalities used to manage the child with a musculoskeletal alteration.
- Design, implement, and evaluate appropriate nursing interventions for the child with altered musculoskeletal function.

CLINICAL REFERENCE

REVIEW OF THE MUSCULOSKELETAL SYSTEM

The nursing care for a child with a musculoskeletal alteration requires an understanding of the structure and function of the musculoskeletal system, comprehension of growth and development, and an awareness of the differences of the musculoskeletal system of infants and children as compared to adults.

Skeletal System

The musculoskeletal system is composed of bones attached to joints, joints connected by ligaments, muscles supported by tendons, and cartilaginous tissues. The function of this system is to provide a skeletal framework to support the body, protect vital organs, and provide movement. It also supplies a storage space for the blood cell production and minerals responsible for regulating resorption and reformation of itself, as well as regulation of mineral and hormonal imbalances in the body (Porth, 2011).

Newborns are born with more bones than adults have, because cranial bones and other small bones, such as bones in the coccyx or sacrum, fuse during infancy and childhood, resulting in the adult complement of 206. The newborn's skeletal structure is mostly cartilaginous at birth, then evolves and ossifies through osteogenesis. There are two distinct types of ossification: intramembranous and endochondral ossification. Intramembranous ossification is the process in which osteoblasts form bone without the cartilaginous stage (Staheli, 2008). Endochondral ossification occurs when the mesenchyme differentiates to cartilage, and cartilage then transforms into bone within primary and secondary ossification centers. Primary ossification occurs in the diaphysis (center of the bone), whereas secondary ossification occurs at the epiphysis (end of the bones). The physis, or growth plate, is formed between the primary and secondary ossification center and allows for longitudinal growth of long bones (Staheli, 2008; Texas Scottish Rite Hospital for Children [TSRHC], 2008). The growth plate absorbs shock and protects the joint surfaces from serious fractures. The metaphysis (above the growth plate) is composed mostly of cartilage and is the area that grows between the diaphysis and epiphysis to form solid bone in adulthood. It is imperative to know the location and the function of these sites of the bone, as these are often the primary sites where infection, neoplasm, fractures, and metabolic and endocrine disorders are identified (Staheli, 2008).

CLINICAL REFERENCE

The periosteum is a vascular connective tissue that lines the outer surface of all bones. It has receptor nerve endings, making it sensitive to manipulation (TSRHC, 2008). The periosteum contributes to bone development by appositional bone growth and has the capability to heal fractures and regenerate bone rapidly in children.

There are five classifications of bones: long bones such as the femur, short bones such as the carpals, irregular bones such as the vertebrae, flat bones such as the ribs, and sesamoid (sometimes classified as short) bones such as the patella. There are also two major divisions to the skeletal system: the axial skeleton, which forms longitudinally and includes the vertebral column and the skull, and the appendicular system, which is attached to the axial and encompasses the pelvis, pectoral girdle, and upper and lower extremities (Porth, 2011).

Articular System

Joints, which are composed of connective tissue and cartilage, connect two or more bones to one another and enable movement. Joints are classified by structure, function, and movement. In general, joints are identified as *synarthrotic* or immovable (e.g., the skull), or synovial *(diarthrotic),* which are freely movable (e.g., the hip) (Porth, 2011).

Alterations in joint movement and swelling require further evaluation. Defective joints are often seen in children with neuromuscular disorders, such as spina bifida and arthrogryposis (Staheli, 2008; TSRHC, 2008). Alterations in joint movement and swelling can also be indicative of trauma, infection, or arthritis.

Muscular System

Muscles help stabilize joints and maintain contact between articular surfaces. Skeletal muscles are attached by tendons to bones. Ligaments bind one bone firmly to another, and the joints are further stabilized by the overlying tendons and muscles. The shape of the two ends of each muscle and of the joint determines the extent of movement or articulation. Skeletal muscles, which are composed of elongated fibers, function voluntarily and produce movement by contraction. Muscle disease in children presents as muscle weakness, spasticity, myoclonus, and myalgia (Staheli, 2008).

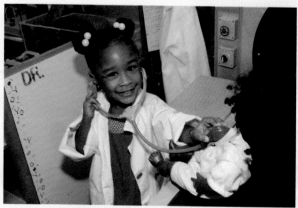

Child with hand differences.

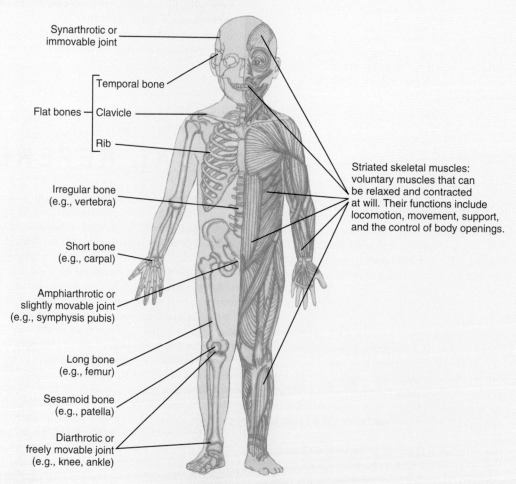

Anatomy of the Musculoskeletal System

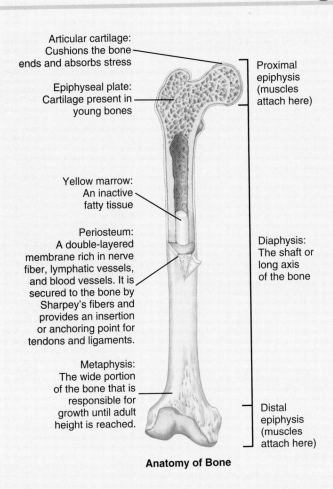

Articular cartilage: Cushions the bone ends and absorbs stress

Epiphyseal plate: Cartilage present in young bones

Yellow marrow: An inactive fatty tissue

Periosteum: A double-layered membrane rich in nerve fiber, lymphatic vessels, and blood vessels. It is secured to the bone by Sharpey's fibers and provides an insertion or anchoring point for tendons and ligaments.

Metaphysis: The wide portion of the bone that is responsible for growth until adult height is reached.

Proximal epiphysis (muscles attach here)

Diaphysis: The shaft or long axis of the bone

Distal epiphysis (muscles attach here)

Anatomy of Bone

PEDIATRIC DIFFERENCES IN THE MUSCULOSKELETAL SYSTEM

- In the fetus, bony tissue begins to develop as closely packed connective tissue. Connective tissue is replaced by cartilage, and cartilage is replaced by mineral salts, which give rise to solid bone. The infant's bones are only 65% ossified at 8 months of age and are neither as firm nor as brittle as those of the older child.
- The periosteum of the child's bone is much stronger than that of adults.
- New bony tissue is produced during periods of growth. The rate of growth varies at different ages. Skeletal growth is stimulated by pituitary growth hormone. Growth of the long bones occurs at the epiphyses, which are located at the ends of the bones and separated from the main portion of the bone by cartilage during the period of growth. Injury to the epiphyses can cause growth disturbances.
- Growing bones produce **callus** and heal quickly, making **internal fixation** of fractures unnecessary in most children. Fractures in children younger than 1 year are unusual due to the large amount of force necessary to break an infant's bone; abuse or underlying pathophysiology is often the cause of fractures in infants.
- The skull is not rigid during infancy, and the sutures of the cranium do not fuse completely until approximately 16 to 18 months of age. Increased intracranial pressure can separate the sutures, causing the infant's head to enlarge.
- Muscle tissue is almost completely developed at birth. Growth occurs because of an increase in size rather than number of the muscle fibers.
- Postural changes during infancy and childhood result from the development of neurologic control, bone and muscle growth, and the laying down of adipose tissue. Postural changes are a good indication of the level of development of the musculoskeletal and neurologic systems.
- Soft tissues are resilient in children, so dislocations and sprains are also less common than in adults.

Cartilage

Cartilage is dense connective tissue that develops at the epiphysis and is capable of withstanding considerable tension. During early fetal development, the skeletal structure is composed mostly of cartilage. In time it will largely convert to bone by ossification. Connective tissue is made up of collagen and proteoglycans (Staheli, 2008). Deficiencies in connective tissues are associated with Marfan syndrome and osteogenesis imperfecta (TSRHC, 2008).

Growth and Development

Knowledge of normal growth and development is essential when assessing, caring for and evaluating the pediatric patient's musculoskeletal system. Infants experience the greatest growth rate. During childhood, growth slows and then increases rapidly again in adolescence with peak height velocity. Peak height velocity is the maximum growth that occurs during puberty. Growth in the length of the long bones continues at the epiphysis until adult height is reached (see Chapter 8).

Pediatric patients should be weighed and measured for length or stature with each visit. The results of these measurements should consistently and correctly be plotted on appropriate growth and development graphs in order to be aware of any variations in height or weight (see Chapter 9). Extreme variations in height and weight can have impact on the child's overall state of health. Childhood obesity, for example, can have a direct impact on children with musculoskeletal problems, such as tibia vara, Blount disease, and slipped capital femoral epiphysis (TSRHC, 2008).

A basic understanding of when children meet their major developmental milestones, especially for gross motor development, is crucial when assessing and treating the child with an alteration of the musculoskeletal system. Failure to meet these milestones in a timely manner may be indicative of hypotonia, cerebral palsy (hemiplegic), or a neuromuscular disorder. See Chapters 5 through 8 for developmental milestones in children of various developmental levels.

Diagnostic and Laboratory Tests

Radiographs are the mainstay of an orthopedic evaluation. They provide important diagnostic evaluation after a clinical assessment when there is concern of a musculoskeletal abnormality. Studies have shown risks of cancer with radiation exposure in a growing child (Brody, Frush, Huda, Brent, & American Academy of Pediatrics [AAP] Section on Radiology, 2007; Gacca, 2008). Several recommendations have been formulated to protect the child. Radiologists and technicians are to use the least and most diagnostically effective radiation exposure on children. In addition, care needs to be taken to shield the gonads, make sure the patient is placed in the correct anatomic position, avoid routine opposite-side radiographs, take single radiographs instead of multiple views, and consult as needed with the provider ordering the radiographs (Brody et al., 2007; Gacca, 2008). It is important to note the pediatric differences in plain films as compared to adults, because the differences can lead to misinterpretation and over- or undertreatment. For example, children have open growth plates at the proximal and distal aspects of the long bones that can easily be confused for fractures. Furthermore, a periosteal reaction in the diaphysis after trauma or infection can be misinterpreted as normal (Staheli, 2008).

CLINICAL REFERENCE

COMMON DIAGNOSTIC PROCEDURES FOR MUSCULOSKELETAL DISORDERS IN CHILDREN

PURPOSE AND DESCRIPTION	NURSING IMPLICATIONS
Radiography (x-ray) *Purpose:* To detect abnormalities or to determine bone age. *Description:* X rays (gamma radiation) are passed through the body, reaching the film on the other side of the body, and creating an image. Different densities of tissue absorb various amounts of radiation. The four densities of x-ray are: Air: appears black Fat: dark gray Water: lighter gray Bone: whitish	Noninvasive Food and fluids are not usually restricted. Clothing and jewelry that may interfere with the study are removed; a paper or cloth gown and shorts without metal are worn. Young children may require assistance for proper positioning and immobilization. Adequate preparation is essential to ensure cooperation.
Ultrasound *Purpose:* To demonstrate body tissue structure or for waveform analysis of Doppler studies. *Description:* The Doppler probe is held over the skin surface or in a body cavity transmitting ultrasound waves to form two-dimensional images of muscles, tendons, cartilaginous tissues, bones, and internal organs.	Noninvasive Food and fluid are not restricted except in small infants, who may be on nothing-by-mouth (NPO) status for 2-3 hr before the procedure so they can eat during the test. Young children may require assistance for proper positioning and immobilization. Adequate preparation is essential to ensure cooperation.
Computed Tomography (CT) *Purpose:* To visualize bony and soft tissue details. *Description:* Narrow-beam x rays in a transverse plane are used to scan an area in successive layers. These images are then reconstructed by computer in the frontal plane and sagittal plane and can even be shown in three-dimensional cross section. *Disadvantages:* Greater radiation exposure, sedation may be required for infants and young children to keep still, and significant costs.	Noninvasive Food and fluids are not restricted. Although the procedure is painless, it may be frightening. Provide developmentally and culturally appropriate preparation and patient education. For example, "The machine looks and sounds like a large clothes dryer or washing machine." Clothing and jewelry that may interfere with the study are removed; a paper or cloth gown and shorts without metal are worn. The child must remain still during procedure, so young children need sedation and may need to be made NPO for food and fluids for safety while sedated. Contrast medium may or may not be used.
Magnetic Resonance Imaging (MRI) *Purpose:* To clearly define organ structures; shows changes in soft tissue, such as edema, blood flow patterns, infarcts. Demonstrates marrow, bone and soft tissue tumors, structure of muscles, ligaments, bones. *Description:* Performed by placing the patient on a moving table, which is pushed into a large cylinder that contains a huge magnet and radio waves that create an energy field that can be translated into a visual image. A variety of noises are heard during the procedure. In contrast to other diagnostic studies, it does not require radiation exposure. *Disadvantages:* Cost.	Noninvasive. Food and fluids are not restricted. Patients are thoroughly screened to assure removal of any metal they might be wearing or have in their possession. The study is not done in children with metal implants, pacemakers, or prostheses. Provide developmentally and culturally appropriate preparation and patient education. Procedure may take 1 hr or more. Adequate preparation, relaxation techniques, and parental presence decrease fear and feelings of claustrophobia. Use of a music headset or video may promote relaxation. The child must remain still during procedure, so young children need sedation and may need to be made NPO for food and fluids for safety while sedated.
Radionuclide Scintigraphy (Bone Scan) *Purpose:* To further investigate trauma with early stress fractures, tumors and cysts to localize the lesion, infections such as osteomyelitis and diskitis, avascular necrosis in Perthes, screen for child abuse in some cases, and pain of unknown origin (Staheli, 2008; TSRHC, 2008). *Description:* A radioactive material (technectium-99m) is administered intravenously and then the body is scanned to evaluate for abnormal uptake after 3-4 hr (Staheli, 2008; TSRHC, 2008).	Encourage fluids 2-4 hr before the test to ensure the child is well hydrated and quickly eliminate radioactive material not absorbed by the bones. Child must void before the scan so that the pelvic bones can be seen. Young children may need sedation.

COMMON DIAGNOSTIC PROCEDURES FOR MUSCULOSKELETAL DISORDERS IN CHILDREN—cont'd

PURPOSE AND DESCRIPTION	NURSING IMPLICATIONS
Arthrography *Purpose:* To evaluate suspected joint damage, such as cartilage tears. *Description:* Dye is injected into the affected joint (usually the knee; sometimes the shoulder or other joint) to further evaluate the cartilaginous structure.	Check for allergies to iodine. Provide developmentally and culturally appropriate preparation and patient education. A local anesthetic is required. The child must remain still during the procedure, so young children may require assistance or sedation for proper positioning and immobilization. If sedated, the child may need to be made NPO for food and fluids. Joint should rest for approximately 12 hr; a compression dressing may be applied after procedure to reduce swelling.
Joint Aspiration Fluid is withdrawn for analysis, usually to detect infection, evaluate arthritis, or relieve pain.	Provide developmentally and culturally appropriate preparation and patient education. A local anesthetic is required. The child must remain still during the procedure, so young children may require assistance or sedation for proper positioning and immobilization. If sedated, the child may need to be made NPO for food and fluids.
Arthroscopy *Purpose:* To image the inside of a joint for diagnosis of injury or minor surgical repairs. Normally arthrography is performed before arthroscopy. *Description:* Fiberoptic endoscope is inserted to examine interior of joint.	Requires local or general anesthesia. The child must be on NPO status if general anesthesia is used; NPO status recommendations for local anesthesia vary with the practitioner. Prepare the child for postoperative dressings, altered mobility, and pain. Assess for infection. Prophylactic antibiotics may be ordered. Use ice postoperatively to reduce swelling.

Clinical laboratory tests are also useful in evaluating the patient with a suspected musculoskeletal alteration. Nurses must have a baseline comprehension of what the normal laboratory values are for each study in order to inform and educate the family about the results. Fasting is not required for these studies.

The hematology workup in orthopedics includes a complete blood count with a differential, C-reactive protein (CRP), and erythrocyte sedimentation rate (ESR) for musculoskeletal conditions such as growing pains, bone pain, stress fractures, hip pain, back pain, and infection (Staheli, 2008; TSRHC, 2008). CRP is a protein that appears in blood during an inflammatory process and is not seen in healthy people. The measurement is nonspecific, merely indicating the presence of inflammation. ESR is the rate at which erythrocytes settle out of unclotted blood, measured in millimeters per hour. Inflammation and necrotic problems cause an elevation in ESR levels.

Chemistry labs assist in the evaluation for metabolic conditions, such as rickets (TSRHC, 2008). These labs include studies of calcium, alkaline phosphatase (ALP), and phosphorus. ALP is an enzyme found mainly in bone, liver, placenta, and kidney. Levels may be elevated in bone disease, fractures, trauma, or liver disease and during periods of rapid growth. Determinations may be ordered to differentiate between bone and liver problems.

Enzyme studies such as creatinine phosphokinase (CPK) may be ordered. CPK is an enzyme found in heart and skeletal muscle; the CPK assay is a specific test for assessing cardiac and muscle damage. Levels are elevated in trauma, myocardial infarction, and muscular dystrophy. Determinations may be ordered to differentiate between cardiac (MB) and skeletal (MM) CPK.

Rheumatoid factor (RF) and a hematology workup are used to evaluate juvenile idiopathic arthritis (Staheli, 2008). RFs are antibodies that may be responsible for the destructive changes associated with rheumatoid arthritis. A positive RF with an elevated CRP and ESR can be indicative of arthritis in children; however, RF is positive in only 5% of these cases (Staheli, 2008).

Musculoskeletal problems affect muscles, bones, joints, and tendons, all of which are necessary for movement and therefore are critical to a child's development. Many musculoskeletal problems occur because of vigorous motor activities that are part of a child's daily life, but the rapid growth of the skeletal system also plays a significant role. Most musculoskeletal problems are short term, but a number of chronic musculoskeletal conditions require long-term treatment and nursing assistance.

The child with a musculoskeletal alteration presents a unique opportunity for nursing care. A general knowledge of the structure and function of the system is required to understand the rationale for the alteration. An awareness of normal versus abnormal growth and development patterns is necessary in order to recognize delays, variations, and medical conditions. An appreciation of the musculoskeletal differences exhibited in the pediatric patient in comparison to the adult is also essential. Nurses should be familiar with the various diagnostic imaging procedures used to assist in the evaluation of patients with musculoskeletal alterations in order to implement nursing considerations. Knowledge of normal laboratory values commonly ordered for patients with musculoskeletal conditions is vital for providing prudent, good-quality, and effective nursing care.

CASTS, TRACTION, AND OTHER IMMOBILIZING DEVICES

Immobilizing a bone or joint helps achieve and maintain a more functional position or rests and protects an affected area during bone healing. Because many musculoskeletal problems require the application of an immobilizing device, the nurse needs to understand general principles of care.

Splints

Splints are used to stabilize and protect or rest an affected area, increase range of motion and function, and decrease pain (TSRHC, 2008). Splints are fabricated of fiberglass, plaster of Paris, metal, or thermoplastic polymers. Splint materials are chosen for drapability, durability, softness, setup time, thickness, capacity for remolding, and color. Splinting may be a safe, effective, and cost-saving alternative to casting for some conditions (Firmin & Crouch, 2009).

Casts

A cast provides support and maintains anatomic position for bone healing or aids in correction of a deformity. Casts may also be used to ensure adherence to treatment protocols or to protect a wound. The age and size of the child, fracture or injury, type of surgery, and amount of weight bearing the extremity can tolerate dictate the type and size of the cast.

Casts are made of synthetic materials, such as fiberglass, semirigid nonfiberglass (softcast), or plaster of Paris (Bakody, 2009). Casting material comes in varied colors and patterns; casts can be wrapped and decorated to appeal to young children. The following equipment is needed for cast application:

- Tubular gauze/stockinette (optional)
- Waterproof lining (optional)
- Cotton under-cast padding material (e.g., Webril)
- Casting material, fiberglass and/or plaster of Paris (rolls and/or strips/splints)
- Water (clarify water temperature with professional applying cast)
- Moleskin
- Waterproof tape
- Scissors
- Cast remover (if needed to trim edges or split cast)

Cast application is usually done by the physician and another trained person, one to hold the extremity in correct alignment and one to apply the cast. It is very important not to move the affected area to be casted while applying the cast. Waterproof liner or stockinette is applied if desired. Waterproof linings for casts have been shown to be as effective as cotton lining for immobilization (Robert, Jiang, & Khoury, 2011). A thin layer of Webril is then applied over the initial lining. The material is rolled in a spiral fashion around the affected area, overlapping each layer by approximately 50%. Additional padding may be placed over bony prominences, making sure there are no wrinkles in any layer. Any wrinkles in the cast padding or cast material become "set" into the cast and may cause skin breakdown. Next, the casting material is dipped in water and applied over the cotton padding, making sure to leave a cotton edge at the top and bottom of the cast for patient comfort and to maintain skin integrity. A chemical reaction between casting material and water makes it feel warm and causes it to harden. The cast should not be covered while warm to prevent a possible burn.

Rough edges of casts must be trimmed to prevent injury. Petaling of cast edges with moleskin or latex-free tape decreases irritation and breakdown of adjacent skin and protects the edges of the cast from excessive wear.

Fiberglass casts dry quickly, usually set within 30 minutes of application. Fiberglass should be rolled on the affected body part without stretching the fiberglass. Fiberglass is less forgiving when swelling is expected, and if the fiberglass is pulled "tight" or stretched during application, neurovascular status may be compromised (TSRHC, 2008).

Fiberglass casts are lighter weight and more durable than plaster (TSRHC, 2008) (Figure 26-1). Fiberglass casts are water resistant, so the hard outer shell will not break down in water; however, the padding underneath the cast material is likely cotton and will absorb and hold water. Therefore, if a fiberglass cast becomes wet, inadequate airflow under the cast will prevent thorough drying of the padding and skin. Damp skin is more susceptible to skin breakdown and infection.

Plaster casts may be used when the physician wants to "mold" the cast to apply corrective forces to a body part, such as in the treatment of a clubfoot or early-onset scoliosis (TSRHC, 2008). Plaster casts will set within 10 to 15 minutes, but will not fully dry for 24 to 48 hours. Plaster is not water resistant and will break down if it gets wet.

Traction

Effective immobilization may also be achieved with traction. Traction is a pull or force exerted on one part of the body. Traction can be applied to the skin or the bone. For treatment, traction may be applied to the spine, pelvis, or long bones of the upper and lower extremities. The angle formed by the placement of the pulley and the angle of the involved joint determine the direction of the pull or force. Once the

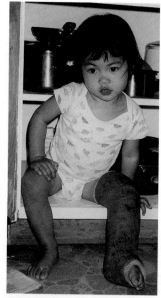

FIG 26-1 Child in a synthetic cast.

direction of the pull or force has been determined, the traction is directed along the long axis of the bone.

An opposing pull or force (countertraction) must be provided at the same time if the traction is to be effective. Countertraction results in a two-way pull that maintains alignment of the affected extremity. The child's weight is usually sufficient to provide the countertraction. If body weight is not sufficient, additional weights may be used. Depending on the age of the child, restraining devices may be needed to maintain countertraction. Some forms of traction, such as halo traction used for severe scoliosis, exert a force without the use of weights.

If traction is being applied while the child is in bed, the part of the bed that holds the traction apparatus is tilted or elevated, thereby assisting with countertraction. For example, if the leg were being placed in traction, the foot of the bed would be elevated. Otherwise, the child would slide in the direction of the traction, disrupting the alignment of the extremity and reducing the effectiveness of treatment. Also, the mattress should be firm, and a foot board or foot plate may be necessary to keep the extremity in the correct position.

Traction can be described as either *continuous* or *intermittent*. Continuous traction exerts a constant pull and is used for fractures and dislocations. Intermittent traction provides a periodic pull or force and is used for contractures, low back pain or muscle spasm. *The nurse should always assume that traction is continuous unless the physician states otherwise.* The removal of traction intended to be continuous could prove harmful to the child. If the force of the traction is altered, the muscles contract and fracture alignment could be disrupted. The tissues around the fracture could also be injured, resulting in poor healing. The nursing care plan should always reflect the frequency and amount of time intermittent traction may be removed. When removing the traction apparatus, the nurse must maintain manual traction and pull on the body part.

The disadvantages of traction include prolonged immobility and the potential need for hospitalization. Currently, early casting and percutaneous pinning are replacing the use of traction for some musculoskeletal conditions (Gosselin, Heitto, & Zirkle, 2009; Hsu, Diaz, Penaranda, et al., 2009).

Skin Traction

Skin traction (Box 26-1) is noninvasive and well tolerated, and application does not require anesthesia (TSRHC, 2008). Skin traction is most effective with children who weigh less than 15 kg or are younger than 2 to 3 years. It can be applied to the pelvis, spine, or extremities (usually the long bones). Skin traction is preferred for conditions in which invasive procedures are contraindicated, such as hemarthrosis (collection of blood in the joint) as a result of hemophilia. Foam rubber straps, adhesive moleskin, elastic bandages, or cloth belts are applied to the skin and then attached to the weights and pulleys. If skin traction to the lower leg is needed, a foam rubber or fabric boot may be used; the fit should be secure.

Skin traction is not appropriate if the child has a skin infection, an open wound, or extensive tissue damage. Skin breakdown may develop as a result of skin traction. Applying tincture of benzoin to the intact skin before the traction is applied may protect against skin irritation.

If the traction has not been set up correctly, neurovascular impairment may occur. Therefore, skin traction is not appropriate for patients with abnormal sensation in the lower extremities (TSRHC, 2008). Hyperextension of the knee and elastic bandages that have been wrapped too tightly are the most common causes of traction-related neurovascular impairment. A thorough assessment of the traction apparatus and the extremity should be conducted at least once each shift.

BOX 26-1 TYPES OF SKIN TRACTION

Buck's Extension

Buck
- *Purpose:* Used to treat some fractures, hip disorders, contractures, and muscle spasms.
- *Description:* Continuous or intermittent boot or circular wrap is applied to the skin. Traction is applied to boot or wrap. Rolled towels are placed on the external surface of the knee to prevent external rotation of the affected leg. Unless otherwise ordered, the mattress should be flexed at the knee (20 to 30 degrees).

Bryant
- *Purpose:* Used to treat very young children (less than 2 years) with femur fractures or developmental dysplasia of the hip.
- *Description:* The child's affected lower extremity or extremities are wrapped. The child lies in bed (or crib) with hips flexed 90 degrees and the knees extended. Traction is applied overhead with just enough weight to elevate the buttock off the surface of the mattress.
- Is continuous for femur fractures, but may be intermittent for children with developmental dysplasia of the hip. Traction may be used for 2 to 4 weeks to loosen muscles before a child goes to the operating room for closed or open reduction for the displaced hip.

Skeletal Traction

Skeletal traction (Box 26-2 and Figure 26-2) exerts greater force than skin traction and can be physiologically tolerated for longer periods. Skeletal traction helps maintain correct alignment of the bony fragments and assists in proper healing. Traction is maintained by a metal device inserted into the bone. The fracture site determines the insertion site of the stainless steel wires, pins, or tongs. Common sites for skeletal traction include the skull, the proximal end of the ulna, and the distal end of the femur, as well as the tibia and heel. General anesthesia is necessary for skeletal traction placement and removal.

The most serious complication associated with skeletal traction is *osteomyelitis*, an infection involving the bone. Organisms gain access to the bone systemically or through the opening created by the metal pins or wires used for traction. Clinical manifestations include localized pain, swelling, warmth, tenderness, unusual odor, fever, and irritability or lethargy in young children. To decrease the risk of infection, pin site care is required at least once per day. Pin site care protocols involve inspecting each site for signs of infection (e.g., tenting or pulling around the pin, redness at the site, purulent drainage) and cleaning the skin around pin sites with one of various cleansing solutions (e.g., chlorhexidine gluconate, plain normal saline, soap and water). A recent evidence-based practice review of pin site care protocols was inconclusive as to the best method for preventing infection at pin sites (Lethaby, Temple, & Santy, 2008).

BOX 26-2   TYPES OF SKELETAL TRACTION

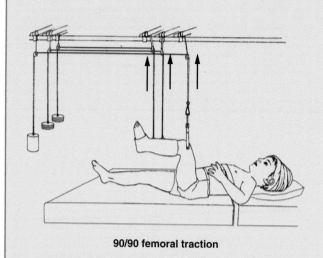

Halo

Halo
- *Purpose:* To stabilize fractures or displaced vertebrae in cervical and thoracic areas. Also used to prepare the spine (muscles, vertebrae, and spinal cord) before spinal fusion, casting, or bracing in younger patients.
- *Description:* The halo is fitted with pins drilled directly into the skull. The halo is then attached by a rope to weights or pulley above the head or to a special vest connected to the halo with rods. When the halo is attached to weights, the center of the curved metal bar over the halo must extend along the same planes as the spinal cord. Traction pull is always along the axis of the spine. The child must maintain straight body alignment.

90/90 femoral traction

90/90 Femoral
- *Purpose:* Most commonly used traction for complicated fractures of the femur; most effective in children older than 6 years. Within 2 to 3 weeks, callus formation is sufficient to allow application of a spica cast.
- *Description:* A pin or wire is inserted through the distal femur.

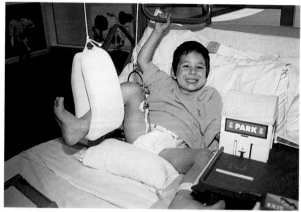

FIG 26-2 Skeletal traction is used to reduce and immobilize fractures and allows greater pull than would be possible with skin traction. Osteomyelitis may be a serious complication because skeletal traction is invasive. (Courtesy Parkland Health and Hospital System, Dallas, TX.)

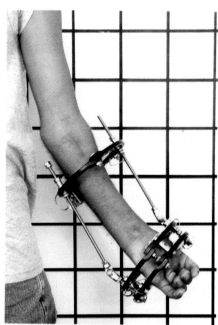

FIG 26-3 Ilizarov external fixator. (Courtesy Shriners Hospitals for Children, Houston, TX.)

External Fixation Devices

External fixation devices may also be used in the treatment of complex fractures, to lengthen bones, and to correct angular deformities that involve bone and soft tissue. These devices provide distraction, keeping the bone ends separated and in alignment so healing can occur. External fixators also allow periodic changes in alignment and bone length. External fixation devices, such as the Ilizarov external fixator (Figure 26-3), consist of pins or wires inserted through skin, soft tissue, and bone and secured on the outer limb surface to a rigid metal frame.

General anesthesia is necessary for placement and removal of external fixation devices.

Because pins or wires of the external fixator pass through the skin to anchor in the bone, meticulous assessment of entry sites for signs of inflammation, infection, or loose pins is necessary. Pin tract infection occurs in approximately 50% of cases (TSRHC, 2008). Pin site care, similar to pin site care for children in traction, is recommended. To prevent injury to the other limb or to others, sharp protrusions from the fixator need to be adequately covered.

Nursing Considerations

Before application of an immobilizing device, assess the child's and parents' knowledge about the procedure. Also assess the child's skin and note the presence of any bruises or abrasions that may be covered by the device.

⚡ SAFETY ALERT

The Child in a Cast or Traction

Tissue ischemia and nerve damage are serious complications that may accompany immobilization in a cast or traction. Skin color and temperature, movement and sensation of the extremity, quality of pulses, and capillary refill time are related to neurovascular status and should be carefully assessed. Problems must be handled quickly to prevent permanent disabilities.

The five *P*s can be used as a guide for assessing neurovascular status (Bakody, 2009):

*P*ain unrelieved by analgesia
*P*allor
*P*ulselessness or lack of capillary refill
*P*aresthesia
*P*aralysis or progressive loss of motion
Assessment that identifies any of these five Ps of neurovascular compromise may indicate tissue ischemia. Prompt referral to a physician and intervention is crucial if neurovascular impairment is to be prevented.

Bakody, E. (2009). Orthopaedic plaster casting: Nurse and patient education. *Nursing Standard, 23*(51), 49-56.

Neurovascular Status

After the device is applied, perform a neurovascular assessment (CSM—*c*irculation, *s*ensation, and *m*otion) at least every 2 hours during the first 48 hours. Assess the strength of the pulse distal to the site, and compare it with the pulse in the uninvolved extremity. A sluggish capillary refill time may indicate neurovascular impairment.

Signs of circulatory impairment include coldness, pallor, blueness of the extremity, swelling, loss of motion, and numbness and tingling of the extremity. Touch the child's skin proximal and distal to the device to assess temperature; ask the child to move the fingers or toes. Paresthesia, or numbness, burning, and tingling, can be assessed by touching the fingers or toes and noting any decrease or loss of feeling. Paresthesia is of serious concern because paralysis can result if the problem is not corrected. Report a child's complaints of a pins-and-needles sensation or of the extremity "feeling asleep." Young children are not always able to describe a feeling or sensation, so avoid questions such as "Do you feel this?" Instead, ask a child to wiggle the fingers or toes to appropriately determine motor impairment.

Special Considerations for the Child in Halo Traction. Children who must be in halo traction have additional neurovascular issues that need to be addressed (Table 26-1).

Assessing and Managing Compartment Syndrome. Serious complications, such as nerve compression, circulatory impairment, or compartment syndrome, can result from swelling caused by trauma or an immobilizing device. The muscles and nerves of the upper and lower extremities are enclosed in compartments that are surrounded by tough, inelastic fascia (comparable to sausage casing). *Compartment syndrome* occurs when swelling causes pressure within these closed fascial compartments to rise, compromising vascular perfusion to the muscles and nerves (Bakody, 2009). Compartment syndrome is a true surgical emergency that requires prompt diagnosis and intervention to prevent paralysis and necrosis of tissues (Bakody, 2009; TSRHC, 2008).

Signs of compartment syndrome include severe pain, often unrelieved by analgesics, and signs of neurovascular impairment (TSRHC, 2008). If extending the fingers or wiggling the toes produces pain, and/or the quality of the radial or pedal pulse is poor to absent, notify the physician. In addition, assess for pallor, paresthesia, and pulselessness as previously described. Paresis and paresthesias are late findings, typically a sign of permanent damage (TSRHC, 2008).

TABLE 26-1 NEUROLOGIC ASSESSMENT FOR PATIENTS REQUIRING HALO TRACTION

Neurologic assessments are usually performed three times per day.
- Obtain and document baseline assessment before first traction application.
- Assess patient in the morning about 30 minutes after the patient goes from bed to wheelchair or walker traction.
- Assess patient again after lunch.
- Assess patient for the third time in the evening after the patient goes from wheelchair or walker traction to bed.

NOTE: All of these checks should be positive, except clonus and the Babinski sign should be negative (but Babinski may be positive up to age 2 years).

Lateral gaze	Check eye movements. Ask patient to follow your finger with the eyes and move your finger side to side.
Tongue movement	(Cranial nerve XII: hypoglossal) Ask patient to stick out tongue and move tongue right, left, up, and down.
Show teeth	(Cranial nerve VII: facial nerve) Ask patient to smile and show teeth.
Swallow	(Cranial nerve IX: glossopharyngeal) Patient should be able to swallow easily and effectively. Should not choke on solids, liquids, or saliva. Should not have difficulty swallowing.
Deltoid-shoulder strength	(Cranial nerve XI: spinal accessory nerve) Have patient abduct and adduct shoulders and move shoulders up against your hands to assess strength.
Grip strength	Have patient grasp your hands and squeeze both right and left hand at the same time.
Quadriceps	While patient is seated with legs dangling over the edge of bed or table, ask patient to extend each leg straight and resist your attempt to bend the leg. You can also check quadriceps strength by asking patient to raise the leg off the bed against your resistance.
Ankle flexion and extension	Ask patient to flex and extend ankle against your resistance.
Big toe	Ask patient to move a big toe down toward the floor and up toward the body—both independently of other toes.
Knee jerk	With leg bent at the knee, firmly tap knee with reflex hammer to elicit response from the lower leg.
Babinski	Using a blunt object (pen or end of a reflex hammer), run object along the sole of foot from the bottom of heel, up along the lateral edge, and over under the big toe. Toes will curl down for a negative Babinski and toes will fan out for a positive result.
Clonus	While holding foot in neutral position with your hand, gently but quickly dorsiflex the ankle. The "jumpy" or "bouncy" feeling you get from the sudden stretching of the Achilles tendon is clonus.

The diagnosis of compartment syndrome is made primarily on physical findings, but if physical findings provoke any question, diagnosis can be aided by measurement of the pressure within the affected compartment. The intracompartmental pressure at which a compartment syndrome exists is unknown, and pressure may vary with the technique of measurement (TSRHC, 2008). If compartment syndrome is suspected, the nurse should immediately elevate the extremity only to the level of the child's heart, loosen any restrictive bandages or dressings (if able), split the cast (if able), notify the physician immediately, and administer pain medication as ordered (Bakody, 2009). The child will need to be kept on nothing-by-mouth (NPO) status for possible emergent surgical management.

Immobility

Children in immobilizing devices are subject to the consequences of immobility. Immobility can affect several body systems. Appropriate assessment and intervention can prevent adverse effects (Table 26-2).

Special Considerations for the Child in Traction

Children who are placed in traction are hospitalized from several days to weeks depending on the underlying condition. It is imperative that the nurse check the amount of traction the patient is receiving against the physician's orders; all weights should be hanging free and not touching the floor or bed, and all ropes need to be appropriately on the pulleys. Elevate the head or foot of the bed as indicated to maintain

TABLE 26-2 CONSEQUENCES OF IMMOBILITY

ASSESSMENT CRITERIA	NURSING DIAGNOSIS	INTERVENTION
Integumentary Red or irritated skin, presence of ulceration or drainage	Impaired Skin Integrity	Reposition the child every 2 hr and as needed; encourage the child in traction to use a trapeze to facilitate movement. Use an egg crate–type or sheepskin mattress for comfort under the back and lower legs. If the child is not capable of any independent repositioning or has decreased sensation, use a pressure relief overlay or mattress. Pay particular attention to the heels to prevent skin breakdown. Wash and thoroughly dry the areas twice a day; refrain from using lotion, powder, or talc, which can retain moisture. Change the untrained child's diapers frequently to prevent skin breakdown. Examine and record the child's skin condition once per shift.
Gastrointestinal Decrease in number or consistency of bowel movements because of decreased gastrointestinal motility	Risk for Constipation	Assess bowel sounds, abdominal distention, elimination pattern; be sure to know the child's normal pattern, usual stool consistency, and words used for defecation. Provide a diet high in roughage and fiber and increase fluid intake with foods and fluids the child likes. Position the child as upright as possible during defecation. Administer laxatives and/or stool softeners if needed.
Respiratory Decreased or altered respirations, shortness of breath, decreased breath sounds, adventitious breath sounds	Ineffective Breathing Pattern	Assess respiratory status at least once per shift. Encourage coughing and deep breathing through the use of games, such as blowing bubbles, pinwheels; older children can use an incentive spirometer. Reposition every 2 hr and as needed.
Genitourinary Decreased urinary output from stasis or retention, concentrated or foul-smelling urine	Impaired Urinary Elimination	Maintain hydration levels. Offer juices (cranberry, apple) and acid-ash foods (cereal, meats) that will acidify the urine. Monitor the child's urinary output.
Musculoskeletal Reduced strength and joint mobility, loss of muscle tone and potential for muscle atrophy, limited range of motion	Impaired Physical Mobility	Test muscle strength and joint mobility every shift and as needed. Encourage active range-of-motion and stretching exercises of unaffected extremities. Plan developmentally appropriate activities that require the use of unaffected extremities. Provide foods high in protein and calcium. Use elastic stockings or thromboembolic disease hose to promote venous return and decrease circulatory stasis.

TABLE 26-2 CONSEQUENCES OF IMMOBILITY—cont'd

ASSESSMENT CRITERIA	NURSING DIAGNOSIS	INTERVENTION
Developmental regression, irritability, anxiety, excessive dependence on others, passive behavior	Powerlessness	Recognize the child's need to regress in response to the immobility; help child regain prior developmental stages when ready.
		Explain all routines and procedures to the child and parents and encourage them to participate in care.
		Provide the opportunity for therapeutic play: modeling clay, paints, remote-control toys (which give the feeling of mobility and control), puppet play, storytelling, role playing.
		Allow the child to use age-appropriate dishes and cups, clothing from home (may have to be adapted to fit over an immobilizing device), transitional object, night-light.
		Determine and follow the child's usual routine.
		Encourage the school-age child and adolescent to keep up with schoolwork and keep in contact with peers.
		Frequently provide a change in environment: move the bed to take advantage of a different view; move the bed into the playroom.
		Allow and encourage the child's autonomy in decision making.

countertraction. It may be necessary to draw a line on the child's bed sheet and ask the parents to keep the child above that line. An older child can pull on an overhead trapeze to maintain proper position and alignment.

Home Care

Most children are discharged home shortly after a cast application. The box, Patient-Centered Teaching: Home Care for the Child in a Cast, presents basic principles for caring for a child in a cast at home. Care for children discharged with an external fixator may involve frequent neurovascular assessments and possibly pin site care. Parents must be able to describe how to care for the cast or fixator, when they need to contact their physician, and how to contact any needed resources in the community (e.g., physical therapy, occupational therapy, school district personnel). The nurse can also help the parents select appropriate clothing and adaptive devices if appropriate. Encourage the parents to promote the child's self-care whenever possible.

FRACTURES

Fractures in children are common and can vary in severity from benign to life threatening. A fracture is a break or disruption in a bone's continuity. Generally fractures occur when excessive or traumatic force exceeds the strength of the bone.

Etiology

Fractures in children usually result from increased mobility and inadequate or immature motor and cognitive skills. They may result from accidental trauma (e.g., falls, motor vehicle crashes, sports injuries), nonaccidental trauma (e.g., child abuse), or pathologic conditions that result in abnormally fragile bones (e.g., osteogenesis imperfecta, tumors, cysts).

Many biochemical and physiologic properties of pediatric bones differ from those of adults. Three essential differences contribute to the understanding of injury, fracture patterns, healing and treatment (Firmin & Crouch, 2009). First, children's bones are less brittle with a higher collagen-to-bone ratio. This difference is protective, making incomplete fractures more likely. Second, children have a stronger

periosteum. This also makes complete fractures less likely or at least limits fracture displacement. The third essential pediatric bone difference is the epiphyseal plate or growth plate. The epiphyseal plate is the weakest part of the growing bone, but often bears the brunt of children's bone injuries.

An understanding of growth and development is helpful when assessing trauma in specific age-groups. For example, fractures in infancy are generally rare because of the cartilaginous quality of the skeleton. Fractures in infants are usually the result of trauma during birth or nonaccidental trauma. Therefore, fractures that occur after the birthing process warrant further investigation to rule out the possibility of child abuse.

Clavicle fractures can occur at any age. Lack of movement or a pseudoparalysis of the upper extremity may be the only sign in an infant who has sustained a fractured clavicle during birth. It is important to assess the infant with clavicle fracture for brachial plexus palsy because the two may be associated. An older child will report pain and show swelling on the clavicle at the site of the fracture. A common mechanism of clavicle injury in older children is blunt trauma from contact sports.

Another major cause of children's fractures is falls. The outstretched arm often receives the full force of the fall, even though this action is the result of the child's protective reflexes (Figure 26-4). Although this force of impact can involve any part of the arm (wrist, elbow, shoulder), the supracondylar humeral fracture of the elbow is most commonly seen with this type of fall. Secondary complications of this injury include circulatory impairment, cellular necrosis, neurovascular damage, ischemic contracture (Volkmann's contracture), or compartment syndrome.

A thorough and timely assessment for a fracture is important to prevent loss of function and disturbance to the bone growth of the pediatric patient regardless of age or type of skeletal injury. Understanding the etiology and location of the fracture is important to prevent complications.

Incidence

Pediatric trauma is the leading cause of death and disability in children and one of the largest challenges to their health (Vitale, 2010). The United States has the highest incidence of pediatric trauma among

Home Care for the Child in a Cast

Check the Edges of the Cast as Follows
- If they appear rough or are irritating the skin, "petal" the cast by overlapping moleskin or adhesive tape (1 to 2 inches in width; 3 to 4 inches in length with one rounded edge) around the cast edges.
- Waterproof tape should be used in the perineal area.

To Assist with Drying the Cast, Do the Following
- Place the child on a firm mattress.
- Support the cast and adjacent joints with pillows.
- For a plaster cast, reposition every 2 to 4 hours to ensure thorough drying.
- Lift the cast with the palms of your hands.
- You may direct a fan toward the cast to facilitate drying.
- Once dry, the cast should sound hollow and be cool to the touch.

Swelling Generally Peaks within 24 to 48 Hours. To Prevent Problems, Do the Following
- Apply bagged ice to the casted area (be sure to keep melting ice from touching the cast or leaking underneath).
- Elevate the extremity at the level of the heart with pillows.
- Apply pressure to the nail bed of the child's casted extremity and count how long it takes for the color to return (it should take no longer than 2 seconds). Repeat every 2 hours for the first 24 to 48 hours.
- The casted extremity should be the same color and temperature as the other extremity.
- Check each finger or toe for sensation and movement several times each day for 2 days.

Protect the Cast as Follows
- If the child is permitted to bathe or shower, be sure to cover the cast with plastic and waterproof tape to keep the cast dry.
- Do not put anything inside the cast. Keep small toys and sharp objects away from the cast. Supervise your child during mealtimes so the child does not get food underneath the cast.

Contact the Physician If Any of the Following Occurs
- The cast feels warm or hot or has an unusual smell.
- Any drainage or blood suddenly appears on the cast.
- Your child reports pain, burning, numbness, or tingling.
- The extremity changes color or temperature, or any swelling persists.
- Any fever above 101.5° F (40° C) taken by mouth.
- Slipping of cast, inability to visualize toes or fingers.

When Preparing to Remove the Cast, Do the Following
- Explain the cast removal to your child. The cast remover works by vibration that creates a warm tickling feeling on the skin and sounds like a vacuum cleaner.
- Allow time for the child to adjust to the cast remover. Ask the technician or physician if your child can examine the cast remover and see how it works ahead of time.
- Once the cast is removed, the skin will be dry and flaky. Wash the area with warm water and soap. Discourage the child from scratching.
- The extremity will be stiff for a while and will look smaller because the muscles have not been used. It may need to be supported with a sling. Normal movement will correct the stiffness.

Fractures and Physeal Growth Plate Injuries

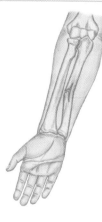

Greenstick
Break occurs through the periosteum on one side of the bone while only bowing or buckling on the other side. Seen most frequently in forearm.

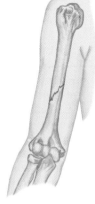

Spiral
Twisted or circular break that affects the length rather than the width. Seen frequently in child abuse.

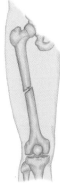

Oblique
Diagonal or slanting break that occurs between the horizontal and perpendicular planes of the bone.

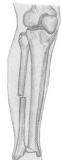

Transverse
Break or fracture line occurs at right angles to the long axis of the bone.

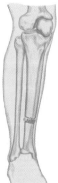

Comminuted
Bone is splintered into pieces. This is a rare occurrence in children.

Pediatric fractures are seldom complete breaks. Rather, children's bones tend to bend or buckle because of increased flexibility. This flexibility is due to a thicker periosteum and increased amounts of immature bone.

PATHOPHYSIOLOGY

Fractures and Physeal Growth Plate Injuries—cont'd

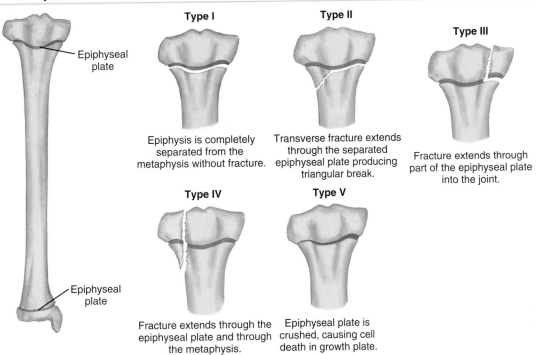

Type I
Epiphysis is completely separated from the metaphysis without fracture.

Type II
Transverse fracture extends through the separated epiphyseal plate producing triangular break.

Type III
Fracture extends through part of the epiphyseal plate into the joint.

Type IV
Fracture extends through the epiphyseal plate and through the metaphysis.

Type V
Epiphyseal plate is crushed, causing cell death in growth plate.

Epiphyseal plate

Epiphyseal plate

Physeal growth plate injuries: Salter-Harris classification. Epiphyseal fractures are common in children.

Fractures result in bone fragmentation and injury to the surrounding tissues. Torn blood vessels cause bleeding from the bone and tissues around the bone fragments. As blood clots at the site, fibrin strands provide a network for healing. Osteoblasts begin forming in immense numbers almost immediately after the injury. This increased osteoblastic activity results in the formation of new bone matrix between the bone fragments. Calcium salts are deposited in the new bone matrix, forming a *callus*. The callus is responsible for stability and support of the fracture while healing occurs. Gradually the callus is formed into new bone. Remodeling, or correction of an injury at the fracture site through the buildup of callus, occurs more rapidly in growing children.

Fractures are referred to as *simple* or *compound*. When the skin is intact, the fracture is classified as *simple* (closed). A simple fracture still requires a thorough nursing assessment because of potential problems associated with this injury. Possible complications include internal hemorrhage, compartment syndrome, or neurovascular compromise.

When the skin, subcutaneous tissue, or muscle has been disrupted, the fracture is classified as *compound* (open). Infection is a risk with this type of fracture because organisms can enter the fracture site through the wound. Children

with compound fractures are at risk for blood loss as a result of external hemorrhage.

Systemic risks associated with fractures, especially multiple fractures or femur fractures, are emboli and shock. Emboli can result from postinjury bleeding with clotting or from fat droplets released from the fractured bone marrow (fat embolism). The emboli enter the circulatory system and may travel to the lungs, heart, or brain. The potential for hypovolemic shock exists with both closed and open fractures.

A break or fracture between the shaft of the bone and epiphyseal plate is referred to as a growth plate injury. In a growing bone, the region of least resistance to stress is the area between the metaphysis and the cartilaginous epiphyseal plate. The amount of growth arrest associated with an epiphyseal injury is determined by the extent of the damage to the epiphyseal plate.* If the germinal cells remain with the epiphysis and appear uninjured, healing is rapid and growth is seldom affected. If the germinal layer is destroyed, however, growth disturbances will occur. The Salter-Harris classification system classifies epiphyseal growth plate injuries and their associated risk of growth disturbance.

*Basener, C. J., Mehlman, C. T., & Dipasquale, T. G. (2009). Growth disturbance after distal femoral growth plate fractures in children: A meta-analysis. *Journal of Orthopaedic Trauma, 23*(9), 663-667.

developing nations; musculoskeletal trauma makes up the largest portion of pediatric injuries, with 25% of children sustaining an injury annually and 10% to 25% of those injuries being fractures (Vitale, 2010).

Fractures are common in children and adolescents because numerous gross motor activities place them at risk for injury. Young children

are acquiring new motor skills, whereas older children and adolescents are participating in risk-taking behaviors as part of their normal growth and development. It is estimated that 40% of boys and 25% of girls will sustain a fracture by 16 years of age (Vitale, 2010). The distal forearm is the most common site to be fractured in children; the clavicle is second.

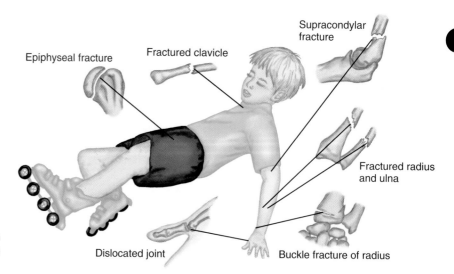

FIG 26-4 Upper extremity fractures in children often occur when the child attempts to break a fall with an outstretched arm.

Manifestations

Presentation of fractures vary with location, type, and cause of injury. General signs and symptoms include pain or tenderness at the site, immobility or decreased range of motion, deformity, and swelling. Other signs and symptoms include crepitus, ecchymosis, erythema, muscle spasm, and inability to bear weight.

The periosteum of children's bones is thicker and stronger than that of adults, and therefore, fractures are less likely to be displaced. Local signs and symptoms of a fracture are not always present, which may make diagnosis of a fracture difficult. Radiography is the most effective tool for determining the type and location of a fracture. Fractures may not be visible on radiographs until healing begins. A radiograph of the unaffected extremity may be obtained for comparison purposes, especially when trying to determine whether a line on the radiograph represents a fracture or merely an epiphyseal line. Radiographs are also obtained after fracture reduction and during the healing process to assess progress.

Therapeutic Management

The goal for managing fractures in children is to maintain function without affecting growth. The key to healing is correct fracture reduction and retention. *Reduction* is the repositioning of the bone fragments into normal alignment. Retention entails the application of a device or mechanism that maintains alignment until healing occurs.

Reduction Methods

Fractures are treated by either closed or open reduction. Closed reduction is accomplished by manual alignment of the fragments followed by immobilization. Simple or closed fractures are treated by closed reduction. Hospitalization is seldom necessary for closed reduction, and most of these fractures heal without complications.

Open reduction entails the surgical insertion of internal or external fixation devices, such as rods, wires, or pins that help maintain alignment while healing occurs. When open reduction is used, hospitalization may be required to assess the child for postoperative complications. Complications after open reduction include delayed healing, nonunion, and infection. Close assessment by the health care team and strict adherence to sterile technique during dressing changes can decrease the risk of postoperative problems and promote healing.

Retention

Once the bone is aligned, the fracture site must be protected and the position of the fragments maintained. This is accomplished through the application of a splint, cast, external fixation device, or traction, which effectively immobilizes the area while healing occurs.

Nursing Considerations

Initial Trauma Assessment

Nursing assessment of the child with a traumatic fracture should begin with a thorough primary survey (see Chapter 10). A complete history of the circumstances surrounding the fracture should be obtained to identify the mechanism of injury and rule out nonaccidental trauma.

Examine the fracture site for bruising, skin lacerations, and swelling. Generally the child will favor the extremity, by cradling or guarding the limb. Often the child will report numbness and tingling distal to the fracture site. Movement and range of motion may be limited. The five Ps of neurovascular status should be assessed carefully and interventions initiated appropriately to prevent impairment.

Assessing and Managing Complications

Fat embolism and resultant respiratory distress are commonly seen in adults with multiple or long bone fractures but are rare in children (Farley & Kay, 2010). Although the cause of fat embolism is unclear, particles of fat escape from the fracture site, are carried through the circulatory system, and lodge in the lung capillaries. Signs and symptoms of fat embolism are the same in a child as in adults. These include axillary petechiae, hypoxemia, and radiographic changes showing pulmonary infiltrates of the lungs (Farley & Kay, 2010). These changes appear within several hours after the fracture. Rarely, fat emboli can lodge in the small capillaries in the brain or other vital organs. Hypoxemia and mental status changes are typically caused by other injuries or from overmedication with opioid analgesics rather than fat embolism. Minimal movement of fractured extremities can prevent or lessen the effects of fat embolism. Treatment is primarily supportive and includes volume resuscitation, respiratory support, and adequate oxygenation.

Another complication that can occur with an orthopedic injury is deep vein thrombosis. The incidence of deep vein thrombosis in children is between 0.2 and 3.3 per 1000 pediatric trauma discharges (O'Brien, Haley, Kelleher et al., 2008). Risk factors include prolonged immobility, obesity, increasing age and long bone trauma (Goel, Buckley, deVries et al., 2009). Prevention includes elevation of the fractured extremity, early ambulation with support, and prompt initiation of postoperative physiotherapy. Pain management is an important adjunct for meeting this goal, as well as for promoting healing and shortening hospital stay. Currently, there is no standard of care for deep vein thrombosis prophylaxis in the pediatric or adolescent trauma patient (O'Brien et al., 2008).

SOFT TISSUE INJURIES: SPRAINS, STRAINS, AND CONTUSIONS

Soft tissue injuries are common among children and are usually related to play or athletic activities.

Etiology

Sprains occur as a result of trauma to a joint in which ligaments are stretched or are partially or completely torn. *Strains,* also known as *pulls, tears,* or *ruptures,* result from an excessive stretch of muscle. *Contusions* occur when soft tissue, muscle, or subcutaneous tissues are damaged. Sprains and contusions frequently accompany each other. Dislocation occurs when a joint is disrupted in such a way that articulating surfaces are no longer in contact.

Incidence

Sprains are not frequently seen in young children because of their poorly developed epiphyseal plates. A twisting or turning injury will more likely result in a fracture at the weak epiphyseal location than a sprain. Sprains and strains are more common in adolescents and are frequently the result of athletic injuries. Anterior cruciate ligament (ACL) tears are one of the most common types of knee injury, especially in adolescent athletes.

Rising participation in sports has been associated with an increase in sports-related injury in young children (Table 26-3). It has been estimated that 3.5 million children age 14 years or younger have received medical treatment for a sports-related injury each year (Andrews, Baker, Bergfeld, & Nelson, 2010).

Manifestations and Diagnostic Evaluation

Manifestations of soft tissue injuries include pain, swelling, localized tenderness, limited range of motion, poor weight bearing, and a pop or snapping sound (sprain). The diagnosis is made on the basis of the clinical picture. A radiographic examination, however, may be ordered to rule out a fracture. An MRI or arthroscopy may be necessary to diagnose knee ligament tears.

Therapeutic Management

The primary goal in managing a soft tissue injury is to control swelling and prevent further injury. External pressure (compression) is most beneficial before edema has accumulated (Draper & Knight, 2010). Swelling can inhibit healing by keeping the ligament ends separated and increasing fibrous scarring. The earlier treatment is initiated, the less severe the swelling and immobility.

The injured area should be immediately wrapped with a compression bandage to support the joint and control the swelling. Ice should be applied to the injured area to reduce swelling for no longer than 20 minutes at a time. The effects of the ice can last as long as 5 to 6 hours, and ice should be used repeatedly for several days. Nonsteroidal antiinflammatory drugs (NSAIDs) help to alleviate pain and reduce inflammation.

For more severe soft tissue injuries, the child should avoid weight bearing for 3 days. Crutches may be necessary to ensure that the child does not bear weight. An *air cast,* which is a plastic, air-filled pressure cuff, may be used over the elastic wrap to support the joint and reduce swelling. The air cast or compression bandage should be worn for several weeks while the joint is healing. The child can begin stretching and isometric exercises to improve joint stability after the swelling and pain have diminished.

Immobilization of the injured joint and cold application are generally effective in the treatment of incomplete ligament tears. A complete rupture could require surgery to prevent excessive scar formation and long-term joint stability problems. Application of a cast or splint for 4 to 5 weeks may also be necessary, especially for knee injuries.

Nursing Considerations

One of the major nursing functions when assessing a sprain is to determine the severity of the injury. Assess the child for neurovascular impairment and for diminished range of motion. The initial examination may reveal localized tenderness over the injured joint, as well as limited joint mobility.

Analgesics, such as ibuprofen or acetaminophen, are appropriate for pain management. Distraction and age-appropriate play activities can be effective in helping children cope with pain.

The nurse needs to keep the extremity elevated at the level of the heart. This position enhances venous return and aids in reducing the swelling. Pillows placed beneath the extremity provide support and comfort. Support and immobilization devices should be snug but not

TABLE 26-3 SPORT-SPECIFIC INJURY RISK					
LOW	**LOW TO MODERATE**	**MODERATE**	**MODERATE TO HIGH**	**HIGH**	**VERY HIGH**
Swimming	Running	Ballet	Ice hockey	Cycling	Trampoline
Tennis	In-line skating	Baseball	Horseback riding	Diving	
	Strength training	Basketball	Skiing	American football	
		Gymnastics	Snowboarding	Skateboarding	
		Soccer		Wrestling	

Data from Staheli, L. T. (Ed.). (2008). *Fundamentals of pediatric orthopedics* (4th ed., pp. 90-92). Philadelphia: Wolters Kluwer Lippincott Williams & Wilkins.

tight. Assess neurovascular status before and after application of any splint, compression wrap, or cast.

For the child who has undergone surgery for any type of knee ligament reconstruction, immediate postoperative use of a cold compression cuff and a continuous passive motion (CPM) machine—a machine that continuously moves the knee joint in flexion and extension—will likely be used. Nursing measures involve regular emptying and refilling of the cuff to maintain the cold temperature. The nurse must also check the settings on the CPM machine to ensure that they match the ordered degree of flexion and extension. Pain control is most important.

Stretching and strengthening exercises are helpful in maintaining joint and muscle integrity. These exercises are done passively at first. As healing progresses, teach the child active stretching and strengthening exercises. The effectiveness of parent and family teaching should be evaluated by return demonstration. Physical therapy referrals may be helpful as well.

The amount of time needed for healing is determined by the severity of the injury. Weight bearing is gradually increased as the pain subsides. More severe injuries may require partial weight-bearing exercises, with full weight bearing introduced once the swelling has resolved. Activities may be restricted as directed by the health care provider.

Review the principles of rest, support, and the application of ice with the parents and child. If wraps, splints, or air casts are used, teach the parents and child how to assess neurovascular status. If crutches are required, review the principles of crutch walking with both the parents and the child. Make sure all family members understand activity and sports restrictions. Discuss follow-up appointments and the importance of adhering to activity restrictions until the injury has healed and the child has been cleared for participation in sports.

⚠ NURSING QUALITY ALERT

The Child with a Soft Tissue Injury

The first 6 to 12 hours after soft tissue injury are the most important in controlling swelling and reducing muscle damage. Treatment of soft tissue injuries is summarized in the acronyms *RICE* and *ICES*:

Rest	**I**ce
Ice	**C**ompression
Compression	**E**levation
Elevation	**S**upport

OSTEOMYELITIS

Osteomyelitis is a serious problem that can be difficult to diagnose and treat. It can result in high morbidity rates and mortality. Osteomyelitis is a bacterial infection of the bone that involves the cortex or marrow cavity. It is classified as *acute, subacute, chronic,* or *chronic recurrent multifocal* (TSRHC, 2008). Osteomyelitis is considered chronic if the infection persists longer than 1 month or does not respond to the initial antibiotic protocol.

Etiology

Bacteria infiltrate the bone through endogenous routes (e.g., skin or respiratory infections, abscessed teeth, acute otitis media) or exogenous routes (e.g., injury, surgical procedures). The infection is usually

the result of vascular spread of the bacteria. Osteomyelitis also may occur as a result of direct entry (open fracture), injury to surrounding soft tissues (cellulitis), external fixation devices, and skeletal traction.

The most common causative organism in all age-groups for osteomyelitis and septic arthritis is *Staphylococcus aureus* (TSRHC, 2008). There have been reported cases of community-acquired methicillin-resistant *S. aureus* osteomyelitis (Geist & Kuhn, 2009). *Streptococcus pyogenes, Haemophilus influenzae* (in unimmunized infants), *Kingella kingae, Escherichia coli,* and group B streptococci (in neonates) may also cause osteomyelitis. When the cause is trauma, the possible organisms include *Pseudomonas aeruginosa* and other organisms found in the soil. *Salmonella* is the most common causative organism for osteomyelitis in children with sickle cell anemia.

PATHOPHYSIOLOGY

Osteomyelitis

Osteomyelitis occurs most frequently in the metaphyseal region of the long bones, especially the femur or tibia. Bacteria enter the metaphysis by small capillaries, and the inflammatory process begins. A preceding trauma can cause rupture of these capillaries, providing a medium for bacterial growth. Pus forms, and because it cannot move from the metaphyseal area into a joint, it spreads toward the medullary canal as well as the cortex of the bone. Pus accumulates under the periosteum and displaces it, causing it to separate and form an abscess.

The underlying blood supply is interrupted, which causes necrotic tissue to form *(sequestrum).* New bone *(involucrum)* develops around the sequestrum, and the inflammatory process continues, causing further damage to surrounding bone tissue. Large sections of sequestrum may eventually become honeycombed with cavities or sinuses that contain infective material. These cavities are so effectively walled off that antibiotic therapy may not be successful. Thus, osteomyelitis may become chronic. Septic arthritis has the same basic pathophysiology, with the bacteria entering the joint.

Incidence

Osteomyelitis typically affects preschoolers (children younger than 6 years). Boys are affected more often than girls, possibly because of more risk-taking behavior that leads to minor trauma (Kaplan, 2011).

Manifestations

The manifestations of osteomyelitis in infants can be vague and nonspecific, such as fever, irritability, lethargy, and feeding difficulties. Some infants demonstrate signs of sepsis. In the older child, the major signs and symptoms include pain, warmth, erythema, and tenderness localized over the site of infection; favoring of the affected extremity; limited range of motion; and systemic manifestations such as fever and lethargy. Pain, usually localized, can radiate to adjacent areas of the body; radiating pain to an adjacent joint necessitates an assessment for possible septic arthritis (TSRHC, 2008).

Diagnostic Evaluation

Imaging studies such as radiography, ultrasonography, radionuclide bone scans, MRI, and CT scans diagnose and monitor the progress of osteomyelitis (TSRHC, 2008). Laboratory evidence of an infectious process, such as elevated ESR, elevated CRP level, and an elevated white blood cell count, is usually present. Blood culture may be positive for the infecting organism. The physician may choose to aspirate the affected area to obtain fluid for culture and sensitivity.

Therapeutic Management

Intravenous antibiotics are usually started based on the probable organism and changed as needed based on culture results. This makes obtaining the child's history a key component of planning the management of the case. Controversy exists regarding the length of time required for antibiotic therapy, the need for IV versus oral antibiotics, and the role of bactericidal antibiotics and therapeutic blood levels. Nevertheless, therapy for osteomyelitis generally requires high-dose parenteral therapy, preferably through a peripherally inserted central catheter (PICC). The organism involved dictates the type of antibiotic and the length of treatment.

Assessment of the child's response to the antibiotics is an integral part of the treatment protocol. Peak and trough serum antibiotic levels are closely monitored. Children receiving aminoglycosides should be periodically assessed for side effects such as ototoxicity and nephrotoxicity. Renal and hepatic function should be monitored and blood cell counts measured frequently to determine bone marrow activity.

Physical activities depend on the child's clinical condition and pain control. Surgical intervention may be necessary if an abscess is present or if the infection does not respond to antibiotics. Invasive procedures include draining the abscess, débriding necrotic tissue, and performing a sequestrectomy (removal of the sequestrum). Osteomyelitis of the proximal femur generally requires some type of surgical decompression because septic arthritis of the hip may accompany this infection.

NURSING CARE OF THE CHILD WITH OSTEOMYELITIS

■ Assessment

Because the organism is frequently transported through the bloodstream, a comprehensive history and physical, including dental history, is indicated. Although the recollection of every injury their child has experienced is difficult for parents, a thorough history of recent falls or traumas may be helpful. The nurse should carefully examine the affected area and note any pain, tenderness, erythema, or swelling. Note if the pain or swelling involves the joint, as this may indicate septic arthritis. Usually the child will appear to protect the extremity, even tensing adjacent muscles and demonstrating reluctance to straighten or move the extremity.

Document the child's neurovascular and pain status at least every 4 hours and more often if indicated. If the child is preverbal or not able to explain, the nurse should consult the parent. During the acute phase, the pain may be quite severe, and the nurse should assess the child's pain level and intervene before activities.

■ Nursing Diagnosis and Planning

The following nursing diagnoses and expected outcomes may be appropriate after assessment of the child with osteomyelitis:

- Acute Pain related to the infectious process.

Expected Outcome. The child will experience a decrease in pain, as evidenced by a decreased pain score on an appropriate pain assessment tool and increased function.

- Impaired Physical Mobility related to the pain.

Expected Outcomes. The child will exhibit full range of motion and participate in self-care.

- Risk for Injury related to complications of antibiotic therapy.

Expected Outcomes. The parenteral insertion site will remain patent and free from signs of infection. The parents will properly store and administer the ordered antibiotics, care for the insertion site, and dispose of IV equipment.

- Deficient Knowledge about home management of long-term antibiotic therapy related to unfamiliarity with the procedures.

Expected Outcomes. The parents will demonstrate the correct administration of antibiotics, verbalize reportable adverse effects, and identify any other concerns or issues regarding home care.

■ Interventions

■ Administering Intravenous Antibiotics. A long-term IV site for antibiotic administration must be maintained. Therefore, the nurse must carefully and frequently monitor the site for signs of complications (see Chapter 14) and flush the line according to protocol.

The nurse should have a thorough knowledge of the antibiotic being given. This includes calculating dosage on the basis of body weight or surface area, reviewing side effects and adverse effects, and determining if therapeutic blood levels are required. If the level of drug in the patient's blood exceeds the therapeutic range, the antibiotic should be withheld and the physician notified. Also notify the physician if the level is below the therapeutic level.

The child may receive multiple antibiotics. The nurse monitors compatibility and the total amount of fluids given. Allergies and any problems the child may have experienced during previous antibiotic administration should be evaluated. The nurse should periodically review current laboratory data to ensure adequate liver and kidney function. A complete blood cell count (CBC), CRP, and ESR should be measured on a regular basis to evaluate the child's response to treatment.

■ Providing Wound Care. Standard Precautions should be maintained at all times. Children with surgical wounds or drains need close monitoring. The color and consistency of the drainage and any unusual odor should be documented in the nurses' notes. A description of the wound should also be included.

■ Maintaining Nutritional Status. Meeting the child's nutritional needs is essential to facilitate growth and development and assist with the healing process. The child should receive a diet high in calories and protein. Frequent small meals and food that has been brought from home are helpful in stimulating the child's appetite.

■ Teaching Home Management. If the child is to receive IV antibiotic therapy at home, teach the parent how to set up the medication, how to maintain the intravenous line, and how to ensure that the infusion is being safely administered. Plan the teaching to fit the parent's schedule, and pay particular attention to signs of frustration or anxiety. Repetitive questions, poor eye contact, and nervous gestures are indicators that anxiety may be interfering with the parent's ability to retain information. Allow the parent to express feelings of concern and give positive feedback as the parent learns procedures. Before discharge, have the designated caregiver return demonstrate giving medications and catheter care. Make a home care referral to assist the family with the IV infusions.

Children who have had a favorable clinical response to IV antibiotics will occasionally be discharged with a course of oral antibiotics. Adherence to the medication regimen must be discussed with the parent. Emphasize the importance of follow-up care.

■ Promoting Optimal Development. Developmental issues need to be addressed by the nurse. Discuss age-appropriate activities that will maintain current developmental levels. If the child is to remain at home for antibiotic therapy, advise and arrange for tutoring as soon as possible. School-age children need to continue with their schoolwork and maintain contact with their friends. Resources available to home-bound children should be explored with the parent. If the child is exhibiting any residual fears or concerns related to hospitalization, therapeutic play activities may be needed.

■ Evaluation

- Is the peripheral intravenous insertion site free from redness or swelling, and does the antibiotic infuse well?
- Can the parent describe and demonstrate proper antibiotic administration, care of the intravenous catheter, and disposal of associated equipment?
- Does the child indicate decreased pain on an appropriate pain assessment scale?
- Can the child exhibit full range of motion?
- Does the child participate in self-care?
- Does the parent provide developmentally appropriate activities for the child?
- Does the child exhibit any signs of developmental regression?
- Can the parent demonstrate all procedures needed for home care?

SCOLIOSIS

Scoliosis is a lateral deviation, or curvature, of the spine, which is defined as a curvature greater than 10 degrees (Goldberg, Moore, Fogarty, & Dowling, 2008), as measured using a Cobb angle measurement, a technique for measuring the extent of a lateral curvature. In addition to the lateral curvature, there is an actual rotation of the vertebral bodies in the spine; therefore, this is a three-dimensional deformity (TSRHC, 2008). As a spinal curvature worsens, rotational structural deformities are seen in the vertebra and rib cage; severe rotational deformities can result in compromised respiratory function. There may also be distortion of the intrathoracic and abdominal

organs in severe deformity; however, this usually does not affect the function of these organs.

Classifications of scoliosis etiologies include congenital, syndromic, neuromuscular, and neural axis abnormalities; spinal tumors; thoracogenic (caused by a thoracotomy approach for surgical repair of an unrelated condition) (Table 26-4); and idiopathic. Idiopathic scoliosis can present at any point during a child's growth and is classified by age at presentation: *infantile* (birth to 3 years of age), *juvenile* (3 to 10 years of age), and *adolescent* (10 years or older).

Early-onset scoliosis (EOS), regardless of cause, occurs in infants and children up to 8 years of age. Children with EOS are at particular risk for *thoracic insufficiency syndrome*, which occurs when progressive rotation of the ribs or lack of thoracic growth (associated with congenital scoliosis) impairs growth of one or both lungs and interferes with respirations (TSRHC, 2008; Wick, Konze, Alexander, & Sweeney, 2009). Children with EOS must be followed frequently to assess any respiratory compromise. Both nonoperative management and operative management are options for these children, with the goals of management being to halt the progression of the curve, facilitate thoracic growth, and improve pulmonary function.

Adolescent Idiopathic Scoliosis (AIS)
Prevalance and Etiology

AIS is the most common type of scoliosis. Radiographic evidence of curves of at least 10 degrees establishes a prevalence of 1.5% to 3% in the general population (TSRHC, 2008). As curves get larger, the ratio of affected females to affected males increases. Females also have more progressive curves (Goldberg et al., 2008; TSRHC, 2008).

To date, there is no defined causative factor for idiopathic scoliosis: the most common research theories are related to central neurologic dysfunction, connective tissue abnormalities, and genetic factors (TSRHC, 2008). There has been evidence of a strong genetic tendency

TABLE 26-4 **CLASSIFICATIONS OF SCOLIOSIS**	
CLASSIFICATION	**CURVE**
Congenital	Deformity occurs during fetal development
	Present at birth
	May have associated organ anomalies
	Defect in vertebral formation and/or segmentation
	Progression is unpredictable
	Surgical management to halt progression
Syndromic	
Idiopathic type (Marfan, neurofibromatosis, osteogenesis imperfecta)	Idiopathic-like or congenital-like curve, depending on specific syndrome
Congenital type (VACTERL [VATER] syndrome, achondroplasia)	Managed with observation and a variety of nonoperative and operative approaches
Neuromuscular	Long, sweeping curve, usually involves whole spine
	Managed with observation, bracing, or fusion using laminar wires (not hooks and screws)
Neural axis abnormalities (syringomyelia [syrinx], tethered cord, diastomatomyelia)	Idiopathic-like curve
	Managed with a variety of nonoperative and operative approaches
Thoracogenic (related to a thoracotomy approach to repair an unrelated diagnosis)	Idiopathic-like curve
	Managed with a variety of nonoperative and operative approaches
Postlaminectomy (typically for tumor removal or trauma) or postirradiation	Curve usually localized to immediate area of laminectomy, but may develop compensatory curve
	Kyphotic deformity more common
	Managed with a variety of nonoperative and operative approaches

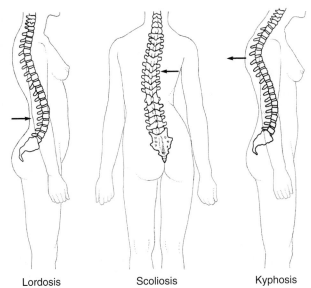

Lordosis   Scoliosis   Kyphosis

FIG 26-5 Most spinal abnormalities in children are abnormal curvatures. In *scoliosis,* the spine curves laterally and the vertebrae rotate, pulling the ribs along. *Kyphosis* is a front-to-back rounding, usually of the thoracic spine; it is often accompanied by scoliosis. *Lordosis* is an exaggerated concave curvature of the spine, usually in the lumbar area.

toward idiopathic scoliosis in some families, as well as apparent autosomal dominant inheritance of adolescent idiopathic scoliosis and linkage between several chromosomes (Wise, Gao, Shoemaker, et al., 2008).

Manifestations

The clinical manifestations of scoliosis include a visible curvature of the spine (Figure 26-5). Other manifestations that may be present are a rib hump when the child is bending forward, asymmetric rib cage, uneven shoulder or pelvic heights, prominence of the scapula, or hip and leg length discrepancy. A difference in the space between the arms and the trunk may be visible when the child is standing. Complaints of back pain are considered atypical and would require a careful history and physical examination by the orthopedist. Impairment of respiratory function is also uncommon, as most patients are treated surgically before the curve progresses to a magnitude that would impair function.

Diagnostic Evaluation

School Screening. The American Academy of Orthopaedic Surgeons (AAOS), the Scoliosis Research Society (SRS), the Pediatric Orthopaedic Society of North America (POSNA), and the AAP recognize the benefit of school screening as a means for earlier detection of scoliosis (SRS, 2010). They recommend that girls be screened twice, at 10 and 12 years of age (grades 5 and 7), and boys once, at age 13 or 14 (grades 8 or 9). Screening should always include the forward bending test, also known as an Adams forward bend test (see Chapter 9). A scoliometer, a small level-type device, may be used during the forward bend test to provide an angle of any vertebral rotation. Referral to an orthopedic surgeon is recommended for scoliometer readings of 7 or greater, indicating a 7-degree angle of trunk rotation. Because no single test is completely reliable for screening, a screening protocol should

also include assessment of shoulder asymmetry, unequal scapular prominence, hip prominence or asymmetry, and head not being centered over the pelvis (see Figure 26-5) (Fong, Lee, Cheung et al., 2010; TSRHC, 2008). If asymmetry is detected, the parents should be informed, and orthopedic referral is recommended.

Physical Examination. The orthopedist will need to view the entire back as well as the shoulders and iliac crests. To preserve the adolescent's modesty, a swimsuit or an examination gown is worn. The examination includes observing the shoulders and iliac crests for presence of asymmetry, flank creases, rib hump, waist asymmetry, limb length discrepancy, and whether the head and/or trunk are centered over the middle of the pelvis. The patient is also assessed from the side to appreciate any decrease or increase in the natural curvature of the sagittal plane of the spine. A basic neurologic examination of strength and reflexes of the extremities will be performed. The patient's abdominal reflexes are assessed to rule out a neurologic cause of the scoliosis (idiopathic patients respond the same on both sides of the abdomen).

Spinal deformity progression is driven by growth; therefore, indicators of skeletal maturity are important factors in analyzing a patient with AIS. For girls, menarche is a crucial indicator; a premenarchal girl is still actively growing, whereas a postmenarchal girl is in the decelerated process of growth and therefore has a lessened chance of curvature progression. The sexual maturity of the patient is assessed by the Tanner system, which classifies breast and pubic hair development (see Chapter 8).

Radiographs. Plain radiographs will be obtained with a coronal and sagittal view, from the head down to the mid-thigh (Figure 26-6). There may be only a single curvature, or a main curvature with secondary or even tertiary curvatures surrounding it. These secondary curves may be structural or compensatory (meaning not a true manifestation of the disease but the body's response in trying to get the head level over the pelvis).

The orthopedist measures the degree of scoliosis seen on the radiographs using the Cobb angle technique. Cobb angle measurements are obtained for all curvatures shown on radiographs in both the coronal and sagittal views. Because scoliosis is a three-dimensional deformity, the amount of vertebral rotation as well as indicators of spinal balance are also assessed on the radiographs.

Radiographs are also examined for signs of skeletal maturity and growth status. An indicator called the Risser sign (grades 1 to 5) can assist with assessing the level of peak height velocity (PHV) (see Chapter 8), and this can determine the probability of whether or not the curve will progress (Nault, Parent, Phan et al., 2010). In general, after skeletal maturity, the rate of curve progression is significantly reduced. Curvature size is also useful in predicting progression, as larger curves have a greater chance of progressing (Tan, Moe, Vaithinathan, & Wong, 2009).

Treatment

Nonsurgical Interventions. Curves less than 25 degrees require observation for progression regardless of skeletal maturity (TSRHC, 2008). Patients closer to 25 degrees who are skeletally immature will require more frequent radiographic observation than a patient with a smaller curvature who is skeletally mature. Progression is defined as a 7- to 10-degree increase in the Cobb angle.

Brace treatment is recommended for patients who present or progress in curve magnitude at 25 degrees or more and are still skeletally immature. The goal of treatment is to prevent further progression; this is accomplished by pads in the brace that push on the curve. Each brace is custom made for the individual patient curve(s) by an orthotist

Video—Spine for Alignment

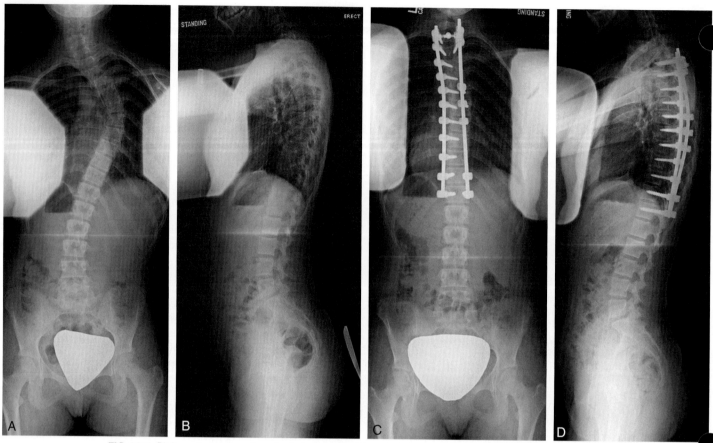

FIG 26-6 Plain radiographs of scoliosis before **(A, B)** and after spinal fusion **(C, D).** (Courtesy Texas Scottish Rite Hospital for Children, Dallas, TX.)

(Figure 26-7). Patients with a lumbar curve typically wear a nighttime-only brace. Other curve patterns require a brace be worn 22 to 23 hours a day. Patients are told to wear a form-fitting T-shirt underneath the brace in order to reduce skin breakdown and irritation. The more adherent the patient is to wearing the brace, the more effective the brace is in preventing progression of the curve (Katz, Herring, Browne et al., 2010).

Radiographs are typically obtained every 4 months during rapid growth, and extended to every 6 months as the patient reaches maturity. The patient is told to not wear the brace the night before the visit to see how the curve is responding. As the patient is growing, adjustments may be needed to the brace, or a new brace may be required. For girls, brace wear is discontinued after the patient is 18 to 24 months postmenarchal, has a Risser grade that suggests near skeletal maturity, and has had no further increase in standing height. For boys, discontinuation is recommended after Risser grade of 5, which is typically in the later teenage years.

Surgical Intervention. Surgery is considered for curvature(s) that reach 40 to 50 degrees. The primary goal is to reduce the size of the curve(s) and obtain a solid fusion of the treated part of the spine. A successful surgery may not completely correct the curvature but will provide the patient with a well-balanced spine that centers the patient's head, shoulders, and trunk over the pelvis (TSRHC, 2008).

Typically, the surgical approach is posterior down the length of the spine to be fused. An anterior approach may be considered for a large, stiff curve; young age; or a curvature limited to the lumbar spine. In a posterior approach, implants, either hooks or screws, are placed on or in the vertebral body. These implants are then attached to two rods that are used to correct the deformity. To achieve a solid fusion of the corrected curvature, additional bone is needed to graft the fixed portion of the spine. Bone graft may be from the patient (autograft). Common graft donor sites are parts of the vertebral body that is removed during surgery, the iliac crest, or ribs. Allograft, frozen bank-stored bone, is becoming increasingly popular as it has proven to be safe, efficacious, and cost effective (Betz, Lavelle, & Samdani, 2010). Bone morphogenetic protein (BMP) is an additive that may be used to speed up and further solidify the fusion.

Surgical Complications. Significant blood loss is common with spinal fusion surgery because of the vascular nature of the vertebrae and spinal canal. Several methods are used to reduce the need for donor blood transfusion intraoperatively; these include preoperative autologous blood donation (children donate their own blood before surgery), controlled hypotensive anesthesia, hemodilution, cell salvage of lost blood, or use of antifibrinolytic agents (aprotinin or Amicar). Clinical indicators, not just hemoglobin values, trigger the decision to transfuse (TSRHC, 2008).

A potential complication of surgical correction can be insult or injury to the spinal cord. Intraoperative neuromonitoring (IONM) of motor and sensory function, with immediate corrective actions by the surgeon or the anesthetist should the changes be severe (Kundnani, Zhu, Tak, & Wong, 2010), can reduce the chance of neurologic injury during surgery.

Other complications include lack of solid bone fusion (pseudoarthrosis), implant failure (which may include rod breakage, or pullout of a hook or screw), continued progression of the deformity, and infection (Carreon, Puno, Lenke et al., 2007). Some infections require only a round of oral antibiotics, whereas others may be extensive and require irrigation, débridement, and total implant removal.

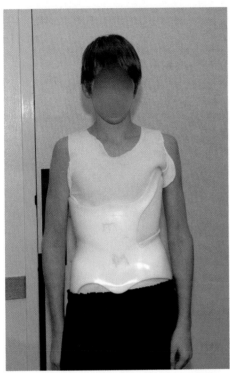

FIG 26-7 Adolescent with scoliosis brace. (Courtesy Texas Scottish Rite Hospital for Children, Dallas, TX.)

Postoperative Management. Postoperative pain management is typically treated by either a patient-controlled analgesia (PCA) pump or epidural analgesia (Milbrandt, Singhal, Minter et al., 2009). These methods of pain management are usually used up to postoperative day 2 or 3, and then the patient is switched to an oral method of pain control. Patients are up in a chair on postoperative day 2 and typically go home by day 4 or 5.

Follow-Up Care. Patients return to the clinic within 1 to 6 weeks, depending on surgeon preference, and are usually followed for 2 or more years postoperatively or until reaching 18 years of age. Most patients return to school after 2 weeks. Patients are released to full activity between 6 months and 1 year postoperatively. Every patient is instructed to avoid tattoos and piercings. Although controversial, some surgeons will also require their patients to have prophylactic antibiotics before dental procedures to reduce the chance of infection (TSRHC, 2008).

KYPHOSIS

Kyphosis is the natural curvature of the thoracic spine in the sagittal plane (see Figure 26-5), although kyphosis can occur in other areas of the spine. Normally, kyphosis ranges between 20 and 45 degrees by Cobb angle measurement. Hyperkyphosis is any angle above 45 degrees. Postural kyphosis is benign and can be corrected by proper posture techniques (actively contracting the erector spinae muscles and tightening the abdominal muscles) (TSRHC, 2008). Typically this is resolved if the patient follows a core muscle strengthening program.

Scheuermann's Kyphosis

Scheuermann's disease is the most common cause of hyperkyphosis in adolescents (TSRHC, 2008). Scheuermann's disease is a fixed angular kyphosis with a characteristic wedging of the anterior vertebra at the apex of the curve (middle). Incidence is reported anywhere from 0.4%

⊚ NURSING CARE PLAN

The Adolescent Undergoing a Spinal Fusion

Focused Assessment

Preoperative Assessment

- Assess anxiety related to surgery, hospitalization, and postsurgical issues (e.g., pain, appearance of the operative site, activity limitations, and altered appearance)

Postoperative Assessment

- Meticulously assess the neurologic status of the lower extremities
- Assess pain, fluid balance, bleeding, and return of bowel function
- Assess and document wound healing, ease of mobility, and nutritional status
- Focus on respiratory assessment if the anterior/thoracic approach has been used and the adolescent has a chest tube
- Determine discharge teaching needs and parent or adolescent understanding of follow-up care

Planning

Nursing Diagnosis

Anxiety (preoperative) related to impending surgery.

Expected Outcome

The adolescent will have reduced anxiety, as evidenced by seeking information about the surgery and postoperative care and by identifying and using effective coping mechanisms to address it.

Intervention/Rationale

1. Determine whether the adolescent is anxious about surgery.
   The adolescent may not be anxious or may be hiding anxiety.
2. Initiate a conversation with the adolescent about what anxiety feels like and how anxiety is a normal response to anticipated surgery.
   The adolescent may need permission to discuss anxiety and may require assistance verbalizing feelings. Adolescents need to be assured that they are normal.
   For example,
   "Many girls facing surgery are nervous about what it will be like to have this operation. Perhaps you would like to know more about what it will be like."
3. Assist the adolescent with identifying positive and effective means for resolving anxiety (e.g., talking with a friend, exercising or engaging in other activities, practicing relaxation techniques).
   By role modeling for the adolescent and discussing various possibilities for coping, the nurse allows the adolescent to find a comfortable means for expressing feelings.
4. Identify and discourage negative behaviors associated with anxiety (e.g., verbal outbursts, physical aggression, withdrawal).
   The adolescent needs to understand that expressing feelings can be done in acceptable and unacceptable ways.

Continued

◎ NURSING CARE PLAN

The Adolescent Undergoing a Spinal Fusion—cont'd

Intervention/*Rationale*—cont'd

Try telling the adolescent,

💬 "It's OK and normal to be anxious about surgery. This is hard for your parents, too. Let's talk about ways you might let your parents know how you are feeling."

5. Reassure the adolescent about specific fears ("Can my parents be with me?" "Will I get a shot?" "Will I have a huge scar?").

   Reassurance and conversation may help resolve some fears.

6. Determine the adolescent's need for specific information, particularly about postoperative care. Explain the reason for the various postoperative interventions:

   a. Neurovascular checks every 2 hours for the first 48 hours and every 4 hours thereafter

   b. Turning by log-rolling every 2 hours

   c. Deep breathing and use of incentive spirometer (chest tube if anterior approach is used)

   d. Wound dressing (if applicable)

   e. Brace application and skin care

   Fears about the unknown may be reduced by increasing knowledge. Adolescents are more cooperative in the postoperative period if they know the reason for interventions.

7. Have the adolescent (or parents and adolescent) demonstrate specific skills (e.g., coughing, recumbent log-rolling).

   Allows the nurse to evaluate learning and allows the adolescent to gain confidence in being able to perform the maneuver; confidence in managing care decreases anxiety.

8. Encourage the adolescent to ask questions and discuss concerns. Correct any inaccurate information.

   Clarification of misperceptions decreases anxiety.

Evaluation

Does the adolescent seek information about the surgery and its postoperative course?

Is the adolescent able to talk about anxiety or fears with parents, friends, or the nurse?

Can the adolescent use appropriate techniques to reduce anxiety?

Planning

Nursing Diagnosis

Acute Pain related to the operative procedure.

Expected Outcomes

The adolescent will indicate decreasing amounts of pain as measured on a pain scale, appear calm and relaxed, and participate in postoperative activities.

Intervention/*Rationale*

1. Frequently monitor the adolescent's pain level by using an appropriate pain rating scale in the postoperative period. (Statements of pain, anxiety, an inability to cough, hyperalertness, reluctance or refusal to move, and sweating may indicate pain.)

   Adolescents may be unable or unwilling to verbalize their pain.

2. Provide prescribed analgesics in a timely manner (children usually receive epidural analgesia or patient-controlled analgesia [PCA] initially after surgery).

   The appropriate and timely use of analgesics provides optimal control of pain. Epidural analgesia provides more constant pain relief and prevents peaks and valleys of pain. Oral analgesics should be given on an around-the-clock schedule to avoid peaks and valleys of pain control from prolonged onset and peak of action.

3. Determine response to pain-relief measures and communicate with the physician about possible adjustments if needed. (See Chapter 15 for a thorough discussion of the nursing care of children and teenagers in pain.)

   Adjustments may be necessary to achieve optimal pain relief.

Evaluation

Can the adolescent use a pain scale to rate pain?

Does the adolescent appear calm and relaxed?

Is the adolescent able to participate in postoperative activities?

Planning

Nursing Diagnosis

Knowledge Deficit related to unfamiliarity with information about spinal fusion and postoperative management at home.

Expected Outcome

The family and adolescent will successfully manage treatment at home, as evidenced by demonstrating procedures, accessing appropriate community resources, and keeping follow-up appointments.

Intervention/*Rationale*

1. Teach the family and adolescent the correct technique for wound care and the signs of wound infection (redness, swelling, drainage, fever); emphasize the role of a well-balanced diet in wound healing.

   Proper wound care and good nutrition promote healing and decrease the chance of infection.

2. Have the adolescent (or parents) demonstrate specific skills (e.g., brace application, skin care, daily exercises, performing activities without bending at the waist).

   Allows the nurse to evaluate learning and encourages the adolescent to gain confidence in the ability to perform the appropriate skills.

3. Discuss home care:

   a. Activity restrictions. (Initially these adolescents will be restricted from participating in sports or gym or lifting more than 10 lb.)

   b. Be alert for signs such as skin breakdown, pain, numbness or tingling in the extremities, and other potential problems.

   Home care instructions reduce the possibility of complications. Activity restrictions are usually maintained for 6 to 9 months depending on the type of surgery and the physician.

4. Provide the name and telephone number of an easily accessible health care provider if questions arise at home. Inform the family about community resources available, including resources for tutoring. Referral to national scoliosis associations (see Evolve website) may be helpful. Schedule a follow-up appointment and emphasize the importance of keeping appointments.

   Access to a health care provider and/or community resources decreases anxiety and improves adherence to treatment. Periodic evaluation is important to recovery.

Evaluation

Can the family demonstrate the procedures necessary to care for the adolescent at home?

Can the adolescent and family demonstrate correct application of the brace (if required), proper wound and skin care, or prescribed exercise regimen?

Is the family aware of sources of help if needed?

Does the family keep follow-up appointments?

to 10% of adolescents between 10 and 14 years of age. There is no defined etiology for the disease.

Patients may complain of pain at the apex of the deformity as well as pain at the base of the neck. The kyphotic apex becomes apparent on an Adams forward bend test. Most patients are given a core strengthening program and need no further intervention, as the natural history of this disease is relatively benign. They may be observed clinically and radiographically on an annual basis.

For patients with a progressive kyphosis and an apex located in the thoracic area, bracing may be advised. However, correction gains made during bracing disappear when bracing is discontinued (TSRHC, 2008). Surgical treatment of Scheuermann's disease is only for patients with documented pain in a rigid curve of more than 70 degrees and a poor sagittal contour clinically. The goal of surgery is to provide a well-balanced spine in the sagittal plane. Typically a posterior spinal fusion is performed in a similar manner to that of an AIS patient. Intraoperative neuromonitoring is key, as the hyperkyphosis presents a more stretched spinal cord than in scoliosis and can increase the risk for spinal cord injury. Potential complications, postoperative care, and follow-up are the same as those defined in operative treatment of AIS (Coe, Smith, Berven et al., 2010).

Other Causes of Hyperkyphosis

Any of the etiologies that have been listed as causing scoliosis can also cause hyperkyphosis. Typically idiopathic-like syndromes, neuromuscular, and neural-axis abnormalities will produce a more global hyperkyphosis, meaning all the thoracic spine and possibly some of the lumbar is involved (TSRHC, 2008). Congenital, postlaminectomy, tubercular, or postirradiation as contributing factors produce a more localized or angular kyphosis, meaning that two to five levels are involved and this can be present in any portion of the spine. In global deformities, surgical intervention will depend on curvature size and amount of growth left in the spine. In angular deformities, surgical intervention is warranted if the curvature is compressing or stretching the spinal cord and causing neurologic symptoms.

LIMB DIFFERENCES

Limb differences are common in children. Most alterations of arms and legs are mild variations of normal posturing. Education and reassurance are the primary nursing interventions for patients with limb differences.

Etiology and Incidence

Limb differences may be physiologic, congenital birth anomalies, or the result of trauma, infection, or radiation. These differences take many forms, including webbing (syndactyly) or extra digits (fingers or toes; polydactyly); genu valgum ("knock-knees") and genu varum (bowlegs); limb length differences; and congenital absence of all or part of an extremity.

Diagnostic Evaluation

Most congenital defects are readily apparent at birth. Mild defects and deformities that develop over time are usually identified by parents or school nurses and are evaluated by specialized clinicians. Radiographs may be necessary to evaluate limb defects fully and assist with developing a treatment plan.

Therapeutic Management and Nursing Considerations

The management and nursing care of children with limb differences is related to the type of difference the child is manifesting.

Femoral Anteversion (Intoeing)

Femoral anteversion is defined by the angle of the femoral neck in relation to the femoral shaft in the coronal plane (TSRHC, 2008). The degree of anteversion is greatest in infancy and gradually decreases as the child approaches skeletal maturity. Femoral anteversion is more prevalent in girls (Jacquemier, Glard, Pomero et al., 2008). An intoeing gait may be noticed when a child first begins to walk. Referral to an orthopedist is unnecessary because most children with femoral anteversion gradually outgrow their intoeing gait (Blackmur & Murray, 2010; TSRHC, 2008). A priority in managing a child who toes in is careful education of the parents (Fabry, 2010a; TSRHC, 2008). Explain that intoeing is a common problem that usually self-corrects. Exercises, braces, modifications of sitting posture, or parental interventions are unnecessary. There are no known serious consequences from having excessive anteversion.

Tibial Torsion

Intoeing and outtoeing may be due to deviations of the rotational alignment of the femur or tibia (TSRHC, 2008). Up to 3 or 4 years of age, tibial torsion is the most common cause of intoeing and outtoeing. This condition is benign. Orthotic management is generally considered unattractive and ineffective. Therefore, observation and parental education are the main forms of tibial torsion treatment.

Genu Varum (Bowlegs)

Genu varum (Figure 26-8) is an extremely common pediatric deformity (TSRHC, 2008). Newborns' legs are typically bowed. The bowing may appear more prominent with weight bearing and often appears to involve both the tibia and femur. Physiologic genu varum spontaneously resolves around 2 years of age. Reevaluation is appropriate if the varus persists beyond 2 years of age or progresses. Determining whether the condition represents physiologic genu varum or a pathologic process, such as rickets, is crucial because the prognosis and treatment differ profoundly.

Tibia Vara (Blount Disease)

Tibia vara is defined as growth retardation at the medial aspect of the tibial epiphysis. Progressive or persistent bowing of the legs results (Jones, Gill, John et al., 2009; Sabharwal, 2009). The infantile form has an onset before the child's third birthday, and the adolescent form has an onset at age 10 years or older (Gilbody, Thomas, & Ho, 2009; Sabharwal, 2009; TSRHC, 2008).

Infantile tibia vara is more common in children of Afro-Caribbean and Scandinavian descent (Sabharwal, 2009). The child with infantile tibia vara appears similar to a child with physiologic genu varum, but there are two major differences (TSRHC, 2008). First, patients with infantile tibia vara exceed the 95th percentile for weight. Obesity is not the cause for tibia vara; however, the two conditions are often related. Weight management will not treat tibia vara. Second, patients with infantile tibia vara often have a clinically apparent lateral thrust to the knee during the stance phase of gait that resembles a limp.

Untreated true infantile tibia vara generally results in a progressive varus deformity, producing joint deformity and growth retardation. Orthotic treatment is recommended and is successful in more than 50% of cases for children with early-stage unilateral Blount disease (TSRHC, 2008). Brace therapy is usually not effective for children older than 3 years, those with bilateral involvement, and those over the 90th percentile for weight (Sabharwal, 2009; TSRHC, 2008). If correction is not achieved by the time the patient is 3 years old, surgical intervention may be recommended. Surgical osteotomy may be performed to straighten the leg.

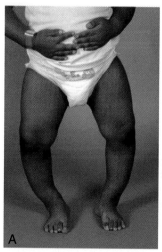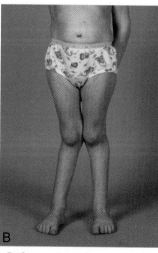

FIG 26-8 **A,** Genu varum (bowlegs). **B,** Genu valgum (knock-knees). In the child with genu varum, or bowlegs, a persistent space is present between the knees when the ankles are together. Genu varum is a normal finding for 1 year after the child begins walking. In the child with genu valgum, or knock-knees, a space is present between the ankles when the knees are together. To remember the terminology, liken the r's and g's: genu va*r*um—knees apa*r*t; genu val*g*um—knees to*g*ether. (Photos courtesy Texas Scottish Rite Hospital for Children, Dallas, TX.)

Treatment of the adolescent form of Blount disease is predominantly surgical (TSRHC, 2008). The goal of surgical treatment is to restore normal physeal growth and prevent degenerative arthritis of the knee. Surgical options include osteotomy (the most common approach), lateral *epiphysiodesis* (surgical manipulation of the growth plate to arrest growth), and gradual realignment with an external fixator. Lateral epiphysiodesis slows the growth on the outside of the leg, thus allowing the inner side of the growth plate to continue growing. It provides satisfactory correction of malalignment 50% to 87% of the time (TSRHC, 2008). External fixation can also be used to gradually align an extremity (Gilbody et al., 2009; Jones et al., 2009; Sabharwal, 2009; TSRHC, 2008). Using an external device includes cutting the bone during surgery and applying an external device. The treatment period is prolonged, and ability to adhere to postoperative care requirements should be considered before surgery.

Genu Valgum (Knock-Knees)

Children between 2 and 8 years of age normally have valgus alignment of the lower extremities, with the maximum amount of physiologic valgus occurring between the ages of 2 and 4 years (TSRHC, 2008). If the deformity persists or increases after 8 years of age, referral is indicated (Fabry, 2010a). Correction also may be indicated when there is gait disturbance, difficulty running, or knee discomfort (TSRHC, 2008). Hemiepiphysiodesis, or slowing the growth on the inside of the growth area, may be considered. This procedure must be done at the appropriate time in the child's growth to avoid overcorrection that would leave the child bowlegged.

Leg Length Discrepancy

Another frequent parental concern is children's leg length inequality (TSRHC, 2008). Asymptomatic leg length inequality is relatively common. Causes may be congenital or acquired. Treatment ranges from no treatment to extensive multistage reconstruction, or even limb ablation and prosthetic fitting. Treatment depends on the severity of the inequality and the function of the limb.

Generally, leg length inequality of 2 to 2.5 cm in someone who is skeletally mature does not require treatment. In theory, any leg length inequality could be managed by placing an appropriate-size lift in a shoe or attaching it to the shoe sole. Shoe lifts are considered when the child starts to walk up on the toes. Toe walking leads to faster fatigue. Using a shoe lift may allow the child to walk longer distances without fatigue. There is little evidence to support the presumption that the use of a shoe lift provides any short- or long-term protective or mechanical benefits.

For leg length differences greater than 2.5 cm, surgical interventions are considered. These include epiphysiodesis on the longer leg in the growing child, or, in a skeletally mature child, femoral shortening. Shortening of the femur is a major procedure requiring internal fixation. Leg lengthening procedures are even more extensive. An expected limb length inequality of 4 cm can be considered a relative indication for a leg lengthening procedure; however, because of potential complications of limb lengthening, there are no absolute indications for a leg lengthening procedure. It is important to counsel the family and child before any lengthening treatment.

Osteochondritis Dissecans

Osteochondritis dissecans of the knee is characterized by cartilage and bone along the femoral articular surface that may be softened, loose, or separated from the rest of the femoral condyle (TSRHC, 2008). The child or adolescent commonly complains of nonspecific knee pain and may report parapatellar aching that is aggravated by sports participation and vigorous activities.

Initial treatment is observation, with enough activity restrictions to allow the symptoms to resolve (TSRHC, 2008). Most stable lesions will spontaneously heal over several months. If symptoms persist, a short period of immobilization in a cast or brace may be tried. Gradual return to activities is allowed after 4 to 6 weeks. If nonoperative treatment fails or symptoms and studies indicate an unstable lesion, arthroscopy is indicated.

Osgood-Schlatter Disease

The classic picture of Osgood-Schlatter disease is bilateral knee pain that is exacerbated by running, jumping, or climbing stairs in the growing child. The child will point to the tibial tubercle as the site of pain, and swelling may be noticed (TSRHC, 2008). Osgood-Schlatter disease is usually seen in adolescents and is more common in boys. Both knees are usually involved. During the adolescent growth spurt, overuse trauma causes inflammation in the tibial tubercle at the tendon insertion site, resulting in tendonitis of the distal infrapatellar tendon. Diagnosis is made based on the clinical and radiographic examination. Treatment is conservative because the disorder is usually self-limiting. Reassure the child and parents that activity can be done to tolerable discomfort, because this is not a progressive or crippling disease. In severe cases, NSAIDs and the use of a knee immobilizer for a few weeks may be helpful. Osgood-Schlatter resolves with skeletal maturity.

DEVELOPMENTAL DYSPLASIA OF THE HIP

Developmental dysplasia of the hip (DDH) describes a variety of disorders that present in different forms at different ages. Dysplasia varies in severity from quite mild to severe dislocation. DDH can be present at birth (congenital), but in some children it develops after birth—hence the term *developmental.*

Etiology and Incidence

The exact cause of DDH is unknown, but genetic factors may play a role (Fan, Shi, & Jiang, 2009). Risk factors include being the first-born child, being female, breech position, and low levels of amniotic fluid in utero (Fabry, 2010b; Stevenson, Mineau, Kerber et al., 2009). Estimates of the incidence of hip instability in the newborn have ranged from as low as 1 per 1000 to a high of 3.4 per 100 births (Stevenson et al., 2009; Walton, Isaacson, McMillan et al., 2010). Higher incidences are reported when screening uses both clinical examination and ultrasonography. There is also distinct geographic and racial variation in the incidence of DDH. Children of African or Chinese descent have a low incidence of DDH, whereas other groups, including Native American children, have a high incidence. One or both hips may be involved.

Manifestations

The symptoms of DDH vary according to age. In neonates, it is characterized by instability of the hip; the femoral head can be displaced partially (subluxated) or fully (dislocated) from the acetabulum by the examiner. The hip may also rest in a dislocated position and be reduced on examination. This can be detected by performing the Ortolani and Barlow tests (Figure 26-9) or by observing significant changes in the morphology of the hip on sonograms.

Infants beyond the newborn period exhibit asymmetry of the gluteal skinfolds when lying with the legs extended against the examining table (or when the infant is held upright with the legs dangling). The affected hip has a limited range of motion, and asymmetric abduction is present when the child is placed supine with the knees and hips flexed. The femur on the affected side appears to be shorter than the other side. The symptoms range from lax ligaments to contractures and stiffness in the affected hip joint or joints.

Any abnormalities in an older child's gait need to be carefully evaluated as possible signs of the condition. Walking children may exhibit limping, toe-walking, or a waddling gait. Bilateral dysplasia is always more difficult to identify than unilateral dysplasia because no normal hip can be used for comparison.

Diagnostic Evaluation

The diagnosis of DDH in the neonate can be difficult to make because the signs and symptoms may be quite subtle. A well-trained nurse or physician screens for DDH at birth and during each routine infant well-child visit by carefully performing the Barlow and Ortolani tests.

An ultrasound of the hip is used to confirm DDH in infants. Ultrasonography shows the soft tissue anatomy of the hip and the relationship of the femoral head and acetabulum (Krul, van der Wouden, Schellevis et al., 2010; Mootha, Saini, Dhillon et al., 2010). Current research supports the concept that ultrasonography is a more sensitive indicator of abnormalities of the infant hip than radiography. However, some authors argue that ultrasonography may be too sensitive and results in overtreatment of hips that would otherwise develop normally.

Plain radiography of the pelvis usually demonstrates a frankly dislocated hip in individuals of any age, but because ossification is not complete in infancy, radiographs may only be diagnostic after 1 year of age. Parents may be concerned about radiation exposure in the course of treating their child's DDH. Reassure them that the increase in carcinogenic risks from the cumulative radiographs taken to manage an average patient with DDH is less than 1% (Bone & Hsieh, 2000). Computed tomography (CT) and magnetic resonance imaging (MRI) are sometimes used in complex cases.

Therapeutic Management

Early diagnosis and treatment of DDH is important to maximize the likelihood of a successful outcome. Treatment depends on the age of the child at the time of diagnosis and on the severity of the dysplasia. The primary goal of treatment in DDH, regardless of age, is to facilitate normal development of the hip socket. This is accomplished through approaches that provide anatomic reduction of the hip and maintenance of the reduction. In newborns and infants younger than 6 months, the treatment of choice for a hip that is dislocated and can be reduced by the examiner is a Pavlik harness. The Pavlik harness maintains the hips in flexion, abduction, and external rotation. The Pavlik harness consists of chest and shoulder straps and foot stirrups

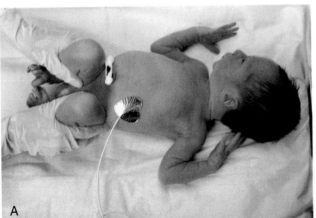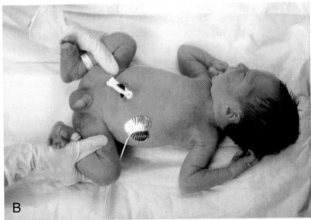

FIG 26-9 Assessment of the hips. Place the fingers over the infant's greater trochanter and thumbs over the femur. Flex the knees and hips. **A,** Barlow test: adduct the hips and apply gentle pressure down and back with the thumbs. In hip dysplasia, the examiner can feel the femoral head move out of the acetabulum. **B,** Ortolani test: abduct the thighs and apply gentle pressure forward over the greater trochanter. A "clunking" sensation indicates a dislocated femoral head moving into the acetabulum. A hip click may be felt or heard, but is usually normal.

PATHOPHYSIOLOGY

Developmental Dysplasia of the Hip

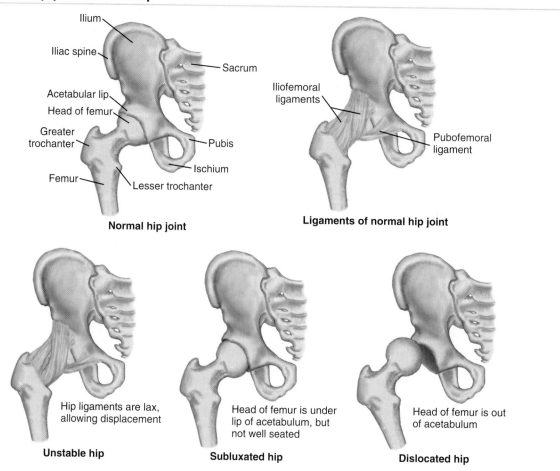

Normal hip joint

Ilium
Iliac spine
Sacrum
Acetabular lip
Head of femur
Greater trochanter
Pubis
Ischium
Femur
Lesser trochanter

Ligaments of normal hip joint

Iliofemoral ligaments
Pubofemoral ligament

Hip ligaments are lax, allowing displacement

Unstable hip

Head of femur is under lip of acetabulum, but not well seated

Subluxated hip

Head of femur is out of acetabulum

Dislocated hip

In the normal infant hip, the head of the femur is well seated in the acetabulum (hip socket) and is stable. Developmental dysplasia of the hip occurs in varying degrees, ranging from instability of the hip joint to frank dislocation, defined as the following:

- *Instability of the hip* is the appropriate term when the head of the femur is located in the acetabulum but may be subluxated (partially dislocated) or even dislocated with manual manipulation.
- *Dislocation of the hip* occurs when the head of the femur lies outside the acetabulum. It can occur as a late stage of developmental dysplasia of the hip, or it can occur in children with certain neuromuscular disorders.
- *Subluxation of the hip* occurs when the head of the femur is positioned under the edge of the acetabulum. It is not well seated in the acetabulum, yet neither is it completely dislocated.

Interestingly, many unstable hips spontaneously resolve. If untreated, only approximately 20% will settle into a dislocated position.

(Figure 26-10). Initially, the harness is worn continuously. This bracing method may be the only treatment necessary to allow the hip to mold and grow normally, promoting development of a functional hip socket and a well-formed femoral head. Hips that remain unstable become progressively deformed as the skeleton matures, resulting in functional disability.

Parents must be taught the proper use of the harness because improper positioning of the infant's hip can cause interruption of the blood supply to the head of the femur, resulting in *avascular necrosis* (tissue damage caused by an inadequate blood supply) or femoral palsy. Teach parents to observe for equal leg extension in and out of the harness. In addition, skin care; techniques for holding, feeding, and diapering; and the importance of vigilant follow-up must be emphasized.

Treatment is more complicated when the condition is diagnosed after the newborn period. Closed or open hip reduction surgery, preceded by home management with Bryant traction (to release muscles and tendons), is usually necessary to manipulate the hip joint (TSRHC, 2008). Positioning and immobilization for 3 months in a spica cast follow the procedure. After reduction of a dislocated hip, the acetabulum begins to remodel in response to the pressure exerted by the femoral head. In some instances, this process may be incomplete, and the acetabulum remains shallow (Fujii, Nakashima, Yamamoto et al., 2010).

Patients may present with hip complaints in adolescence. The affected patient may complain of groin pain (indicating pain coming from the hip joint) or lateral hip pain (usually indicating lateral abductor fatigue pain). For children with residual dysplasia and acetabular dysplasia diagnosed during adolescence, one of various types of

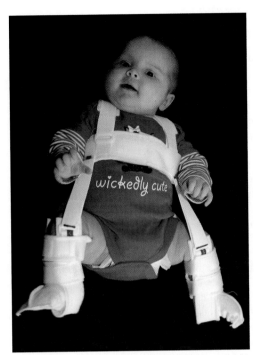

FIG 26-10 An infant in a Pavlik harness to treat developmental dysplasia of the hip. (Courtesy Texas Scottish Rite Hospital for Children, Dallas, TX.)

osteotomy procedures (surgical cutting of the bone) and repositioning of the femur is recommended (Javid & Wedge, 2009; Spence, Hocking, Wedge, & Roposch, 2009; Sucato, Tulchin, Shrader et al., 2010; Thawrani, Sucato, Podeszwa, & Delarocha, 2010). After certain surgeries, long-term immobilization in a spica cast is necessary until healing is achieved. Radiographs show the progress achieved with treatment. Follow-up monitoring is essential.

NURSING CARE OF THE CHILD WITH DEVELOPMENTAL DYSPLASIA OF THE HIP

■ Assessment

All infants should be assessed for DDH during routine neonatal and well-child visits to ensure prompt diagnosis and treatment. Assessment procedures vary with the age of the child. Once the diagnosis is established, nursing assessment is directed to the parents' knowledge level, their anxiety and coping abilities, and ensuring that the treatment regimen is followed.

Because the needs of children with musculoskeletal disorders are often long term, parents usually have a good understanding of their child's progress. Questions such as "What concerns do you have about your child's progress today?" or "How are you doing at home?" acknowledge that the parents' feelings and ideas are valued and important. Information generated by such questions can become the focus for assessment and further intervention.

Monitor the skin integrity of an infant in a Pavlik harness or spica cast. When surgery becomes necessary, nursing priorities shift to an assessment of lower extremity circulation and pain.

■ Nursing Diagnosis and Planning

The nursing diagnoses and expected outcomes that may be appropriate for the child with DDH and the child's family include the following:

- Deficient Knowledge related to confusion regarding child's condition and ongoing treatment.

Expected Outcomes. The parents will demonstrate understanding of DDH and the therapeutic use of a Pavlik harness (or spica cast). The parents will describe and demonstrate how to care for their child in a Pavlik harness (or spica cast). The parents can describe adverse effects, complications of treatment, and whom to contact with questions and concerns.

- Anxiety (Parental) related to guilt (for having a less-than-perfect child) and the need to provide complex care for an extended period.

Expected Outcome. The parents will feel less anxious, as evidenced by being able to describe DDH and its treatment in lay terms to other family members; carry out treatment regimens; demonstrate increased self-confidence in the care of their child; treat the child as normally as possible; and interact with health care providers and others in a calm and friendly manner.

- Risk for Impaired Skin Integrity related to skin chafing by the Pavlik harness or spica cast.

Expected Outcomes. On follow-up visits, the cast will be reasonably clean and dry and the child's skin will be clear and intact, without abrasions or sores.

- Ineffective Peripheral Tissue Perfusion (Lower Extremities) related to impaired circulation as a result of bracing, casting, or surgery.

Expected Outcome. The circulation to the child's feet and toes will remain adequate as evidenced by capillary refill time less than 2 seconds and toes that are pink and warm.

- Risk for Injury related to improper positioning of a child in a Pavlik harness or spica cast.

Expected Outcomes. The child will be safe from falls and will be adequately restrained when traveling in an automobile.

■ Interventions

■ Teaching about the Pavlik Harness. Demonstrate and teach the parents the proper care and application of the Pavlik harness, including how to position and fasten the chest halter (leave room for two fingers to rotate under this strap), fasten the shoulder straps (crossed in back) over each shoulder (leave room under the top of each shoulder strap for one finger), place the child's leg and foot into the stirrup and straps, and connect the straps to the chest halter. The requirements for harness use may change during therapy, so teaching, demonstration, and return demonstration are essential at every visit. Leg straps should be secure enough to keep the child's hips flexed without being tight. The harness should be worn 23 hours per day and should be removed only according to the physician's recommendation. Encourage the parents to hold and cuddle the infant as much as possible. An infant in a Pavlik harness can be fed in the usual positions.

Teach the parents to protect the child's skin and legs under the harness. A long T-shirt ("onesie") under the halter reduces harness rubbing. The diaper should go under the harness. Teach the parents to inspect the child's skin frequently for reddened or irritated areas and to reposition the child often.

■ Teaching about Spica Cast Care. Caring for a child in a spica cast is similar to caring for a child in any other type of cast (as previously discussed), with some additional adaptations. Because the cast covers the entire lower half of the child's body with only a limited perineal opening, managing the child's elimination is a challenge. Excess urine can trickle under the cast, irritating and macerating the skin, resisting drying, and becoming malodorous. Advise the family to tuck a disposable diaper underneath the cast edges at the circular perineal opening;

advise parents not to use sheet plastic under the cast, which can cause pooling of urine beneath the cast and subsequent skin breakdown. Place a sanitary napkin within the diaper that is tucked under the cast edges. Elevating the head of the bed helps urine and feces drain downward and away from the cast.

Monitor the child's neurovascular status frequently (Figure 26-11), and teach the family the signs of neurovascular compromise. Fever, wound drainage, and discomfort may be signs of infection and should be reported promptly. Teach the family ways to provide environmental and developmental stimulation (e.g., by moving the child to different areas during the day, placing appropriate toys within reach, and providing age-appropriate activities). Teach the family to ensure that the extremities within the cast are always supported with pillows, rolled-up towels, or "bean bag" chairs. Explain the importance of feeding the child a diet high in fluids, calories, calcium, protein, and fiber, and instruct parents to keep the child in an upright position for a minimum of 30 minutes after feeding. Explain ways to dress the child to accommodate climate, style, and other needs (e.g., by fitting socks over the toes of the cast, using Velcro closures on pants and shorts, or using clothing made of stretch fabrics). Give the parents the name and telephone number of an easily accessible health care provider in case questions arise at home.

■ **Alleviating Anxiety.** Communicate information to parents in a clear, kind, and straightforward manner because complex or ambiguous messages raise anxiety. Adjust teaching to accommodate parents' need for information and support. Reduce waiting time during follow-up visits and express interest in the child and parents. Preoperative teaching should include pictures of children in spica casts and showing a doll in a sample spica cast. Providing reliable, respectful, and empathetic care builds trust and reduces stress.

■ **Preventing Injury.** Assume a proactive role, and advise parents of the potential for injury and the importance of taking safety precautions. Most infant-carrying devices are not suitable or safe for infants in spica casts. Assist parents in identifying strategies for transporting their infant in a safe and comfortable manner, including the use of a car seat that can accommodate the wide leg spread caused by the spica cast or a car vest restraint for older children (Figure 26-12). During waking hours, teach parents to vary the child's position at least every 2 hours throughout the day. Remind parents that the child must never be left unattended; infants and young children often develop a surprising ability to move despite the restrictions imposed by a cast.

■ **Evaluation**

- Do the parents demonstrate the use of the Pavlik harness or spica cast in a safe and therapeutic manner?
- Can the parents describe adverse effects or complications of treatment?
- Can the parents describe DDH and its treatment in lay terms to other family members, carry out the prescribed therapy to the greatest extent possible, and treat the child as a normal developing child?
- Do the parents and child appear calm and able to participate in care?
- Do the parents seek recommended health care and keep follow-up appointments?
- Is the child's skin clear and free of lesions or breakdown?
- Are the child's toes warm and pink, with capillary refill time less than 2 seconds, and can the child move the toes freely?
- Does the child remain injury free?
- Can the parents describe home care adaptations, and are these appropriate for the child's developmental level?

LEGG-CALVÉ-PERTHES DISEASE

Legg-Calvé-Perthes disease is a condition in which an avascular event affects the epiphysis of the femur and prevents further growth of the ossific nucleus, resulting in increased bone density. As the bone is subsequently reabsorbed and replaced by new bone, the femoral head tends to flatten and enlarge. The child usually complains of a painful limp that is exacerbated by activities such as walking or running.

Etiology and Incidence

The cause of Legg-Calvé-Perthes disease is unknown, but it is widely accepted to be a growth disorder. Children with Legg-Calvé-Perthes disease are usually shorter-than-average height, and many were low-birth-weight infants (less than 2.5 kg). Abnormalities in certain clotting mechanisms (tendency to develop or failure to lyse thrombi) may also contribute to this condition (TSRHC, 2008). Studies have

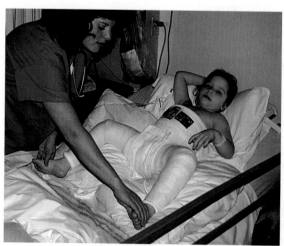

FIG 26-11 Regular assessment of circulation, sensation and movement in the lower extremities is essential when a child has a hip spica cast.

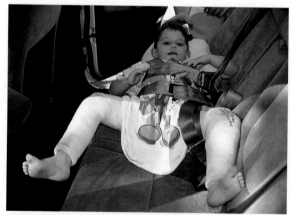

FIG 26-12 Use a car seat that can accommodate the wide leg spread caused by the spica cast or a car vest restraint for older children.

identified other factors related to the etiology of the disorder based on findings of abnormal growth and development, including trauma, hyperactivity, hereditary influences, and environmental factors (Krul et al., 2010; Nelitz, Lippacher, Krauspe, & Reichel, 2009; Vosmaer, Pereira, Koenderman et al., 2010).

Legg-Calvé-Perthes disease occurs in approximately 15 of every 100,000 children. The ratio of affected boys to girls is 5:1. Legg-Calvé-Perthes disease is most commonly seen in children between 4 and 10 years of age, but can occur in children 2 to 12 years of age (Nelitz et al., 2009). The earlier the condition is identified, the better the long-term prognosis (Sankar, Horn, Wells, & Dormans, 2011a). Unilateral hip involvement is more common than bilateral involvement. This disease is rare in African-Americans and Asians.

PATHOPHYSIOLOGY

Legg-Calvé-Perthes Disease

The disorder is classified by the extent of femoral head involvement and disease stage. The disorder usually progresses through five stages over a 1- to 2-year period. During *stage 1*, the epiphysis begins to show the results of ischemia. Synovitis produces stiffness and pain. Necrosis begins; radiographs show a reduction in size and increased density of the femoral head. Once necrosis occurs *(stage 2)*, the bone weakens and dies, causing collapse of the femoral head. *Stage 3* is the fragmentation stage, in which avascular bone is reabsorbed. Healing occurs as new bone is formed. During the reossification stage, *stage 4*, the femoral head and neck begin to re-form. *Stage 5*, or the stage of reconstitution, results in final healing.

Manifestations

The most common symptom of Legg-Calvé-Perthes disease is persistent pain of the hip that worsens with movement. Pain may be intermittent over a period of weeks or months and can be felt in other parts of the leg, such as groin, thigh, or knee. Patients may have a limp or limited range of motion.

The most serious complication of Legg-Calvé-Perthes disease is permanent deformity. If the femoral head protrudes outside the acetabulum and the healing process within the femoral head is incomplete, the femoral head will flatten over time and take on a misshapen appearance.

Diagnostic Evaluation

In the majority of cases, plain radiographs of the femoral head will disclose the condition. A bone scan or MRI study may reveal necrosis and irregularity of the femoral head.

Therapeutic Management

Treatment goals are to prevent deformity of the hip and delay the onset of arthritis and degenerative joint disease. The femoral head is contained and maintained in the acetabulum and protected from the stress of weight bearing during the healing process. Some physicians, however, do not believe that weight bearing is harmful as long as the femur remains in the acetabulum.

Initial treatment includes antiinflammatory medications (such as ibuprofen), range-of-motion exercises, and bed rest. If improvement is not seen within 7 to 10 days and the child is still unable to abduct the hip, alternative methods of treatment are considered. Traction, Petrie casts, or abduction braces may be recommended.

For children with severe necrosis, the femoral head is abducted and internally rotated in relation to the acetabulum through a type of containment device that uses the acetabulum to maintain the spherical shape of the femoral head. Containment prevents the acetabulum from rubbing against the weakened portion of the femoral head and creating a flat shape. Surgical procedures include an osteotomy, which places the femur more securely into the acetabulum, or an acetabular osteotomy, which rotates the acetabulum to cover the femoral head completely. Many physicians recommend surgical intervention because it reduces treatment time and eliminates problems with adherence to treatment.

NURSING CARE OF THE CHILD WITH LEGG-CALVÉ-PERTHES DISEASE

■ Assessment

Assessment of a child with Legg-Calvé-Perthes disease reveals loss of internal hip rotation and limited abduction. The nurse determines how long the child has been limping, as well as the pattern, timing, and severity of the pain. The pain may be referred to the thigh or knee. The child will describe the pain as increasing with activity and decreasing with rest. Physical examination of the extremity may reveal muscle wasting of the thigh and buttock—a reflection of disuse. Shortening of the extremity on the affected side indicates collapse of the femoral head.

■ Nursing Diagnosis and Planning

The following nursing diagnoses and expected outcomes may be appropriate after assessment of the child with Legg-Calvé-Perthes disease:

- Impaired Physical Mobility related to activity restrictions.
Expected Outcomes. The child will maintain mobility and strength of all unaffected joints and tolerate activity restrictions.
- Anxiety related to knowledge deficit about the condition and home management.
Expected Outcomes. The family will provide safe home care and provide age-appropriate activities for their child.

■ Interventions

■ **Facilitating Appropriate Activity.** Activity restrictions are one of the most problematic areas in the care of a child with Legg-Calvé-Perthes disease. The child may become frustrated and angry when unable to meet the physical and social demands of peers. Initially, the child may appear to adjust to the lifestyle restrictions, but the nurse must be alert to subtle indicators of rebellion and uncooperative behavior. Other children will adapt quickly. Do not construe a child's refusal to adhere to treatment regimens as maladaptive behavior. The demand to keep up with their peers is sometimes so great that children are simply unable to make appropriate choices regarding their health.

If a brace is prescribed, returning to school with a brace poses unique problems. The school nurse and the child's teacher should be involved in the discharge planning. The child should participate in as many school-related activities as possible. Acknowledging the child's mobility limitations and working with school officials to identify appropriate alternatives will ensure a successful school re-entry. Emphasizing hobbies and other creative activities provides ways for the child to excel and feel a sense of accomplishment.

■ **Teaching Home Management.** Because the child will receive the majority of treatment as an outpatient, nursing care should focus on home care management. The family must clearly understand the need for care adherence and the role it will play in the healing process. Teach parents to perform neurovascular assessments. The nurse should also help parents identify skin and safety issues related to the child's mobility restrictions and the use of a brace. Physical and occupational therapists are important resources for the parents.

■ Evaluation

* Does the child exhibit normal joint and muscular integrity, and does the child adhere to the treatment plan?
* Does the child participate in age-appropriate peer and school-related activities within activity limitations?
* Can the child appropriately express frustration or feelings about being different?
* Are the parents able to provide developmentally appropriate activities for their child?
* Can the parents describe and demonstrate brace care (if applicable) and neurovascular assessments?

SLIPPED CAPITAL FEMORAL EPIPHYSIS

Slipped capital femoral epiphysis (SCFE) is a condition that occurs during a period of rapid growth in adolescence. Shearing stress causes the femoral capital epiphysis to displace from its normal position relative to the femoral neck.

Etiology and Incidence

The cause of slipped capital femoral epiphysis is unknown. Slippage appears to be related to increased stress on the proximal femur at a time when the epiphyseal plate is preparing for eventual closure. The weakness of the growth plate may be related to adolescent hormonal imbalance combined with mechanical stress on the hip during growth (Sankar, Horn, Wells, & Dormans, 2011b). SCFE most frequently occurs in adolescent boys who are overweight; the majority of affected adolescents exceed the 90th percentile for weight (Sankar et al., 2011b).

The incidence is approximately 2 per 100,000, although this rate varies according to race, sex, and geographic location (Koteles & Lewi, 2010; Larson, Yu, Melton et al., 2010; Yildirim, Bautista, & Davidson, 2008). SCFE occurs approximately two to three times more in young boys than young girls, and families may have an increased incidence. Although initially the condition is unilateral, approximately 25% become bilateral.

Pathophysiology

The epiphyseal plate begins to thin in response to hormonal influences during adolescence. Increased body weight and height place more stress on the epiphysis, causing a relative displacement (slip) of the femoral neck from the femoral head. The epiphyseal movement appears to be in a posterior and inferior direction. The usual deformity consists of an upward and anterior movement of the femoral neck on the capital epiphysis. The slip can occur gradually, acutely without prior symptoms, or acutely after an extended period of mild symptoms. SCFE requires immediate medical treatment.

Manifestations and Diagnostic Evaluation

The classic symptoms of SCFE include a limp and pain. The pain usually is in the groin, thigh, or knee; it is intermittent and worsens with activity. Because the adolescent may complain of knee pain, hip involvement may be overlooked. The leg often is externally rotated. Presenting symptoms along with characteristic growth signs suggest the diagnosis. Radiographs confirm the diagnosis. Radiographs are obtained with the legs in a frog-leg position.

Therapeutic Management and Nursing Considerations

As soon as the diagnosis is made, the adolescent is admitted to the hospital and placed on bed rest to prevent exacerbation of the slip. Treatment is usually internal fixation: a pin or screw inserted across the growth plate secures the femoral head and prevents further slippage. More severe slips may require reconstruction of the femoral head, followed by pinning. Postoperatively, the adolescent uses crutches with partial weight bearing for 4 to 6 weeks. Depending on the severity of the slip and extent of the osteotomy, some adolescents may be required to be non–weight-bearing for 4 to 6 weeks, with transfers to a wheelchair only. The screw or pin may be removed after several years.

The nurse should assess adolescents for SCFE any time an adolescent reports knee or thigh pain. Interventions are similar to those for any child in traction or undergoing surgery. Postoperatively, the adolescent needs to be taught isometric exercises and crutch walking. Weight control may be an issue; the overweight adolescent needs to learn to develop good nutritional habits and avoid high-calorie foods. Referral to a dietitian may be helpful. Provide the adolescent and parent with written instructions before discharge.

❓ CRITICAL THINKING EXERCISE 26-1

Children often come to the ambulatory care setting reporting hip or knee pain and walking with a limp. Compare and contrast the three common hip disorders in children.

CLUBFOOT

Clubfoot (*talipes equinovarus*) is characterized by rigid midfoot *C*avus, forefoot *A*dduction, heel *V*arus, and ankle *E*quinus (CAVE).

Etiology and Incidence

Clubfoot represents a congenital dysplasia of all tissue (bone, muscle, ligaments, nerves, and blood vessels) below the knee. The incidence of clubfoot is 1 in 1000 live births, both feet are affected in nearly 50% of patients, and it is seen more commonly in males by over a 2:1 ratio (Sorbie, 2008). Although the means of transmission remains unknown, heredity and race, not environment (i.e., intrauterine packing), seem to play a factor in the occurrence of clubfoot. One affected child increases the probability of another sibling having clubfoot by 20% to 30%, and a family history of clubfoot is noted in approximately 24% of affected individuals (Kruse, Dobbs, & Gurnett, 2008). Clubfoot is seen least frequently in the Asian population (0.39:1000) and most frequently in the Polynesian population (6.8:1000). Although clubfoot can be seen as a part of some syndromes, such as arthrogryposis or spina bifida, it is frequently identified as an isolated birth defect (Canto, Cano, Palau, & Ojeda, 2008). Many etiologic theories have been proposed, but none can fully explain this complex deformity. The cause is likely multifactorial (TSRHC, 2008).

Manifestations and Diagnostic Evaluation

Clubfoot can be diagnosed prenatally by ultrasound. However, radiographs, ultrasound, or MRI imaging is rarely used or necessary for assessment of a clubfoot. The deformity is easily recognized on clinical examination (Figure 26-13) (Anand & Sala, 2008; Canto et al., 2008).

Therapeutic Management

The primary goal of treatment of a child with a clubfoot is to reduce or eliminate all of the components of the deformity so the child has a

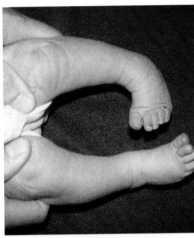

FIG 26-13 An infant with left clubfoot. Note the positional difference between the two feet.

functional, structural, mobile, pain-free foot (Forster & Fraser, 2007). Secondary goals for treatment include a satisfactory appearance, ability to wear normal shoes, and the avoidance of unnecessary or prolonged treatment.

Until the mid-1990s, the preferred treatment for clubfoot in the United States was predominantly surgical. Because long-term complications and recurrence were found to occur after surgical correction, nonoperative treatment modalities are now used. The Ponseti casting method and the French physiotherapy method greatly decrease the need for extensive surgery in these patients (Zionts, Zhao, Hitchcock, et al., 2010).

The French physiotherapy method, used by only experienced physical therapists and in a few treatment centers, involves daily sequential stretching, strengthening, and mobilization of the foot followed by taping and splinting to allow for gradual correction of the deformity (Anand & Sala, 2008). Most of the correction is obtained by the physical therapist within the first 3 months of treatment, with full correction expected within 5 months. Committed, well-trained parents are an integral part of the technique, with parents being taught the technique early on and home therapy continued until walking age. Splinting continues until 2 or 3 years of age in an effort to prevent recurrence of the deformity (Anand & Sala, 2008; TSRHC, 2008).

Ponseti Casting Method

By far, the standard of care for clubfoot treatment is the Ponseti casting method (Ponseti, 1992), developed in the 1940s and essentially unchanged to this day. This method requires weekly, gentle stretching and manipulation of the misaligned bones followed by application of a well-molded long-leg plaster cast (TSRHC, 2008). The cast maintains the correction obtained by the orthopedist and allows for further relaxation and softening of the tissues with atraumatic remodeling of the abnormal joint surfaces. Unlike other forms of nonoperative treatment, the Ponseti method corrects all the components of the deformity simultaneously, with the exception of the equinus, which is corrected last. Correction of the deformity is usually obtained within 6 to 8 weeks of casting, with a percutaneous tendoachilles lengthening (TAL) being frequently performed before the final cast application to correct the equinus contracture (Anand & Sala, 2008). The TAL is generally performed in the clinic setting using a topical anesthetic cream (EMLA)

or needleless injectable lidocaine (J-Tip) (TSRHC, 2008). A final cast is applied and maintained for 3 weeks. On completion of casting, the foot will appear overcorrected. Correction is maintained through the use of an abduction orthosis fulltime for 3 months followed by 12-hour nightly use until at least 2 years of age in an effort to prevent recurrence of the deformity.

Clubfoot Recurrence

Despite the differences in the Ponseti casting and French physiotherapy methods, both have been shown by MRI to be effective in achieving and sustaining normal bone and joint alignment in the foot. Both have demonstrated satisfactory short-term outcomes with reduction in the need for extensive surgery, and to date, neither has been shown to be superior to the other (Faulks & Richards, 2009). Unfortunately, there are still clubfeet that ultimately require surgical intervention. Surgical correction may involve a limited posterior release, anterior tibialis tendon transfer, lateral column release, or complete posteromedial release (TSRHC, 2008).

Nursing Considerations

Regardless of the method of treatment used, patients and their families will encounter many similar challenges that can be effectively managed with good nursing care. Nursing interventions include education and anticipatory guidance, reduction of infant discomfort and pain, and patient advocacy (Forster & Fraser, 2007).

Education and Anticipatory Guidance

Information about their child's clubfoot and treatment protocol can be helpful in reducing the anxiety and guilt experienced by many parents and facilitates treatment adherence, which leads to improved patient outcomes. When talking with families, use descriptive rather than scientific terms. Explain that the cause of clubfoot remains unknown and that children with idiopathic clubfoot are expected to develop normally and participate in normal activities. Prepare the families for expected disruptions in their child's care such as difficulties with dressing, sleep, and play often seen with the initiation of casting and bracing. Knowledge that their child will adapt, usually within 24 to 48 hours, is helpful to families. Families must receive thorough and ongoing education about proper neurovascular, skin, and pain assessment to help prevent potential problems. Positioning, bathing, and skin care must be addressed with clear verbal and written instructions. Inform families whom to contact with questions or concerns.

Reduction of Discomfort and Pain

Best results occur in both the Ponseti casting and French physiotherapy treatment methods when the infant is relaxed during manipulation of the foot. Timing of infant feeding should coincide with the treatment session to aid in infant distraction and relaxation. This may require alterations in feeding routines and may necessitate breastfeeding mothers to pump or supplement with formula or a pacifier and 24% sucrose during casting sessions. Providing a calm, quiet, warm environment with dimmed lights, soft music, and parental involvement is comforting to infants and helps them relax, or even sleep during the session. If a TAL is required, premedication with a local anesthetic is indicated to decrease procedural discomfort (Forster & Fraser, 2007; TSRHC, 2008).

If surgery is needed, the nurse oversees pain management in the immediate postoperative period. Elevate the child's feet postoperatively to reduce swelling and pain. Administer analgesics. Assess the neurovascular status of the toes at least every 2 hours in the immediate postoperative period.

Patient Advocacy

Family involvement and commitment to the treatment is critical for a successful outcome. Nurses can advocate for their young patients and help improve family adherence through frequent reinforcement of treatment protocol and parental encouragement with ongoing education, phone calls to the home to address problems and concerns, frequent follow-up appointments and facilitation of a parent support network.

SYNDROMES AND CONDITIONS WITH ASSOCIATED ORTHOPEDIC ANOMALIES

Several syndromes and other conditions have been associated with various orthopedic anomalies. Table 26-5 describes these. Because people unfamiliar with osteogenesis imperfecta may assume that the child's fractures and old fractures are the result of child abuse, the nurse needs to be particularly careful with nursing assessments for all children with unexplained fractures.

MUSCULAR DYSTROPHIES

Muscular dystrophies include more than 30 genetic diseases (National Institute of Neurological Disorders and Stroke [NINDS], 2009a). These are progressively degenerative, inherited diseases that affect the muscle cells of specific muscle groups, causing weakness and atrophy.

Etiology

Muscular dystrophies vary in pattern of inheritance and age at onset, but most are identified in early childhood (Table 26-6).

Incidence

Duchenne muscular dystrophy is the most common muscular dystrophy, occurring in 1 in 3500 male children (NINDS, 2009b). This disease accounts for approximately 50% of all cases of muscular dystrophy.

Pathophysiology

Despite differences in genetic transmission, age at onset, distribution of involvement, and clinical course, changes in muscles are similar across all forms of muscular dystrophies (TSRHC, 2008). Early in this process, muscle fibers begin to leak the protein creatine kinase and take on excess calcium, causing further harm to muscle fibers. Over time, muscle fibers degenerate and are replaced by fat and connective tissue. As muscle fibers die, progressive weakness and wasting of symmetrical groups of skeletal muscles result in increasing disability and deformity.

Manifestations

In children with Duchenne muscular dystrophy, progressive, symmetrical muscle wasting and weakness without loss of sensation first appear after walking is achieved (usually 3 to 7 years). The child must use the Gower maneuver to rise from the floor (child puts hands on knees and moves the hands up legs until standing erect) (TSRHC, 2008). The child has a waddling, wide-based gait. The calf muscles are characteristically weak but hypertrophied. The muscles of the pelvis and shoulders are also affected. Increasing disability and deformities include hip and knee contractures, foot deformities, scoliosis, and lordosis. Walking ability is lost by age 9 to 12 years. Associated signs and symptoms include moderate obesity, cognitive disability, cardiomyopathy, and shortened life span. Other forms of muscular dystrophy also affect the cardiopulmonary and gastrointestinal systems, eyes, brain, and other organs (NINDS, 2009b). Cardiopulmonary complications are the most common cause of death.

Diagnostic Evaluation

The gene loci for many muscular dystrophies have been identified, which makes carrier status for women easier to determine. Children with a positive family history are especially at risk for muscular dystrophy and should be monitored for clinical symptoms. Serum creatine kinase (CK) levels are elevated in the early stages of the disease and then decrease as muscle bulk decreases. Electromyography and muscle biopsy may also assist with the diagnosis.

Therapeutic Management

The therapeutic management of the child with a muscular dystrophy is aimed at maintaining ambulation and independence for as long as possible as muscle weakness progresses. Contractures further reduce mobility and independence. Surgery, bracing, and physical therapy contribute to keeping the child as mobile as possible. Later therapy is directed toward maximizing sitting capabilities, respiratory function, and self-care. The prevention of obesity to facilitate mobility and care is a priority. Prompt attention to infection, especially of the respiratory tract, is essential.

Nursing Considerations

When muscular dystrophy is present in the family history, infants and young children need to be monitored carefully for its occurrence. When a diagnosis is made, nursing interventions can become a major source of support for these children and their families. Nursing interventions for the child with muscular dystrophy include coordinating a variety of health care services. Anticipating the child's future needs requires a sensitive yet knowledgeable approach. The family's ability to cope with chronic illness and the poor prognosis of muscular dystrophy needs to be assessed. Over time, the child's mobility and self-care abilities should be monitored to ensure independence for as long as possible. Maintenance of activity and self-care functions is important to the child and the family, and independence must be fostered within the limits of safety. Activities such as swimming that promote range of motion and mobility for as long as possible are helpful. As the disease progresses and movement is increasingly restricted, the nurse can suggest activities that take less energy but keep the child involved with peers. The potential for weight gain and respiratory tract infection and the adequacy of support systems must be regularly assessed.

Children in the late stages of muscular dystrophy have difficulty moving. The nurse and family should assist with position changes every 2 hours to prevent injury to the skin and other tissues from prolonged pressure. Adequate fluid intake must be encouraged to prevent urine stasis. A bowel regimen, including stool softeners or laxatives, may be necessary.

The home environment, including bathing and toileting facilities, may need to be modified to allow wheelchair mobility. Creative approaches to clothing can simplify dressing while meeting the needs of a child trying to fit in with peers.

Specific suggestions about dietary modifications to control weight may be necessary. The nurse can educate families about how to make dietary changes without making food a source of controversy. To reduce the chance of life-threatening respiratory infections, the child needs to be protected from children with respiratory and contagious diseases. As disability progresses, pulmonary hygiene and respiratory exercises are needed to maintain respiratory function.

TABLE 26-5 **SYNDROMES AND CONDITIONS WITH ASSOCIATED ORTHOPEDIC ANOMALIES**

SYNDROME OR CONDITION	INCIDENCE	ORTHOPEDIC ANOMALIES

Achondroplasia	Most common form of dwarfism 1.3 in 100,000 to 1.5 in 10,000 live births	Angular deformity of lower extremities: genu varum and tibia vara more common than valgus
		Cranial cervical stenosis
		Mortality rate as high as 7.5%
		Symptoms include hypotonia and sleep apnea
		Elbow deformity: lack of full extension
		Short stature
		Spinal stenosis
		  • $\frac{1}{3}$ of patients with symptoms by 15 years
		  • Symptoms include pain in lower back and legs exacerbated by activity
		Thoracolumbar kyphosis: surgery indicated for persistent kyphosis

Arthrogryposis	1 in 3000 live births	Congenital joint stiffness, typically all four extremities are involved Varying degrees of muscle weakness Normal to above normal intelligence Goals of treatment: independent ambulation and function of upper extremities for activities of daily living

Down syndrome (see Chapter 30)	Genetic condition associated with intellectual disability 1 in 800 live births 40% have congenital heart defects	Hypermobility of the upper cervical spine
		  • Atlantoaxial (C1-C2), screen for instability before athletic or Special Olympics participation
		  • Occipital-atlanto, reported incidence varies widely
		  • Only indication for surgery is neurologic symptoms
		Hypermobility and ligamentous laxity of hips
		  • 7.9% have some form of hip abnormality
		  • Recurrent, usually painless dislocations (see DDH) occur in nearly 5%, typically between 2 and 10 yr of age
		  • Slipped capital femoral epiphysis
		  • Avascular necrosis
		Patella femoral disorders
		Clubfeet, may be resistant to nonoperative treatment
		Flat feet

Marfan	Autosomal dominant Prevalence: 1 in 5000 live births More may have subtle variations	Tall, lanky, abnormally long arms with reduced extension of the elbows Generalized joint laxity Protrusio acetabuli (increased depth of the acetabulum) Arachnodactyly (long, slender, spider-like fingers) Scoliosis, spondylolisthesis Chest wall deformity, pectus deformities Developmental dysplasia of the hips Extreme myopia Loud cardiac murmur; may have aortic dilation, an aortic aneurysm, and mitral valve prolapse
Neurofibromatosis	Hereditary	Neurofibromatosis-1 associated with orthopedic conditions Orthopedic conditions rare for children with neurofibromatosis-2 Spinal deformities, typically thoracic Hemihypertrophy Congenital pseudoarthosis of the tibia

Osteogenesis imperfecta	Autosomal dominant or recessive, or spontaneous mutation Incidence Type 1: 1 in 30,000 live births Type 2: 1 in 62,000 live births Type 3: Very rare Type 4: Unknown	Characterized by connective tissue defects and extreme bone fragility
		90% of those affected have a genetic defect in type I collagen formation
		  • Most common manifestation is frequent fractures with even the slightest injury; the earlier the fracture occurs, the more severe the disease
		  • Short stature
		  • Spinal and long bone deformities, frequently require surgical intervention
		  • Osteoporosis
		  • Blue sclera
		  • Discolored teeth
		  • Conductive hearing loss
		Infants with type 2 usually die during the perinatal period or early infancy
		Older children need gentle handling and movement, injury prevention, nutritional management; enhance family and child coping with chronic condition
		IV bisphosphonate may increase bone density

TABLE 26-6 MUSCULAR DYSTROPHIES OF CHILDHOOD

ONSET AND PROGRESSION	INHERITANCE AND INCIDENCE	CLINICAL MANIFESTATIONS
Duchenne Onset: usually before 3 yr, manifests between 3-6 yr Rapidly progressive; loss of walking by 9-12 yr; death in late teens from respiratory failure, heart failure, pneumonia	X-linked recessive Most common hereditary neuromuscular disease; affects all races Incidence: 1 in 3600 male infants	Progressive generalized weakness and muscle wasting affecting limb and trunk muscles first; calves often enlarged; waddling gait; lordosis; cardiomyopathy; Gower maneuver; cognitive disability common
Becker Onset: usually 7-11 yr Slowly progressive; maintain walking past early teens; life span into third decade	X-linked recessive Incidence: 1 in 20,000 male births	Almost identical to Duchenne but less severe; child is mobile at least until late teens; normal intelligence
Congenital Myotonic Severe neonatal form Onset: birth Weakness at birth, may have paralysis of diaphragm If child survives early weeks of life, steady improvement in motor function over the first decade, usually developing ability to walk; often survive to late adulthood	Autosomal dominant Incidence: 1 in 30,000 births	In the severe neonatal form, hypotonia and muscle weakness (especially of the face) at birth; difficulty swallowing, sucking, impaired breathing, absence of reflexes, skeletal deformities, such as clubfeet
Steinert Onset: late adolescence to early adulthood	Autosomal dominant Incidence: 1 in 8000 births	May appear normal at birth; mild weakness in first few years, with progressive wasting of distal muscles; myotonia worsened by cold, fatigue, stress; cognitive disability in approximately half of cases
Facioscapulohumeral (FSH, or Landouzy-Dejerine Disease) Onset: usually late teens to early 20s Slowly progressive loss of walking in later life; variable life expectancy; disease may span many decades	Autosomal dominant or recessive Incidence: 3-10 per 1 million births	Earliest and most severe weakness occurs in facial and shoulder girdle muscles; may be unable to pucker lips, whistle, close eyes completely during sleep; may be mild, causing minimal disability; normal intelligence
Scapuloperoneal or Scapulohumeral (Emery-Dreifuss) Onset: middle childhood to early teens Progression is quite slow; many survive to late adulthood	X-linked recessive Incidence: rare	Contractures of elbows and ankles develop early; shoulder muscles become wasted; slowly progressive, with eventual cardiac abnormality
Congenital Onset: birth to before 2 yr Typically slow but variable; many do not attain walking; shortened life span	Autosomal recessive Incidence: rare	Generalized muscle weakness with possible joint deformities and contractures; scoliosis, foot deformities, respiratory and swallowing difficulties, hypotonia; normal to severe cognitive disability; may affect central nervous system causing seizures, vision, and speech problems

Data from The Texas Scottish Rite Hospital for Children. (2008). In J. A. Herring (Ed.), *Tachdjian's pediatric orthopaedics* (4th ed.), Philadelphia: Elsevier Saunders; National Institute of Neurological Disorders and Stroke (2009). *Muscular dystrophy: Hope through research.* Retrieved from www.ninds.nih.gov/disorders/md/detail_md.html.

Regular monitoring by a multidisciplinary team helps meet the varying needs of the child and family as the child's condition changes. Therapy is individualized to address the child's specific needs. Genetic screening and counseling are recommended for parents and siblings of children with muscular dystrophy.

Parents need to be taught how to perform basic nursing tasks and be referred to agencies that can assist with home care and equipment, such as a motorized wheelchair. Extended family and support groups, such as the Muscular Dystrophy Association of America (see Evolve website), can provide needed emotional support and specific assistance

as parental energies are exhausted. In addition, the needs of the grieving family should be addressed.

JUVENILE IDIOPATHIC ARTHRITIS

Juvenile idiopathic arthritis (JIA), formerly known as *juvenile rheumatoid arthritis*, is an autoimmune inflammatory disease with no known cause. The term *juvenile rheumatoid arthritis* is misleading because it implies a positive rheumatoid factor (RF). However, only approximately 5% of children with JIA have a positive rheumatoid factor.

TABLE 26-7   MAJOR TYPES OF JUVENILE IDIOPATHIC ARTHRITIS

SUBTYPE OF JIA	GENDER	AGE	JOINTS AFFECTED	OTHER MANIFESTATIONS
Oligoarticular, early onset	Females > males	1-4 yr	Four or fewer joints affected; in ⅓ of patients involve single joint	ANA (+) in approximately 60% (increased risk of uveitis)
Enthesitis-related arthritis (late-onset oligoarticular)	Males > females	9-12 yr	Often have four or fewer joints involved but can have a polyarticular course; possible sacroiliitis	May carry the *HLA-B27* gene, enthesitis
RF(−) polyarticular	Females > males	1-4 yr	Affects five or more joints, combination of small and large joints, often symmetrical involvement	RF(−)
RF(+) polyarticular	Females > males	9-16 yr	Affects five or more joints, combination of small and large joints, often symmetrical involvement	RF(+), rheumatoid nodules, risk of bony erosions
Systemic-onset JIA	Females = males		Usually polyarticular involvement	High daily or twice-daily spiking fevers, rash, risk of pericarditis, lymphadenopathy, hepatosplenomegaly

Arthritis in children can appear in a number of different forms, each with a different treatment protocol and prognosis.

The term *arthritis* refers to swelling in a joint. There are many causes of joint swelling, such as trauma or infection. To diagnose JIA, the child must be younger than 16 years of age and have joint swelling in at least one joint for at least 6 weeks that is not the result of trauma, infection, or malignancy (Dannecker & Quartier, 2009).

JIA is one of the more common chronic diseases in children and the leading cause of childhood disability. With ongoing research and advances in treatment, the prognosis has improved over the past decade.

Etiology

Despite extensive research, the cause of JIA remains unknown. The cause is most likely multifactorial, including genetic predisposition, abnormal immune response, and environmental triggering factors such as infection or trauma.

PATHOPHYSIOLOGY

Juvenile Idiopathic Arthritis

The synovial joints are the primary structures involved in this process. Normally joints are movable and contain synovium, a highly vascular tissue that produces a clear, viscous synovial fluid that nourishes and lubricates articular cartilage. In JIA, immune complexes in blood and synovial tissue initiate the inflammatory response, producing inflammatory cytokines. Phagocytosis and accumulation of immune complexes cause chronic inflammation and joint destruction.

As the synovium becomes inflamed, excessive fluid is produced. Unlike normal synovial fluid, this fluid is thin and watery. The synovium swells, and thickened villi and nodules protrude into the joint cavity. *Pannus* (inflamed granulating tissue) formation occurs over the articular cartilage. With further deterioration, the articular cartilage and contiguous bone become eroded and are destroyed.

Incidence

JIA affects approximately 100,000 children in the United States. The most common age of onset is between 2 and 4 years of age and for the most common subtype of JIA (pauciarticular) girls are three times more likely to experience the condition than boys (Wu, Van Mater, & Rabinovich, 2011).

Manifestations

Persistent joint swelling in one or more joints that lasts 6 weeks or longer suggests JIA. The joints may be, stiff, swollen, warm to the touch, erythematous, and with limited range of motion. Stiffness is worse in the morning or after a prolonged period of rest. This is referred to as the "gel phenomenon" because the joints seem to gel in place. Identification of subtype will guide management and prognosis. Table 26-7 lists associated signs and symptoms of the JIA subtypes (Dannecker & Quartier, 2009). If untreated, *uveitis*, or inflammation of the eye structures in the uveal tract, can lead to vision loss.

Diagnostic Evaluation

The early diagnosis of JIA depends on a comprehensive history and physical examination. The character, frequency, and severity of the systemic and articular manifestations are critical to the diagnosis and treatment. Laboratory markers such as the rheumatoid factor (RF), antinuclear antibody (ANA), *HLA-B27* gene, and anti-cyclic citrullinated peptide (anti-CCP) antibody may be helpful in identifying the subtype of JIA. CBC, ESR, and CRP can be useful in identifying the presence of inflammation. In addition, children with JIA need routine slit-lamp eye exams to screen for uveitis, which occurs more frequently in the presence of a positive ANA.

Therapeutic Management

This is no known cure for JIA. Therapeutic management is directed toward preserving joint function, controlling the inflammatory process, minimizing deformity, and reducing the impact of the disease on the child's development (Shenoi & Wallace, 2010). Management includes medication, physical and occupational therapy, family education, home care, and encouragement of age-appropriate activities as tolerated.

Drug Therapy

The medication treatment is dependent on severity of the disease and number of joints involved. Although NSAIDs such as ibuprofen, naproxen sodium (Naprosyn), sulindac (Clinoril), and celecoxib (Celebrex) are the first line of treatment, other medications are often needed. If the child's condition does not improve after 4 to 6 weeks, methotrexate, a disease-modifying antirheumatic drug (DMARD) is added to the medication regimen. However, methotrexate may be started at the time of diagnosis if the arthritis is considered moderate to severe. Additional medications, commonly referred to as biologics, may be needed in order to completely control the child's arthritis. These include etanercept (Enbrel), adalimumab (Humira), and infliximab (Remicade). Anakinra (Kineret) is a newer medication used in children with systemic-onset juvenile arthritis. Local corticosteroid injections are often used to reduce inflammation in selected joints.

Physical and Occupational Therapy

In addition to drug therapy, physical and occupational therapy are also important interventions to preserve muscle integrity and joint mobility. Active disease processes can place the child with JIA at risk for impaired mobility, contractures, and altered growth and development. Rehabilitation is designed to prevent such problems from occurring. Depending on the disease process, a program of rest, proper positioning, exercises, and ADL (activities of daily living) modifications will be developed by occupational and physical therapists. To ensure effectiveness and cooperation, an individualized therapy program will take into consideration the child's limitations, abilities, home/school environment, and interests.

Exercise programs consist of gentle active and/or passive range of motion and strengthening. Active range of motion and rest are indicated during times of increased synovitis and pain. Gentle movement through available range will maintain joint mobility. Rest or frequent rest breaks will increase overall endurance and limit joint impact throughout the day. Inactivity could lead to loss of joint motion and decrease in muscle strength. Passive range of motion is not indicated in early stages of the disease or during times of active inflammation; instead, it will be more advantageous to encourage play activities to increase active range. A child may begin gradual strengthening once the synovitis is well controlled and functional range of motion is obtained. Examples of low-impact strengthening activities are swimming and riding a bicycle.

In addition to exercise, modalities such as heat and splinting are helpful in reducing pain and maintaining range during painful episodes. Hot baths, whirlpools, moist hot packs, and paraffin baths are all examples of heat that can be used at home or in conjunction with therapy. Heat will also reduce joint stiffness and increase the elasticity of tissues surrounding the joints, making stretching more effective. Splinting is used to rest the joint, decrease pain, and align the joint in the proper position; it may also be helpful as a support when the child becomes more active.

The goal of rehabilitation is to maintain functional mobility and allow affected children to keep up with their peers. Children are naturally active, and children with JIA are no different. Activity that helps maintain normal muscle and joint integrity should be encouraged but may need to be modified.

Surgical Treatment

Surgical intervention, although rare, is considered when the child or adolescent is having problems with joint contractures, micrognathia, or unequal growth of extremities.

NURSING CARE OF THE CHILD WITH JUVENILE IDIOPATHIC ARTHRITIS

■ Assessment

The nursing assessment focuses on the status of affected joints, the child's physical limitations, the level and intensity of the pain, and the child's and family's response to the disease process. The nurse assesses the affected joints for warmth, tenderness, pain, and limited range of motion. Be alert for guarding of painful joints, refusal to bear weight, limping, and facial expressions of discomfort. The parent may describe the child as fussy and irritable in the morning. The young child may be reluctant to walk and want to be carried.

DRUG GUIDE

Naproxen, Naproxen Sodium

Classification
NSAID

Action
Unknown; reduces inflammation and fever, possibly by inhibiting prostaglandin synthesis.

Indication
JIA

Dosage and Route
10 mg/kg/day orally in two divided doses; medication comes in tablet or liquid suspension (125 mg/5 mL).

Absorption
Absorbed rapidly from the gastrointestinal tract with peak action in 1 to 4 hours.

Excretion
Effects last approximately 7 hours; eliminated primarily by the kidneys.

Contraindications
Contraindicated in any child who has had an allergic reaction to this drug or similar drugs or in children with a syndrome of asthma, rhinitis, and nasal polyps; naproxen should not be administered concurrently with naproxen sodium.

Precautions
Can prolong bleeding time, alter liver functions, and contribute to renal toxicity. Use cautiously if the child is also taking methotrexate, aspirin, anticoagulants, probenecid, or steroids.

Adverse Reactions
Primarily gastrointestinal irritation (gastrointestinal ulceration with bleeding from prolonged use); edema; headache, drowsiness, or dizziness; tinnitus; pruritus or skin rash; risk for renal failure.

Nursing Considerations
Assess for adverse reactions, particularly if the child is receiving long-term therapy. Advise the child to take the medication with food or milk to minimize gastrointestinal upset. Be aware that antiinflammatory medications can mask signs of infection. Teach the child and family signs of gastrointestinal bleeding.

Assess joint stiffness, including the duration of the stiffness and the child's description of how difficult movement is after periods of inactivity. Assess the child for any indication of systemic involvement, such as history of temperature elevations, especially in the late afternoon or evening. Determine whether a rash occurs with the fever. Also assess for anorexia, weight loss, and failure to grow.

■ Nursing Diagnosis and Planning

The following nursing diagnoses and expected outcomes may be appropriate to the child with juvenile arthritis and the child's family:
- Chronic Pain related to the inflammatory process.

Expected Outcome. The child's pain will decrease, as evidenced by increased participation in usual activities and verbal report of decreased pain.

- Impaired Physical Mobility related to inflammation of the joint and associated muscle weakness.

Expected Outcomes. As a result of appropriate activity and an ongoing exercise program, the child's joints will remain mobile. The child will correctly use any appropriate adaptive equipment to accomplish activities of daily living (ADLs) and participate in a regular exercise program. The child will show no signs of the hazards of immobility.

- Delayed Growth and Development related to activity intolerance.

Expected Outcomes. The child will exhibit age-appropriate behaviors. The parents will support and maintain appropriate developmental activities for their child.

- Disturbed Body Image related to activity intolerance.

Expected Outcomes. The child will maintain relationships with peers and participate in age-appropriate activities when able.

- Deficient Knowledge about the care and treatment of JIA related to unfamiliarity with the condition.

Expected Outcome. The parents will demonstrate safe home care and adherence to the treatment regimen and the prescribed exercise program.

Interventions

Managing Pain. Teach parents to identify both verbal and nonverbal pain indicators. Nonverbal cues are more difficult to recognize but may include restlessness, withdrawal, decreased attention span, increased crying, and decreased sleep. Maintaining a therapeutic blood level of pain medication is the most effective way to ensure maximal comfort. The nurse needs to teach parents the side effects of the prescribed medications and advise that most NSAIDs should be given with food or milk to prevent gastrointestinal irritation. Non-pharmacologic pain-relief measures such as diversion, splinting, heat or cold application, imagery, and meditation can be useful for some children.

Promoting Mobility. Teach positioning of inflamed joints, appropriate application of heat or cold, and how to support and protect the affected joints. Encourage families to be consistent with exercise programs prescribed by the physical and/or occupational therapist. Emphasize that isometric exercises and passive range-of-motion exercises will prevent contractures and deformities. Help the family to identify when there may be a flare in the child's condition, thus necessitating activity modification. If there are no restrictions per therapy, parents should promote the child's participation in age-appropriate activities.

The child may need more time than average to begin morning activities. Teach the parents to allow plenty of time for the child to awaken, take a warm shower or bath, and relieve morning joint stiffness. Keeping the child's room or bed warm is important. Administering the child's NSAID with a snack first thing in the morning and allowing the medication to take effect before the child arises may help reduce pain and stiffness.

Managing Potential Infections. Some of the medications used to treat JIA cause immunosuppression, so teach the parents to recognize the signs of possible infection and whom to notify. Medications may need to be temporarily withheld if the child is actively infected. Live-virus vaccinations, including varicella, MMR, and flu-mist, must be held while the child is on any DMARD or biologic medication. Encourage yearly flu vaccination with the injectable form.

Facilitating Emotional and Social Development. Acknowledge the child's and family's anxiety and allow family members to express concerns. Encourage expressive therapeutic activities such as doll play,

pounding boards, bean bags, clay, painting, and story composing. Therapeutic play provides a safe and effective mechanism for reducing the stress. The nurse should recognize that age, sex, and self-concept play a role in a child's adjustment to chronic illness. Use anticipatory guidance to help the child develop coping mechanisms that will foster the development of optimism and a sense of personal competence. Help the child identify strengths and areas of accomplishments to increase self-esteem. Identify creative hobbies or activities that will enhance the child's sense of self-worth.

Communicate with the school nurse about scheduling necessary rest periods for the child during the school day. The child might enjoy a short period of quiet activity in the school health office if allowed to bring a friend. School nurses can help with the child's transition to school by communicating with teachers about the child's needs.

Family Education. As part of the multidisciplinary approach, the nurse must take an active part in helping the child and parents learn how to cope with and adapt to the limitations of the disease. This includes referring them from the onset to sources of accurate information about the condition and its associated care. Information should be in a variety of types and appropriate for the child's developmental level. The Arthritis Foundation can provide information to parents and children. Parents also want to ensure that others in the community have an understanding of JIA. Increased understanding by others in the child's environment will increase the affected child's ability to maintain a normal, developmentally appropriate lifestyle.

Because most of the child's care takes place in the home, the success of the therapeutic plan will be determined by the parents. Planning begins as soon as possible in the course of the illness. The parents should be involved in as many nursing activities as possible. This will reduce their anxiety and increase their sense of control over difficult situations. Provide verbal and written instructions and use return demonstration to ensure parental understanding of procedures. Coordinate referrals and physical therapy with the child's and parents' routines and schedules.

Encourage the parents to provide a diet high in fiber, protein, and calcium and an adequate fluid intake. If the child has anorexia or pain while eating, consider smaller, more frequent high-calorie foods.

Emphasize regular visits to the ophthalmologist to evaluate the eyes for inflammation. Children with JIA should be referred to an ophthalmologist at diagnosis and for recommended periodic follow-ups (Wu et al., 2011).

Evaluation

- Does the child experience pain control, as evidenced by report of decreased pain, increased sleep, decreased restlessness and irritability, and increased participation in age-appropriate activities?
- Is the child free from joint inflammation, and does the child demonstrate age-appropriate range of motion and muscle strength?
- During an exacerbation, is the child able to accept activity restrictions and participate in the exercise program?
- Is the child free from respiratory problems or other problems associated with immobility?
- Is the child able to perform age-appropriate self-care activities?
- Do the parents demonstrate the ability to facilitate the child's growth and development within the limitations posed by the child's disease?
- Does the child demonstrate age-appropriate behaviors, increased social interactions with friends, and appropriate adaptation to school?
- Are the parents able to articulate and demonstrate solutions to care for problems encountered in the home?

KEY CONCEPTS

- The neurovascular assessment of a child in traction or a cast includes assessment of skin color, capillary refill time, temperature, sensation, and movement of digits in casted hand or foot, if exposed. The quality of the pulse distal to the site should also be evaluated and compared with that of the uninvolved extremity.

- When evaluating neurovascular status, remember to assess for the five Ps of ischemia—pain, pallor, pulselessness, paresthesia, and paralysis.

- Consequences of immobility include alterations in the integumentary, gastrointestinal, respiratory, genitourinary, and musculoskeletal systems as well as children's growth and psychological development.

- Musculoskeletal problems are frequently caused by trauma. Nonaccidental trauma or child abuse may be involved. Therefore, nursing assessment should always begin with a primary emergency survey.

- Treatment of fractures involves repositioning the bone fragments (reduction) and applying a cast or traction to maintain alignment (retention) until healing occurs.

- Nursing care of the child with osteomyelitis includes assessment and documentation of the child's status, pain management, and administration of antibiotics without iatrogenic injury.

- Frequently seen musculoskeletal developmental disorders include scoliosis, limb differences, developmental dysplasia of the hip (DDH), Legg-Calvé-Perthes disease, slipped capital femoral epiphysis (SCFE), and clubfoot. Each often requires splinting, traction, bracing, casting, or a combination. Similar approaches are used in the management of orthopedic anomalies related to various childhood syndromes.

- Nursing outcomes for a child with muscular dystrophy include maintaining physical activity, promoting respiratory function, managing weight, and reducing the impact of the disease on the child's development.

- Nursing outcomes for a child with JIA include keeping the child free from injury, controlling pain, enhancing physical mobility, and promoting age-appropriate developmental behaviors.

REFERENCES

Allen, S., Parent, E., Khorasani, M., et al. (2008). Validity and reliability of active shape models for the estimation of Cobb angle in patients with adolescent idiopathic scoliosis. *Journal of Digital Imaging, 21*(2), 208-218.

Anand, A., & Sala, D. A. (2008). Clubfoot: Etiology and treatment. *Indian Journal of Orthopaedics, 42*(1), 22-28.

Andrews, J. R., Baker, C. L., Bergfeld, J. A., & Nelson, B. J. (2010). Prevention and misconception are chief concerns in battling youth sports injuries. *Orthopedics Today, 30*(5), 9-12.

Bakody, E. (2009). Orthopaedic plaster casting: Nurse and patient education. *Nursing Standard, 23*(51), 49-56.

Basener, C. J., Mehlman, C. T., & Dipasquale, T. G. (2009). Growth disturbance after distal femoral growth plate fractures in children: A meta-analysis. *Journal of Orthopaedic Trauma, 23*(9), 663-667.

Betz, R. R., Lavelle, W. F., & Samdani, A. F. (2010). Bone grafting options in children. *Spine, 35*(17), 1648-1654.

Blackmur, J. P., & Murray, A. W. (2010). Do children who in-toe need to be referred to an orthopaedic clinic? *Journal of Pediatric Orthopaedics, 19*(5), 415-417.

Bone, C. M., & Hsieh, G. H. (2000). The risk of carcinogenesis from radiographs to pediatric orthopaedic patients. *Journal of Pediatric Orthopaedics, 20*, 251.

Brody, A. S., Frush, D. P., Huda, W., Brent, R. L., & American Academy of Pediatrics Section on Radiology. (2007). Radiation risk to children from computed tomography. *Pediatrics, 120*(3), 677-681.

Canto, M. J., Cano, S., Palau, J., & Ojeda, F. (2008). Prenatal diagnosis of clubfoot in low-risk population: Associated anomalies and long-term outcome. *Prenatal Diagnosis, 28*(4), 343-346.

Carreon, L. Y., Puno, R. M., Lenke, L. G., et al. (2007). Nonneurologic complications following surgery for adolescent idiopathic scoliosis. *Journal of Bone and Joint Surgery, 89*(11), 2427-2432.

Coe, J. D., Smith, J. S., Berven, S., et al. (2010). Complications of spinal fusion for Scheuermann kyphosis: A report of the Scoliosis Research Society Morbidity and Mortality Committee. *Spine, 35*(1), 99-103.

Dannecker, G. E., & Quartier, P. (2009). Juvenile idiopathic arthritis: Classification, clinical presentation and current treatments. *Hormone Research, 72*(1), 4-12.

Draper, D. O., & Knight, K. L. (2010). The relative importance of compression in RICES injury treatment. *Athletic Therapy Today, 15*(3), 23-25.

Fabry, G. (2010a). Clinical practice: Static, axial, and rotational deformities of the lower extremities in children. *European Journal of Pediatrics, 169*(2), 529-534.

Fabry, G. (2010b). Clinical practice: The hip from birth to adolescence. *European Journal of Pediatrics, 169*(2), 143-148.

Fan, J., Shi, D., & Jiang, Q., et al. (2009). Progress in researches on the molecular genetics of developmental dysplasia of the hip. *Chinese Journal of Medical Genetics, 26*(6), 674-677.

Farley, F. A., & Kay, R. M. (2010). Management of the multiply injured child. In J. H. Beaty & J. R. Kasser (Eds.), *Rockwood and Wilkins' fractures in children* (7th ed.). Philadelphia: Lippincott Williams & Wilkins.

Faulks, S., & Richards, B. S. (2009). Clubfoot treatment: Ponseti and French functional methods are equally effective. *Clinical Orthopaedics and Related Research, 467*(5), 1278-1282.

Firmin, F., & Crouch, R. (2009). Splinting versus casting of "torus" fractures to the distal radius in the paediatric patient presenting at the emergency department (ED): A literature review. *International Emergency Nursing, 17*, 173-178.

Fong, D. Y., Lee, C. F., Cheung, K. M., et al. (2010). A meta-analysis of the clinical effectiveness of school scoliosis screening. *Spine, 35*(10), 1061-1071.

Forster, E., & Fraser, J. (2007). Turning around talipes: Nursing considerations. *Neonatal, Paediatric & Child Health Nursing, 10*(1), 27-32.

Fujii, M., Nakashima, Y., Yamamoto, T., et al. (2010). Acetabular retroversion in developmental dysplasia of the hip. *Journal of Bone and Joint Surgery, 92*(4), 895-903.

Gacca, A. M. (2008). Radiation protection and safety in pediatric imaging. *Pediatric Annals, 37*(6), 383-387.

Geist, A., & Kuhn, R. (2009) Pharmacological approaches for pediatric patients with osteomyelitis: Current issues and answers. *Orthopedics, 32*(8), 573-577.

Gilbody, J., Thomas, G., & Ho, K. (2009). Acute versus gradual correction of idiopathic tibia vara in children: A systematic review. *Journal of Pediatric Orthopaedics, 29*(2), 110-114.

Goel, D. P., Buckley, R., deVries, G., et al. (2009). Prophylaxis of deep-vein thrombosis in fractures below the knee. *Journal of Bone and Joint Surgery, 91-B*(3), 388-394.

Goldberg, C. J., Moore, D. P., Fogarty, E. E., & Dowling, F. E. (2008). Scoliosis: A review. *Pediatric Surgery International, 24*(2), 129-144.

Gosselin, R. A., Heitto, M., & Zirkle, L. (2009). Cost-effectiveness of replacing skeletal traction by interlocked intramedullary nailing for femoral shaft fractures in a provincial trauma hospital in Cambodia. *International Orthopaedics, 33*, 1445-1448.

Hsu, A. R., Diaz, H. M., Penaranda, N. R. P., et al. (2009). Dynamic skeletal traction spica casts for paediatric femoral fractures in a resource-limited setting. *International Orthopaedics, 33*, 765-771.

Jacquemier, M., Glard, Y., Pomero, V., et al. (2008). Rotational profile of the lower limb in 1319 healthy children. *Gait & Posture, 28*, 187-193.

Javid, M., & Wedge, J. H. (2009). Radiographic results of combined Salter innominate and femoral osteotomy in Legg-Calvé-Perthes disease in older children. *Journal of Children's Orthopaedics, 3*(3), 229-234.

Jones, J. D., Gill, L., John, M., et al. (2009). Outcome analysis of surgery for Blount disease. *Journal of Pediatric Orthopaedics, 29*(7), 730-735.

Kaplan, S. (2011). Osteomyelitis. In R. Kliegman, B. Stanton, J. St. Geme, et al. (Eds.), *Nelson textbook of pediatrics* (19th ed., pp. 2394-2398). Philadelphia: Elsevier Saunders.

Katz, D. E., Herring, J. A., Browne, R. H., et al. (2010). Brace wear control of curve progression in adolescent idiopathic scoliosis. *Journal of Bone and Joint Surgery, 92*(6), 1343-1352.

Koteles, M. R., Jr., & Lewi, J. E. (2010). Slipped capital femoral epiphysis (SCFE) attributable to primary hypothyroidism. *Endocrine Practice, 16*(2), 340.

Krul, M., van der Wouden, J. C., Schellevis, F. G., et al. (2010). Acute non-traumatic hip pathology in children: Incidence and presentation in family practice. *Family Practice, 27*(2), 166-170.

Kruse, L. M., Dobbs, M. B., & Gurnett, C. A. (2008). Polygenic threshold model with sex dimorphism in clubfoot inheritance: The Carter effect. *Journal of Bone and Joint Surgery, 90*(12), 2688-2694.

Kundnani, V. K., Zhu, L., Tak, H. H., & Wong, H. K. (2010). Multimodal intraoperative neuromonitoring in corrective surgery for adolescent idiopathic scoliosis: Evaluation of 354 consecutive cases. *Indian Journal of Orthopaedics, 44*(1), 64-72.

Larson, A. N., Yu, E. M., Melton, L. J., 3rd, et al. (2010). Incidence of slipped capital femoral epiphysis: A population-based study. *Journal of Pediatric Orthopaedics*, 19(1), 9-12.

Lethaby, A., Temple, J., & Santy, J. (2008). Pin site care for preventing infections associated with external bone fixators and pins. *Cochrane Database of Systematic Reviews*, 4, Art. No. CD004551.

Milbrandt, T. A., Singhal, M., Minter, C., et al. (2009). A comparison of three methods of pain control for posterior spinal fusions in adolescent idiopathic scoliosis. *Spine*, 34(14), 1499-1503.

Mootha, A. K., Saini, R., Dhillon, M., et al. (2010). Do we need femoral derotation osteotomy in DDH of early walking age-group? A clinico-radiological correlation study. *Archives of Orthopaedic and Trauma Surgery*, 130(7), 853-858.

National Institute of Neurological Disorders and Stroke. (2009a). *NINDS muscular dystrophy information page*. Retrieved from www.ninds.nih.gov/disorders/md/detail_md.html.

National Institute of Neurological Disorders and Stroke. (2009b). *Muscular dystrophy: Hope through research*. Retrieved from www.ninds.nih.gov/disorders/md/detail_md.html.

Nault, M. L., Parent, S., Phan, P., et al. (2010). A modified Risser grading system predicts the curve acceleration phase of female adolescent idiopathic scoliosis. *Journal of Bone and Joint Surgery*, 92(5), 1073-1081.

Nelitz, M., Lippacher, S., Krauspe, R., & Reichel, H. (2009). Perthes disease: Current principles of diagnosis and treatment. *Deutsches Ärzteblatt International*, 106(31-32), 517-523.

O'Brien, S. H., Haley, K., Kelleher, K. J., et al. (2008). Variation in DVT prophylaxis for adolescent trauma patients: A survey of the Society of Trauma Nurses. *Journal of Trauma Nursing*, 15(2), 53-57.

Ponseti, I. (1992). Current concepts review: Treatment of congenital clubfoot. *Journal of Bone and Joint Surgery*, 74-A, 448-454.

Porth, C. (2011). *Essentials of pathophysiology* (3rd ed.). Philadelphia: Wolters Kluwer.

Ramirez, N., Flynn, J. M., Serrano, J. A., et al. (2009). The Vertical Expandable Prosthetic Titanium Rib in the treatment of spinal deformity due to progressive early onset scoliosis. *Journal of Pediatric Orthopaedics*, 18(4), 197-203.

Robert, C., Jiang, J., & Khoury, J. (2011). A prospective study on the effectiveness of cotton versus waterproof cast padding in maintaining the reduction of pediatric distal forearm fracture. *Journal of Pediatric Orthopaedics*, 31(2), 144-149.

Sabharwal, S. (2009). Blount disease. *Journal of Bone and Joint Surgery*, 91,1758-1776.

Sankar, W., Horn, D., Wells, L., & Dormans, J. (2011a). Legg-Calvé-Perthes disease. In R. Kliegman, B. Stanton, J. St. Geme, et al. (Eds.), *Nelson textbook of pediatrics* (19th ed., pp. 2361-2363). Philadelphia: Elsevier Saunders.

Sankar, W., Horn, D., Wells, L., & Dormans, J. (2011b). Slipped capital femoral epiphysis. In R. Kliegman, B. Stanton, J. St. Geme, et al. (Eds.), *Nelson textbook of pediatrics* (19th ed., pp. 2363-2365). Philadelphia: Elsevier Saunders.

Schwartz, D. M., Auerbach, J. D., Dormans, J. P., et al. (2007). Neurophysiological detection of impending spinal cord injury during scoliosis surgery. *Journal of Bone and Joint Surgery*, 89A(11), 2440-2449.

Scoliosis Research Society. (2010). *SRS/AAOS position statement: Screening for idiopathic scoliosis in adolescents*. Retrieved from www.srs.org/professionals/positions/?id=62.

Shannon, E. G., Difazio, R., Kasser, J., et al. (2005). Waterproof casts for immobilization of children's fractures and sprains. *Journal of Pediatric Orthopaedics*, 25(1), 56-59.

Shenoi, S., & Wallace, C. A. (2010). Remission in juvenile idiopathic arthritis: Current facts. *Current Rheumatology Reports*, 12, 80-86.

Sorbie, C. (2008). Blue notes. Clubfoot: Rising incidence—why? *Orthopedics*, 31(12), 1175.

Spence, G., Hocking, R., Wedge, J. H., & Roposch, A. (2009). Effect of innominate and femoral varus derotation osteotomy on acetabular development in developmental dysplasia of the hip. *Journal of Bone and Joint Surgery*, 91(11), 2622-2636.

Staheli, L. T. (2008). *Fundamentals of pediatric orthopedics* (4th ed., pp. 1-56, 90-92). Philadelphia: Wolters Kluwer Lippincott Williams & Wilkins.

Stevenson, D. A., Mineau, G., Kerber, R. A., et al. (2009). Familial predisposition to developmental dysplasia of the hip. *Journal of Pediatric Orthopedics*, 29(5), 463-466.

Sucato, D. J., Tulchin, K., Shrader, M. W., et al. (2010). Gait, hip strength and functional outcomes after a Ganz periacetabular osteotomy for adolescent hip dysplasia. *Journal of Pediatric Orthopedics*, 30(4), 344-350.

Tan, K. J., Moe, M. M., Vaithinathan, R., & Wong, H. K. (2009). Curve progression in idiopathic scoliosis: Follow-up study to skeletal maturity. *Spine 34*(7), 697-700.

Texas Scottish Rite Hospital for Children. (2008). In J. A. Herring, (Ed.), *Tachdjian's pediatric orthopaedics* (4th ed.). Philadelphia: Elsevier Saunders.

Thawrani, D., Sucato, D. J., Podeszwa, D. A., & Delarocha, A. (2010). Complications associated with the Bernese periacetabular osteotomy for hip dysplasia in adolescents. *Journal of Bone and Joint Surgery*, 92(8), 1707-1714.

Vitale, M. (2010). Epidemiology of fractures in children. In J. H. Beaty & J. R. Kasser (Eds.), *Rockwood and Wilkins' fractures in children* (7th ed.) Philadelphia: Lippincott Williams & Wilkins.

Vosmaer, A., Pereira, R. R., Koenderman, J. S., et al. (2010). Coagulation abnormalities in Legg-Calvé-Perthes disease. *Journal of Bone and Joint Surgery*, 92(1), 121-128.

Walton, M. J., Isaacson, Z., McMillan, D., et al. (2010). The success of management with the Pavlik harness for developmental dysplasia of the hip using a United Kingdom screening programme and ultrasound-guided supervision. *Journal of Bone and Joint Surgery*, 92(7), 1013-1016.

Wick, J. M., Konze, J., Alexander, K., & Sweeney, C. (2009). Infantile and juvenile scoliosis: The crooked path to diagnosis and treatment. *AORN Journal*, 90(3), 347-380.

Wise, C. A., Gao, X., Shoemaker, S., et al. (2008). Understanding genetic factors in idiopathic scoliosis, a complex disease of childhood. *Current Genomics*, 9(1), 51-59.

Wu, E., Van Mater, H., & Rabinovich, C.E. (2011). Juvenile idiopathic arthritis. In R. Kliegman, B. Stanton, J. St. Geme, et al. (Eds.), *Nelson textbook of pediatrics* (19th ed., pp. 829-839). Philadelphia: Elsevier Saunders.

Yildirim, Y., Bautista, S., & Davidson, R. S. (2008). Chondrolysis, osteonecrosis, and slip severity in patients with subsequent contralateral slipped capital femoral epiphysis. *Journal of Bone and Joint Surgery*, 90(3), 485-492.

Zionts, L. E., Zhao, G., Hitchcock, K., et al. (2010). Has the rate of extensive surgery to treat idiopathic clubfoot declined in the United States? *Journal of Bone and Joint Surgery*, 92(4), 882-889.

The Child with an Endocrine or Metabolic Alteration

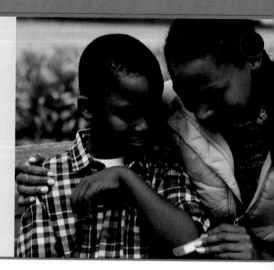

evolve WEBSITE

http://evolve.elsevier.com/James/ncoc

LEARNING OBJECTIVES

After studying this chapter, you should be able to:

- List the major hormones of the endocrine system.
- Describe negative feedback.
- Discuss nursing strategies to improve adherence with medication administration.
- Discuss and describe endocrine problems seen in the neonate.
- Describe the signs and symptoms of hypothyroidism versus hyperthyroidism.
- Compare and contrast diabetes insipidus and syndrome of inappropriate antidiuretic hormone as they relate to fluid and electrolyte balance.
- Describe the psychosocial issues concerning children with precocious puberty.
- Identify the role of insulin in the metabolism of carbohydrates, fats, and proteins in both the fasting and postprandial states.

- Compare and contrast type 1 diabetes mellitus and type 2 diabetes mellitus.
- Identify management goals and nursing implications of insulin therapy, diet therapy, exercise, self-monitoring of blood glucose, and urine ketone monitoring in the care of the child with type 1 diabetes.
- Describe the signs, symptoms, causes, and treatment of hypoglycemia and hyperglycemia in the child with diabetes.
- Identify the pathophysiology of diabetic ketoacidosis, and describe the management and nursing care of the child in diabetic ketoacidosis.
- Identify management goals and nursing implications of medication, diet therapy, exercise, and self-monitoring of blood glucose in the care of the child with type 2 diabetes.

CLINICAL REFERENCE

REVIEW OF THE ENDOCRINE SYSTEM

The endocrine system is composed of various tissues that produce and secrete chemicals called hormones. The hormones stimulate and regulate the actions of other tissues—the target tissues.

The endocrine system and the autonomic nervous system function in tandem to regulate growth, metabolism, and reproduction. The hypothalamic-pituitary axis controls their activities. The autonomic nervous system reacts to a stimulus, transmitting its message to the hypothalamus. In turn, the hypothalamus manufactures and secretes the appropriate hormonal factors. These are transmitted to the anterior pituitary gland, which then stimulates or inhibits the release of the involved hormones.

PEDIATRIC DIFFERENCES IN THE ENDOCRINE SYSTEM

The endocrine system is less developed at birth than any other body system. Hormonal control of many body functions is lacking until 12 to 18 months of age. As a result, infants may manifest imbalances in the concentration of fluids, electrolytes, amino acids, glucose, and trace substances.

The principle of feedback control is involved in hormone production and secretion. In negative feedback, increasing levels of a specific hormone begin to inhibit the system responsible for releasing that hormone. As the hormonal secretion rises, the secretion and production of its stimulating hormone decrease. Conversely, when too little

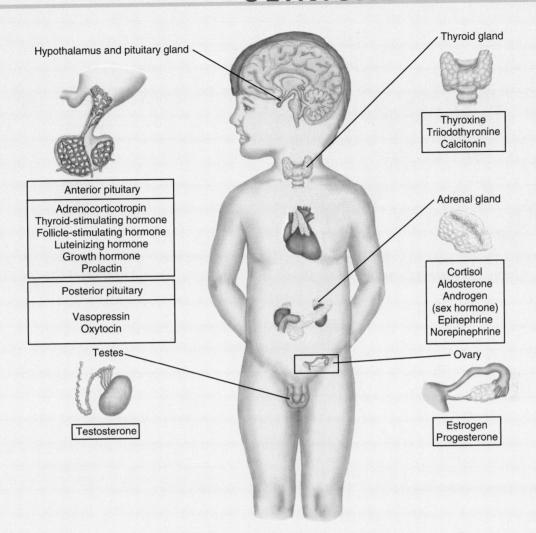

Hypothalamus and pituitary gland

Thyroid gland

Thyroxine
Triiodothyronine
Calcitonin

Anterior pituitary
Adrenocorticotropin
Thyroid-stimulating hormone
Follicle-stimulating hormone
Luteinizing hormone
Growth hormone
Prolactin

Posterior pituitary
Vasopressin
Oxytocin

Adrenal gland

Cortisol
Aldosterone
Androgen
(sex hormone)
Epinephrine
Norepinephrine

Testes

Ovary

Testosterone

Estrogen
Progesterone

Tissues and Hormones of the Endocrine System

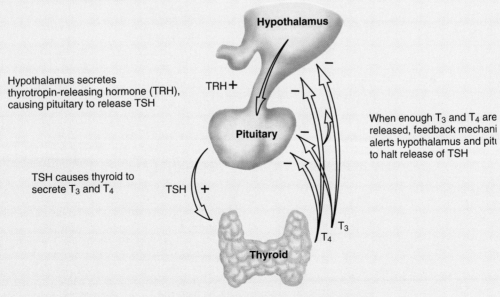

Hypothalamus

Hypothalamus secretes thyrotropin-releasing hormone (TRH), causing pituitary to release TSH

TRH +

−

Pituitary

When enough T_3 and T_4 are released, feedback mechani alerts hypothalamus and pit to halt release of TSH

−

TSH causes thyroid to secrete T_3 and T_4

TSH +

−

T_3

T_4

Thyroid

Feedback Control in Hormone Production

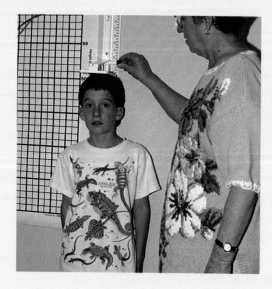

Fetal endocrine systems develop and function in utero. Portions of the endocrine system may be immature at birth but transition to more mature function after delivery.

DIAGNOSTIC TESTS AND PROCEDURES

Diagnosing endocrine dysfunction usually involves laboratory testing. Serum hormone levels are measured to determine if the amounts are adequate, deficient, or excessive. Laboratory screening is useful for diagnosing disease and monitoring children on hormone therapy.

Normal hormone levels are related to the child's age and stage of puberty. Because hormones are secreted at various times during the day or on a circadian rhythm, random blood samples may be difficult to interpret. Stimulation testing frequently demonstrates more accurate and definitive test results. With stimulation testing, a releasing factor or other agent is given to trigger the release or inhibition of a specific hormone. Serial blood sampling identifies the peak or trough level of the hormone, aiding in more accurate interpretation. A list of the common stimulation studies is provided in the accompanying table.

Other diagnostic tests include radiography and imaging techniques. Bone age radiographs can determine bone maturation, and from this, growth potential can be determined. Computed tomography (CT) scans and magnetic resonance imaging (MRI) are used to determine the presence of tumors or congenital malformations affecting the hypothalamus, pituitary, or target glands.

Accurate measurements of height and weight are essential when assessing the child for endocrine function. Evaluation of sexual development according to Tanner stages is also a part of the diagnostic workup (see Chapter 8). Developmental milestones and school performance should also be monitored because delays may be associated with endocrine disorders.

circulating hormone is present, the target gland is stimulated to secrete additional hormone.

The pituitary gland is composed of an anterior lobe and a posterior lobe. The anterior lobe secretes adrenocorticotropic hormone (ACTH), thyroid-stimulating hormone (TSH), follicle-stimulating hormone (FSH), luteinizing hormone (LH), growth hormone (GH), and prolactin. Four of these hormones (ACTH, TSH, LH, and FSH) in turn stimulate their target glands to secrete the appropriate specific hormones. The posterior pituitary lobe stores and releases antidiuretic hormone (ADH) and oxytocin, which are synthesized by the hypothalamus.

Congenital malformations, infections, and neoplastic or autoimmune processes may disrupt normal endocrine function of the hypothalamus, pituitary gland, or target gland.

COMMON LABORATORY AND DIAGNOSTIC TESTS OF ENDOCRINE FUNCTION

DESCRIPTION	NORMAL FINDINGS	INDICATIONS	PREPARATION AND NURSING CONSIDERATIONS
GH Test An agent (e.g., insulin, arginine, clonidine) is given to stimulate release of GH.	One or more peak levels of GH >7-10 ng/mL	Evaluate GH production. Identify GH deficiency.	Time specific; specimens must be drawn accurately. NPO after midnight. Notify physician if hypoglycemia or hypotension develops.
Cortrosyn Test Cortrosyn (ACTH) is given after baseline laboratory values have been obtained and 1 hr later. Tests adrenal glands' ability to function.	Cortisol should rise at least double the baseline Cortisol <18 mcg/dL suggests adrenal insufficiency	Evaluate adrenal production of cortisol. Identify infants with congenital adrenal hyperplasia.	Time specific; laboratory samples must be drawn before and 1 hr after Cortrosyn administration.
Factrel (Gonadorelin) Test GnRH is administered IV or subcutaneously to test the pituitary-ovarian axis for central precocious puberty.	For IV test, less than fourfold to fivefold rise in LH is observed For subcutaneous test, LH rises less than 8 ng/mL	Evaluate for central precocious puberty. Identify premature thelarche (breast development).	Time specific; specimens must be drawn accurately. IV test with serial sampling of LH and FSH. One laboratory sample drawn at 40 min for subcutaneous test.

ACTH, Adrenocorticotropic hormone; *FSH*, follicle-stimulating hormone; *GH*, growth hormone; *GnRH*, gonadotropin-releasing hormone; *LH*, luteinizing hormone.

COMMON LABORATORY AND DIAGNOSTIC TESTS OF ENDOCRINE FUNCTION—cont'd

DESCRIPTION	NORMAL FINDINGS	INDICATIONS	PREPARATION AND NURSING CONSIDERATIONS
Water Deprivation Test Child deprived of water and fluids for 7-8 hr.	Decreased urine output Increased urine specific gravity Normal serum sodium and osmolality	Confirm diagnosis of diabetes insipidus.	Strict monitoring of serum sodium and serum and urine osmolality. Weigh child before, during, and after test. Stop test if significant weight loss or change in vital signs or neurologic status develops.
hCG Test Intramuscular hCG is administered serially to stimulate testicular production of testosterone. Allows test for conversion of testosterone to DHT. Tests function of undescended testes.	Low levels of testosterone and DHT in prelaboratory samples Elevated levels of both testosterone and DHT—compare with known standards	Confirm testicular insufficiency. Confirm 5-alpha-reductase deficiency. Undescended testes may descend.	Time specific; draw samples before and after hCG. Monitor for testicular descent and increase in phallic length.

DHT, dihydrotestosterone; *hCG*, human chorionic gonadotropin.

Pediatric endocrine disorders are generally managed in the outpatient setting. Most endocrine disorders are chronic conditions requiring long-term nursing management. The nurse assumes a role of both educator and advocate for the child. Also important for the care of children with chronic medical problems is a careful psychosocial evaluation on a regular basis.

NEONATAL HYPOGLYCEMIA

Hypoglycemia is an abnormally low level of glucose (sugar) in the blood. It can result from an excessive rate of removal of glucose from the blood or from decreased secretion of glucose into the blood. Hypoglycemia in the neonate is defined as a plasma glucose concentration of less than 40 mg/dL.

Etiology

There are a number of risk factors for hypoglycemia in the neonate (Box 27-1). Hypoglycemia in some neonates results from hyperinsulinism, a genetic defect that affects beta cell regulation of insulin secretion (Cranmer & Shannon, 2009). Postterm and large-for-gestational-age (LGA) neonates are at higher risk than appropriate-for-gestational-age (AGA) term infants. Neonates who are most likely to have hypoglycemia are premature infants and infants who are small for gestational age (SGA). The SGA infant has a higher risk for hypoglycemia because of lower glycogen stores, decreased muscle protein, and decreased body fat (Cranmer & Shannon, 2009).

Incidence

The incidence of hypoglycemia varies with the infant's gestational age at birth and appropriateness of growth. In general, the incidence is 1.3 to 3 in 1000 live births (Cranmer & Shannon, 2009). The incidence is much higher in SGA infants.

BOX 27-1 RISK FACTORS FOR NEONATAL HYPOGLYCEMIA

- Prematurity
- Postmaturity
- Intrauterine growth restriction
- Large or small for gestational age
- Asphyxia
- Cold stress
- Problems at birth
- Maternal diabetes
- Maternal intake of terbutaline

Manifestations

Many infants with hypoglycemia are asymptomatic and are diagnosed because risk factors in their history have prompted glucose monitoring. The symptomatic neonate may demonstrate jitteriness, poor feeding, lethargy, seizures, respiratory alterations including apnea, hypotonia, high-pitched cry, bradycardia, cyanosis, and temperature instability.

Diagnostic Evaluation

Neonates who demonstrate risk factors for hypoglycemia are screened. A blood glucose concentration can be determined by a laboratory chemical test. Although this method is the most accurate, it is lengthy. For this reason, screening tests are used in most nurseries even though the results can vary. A blood glucose monitor is used to test a drop of blood, which can be obtained by a heel stick. Severely low readings are often verified by laboratory determinations, but intervention is initiated before the results are available because of the potential for sequelae

PATHOPHYSIOLOGY

Neonatal Hypoglycemia

Glucose is the major source of energy for the fetus and is transported from the mother across the placenta to the fetus. Glucose is used to support the rapid growth taking place. In the last weeks of gestation, excess glucose is stored in the liver and skeletal muscle as glycogen or converted to fatty acids and then stored as triglycerides in fat cells. Insulin is not transported across the placenta, requiring the fetus to produce insulin.

With the steady source of glucose from mothers stopped by the clamping of umbilical cords at delivery, infants must depend on their own hepatic glycogen stores and glucoregulatory mechanisms to mobilize and use glucose. Neonates undergo a decrease in glucose concentration, reaching the nadir (lowest level) at 1 to 3 hours of postnatal age.

The neonate's requirement for glucose is increased because of several factors. High energy needs postnatally result from increased metabolic and motor activity. The larger brain in proportion to body size requires glucose as its fuel source. Access to glucose is limited because of the neonate's immature liver enzyme system, including a decreased response to glucagon, the hormone that promotes the release of glucose from glycogen stores.

from prolonged hypoglycemia. Urinalysis may be performed to test for ketones, which are not present if the infant has hyperinsulinism. Other tests may be done to rule out underlying metabolic disorders.

Therapeutic Management

Infants who are hypoglycemic but asymptomatic may be fed breast milk, formula, or dextrose 5% in water. Frequent glucose checks are needed to monitor response. Neonates who are lethargic and not interested in nipple feeding can be gavage fed. If the blood glucose level is less than 20 to 25 mg/dL, intravenous (IV) glucose is given, first by bolus (dextrose 10% in water, 2.5 mL/kg) and then by continuous drip. The goal is to maintain a blood glucose level of at least 45 mg/dL (Cranmer & Shannon, 2009).

In some cases of intractable hypoglycemia, steroids may be used to stimulate gluconeogenesis from noncarbohydrate sources. Diazoxide may be given to suppress pancreatic insulin secretion in infants with hyperinsulinism.

Nursing Considerations

The assessment begins at the time of birth. Risk factors such as maternal diabetes, sepsis, shock, or perinatal asphyxia alert the nurse that the infant may be at risk for hypoglycemia. Determination is also made of gestational age and appropriateness of growth. Delays in enteral feedings or in the initiation of IV fluids also place the infant at higher risk. Inappropriate behavior or changes in behavior, including other commonly associated clinical signs and symptoms of hypoglycemia, are monitored.

Some infants may be asymptomatic. Infants at risk should be identified by obtaining a complete perinatal history to identify factors such as maternal hypertension, maternal diabetes, fetal distress, intrauterine growth retardation, or perinatal asphyxia. Because preterm, LGA, and SGA infants are at increased risk for hypoglycemia, a gestational age assessment should be performed. The infant's weight, length, and head circumference should be plotted on a growth curve to determine appropriateness of growth.

If an infant is at risk, a blood glucose level should be obtained with a screening strip (e.g., Dextrostix, Chemstrip bG) by 2 hours of age.

The puncture site is cleansed with an appropriate antiseptic solution and allowed to dry before the puncture (see Chapter 13). Blood glucose levels of less than 60 mg/dL should be reported.

Enteral feedings are provided by nipple or gavage, if required. The compromised infant may be unable to nipple feed safely as a result of respiratory distress or lethargy. The nurse monitors the IV site for signs of infiltration and treats an IV infiltrate with hyaluronidase, because glucose infiltration can cause severe extravasation.

Since hypothermia increases glucose requirements, the risk of hypoglycemia can be decreased by providing the infant with a neutral thermal environment. If signs and symptoms of hypoglycemia persist, the nurse notifies the physician according to protocol. Persistent hypoglycemia can require extensive medical evaluation and treatment.

NEONATAL HYPOCALCEMIA

Hypocalcemia results from inadequate stores of calcium, ineffective calcium homeostasis because of immature hormonal control, the inability to mobilize calcium, or interference with calcium usage. Neonatal hypocalcemia is defined as total serum calcium concentration of less than 7 mg/dL. Neonatal hypocalcemia occurs most often in infants of diabetic mothers because maternal diabetes causes functional hypoparathyroidism in the neonate (Singhal & Campbell, 2010). Other causes include birth asphyxia and SGA.

Neonates may experience twitching or tremors, irritability, jitteriness, electrocardiogram (ECG) changes, and, rarely, seizures. Some infants are asymptomatic but are screened because of history.

Ionized serum calcium levels are measured. Normal levels for blood ionized calcium range from 4 to 5 mg/dL. Initiation of feedings is often the only treatment necessary to correct early hypocalcemia. In infants who are limited in their enteral intake or who have significant hypocalcemia, therapy includes both oral and parenteral calcium administration. Oral supplements are given with enteral feedings. IV supplementation may be given as bolus doses or continuous infusion with IV fluids. If oral calcium is ordered, the nurse gives the medication with enteral feedings because it may cause gastric irritation. The IV site should be observed for signs of infiltration, and hyaluronidase is used to treat infiltrates. Extravasation of calcium-containing fluid can produce necrosis and ulceration. Many medications precipitate with calcium ions and should not be mixed together in IV lines. The nurse must not mix calcium with sodium bicarbonate because this combination also will form a precipitate in IV fluids. Persistent hypocalcemia requires further diagnostic evaluation.

PHENYLKETONURIA

Phenylketonuria (PKU) is a genetic metabolic disorder that results in central nervous system (CNS) damage from toxic levels of phenylalanine in the blood. PKU is characterized by a deficiency of phenylalanine hydroxylase, the enzyme needed to convert phenylalanine to tyrosine.

Etiology

PKU is an autosomal recessive disorder and is manifested only in the homozygote (individual who inherited two identical genes for a specific trait). With both parents carrying the recessive gene, each pregnancy has a 25% chance that the child will have PKU.

Incidence

PKU occurs in approximately 1 in 15,000 births in the United States (Arnold, 2009). It is more prevalent in some European countries.

Manifestations

The underlying metabolic alterations begin to have an immediate effect on the infant, although signs may not be apparent until the infant is approximately 3 months old. The first sign may be digestive problems with vomiting. These infants also may have a musty or mousy odor to the urine, infantile eczema, hypertonia, and hyperactive behavior. Older children may have hypopigmentation of the hair, skin, and irises; they are commonly blond with light blue eyes. Intellectual impairment is a long-term consequence of untreated PKU.

Diagnostic Evaluation

Routine neonatal screening for PKU is mandatory in all 50 states of the United States. With early postpartum discharge, screening is often performed at less than 2 days of age because of the concern that the infant will be lost to follow-up. Because the test depends on the accumulation of phenylalanine, screening done before the third day of life has a higher risk of a false-negative outcome. For this reason, testing should be done after the infant is 48 hours old, or, if done earlier, the test should be repeated at several days of age. Small quantities of blood are collected on filter paper cards. Screening is done by bacterial inhibition (Guthrie test) or chromatographic or fluorometric assays. A positive result is not diagnostic but indicates which infants should be evaluated further. PKU is characterized by serum phenylalanine levels greater than 20 mg/dL (normal level 2 mg/dL) (Arnold, 2009).

PATHOPHYSIOLOGY

Phenylketonuria

Phenylketonuria (PKU) refers to a group of biochemical diseases associated with enzymatic blocks in the conversion of the essential amino acid *phenylalanine* to *tyrosine*. Classic PKU consists of the absence of the enzyme *phenylalanine hydroxylase*. This deficiency results in the toxic accumulation of phenylalanine in the bloodstream after the ingestion of protein containing phenylalanine. Phenylalanine can adversely affect the myelinization process in CNS development. Most of that process takes place during the first decade of life. Intellectual impairment occurs and progresses if treatment is not implemented.

Therapeutic Management

Treatment should be instituted as soon as the diagnosis is confirmed because the best results are obtained with early treatment. Infants and children with PKU are treated with a special diet that restricts phenylalanine intake. Phenylalanine tolerance varies according to the infant and the severity of the enzyme deficiency. The goal of therapy is to keep the serum phenylalanine level at 2 to 6 mg/dL in infants and young children and 2 to 15 mg/dL in children older than 12 years of age. Phenylalanine intake should be limited while providing enough of this essential amino acid to meet the baby's growth requirement. Dietary management must be started early in neonatal life because the untreated infant will show evidence of CNS damage by several weeks of age. The age at which the diet may be discontinued is a point of controversy. Most health care facilities in the United States recommend lifelong continuation of the diet (Arnold, 2009). Cofactor tetrahydrobioprotein (Kuvan), a medication that can lower blood phenylalanine level, may be appropriate for some individuals with PKU (Arnold, 2009).

Another consideration is genetic counseling for women with PKU who become pregnant. Adolescent girls and women of childbearing age require counseling about fetal risks including mental deficiency,

microcephaly, retarded growth, seizures, and an increased incidence of structural defects. The goal is to control phenylalanine levels before conception and maintain strict control during the pregnancy.

Nursing Considerations

Although a family history of PKU would alert the caregiver to an infant at risk, most infants with PKU are not identified at birth. Neonatal symptoms are usually not present. A screening test, part of the newborn screen done in all states, is the first diagnostic procedure. Newborn screenings usually include testing for PKU and congenital hypothyroidism, as well as any other screening tests mandated by local and state public health departments, such as sickle cell trait, galactosemia, and maple syrup urine disease. A positive screening result requires further diagnostic evaluation to verify the diagnosis.

A low-phenylalanine diet is begun immediately; the infant with PKU is fed a low-phenylalanine formula and, as foods are introduced, the child must follow a protein-restricted diet. The child must avoid high-protein foods such as meats, fish, eggs, cheese, milk, and legumes. Because protein is also present in grains, low-protein breads, cereals, and pastas are used. Dietary staples are vegetables, fruits, and starches. To avoid the consequences of insufficient protein for growth, children with PKU may take a phenylalanine-free protein supplement. The growth pattern and neurobehavior of the affected child must be monitored.

Follow-up is provided for all infants if the initial screening result is abnormal. The nurse assists with referral to a genetic center that is capable of diagnosing and treating the infant.

Phenylalanine requirements change rapidly in the first months of life. Parents are encouraged to adhere to monitoring requirements for the infant diagnosed with PKU. Rigid regimens for diet control will not be successful unless the family accepts the changes required. The nurse helps the family deal with lifestyle changes by initiating referrals as needed (e.g., to social service agencies, registered dietitian, support groups). On-line support groups and chat rooms provide ideas for adapting recipes; specialized cookbooks are also available.

The nurse encourages the parents to express their feelings about the infant's diagnosis and the risk of PKU in future children. Family members need support to recognize the problems caused by the disease and identify strategies for dealing with the stress of having a child with a chronic illness. Physical measurements and neurologic and intellectual development should be documented through standardized testing. If control of the phenylalanine level is established early, normal infant growth and development should occur.

INBORN ERRORS OF METABOLISM

In addition to PKU, there are other genetically transmitted metabolic diseases that rarely occur in newborns (Table 27-1). Nurses should create a climate in which parents can express their feelings about the lifelong care of their child, as well as concerns for future pregnancies. Families with affected infants are referred to genetic counseling centers. Many of these infants are identified through universal newborn screening or screening specific for at-risk infants. Additional nursing care is related to the particular disorder but is similar to that for the child with PKU.

CONGENITAL ADRENAL HYPERPLASIA

Congenital adrenal hyperplasia (CAH) is a group of disorders in which the adrenal gland is not able to manufacture adequate glucocorticoid and, while working to make glucocorticoid, produces excess

TABLE 27-1   INBORN ERRORS OF METABOLISM

DESCRIPTION	MANAGEMENT
Galactosemia A deficiency of galactose-1-phosphate uridyltransferase prevents the conversion of galactose to glucose in lactose digestion. Infants cannot properly digest milk or sugar. Although rare (1 in 40,000-60,000 live births), infants exhibit intrauterine growth retardation, hypotonia, liver damage, cataracts, and infections. The urine contains reducing substances. Vomiting and diarrhea occur after feedings.	The child is on a lifelong lactose-restricted diet and close monitoring for and treatment of infections. If untreated, the infant usually dies; infants who have been treated may have developmental or learning deficits. The condition is genetically transmitted through an autosomal recessive inheritance pattern; referral to a genetic counseling center is warranted.
Maple Syrup Urine Disease This is a very rare (1 in 250,000-300,000 live births) autosomal recessive inherited condition that affects metabolism of certain amino acids. Buildup of acids causes ketoacidosis, which appears 48-72 hr after birth. The infant is lethargic and can display poor feeding, vomiting, weight loss, seizures, and loss of reflexes. The urine smells like maple syrup.	Dialysis is needed to reduce accumulated acids. The child must be on a lifelong low-protein, limited amino acid diet. If untreated, the child can die quickly; children who have been treated can have neurologic deficits. Referral to a genetic counseling center is warranted.
Tay-Sachs Disease A genetic condition that affects primarily infants in the Ashkenazi Jewish population. It is caused by an abnormal buildup of gangliosides (normal constituents in nerve synapse membrane) in the neurons. After a 6-month period of relatively normal development, the infant begins to demonstrate developmental delay and progressive neurologic deterioration. The infant usually exhibits macrocephaly, seizures, blindness, and deafness; death occurs during early childhood.	Management is symptomatic and supportive to the child and family. Referral to a genetic counseling center is essential.

Data from Rezvani, I., & Rezvani, G. (2011). An approach to inborn errors of metabolism. In R. Kliegman, B. Stanton, J. St. Geme, et al. (Eds.), *Nelson textbook of pediatrics* (19th ed., pp. 416-418). Philadelphia: Elsevier Saunders.

androgens. CAH is caused by a defect in the enzymatic pathway of adrenal steroid production. Diminished glucocorticoid production prompts increased ACTH production, further increasing adrenal androgen excess. Mineralocorticoid production may be normal or low.

Etiology

Infants with diminished mineralocorticoid production will waste salt through the kidneys, resulting in a "salt-wasting" crisis. This occurs with the more life-threatening form of CAH, which makes up 50% of cases and is the most common type (Wilson, 2010). Salt-wasting crisis results in hypovolemia, low serum sodium levels, hypotensive crisis, and hyperkalemia. Several enzymatic defects have been identified, the most common being 21-hydroxylase deficiency (CYP21). CAH is an autosomal recessive condition.

Manifestations

CAH is marked by ambiguous genitalia of the newborn female infant; postnatal virilization in both sexes; and salt-wasting crisis (in the first few weeks of life) with low serum sodium, high serum potassium, hypovolemia, and hypotensive crisis. Simple virilizing CAH is not associated with a salt-wasting crisis and manifests with a muscular body, advanced bone age, and premature pubic hair. Typically this form is seen later in infancy or early childhood. Untreated or poorly treated CAH can result in an advanced bone age with ultimate adult short stature. A milder form of CAH, 3-beta-hydroxysteroid dehydrogenase (3β-HSD), may become symptomatic during childhood or adolescence, with the child manifesting hirsutism, menstrual irregularities, or delayed menses.

Diagnostic Evaluation

The finding of ambiguous genitalia in the newborn infant should raise the possibility of CAH. The diagnosis is confirmed by elevated values of 17-hydroxyprogesterone, a glucocorticoid precursor. CAH is a part of newborn screening in many states. An appropriate evaluation includes obtaining serum electrolyte carbon dioxide, and renin levels, and performing a physical examination. Serum sodium levels in the infant suspected of CAH will be low, with elevated serum potassium. Serum renin levels will be elevated, indicating mineralocorticoid deficiency. A karyotype to determine genetic sex may be indicated depending on the degree of genital ambiguity.

Therapeutic Management

An accurate diagnosis and prompt treatment of fluid and electrolyte abnormalities may avert a salt-wasting crisis. The child with CAH requires lifelong glucocorticoid therapy. An oral glucocorticoid (hydrocortisone acetate, cortisone acetate) dosage is prescribed on the basis of body size and is given two or three times per day in either a liquid suspension or tablet form. For children with salt-wasting CAH, mineralocorticoid replacement therapy is required using fludrocortisone acetate (Florinef) which is taken once or twice daily. Therapy effectiveness is evaluated with serum electrolyte, 17-hydroxyprogesterone level, and renin levels. Special sick-day instructions should be provided to the family. The glucocorticoid dosage is usually doubled or tripled when the child is ill, has a broken bone, or is undergoing a surgical procedure. Bone age radiographs are performed yearly to assess skeletal maturity; poor adherence to the medication regimen or undertreatment can result in advanced bone age and decreased final adult height.

Nursing Considerations

All newborn girls should be assessed for ambiguous genitalia; fused labia, enlarged clitoris, or migration of urethral opening. Infant boys with unexplained dehydration and low serum sodium levels should be considered to have adrenal insufficiency, and undergo careful assessment of fluid and electrolyte status.

Infant girls with ambiguous genitalia might require reconstructive surgery. Depending on degree of virilization, surgical correction may

Congenital Adrenal Hyperplasia

- Children with salt-wasting congenital adrenal hyperplasia (CAH) require glucocorticoid replacement to survive.
- In the event of significant stress, such as fever, broken bone, or surgery, children with CAH will require "stress dose" medical therapy.
- If the child with CAH begins to vomit, the glucocorticoid must be administered parenterally.
- Mineralocorticoid therapy is required in salt-wasting CAH.
- Supplemental sodium occasionally may also be required.

be recommended in infancy or in early puberty. When appropriate, the nurse reassures the parents that the infant has appropriate internal structures and that external structures can be corrected surgically. Parents are encouraged to express their concerns. The nurse helps to facilitate parent-infant attachment.

Older children receiving glucocorticoid replacement therapy are assessed for linear growth and signs of early puberty. Serial height measurements can provide data about the adequacy of glucocorticoid supplementation. In children with salt-wasting CAH, serum renin levels should be closely monitored; effective treatment with mineralocorticoids will maintain these levels in or near the normal range (White, 2011). Nonadherence can cause early virilization, increased growth velocity, diminished final adult height, and menstrual irregularities in girls. Blood pressure monitoring is important for children receiving mineralocorticoid replacement therapy.

The nurse carefully instructs the parents about replacement hormone administration and the timing of medication. Parents are included in the development of a plan for sick-day dosages of medications. The infant with salt-wasting CAH may require salt supplements; the family needs instruction on preparation of these supplements.

Follow-up evaluations with the endocrinologist are scheduled every 2 to 3 months in infancy and every 4 to 6 months in the older child. Parents of the child with CAH should be referred to a genetic counselor if they plan more pregnancies because future children are at risk for CAH. In utero treatment is available to prevent virilization of the female fetus. If effective, this prenatal treatment eliminates the need for surgical correction of ambiguous genitalia in the affected female infant.

Adolescents are encouraged to assume increasing responsibility for medication administration. The nurse strongly emphasizes the importance of compliance. Surgical reconstruction of the genitalia and vaginal dilation may be required in the adolescent years. Careful explanations and preparation for these procedures will reassure affected adolescents and help them understand the expected outcomes following the procedures.

CONGENITAL HYPOTHYROIDISM

Congenital hypothyroidism is a condition in which the thyroid gland does not produce sufficient thyroid hormone to meet the body's metabolic needs. The condition is present from birth and, if not treated, can lead to intellectual impairment.

Etiology

Congenital hypothyroidism is caused by an absent (aplastic), under-developed, or ectopic thyroid gland. This group of congenital defects is referred to as *thyroid dysgenesis.* For unknown reasons, the fetal

thyroid gland fails to develop properly or fails to migrate to the appropriate location. Other rare causes are hypothalamic or pituitary disorders in which TSH secretion is insufficient to stimulate the thyroid gland. Biochemical defects in thyroid hormone production also cause congenital hypothyroidism. Maternal intake of medications such as propylthiouracil (PTU) during pregnancy to control maternal hyperthyroidism can cause transient hypothyroidism in the infant. Transfer of maternal antibodies to the fetus may also cause transient hypothyroidism (Postellon, 2010).

PATHOPHYSIOLOGY

Congenital Hypothyroidism

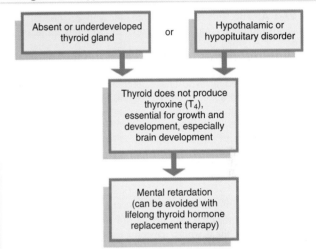

The thyroid gland is a butterfly-shaped gland located in front of the neck. Thyroid stimulating hormone (TSH), secreted by the pituitary, induces the thyroid to produce T_4 (thyroxine) and T_3 (triiodothyronine). The thyroid traps iodine and produces T_4, which is essential for normal growth and development, especially brain development, in the first 2 years of life. Immediately after delivery, TSH increases dramatically, likely related to the stress of the birth process. Within the first week of life, the TSH level gradually falls.

Underdevelopment of the thyroid gland or a hypothalamic or pituitary disorder causes inadequate production of T_4, which is essential for brain development. If not treated, this can cause intellectual impairment in the developing child. An infant with congenital hypothyroidism has elevated TSH and low T_4 levels.

Incidence

The incidence of congenital hypothyroidism in the United States is approximately 1 in 4000 live births (Postellon, 2010). Because untreated hypothyroidism causes mental retardation, all states have mandatory newborn screening programs to diagnose hypothyroidism before symptoms occur. Early detection and treatment favor increased intellectual function. Most occurrences are spontaneous, with a smaller percentage having a genetic (autosomal recessive) inheritance that results in defective thyroxine synthesis (Postellon, 2010).

Manifestations

The infant with congenital hypothyroidism often displays signs of (Figure 27-1) skin mottling, a large fontanel, a large tongue, hypotonia, slow reflexes, and a distended abdomen. Other signs and symptoms include prolonged jaundice, lethargy, constipation, feeding problems,

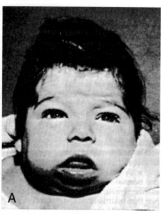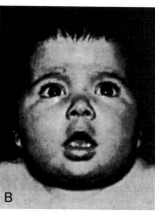

FIG 27-1 A, This untreated 6-month-old with congenital hypothyroidism fed poorly and was constipated. She was lethargic and had no social smile or head control. Note her puffy face, large tongue, dull expression, and excessive hair growth (hirsutism) on the forehead. **B,** The same infant 4 months after treatment. Note the decreased facial puffiness, decreased forehead hirsutism, and an alert appearance. (From LaFranchi, S. [2011]. Hypothyroidism. In R. Kliegman, B. Stanton, J. St. Geme, et al. [Eds.], *Nelson textbook of pediatrics* [19th ed., p. 1898]. Philadelphia: Elsevier Saunders.)

coldness to touch, umbilical hernia, hoarse cry, and excessive sleeping. The infant with congenital hypothyroidism may have none of these signs or symptoms; the newborn screening test is essential to recognize these infants.

Diagnostic Evaluation

Congenital hypothyroidism is usually diagnosed by testing of the serum T_4 level with newborn screening. Ideally, testing should be performed at 2 to 6 days of age. Tests performed sooner than 48 hours after delivery may be falsely interpreted because of the rise in TSH immediately after birth as part of the normal newborn transition. For a newborn with a low T_4 value, a TSH level will be obtained. A low T_4 level with TSH elevation is indicative of congenital hypothyroidism; further testing is often done to determine the cause (LaFranchi, 2011b). Thyroid scans can identify any functioning thyroid tissue. Treatment should never be delayed while waiting for scan results.

Therapeutic Management

Treatment of children with congenital hypothyroidism consists of lifelong thyroid hormone replacement, usually in the form of levothyroxine. It is given as a single daily oral dose that varies with the weight and age of the child or adult (Postellon, 2010). The dosage is titrated to maintain TSH and thyroxine (T_4) in a normal range.

NURSING CARE OF THE INFANT WITH CONGENITAL HYPOTHYROIDISM

■ Assessment

Nursing care of the infant with congenital hypothyroidism involves assessing growth and development and ensuring adherence to the prescribed medication regimen. Nurses can play a major role in recognizing the infant with hypothyroidism. Intellectual impairment

caused by untreated hypothyroidism cannot be reversed, but it can be prevented through early identification and proper treatment. In general, infants with hypothyroidism are evaluated every 1 to 2 months for the first year of life and then every 3 to 6 months thereafter. The nurse should obtain accurate measurements of height, weight, and head circumference at each visit. Frequent developmental assessments are also essential.

■ Nursing Diagnosis and Planning

The following nursing diagnoses and expected outcomes may be appropriate for the infant with congenital hypothyroidism and the infant's parents:

- Deficient Knowledge related to unfamiliarity with the congenital disorder.

Expected Outcomes. The parents will demonstrate the ability to monitor their infant for signs and symptoms of hypothyroidism and hyperthyroidism and give thyroid medication properly. The parents will verbalize an understanding of normal growth and developmental milestones and their child's lifelong needs for care and follow-up.

- Delayed Growth and Development related to disease process.

Expected Outcome. As a result of appropriate disease management, the infant will demonstrate growth and developmental milestones appropriate for age.

- Ineffective Thermoregulation related to decreased basal metabolic rate.

Expected Outcome. As a result of disease management, the infant will maintain a temperature within normal range.

■ Interventions

The nurse instructs family members on the importance of medication adherence emphasizing that the medication is necessary for the child's growth, especially for the rapidly developing brain.

The family is taught how to administer levothyroxine orally as a single daily dose. It can be dissolved in a small amount of water and given by syringe or placed into the nipple of a baby bottle (see Chapter 14). When the infant is older, the medication can be given in a spoonful of baby food. Toddlers can usually chew tablets without difficulty. If the infant or child vomits within 1 hour of taking medication, the dose should be readministered. Frequently missed doses can lead to developmental delays and poor growth.

> ### ! NURSING QUALITY ALERT
> #### *The Child with Congenital Hypothyroidism*
>
> - Untreated hypothyroidism leads to intellectual impairment.
> - T_4 and TSH levels vary with age, but any infant with a low T_4 and an elevated TSH value rising to greater than 100 mU/L, is considered to have primary hypothyroidism until proven otherwise.*

*LaFranchi, S. (2011). Hypothyroidism. In R. Kliegman, B. Stanton, J. St. Geme, et al. (Eds.), *Nelson textbook of pediatrics* (19th ed., pp. 1895-1903). Philadelphia: Elsevier Saunders.

The nurse also teaches the parents the signs and symptoms of both hypothyroidism and hyperthyroidism and when to notify the physician if symptoms occur. Hyperthyroidism can develop in infants receiving too much medication. Parents need to be taught to count their child's pulse and notify their health care provider if the rate is greater than the recommended parameter.

Because hypothyroidism is a lifelong condition, school-age children and teenagers should be made aware of the importance of taking their medication and of keeping regular follow-up appointments with the physician.

■ Evaluation

*   Have the parents demonstrated the ability to monitor the child's signs and symptoms, recognize growth and developmental problems, administer the medication, and discuss the child's lifelong needs for care and follow-up?
*   Is the child developing appropriately for age according to growth charts and formalized developmental screening tests?
*   Does the child have normal results on thyroid function tests?
*   Is the child's body temperature within normal limits?

ACQUIRED HYPOTHYROIDISM

Hypothyroidism is a condition in which the thyroid gland produces an inadequate amount of thyroid hormone to meet the body's metabolic needs.

Etiology

Hashimoto's thyroiditis, a common cause of acquired hypothyroidism, is usually associated with a goiter. It is the result of an autoimmune process. Other causes of acquired hypothyroidism include surgical thyroidectomy, radioactive iodine therapy for hyperthyroidism, radiation therapy for malignancies, and excessive iodine ingestion. Less frequently, decreased TSH secretion by the pituitary gland or decreased thyrotropin-releasing hormone (TRH) secretion by the hypothalamus causes hypothyroidism.

Autoimmune thyroiditis is the most common cause of acquired hypothyroidism in children and adolescents (LaFranchi, 2011b). It often occurs in families with a history of thyroid disease. Other family members may have positive thyroid antibodies. Thyroiditis is more common in girls, with as many as 10% of young girls exhibiting signs of autoimmune thyroid dysfunction, most often chronic lymphocytic thyroiditis (Ferry & Bauer, 2010).

Pathophysiology

Circulating autoantibodies known as *thyroid-blocking immunoglobulins* decrease thyroid gland production of triiodothyronine (T_3) and T_4. These antibodies bind at the TSH receptor sites on the thyroid gland, resulting in decreased thyroid hormone production. The cause of antibody production is unknown.

In contrast to congenital hypothyroidism, adverse effects from hypothyroidism acquired after 2 to 3 years of age are often reversible. Goiter, an enlarged thyroid gland, occurs in response to increased TSH secretion, autoimmune attack of the thyroid gland, or goitrogens.

Manifestations

Clinical manifestations of hypothyroidism include goiter (one lobe frequently larger than the other); dry, thick skin; coarse, dull hair; fatigue; cold intolerance; constipation; weight gain; decreased linear growth; edema of face, eyes, and hands; and irregular or delayed menses (see Box 27-2).

Diagnostic Evaluation

Elevated TSH and low T_4 levels are diagnostic of hypothyroidism. Elevated TSH level is the most sensitive indicator of primary hypothyroidism.

Thyroiditis is diagnosed by the presence of circulating thyroid antibodies and is usually associated with a firm goiter. Initially TSH is elevated with normal T_4 levels, although T_4 decreases over time. With secondary or tertiary hypothyroidism, TSH is not elevated; therefore, thyroid-releasing hormone stimulation testing is usually required for diagnosis.

Therapeutic Management

Management of the child with hypothyroidism involves thyroid hormone replacement, usually with levothyroxine. Dosage varies according to the child's age and weight and is given as a single daily dose. The dose is titrated to maintain T_4 in the upper half of the normal range and to maintain TSH in the normal range for age.

NURSING CARE OF THE CHILD WITH ACQUIRED HYPOTHYROIDISM

■ Assessment

Care of the child with acquired hypothyroidism includes assessing response to treatment and adherence to the medication regimen. With treatment, the goiter should decrease in size. Signs and symptoms of hypothyroidism should also resolve with adequate thyroid hormone replacement. Monitoring height and weight, and conducting developmental screening at each clinic visit assesses the child's growth and development. The nurse should monitor school performance as well and maintain contact with the school nurse.

■ Nursing Diagnosis and Planning

The following nursing diagnoses and expected outcomes may be appropriate for a child with acquired hypothyroidism:

*   Constipation related to decreased basal metabolic rate as a result of hypothyroidism.

Expected Outcome. The child will maintain regular bowel movements of normal consistency as basal metabolic rate improves.

*   Activity Intolerance related to fatigue.

Expected Outcome. The child will maintain normal energy levels for age, as evidenced by the ability to exercise at the same level as peers.

*   Disturbed Body Image related to weight gain/obesity.

Expected Outcomes. The child will verbalize feelings about body changes and will accept reassurances that changes will resolve with treatment.

*   Ineffective Thermoregulation related to decreased basal metabolic rate secondary to hypothyroidism.

Expected Outcome. As a result of appropriate disease management, the child will maintain normal body temperature.

■ Interventions

Parents and children who are school age or older should be instructed on the correct dose and timing of thyroid medication. Thyroid hormone levels are usually checked every 3 to 6 months. Laboratory values within the normal range indicate good response to therapy. The nurse educates the older child and parents on the signs and symptoms of hypothyroidism and hyperthyroidism and to notify the physician if symptoms occur. The child is reassured that signs such as constipation, fatigue, and weight gain will resolve as the medication becomes effective.

■ Evaluation

*   Has the child maintained regular bowel movements of normal consistency?

- Can the child tolerate exercise at the same level as peers?
- Does the child express feelings related to body changes and accept reassurances that problems will resolve?
- Has the child maintained normal body temperature?

HYPERTHYROIDISM (GRAVES DISEASE)

Graves disease is an autoimmune condition in which excessive thyroid hormones are produced by an enlarged thyroid gland. It is the most common cause of hyperthyroidism in children.

Incidence

The incidence of Graves disease in children is approximately 1 in 5000, with girls being five times more likely than boys to acquire the condition. Peak age for acquiring the condition is between 10 and 14 years (Ferry & Levitsky, 2010). Graves disease may also have a familial tendency (Ferry & Levitsky, 2010). Children with autoimmune disease are at risk for other autoimmune disorders. Neonatal Graves disease is associated with maternal hyperthyroidism and is relatively uncommon.

Pathophysiology

Circulating autoantibodies known as *thyroid-stimulating immunoglobulins* (TSIs) stimulate the thyroid gland to make T_3 and T_4. These antibodies bind to the TSH receptor sites on the thyroid gland, resulting in excessive thyroid hormone production. The cause of antibody production is unknown. In newborns, maternal TSI is transferred through the placenta to the fetus. TSIs bind to the TSH receptor, causing neonatal hyperthyroidism.

Manifestations

Goiter, increased appetite, weight loss, nervousness, diarrhea, increased perspiration, heat intolerance, increased heart rate, muscle weakness, palpitations, tremors, exophthalmos, poor attention span, and behavior or school problems are common in Graves disease (Box 27-2). In the neonate, irritability, tachycardia, hypertension, voracious appetite with poor weight gain, flushing, prominent eyes, and thyroid enlargement are major signs. These are self-limiting signs, but cardiac failure and death can occur if the signs are unrecognized or poorly treated.

BOX 27-2	INDICATORS OF HYPOTHYROIDISM OR HYPERTHYROIDISM	
HYPOTHYROIDISM	**HYPERTHYROIDISM**
Fatigue	Emotional lability, anxiety
Constipation	Diarrhea
Cold intolerance	Heat intolerance
Weight gain	Weight loss, increased appetite
Dry, thick skin	Smooth, velvety skin
Edema of face, eyes, hands (myxedema)	Prominent eyes
Decreased growth, delayed skeletal maturation and puberty	Accelerated linear growth
Decreased activity and energy	Hyperactivity
Muscle hypertrophy (psydodystrophy)	Muscle weakness
Decreased heart rate	Increased heart rate
Increased need for sleep	High blood pressure
Ataxia	Tremor

Diagnostic Evaluation

Elevated serum T_4 levels and suppressed TSH levels, associated with signs and symptoms of hyperthyroidism, suggest Graves disease. Autoantibodies to thyroid tissue usually are positive. Thyroid uptake of radioactive iodine is increased.

Therapeutic Management

The three approaches to the management of Graves disease are antithyroid drug therapy, radioactive iodine, or surgery. Antithyroid drug therapy with methimazole is the treatment of choice for childhood hyperthyroidism. Propylthiouracil (PTU), because of its increased risk for liver toxicity, should only be used in children who are allergic to methimazole (Ferry & Levitsky, 2010). These drugs act by blocking thyroid hormone production by the thyroid gland (Ferry & Levitsky, 2010). The medications usually are given three times per day, and they lower thyroid hormone levels in several weeks. Minor adverse effects include arthralgia, skin rash, pruritus, and gastric intolerance. Major adverse effects may include neutropenia, hepatotoxicity, and hypothyroidism.

A second approach to management is oral radioactive iodine treatment. Radioactive iodine (^{131}I) is given as an oral solution. It is typically used in children older than 10 years. With this therapy, the radioactive iodine is absorbed and concentrated by the thyroid gland, destroying the thyroid tissue in approximately 6 to 18 weeks. Hyperthyroid symptoms may intensify briefly after treatment. Hypothyroidism can result once the thyroid gland is irradiated, necessitating thyroid replacement therapy.

Subtotal or partial thyroidectomy, the surgical removal of thyroid gland tissue, is the third form of management. Lugol's solution (potassium iodide), given 10 to 14 days before surgery, decreases the gland's vascularity. Surgery carries the risk of injury to the parathyroid glands, resulting in hypocalcemia. Calcium levels are monitored after surgery.

Recurrence of hyperthyroidism is uncommon but possible. Affected children also have a 60% to 80% chance for developing hypothyroidism, which can be treated with thyroid replacement therapy.

Follow-up evaluations correlate with response to therapy. As thyroid functions normalize, follow-up endocrine evaluations are recommended once or twice per year.

NURSING CARE OF THE CHILD WITH HYPERTHYROIDISM

■ Assessment

The treatment goals consist of normalizing thyroid hormone levels, alleviating symptoms of hyperthyroidism, and decreasing the goiter.

The nurse should assess for adherence to medical therapy and determine if the family understands that medical therapy might take several weeks to decrease thyroid hormone action. The child is closely monitored for adrenergic signs and symptoms. Propranolol, a beta-adrenergic blocker, may be prescribed to decrease adrenergic signs and symptoms (tachycardia, heat intolerance, tremor) until the antithyroid medication takes effect.

A child being treated with propylthiouracil has an increased risk of neutropenia and hepatotoxicity; regular blood counts and liver function studies are done to assess these risks. The nurses assesses the child for fever, joint pain, edema, rash, or excessive bruising. A child who acquires a fever or sore throat while receiving propylthiouracil should be evaluated by a physician and a complete blood count obtained.

■ Nursing Diagnosis and Planning

The following nursing diagnoses and expected outcomes may be appropriate for a child with hyperthyroidism:

- Ineffective Family Therapeutic Regimen Management related to nonadherence to the medication regimen.

Expected Outcome. The family will adhere to the medication regimen, as evidenced by normal thyroid hormone levels.

- Diarrhea related to increased basal metabolic rate secondary to hyperthyroidism.

Expected Outcomes. The child will be euthyroid, as evidenced by normal results on thyroid function tests. The child will have normal bowel movements.

- Risk for Activity Intolerance related to loss of muscle mass from increased basal metabolic rate secondary to hyperthyroidism.

Expected Outcome. The child will be able to exercise at the same level as peers as basal metabolic rate returns to normal.

- Disturbed Sleep Pattern related to increased basal metabolic rate secondary to hyperthyroidism.

Expected Outcome. The child will sleep the appropriate amount of time for age as basal metabolic rate returns to normal.

- Ineffective Thermoregulation related to increased basal metabolic rate secondary to hyperthyroidism.

Expected Outcome. The child will regain normal body temperature as basal metabolic rate returns to normal.

■ Interventions

The antithyroid drug propylthiouracil is usually given two or three times per day, whereas methimazole can be given once daily (LaFranchi, 2011a). A multiple-times-a-day medication regimen may be difficult for some children and parents to follow. Use of pill dispensers and a watch with an alarm to remind the child to take the medication at specific times enhances compliance. The endocrinologist should evaluate the child and monitor thyroid function every 2 to 4 months while the child is undergoing treatment. Normal values for thyroid function tests and alleviation of symptoms indicate appropriate responses to therapy.

Once the child is euthyroid and asymptomatic, the child should be evaluated once or twice a year. Medication dosages may be tapered after 2 to 3 years to evaluate for remission. Contact sports should be limited while the child is being treated to decrease the possibility of damage to the liver. Collaboration with the school nurse to facilitate medication administration is an important nursing function.

■ Evaluation

- Does the child have normal results on thyroid function tests?
- Has the basal metabolic rate returned to normal?
- Does the child demonstrate normal bowel movements?

- Is the child able to exercise at an age-appropriate level?
- Does the child obtain an appropriate amount of sleep?
- Has the child maintained a normal body temperature?

DIABETES INSIPIDUS

Diabetes insipidus (DI) is an inability to concentrate urine. In central DI, there is a deficiency of vasopressin, also known as *antidiuretic hormone* (ADH). In nephrogenic DI, the kidneys are insensitive to vasopressin (Breault & Majzoub, 2011a).

Etiology

Both forms of diabetes insipidus can occur from inherited defects or acquired conditions (Breault & Majzoub, 2011a). Central DI frequently results from head trauma, tumors, or infection in the area of the hypothalamus. The most common type of tumor involving the hypothalamus that causes diabetes insipidus is craniopharyngioma. Cranial radiation for treatment of tumors may lead to ADH deficiency. Other causes include infections of the CNS such as meningitis or encephalitis, and congenital malformations such as septo-optic dysplasia or isolated pituitary malformation or ectopy. Several genetic mutations in the vasopressin gene causing DI have been identified (Cooperman, 2010). DI may also be idiopathic.

Incidence

Diabetes insipidus is not common in the United States, occurring in 1 of every 25,000 individuals. Head trauma and cranial surgery account for the largest percentage of cases of diabetes insipidus. Thirty percent of cases are classified as idiopathic (Cooperman, 2010).

Manifestations

Increased urination (polyuria) and excessive thirst (polydipsia) are the classic manifestations of diabetes insipidus. Other signs and symptoms include nocturia and dehydration (Box 27-3).

Diagnostic Evaluation

Diagnostic criteria include polyuria with associated hypernatremia (greater than 150 mEq/L) and low urine specific gravity (less than 1.005) in the absence of hyperglycemia. Urine should be checked for glucose to rule out hyperglycemia as a cause of increased urine output.

A water deprivation test may also be necessary to confirm the diagnosis. In this 7- to 8-hour procedure, the child is deprived of all

BOX 27-3 INDICATORS OF DIABETES INSIPIDUS OR SIADH	
DIABETES INSIPIDUS (HIGH AND DRY)	**SIADH (LOW AND WET)**
Increased urination (polyuria)	Decreased urination
Nocturia	Hypertension
Increased thirst (polydipsia)	Weight gain
Dehydration	Fluid retention
Hypernatremia	Hyponatremia
Urine specific gravity <1.005	Urine specific gravity >1.030
Elevated serum osmolality (>300 mOsm/kg)	Decreased serum osmolality (<280 mOsm/kg)
Decreased urine osmolality	Increased urine osmolality

fluid intake. A normal response is decreased urine output with a high urine specific gravity and no change in serum sodium. In diabetes insipidus, when fluid is restricted, the child continues to have large amounts of dilute urine (low urine specific gravity). The serum sodium level also increases. To ensure the child's safety, this test is done in a hospital setting with frequent monitoring of serum sodium, hematocrit, and osmolality. Urine osmolality and output are also measured. The child is weighed at the beginning, middle, and conclusion of the water deprivation test. Water deprivation should be stopped if the child loses 3% to 5% of baseline body weight, becomes dehydrated, or demonstrates a significant change in vital signs or neurologic status.

Therapeutic Management

Treatment for central DI involves maintaining fluid balance and administering synthetic vasopressin (1-deamino-8-D-arginine vaso-pressin [DDAVP]). The dosage of DDAVP ranges from 5 to 30 mcg/day (intranasal) or 2 to 4 mcg/day (IV/subcutaneous), divided into one or two doses per day. It is generally administered either intranasally, through a soft, flexible tube (rhinal tube) or metered spray, or by subcutaneous injection. The concentration of intranasal DDAVP is 100 mcg/mL; the concentration of subcutaneous DDAVP is 4 mcg/mL. The oral form of DDAVP is used primarily for nocturnal enuresis, though it has also been used in the treatment of diabetes insipidus.

PATHOPHYSIOLOGY

Diabetes Insipidus

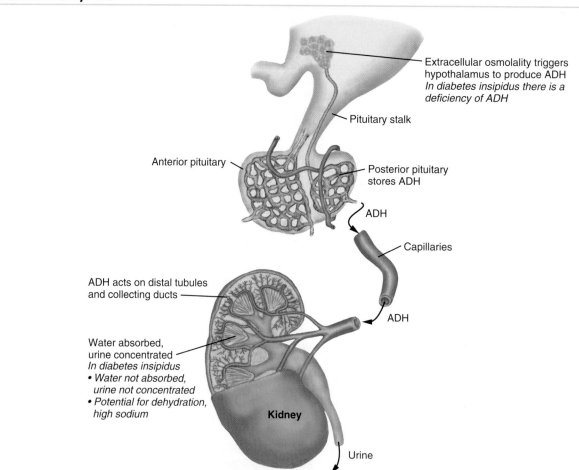

Extracellular osmolality triggers hypothalamus to produce ADH
In diabetes insipidus there is a deficiency of ADH

Pituitary stalk

Anterior pituitary

Posterior pituitary stores ADH

ADH

Capillaries

ADH

ADH acts on distal tubules and collecting ducts

Water absorbed, urine concentrated
In diabetes insipidus
• *Water not absorbed, urine not concentrated*
• *Potential for dehydration, high sodium*

Kidney

Urine

Antidiuretic hormone (ADH) is produced in the hypothalamus, transported through the pituitary stalk, and stored in the posterior pituitary. It is carried through the blood to the kidneys, where it acts on the distal tubules and collecting ducts to increase reabsorption of free water, thereby concentrating urine and decreasing urinary output.

ADH is under the control of osmoreceptors in the anterior pituitary. These osmoreceptors operate on a negative feedback system based on serum osmolality, particularly sodium concentration. When the serum osmolality is low, production of ADH decreases, causing increased urine output and normalizing osmolality; conversely, when serum osmolality is increased, ADH production increases, causing water retention and decreasing urine output. In diabetes

insipidus, a deficiency of ADH makes the body unable to conserve water, which results in the excretion of large volumes of dilute urine. Loss of free water leads to an increase in serum sodium concentration. If the child has an intact thirst center, increasing oral intake might compensate for the large fluid loss. If the thirst drive is not intact or the child is unable to drink enough, the child may become dehydrated and develop a high serum sodium level.

A child with an intact thirst center is able to self-regulate fluid needs and intake. An infant who is too young or a child who had head trauma or surgery may not be able to recognize thirst; the physician should prescribe a 24-hour fluid intake requirement to ensure adequate hydration.

Oral dosages range from 25 to 300 mcg every 8 to 12 hours (Cooperman, 2010).

Dosage is individualized on the basis of the child's age, size, urine output, and urine specific gravity. The duration of action varies from 8 to 24 hours. Doses are timed so that before the next dose, the child is allowed to have mildly increased urination. This helps prevent overtreatment and water retention. Parents are often taught to measure urine specific gravity at home to monitor effectiveness of treatment.

! NURSING QUALITY ALERT

Diabetes Insipidus

- Hypernatremia (sodium >150 mEq/L) and low urine specific gravity in the absence of hyperglycemia are diagnostic of diabetes insipidus.
- DDAVP is the only therapy for central diabetes insipidus.
- Overtreatment with DDAVP will result in fluid retention and dilutional hyponatremia. If the hyponatremia is severe enough, seizures may occur.

The goals for the management of nephrogenic DI are to prevent severe dehydration and provide adequate calories for growth. With acquired disease, treatment is focused on eliminating the underlying cause; congenital nephrogenic DI is very difficult to treat (Breault & Majzoub, 2011a).

Nursing Considerations

Nursing care involves assessing the understanding of the child and parents about diabetes insipidus. The nurse educates the family about the basic pathophysiology of water metabolism and the cause of diabetes insipidus. This includes a description of signs and symptoms (increased thirst, polyuria, dehydration) and how they indicate the need for DDAVP, as well as signs and symptoms of excessive DDAVP administration (decreased urine output, headaches, water retention). The child must be closely monitored for signs and symptoms of dehydration and the parents must know the appropriate actions to take if this occurs.

The family is taught how to correctly administer DDAVP and then provides a return demonstration of medication administration. If appropriate, the nurse instructs the family in the use of a refractometer to measure urine specific gravity. The child should wear a medical alert bracelet noting the diagnosis of diabetes insipidus. School personnel need to be aware of the diagnosis and must allow the child free access to water and toilet facilities.

SYNDROME OF INAPPROPRIATE ANTIDIURETIC HORMONE

The syndrome of inappropriate antidiuretic hormone (SIADH) results from excessive production or release of ADH, or vasopressin.

Etiology

Childhood SIADH is rare and usually related to an underlying cause. The most frequent cause is excessive use of vasopressin in the treatment of central diabetes insipidus (Breault & Majzoub, 2011b). Other causes include CNS infections (e.g., encephalitis and meningitis), head trauma, brain tumors, and generalized seizures (see Chapter 28). SIADH is usually transient and resolves when the underlying condition is corrected. However, brain surgery in the region of the hypothalamus or pituitary gland may cause the child to have transient SIADH but

permanent diabetes insipidus. A triple response may occur after surgery; the child has diabetes insipidus, then the child experiences temporary SIADH, and finally the child may return to permanent diabetes insipidus (Breault & Majzoub, 2011a).

Manifestations

Manifestations that occur with SIADH include hyponatremia, decreased urine output, increased urine specific gravity, fluid retention with slightly elevated plasma volume, weight gain, and increased urine osmolality (see Box 27-3).

PATHOPHYSIOLOGY

Syndrome of Inappropriate Antidiuretic Hormone

Excessive ADH results in the kidney reabsorbing too much free water. This causes decreased output of concentrated urine, evidenced by a high urine specific gravity (greater than 1.030). The excess water also causes a slightly expanded intravascular fluid volume and a low serum sodium level. Once the sodium level falls below 125 mEq/L, the child can become symptomatic and have anorexia, nausea, weakness, weight gain, confusion, irritability, and seizures.

Diagnostic Evaluation

SIADH should be suspected in children with CNS involvement, such as infections or head trauma, who have decreased urine output despite adequate intake. Laboratory diagnosis includes evidence of hyponatremia, hypochloremia, and low serum osmolality. Urine osmolality is usually greater than serum osmolality. Urine specific gravity is more than 1.030. Adrenal, thyroid, and renal function studies can rule out other causes of hyponatremia.

Therapeutic Management

Initial treatment is correction of the underlying cause. The physician orders fluid restriction to correct hyponatremia (Ferry & Pascual-y-Baralt, 2010). A child with severe hyponatremia may need an IV infusion of sodium chloride. Drug therapy usually is not indicated for transient SIADH. Medications such as lithium and demeclocycline block the action of ADH at the renal collecting tubules and have been used in the management of chronic SIADH.

Nursing Considerations

The nurse should assess the child with SIADH for signs and symptoms of fluid overload, including edema, weight gain, and urine specific gravity more than 1.030, and for dilutional hyponatremia by checking serum electrolyte levels frequently. The child with hyponatremia is at risk for injury related to seizures. The child's neurologic status is closely monitored every 2 to 4 hours by assessing and recording level of consciousness and observing for headache, irritability, or seizures (Box 27-4). The physician is alerted immediately if any changes in neurologic status occur. The nurse initiates seizure precautions if the serum sodium level drops below 125 mEq/L.

Additional interventions are directed toward maintaining fluid and electrolyte balance. The child's hydration status is carefully assessed. Intake and output are accurately measured and recorded. The child is weighed at least daily to monitor fluid retention. Fluid restrictions are strictly maintained. The child may have difficulty adhering to a decrease in fluid intake. The nurse explains to the child and parents the reasons for limiting fluids and that the restrictions are temporary. The nurse

---

BOX 27-4 SIGNS OF HYPONATREMIA

MILD (EARLY)	MODERATE	SEVERE
Anorexia	Confusion	Seizures
Nausea	Lethargy	Coma
Headache	Irritability	
Vomiting	Altered level of consciousness	

may give the child hard sugarless candies or apply wet washcloths to help keep mucous membranes moist.

! NURSING QUALITY ALERT

SIADH

- SIADH is characterized by low serum sodium (125 mEq/L or lower) and high urine specific gravity, as well as decreased serum osmolality and increased urine osmolality.
- Seizures may develop with hyponatremia.
- Treatment depends on strict fluid restriction to maintain serum sodium in a near-normal range. Frequent and precise measurements and recording of intake and output along with daily weights are critical to the evaluation and management of the child with SIADH.

Diet for the child with hyponatremia should include foods with high sodium content because extra sodium can help correct this problem. However, salty foods such as chips may make the child thirsty.

Evaluation of the child with SIADH should address a balanced intake and output, stable weight, and normal serum sodium levels. Urine specific gravity should be maintained between 1.010 and 1.020.

PRECOCIOUS PUBERTY

Precocious puberty refers to early onset of puberty. Traditionally this has been viewed as the onset of puberty before 8 years of age in girls and before 9 years of age in boys. It is defined as the premature appearance of secondary sexual characteristics, accelerated growth rate, and advanced bone maturation (Garibaldi & Chemaitilly, 2011). The major consequence of precocious puberty is rapid bone growth, which causes early growth plate fusion and ultimately short stature in adulthood compared with genetic height potential.

Etiology

Central precocious puberty can be idiopathic or caused by CNS tumors (including benign hamartomas), head trauma, or cranial radiation (Garibaldi & Chemaitilly, 2011). CNS abnormalities are seen with much greater frequency in boys than girls (Kaplowitz, 2010). In girls, precocious puberty is idiopathic in 90% of cases (Garibaldi & Chemaitilly, 2011). Factors that may contribute to precocious puberty in girls include obesity, ethnicity, genetic predisposition, psychosocial stress, and exposure to certain environmental chemicals that disrupt endocrine function (Cesario & Hughes, 2007).

The causes of the much less common precocious pseudopuberty (peripheral) include congenital adrenal hyperplasia (CAH); other abnormalities or tumors of the adrenal glands, ovaries, or testes; McCune-Albright syndrome in girls; and the genetic disorder *familial testotoxicosis* in boys (Ferry & Fenton, 2009).

Incidence

Precocious puberty affects 1 in every 5000 children and is 10 times more likely to occur in girls than boys (Cesario & Hughes, 2007). There is growing evidence that the number of girls diagnosed with precocious puberty has increased over the past 30 years and that African American girls mature earlier than white girls of the same age (Cesario & Hughes, 2007). Some experts have recommended that precocious puberty be redefined as the appearance of secondary sexual characteristics in white girls under age 7 years and African-American girls under age 6 years.

Manifestations

Manifestations of precocious puberty reflect gender differences:

Girls	Boys
Breast development	Testicular enlargement
Pubic and axillary hair	Penile enlargement
Enlargement of vagina, uterus, and ovaries	Pubic hair
Growth spurt	Facial hair
Acne	Acne
Adult body odor	Adult body odor
Onset of menstrual periods	Deepening of voice
Moodiness	Moodiness

Diagnostic Evaluation

Diagnosis of precocious puberty begins with a thorough history, including onset of secondary sexual characteristics, and a physical examination. Blood tests are performed to evaluate for elevated levels of LH, FSH, testosterone, and estrogen. Unfortunately, because these hormones are released in small bursts during the day, random samples may not be adequate.

The gonadotropin-releasing hormone (GnRH) stimulation test is a definitive test to delineate between central (gonadotropin dependent) and peripheral (gonadotropin independent) causes of precocious puberty (Kaplowitz, 2010). Synthetic GnRH is administered IV or subcutaneously to stimulate the release of LH and FSH from the pituitary gland. Serial samples of LH and FSH are then obtained over a 2-hour period after IV administration. With subcutaneous administration, a single sample of LH and FSH may be obtained with the use of an ultrasensitive assay. Before the onset of puberty, the FSH peak is higher than the LH peak. With the onset of puberty, the LH peak is higher than the FSH peak.

Radiographic studies also support the diagnosis of precocious puberty. Radiographs of the wrist determine bone age and maturation and can assist in predicting final adult height. Skull radiographs screen for CNS lesions, although CT scans and MRI are more accurate in visualizing tumors. Abdominal ultrasound and pelvic ultrasound are beneficial in diagnosing adrenal and ovarian tumors or cysts. Pelvic ultrasound also provides evidence of pubertal changes in the uterus and ovaries. Finally, isolated pubic hair development and elevated androgen hormone levels suggest an adrenal origin for premature hair growth.

Therapeutic Management

Treatment of the child with precocious puberty aims to stop or reverse the development of secondary sexual characteristics and to maximize adult height. Current therapy for central precocious puberty involves administration of a GnRH agonist, or blocker. GnRH blockers inhibit the binding of GnRH to the pituitary gland, causing decreased production of the pubertal hormones and slowing or reversing sexual development.

Several commercially available GnRH agonists can be administered either intranasally or by a monthly intramuscular injection. Once therapy is initiated, GnRH secretion is suppressed within 2 to 4 weeks. The accelerated growth rate and bone maturation will slow, and some secondary sexual characteristics will regress within the first year of treatment. Nonadherence with medication therapy, such as missed or delayed administration of injections, can promote pubertal changes rather than suppress puberty.

No evidence suggests that GnRH agonist therapy interferes with the child's reproductive function in the future. Once therapy is discontinued, pubertal progression resumes. For children with peripheral precocious puberty, treatment is aimed at correcting the underlying cause.

NURSING CARE OF THE CHILD WITH PRECOCIOUS PUBERTY

■ Assessment

Nursing care of the child with precocious puberty addresses the physical and behavioral changes associated with puberty. A nurse working with these children may note that they feel more comfortable around

PATHOPHYSIOLOGY

Precocious Puberty

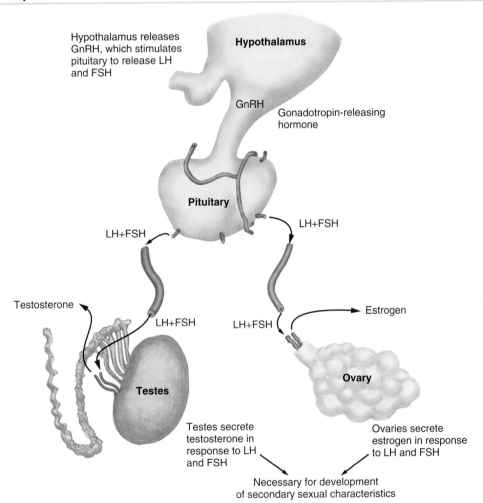

Hypothalamus releases GnRH, which stimulates pituitary to release LH and FSH

Hypothalamus

GnRH

Gonadotropin-releasing hormone

Pituitary

LH+FSH

LH+FSH

Testosterone

LH+FSH

LH+FSH

Estrogen

Testes

Ovary

Testes secrete testosterone in response to LH and FSH

Ovaries secrete estrogen in response to LH and FSH

Necessary for development of secondary sexual characteristics

Puberty occurs when the hypothalamus releases gonadotropin-releasing hormone (GnRH). This stimulates the pituitary gland to release luteinizing-hormone (LH) and follicle-stimulating hormone (FSH). In girls, FSH stimulates formation of ovarian follicles to produce estrogen. Estrogen is necessary for the development of secondary sexual characteristics, such as breast development and maturation of the vagina and labia. LH is involved in the process of ovulation. In boys, FSH triggers the testes to support the development of sperm. LH stimulates the production of testosterone, which is necessary for the development of sexual characteristics and sperm production. Puberty development is classified according to Tanner stages 1 through 5 (see Chapter 8). The adrenal glands

produce the hormone dehydroepiandrosterone (DHEA), which causes pubic and axillary hair growth. During puberty the growth rate increases, called a "growth spurt," in which a child grows an average of 4 to 6 inches per year.

In precocious puberty the sex hormones that accelerate growth also cause the bone plates (epiphyseal plates) to close early. Usually the epiphyseal plates fuse at 14 years of age for girls and 17 years for boys; premature closure can lead to decreased linear growth with reduced adult height. With true precocious puberty, children have hormonal changes that mimic the onset of normal puberty. These hormonal changes may be central, arising from the hypothalamus, or peripheral, arising from the ovaries, testes, or adrenal glands.

older children rather than peers their own age. They often experience teasing about their bodies and may limit social activities, such as swimming. Boys often exhibit aggressive behavior. Children who go through early puberty appear older than their chronologic age and are often treated accordingly by adults. Because of their mature appearance, girls with precocious puberty are potentially at greater risk for sexual abuse and exploitation (Zuckerman, 2009).

💬 If a child appears embarrassed or uncomfortable when being interviewed about sexual development, the nurse should explain to the child, "Everyone goes through body changes when growing up; it's just that these changes are happening to you sooner than most children. Can you tell me in your own words how you feel about your body?"

▪ Nursing Diagnosis and Planning

The following nursing diagnoses and expected outcomes may be appropriate for the child with precocious puberty:

- Deficient Knowledge about medication administration related to inadequate understanding of intramuscular or intranasal GnRH agonist.

Expected Outcomes. The parents will explain the need for the medication and will give an appropriate return demonstration of medication administration technique.

- Disturbed Body Image related to early sexual development.

Expected Outcomes. The child will describe the relationship between early sexual development and the underlying condition, express feelings about early sexual development, and verbalize acceptance of body appearance.

- Impaired Social Interaction related to appearing older than chronologic age.

Expected Outcome. The child will adjust socially to body changes, as evidenced by exhibiting age-appropriate behaviors and social interactions.

! NURSING QUALITY ALERT

Precocious Puberty

- Children with precocious puberty appear older than their chronologic age. Although they tend to be treated as older children, they should be treated according to their chronologic age.
- Other children often tease children with precocious puberty.
- Precocious puberty may occur in infancy or childhood.

▪ Interventions

Many parents may not be comfortable with their child's early development. The nurse explains the stages of puberty and each stage's associated behavioral changes. The nurse teaches parents that the child is experiencing normal changes at an earlier time than expected.

Explanations given to the child should be geared to the level of intellectual development. The nurse can direct the parent to books that explain sexual maturation in terms the child can understand. Psychological counseling might be necessary to help the family deal with the sensitive issues of sexuality.

The nurse also teaches the family about the prescribed medication regimen. In some instances, the parent is taught how to administer the injections. These might be stressful for the young child. The nurse demonstrates appropriate injection technique and teaches the child coping strategies to be used when the injection is given.

▪ Evaluation

- Can the parents explain the need for the medication and demonstrate proper medication administration?
- Is the child able to relate the body changes to the underlying condition?
- Have the child and parents verbalized any concerns about the child's early sexual development?
- Is the child exhibiting age-appropriate social interactions?

GROWTH HORMONE DEFICIENCY

Growth hormone (GH) deficiency results from inadequate production or secretion of GH, causing poor growth and short stature. Hypoglycemia may be a manifestation of GH deficiency.

Etiology

GH deficiency may be isolated or may be associated with an underlying cause. Such causes include hypopituitarism, congenital malformations of the pituitary gland, brain tumors (most commonly craniopharyngioma), and cranial irradiation. Other disorders associated with short stature that may respond to GH therapy include Turner syndrome, Prader-Willi syndrome, and chronic illnesses such as renal disease and inflammatory bowel disease.

Incidence

A study of 80,000 children in the United States demonstrated a growth hormone deficiency incidence of 1 in every 3500 children (Kemp, 2010). No racial differences in incidence are apparent. Boys are much more likely to be diagnosed and treated for GH deficiency than girls; it is uncertain if this is because of referral bias by parents and practitioners (Kemp, 2010).

Manifestations

Manifestations typical of GH deficiency include height less than 5th percentile for age and gender, diminished growth rate (less than 2 standard deviations below the mean for age and gender), immature or cherubic facies, delayed puberty, hypoglycemia, diminished muscle mass with relatively increased body fat (adiposity), and micropenis (associated with hypopituitarism).

PATHOPHYSIOLOGY

Growth Hormone Deficiency

Growth hormone (GH), thyroxine, cortisol, and sex hormones all influence growth. The hypothalamus secretes GH-releasing factor, which stimulates the pituitary gland to release GH. This hormone is secreted in pulses, with increased secretion during the night. In the presence of hypoglycemia, GH is secreted to counteract insulin and raise the blood glucose level. Many children with GH deficiency may have hypoglycemia.

Most children with short stature have constitutional growth delay. Children with short stature or poor growth rates may also be deficient in other hormones. Normal thyroid function is essential for growth; therefore, hypothyroidism may cause short stature. Sex hormones are required for the growth spurt and sexual maturation that occur with puberty. Children lacking more than one hormone produced by the pituitary gland are referred to as having *hypopituitarism*. Rate of growth and final adult height depend on factors such as genetics (family heights), nutrition, and general health. Any child growing less than 5 cm per year should be referred to an endocrinologist for further evaluation.

Diagnostic Evaluation

Diagnosis of GH deficiency begins with careful measurements of growth over an extended period (usually 6 to 12 months). Height should be measured on a consistent scale, preferably with a calibrated stadiometer. Diagnosis is made during two age peaks: 5 years and 10 to 13 years for girls or 12 to 16 years for boys (Kemp, 2010). Initial screening involves thyroid function tests, electrolytes, blood urea nitrogen (BUN), creatinine, complete blood count, insulin-like growth factor 1 (IGF-1) and IGF binding proteins (IGFBP-3), and a bone age radiograph. Normal thyroid function is essential for adequate growth; thyroid studies are essential when evaluating for short stature. Complete blood count and other specific blood screening for any systemic or chronic illness should be done. Electrolytes and renal function studies eliminate primary kidney dysfunction as a cause of poor growth. A karyotype (chromosomes) may be performed for girls to rule out Turner syndrome.

Because GH is normally secreted in pulses throughout the day and night, stimulation testing is necessary to confirm the diagnosis of GH deficiency. Agents used in provocative testing to stimulate GH production include insulin, arginine, clonidine, glucagon, and levodopa (L-dopa). Once the stimulating agent is given, serial GH levels are drawn. Although diagnostic criteria vary, most clinicians accept a GH level less than 10 ng/mL as indicative of GH deficiency. Generally, two positive tests are required for diagnosis.

Therapeutic Management

A child with GH deficiency requires replacement therapy. Synthetic GH comes in a powdered form that must be diluted for administration or a premixed liquid form. It is given as a subcutaneous injection six or seven times per week, usually at bedtime. An alternative form of administration is a subcutaneous deposition of time-release GH, designed to last 2 to 4 weeks. Dosage ranges from 0.18 to 0.3 mg/kg/week, depending on the child's age, pubertal stage, and response to therapy (Parks & Felner, 2011). Once diluted, GH must be stored at 36° to 46° F (2.2° to 7.7° C). With treatment, many children experience linear growth of 4 inches (10 cm) or more the first year and then at least 3 inches (8 cm) per year for 2 more years, after which the growth rate slows (Kaneshiro, 2010). When treatment is started at a younger age, the child's height potential is increased. GH therapy continues until the child's growth plates close or the child reaches an acceptable or predicted final height.

NURSING CARE OF THE CHILD WITH GROWTH HORMONE DEFICIENCY

■ Assessment

Nursing care of the child with GH deficiency includes assessment of family attitudes and perceptions. Parental attitudes regarding the child's size can influence the child's self-esteem. Assessment of the child's attitude about height is essential. The nurse determines if height and growth concerns are voiced more by the parents or by the child. If parents place excessive emphasis on height, the child may be more self-conscious or demonstrate low self-esteem. Height issues may adversely affect a child's psychosocial adjustment, as demonstrated by poor school performance and lack of involvement in extracurricular activities. Often short children appear younger and are treated as such by adults. They may be teased by their peers. The nurse might ask, "Have you ever been teased or been in any fights at school because of your height?" Once the child is receiving therapy, the nurse assesses adherence to the medication regimen, injection technique, and

medication preparation and storage. These should be reviewed periodically and with each dosage change. As the child matures, self-injection techniques can be taught.

■ Nursing Diagnosis and Planning

The following nursing diagnoses and expected outcomes may be appropriate for the child with GH deficiency:

- Delayed Growth and Development related to GH deficiency.

Expected Outcomes. The child will receive and respond to treatment, as evidenced by increased linear growth rate.

- Disturbed Body Image related to short stature.

Expected Outcome. The child will demonstrate acceptance of body image, as evidenced by verbalization of acceptance of ultimate height.

- Situational Low Self-Esteem related to short stature.

Expected Outcome. The child will accept short stature, as evidenced by verbalizing appropriate feelings of self-esteem.

- Ineffective Family Therapeutic Regimen Management related to nonadherence to daily injection.

Expected Outcome. The child and parents will adhere to the injection schedule, as evidenced by appropriate record keeping and the child's steady growth.

! NURSING QUALITY ALERT

Criteria for Suspecting Growth Hormone Deficiency

- Consistently poor growth (<5 cm per year)
- Growth rate more than 2 standard deviations below the mean for age
- Downward deviation from the previous growth curve

■ Interventions

The nurse reassures the child and parents that adherence to the injections will improve growth rate. Reminders that the injections are temporary and are helping the child to grow are also helpful. Keeping a growth chart at home and noting the need for larger clothing sizes are physical signs the child can use to monitor growth. These indicators also can assist with adherence.

The nurse has an important role in educating children and families about the proper dilution and administration of the GH. The nurse demonstrates the injection technique to the parents (and child if age appropriate) and requests a return demonstration.

Effectiveness of therapy is evidenced by the child's growth rate. Children are evaluated approximately every 3 to 4 months by an endocrinologist; accurate measurements of height are essential. The use of a growth chart helps identify growth velocity. GH therapy is continued until the child reaches an acceptable adult height or radiographic evidence shows growth plate fusion.

? CRITICAL THINKING EXERCISE 27-1

Parents of young adolescent boys often are concerned about their child's current and eventual adult height. Boys who are significantly shorter than their peers during early adolescence can experience altered self-esteem.

How should a nurse respond if parents ask whether giving growth hormone (GH) to their 13-year-old son with short stature will increase his eventual adult height?

■ **Evaluation**

- Has the child exhibited increased linear growth rate?
- Does the child verbalize positive feelings regarding body image and self-esteem?
- Do the child and family adhere to the injection schedule?

DIABETES MELLITUS

Type 1 and type 2 diabetes are chronic diseases requiring life-long management and care (see Chapter 12). Both types involve abnormal carbohydrate metabolism and hyperglycemia. Evidence has been accumulating that demonstrates a worldwide increase in the incidence of type 1 diabetes mellitus, with the annual incidence in the United States rising to 24.3 cases per 100,000 population (Lamb, 2010). Though incidence increases with age until mid-puberty, type 1 diabetes mellitus can occur at any age including infancy.

Type 1 diabetes cases are significantly higher in white children (Lamb, 2010). The incidence of type 2 diabetes has also risen dramatically in children, particularly in minority populations (Pozzo, 2010).

Type 1 Diabetes Mellitus

Type 1 diabetes mellitus results when the pancreas is unable to produce and secrete an adequate amount of insulin. This form of diabetes, the most common childhood endocrine disorder, presents challenges in the areas of teaching, management, and adherence. Because of recent changes in the health care delivery system, meeting the needs associated with management of type 1 diabetes mellitus has become more complicated. Unless the newly diagnosed child is in diabetic ketoacidosis (DKA), the child may not be hospitalized. The nurse must develop a plan of care that involves child and family education and support, in either an inpatient or outpatient setting.

Etiology

Type 1 diabetes mellitus is an inflammatory process in the insulin-secreting islet cells of the pancreas and results from an autoimmune process that causes their eventual destruction. Although multiple genes are thought to play a role in the genetic predisposition to type 1 diabetes, an environmental trigger is thought to initiate the autoimmune destructive process. Possible triggers include viral infections, dietary toxins, history of obesity, and certain chemicals (Lamb, 2010). Current research is focused on identifying factors that increase susceptibility and exploring methods of interrupting or preventing the autoimmune response in susceptible individuals (first-degree relatives of a person with diabetes). At this time no prevention or cure is available; however, several different types of islet cell and pancreas transplantation are being explored. Children with type 1 diabetes mellitus are prone to developing other autoimmune conditions, such as Graves disease, Hashimoto thyroiditis, and celiac disease (see Chapter 19).

Incidence

More than 25 million children and adults in the United States have diabetes (American Diabetes Association [ADA], 2011). Approximately 215,000 people younger than 20 years have diabetes—0.26% of the population in this age-group. Type 1 diabetes is diagnosed in approximately 1 of every 400 children and adolescents (ADA, 2011). Incidence peaks in early childhood (age 4 to 6 years) and then a much greater peak occurs during early adolescence (age 10 to 14 years) (Lamb, 2010).

Manifestations

Type 1 diabetes mellitus is manifested by the classic initial signs of hyperglycemia, known as the three *P*s; *p*olyuria (or enuresis in a

TABLE 27-2	**ACTIONS OF INSULIN**	
ANABOLIC ACTIONS OF INSULIN	**CATABOLIC CONSEQUENCES OF INSULIN DEFICIT**
Promotes glucose as a fuel source	Promotes fats and proteins as fuel sources
Promotes storage of glucose as glycogen	Allows glycogen stores to be broken down
Prevents breakdown of fat stores	Allows fat stores to be depleted
Increases protein synthesis	Allows protein breakdown into amino acids

toilet-trained child), *p*olydipsia, and *p*olyphagia. The child's other symptoms include weight loss (despite increased food intake), fatigue, and blurred vision.

If the condition progresses without intervention, the child can exhibit signs and symptoms of DKA: nausea and vomiting, abdominal pain, acetone (fruity) odor to breath, dehydration, increasing lethargy, Kussmaul respirations, and coma.

Children who receive insulin for treatment of type 1 diabetes mellitus can have hypoglycemia. Table 27-2 lists the actions of insulin, and Table 27-3 compares hypoglycemia, hyperglycemia, and ketoacidosis.

Diagnostic Evaluation

Diagnosis of type 1 diabetes mellitus is made on the basis of a clinical picture of hyperglycemia (and acidosis) combined with the laboratory data of a fasting blood glucose (FBG) exceeding 126 mg/dL and a random serum glucose of 200 mg/dL or greater (Lamb, 2010). Ketonuria, although not diagnostic, is a frequent finding, as is glycosuria. Glucose tolerance testing is rarely used in diagnosing type 1 diabetes mellitus. The glycosylated hemoglobin (HbA$_{1c}$) value is elevated in response to prolonged elevations of blood glucose.

Therapeutic Management

The American Diabetes Association (2008b) recommends that children newly diagnosed with diabetes mellitus be managed and educated by a multidisciplinary team of experts in pediatric diabetes. Children diagnosed with type 1 diabetes will be started on insulin therapy to reverse metabolic imbalances (Lamb, 2010). At the time of their initial type 1 diagnosis, 15% to 67% of children are in DKA (Weitzel, Pfeffer, Dost et al., 2010) and require management in a pediatric intensive care unit (Lamb, 2010).

The goals of diabetes management for children with type 1 diabetes mellitus include the following:

- Facilitating appropriate growth (height, weight)
- Maintaining an age-appropriate lifestyle
- Achieving age-related near-normal HbA$_{1c}$ with minimal episodes of hypoglycemia
- Preventing acute complications (hypoglycemia, hyperglycemia, DKA)

Insulin Therapy

The child with type 1 diabetes mellitus loses the ability to make insulin because of autoimmune destruction of the insulin-producing cells, the beta cells. Symptoms of hyperglycemia become evident when most of the beta cells are destroyed. After initiation of insulin therapy, the child may have a "honeymoon" phase characterized by hypoglycemia and

TABLE 27-3   COMPARISON OF HYPOGLYCEMIA, HYPERGLYCEMIA, AND KETOACIDOSIS

HYPOGLYCEMIA	HYPERGLYCEMIA	KETOACIDOSIS
Onset		
Rapid	Slow	Slow
Signs and Symptoms		
Adrenergic signs:	Increased urination	*Hyperglycemia signs plus:*
Trembling	Increased thirst	Abdominal pain
Sweating	Fatigue	Chest pain
Tachycardia	Weight loss (gradual, over several weeks)	Kussmaul respirations
Pallor	Blurred vision	Nausea and vomiting
Clammy skin		Acetone (fruity) breath odor
		Signs and symptoms of dehydration:
		Dry lips and mucous membranes
		Sunken eyes
		Sudden weight loss
		Decreased urination
Alterations in Sensorium		
Neuroglycopenic symptoms:	Emotional lability	Increasing lethargy
Personality change	Headache	Decreasing level of consciousness
Irritability	Hunger	Coma
Drunken behavior		
Slurred speech		
Decreased level of consciousness to total loss of consciousness		
Seizure activity		
Laboratory Data		
Blood glucose <60 mg/dL	Blood glucose >160 mg/dL	Blood glucose ≥300 mg/dL
		Urinary ketones positive
		Serum pH <7.30
		Bicarbonate 15 mEq/L
		Serum ketones positive
Causes		
Too much insulin	Excessive intake of carbohydrate	Inadequate amount of insulin
Excessive activity without eating extra carbohydrates	Little or no exercise	Excessive stress
Missed or delayed meal	Inadequate amount of insulin	
	Increased stress, either emotional or physical	
Treatment		
15 g of carbohydrate	Insulin	IV fluids
For loss of consciousness or seizure activity:	Exercise	IV insulin
Glucagon subcutaneous or intramuscular	Increased oral fluids	Electrolyte replacement
IV glucose		Generalized supportive care

a decreasing need for insulin. This may last from a few weeks to 1 year or longer. The nurse should prepare the child and family for the possibility of a honeymoon phase, both to avoid the misconception that the diabetes is "going away" and to provide instruction on recognition and treatment of hypoglycemia.

The goal of insulin therapy is to replace the insulin the child is no longer able to make in an acceptable physiologic pattern. Synthetic human insulin, made by recombinant deoxyribonucleic acid (DNA) technology, is free of animal impurities and is recommended for children. Oral hypoglycemic agents, although useful in the treatment of type 2 diabetes, are not effective in the treatment of type 1 diabetes.

The choice of insulin types and schedule of injections are determined on the basis of the child's needs (Table 27-4). Daily self-monitoring of blood glucose aids in defining insulin requirements. The child in the honeymoon phase needs less insulin than the child who makes no endogenous insulin. The pubertal child requires a larger insulin dosage.

Schedule. Insulin requirements are commonly based on age, body weight, and pubertal status. In general, children who are newly diagnosed with type 1 diabetes typically need an initial total daily dose of approximately 0.5 to 1 unit/kg. Because dosages for infants and toddlers frequently are less than 1 unit, the insulin is diluted with an approved diluent to increase the volume to be administered and improve accuracy

PATHOPHYSIOLOGY
Type 1 Diabetes Mellitus

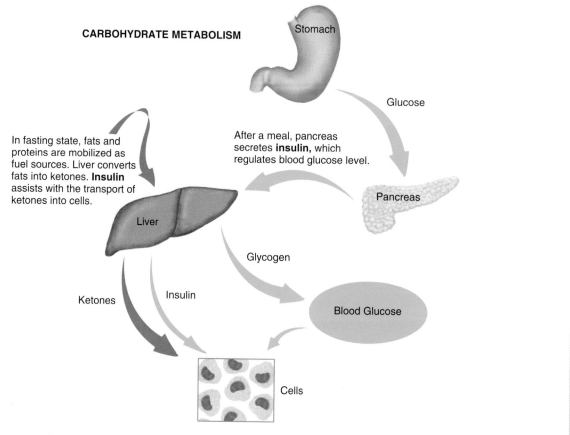

CARBOHYDRATE METABOLISM

Stomach

Glucose

After a meal, pancreas secretes **insulin,** which regulates blood glucose level.

Pancreas

In fasting state, fats and proteins are mobilized as fuel sources. Liver converts fats into ketones. **Insulin** assists with the transport of ketones into cells.

Liver

Glycogen

Ketones

Insulin

Blood Glucose

Cells

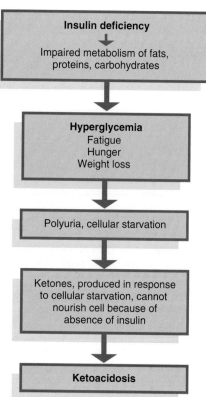

Insulin deficiency
↓
Impaired metabolism of fats, proteins, carbohydrates

↓

Hyperglycemia
Fatigue
Hunger
Weight loss

↓

Polyuria, cellular starvation

↓

Ketones, produced in response to cellular starvation, cannot nourish cell because of absence of insulin

↓

Ketoacidosis

Glucose is the primary source of energy for body cells. Any extra glucose taken in by the body can be stored as glycogen in muscle or liver cells or in the form of fatty tissues. Glucose can be extracted from glycogen for periods of fasting (e.g., overnight). Once glycogen stores have been depleted, new glucose (gluconeogenesis) is made from amino acids released from muscle into the bloodstream. The energy for gluconeogenesis is supplied by the breakdown of stored fats.

Insulin, a hormone, is secreted by the beta cells of the pancreas. Its main function is to regulate the blood glucose level by controlling the rate of glucose uptake by cells. Little or no insulin is secreted by the beta cells when a person is in the fasting state; greater quantities are secreted after the person has eaten a meal. In the fasting state, with relatively small quantities of available insulin, the body mobilizes fats and proteins to be used as fuel sources. The liver then converts the fats into **ketoacids,** or ketones. With the assistance of insulin, ketones are transported into the cells and are used as an alternative source of fuel for cellular energy. This process ensures an energy source during long periods of fasting. Not all cells in the body are capable of using ketone bodies and require glucose as their primary fuel (see Table 27-2).

In the absence of insulin, the metabolism of fats, proteins, and carbohydrates is impaired. Glucose is unable to move into the intracellular space, resulting in hyperglycemia. As blood glucose levels exceed the renal threshold, glucose is "spilled" into the urine causing osmotic diuresis and subsequent polyuria. Excessive thirst follows in response to fluid loss. Fatigue, hunger, and weight loss also accompany the onset of type 1 diabetes mellitus because cellular starvation continues in the absence of insulin.

Ketones (ketoacids), manufactured by the liver from adipose tissue, are produced in response to cellular starvation. In the absence of insulin, ketones are also unavailable to the cell for nourishment. Increasing blood levels of ketones (ketonemia) result in ketoacidosis.

TABLE 27-4   INSULIN ACTION BY TYPE

NAME	TYPE	ONSET	PEAK	DURATION
Lispro/aspart	Rapid-acting	5-15 min	30-90 min	5 hr
Regular	Short-acting	30-60 min	2-3 hr	5-8 hr
Isophane (NPH)	Intermediate-acting	2-4 hr	4-10 hr	10-16 hr
Glargine (Lantus)	Long-acting	2-4 hr	No peak	20-24 hr

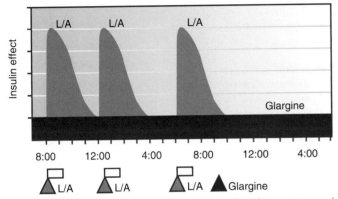

FIG 27-2 Peak action of insulin injections is timed to correspond with the child's usual meal and snack times to minimize the chance of hypoglycemia. *L/A*, Lispro/aspart (rapid-acting insulin). (Data from Alemzadeh, R., & Ali, O. [2011]. Type 1 diabetes mellitus (immune mediated). In R. Kliegman, B. Stanton, J. St. Geme, et al. [Eds.], *Nelson textbook of pediatrics* [19th ed., pp. 1969-1990]. Philadelphia: Elsevier Saunders.)

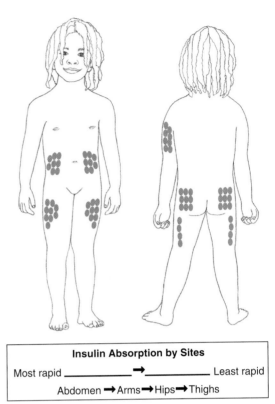

Insulin Absorption by Sites

Most rapid _____⟶_____ Least rapid

Abdomen ⟶ Arms ⟶ Hips ⟶ Thighs

FIG 27-3 Subcutaneous insulin injection sites most commonly used. Rate of absorption varies by site. (Chart modified from Albisser, A. M., & Sperlich, M. [1993]. Adjusting insulins. *Diabetes Educator, 18*[3], 211-227.)

in dosing. Many children are managed through administration of insulin by three or more injections per day. A combination of intermediate or long-acting insulin (basal) and rapid or short-acting insulin (bolus) injected multiple times per day before meals and snacks, is used. More children are now receiving insulin by a continuous subcutaneous insulin infusion (CSII) pump. The insulin administration schedule is individually prescribed according to the child's age-related glycemic targets. The peak actions of these insulins are timed to correspond to the child's usual mealtimes and snack times to minimize the possibility of hypoglycemia. To prevent hypoglycemia, a child must eat within 15 minutes of administration of rapid-acting insulin.

A recent option for the basal/bolus insulin regimen is using both rapid-acting analogs and a long-acting insulin that has no peak action time. Glargine (Lantus), a long-acting peakless analog, has been approved for children ages 6 years and older and is given in the evening as the basal insulin, and complemented during the day by a rapid-acting insulin (lispro or aspart) when the child eats carbohydrates (Lamb, 2010). This schedule provides improved glycemic control (Figure 27-2) (ADA, 2008b). Lantus insulin is not mixed in the same syringe with other types of insulin or solutions. Rapid-acting insulin analogs are also beneficial in the management of issues related to insulin resistance during puberty.

Administration. Because insulin is a protein and would be digested if taken orally, it is given parenterally. Insulin is administered by subcutaneous injection using a specialized insulin syringe into the adipose tissue over large muscle masses. Preferred sites include the back of the upper arms, the top and outer portion of the thighs, the abdomen, and the hip (Figure 27-3). To avoid injecting into the muscle

or vascular space, a 45-degree angle of injection is used with a ½-inch needle or a 90-degree angle with a ⅜-inch needle. Rotation of injection sites helps prevent areas of adipose hypertrophy (fatty lumps), which interfere with insulin absorption. Various injection sites absorb insulin at slightly different rates. Absorption is also affected by body temperature and the level of muscle activity (exercise) under a given injection site. To help decrease variations in absorption, the child should use different locations within a major injection site for one day. For example, the child would inject insulin in one location on the back of the upper right arm for the morning injection, then rotate to another location on the back of the upper right arm for the afternoon injection, and a third location again on the upper right arm for the evening injection. The next day, another major site such as the top, outer portion of the right thigh may be used, depending on the site rotation schedule.

Insulin can be administered by an insulin syringe, air injector, or insulin pump. Disposable syringes are to be used only one time and then safely discarded (with the syringe/needle placed in a puncture-resistant, opaque container before placing in the trash). The air injector uses compressed air to deposit the insulin within the fatty tissue without the use of a needle. The child or family must learn to use the air injector device by correctly loading insulin, adjusting pressure settings to avoid intramuscular delivery, and cleaning.

The insulin pump is a battery-operated device that provides a continuous infusion of rapid-acting insulin (Skyler, Ponder, Kruger et al., 2007). Use of the pump in the pediatric population continues to increase. Evidence suggests that the insulin pump provides tighter control of blood sugar levels and more flexibility in lifestyle. The pump

Animation—Insulin Injection

is a mechanical device, approximately the size of a pager, which is often worn on a belt or in a pocket. It delivers insulin to the body through an infusion set consisting of thin plastic tubing attached to a cannula or needle inserted into the subcutaneous tissue of the thigh, abdomen, or buttocks. A continuous basal rate of insulin infusion is maintained, and bolus dosages are infused as determined by blood glucose testing.

The pump most closely mimics physiologic delivery of insulin (Sherr, Cengiz, & Tamborlane, 2009). A candidate for insulin pump therapy must be confident in diabetes management, willing to measure blood glucose meticulously (at least four glucose checks per day), be able to count carbohydrates and calculate appropriate insulin coverage, and have a supportive home environment. Parents and/or other care-givers are responsible for the insulin pump when used by infants and toddlers. Dietary recommendations are different for children or adolescents using an insulin pump and are based on carbohydrate counting.

Nutrition Therapy

The goal of nutrition therapy is to promote normal growth, encourage healthy nutrition, prevent complications, and maintain near-normal blood glucose levels. Because the insulin dosage is balanced with food intake, the diet plan should stress a consistent intake, particularly of carbohydrate food products. The diet therapy chosen should be easy to understand and help the child and family learn to make healthy food choices. The individualized meal plan is based on the child's diet history and is tailored to food preferences, physical activity, cultural aspects, and schedules. As the child grows, the meal plan is tailored to meet changing dietary needs.

Physical Activity

Exercise is an important aspect of diabetes management. Exercise enhances the action of insulin in lowering blood glucose levels. In addition, exercise promotes a greater sense of well-being, improves physical and cardiovascular fitness, and contributes to an improved lipid profile. The child with diabetes should be encouraged to participate in age-appropriate sports. Early enjoyment of a sport or activity can promote a lifelong active lifestyle. Because exercise lowers glucose levels, the child must be taught how to prevent hypoglycemia. The child should try to schedule activities to avoid exercising when an insulin dose is peaking. Proper hydration must be maintained while exercising.

The child and family are taught to add extra carbohydrate snacks that correlate to duration of exercise. Coaches and teammates should be taught how to recognize and treat hypoglycemia. Delayed or nocturnal hypoglycemia can occur after strenuous activity. Additional carbohydrate intake might be required after exercise to maintain blood glucose levels. The child should always wear medical alert identification.

Blood Glucose Monitoring

Self-monitoring of blood glucose (SMBG) provides an objective tool to assist with diabetes control. Monitoring is recommended before meals and before the bedtime snack. More frequent monitoring may be used during prolonged exercise, during an illness, or if nighttime hypoglycemia is suspected.

Blood glucose goals must be tailored to the abilities of the caregivers and the age of the child. For example, goals for the infant or toddler are usually liberalized to help prevent severe hypoglycemia. The identified goals are a target range; not all glucose levels fall in this range, even in the child with excellent diabetes control. Preprandial (before meal) blood glucose goals are as follows (ADA, 2008b):

! **NURSING QUALITY ALERT**

Managing the Child with Type 1 Diabetes Mellitus

Insulin
- Store insulin in a cool, dry place. Do not freeze or expose to excessive heat.
- Do not shake insulin. It is recommended to roll the vial back and forth to mix.
- Check the expiration date on the vial before using.
- Once opened, date the vial and discard as recommended.
- When mixing two different types of insulin in the same syringe, inject the appropriate amount of air into both vials, withdraw the short-acting (clear) insulin *first*, and then withdraw the intermediate-acting (cloudy) insulin.

Nutrition
- Meals and snacks are balanced with insulin action.
- Both the timing of the meal or snack and the amount of food are important in avoiding hyperglycemia or hypoglycemia.
- Adherence to a daily schedule that maintains a consistent food intake combined with consistent insulin injections aids in achieving metabolic control.

Exercise
- Avoid exercising during insulin peak times.
- Add extra 15- to 30-g carbohydrate snacks for each 45-60 min of exercise.

Blood Glucose Monitoring
- Record blood glucose results in a diary.
- A 3- to 4-day alteration in glucose levels requires an adjustment of insulin doses.

- Nondiabetic: 70 to 110 mg/dL
- Children with type 1 diabetes mellitus: 90 to 180 mg/dL
- Infants and toddlers with type 1 diabetes mellitus: 100 to 180 mg/dL

Glucose test results should be recorded in a diary or record book. Patterns or trends in blood glucose levels outside the target range indicate a need to adjust the insulin dose. Three or four days of a consistent pattern of elevated glucose values (e.g., 200 mg/dL before the evening meal for 3 consecutive days) indicates a need to increase the dose of the appropriate insulin. The health care team may provide the family with guidelines for increasing insulin doses on the basis of blood glucose patterns.

A majority of blood glucose meters can store multiple monitoring results so blood glucose patterns can be evaluated. Blood glucose meters are accurate only if used according to manufacturer recommendations. Regardless of the brand selected, quality control procedures must be performed as recommended. Test supplies must be stored according to manufacturer specifications and discarded when outdated.

Developmental Issues

Infant and Toddler. The infant or toddler with type 1 diabetes poses special challenges for diabetes management. The parents must adapt to the diagnosis and master the daily management needs of the child. Severe hypoglycemia occurs most often in this age-group so glucose target levels are liberalized.

Achieving consistency in dietary intake can be difficult. Inconsistent intake, particularly of carbohydrates, contributes to blood glucose variability. Food control issues can easily become a battleground between the child and the parent. A diet strategy that stresses carbohydrate consistency rather than specific food groups offers more flexibility.

Allowing the toddler to participate in making food choices (from perhaps two or three options) can provide the child a sense of control. The signs and symptoms of hypoglycemia are difficult to recognize in the infant or may be mistaken for a toddler's temper tantrum. Establishing rituals and routines also helps the toddler feel more in control. Parents are encouraged to have a specific place to perform blood tests and to safely store supplies. Toddlers need to be able to predict when care activities will occur as well as participate according to their developmental level (Table 27-5).

Preschooler. The preschool years are characterized by increasing motor maturity, a widening social circle, and magical thinking. The preschooler can understand simple explanations regarding diabetes. Such explanations help allay fears that the diabetes was caused by the child being "bad." Play therapy with dolls and diabetes equipment helps the preschooler express concerns regarding injections and finger sticks.

The preschooler has a more predictable appetite than the toddler and is frequently willing to try new foods. Nonetheless, supervision is necessary to ensure that meals and snacks are eaten, especially if the child is in a daycare setting with many distractions.

The preschooler may be able to identify the feelings associated with hypoglycemia. It is important to use the child's description as a code word for the onset of hypoglycemia symptoms. Preschoolers' preferences for high-energy activities puts them at risk for hypoglycemia. The parents and other caregivers should be prepared with readily available carbohydrate foods, as well as emergency medications.

School-Age Child. The school-age child and family face the challenge of incorporating diabetes care within a busy school day. To avoid singling out the child, the diabetes care should be as unobtrusive as possible while still maintaining a safe environment for the child. Children with type 1 diabetes mellitus fall under the Individuals with Disabilities Education Act and, as such, are entitled to services within the school setting. The child should have a diabetes management plan that specifically describes frequency of blood glucose testing, insulin doses, nutrition, and any other therapy or modifications associated with the diabetes (Funnell, Brown, Childs et al., 2008). The family should communicate with school personnel about the child's diabetes. A school nurse or health aide should be identified to supervise before-lunch blood glucose monitoring, assist with insulin injections, and educate other school personnel in recognizing and treating hypoglycemia. Schools vary on the availability of nursing services. Parents may have to work with school personnel to identify appropriate staff to supervise their child's diabetes care.

Planning ahead for field trips, school parties, and athletic events allows the child with diabetes to participate safely in age-appropriate

TABLE 27-5 EXAMPLES OF DIABETES MANAGEMENT TASKS DELEGATED TO CHILD (WITH SUPERVISION)

DEVELOPMENTAL CHARACTERISTICS	MANAGEMENT TASK	DIET TASK
Toddler or Preschooler Likes rituals Finicky eater Not yet able to understand need for insulin	Chooses and cleans finger for puncture Helps by holding still for injection Identifies a word or phrase to describe a feeling of hypoglycemia	Helps by choosing foods
School-Age Child Present oriented Spends large amounts of time away from parents Begins to develop self-concept	Performs finger puncture and blood glucose test Chooses injection site according to rotation schedule Pushes plunger on insulin syringe after the needle is inserted by parent or gives own injection Performs ketone urine test	Recognizes need to eat on time to avoid hypoglycemia Knows treatment for hypoglycemia
Early Adolescent Looks to peer group for identity Needs to conform to peer-group norms Increased risk-taking behaviors	Records blood glucose values in diary Draws up insulin with supervision Performs insulin injection Begins to manage insulin pump and carbohydrate counting	Knows meal plan Can choose correct foods for snack Adds extra snack for increased activity
Middle or Late Adolescent Future oriented Wants to take charge of life Able to recognize consequences of behaviors and choices Emotional separation from parents	Draws up and injects insulin Looks for patterns in blood glucose values Recognizes when to test for ketones in urine Initiates treatment for ketones (fluids)	Can plan meals and snacks based on meal plan Can choose appropriate foods at a party or when eating out

activities. For example, the child who has soccer practice three afternoons per week needs to plan how to prevent hypoglycemia during practice.

Adolescent. The adolescent's developmental milestones are often in conflict with the recommendations for achieving diabetes control. The young adolescent is concerned with body image and peer-group acceptance and is moving away from the family for support and identity. Clothing, diet, lifestyle, and speech are areas in which the early adolescent strives to conform to peers.

The child in mid-adolescence may engage in risk-taking behaviors and more openly challenge parental authority. By late adolescence, the individual becomes more future oriented, with behaviors based more on abstract reasoning and less on peer-group demands.

These normally recognized milestones become dilemmas when diabetes control is affected. Missed injections, omitted blood tests, irregular meals, and dietary splurges are frequent complaints of parents of diabetic adolescents.

Parents and their adolescents must accept that diabetes management responsibility increasingly shifts to the adolescent. Parents are encouraged to work as partners with the adolescent to achieve diabetes control. It is essential to identify what is important to the adolescent, and use that information to motivate adherence. The adolescent is not motivated by predictions of complications in the distant future. Rather, motivation should focus on issues of current significance to the adolescent such as personal appearance, athletic ability, strength and muscle mass, endurance, or ideal weight.

◎ NURSING CARE PLAN

The Child with Type 1 Diabetes Mellitus in the Community Setting

Focused Assessment
- Obtain history from family of signs and symptoms of hyperglycemia:
  - Polydipsia: requests water through the night
  - Polyuria: increased frequency of urination
  - Enuresis (if previously toilet trained)
  - Polyphagia
  - Weight loss
  - Fatigue
  - Nausea and vomiting
- Ask family about all medications the child is taking
  - Certain drugs can cause hyperglycemia
- Perform a physical assessment and look for signs and symptoms of:
  - Dehydration
  - Acidosis
  - Infection
- Assess the child's and family's knowledge and ability to carry out the diabetes home management plan
- Assess the child's and family's ability to cope with the diagnosis of a chronic illness

Planning
Nursing Diagnosis
Deficient Knowledge related to unfamiliarity with home care needs of the child with type 1 diabetes mellitus.

Expected Outcome
The child and family will be able to successfully manage diabetes, as evidenced by demonstration of skills and verbalization of concepts necessary for home care (see Patient-Centered Teaching: Home Management of Type I Diabetes Mellitus box).

Intervention/Rationale
1. Identify potential barriers to learning home care information and performing diabetes management skills. Specifically address language, literacy, manual dexterity, stressors, and fears.
   Identifying and addressing these issues before education begins will optimize the family's learning. Additional resources may be needed such as translator services or counseling.
2. Assess the family's knowledge of diabetes. Identify learning objectives with the child and family.
   The education plan needs to be individualized. Specific objectives guide the learning process.

3. Prepare the family to participate in diabetes education.
   The child and family must learn home care strategies and skills.
4. Present information that is suitable for the child's age and developmental level.
   The child needs to understand diabetes and the management plan to engage in self-care at a developmentally appropriate level.

Evaluation
Can the child and family successfully manage care, as evidenced by return demonstrations of knowledge and skills necessary to provide home care?
Are the child and family able to describe principles of diabetes management?

Planning
Nursing Diagnosis
Interrupted Family Processes related to the chronic health care needs of a child with type 1 diabetes mellitus.

Expected Outcome
The child and family will cope with managing diabetes, as evidenced by recognizing stresses and constructing strategies for dealing with the stress of a chronic disease.

Intervention/Rationale
1. Help the family identify diabetes management responsibilities appropriate to delegate to the child and those the parents must assume.
   Delegation of responsibilities to the child occurs when the child is able to both perform the skill and understand the implications. Parental support and supervision are essential for all children.
2. Help the child and family identify behaviors that the child recognizes as supporting adherence to the diabetes management plan.
   Family communication and participation facilitates adherence (i.e., all family members follow the child's meal plan).
3. Identify community support systems available for the child and family (i.e., summer diabetes camp, peer and parents support groups, community agencies, and financial resources).
   ⊖ *Community resources offer a variety of services (see Evolve website). Peer support groups for the diabetic child and the family build motivation and self-esteem.*
4. Identify alternative care options that allow the primary caregiver to take a break from diabetes management responsibilities.
   Taking care of a child with diabetes is very stressful and demanding. Sharing responsibilities among family members and other caregivers helps decrease stress.

Additional Resources—Resources for Health Care Providers and Families

◎ NURSING CARE PLAN

The Child with Type 1 Diabetes Mellitus in the Community Setting—cont'd

Evaluation

Can the child and family verbalize a plan for sharing diabetes management responsibility?

Planning

Nursing Diagnosis

Imbalanced Nutrition: Less Than Body Requirements related to insulin deficit.

Expected Outcomes

The family and child will maximize nutritional status, as evidenced by demonstrating the ability to administer insulin, control diet and exercise, and perform blood glucose monitoring.

The child will be in nutritional balance, as evidenced by appropriate glucose levels and expected growth.

Intervention/Rationale

1. Teach the child and family how food intake affects blood glucose level (i.e., carbohydrates raise blood glucose; fats and proteins have minimal effects).
   Understanding the relationship of food to blood glucose levels provides the child and family the rationale for adhering to the diet plan.

2. In conjunction with the child and family, develop an eating schedule for meals and snacks that also includes times for blood glucose testing, medications, and exercise.
   The consistent timing of meals and snacks in relation to insulin injections and exercise is essential. Child and family involvement in schedule planning provides a sense of control and promotes adherence to the schedule.

3. Ask the child to identify favorite foods and demonstrate how these can be incorporated into the meal plan.
   Most foods can be incorporated into the meal plan, even if only in small amounts. Allowing some quantity of favorite foods encourages adherence.

4. Observe whether the child's hunger is satisfied on the prescribed diet and adjust meal plan as needed.
   The meal plan is tailored to the child's nutritional needs and activity level.

5. Record height and weight measurements on the appropriate growth charts.
   Monitoring the child's growth indicates whether the meal plan is meeting nutritional needs.

6. Identify ideal blood glucose levels for the child. Ask the child and family to identify what changes could be made to diet, insulin, and/or exercise if the blood glucose level is out of the ideal range.
   Diet, exercise, and insulin therapy are diabetic management tools that the child and family must learn how to use to attain ideal blood glucose levels.

Evaluation

Do the child and family demonstrate appropriate insulin administration, diet therapy, and glucose monitoring?

Do the child and family adhere to the schedule for blood glucose testing, insulin injections, food intake, and exercise?

Do the child and family adhere to the meal plan?

Are the child's height and weight appropriate for age compared with growth chart percentiles?

Planning

Nursing Diagnosis

Risk for Injury related to hypoglycemia or hyperglycemia.

Expected Outcomes

The child will remain injury free as a result of appropriate recognition and management of hypoglycemia or hyperglycemia.

Family members will demonstrate knowledge of the signs, symptoms, and treatment of hypoglycemia and hyperglycemia and will initiate appropriate treatment.

Intervention/Rationale

For hypoglycemia (blood glucose level less than 60 mg/dL):

1. Teach the child and family to recognize the signs and symptoms of hypoglycemia (see Table 27-3). Involve the daycare workers for young children and the school nurse, teachers, and other personnel in the care of a school-age child or adolescent.
   Recognition of hypoglycemia signs and symptoms prompts the child, parent or school personnel to perform a blood glucose check and rapidly initiate treatment for hypoglycemia if indicated.

2. Teach the child and family (as well as daycare and school personnel) to treat hypoglycemia immediately with oral intake of 15 g of easily digested (simple) carbohydrates. In 15 minutes, if symptoms are not relieved or blood glucose is 80 mg/dL or lower, repeat treatment. If the hypoglycemia occurs during the night, treat with 30 g of carbohydrate ($\frac{1}{2}$ simple and $\frac{1}{2}$ complex) and with protein.
   Early treatment reduces the possibility of a more severe reaction. There are 15 g of carbohydrates in 4 oz of 100% fruit juice.

3. Teach the family as well as daycare and school personnel how to treat severe hypoglycemia for a child who is unconscious or having seizures. Place the child in the side-lying position. Rub glucose gel, frosting, or honey on the child's inner cheek and gums. If prescribed, glucagon can be injected subcutaneously or IM (onset of action is 10 to 15 minutes).
   Urgent treatment is essential if a hypoglycemic child is unconscious or seizing. The child is positioned on the side to prevent aspiration. Glucose is rapidly absorbed through mouth epithelial tissues into the bloodstream. Glucagon is a pancreatic hormone that opposes the action of insulin and promotes conversion of liver glycogen to blood glucose.

4. Help the child and family identify strategies to prevent and, if needed, treat hypoglycemia. Have the child wear medical alert identification at all times.
   Many episodes of hypoglycemia can be averted by better planning of food intake and avoiding late or missed meals, excess insulin, or extra exercise. A diabetes box with hypoglycemia treatment instructions and supplies should be available at home and at daycare or school.

For hyperglycemia (blood glucose level higher than target range):

1. Teach the child and family (as well as daycare and school personnel) to recognize the signs, symptoms, and causes of hyperglycemia (see Table 27-3).
   Being aware of situations that may result in hyperglycemia can help distinguish the signs and symptoms of hyperglycemia versus hypoglycemia. The child's blood glucose level must be checked before starting treatment.

2. Teach the child and family the correct procedure to test for ketones in the urine when the child is ill or the blood glucose level exceeds 250 mg/dL.
   Ketones are formed in response to insulin deficit. Early recognition of ketonuria and treatment can prevent acute complications including diabetic ketoacidosis (DKA).

Continued

◎ NURSING CARE PLAN

The Child with Type 1 Diabetes Mellitus in the Community Setting—cont'd

Intervention/*Rationale*—cont'd

3. Teach child and family how to treat hyperglycemia. Administer calorie-free oral fluids and additional short-acting insulin subcutaneously as ordered by the physician.

   Fluids and insulin remove excess ketones. A child with nausea and vomiting cannot be treated with oral fluids; the physician must be notified because of the risk of dehydration.

4. Instruct family on sick-day diabetes management. Explain to the family how and when a diabetes health care team member should be contacted (Box 27-5).

   Stress resulting from infection or other causes can result in uncontrolled diabetes. Sick-day management is an effective prevention strategy.

5. Evaluate the child's dosages and types of insulin prescribed and the administration schedule.

   Persistent hyperglycemia may indicate the need to adjust the insulin regimen. The growing child will need periodic increases in baseline insulin dosages.

6. Evaluate the family's diabetes home management knowledge, adherence to the recommended plan, home supervision of the child, and coping skills.

   Frequent episodes of hyperglycemia (and DKA) may reflect a lack of understanding or nonadherence to the home management plan, inadequate child supervision, and ineffective coping strategies.

7. Help the child and family identify strategies to prevent hyperglycemia. Provide additional interventions or refer to support services, as indicated.

   Consistency in diet, exercise, and insulin injection times helps prevent hyperglycemia. The child and family may need additional services to successfully manage the child's chronic illness.

Evaluation

Does the child remain injury free?

Are the child and family able to recognize and correctly and promptly treat hypoglycemia and hyperglycemia?

Is the child free of episodes of severe hypoglycemia or hyperglycemia?

PATIENT-CENTERED TEACHING

Home Management of Type 1 Diabetes Mellitus

The child and family are understandably overwhelmed with questions and fears about the diagnosis. Encourage all family members to participate in the educational process. Choose a comfortable location subject to few interruptions. Provide appropriate literature and materials for family members. DVDs, booklets, and pamphlets should be developmentally appropriate. Educational materials for the parents should also match the parents' literacy skills.

The following checklist of outcomes evaluates the family's understanding of the pertinent information:

- General information about type 1 diabetes mellitus
- How to administer and store insulin
- How to monitor blood glucose levels and use the equipment properly
- Signs and management of hypoglycemic episodes
- Signs and management of hyperglycemia
- Strategies for when the child is ill
- Nutrition and exercise principles
- Potential long-term complications
- Available resources for community services and emotional support

All family members should be given the opportunity to practice skills taught. Practicing procedures on themselves or each other helps allay fears and allows the child to supervise as a family member performs the procedure. Help develop problem-solving skills by using various scenarios that encourage decision making. Because education is an ongoing process, the family needs a contact person to whom they can turn for advice and support.

Outcomes

General Information

The child and family will be able to do the following:

1. Describe the action of insulin in the body.
2. Describe the characteristics of type 1 diabetes.
3. Identify three factors that can be used to control blood glucose levels.

Medication Therapy

The child and family will be able to do the following:

1. Name the types of insulin the child is using and identify the onset, peak, and duration of action for each.
2. State the storage recommendations for insulin.
3. State the recommended expiration date of the insulin.
4. Demonstrate accurate syringe or air injector preparation for a single type of insulin.

5. Demonstrate syringe preparation for two types of insulin.
6. Demonstrate subcutaneous insulin injection technique with syringe/needle or air injector.
7. Identify insulin injection sites and describe a pattern of rotation.
8. Identify a plan for safe syringe and needle disposal.
9. Identify recommended insulin dosages and injection times.
10. Describe the function and management associated with an insulin pump. Demonstrate set-up and use of an insulin pump, if applicable.

Home Glucose Monitoring

The child and family will be able to do the following:

1. Identify nondiabetic blood glucose levels and target goals for good glucose control.
2. Demonstrate the use, calibration, control testing, and cleaning of the blood glucose monitor.
3. Demonstrate finger-stick technique to obtain the blood sample.
4. Identify a plan for recording blood glucose values.

Hypoglycemia

The child and family will be able to do the following:

1. Identify the signs and symptoms of a hypoglycemic reaction.
2. Describe appropriate treatment for both a mild and a severe hypoglycemic reaction.
3. Identify three potential causes of a hypoglycemic reaction.
4. Identify the importance of medical emergency identification.
5. Describe typical blood glucose trends during the honeymoon phase.

Hyperglycemia

The child and family will be able to do the following:

1. Identify the signs and symptoms of hyperglycemia.
2. Identify strategies to control hyperglycemia.
3. Describe the possible effects of stress or illness on diabetes control.
4. Demonstrate the procedure for ketone (urine, serum) testing.
5. State when to test for ketones.
6. State basic treatment if the child tests positive for ketones.
7. Describe the signs and symptoms requiring physician or other health care team contact.

PATIENT-CENTERED TEACHING—cont'd

Nutrition/Exercise

The child and family will be able to do the following:

1. State the effect of exercise on blood glucose levels.
2. State the benefits of an appropriate nutrition plan and describe precautions for exercise.
3. Identify the correlation of diet, exercise, and insulin with blood glucose control.
4. Generate a home schedule that identifies mealtimes and snack times, blood test times, and insulin injection times.

Complications

The child and family will be able to do the following:

1. Identify the role of glucose control in the prevention or delay of diabetes-related complications.
2. Identify appropriate health care follow-up for the child with diabetes.

Psychological Adjustment and Family Involvement

The child and family will be able to create a plan for the entire family to participate in diabetes care and management.

Community Resources

The child and family will be able to identify available community resources for ongoing diabetes services, education and support.

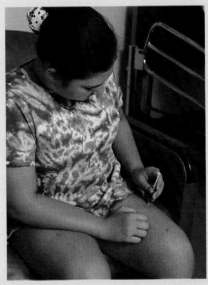

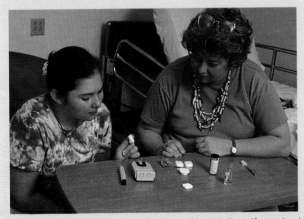

The school-age child is usually able to perform daily self-monitoring of blood glucose with parental help. However, the child should not be expected to adjust the insulin dose based on the reading. By early adolescence, the child can be in charge of recording blood glucose values in the diary.

When other parts of the treatment regimen have become familiar, the injection technique can be taught. Initially, self-injecting insulin may be frightening for the school-age child, so the parent may insert the needle and have the child then push the plunger. The child can then progress to performing self-injection.

BOX 27-5   SICK-DAY MANAGEMENT FOR THE CHILD WITH TYPE 1 DIABETES MELLITUS

1. Always give insulin injections, even if the child does not want to eat. If concerned that the child will become hypoglycemic with the usual dose, contact a diabetes health care team member for instructions. If ordered, use sliding scale, rapid- or short-acting insulin for hyperglycemia every 3 to 4 hours.
2. Test blood glucose level at least every 4 hours or more often if hypoglycemic or hyperglycemic.
3. Test for urine ketones with each voiding. Notify diabetes team member if moderate or large amounts of urine ketones are present. Additional regular insulin may be ordered.
4. Encourage intake of calorie-free liquids. Liquids aid in clearing ketones from the blood.

5. Follow the child's usual meal plan. If the child has a poor appetite, a sick-day diet replacing the usual grams of carbohydrate with simple carbohydrate foods is used.
6. Encourage rest. Exercising while ketones are present results in increased ketone formation.
7. Notify the diabetes health care team member of the following:
   - Nausea and vomiting
   - Fruity odor to the breath
   - Deep, rapid respirations
   - Decreasing level of consciousness
   - Moderate or high urine ketones
   - Persistent hyperglycemia

Delegating Diabetes Management Responsibilities

Children with diabetes are functionally able to perform diabetes management tasks far sooner than they can cognitively understand the implications of the action or consequences of omitting the action. Transfer of responsibility from the parents to the child should be on a step-by-step basis, according to the child's cognitive understanding and functional abilities. Diabetes management shifts from full parental responsibility to a partnership between parent and child and then to the acceptance of full responsibility by the young adult. Delegation of management responsibility to the child too soon may result in poor diabetes control and frequent DKA episodes. Ongoing parental support and supervision is essential (see Table 27-5).

DIABETIC KETOACIDOSIS

DKA is the metabolic consequence of a severe insulin deficit leading to hyperglycemia and presence of ketone bodies in the blood, followed by metabolic acidosis. For individuals with type 1 diabetes, DKA is seen more frequently in young children and adolescents than in adults (Hamdy, 2009).

Etiology

DKA results from an absolute or relative insulin deficit. In the younger diabetic child, the most common cause is insulin resistance, such as a stress response initiated by an infection. In the adolescent, the most common cause is one or more missed insulin injections.

Manifestations

Table 27-3 lists signs and symptoms of DKA, which include abdominal and chest pain, nausea and vomiting, fruity breath smell, decreased level of consciousness (LOC), Kussmaul respirations, and symptoms of dehydration.

Diagnostic Evaluation

Diabetic ketoacidosis is confirmed by the following test results:
- Blood glucose: Elevated
- Arterial or venous pH: Low
- Urine ketones: Large
- Serum ketones (beta-hydroxybutyric acid, acetone): Elevated
- Serum potassium: Elevated, normal, or low
- Serum phosphorus: Low
- White blood cell count (WBC): Elevated as a result of stress demargination (higher with infection)
- Serum carbon dioxide: Low

Therapeutic Management

The child in DKA usually is admitted to an intensive care unit. Management includes hourly glucose monitoring, hourly vital signs and neurologic checks, strict intake and output measurements, frequent assessment of fluid and electrolyte status, IV fluid replacement, potassium replacement if needed, and administration of continuous IV insulin (Orlowski, Cramer, & Fiallos, 2008).

◎ NURSING CARE PLAN

The Child in Diabetic Ketoacidosis (DKA)

Focused Assessment
- Assess for signs and symptoms related to:
  - Respiratory status
  - Level of consciousness
  - Hydration status
  - Electrolyte and acid-base balance
- Obtain the following history data from family:
  - Most recent blood glucose values
  - Urinary ketones test results and treatment
  - Time and amount of last insulin injection
  - Time and amount of last food eaten
  - Routine daily management plan (insulin dose/schedule, blood glucose checks, diet, and exercise)
  - Sick-day management plan
  - Family's understanding of diabetes management plan

Planning
Nursing Diagnosis
Deficient Fluid Volume related to abnormal fluid losses through diuresis and emesis.

Expected Outcome
The child will be safely rehydrated, as evidenced by normal weight, good skin turgor, appropriate urine output for age, and moist mucous membranes.

Intervention/Rationale
1. Determine the child's hydration status, evaluating weight, skin turgor, mucous membranes, and urine output.
   This identifies current hydration status. A comparison of the child's usual weight with the admission weight provides an estimation of percent body fluid loss.
2. Encourage intake of calorie-free fluids if the child is not nauseated. Administer IV fluids as ordered (normal saline is given initially).
   Rehydration is the initial step in resolving DKA. Fluid losses occur primarily from the osmotic diuresis with hyperglycemia. If acidosis has resulted in nausea and vomiting, IV fluids are required.

3. Maintain strict intake and output monitoring.
   Accurate intake and output records are essential in determining rehydration status.
4. Observe for edema or pulmonary congestion.
   These signs indicate overhydration.
5. Weigh child on admission and every 8 to 12 hours.
   Comparing admission weight to the child's usual weight indicates initial hydration status. Follow-up weights provide ongoing assessment.

Evaluation
Is the child safely rehydrated, as evidenced by normal weight, urine output appropriate for age, good skin turgor, and moist mucous membranes?

Planning
Nursing Diagnosis
Risk for Injury from altered acid-base balance leading to ketone production and acidosis related to lack of insulin.

Expected Outcome
The child will have a resolution of ketosis and acidosis, as evidenced by laboratory results and clinical assessment.

Intervention/Rationale
1. Test all urine samples for the presence of ketones. Monitor the child's breath for acetone. Observe for Kussmaul respirations.
   Urinary ketones indicate possible acidosis. Serum ketone analysis, or beta-hydroxybutyric acid, is a direct measurement. When acetone, a ketoacid, is expelled, the child's breath has a fruity smell. High acid levels trigger rapid and deep breaths (Kussmaul respirations).
2. Encourage calorie-free fluids if the child is able to drink. If ordered, begin IV fluids.
   Fluids are essential in flushing ketones out of the blood.
3. Initiate continuous IV infusion of regular insulin as ordered. Titrate to maintain blood glucose in safe range.
   Insulin therapy starts after rehydration is underway. Blood glucose should drop no more than 80 to 100 mg/dL/hr to prevent rapid fluid shifts.

◎ NURSING CARE PLAN

The Child in Diabetic Ketoacidosis (DKA)—cont'd

Intervention/Rationale—cont'd

4. Monitor blood glucose every hour during IV insulin infusion.
   IV insulin acts quickly and can suddenly cause hypoglycemia.
5. Provide glucose-containing IV fluids as ordered.
   Insulin inhibits the production of ketones. When blood glucose reaches 230 to 300 mg/dL, glucose is added to the IV fluids to prevent hypoglycemia. Insulin infusion continues until serum ketones are cleared.

Evaluation

Within 24 hours of admission, does the child display any evidence of ketosis (ketonuria, fruity breath, elevated blood glucose)?

Planning

Nursing Diagnosis

Risk for Injury related to electrolyte imbalance from emesis and acidosis.

Expected Outcome

The child will remain free from adverse consequences of electrolyte abnormalities, as evidenced by normal serum sodium and potassium values.

Intervention/Rationale

1. Monitor potassium levels every 1 to 2 hours initially; look for signs and symptoms of hyperkalemia (bradycardia, muscle weakness, hyperreflexia, cardiac or respiratory arrest) and hypokalemia (muscle weakness, fatigue, hypotension). Monitor serum sodium levels at intervals.
   During acidosis, potassium moves out of the cells to the intravascular space and then is excreted through diuresis. Initially, serum potassium levels may be acceptable; this does not reflect intracellular losses. With rehydration and correction of acidosis, potassium moves back into the cells, resulting in lower serum levels (see Chapter 16).
2. Maintain child on a cardiac monitor to watch for abnormal electrocardiogram findings. Prepare for a rapid response if a medical emergency occurs.
   Hypokalemia produces prolonged ST segments; notched, flat, or inverted T waves; and arrhythmias. Hyperkalemia produces flattened P waves or peaked T waves and ventricular fibrillation.

3. Administer potassium as ordered, if child has urine output. If anuric, notify physician and *do not* give potassium.
   Renal failure can result from severe dehydration. With anuria, potassium is retained, resulting in hyperkalemia.

Evaluation

Does the child maintain a stable fluid and electrolyte balance, with serum sodium and potassium levels within normal limits?

Planning

Nursing Diagnosis

Risk for Injury related to cerebral edema from resolving DKA.

Expected Outcome

The child will remain free from adverse consequences of cerebral edema, as evidenced by appropriate level of consciousness, pupils equal and reacting to light, and absence of headache.

Intervention/Rationale

1. Perform neurologic checks every 1 to 2 hours and observe for signs of cerebral edema (headache; decreased level of consciousness; nonreactive to light, unequal, or dilated pupils). Notify physician immediately of any neurologic changes.
   Cerebral edema is a complication of resolving DKA that can result in brain damage or death. Causes are unclear; may be related to overhydration, rapid fluid shifts, and electrolyte imbalances. Prompt recognition and treatment may prevent neurologic injury (see Chapter 28).

Evaluation

Is the child alert, with equal and reactive pupils and without reports of headache?

LONG-TERM HEALTH CARE NEEDS FOR THE CHILD WITH TYPE 1 DIABETES MELLITUS

Serious complications are associated with long-term type 1 diabetes including retinopathy, nephropathy, neuropathy, and cardiovascular disease. Studies have demonstrated that strict metabolic control of diabetes may decrease the severity of complications and/or delay onset. A team approach to diabetes management can best provide the tools to achieve metabolic control. The team includes the physician specialist, nurse educator, dietitian, and behavioral specialist. Regular checkups and frequent telephone communication between the diabetes team and the parents—and the child, if age-appropriate—are essential to address the needs of the growing child.

Glycemic control over time (3 months or longer) as assessed by HbA$_{1c}$ is critically important for children to reduce the cognitive sequelae of hypoglycemic episodes (ADA, 2008b). Although the normal HbA$_{1c}$ for adults is considered to be approximately 7% or less, recommendations are less restrictive for children and adolescents. HbA$_{1c}$ levels between 7.5% and 8.5% are considered acceptable during early childhood and HbA$_{1c}$ levels less than 7.5% are considered acceptable for adolescents (ADA, 2008b).

Older children with type 1 diabetes should be screened to prevent long-term complications. The ADA (2008b) recommends that children older than 10 years and those who are symptomatic be screened for microscopic albuminuria, autoimmune thyroid disease, retinopathy, hypertension, dyslipidemia, and celiac disease. Early identification of and treatment for these conditions can minimize serious complications in adulthood.

Routine health care for the child with diabetes should also include yearly dental and ophthalmologic evaluations, as well as prophylactic interventions such as influenza vaccinations. Children and their families should be referred to other health care providers, counselors, other service providers, and community resources as specific needs are identified.

Diabetes research is aimed at preventing diabetes and finding a cure after diagnosis. Multiple immune intervention strategies are being identified and tested. In addition, pancreas and islet cell transplantation continues to be researched as a potential cure in the future.

TYPE 2 DIABETES MELLITUS

Type 2 diabetes is an emerging problem in the pediatric population. The rise in the incidence of overweight and obese children is directly related to the increased number of children diagnosed with type 2 diabetes (Pozzo, 2010). At the time of diagnosis, approximately 50% of the beta cells in the pancreas of children with type 2 diabetes are still producing insulin. These children have a combination of insulin resistance and decreased insulin secretion (Pozzo, 2010).

Etiology

The majority of children with type 2 diabetes are at risk for being overweight (body mass index [BMI] between 85th and 95th percentile) or are overweight (BMI greater than 95th percentile) at diagnosis and have glycosuria without ketonuria, absent or mild polydipsia and polyuria, and no or little recent weight loss. Type 2 diabetes is not caused by an autoimmune response. The pancreas still produces insulin, but in an amount insufficient to overcome persistent hyperglycemia. Genetics and familial factors, race/ethnicity, maternal gestational diabetes, and intrauterine growth retardation, along with a lack of physical activity in childhood and adolescence, seem to be crucial factors in the development of type 2 diabetes in children (ADA, 2008b).

Incidence

Type 2 diabetes represents 8% to 45% of all new cases of diabetes diagnosed in children and adolescents, a substantial increase in the past two decades (Pozzo, 2010). Mean age of type 2 diabetes onset is 12 to 16 years (Pozzo, 2010). In the United States, the SEARCH for Diabetes in Youth Study found that in 15- to 19-year-olds, the highest incidence of type 2 diabetes occurs in American Indians followed by Asian-Pacific Islanders and African-Americans (Dabelea, Bell, D'Agostino et al., 2007).

Manifestations

Children with type 2 diabetes are typically overweight and have acanthosis nigricans, a velvety darkening of the skin around the back and sides of the neck and other areas including inguinal folds, axilla, umbilicus, knees, antecubital fossa, and backs of the hands. It is a marker for metabolic syndrome, also known as insulin resistance syndrome (Pozzo, 2010). Other possible symptoms include fatigue, yeast infections, blurred vision, and frequent urination. Hypertension, elevated triglyceride and low-density lipoprotein levels, and polycystic ovary syndrome may be presenting signs.

Diagnostic Evaluation

Diagnosis of type 2 diabetes depends on careful physical examination, elevated endogenous insulin levels, and no evidence of serum autoantibodies. A fasting blood glucose over 126 mg/dL or a random serum glucose level of 200 mg/dL or more indicates diabetes, either type 1 or type 2. The fasting C-peptide level is usually elevated in type 2 diabetes (Pozzo, 2010).

Therapeutic Management

The mainstays of treatment for children with type 2 diabetes are nutritional interventions for weight maintenance or weight loss (depending on age) and regular, moderate-intensity physical exercise (Pozzo, 2010).

Any child with severe hyperglycemia, ketonemia, and metabolic abnormalities, whether diagnosed with type 1 or type 2 diabetes, will need insulin therapy to reverse metabolic imbalances. Some children with type 2 diabetes may require insulin; however, most are managed with oral agents that decrease insulin resistance or augment endogenous insulin production. Blood glucose monitoring and diet management are important aspects of therapy. If these children lose weight, some can be managed with diet and exercise alone.

The goals of type 2 diabetes management for children include the following (Pozzo, 2010):
- Achieving near-normal glycemic control (acceptable HbA_{1c} according to age)
- Facilitating reasonable weight for height
- Achieving normal blood glucose levels
- Prevention of hyperlipidemia and hypertension
- Decreasing the frequency of microvascular and cardiovascular complications

Medication Therapy

For the child with type 2 diabetes mellitus, oral hypoglycemic agents may be used if the diabetes cannot be managed with diet and exercise. At present, metformin is the only type 2 diabetes medication approved by the U.S. Food and Drug Administration for use in children ages 10 years and older (Pozzo, 2010). It is commonly prescribed as the initial oral hypoglycemic medication if severe hyperglycemia is not present. Reduced serum triglyceride and cholesterol levels and weight stabilization or decrease are other effects of metformin use.

Nutrition Therapy

Nutrition therapy goals for children and adolescents with type 2 diabetes are individualized, with emphasis on improved glycemic control and weight maintenance or loss through a reduced intake of calories. A dietary pattern that encourages consumption of fruits, vegetables, whole grains, legumes, and low-fat milk is recommended (ADA, 2008a). Improved glycemic control can be achieved through carbohydrate counting. Reducing foods containing saturated and trans fatty acids, cholesterol, and sodium may lead to improvement in dyslipidemia and lower blood pressure (ADA, 2008a). Participation of the entire family in a weight management program, which incorporates behavior modification strategies, is a key to success.

Physical Activity

Increased physical activity by individuals with type 2 diabetes can improve glycemic control, decrease insulin resistance, and reduce cardiovascular disease risk factors (ADA, 2008a). For children with type 2 diabetes, 60 to 90 minutes of moderate physical activity daily and less than 60 minutes per day of "screen time" sedentary activities (TV, computer, video games) are required for prevention and management of type 2 diabetes (Pozzo, 2010).

Blood Glucose Monitoring

The frequency of blood glucose testing for a child with type 2 diabetes is based on blood glucose goals, as well as the child's and family's willingness and ability to perform the tests. Ideally, blood glucose levels should be checked two or three times daily and HbA_{1c} levels monitored every 3 months (Pozzo, 2010).

Prevention

The American Diabetes Association (2008b) recommends routine monitoring for the presence or development of type 2 diabetes in children who are overweight and have two or more risk factors. Risk factors include a family history of type 2 diabetes, member of at-risk race/ethnic group (African-American, Latino/Hispanic, Native-American Indian, Asian-American, Pacific Islander), signs of insulin resistance or associated conditions (hypertension or dyslipidemia), and a mother who had gestational diabetes or diabetes starting at age 10 years or younger (with the onset of puberty). These children should have fasting blood glucose testing done every 2 years (ADA, 2008b).

Metabolic syndrome predicts the development of both type 2 diabetes mellitus and cardiovascular disease in adults (De Ferranti, Gauvreau, Ludwig et al., 2004). An individual with at least three of these characteristics is considered to have metabolic syndrome:

hypertension, low HDL (high-density lipoprotein) cholesterol, high serum triglycerides, elevated fasting blood glucose, and central obesity with increased waist circumference. Research has revealed that 4% to 9.5% of all adolescents and 29% of overweight adolescents have metabolic syndrome (Cook, Weitzman, Auinger et al., 2003; Jago, Baranowski, Buse et al., 2008). Children and adolescents must be identified and early interventions provided to reduce their risk of developing chronic, debilitating diseases as adults.

KEY CONCEPTS

- The six major hormones of the endocrine system secreted by the anterior pituitary gland are ACTH, TSH, FSH, LH, GH, and prolactin.
- The pituitary gland secretes stimulating hormones that cause target organs to produce specific hormones. Per the negative feedback system, when hormone levels are sufficient, secretion of stimulating hormones decreases.
- Pill dispensers and reminder watch alarms can improve adherence to daily medication regimens.
- Metabolic and endocrine conditions that affect newborns are often genetic and may require long-term management.
- Some signs and symptoms of hypothyroidism (fatigue, weight gain, constipation, cold intolerance) are opposite of those for hyperthyroidism (nervousness, weight loss, diarrhea, heat intolerance).
- Diabetes insipidus is caused by deficient ADH leading to high output of unconcentrated urine and hypernatremia. SIADH occurs with excessive production of ADH and results in decreased output of concentrated urine and hyponatremia.
- Children with precocious puberty may experience psychosocial issues including self-consciousness about their bodies, being treated as older than their chronologic age, and aggressive behavior by boys.

- Without insulin, metabolism is impaired and glucose does not move into the intracellular space, resulting in hyperglycemia.
- Both type 1 diabetes mellitus and type 2 diabetes mellitus involve abnormal carbohydrate metabolism and hyperglycemia; however, causes, risk factors, treatment, and prevention differ significantly.
- The goals of diabetes management are to maintain glycemic control, reasonable weight for height, and an age-appropriate lifestyle as well as prevent acute and long-term complications.
- Hypoglycemia results from too much insulin with neuroglycopenic symptoms (personality changes, slurred speech, decreased LOC) and adrenergic signs (trembling, sweating, tachycardia, pallor, clammy skin); treat with ingestion of 15 g of easily digested carbohydrate.
- Hyperglycemia is caused by excessive carbohydrate intake and inadequate insulin, with signs and symptoms of increased urine output, thirst, and hunger as well as fatigue, blurred vision, headache, and emotional lability; treat with insulin and increased fluid intake.
- DKA occurs as a result of severe hyperglycemia with ketones in the blood and metabolic acidosis. Management often requires intensive care to lower blood glucose, reverse acidosis, and correct fluid and electrolyte imbalances.

REFERENCES

American Diabetes Association. (2008a). Nutrition recommendations and interventions for diabetes. *Diabetes Care, 31*(Suppl. 1), S61-S78.

American Diabetes Association. (2008b). Standards of medical care in diabetes—2008. *Diabetes Care, 31*(Suppl. 1), S12-S54.

American Diabetes Association. (2011). *Diabetic statistics.* Retrieved from www.diabetes.org/diabetes-basics/diabetes-statistics.

Arnold, G. (2009). Phenylketonuria. Retrieved from http://emedicine.medscape.com/article/947781-overview.

Breault, D., & Majzoub, J. (2011a). Diabetes insipidus. In R. Kliegman, B. Stanton, J. St. Geme, et al. (Eds.), *Nelson textbook of pediatrics* (19th ed., pp. 1881-1884). Philadelphia: Elsevier Saunders.

Breault, D., & Majzoub, J. (2011b). Other abnormalities of arginine vasopressin metabolism and action. In R. Kliegman, B. Stanton, J. St. Geme, et al. (Eds.), *Nelson textbook of pediatrics* (19th ed., pp. 1884-1886). Philadelphia: Elsevier Saunders.

Cesario, S., & Hughes, L. (2007). Precocious puberty: A comprehensive review of literature. *Journal of Obstetric, Gynecologic, and Neonatal Nursing, 36*(3), 263-274.

Cook, S., Weitzman, M., Auinger, P., et al. (2003). Prevalence of a metabolic syndrome phenotype in adolescents. *Archives of Pediatric and Adolescent Medicine, 157*(8), 821-827.

Cooperman, G. (2010). *Diabetes insipidus.* Retrieved from http://emedicine.medscape.com/article/117648-overview.

Cranmer, H., & Shannon, M. (2009). *Pediatrics, hypoglycemia.* Retrieved from http://emedicine.medscape.com/article/802334-overview.

Dabelea, D., Bell, R., D'Agostino, R., et al. (2007). Incidence of diabetes in youth in the United States. *JAMA, 297*(24), 2716-2724.

De Ferranti, S., Gauvreau, K., Ludwig, D., et al. (2004). Prevalence of the metabolic syndrome in American adolescents. *Circulation, 110*(16), 2494-2497.

Ferry, R., & Bauer, A. (2010). *Hypothyroidism.* Retrieved from http://emedicine.medscape.com/article/922777-overview.

Ferry, R., & Fenton, C. (2009). *Precocious pseudopuberty.* Retrieved from http://emedicine.medscape.com/article/923876-overview.

Ferry, R., & Levitsky, L. (2010). *Graves disease.* Retrieved from http://emedicine.medscape.com/article/920283-overview.

Ferry, R., & Pascual-y-Baralt, J. (2010). *Syndrome of inappropriate antidiuretic hormone secretion.* Retrieved from http://emedicine.medscape.com/article/924829-overview.

Funnell, M., Brown, T., Childs, B., et al. (2008). National standards for diabetes self-management education. *Diabetes Care, 31*(Suppl. 1), S97-S104.

Garibaldi, L., & Chemaitilly, W. (2011). Central precocious puberty. In R. Kliegman, B. Stanton, J. St. Geme, et al. (Eds.), *Nelson textbook of pediatrics* (19th ed., pp. 1887-1889). Philadelphia: Elsevier Saunders.

Hamdy, O. (2009). *Diabetic ketoacidosis.* Retrieved from http://emedicine.medscape.com/article/118361-overview.

Jago, R., Baranowski, J., Buse, S., et al. (2008). Prevalence of the metabolic syndrome among a racially/ethnically diverse group of U.S. eighth-grade adolescents and association with fasting insulin and homeostasis model

assessment of insulin resistance levels. *Diabetes Care, 31*(10), 2020-2025.

Kaneshiro, N. (2010). *Growth hormone deficiency—children.* Retrieved from www.ncbi.nlm.nih.gov/pubmedhealth/PMH0002159.

Kaplowitz, P. (2010). *Precocious puberty.* Retrieved from http://emedicine.medscape.com/article/924002-overview.

Kemp, S. (2010). *Growth hormone deficiency.* Retrieved from http://emedicine.medscape.com/article/923688-overview.

LaFranchi, S. (2011a). Hyperthyroidism. In R. Kliegman, B. Stanton, J. St. Geme, et al. (Eds.), *Nelson textbook of pediatrics* (19th ed., pp. 1909-1913). Philadelphia: Elsevier Saunders.

LaFranchi, S. (2011b). Hypothyroidism. In R. Kliegman, B. Stanton, J. St. Geme, et al. (Eds.), *Nelson textbook of pediatrics* (19th ed., pp. 1895-1903). Philadelphia: Elsevier Saunders.

Lamb, W. (2010). *Diabetes mellitus, type 1.* Retrieved from http://emedicine.medscape.com/article/919999-overview.

Orlowski, J., Cramer, C., & Fiallos, M. (2008). Diabetic ketoacidosis in the pediatric ICU. *Pediatric Clinics of North America, 55*(3), 577-587.

Parks, J., & Felner, E. (2011). Hypopituitarism. In R. Kliegman, B. Stanton, J. St. Geme, et al. (Eds.), *Nelson textbook of pediatrics* (19th ed., pp. 1876-1881). Philadelphia: Elsevier Saunders.

Postellon, D. (2010). *Congenital hypothyroidism.* Retrieved from http://emedicine.medscape.com/article/919758-overview.

Pozzo, A. (2010). *Diabetes mellitus, type 2.* Retrieved from http://emedicine.medscape.com/article/925700-overview.

Sherr, J., Cengiz, E., & Tamborlane, W. (2009). From pumps to prevention: Recent advances in the treatment of type 1 diabetes. *Drug Discovery Today, 14*(19-20), 973-981.

Singhal, A., & Campbell, D. (2010). *Hypocalcemia*. Retrieved from http://emedicine.medscape.com/article/921844-overview.

Skyler, J., Ponder, S., Kruger, D., et al. (2007). Is there a place for insulin pump therapy in your practice? *Clinical Diabetes, 25*(2), 50-56.

Weitzel, D., Pfeffer, U., Dost, A., et al. (2010). Initial insulin therapy in children and adolescents with type 1 diabetes mellitus. *Pediatric Diabetes, 11*(3), 159-165.

White, P. (2011). Congenital adrenal hyperplasia due to 21-hydroxylase deficiency. In R. Kliegman, B. Stanton, J. St. Geme, et al. (Eds.), *Nelson textbook of pediatrics* (19th ed., pp. 1930-1935). Philadelphia: Elsevier Saunders.

Wilson, T. A. (2010). *Congenital adrenal hyperplasia*. Retrieved from http://emedicine.medscape.com/article/919218-overview.

Zuckerman, D. (2009). *Early puberty in girls. National Research Center for Women and Families*. Retrieved from www.center4research.org/2010/04/girls-to-women.

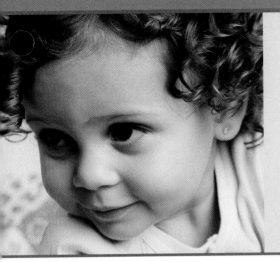

CHAPTER

28

The Child with a
Neurologic Alteration

⊖volve WEBSITE

http://evolve.elsevier.com/James/ncoc

LEARNING OBJECTIVES

After studying this chapter, you should be able to:

- Describe the embryologic development of the nervous system.
- Describe the anatomy and physiology of the nervous system.
- Describe the normal compensatory mechanisms that keep intracranial pressure within a constant range.
- Identify the neurologic differences among the infant, child, and adult.
- Be able to perform a neurologic assessment of a child and record findings.
- Use the nursing process to assess, plan, and provide nursing care to children with common neurologic alterations.

- Discuss the nursing implications of medications frequently used in the management of neurologic disorders.
- Describe teaching strategies that can be used for the child with neurologic problems and the child's family.
- List the measures used to keep a child safe during a seizure.
- List the measures used to prevent or treat cerebral edema.
- Differentiate between abnormal flexion and extension posturing and discuss the significance of each.
- List the compensatory mechanisms that affect intracranial blood flow and extravascular fluid volume if hydrocephalus develops.

CLINICAL REFERENCE

REVIEW OF THE CENTRAL NERVOUS SYSTEM

Embryologic Development

The nervous system is one of the first systems to form in utero. A neural tube remains hollow throughout development and eventually becomes the central nervous system. By the 4th week of gestation, the neural tube has closed at the anterior end to form the brain and at the posterior end to form the spinal cord.

During the 2nd month of gestation, the brain becomes the prominent body structure. It grows rapidly and continues to grow until approximately the 5th year of life. Two periods of rapid brain cell growth appear to occur during gestation. Between the 15th and 20th weeks of gestation, the number of neurons increases significantly. At 30 weeks, the number of neurons increases again, continuing through 1 year of age. Appropriate prenatal care during periods of rapid neuronal increase can prevent developmental neurologic deficits.

The Myelin Sheath

Myelin is the fatty substance that surrounds the nerves of both the central and the peripheral nervous systems. The myelin begins to form at approximately the 16th week of gestation. Myelin insulates the nerves and helps conduct electrical impulses. Coordination of fine and gross motor skills progresses with the deposition of the myelin sheath. Nerve fibers can conduct impulses in the absence of myelin; however, the impulses travel more slowly. Gross motor skills develop before fine motor skills as coordination and control advance throughout childhood. The myelin sheath can be destroyed by disease, drugs, and the aging process.

The Neural System

The neural system develops multiple connections among the areas of the brain that control specific functions, including vision, hearing, motor function, sensation, coordination, and speech. Each function is under the control of a specific area of the brain. The right half, or

733

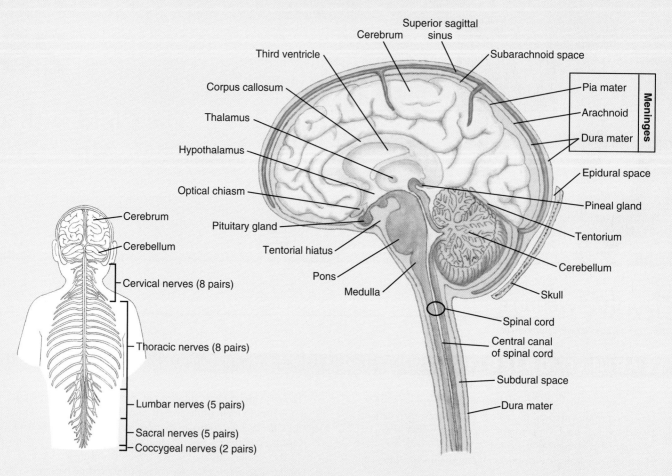

Anatomy of the Central Nervous System

PEDIATRIC DIFFERENCES IN THE CNS

- The brain constitutes 12% of a newborn's body weight compared with only 2% of an adult's body weight.
- The brain of a term infant is two thirds the weight of an adult's brain. By age 1 year, it weighs 80% as much as an adult's brain, and by age 6 years it weighs approximately 90% as much as an adult's brain.
- An infant has approximately 50 mL of CSF compared with 150 mL in an adult.
- The peripheral nerves are not completely myelinated by birth. As myelinization progresses, so do the child's coordination and fine muscle movements.
- The head circumference in a term infant is 34 to 35 cm. By age 6 months the head circumference is 44 cm, and by age 12 months it is 47 cm.
- Papilledema rarely occurs in infancy because of the open fontanels and sutures, which can expand with increased intracranial pressure.
- The primitive reflexes of Moro, grasp, and rooting, present at birth, disappear at various times during the first 5 months. These primitive reflexes may reappear with neurologic disease.

The neonate's neurologic system functions at a subcortical level. Spinal cord reflexes, such as sucking and cardiorespiratory functions, are present. Cortical functions, including memory and coordination, are only partially developed.

The Axial Skeleton

The axial skeleton protects the underlying structures of the central nervous system (CNS). For convenience of study, the bones of the skull and the vertebral column are divided into regions that form the wall of the cranial cavity and the spinal column. The frontal, occipital, temporal, and parietal bones form the cranial vault. The floor of the cranial vault is composed of three compartments, or fossae—the anterior, middle, and posterior fossae. The anterior fossa houses the frontal lobes of the brain, the middle fossa contains the upper brainstem and the pituitary gland, and the posterior fossa contains the lower brainstem. Blood vessels and cranial nerves enter and leave the skull through the foramina.

At birth, the skull plates are not fused but are separated by nonossified spaces called fontanels. The posterior fontanel usually fuses by age 2 months and the anterior fontanel by 16 to 18 months. The fontanels allow the cranium to expand in response to rapid brain growth. Before fusion of the fontanels and sutures, an increase in intracranial pressure (ICP) will produce an increase in head circumference and may result in macrocephaly.

Because brain growth is rapid during infancy, the long-term sequelae of neurologic insults that occur to infants are difficult to

hemisphere, of the brain controls the left side of the body and is concerned with the social aspects of perception, intuition, and experience. The left hemisphere controls the right side of the body and is largely concerned with language acquisition and use and logical verbal reasoning.

predict. Brain growth can be assessed by head circumference measurements. These measurements are an important part of the routine physical examination of children and should be plotted on a growth chart. Insufficient or excessive head and brain growth could indicate a potential neurologic problem. Premature closing of the fontanels or sutures can cause massive neurologic damage, and continued evaluation by the physician is needed.

The Meninges

The meninges are the membranes that surround the brain and spinal column. The outer layer is the dura mater, a fibrous connective tissue structure containing many blood vessels (Atabaki, 2007). The dura mater consists of two layers having outer and inner meningeal components. Between the periosteum of the bone and the dura mater lies the epidural space. Sheets of dura also extend downward and inward to form partitions within the cranium. The falx cerebri separates the cerebral hemispheres, and the falx cerebelli separates the cerebellar hemispheres.

The tentorium is a tentlike structure that separates the cerebellum from the occipital lobe of the cerebrum. The large gap through which the brainstem passes is the tentorial hiatus.

The middle meningeal layer is the arachnoid, a delicate, avascular, weblike, serous membrane loosely covering the brain. Between the arachnoid and the dura lies the subdural space, which contains a small amount of fluid, just sufficient to prevent adhesion of the two membranes.

The innermost layer is the pia mater. It is a delicate, transparent membrane that adheres closely to the outer surface of the brain. The pia mater is a vascular membrane, consisting of arteries and veins.

Between the pia mater and the arachnoid is the subarachnoid space, which is filled with cerebrospinal fluid (CSF). The CSF acts as a cushion to reduce the force of trauma on the brain. Endothelial cells within the brain form a semipermeable blood-brain barrier that allows some substances to pass to the brain and prevents others from entering. The blood-brain barrier provides protection for the brain.

The Brain

The three sections of the brain are the cerebrum, the cerebellum, and the brainstem. The cerebrum is the largest component, filling the upper portion of the skull. It is divided into two hemispheres, right and left, which are separated by a longitudinal fissure. The two hemispheres are joined by a band of commissural fibers called the *corpus callosum*. The cerebral hemispheres are further divided into lobes in relation to the cranial bones: frontal, parietal, temporal, and occipital. The cerebrum also includes part of the thalamus, the hypothalamus, the basal ganglia, and the olfactory and optic nerves.

The cerebellum is composed of white matter and gray matter. The gray matter is often referred to as the cerebral cortex. It is attached to the brainstem by paired bundles of fibers. The brainstem consists of the midbrain, the pons, the medulla, the thalamus, and the third ventricle.

The Cranial Nerves

Twelve pairs of cranial nerves arise from the brain and brainstem, each with a specific function. Testing these nerves can indicate the location and degree of CNS injury (see Chapter 9).

The Spinal Cord

The spinal cord is described as segmented into the cervical, thoracic, lumbar, and sacral regions. The spinal nerves are named for their corresponding vertebral segments.

The spinal cord transmits signals to and from the brain and responds to local sensory information through automatic motor responses called reflexes. The simplest type of spinal cord response is the reflex arc. Sensation is transmitted to the spinal cord from a sensory nerve fiber. It synapses with a motor neuron in the same cord segment, causing a muscle or tendon contraction in the corresponding motor nerve. Deep tendon reflexes are examples of the reflex arc.

Sensory innervation occurs as sensory nerves carrying body sensations enter the spinal cord on the dorsal surface. Most sensory fibers for pain and temperature ascend to the brain by lateral spinal tracts. Sensory fibers for touch and pressure ascend through anterior tracts. Almost all sensory fibers pass through the thalamus, where the perceptions of touch, pressure, and temperature are interpreted. Perceptions of texture, size, and weight are interpreted in the cortex.

Motor nerves are stimulated to respond after the brain receives a signal from a sensory nerve. The motor nerves cross over to the contralateral (opposite) side of the spinal cord from which they originate and then exit on the ventral surface of the spinal cord. The side of the body contralateral to the injured side of the brain will be the side affected by injury.

Functional differences exist between the upper and lower motor neurons. The outcome of a spinal cord injury is affected by the site of the injury. An injury between the brain and the dendrites (the nerve fibers that carry impulses toward the cell body) will render the brain incapable of signaling the muscle cells to cease responding reflexively, and the muscle will become contracted, or spastic. If the injury is to a section of the nerve between the muscle and axons (the nerve fibers that carry impulses away from the cell body), the muscles will become incapable of responding reflexively, causing them to become flaccid.

CSF ANALYSIS IN CHILDREN: NORMAL FINDINGS

PARAMETER	NEONATE PRETERM	NEONATE TERM	CHILD OLDER THAN 6 MONTHS
WBCs (per mm^3)	≤25	≤19 (infants ages 6-28 days)	≤5
		≤9 (infants ages 29-56 days)	
Protein (mg/dL)	<150	<170	<45
Glucose (mg/dL)	>30	>60	>40
Pressure (mm Hg)	50-80	50-80	100-280

Cerebrospinal Fluid

CSF is a clear liquid produced in the choroid plexus of the ventricles at approximately 0.3 to 0.4 mL/minute. The CSF aids in protecting the brain, spinal cord, and meninges by acting as a watery cushion surrounding them to absorb the shocks to which they are exposed. CSF also functions to maintain homeostasis as it drains unwanted substances away from the brain. It is reabsorbed through the arachnoid villi into the venous sinuses. The total volume of CSF is renewed approximately three times or more each day.

Cerebral Blood Flow and Intracranial Regulation

The internal carotid arteries supply blood to all parts of the brain. Approximately 17% of cardiac output and 20% of body oxygen are transported to the brain. The brain requires approximately 10 times the oxygen used by the rest of the body.

CLINICAL REFERENCE

Cerebral blood flow (CBF) is controlled by cerebral perfusion pressure (CPP), which is the difference between the mean arterial blood pressure (MBP) and ICP.

Autoregulation, or self-regulation, is a unique physiologic ability. It allows cerebral arteries to change diameter in response to changes in the CPP. The cerebral vessels can maintain a steady blood flow to the brain during alterations in blood pressure and perfusion. However, autoregulation fails when the limits of cerebrovascular dilation are reached.

Autoregulation may be impaired as a result of trauma, ischemia, or increased intracranial pressure. It is influenced significantly by changes in partial pressure of oxygen in arterial blood (PaO_2) and partial pressure of carbon dioxide in arterial blood ($PaCO_2$). An increase in $PaCO_2$ (above 40 mm Hg) produces cerebral vasodilation and an increase in CBF. A decrease in $PaCO_2$ (25 to 30 mm Hg) causes cerebral vasoconstriction and thus reduces blood flow to the brain. Alterations in PaO_2 between 80 and 100 mm Hg have little effect on CBF, although hypoxia will dramatically increase CBF.

CSF ANALYSIS: FINDINGS IN PATHOLOGIC CONDITIONS

CONDITION	APPEARANCE	PRESSURE	CELLS	PROTEIN	GLUCOSE/OTHER
Traumatic tap	Bloody; supernatant fluid clear	Normal	Any red blood cells	4 mg/dL rise per 5000 red cells	Not applicable
Acute bacterial meningitis	Cloudy to milky or yellow (xanthochromatic)	Usually elevated	Polymorphonuclear cells: ≥100/mm³	100-500 mg/dL	Decreased compared with blood glucose
Viral meningitis	Clear	Normal or increased	Zero to a few hundred per mm³, mostly leukocytes	50-200 mg/dL	Normal
Encephalitis	Clear, colorless	Normal or slightly increased	Normal or increased	50-200 mg/dL	<40 mg/dL
Subdural hematoma	Yellow to clear, colorless	Increased	Normal	Normal or increased	Normal
Diabetic coma	Clear, colorless	Decreased	Normal	Normal or slightly increased	May be 200-300 mg/dL
Guillain-Barré syndrome	Clear	Normal	<10 white blood cells per mm³	More than 2× normal	Normal

COMMON DIAGNOSTIC TESTS AND PROCEDURES FOR NEUROLOGIC DISORDERS

TEST	DESCRIPTION	PURPOSE	NURSING CONSIDERATIONS
CT scan	Produces computer image of horizontal and vertical cross sections of brain at any axis.	To identify abnormal tissue and structures, such as in brain tumor, bleeding, or hydrocephalus.	Insert IV line if contrast medium is used. Notify the radiologist if the child is allergic to iodine. May need to sedate child. Consider number of previous CT scans and risk of radiation exposure, MRI may be preferred.
Angiography	After IV contrast dye is injected, a clear image of the vessels is obtained; view of all other tissues not infused with dye is eliminated.	To reveal vascular abnormalities.	Child may have nothing-by-mouth order. Notify the radiologist if the child is allergic to iodine. Obtain signed permission form. Some restrictions on activity necessary after the test.
Echoencephalography	Echoes from ultrasonic waves are recorded as they reflect off various surfaces of the skull.	To identify abnormal structure, position, and function.	Painless procedure. No preparation.
EEG	Electrodes placed on the scalp conduct and amplify electrical activity; electrical potential of the brain is measured and recorded.	To identify abnormal electrical brain discharges, such as in seizures.	Child may have regular diet or fluids but no caffeine or stimulants. Hair should be clean. May include sleep EEG; in this case, child should be sleep deprived the night before test. The procedure is painless.
Long-term video EEG	Continuous EEG with video of physical symptoms. Process can last 24 hr to several days.	To enable clinical events to be recorded and played back for in-depth review, as well as correlated with the presence of abnormal electrical activity.	Electrodes are secured with skin glue. Electrode sites should be evaluated and documented every shift. Child will have to stay in a small area during testing. Age-appropriate toys and activities are made available.
Lumbar puncture	CSF pressure is measured and a specimen obtained as a needle is inserted into the subarachnoid space between L3 and L4.	To determine pressure and analyze CSF. Can identify hemorrhage or infections. Procedure may be used to administer medications.	Obtain signed consent. Instruct the child to lie on the side with the knees up to chest. After the procedure, the child lies flat. If not fluid restricted, encourage fluids after the procedure. Use a topical anesthetic at needle insertion site to decrease pain, whenever possible.

COMMON DIAGNOSTIC TESTS AND PROCEDURES FOR NEUROLOGIC DISORDERS—cont'd

TEST	DESCRIPTION	PURPOSE	NURSING CONSIDERATIONS
MRI	Produces computer images of the brain by radiofrequency emissions from certain elements.	To demonstrate morphologic features of tissue and structures with high degree of detail.	The procedure is painless, but the child must not move; sedation may be necessary. Inform child that loud clicking noises will be heard. The child's head will be restrained.
Nuclear brain scan (single-photon emission computed tomography [SPECT])	A radioactive substance is injected IV. Abnormal uptake indicates abnormal tissue or structure.	To identify focal brain lesions by allowing the visualization of blood flow through the brain.	The child needs to remain still during the test. An IV line is needed. The amount of the substance injected is measured and recorded.

LUMBAR PUNCTURE: EDUCATING THE FAMILY

If the child is old enough to understand, explain the following:
- The child will need to lie on his or her side with body bent and knees and chin touching. Explain that you will help hold the child in that position by "hugging" the knees to the chin. If there is time, allow the child to practice the position. (An infant can be in a side-lying position or a sitting position with the infant facing you and your thumbs across the infant's scapulae; steady the infant's head against your body.) For an older child, consider demonstrating the procedure on a stuffed animal or doll.

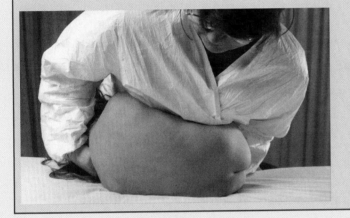

- Tell the child that the physician will wash the child's back with a cool liquid. After that, the child might feel a "pinch" or "sting" as the needle is inserted. A topical anesthetic should be used whenever possible to decrease the pain caused by the needle. The child must remain still.
- Encourage the child to relax, sing, take deep breaths, or use guided imagery throughout the procedure to help decrease anxiety. The collection of CSF samples and pressure measurement usually takes several minutes. When the needle is withdrawn, the child will feel light pressure and the application of a small dressing.

Remember to do the following:
- Monitor the child's cardiorespiratory status throughout the procedure.
- Help the parents comfort the child during and after the procedure.

For the lumbar puncture: Place one hand farther down, under the child's neck. Your forearm moves behind the child's head to support the neck. Place the other arm farther under the child's upper thighs and curl the child's body by bringing the knees up to the head. Note that this nurse's weight is supported on the edge of the examination table, and the nurse leans slightly over the child, controlling the arms and legs. Because direct visibility of the child's respiratory status is limited in this position, a cardiorespiratory monitor must be used for the child. (Photo courtesy Cook Children's Medical Center, Fort Worth, TX. © Bob Lukeman, photographer.)

Animation—Lumbar Puncture

Care of the child with a neurologic problem requires knowledge of neuroanatomy, neurophysiology, and normal growth and development. The nurse plays an important role in the early recognition of pediatric neurologic problems, some of which have the potential for devastating long-term outcomes. The nurse assesses the child's condition by comparing the child's normal behavior with current behavior. The family is an invaluable source of information about the child's normal behavior and how current behavior deviates from that norm. The child and the family need support and understanding because the child's condition represents a crisis in their lives. The family's ability to respond and influence the child's coping mechanisms directly influences the recovery and adaptation process.

Many conditions of the neurologic system share common assessment data, diagnoses, and interventions. Principles of nursing care for the child with a neurologic system disorder can be applied to a variety of situations.

INCREASED INTRACRANIAL PRESSURE

Increased ICP reflects the pressure exerted by the blood, brain, CSF, and any other space-occupying fluid or mass. Increased ICP results from a disturbance in autoregulation and is defined as pressure sustained at 20 mm Hg or higher for 5 minutes or longer.

Etiology

Alterations in the brain can result from a space-occupying lesion, such as a brain tumor or hematoma. The brain can swell as a result of head trauma, infection, or a hypoxic episode. Overproduction of fluid,

NURSING CARE PLAN

The Child with a Neurologic System Disorder

Focused Assessment

- Assess child's level of consciousness using the Glasgow Coma Scale (GCS) modified for children
- Assess child's orientation, mood, and behavior
  - Compare with normal developmental milestones for age
  - Observe interactions with family and environment
  - Note lethargy, drowsiness, hyperactivity, tremors or jitteriness
- Assess motor skills, balance, and coordination
  - Observe child dressing, playing, throwing a ball, using a pencil, or touching finger to nose
  - Observe child walking to assess gait (look for hemiplegia, scissors gait, wide-spaced gait)
  - Check muscle development, strength, and tone
- Determine range of motion for all joints
- Test deep tendon reflexes; comparing side to side
- Assess for sensory function and symmetry of both sides of face, trunk, arms and legs
  - Test for vibration, superficial tactile sensation, superficial pain, and temperature

Planning

Nursing Diagnosis

Risk for Ineffective Tissue Perfusion (cerebral) related to alteration of arterial or venous blood flow, cerebral infarction, hemorrhage, hematoma, increased ICP, cerebral edema, seizures, hypoventilation, or increased cerebral metabolism.

Expected Outcomes

The child will have improved cerebral perfusion, as evidenced by absence of cranial nerve deficits, improved or normal level of consciousness, vital signs in baseline normal, and GCS score within normal limits.

The child will demonstrate appropriate behavior or thought patterns for age.

Intervention/Rationale

1. Determine the child's baseline age and developmental level.
   Baseline age and developmental level will help the nurse gauge changes in neurologic status.
2. Perform a baseline neurologic and level of consciousness (LOC) assessment and measure vital signs on admission.
   Changes in neurologic signs can indicate deterioration or improvement in status. Changes are compared with baseline.
3. Monitor factors that may further increase cerebral edema and ICP (hypoxia, fever, seizures, hypotension, hypercapnia).
   Monitoring these factors allows for correction of conditions that increase ICP and keeps cerebral metabolic needs to a minimum.
4. Maintain head of bed at a 30- to 45-degree angle.
   Venous outflow drainage of the brain is facilitated by gravity.
5. Avoid the prone or flat, supine position, neck flexion, or hip flexion.
   These positions tend to increase ICP. Neck flexion can partially occlude the jugular vein and impairs drainage. Hip flexion can increase intraabdominal or intrathoracic pressure, thus increasing ICP.
6. Organize nursing care around periods of low ICP. Decrease stimulation (noise, bright lights, touch, movement, pain) and avoid activities as much as possible that cause agitation and may increase ICP.
   Nursing care such as suctioning, bathing, and repositioning, and other stimuli increase ICP; minimizing stimuli will decrease ICP.
7. Monitor pupil size and reactivity to light every hour as needed or as ordered.
   An increase in pupil size and no or sluggish constriction in response to light may indicate an increase in ICP.

8. Monitor vital signs every 1 to 2 hours.
   Acute changes in vital signs may indicate increased ICP.
9. Measure head circumference daily or more often as needed, and record on age-appropriate growth chart.
   If fontanels are open, cranial expansion takes place when the CSF is under pressure.
10. Palpate the anterior fontanel every 8 hours if age appropriate.
    An increase in fontanel size and tenseness may indicate an increase in CSF accumulation.
11. Palpate the cranial suture lines every 8 hours if age appropriate.
    The cranial sutures may separate with an increase in CSF volume or pressure.
12. Observe the infant for irritability, lethargy, feeding intolerance, and decreasing GCS score.
    These are signs of increasing ICP and deteriorating neurologic status.
13. Place emergency equipment (oxygen, suction, bag-valve-mask) near the child's room or at the bedside.
    Increased ICP can cause apnea and may lead to cardiopulmonary arrest.

Evaluation

Does the child demonstrate an improved LOC?

Are vital signs within normal limits?

Does the child show intact cranial nerve function, an optimum level on the GCS, and behavior and thought patterns appropriate for age?

Planning

Nursing Diagnosis

Imbalanced Nutrition: Less Than Body Requirements related to restricted intake, neurologic impairment, swallowing or chewing difficulty, risk for aspiration, nausea, or vomiting.

Expected Outcome

The child will have adequate nutritional intake, as evidenced by maintaining stable or normal weight for age and height; exhibiting normal serum protein levels, moist mucous membranes, and adequate urine output; and being free of nausea and vomiting.

Intervention/Rationale

1. Determine the child's LOC before giving liquids.
   A decreased LOC increases the risk of aspiration with swallowing.
2. Weigh the child daily on the same scale, at the same time of day, and in the same clothes. Record on a growth chart.
   Changes in weight indicate alterations in fluid balance and nutritional status. Being consistent with timing and type of clothing enhances accurate comparison. The nurse should weigh the child only if the procedure does not increase ICP.
3. Monitor skin turgor, mucous membranes, eye orbits, urine output, urine specific gravity, and serum and urine electrolyte values.
   These are indicators of fluid and electrolyte status.
4. Consult a registered dietitian.
   The dietitian will advise how best to meet metabolic demands and plan the most efficient way to provide the child with calories.
5. Position the child or infant upright after feedings. If the child is old enough and the ICP is not elevated, the head should be slightly flexed and facing forward. Arms should be positioned forward with feet placed on a firm surface.
   Proper positioning will decrease the risk of aspiration, enhance comfort, prevent contractures, and provide for safety while feeding/eating.

NURSING CARE PLAN

The Child with a Neurologic System Disorder—cont'd

Intervention/*Rationale*—cont'd

6. Verify placement of any oral or nasogastric tube before tube feedings are initiated.
   Incorrect placement of a nasogastric tube will result in placing feedings into the lungs (see Chapter 13).
7. Provide a flexible feeding schedule with small feedings of favorite foods.
   These techniques facilitate digestion, voluntary food intake by the child, and the ability to maintain adequate caloric intake.
8. Minimize handling around feeding times.
   Minimal handling during feeding decreases the likelihood of vomiting and aspiration.
9. If swallowing is impaired, assist the child with chewing by holding the child's chin and jaw.
   Swallowing may be facilitated by this method, because it keeps the child's head stabilized in an appropriate anatomical position.
10. Obtain order to medicate for nausea and vomiting if necessary.
    The child will be more likely to tolerate feedings when nausea is controlled.

Evaluation

Does the child show normal growth for age, with no weight loss?
Does the child have age-appropriate caloric intake daily?
Does the child have proper hydration with moist mucous membranes and age-appropriate urine output for age?
Is the child free from nausea and vomiting?

Planning
Nursing Diagnosis

Risk for Impaired Skin Integrity related to neuromuscular impairment, decreased level of consciousness, inadequate physical activity, immobility, or improper fluid or nutritional intake.

Expected Outcome

The child's skin will remain intact and free from pressure breakdown.

Intervention/*Rationale*

1. Use pressure-equalizing mattress or special flotation mattress to protect bony prominences. Reposition every 2 hours and as needed. Check for redness and pressure areas.
   The child with a depressed LOC may not be active, and immobility can lead to skin breakdown.
2. Observe skin condition every 2 hours with the repositioning of the child or infant.
   Prolonged pressure on the skin will quickly lead to breakdown.
3. Avoid putting temperature probes, cardiac monitor leads, or excessive tape over a ventriculoperitoneal shunt site.
   Irritation from adhesives will contribute to skin breakdown and possible infection.
4. Encourage parents to participate in passive range-of-motion exercises for the child if appropriate.
   Participating in the child's care enhances the parents' sense of control and the child's sense of well-being. Passive range-of-motion exercises provide emotional and physical support for the child and increase the child's activity.
5. If braces or splints are used, assess the skin before and after the splints or assistive devices are put on and taken off.
   Correct application of braces will minimize pressure points and reduce skin breakdown.

6. Implement a daily skin care regimen. Teach parents or family to check skin frequently.
   Bathing, moisturizing, and inspecting the skin will preserve skin integrity.

Evaluation

Does the child have intact, clean, dry skin without pressure areas or sores?

Planning
Nursing Diagnosis

Anxiety (parental) related to change in the child's health status; the child's behavior changes, possible injury, seizures, neurologic impairment; threat to parental role identity, social isolation, or lack of privacy.

Expected Outcome

The parents will demonstrate management of anxiety, as evidenced by maintaining social and personal relationships, verbalizing relaxation, verbalizing feelings about the child's neurologic impairment, and demonstrating effective coping skills.

Intervention/*Rationale*

1. Keep the parents informed of the child's progress, prognosis, and plan of care. Encourage parents to talk about concerns and ask questions. Allow parents to make decisions when possible.
   Control over any event in the child's care helps the parents feel they are part of the caregiving team and lessens their anxiety.
2. Encourage parents to participate actively in activities of daily living (e.g., oral hygiene, bathing, feeding), as the child's condition permits.
   Touching the child and actively participating in the child's care lower parental anxiety.
3. Orient the parents to hospital routine, and refer to clergy, social worker, and other team members.
   A familiar environment is less threatening and will enable the family to more positively deal with the child's condition and prognosis.
4. Encourage rooming-in when possible.
   Rooming-in will involve the parents more in the child's care, facilitate collaboration with the health care team, and decrease the child's anxiety.
5. Assist with anxiety-reduction techniques such as relaxation techniques, music, and guided imagery.
   Such techniques facilitate coping and stress reduction.

Evaluation

Are the parents able to discuss concerns and fears?
Do the parents plan with the team for the child's future and participate in decision making?
Are the parents able to state reduced feelings of anxiety?
Do the parents demonstrate coping and problem-solving skills?

Planning
Nursing Diagnosis

Deficient Knowledge related to unfamiliarity with infectious process, disease process, medication regimen, dietary or fluid needs, measures for prevention, or chronic illness of a child or infant.

Expected Outcomes

The child and parents will verbalize and demonstrate an understanding of the child's disease process, as evidenced by stating age-appropriate, realistic factors about the child's condition; listing factors to decrease neurologic deficits and measures to prevent further occurrences of illness; and demonstrating medication administration and nutritional adaptations.

Continued

NURSING CARE PLAN

The Child with a Neurologic System Disorder—cont'd

Intervention/Rationale

1. Allow time for family education. If the child is to undergo surgery, provide preoperative teaching for the child and parents.

   Teaching answers questions and reinforces information given to the parents by the physician. It includes the parents in the learning experience.

2. Determine the parents' understanding of the child's condition, including the child's need for physical, speech, or occupational therapy.

   Parents need to understand their child's intellectual and physical abilities and challenges in order to give informed consent or reinforce the need for rehabilitative therapies.

3. Refer the parents to community and web-based support groups.

   Support can be gained by seeing or hearing how others coped with similar situations.

4. Supply the parents with telephone numbers to call for needed information once they are home.

   Health care providers can help parents feel in touch and educate them at the same time by discussing the child's condition on the telephone.

5. Teach the parents important signs and symptoms to monitor related to their child's condition, side effects of medications, and when to call the physician or nurse. Provide written instructions.

   The parents need to state important signs and symptoms that indicate a change in the child's condition and be aware of when to seek medical

attention. Anxiety reduces learning and attention span. A written copy of signs and symptoms and instructions provides an ongoing resource that can be referred to later.

6. Review the signs and symptoms of wound infection.

   Until the surgical incision is healed, the risk of infection is present.

7. Instruct the parents to watch for signs and symptoms of urine retention or urinary tract infection.

   Because of retention and reflux, the child may be at risk for urinary tract infections. Parents must seek treatment for the child if signs and symptoms of retention or infection are observed.

8. Provide reliable and credible Internet resources for parents.

   Credible Internet resources provide enhanced knowledge for parents and are available when parents are ready to learn more about their child's condition.

Evaluation

Can the parents discuss the child's care appropriately?

Are the parents able to list situations in which the child should be seen by the physician or nurse?

Do the parents know how to contact community support?

Can the parents demonstrate an understanding of their child's disease and care requirements?

---

malabsorption of fluid, or a communication problem within the system can disrupt CSF dynamics. Aneurysms within the brain and acute liver failure can also lead to increased ICP.

Manifestations

Signs and symptoms of increased ICP differ according to the child's developmental level (Box 28-1).

Level of Consciousness

Children with increased ICP often have an altered level of consciousness. The Glasgow Coma Scale (GCS) is a standardized scale that, in a modified form, is frequently used to assess level of consciousness in infants and children. It consists of a three-part assessment: eye opening, verbal response, and motor response (Table 28-1). Each level of response is assigned a number value. When the assessment of each response is complete, the scores are totaled, providing an objective measure of the child's level of consciousness. The total numeric scores range from 15, indicating no change in level of consciousness, to 3, indicating a deep coma and poor prognosis. A modified version of the GCS is available and is a reliable tool for assessing level of consciousness and predicting the need for acute medical interventions when properly administered (Kirkham, Newton, & Whitehouse, 2008).

Behavior

Changes in the child's normal behavior pattern may be an important early sign of increased ICP. Parents often are the first to notice a change in the child's behavior; therefore a parent's comment that "he isn't acting like himself" should be taken seriously. Irritability, mild confusion, and agitation are symptoms that warrant further assessment. The child who no longer recognizes parents, cannot follow commands, or has minimal response to pain is deteriorating. Decreased responsiveness to painful stimuli is a significant sign of alteration in level of consciousness.

BOX 28-1 DEVELOPMENTAL MANIFESTATIONS OF INCREASED ICP

INFANT	CHILD
• Poor feeding or vomiting	• Headache
• Irritability or restlessness	• Diplopia
• Lethargy	• Mood swings
• Bulging fontanel	• Slurred speech
• High-pitched cry	• Papilledema (after 48 hr)
• Increased head circumference	• Altered level of consciousness
• Separation of cranial sutures	• Nausea and vomiting, especially in the morning
• Distended scalp veins	
• Eyes deviated downward ("setting-sun" sign)	
• Increased or decreased response to pain	

Pupil Evaluation

As ICP rises, compression of the third cranial nerve occurs, resulting in pupil dilation with sluggish or absent constriction in response to light. A fixed, dilated pupil is an ominous sign in an unconscious child. This suggests a herniation of the center section of the brain (also known as a transtentorial herniation). Other eye dysfunctions associated with increased ICP include ptosis and ovoid pupil. Older children may complain of blurry vision, diplopia, or decreased visual acuity.

Motor Function

The child with increased ICP exhibits changes in motor function. Purposeful movement will decrease, and abnormal posturing may be observed. Flexion, or decorticate posturing, refers to flexion of the

PATHOPHYSIOLOGY

Increased ICP

The major pathophysiologic changes associated with increased ICP result from alterations in the brain, CSF dynamics, and cerebral blood flow. To maintain cerebral pressure and volume within normal range, changes in one or more of the contents of the cranium must be compensated for by changes in the others; this is referred to as the Monro-Kellie doctrine.

Compensatory mechanisms include a reduction in CSF production, an increase in CSF absorption, and a reduction in cerebral mass as a result of fluid displacement. Once the limits of compensation are reached, any further increase in volume or pressure will cause a sudden increase in ICP and an associated decline in the child's clinical status. Ultimately, increased ICP will compromise cerebral perfusion and produce shifting of brain tissue, causing herniation. The consequences of herniation depend on its severity and location.

Herniation is classified into four types:

- *Transtentorial herniation* occurs when part of the brain herniates downward and around the tentorium cerebelli. It may be unilateral or bilateral and may involve anterior or posterior portions of the brain. If a large amount of tissue is involved, it may cause death because vital brain structures are compressed and become unable to perform their functions.
- *Temporal lobe herniation,* or uncal herniation, refers to a shifting of the temporal lobe laterally across the tentorial notch. This produces compression of the third cranial nerve and ipsilateral pupil dilation. If pressure continues to rise, flaccid paralysis, pupil dilation, pupil fixation, and death will result.
- *Tonsillar herniation* occurs when the cerebellar tonsils herniate through the foramen magnum. The child will develop nuchal rigidity, shoulder or arm numbness, and changes in heart and respiratory rates and patterns. Arnold-Chiari malformation, a condition sometimes associated with hydrocephalus, includes herniation of the cerebellar tonsils.
- *Brainstem herniation* through the foramen magnum results in death as a result of compression of vital cardiorespiratory centers.

Infants are somewhat able to compensate for increasing ICP because their cranial sutures remain open. *Craniosynostosis* is premature closure of the cranial sutures. This abnormal skull development causes an abnormally shaped skull. In some cases, craniectomy is needed to manage the increased ICP.

TABLE 28-1	GCS MODIFIED FOR CHILDREN
CHILD	**INFANT**
Eyes	
4 = Opens eyes spontaneously	4 = Opens eyes spontaneously
3 = Opens eyes to speech	3 = Opens eyes to speech
2 = Opens eyes to pain	2 = Opens eyes to pain
1 = No response	1 = No response
	____ = Score (Eyes)
Motor	
6 = Obeys commands	6 = Spontaneous movements
5 = Localizes	5 = Withdraws to touch
4 = Withdraws	4 = Withdraws to pain
3 = Flexion	3 = Flexion (decorticate)
2 = Extension	2 = Extension (decerebrate)
1 = No response	1 = No response
	____ = Score (Motor)
Verbal	
5 = Oriented	5 = Coos and babbles
4 = Confused	4 = Irritable cry
3 = Inappropriate words	3 = Cries to pain
2 = Incomprehensible words	2 = Moans to pain
1 = No response	1 = No response
	____ = Score (Verbal)

Reprinted from James, H. E., Anas, N. G., & Perkin, R. M. (1985). *Brain insults in infants and children.* Orlando, FL: Grune & Stratton. Total scores will range from 3 to 15.

upper extremities (elbows, wrists) and extension of the lower extremities. Plantar flexion of the feet may also be observed. This type of posturing implies an injury to the cerebral hemispheres. Extension, or decerebrate posturing, involves extension of the upper extremities with internal rotation of the upper arm and wrist. The lower extremities will extend, with some internal rotation noted at the knees and feet. This type of posturing indicates damage to more areas of the brain, such as the diencephalon, midbrain, or pons. The progression from flexion to extension posturing usually indicates deteriorating neurologic function and warrants physician notification (Figure 28-1). Flaccid paralysis indicates further deterioration in the child's condition.

Vital Signs

Temperature elevation may occur in children with increased ICP. Cushing's response, which consists of an increased systolic blood pressure with widening pulse pressure, bradycardia, and a change in respiratory rate and pattern, is usually apparent just before or at the time of brainstem herniation. This usually indicates an alteration in brainstem perfusion, with the body attempting to improve cerebral blood flow by increasing blood pressure. In children, Cushing's response is a late sign of increased ICP.

As ICP rises, the child's baseline respiratory pattern may change, exhibiting Cheyne-Stokes respiration, central neurogenic hyperventilation, or apneustic breathing. *Cheyne-Stokes respiration* refers to a pattern of breathing characterized by increasing rate and depth and then decreasing rate and depth with a pause of variable length.

Flexion Posturing

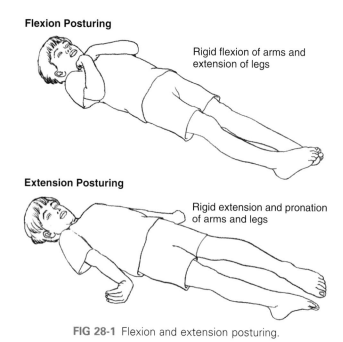

Rigid flexion of arms and extension of legs

Extension Posturing

Rigid extension and pronation of arms and legs

FIG 28-1 Flexion and extension posturing.

The cycle will be repeated again and again. *Central neurogenic hyperventilation* is identified by a rapid rate despite normal arterial blood gas values. This type of breathing pattern usually indicates midbrain or pontine involvement. *Apneustic breathing* occurs when the child demonstrates prolonged inspiration and expiration. As Cushing's response occurs, the child will develop apnea. Late signs of increased ICP include tachycardia that leads to bradycardia, apnea, systolic hypertension, widening pulse pressure, and flexion or extension posturing.

Diagnostic Evaluation and Therapeutic Management

Diagnostic tests for increased ICP include computed tomography (CT), magnetic resonance imaging (MRI), lumbar puncture, serum and urine electrolytes, arterial blood gas determinations, a complete blood cell (CBC) count, electroencephalography (EEG), and radiography. Normal blood gas levels are PaO_2 greater than 80 mm Hg and $PaCO_2$ less than 45 mm Hg in a child with normal ICP.

The management of increased ICP is multimodal and is directed toward treating its underlying cause, reducing the volume of the CSF, preserving cerebral metabolic function, and avoiding situations that increase ICP. An intraventricular catheter may be utilized to measure ICP, drain CSF, and/or administer medications (Box 28-2).

The head of the child's bed should be elevated 30 degrees, and normothermia should be maintained. The child may be given an osmotic diuretic (e.g., mannitol), sedation and analgesia, and anticonvulsant medications (May, 2009). Blood glucose levels are closely monitored to maintain normal levels and prevent further increases in metabolic demands. Hypertonic intravenous solutions are considered for children with hypovolemia (May, 2009). Aggressive passive hyperventilation should be avoided because this intervention may lead to cerebral vasoconstriction with a resultant decrease in cerebral blood flow to ischemia levels (Dumont, Visioni, Rughani et al., 2010; Neumann, Chambers, Citerio et al., 2008). Corticosteroids are no longer used in the treatment of increased ICP due to traumatic brain injury (TBI). In fact, high doses of corticosteroids have been associated with increased mortality for patients with TBI (Tang & Lobel, 2009).

BOX 28-2 INSTRUMENTS FOR MONITORING INCREASED ICP

SUBARACHNOID BOLT	INTRAVENTRICULAR CATHETER
The end of the bolt is placed in the subarachnoid space. The top of the bolt is attached to a transducer to conduct a waveform to the monitor. The neurosurgeon adjusts the transducer to produce a waveform on the monitor.	The catheter is placed in the lateral ventricle or subarachnoid space. The catheter provides a method for measuring pressure, as well as a conduit to drain off extra fluid into the drainage bag. The manometer and drainage bag are part of a sterile closed system.

! NURSING QUALITY ALERT
Standard Terms for Level of Consciousness

Level of consciousness should be described by the nurse using standard terminology:
- *Full consciousness:* Awake, alert, oriented, interacts with environment
- *Confused:* Lacks ability to think clearly and rapidly; usually oriented to person
- *Delirious:* Not oriented to person, place, or time; impairment of reality with auditory or visual hallucinations possible
- *Disoriented:* Lacks ability to recognize place or person
- *Lethargic:* Very drowsy and needs increased stimuli to be awakened
- *Obtunded:* Sleeps unless aroused; once aroused has limited interaction with the environment; answers questions with minimal response
- *Stupor:* Requires vigorous stimulation to arouse
- *Coma:* Vigorous stimulation produces no motor or verbal response

---

SPINA BIFIDA

Spina bifida is a congenital neural tube defect characterized by incomplete closure of the vertebrae and neural tube during fetal development. Spina bifida is classified as spina bifida occulta and spina bifida cystica (Figure 28-2). Spina bifida occulta usually occurs between the L5 and S1 vertebrae, with failure of the vertebrae to completely fuse. The child may have no sensory or motor defects. The only clinical manifestation may be a dimple, a small tuft of hair, a hemangioma, or a lipoma in the lower lumbar or sacral area, detected accidentally on routine radiographs. Spina bifida cystica is a more extensive defect with a range of sensory and motor impairments.

Etiology and Incidence

The cause of spina bifida is unknown in most cases. Evidence suggests a possible genetic predisposition. Maternal folic acid deficiency has been strongly linked to neural tube defects. Daily consumption of 0.4 mg of folic acid by all women of childbearing age is recommended. Evidence of a viral origin has prompted research, but other than folic acid, no cause or preventive measures have been identified.

Manifestations

In addition to the appearance of the lesion, manifestations relate to the degree of deficit, which is determined by the level of the lesion (Figure 28-3).

EVIDENCE-BASED PRACTICE

Assessment Accuracy Using the Glasgow Coma Scale (GCS)

The GCS (see Table 28-1) is one of the most widely used assessment tools for determining and monitoring changes in level of consciousness in patients who have sustained neurologic insult. First introduced in the mid-1970s, its original purpose has been expanded in general use to include assessing diagnostic and prognostic criteria for individuals with traumatic brain injury.[*][†] Because the *best verbal response* of the GCS was particularly difficult to assess in preverbal infants and children, as well as in intubated children and adults, various modifications of the scale for use with these populations have been presented in the literature.

Research relating to reliability and validity of the original GCS has demonstrated varying results.[‡] Kirkham and colleagues recognized the limitations associated with verbal scoring, particularly in children under 5 years of age.[*] Chieregato and colleagues concluded that the use of sedation may cause practitioners to underestimate scores.[§] Nurses in clinical practice should be certain the scale is used in a trustworthy manner and with high interrater reliability.

Several in-depth reviews of research on the GCS have suggested the following limitations that apply to clinical practice for nurses:

- Experienced personnel are more accurate and consistent in application of the scale criteria than are inexperienced personnel.
- Several conditions (e.g., sedation, endotracheal intubation, fractures) interfere with accurate observation of parts of the scale and therefore rely on individual clinician judgment for scoring.
- When assessing response to painful stimuli, nurses use a variety of methods to elicit the pain response, thus calling into question the consistency, accuracy, and reliability of the assessment.

What implications do these pieces of research have for clinical practice? The GCS is only one part of an overall neurologic assessment. Correlation of the patient's history, symptoms, and radiology study results are imperative components of a complete neurologic evaluation.[§] Furthermore, because evidence suggests that experience increases accuracy, clinical agencies should consider first establishing a consistent and written procedure for assessing all components of the scale, then pairing inexperienced nurses with experienced nurses to ensure appropriate training and execution of the assessment procedure. Consistency of scores may be ensured at hand-off when two nurses conduct a neurologic assessment and score the patient together.[‡]

[*]Kirkham, F. J., Newton, C., & Whitehouse, W. (2008). Paediatric coma scales. *Developmental Medicine & Child Neurology, 50*(4), 267-274. Retrieved from http://onlinelibrary.wiley.com/doi/10.1111/j.1469-8749.2008.02042.x/full.

[†]Neumann, J. O., Chambers, I. R., Citerio, G., et al. (2008). The use of hyperventilation therapy after traumatic brain injury in Europe: An analysis of the BrainIT database. *Intensive Care Medicine, 34*(9),1676-1682. Retrieved from https://springerlink3.metapress.com/content/v81rjq5p55n00327/resource-secured/?target=fulltext.html&sid=mypppaqvod3gme454bh3byzw&sh=www.springerlink.com.

[‡]Caton-Richards, M. (2010). Assessing the neurologic status of patients with head injuries. *Emergency Nurse, 17*(10), 28-31. Retrieved from http://emergencynurse.rcnpublishing.co.uk/resources/archive/GetArticleById.asp?ArticleId=7617.

[§]Chieregato, A., Martino, C., Pransani, V., et al. (2010). Classification of a traumatic brain injury: The Glasgow Coma Scale is not enough. *Acta Anaesthesiologica Scandinavica, 54*(6), 696-702. Retrieved from http://onlinelibrary.wiley.com/doi/10.1111/j.1399-6576.2010.02234.x/full.

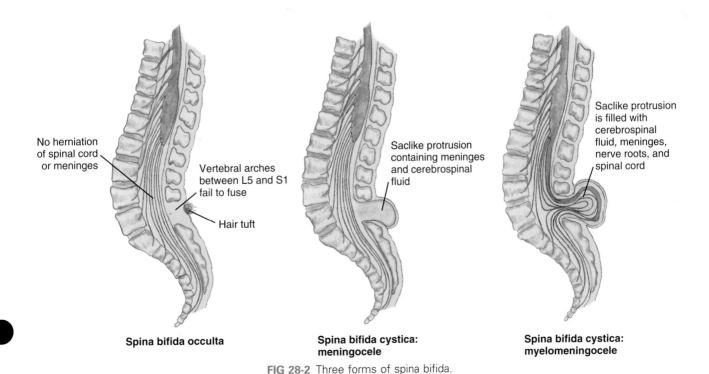

No herniation of spinal cord or meninges

Vertebral arches between L5 and S1 fail to fuse

Hair tuft

Spina bifida occulta

Saclike protrusion containing meninges and cerebrospinal fluid

Spina bifida cystica: meningocele

Saclike protrusion is filled with cerebrospinal fluid, meninges, nerve roots, and spinal cord

Spina bifida cystica: myelomeningocele

FIG 28-2 Three forms of spina bifida.

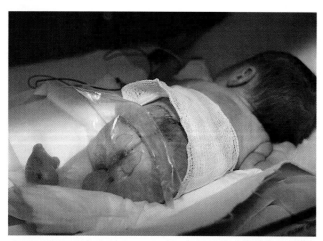

FIG 28-3 This infant has a repaired myelomeningocele. Note the left clubfoot. This deformity often accompanies the defect because normal intrauterine movement does not occur in the fetus with spina bifida, interfering with the development of the extremities. The legs are flaccid, and normal neonatal flexion is absent. The infant also dribbles stool and urine constantly. Hydrocephalus commonly accompanies these neural tube defects. (Courtesy Parkland Health and Hospital System, Dallas, TX.)

T12	Flaccid lower extremities, decreased sensation, and bowel and bladder incontinence
L1 to L3	Hip flexion, flail feet
L2 to L4	Hip adduction
L3 to S2	Hip adduction, hip extension, knee flexion
S3 and below	No motor impairment
Sacral roots	Plantar flexion

Children with spina bifida are at high risk for developing latex allergies because of frequent exposure to latex during catheterizations, shunt placements, and other operations. Latex allergy is estimated to occur in approximately 73% of children with spina bifida (Spina Bifida Association, 2009a). Allergic reactions can range from mild signs and symptoms to anaphylactic shock. Children should be tested for latex allergy, and precautions should be taken from birth to decrease exposures. The nurse should check equipment and supplies for latex and select non-latex alternatives for use.

Diagnostic Evaluation

Diagnostic tests include determining alpha-fetoprotein (AFP) levels in blood at 16 to 18 weeks of gestation. If the AFP screen is elevated, amniocentesis and fetal ultrasound are performed. After delivery, the infant may undergo a CT scan or myelography.

Therapeutic Management

Prenatal microsurgical closure of the myelomeningocele, performed at approximately 19 to 25 weeks of gestation, shows promise for reducing the severity of Chiari type II malformations and incidence of hydrocephalus (Fichter, Dornseifer, Henke et al., 2008). Furthermore, there may be long-term orthopedic benefits associated with prenatal closure (Danzer, Gerdes, Bebbington et al., 2009). Risks associated with prenatal surgery include premature birth, with its associated consequences, and possible fetal death. Maternal risks (e.g., abruptio placentae, preterm membrane rupture, preterm labor, wound infection, chorioamnionitis, uterine hemorrhage, loss of uterus, and damage to adjacent organs) are directly related to the hysterotomy (Kunisaki & Jennings, 2008).

PATHOPHYSIOLOGY
Spina Bifida

Spina bifida occurs during the 4th week of gestation (days 24 to 28), when ventral induction of the neural tube fails to occur. The degree of impairment corresponds to the level of the defect on the spinal cord and the size of the defect. Ninety percent of spinal cord lesions are at or below the L2 vertebra. The lesion results in paralysis, partial paralysis, or varying sensory defects. Clubfeet, scoliosis, and contracture and dislocation of the hips may be associated with the defect. Hydrocephalus and Arnold-Chiari malformation can occur in conjunction with spina bifida. Spina bifida cystica results in incomplete closure of the vertebrae and neural tube, evidenced by a saclike protrusion in the lumbar or sacral area with varying degrees of nervous tissue involvement. Spina bifida cystica is further described as meningocele, myelomeningocele, lipomeningocele, and lipomyelomeningocele. Meningocele is a saclike protrusion filled with spinal fluid and meninges. The most severe form is myelomeningocele, in which the sac is filled with spinal fluid, meninges, nerve roots, and spinal cord.

The incidence of myelomeningocele is 1 in 4000 live births. In the United States, this number is declining. Awareness of the importance of folic acid supplementation during pregnancy and prenatal diagnosis techniques have contributed to a reduction in children born with this defect.* Nearly 80% of infants with myelomeningocele will require shunting to treat associated hydrocephalus.†

*Bowman, R. M., Boshnjaku, V., & McLone, D. G. (2009). The changing incidence of myelomeningocele and its impact on pediatric neurosurgery: A review from the Children's Memorial Hospital. *Child's Nervous System, 25*(7), 801-806. Retrieved from www.springerlink.com/content/k0q1h238135k4077.
†Pinto, F. C. G., Matushita, H., Furlan, A. L. B., et al. (2009). Surgical treatment of myelomeningocele carried out at "time zero" immediately after birth. *Pediatric Neurosurgery, 45*(2),114-118.

Following birth, immediate surgical closure of the defect decreases the risk of infection, morbidity, and mortality. Other benefits are improved prognosis without further cord deterioration, and earlier and easier physical handling and bonding between the newborn and the parents.

The child will need lifelong management of neurologic, orthopedic, and urinary problems and is best managed in a multispecialty outpatient setting. Urodynamic studies are performed early, and a bladder-emptying program is initiated, with close monitoring of the child's urinary tract infection status. In most instances, the child will require orthopedic bracing and possibly orthopedic surgery to maximize the child's mobility.

HYDROCEPHALUS

Hydrocephalus develops as a result of an imbalance between the production and absorption of CSF. As excess CSF accumulates in the ventricular system, the ventricles become dilated and the brain is compressed against the skull. This results in enlargement of the skull if the sutures are open; it results in signs and symptoms of increased ICP if the sutures are fused.

Etiology

Hydrocephalus may be congenital, acquired, or of unknown etiology. In infancy, hydrocephalus is most often congenital or related to prematurity. Congenital hydrocephalus results from developmental defects such as Arnold-Chiari malformations, congenital arachnoid cysts, congenital tumors, or aqueductal stenosis. In premature infants, neonatal meningitis or subarachnoid hemorrhage may result in hydrocephalus. Hydrocephalus is often associated with myelomeningocele. Intrauterine infection and perinatal hemorrhage cause hydrocephalus in some infants. In older children, hydrocephalus is usually acquired as a complication of meningitis, tumor, or hemorrhage.

Incidence

In general, the estimated prevalence of hydrocephalus is 1 in every 500 children in the United States (National Institute of Neurological Disorders and Stroke [NINDS], 2010b). The incidence of hydrocephalus with spina bifida is considered to be 3 to 4 in 1000 live births. Obstructive, or noncommunicating, hydrocephalus accounts for nearly all cases of hydrocephalus in children.

Manifestations and Diagnostic Evaluation

Because of anatomic differences between infants and children, manifestations of hydrocephalus differ according to developmental stage (Table 28-2).

Diagnostic tests for hydrocephalus include serial measurements of head circumference, CT, MRI, ultrasonography, and lumbar puncture with pressure monitoring.

Therapeutic Management

Therapy is aimed at preventing further CSF accumulation and reducing disability and death. The objective is to bypass the blockage and drain the fluid from the ventricles to an area where it may be reabsorbed into the circulation. A *ventriculoperitoneal shunt,* a tube leading from the ventricles out of the skull and passing under the skin to the peritoneal cavity, accomplishes this (Figure 28-4). An alternative shunt, the *ventriculoatrial shunt,* which is used in older children, drains the fluid from the ventricles to the right atrium of the heart.

The shunt may need to be revised as the child grows. Long-term follow-up is essential. The child may exhibit mild learning challenges and may have accelerated pubertal development (Spina Bifida Association, 2009b).

A surgical procedure, endoscopic third ventriculostomy, facilitates the rerouting of CSF around the obstructed ventricular system (Bhatia, Tahir, & Chandler, 2009). This technique has become increasingly popular over the past 20 years. For this procedure, the surgeon creates a small burr hole in the skull through which an endoscope is passed. The third ventricle is visualized and a small opening is created in its floor. This allows the CSF to bypass the fourth ventricle and return to circulation, where it is reabsorbed. The procedure is 50% to 80% successful in children older than 2 years. Other surgical techniques for treating hydrocephalus may be preferred in some children, particularly those under age 2, because surgical outcomes from the

Animation—Ventriculoperitoneal Shunt

PATHOPHYSIOLOGY

Hydrocephalus

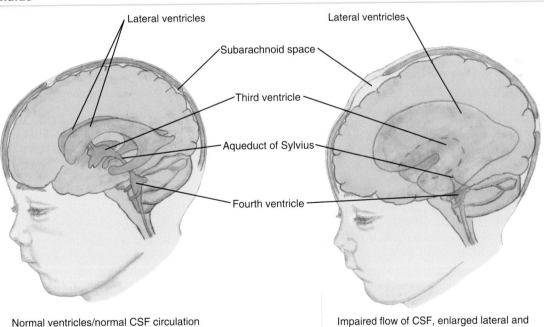

Normal ventricles/normal CSF circulation

Impaired flow of CSF, enlarged lateral and third ventricles, stenosis of aqueduct

Cerebrospinal fluid is produced primarily by the choroid plexus, which lines the lateral ventricles. CSF circulates through the ventricular system and flows into the subarachnoid space around the brain and the spinal cord. It is then reabsorbed within the subarachnoid space.

Hydrocephalus results when either of the following conditions is present: (1) impaired absorption of CSF within the subarachnoid space *(communicating hydrocephalus)* or (2) obstruction of CSF flow within the ventricles that prevents CSF from circulating around the spinal cord and the subarachnoid space *(noncommunicating hydrocephalus).* In rare cases, hydrocephalus may be caused by overproduction of CSF because of a tumor of the choroid plexus.

TABLE 28-2	EARLY AND LATE MANIFESTATIONS OF HYDROCEPHALUS

EARLY	LATE
Infant	
Rapid head growth—increase in head circumference above the normal growth curve	Setting-sun sign; sclera visible above the iris
Full, bulging anterior fontanel	Frontal bone enlargement or bossing
Irritability	Vomiting; difficulty feeding and swallowing
Poor feeding	Increased blood pressure, decreased heart rate
Distended, prominent scalp veins	Altered respiratory pattern
Widely separated cranial sutures	Shrill, high-pitched cry
	Sluggish or unequal pupillary response to light
Child	
Strabismus	Seizures
Frontal headache that occurs in the morning and is relieved by emesis or by sitting upright	Increased blood pressure
	Decreased heart rate
Nausea and vomiting (may be projectile)	Alteration in respiratory pattern
	Blindness from herniation of the optic disc
Diplopia	Decerebrate, extension posturing and rigidity
Restlessness	
Changes in ability to do schoolwork	
Behavior or personality changes	
Ataxia	
Papilledema	
Irritability	
Sluggish and unequal pupillary response to light	
Confusion	
Lethargy	

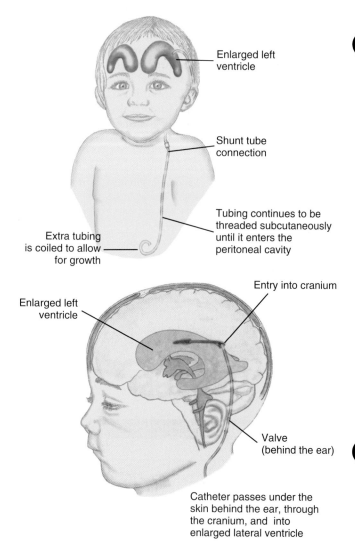

FIG 28-4 A ventriculoperitoneal shunt may be implanted in the child with hydrocephalus to prevent excess accumulation of CSF in the ventricles. The tubing diverts the CSF from the ventricles into the peritoneal cavity, where it is reabsorbed. Nursing care includes monitoring for infection, obstruction, and pain, administering antibiotics and pain medications as ordered, and teaching the family how to change dressings and how to recognize shunt blockages or other problems.

third ventriculostomy approach are poor for this age-group (Ogiwara, Dipatri, Alden et al., 2010).

CEREBRAL PALSY

Cerebral palsy is a chronic, nonprogressive disorder of posture and movement (O'Shea, 2008). It is characterized by difficulty in controlling the muscles because of an abnormality in the extrapyramidal or pyramidal motor system (motor cortex, basal ganglia, cerebellum). Co-morbidities such as cognitive, hearing, speech, and visual impairments, as well as seizures, are common but vary widely from one affected child to another (Straub & Obrzut, 2009).

Etiology and Incidence

The damage to the motor system can occur prenatally, perinatally, or postnatally (Box 28-3). Cerebral palsy (CP) is one of the most common chronic neurologic impairments in children, and more that 500,000 Americans are affected. The rate of cerebral palsy is 1.1 per 1000 live births. Problems associated with prematurity and low birth weight are related to the occurrence of cerebral palsy. Aggressive neonatal intensive care, administration of surfactant to mature infant lungs, and administering steroids to the mother before delivery have improved

survival rates to as high as 85% for a 26-week-gestation premature infant, and also resulted in an increased prevalence of CP (Marsal, 2009). Infants with the lowest birth weights (less than 1000 g) may be at increased risk for cerebral palsy because of intracerebral hemorrhage or periventricular leukomalacia (Fukuda, Yokoi, Kitajima et al., 2009). In general, however, children diagnosed with cerebral palsy are born at term and after a normal labor and delivery (Shankaran, 2008).

Manifestations

The manifestations of cerebral palsy vary widely from one child to another. A child with CP may have persistence of primitive reflexes, delayed gross motor development, abnormal muscle tone, and lack of progression through developmental milestones. Abnormal posturing with inability to maintain normal posture and balance may be present, as well as spasticity or uncontrollable movements in the extremities. Also seen are disturbances of gait (particularly ataxia and toe walking),

BOX 28-3   FACTORS ASSOCIATED WITH CEREBRAL PALSY

Prenatal
- Maternal diabetes
- Rh or ABO blood type incompatibility
- Rubella in the first trimester
- Genetic causes
- Intrauterine ischemic event
- Toxoplasmosis
- Cytomegalovirus
- Congenital brain abnormality
- Prenatal exposure to maternal infection
- Precipitous delivery
- Pregnancy-induced hypertension
- Birth trauma
- Anoxia
- Prolonged labor
- Perinatal metabolic condition (diabetes)
- Intracranial hemorrhage
- Other congenital anomalies

Perinatal
- Asphyxia
- Low birth weight
- Prematurity

Postnatal
- Infections
- Trauma
- Stroke
- Poisoning

PATHOPHYSIOLOGY

Cerebral Palsy

A number of neuromuscular disabilities are associated with cerebral palsy. The alteration in voluntary muscular control is related to a cerebral insult. The area of the brain that is affected determines the type of neuromuscular disability.

The five classifications of cerebral palsy are dyskinetic, spastic, ataxic, rigid, and mixed:

- *Dyskinetic (athetoid) palsy* refers to a disorder in the basal ganglia. Slow, writhing, uncontrolled, involuntary movements involving all extremities characterize this type.
- *Spastic cerebral palsy* is the most common type. The affected area of the brain is the cortex. Spastic cerebral palsy is characterized by increased deep tendon reflexes, hypertonia, flexion, and sometimes contractures. The child's muscles are very tense, and any stimulus may cause a sudden jerking movement. The child has to make a conscious effort to relax. Scissors gait, hip flexion with adduction and internal rotation, or toe walking because of tight heel cords may be present.
- In *ataxic cerebral palsy,* the affected area of the brain is the cerebellum. This type of cerebral palsy is characterized by a loss of coordination, equilibrium, and kinesthetic sense. Overall, the child appears clumsy.
- *Rigid (tremor, atonic) cerebral palsy* is relatively rare in children. The child has rigidity of both flexor and extensor muscles. In a child with tremors, the tremors are apparent both at rest and during movement. The prognosis for a child with this type of cerebral palsy is poor because of associated deformities and lack of active movement.
- *Mixed* is more than one type of cerebral palsy. A common combination is spastic and dyskinetic.

Approximately half of children with cerebral palsy have other disabilities including epilepsy, a cognitive disability, learning problems, poor attention span, hyperactivity, hearing or visual impairment, and emotional problems. Gastroesophageal reflux may occur (see Chapter 19). Intense movements that cause a high expenditure of calories along with feeding challenges, may lead to a calorie deficit and poor nutritional status.

seizures, attention-deficit disorder, sensory impairment, failure of automatic reactions (equilibrium), and speech and swallowing impairments.

Diagnostic Evaluation and Therapeutic Management

A diagnostic evaluation includes EEG, CT scan or MRI, electrolyte levels, metabolic workup, a thorough history, and a complete neurologic examination. The Gross Motor Function Classification System (GMFCS) is a valid tool to classify severity of CP and assess acquisition of future motor skills (Rosenbaum, Palisano, Bartlett et al., 2008).

The goal of managing the child with cerebral palsy is early recognition and intervention to maximize the child's abilities. Cerebral palsy often is not diagnosed before the child is 2 years old. Before age 2, the child may be diagnosed with *static encephalopathy,* a nonspecific term referring to permanent brain damage. Repetition of motor activities facilitates development of new brain pathways through alternative receptor sites and enhances appropriate motor function. The child may be intellectually intact, but this may be overlooked because of the child's physical limitations. Intrathecal baclofen, a skeletal muscle relaxant, administered via an infusion pump can be used to treat severe spasticity in children with cerebral palsy. Close monitoring of the child for infection and the pump for malfunction, as well as correct pump assembly and programming, are required (Keenan, 2010; Ward, Hayden, Dexter, & Scheinberg, 2009).

A multidisciplinary health care team approach is necessary to meet the many needs of the child with cerebral palsy. The team includes the child and family, pediatrician, neurologist, orthopedic surgeon, nurse, speech and hearing therapists, social worker, occupational therapist, physical therapist, educators, physiatrist, neurosurgeon, and orthotist.

HEAD INJURY

Head injury refers to the pathologic result of any mechanical force to the scalp, skull, meninges, or brain.

Types of Head Injuries

Types of head injury include the following:
- *Closed head injury:* Nonpenetrating injury to the head in which no break occurs in the integrity of the barrier between the outside environment and the intracranial cavity
- *Open head injury:* Penetrating injury to the head in which there is a break in the integrity of the barrier (skull, meninges) between the outside environment and the intracranial cavity; infection is a major concern
- *Coup injury:* Cerebral injury sustained directly below the site of impact
- *Contrecoup injury:* Cerebral injury sustained in the region or pole opposite the site of impact; caused by the rapid movements of the semisolid brain within the cranial vault

◎ NURSING CARE PLAN

The Child with Cerebral Palsy in the Community Setting

Focused Assessment

- Monitor at-risk infants for indications of cerebral palsy
  - Irritability, feeding difficulties, delayed development, poor motor development, abnormal posturing, persistent primitive reflexes, poor muscle tone, and ataxic gait
- Assess infants and children for delays in reaching developmental milestones (key indicator of cerebral palsy)
- For children with cerebral palsy, assess response to therapy
  - Monitor and document progress or lack of progress
- For school-age children with cerebral palsy, assess need for physical and learning adaptations in the school setting
  - Consider use of assistive devices (i.e., wheelchairs, walkers, communication boards, and computers)
  - Provide assessment on regular basis; school nurse is member of educational team that develops the child's individual learning plan

Planning
Nursing Diagnosis

Impaired Physical Mobility related to spasticity and muscle weakness.

Expected Outcomes

The child will maximize ability for movement, as evidenced by freedom from contractures or injuries and no complications from immobility.

The parents will demonstrate how to do the child's exercises and notify the school nurse if any changes are made in the child's plan.

Intervention/Rationale

1. Reinforce physical therapy exercises to strengthen and help coordination of muscles. These exercises may have to be performed in the school setting.
   Early intervention and consistent therapy facilitate proper posture and circumvent the development of contractures.
2. Encourage parents to be active in the child's daily physical and occupational therapies.
   Active involvement in the child's care empowers the parents.
3. Observe and record the child's response to physical therapy.
   Changes in therapy may be made in a timely fashion for a higher degree of success.
4. Determine the need for special equipment for reading, writing, eating, and mobility. Convey this information to the school evaluation team.
   The use of special equipment improves the chance for successful self-care. Incorporating this into the child's education plan will maximize learning potential.
5. Monitor the child for chronic pain resulting from surgical procedures and other interventions used to improve mobility and decrease spasticity.*
   Chronic pain can contribute to lack of well-being for the child and family.

Evaluation

Have the child's joints remained mobile and free from contractures?

Does the child demonstrate improved mobility and self-care?

Can the parents demonstrate physical therapy techniques used for their child?

Have the parents notified the school about any changes in the child's plan of care?

Planning
Nursing Diagnosis

Delayed Growth and Development related to neuromuscular impairment.

Expected Outcome

The child will maximize potential for meeting growth and developmental milestones, as evidenced by participation in family, social, and school activities.

Intervention/Rationale

1. Monitor the child's developmental level and cognitive abilities using specific and sensitive developmental screening tests, both on a routine basis and as needed.
   The child with cerebral palsy should be given opportunities to learn and should be exposed to new experiences to maximize developmental progress.
2. Encourage early intervention and refer for early intervention community programs. Promote participation in school programs including play/social activities involving peers.
   Interventions by multidisciplinary providers will maximize the child's potential for learning. Involvement with peers is essential to achieving developmental milestones.
3. Communicate and interact with the child at the child's functional level, not chronological age.
   A child with normal cognitive abilities can understand age-appropriate communication and speech, but a child with a decreased cognitive level may have different understanding than the chronological age would indicate.

Evaluation

Do the parents encourage social and developmental activities that maximize the child's potential?

Does the child attend public school and play with peers when possible?

Does the child participate in physical, speech, and occupational therapy at school?

Planning
Nursing Diagnosis

Risk for Injury related to spasticity, uncontrolled muscle movements, or seizures.

Expected Outcomes

The child will have a safe environment, as evidenced by freedom from injuries.

The parents will describe ways to adapt the child's environment to maximize safety.

Intervention/Rationale

1. Teach the family principles for providing a safe environment (e.g., remove sharp objects and toys, pad sharp furniture edges).
   A safe environment will reduce the risk of injury.
2. Have the child wear a protective helmet and pads if the child falls frequently.
   A helmet protects against head injury.

*Swiggum, M., Hamilton, M., Gleeson, P., & Roddey, T. (2010). Pain in children with cerebral palsy: Implications for pediatric physical therapy. *Pediatric Physical Therapy, 22*(1), 86-92.

◎ NURSING CARE PLAN

The Child with Cerebral Palsy in the Community Setting—cont'd

Intervention/*Rationale*—cont'd

3. If the child is hospitalized, implement bedside seizure precautions. (Do not pad the rails with pillows.)
   Keeping suction, oxygen, and airway equipment at the bedside and padding the side rails help prevent injury and allow for resuscitation of the child if necessary. Pillows should not be used as pads because they may cause suffocation.
4. Provide safe toys that are appropriate for age and developmental level.
   No sharp, very small, or easily shattered toys should be allowed for the child who may fall because of erratic movements.
5. Position the child upright during and after meals.
   An upright position prevents aspiration from gastroesophageal reflux.

Evaluation

Does the child remain free from injury?
Do the parents demonstrate safety measures for their child?
Have the parents adapted the child's environment to be safe and secure?

Planning

Nursing Diagnosis

Impaired Verbal Communication related to neuromuscular impairment and difficulty with articulation.

Expected Outcome

The child will maximize communication ability, as evidenced by appropriately expressing needs and developing methods for communicating with others.

Intervention/*Rationale*

1. Use the child's usual mode of communicating, such as flash cards and talking boards, to facilitate communication.
   Teaching aids help reinforce language and speech development and increase self-esteem.
2. Refer the child to a speech therapist.
   Early intervention maximizes speech capabilities.
3. Encourage and reinforce speech therapy techniques, nonverbal methods of communication, and jaw control.
   These techniques facilitate communication and decrease the child's frustration at not being understood.
4. Encourage parents to convey in detail the child's communication techniques any time the child is in a new situation.
   Sharing the child's communication techniques helps the child adjust to new situations.

Evaluation

Does the child participate in groups using appropriate communication?
Does the child use various methods to communicate?
Do the parents allow time for the child to respond to questions and conversations?
Have the parents learned the same communication method that the child uses?

- *Missile injury:* Penetrating injury of the skull or brain, most often caused by a bullet
- *Impalement injury:* Penetrating injury caused by piercing of the scalp, skull, or brain by a sharp object

Skull Fractures

Skull fractures include the following types:
- *Linear:* Straight-line fracture; dura not involved
- *Depressed:* Bone pressing downward, indented
- *Basilar:* Fracture of the base of the skull; symptoms are Battle sign, raccoon eyes, rhinorrhea, otorrhea, and hemotympanum (blood behind the eardrum)
- *Comminuted:* Fragmentation of the bone into many pieces or a multiple fracture line

Contusion

Contusions are petechial hemorrhages along the superficial aspects of the brain. They may occur at the site of impact or in association with a lesion remote from the site of direct impact.

Concussion

A concussion is transient and reversible neuronal dysfunction, with instantaneous loss of awareness and responsiveness.

Intracranial Hemorrhage

Intracranial hemorrhages are defined as the following two types:
   Epidural: Blood accumulates between the dura and the skull. Arterial damage is the usual type of injury, and the hemorrhage therefore develops rapidly (Figure 28-5).

   Subdural: Blood accumulates between the dura and the cerebrum. A subdural hemorrhage is usually caused by an injury to a vein and can be acute or chronic.

Incidence

Multiple trauma is the leading cause of death in children beyond infancy. In the United States, nearly 500,000 children between infancy and 14 years of age are seen in emergency departments for assessment and treatment of traumatic brain injury; falls and motor vehicle crashes are the primary cause of traumatic brain injury in this age-group (Centers for Disease Control and Prevention, 2010a). Other causes of head injuries include bicycle collisions, sports injuries, child abuse, and gunshot wounds.

Manifestations

Head injuries are classified as minor, moderate, or severe as correlated with the GCS. Children with minor head injuries may have a change in level of consciousness, and also exhibit transient periods of confusion, irritability, vomiting, somnolence, and headache. Moderate to severe head injuries are marked by a decreased level of consciousness, vital signs changes, signs of increased ICP, retinal hemorrhage, hemiparesis, and papilledema (Box 28-4).

Diagnostic Evaluation

A complete history of the event helps determine the mechanism of injury and whether the child lost consciousness. Spinal radiographs are obtained to ascertain any cervical spinal cord injury; these are followed by a complete neurologic examination. Any indication of increased ICP is quickly reported to the physician. CT scan or MRI is the most

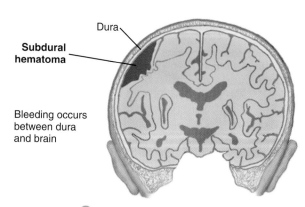
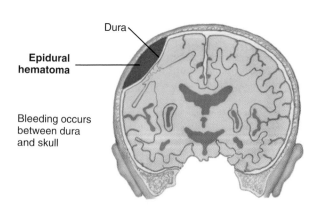

FIG 28-5 Epidural and subdural hematomas are the two most common cranial hematomas, occurring in 6% to 7% of all children with head injuries. With *epidural hematoma*, a rapid decline in neurologic function may occur 4 to 8 hours after a brief period of lucidity. If untreated, the increased ICP can cause death in a short time. A *subdural hematoma* is often caused when the head strikes an immovable object. In an infant, a subdural hematoma (along with retinal hemorrhage) may result from aggressive shaking (shaken baby syndrome, a form of child abuse).

BOX 28-4 CLASSIFICATION OF SEVERITY OF HEAD INJURIES BASED ON GLASGOW COMA SCALE (GCS)*

Minor (mild) head injury: GCS score = 13-15
Moderate head injury: GCS score = 9-12
Severe head injury: GCS score = 3-8

*Data from Atabaki, S. M. (2007). Pediatric head injury. *Pediatrics in Review, 28*(6), 215-224.

---

precise study with which to diagnose the specific kind of head injury sustained. A scalp hematoma in an infant may be a presenting symptom of skull fracture and necessitates additional evaluation (Matschke, Voss, Obi et al., 2009). Seizures may be a presenting sign in an infant with nonaccidental head trauma as well (Fanconi & Lips, 2010).

Therapeutic Management

Initial management of the child with a head injury includes assessment of airway, ventilatory function, neurologic status, and any other injuries present (see Chapter 10). Interventions to maintain vital functions, including adequate oxygenation and perfusion, are provided until all injuries are determined. Increased ICP or seizures may develop in a child with a head injury. In children with traumatic brain injury, the presence of hypoventilation, hypoxemia, and hypotension is concerning and is correlated with increased mortality (Swaminathan, Levy, & Legome, 2009).

Because their brains are still developing, children and adolescents who suffer concussions are at risk for long-term complications necessitating appropriate management (Halstead & Walter, 2010). Recommendations from the American Academy of Pediatrics (Halstead & Walter, 2010) state that all young athletes who have sustained a sport-related concussion must do the following:

- Be evaluated by a physician.
- Be restricted from physical activity until they are asymptomatic at rest and with exertion.
- Be allowed a minimum of 7 to 10 days and up to weeks and months to fully recover.
- Be provided neuropsychologic testing to obtain objective data.

- Be informed there is no evidence that treatment with medications is safe or effective.
- Be told to consider retirement from contact sports if multiple concussions have been sustained or if postconcussion symptoms have persisted for over 3 months.

Under no circumstances should a child or adolescent resume playing a sport the same day of the concussion; protocols have been developed to guide the gradual return of the young athlete to "return to play" after a concussion (Halstead & Walter, 2010). Several states have enacted or are considering legislation that requires school districts to have guidelines regarding concussion prevention and management.

Nursing Considerations

Initial and ongoing assessment of the child with a head injury includes evaluation of the *ABCDEs*; *a*irway, *b*reathing, *c*irculation, *d*isability (level of consciousness), and *e*xposure (see Chapter 10). The child's neck must be immobilized because there is a higher incidence of associated cervical spine injury with head trauma. The nurse obtains and records baseline vital signs, as well as other data as indicated by the child's clinical condition. A complete history and comprehensive neurologic examination should be performed. The child's level of consciousness (using the GCS), pupil size, and pupil reactivity to light are assessed frequently.

Cranial nerve function is tested to identify deficits resulting from the injury and monitor for increased ICP. The clinical signs and symptoms of increased ICP, with or without actual measurement of the ICP, determine both the child's clinical status and medical and nursing interventions. Nasotracheal suctioning or placement of a nasogastric tube is contraindicated in a child with a basilar skull fracture; because of the nature of the injury, the suction catheter or tube could be introduced into the brain. CSF may leak from the nose or ears; packing or blowing of the nose is contraindicated.

Nursing care of the child with a head injury is similar to nursing care of any child with increased ICP. The nurse must closely monitor for signs and symptoms of increased ICP as well as avoid activities and stimuli that can elevate ICP. Positioning the child with the head of the bed elevated 30 to 45 degrees promotes venous drainage (see Nursing Care Plan: The Child with a Neurologic System Disorder).

Any child with a head injury needs to be assessed for fluid and electrolyte alterations. The child with a head injury can have a

PATHOPHYSIOLOGY

Head Injury

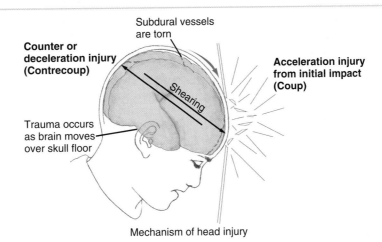

Counter or
deceleration injury
(Contrecoup)

Subdural vessels
are torn

Acceleration injury
from initial impact
(Coup)

Shearing

Trauma occurs
as brain moves
over skull floor

Mechanism of head injury

The cranium is a rigid structure that contains blood, brain tissue, and CSF. The pressure exerted by these components on the cranium is between 2 and 10 mm Hg, depending on the age and activity level of the child.* According to the Monro-Kellie doctrine, an increase in one of these components must be accompanied by a decrease in one of the other components to maintain ICP within normal range. Cerebral function depends on adequate delivery of nutrients such as oxygen, glucose, and other substrates; an abnormal increase in ICP interferes with the balance and delivery of these nutrients.

Head injuries are either primary or secondary. *Primary head injuries* are those in which damage is sustained at the time of injury; *secondary head injuries* refer to the consequences of the primary injury, particularly increased ICP.

The severity of the injury depends on the amount of stress to the cranium and brain. Head injuries include concussions, contusions, lacerations, fractures, and hematomas.

Motor vehicle collisions, falls, sports injuries, and child abuse cause most head injuries in children. *Acceleration-deceleration* is the term used to describe the mechanism of injury. The shearing force of the initial impact moves the brain forward in the brain, followed by a countering, backward movement of the brain in the skull. The shearing force produces bruising, tearing, and bleeding. "Shaken baby syndrome" is a type of child abuse that may result in epidural hematomas and retinal hemorrhages (see Chapter 29).

*Inoue, K. (2010). Caring for the perioperative patient with increased intracranial pressure. *AORN Journal, 91*(4), 511-518.

postinjury alteration in antidiuretic hormone (ADH). Possibly as a result of injury to the hypothalamus or posterior pituitary, the child can exhibit signs of excess ADH (syndrome of inappropriate antidiuretic hormone [SIADH]) or deficient ADH (diabetes insipidus) (see Chapter 27). The nurse must carefully monitor intravenous and oral fluid intake, determine hourly fluid output, document all data, and evaluate the child's fluid balance status. Laboratory data for serum electrolytes should be checked frequently and abnormalities reported to the physician. If the child develops SIADH, fluids may be restricted to reduce the risk of increasing ICP from cerebral edema. Fluid restriction is a nursing challenge because it involves the cooperation of parents and others involved in the child's care. Placing a sign at the child's bedside to alert others of the restriction is useful. The nurse should select fluids the child likes and distribute the allocated amounts over the course of the child's waking hours.

If the child is discharged from the emergency department, written instructions should be given to parents for home monitoring, signs and symptoms to immediately report to the physician, and follow-up care. Children with severe head injuries may require surgical intervention, intensive care, prolonged acute-care hospitalization, and multidisciplinary rehabilitative care in a specialized unit or facility.

SPINAL CORD INJURY

Spinal cord injury can result from any trauma or injury to the spinal cord or its vascular supply or venous drainage.

Etiology

Spinal cord injuries in children are usually caused by motor vehicle crashes, falls, diving accidents, sports injuries, tumor, congenital anomalies, gunshot or knife wounds, or attempted suicide. In the infant, a common cause of spinal cord injury is intentional, aggressive shaking by an older person.

Incidence

Spinal cord injuries are less common in children than in adults, with spinal cord injuries occurring in 1% to 13% of children who sustain spinal injuries (Lee, Sung, Kang, & Park, 2009). Most spinal cord injuries in children occur in the cervical spine, between the occiput and C6. Young children are more susceptible to upper spinal cord injury because of their larger head size in relation to body size. As the child grows older, the likely site of the spinal cord injury moves distally. Seventy-five percent of children who sustain spinal cord injuries from motor vehicle accidents were not wearing seatbelts (Dawodu, 2008).

Manifestations

Manifestations of spinal cord injury include loss of some or all movement or sensation below the level of injury, respiratory depression or apnea, hypotension and bradycardia, hypothermia, and neck pain. These signs vary with the level of injury as well as whether the spinal cord injury is complete or incomplete. If complete, the cord is completely severed and no spinal innervation is present below the injury. For example, with a complete injury at the C2 level (cervical vertebrae 2),

PATIENT-CENTERED TEACHING

Guidelines for the Child with a Head Injury*

After the injury, apply cold (cool pack wrapped in a towel or cool wet compresses) to the site for 20 minutes to prevent or reduce swelling. Clean any scrapes or cuts with soap and water. Encourage the child to rest and limit foods if the child is vomiting. You will need to watch your child closely for the first 24 to 48 hours after the injury in case the child develops a problem and needs to be taken to the health care provider. Follow your health provider's directions as to whether the child needs to be awakened at night. Some providers suggest waking the child every few hours to be sure the child becomes alert and answers questions appropriately.

The following are signs of more serious injury, and you should call the physician or emergency transport immediately after the injury if the child demonstrates the following:

- Has bleeding that does not stop after pressure has been applied for 10 minutes, or is oozing from the nose or ears
- Needs sutures
- Is younger than 2 years
- Has trouble breathing
- Vomits or complains of a severe headache that does not go away
- Had a seizure after the head injury
- Was unconscious or confused
- Has a severe headache or vomiting
- Has slurred speech or blurred vision
- Has blood or watery fluid coming from the ear or nose
- Has unequal pupils or crossed eyes
- Has difficulty walking or crawling or weakness in the arms
- Becomes hard to wake up
- Becomes pale and remains that way for more than an hour
- Has other symptoms that concern you

Postconcussion Syndrome

Some children who have had a head injury can have an after effect called *postconcussion syndrome*. If your child has this condition, your child may be upset easily and may be irritable if tired or stressed. Memory problems are common, as are learning difficulties, double vision, dizziness, headaches, fatigue, and light sensitivity. These symptoms may last many months.

Second Impact Syndrome

If your child is diagnosed with concussion, a second concussion may cause more harm to the brain and may even lead to death. Be sure to talk with your health provider about whether and when the child can return to activities or sports.†

*Atabaki, S. M. (2007). Pediatric head injury. *Pediatrics in Review, 28*(6), 215-224.
†Bey, T., & Ostick, B. (2009). Second impact syndrome. *Western Journal of Emergency Medicine, 10*(1), 6-10. Retrieved from www.ncbi.nlm.nih.gov/pmc/articles/PMC2672291.

the child is apneic and requires ventilatory support. With an incomplete spinal cord injury, the cord has some function remaining below the level of injury (NINDS, 2011).

Diagnostic Evaluation

After the nurse takes the history of the injury and performs a complete neurologic examination, the extent of the spinal cord injury is determined by radiography or MRI. The extent of the motor or sensory deficit may resolve somewhat as spinal shock resolves. Spinal cord injury without radiologic abnormalities (SCIWORA) is a neurologic

PATHOPHYSIOLOGY

Spinal Cord Injury

Spinal cord injuries occur in children when vertebral bodies are fractured or subluxation of the vertebra occurs. Subluxation results in malalignment of contiguous vertebrae so that the spinal cord is compressed. The cord may be crushed, stretched beyond tolerance, or completely divided. All neurons carrying sensations from those parts of the body below the lesion are unable to pass their message on to the brain. A cord injury causes complete paralysis and complete loss of sensation below the level where the spinal cord was severely damaged or severed.

Flaccid paralysis of the affected limbs immediately follows a spinal cord injury. Paralysis is caused by spinal shock, which can last 4 to 6 weeks or longer. The flaccidity changes to spasticity when the spinal shock resolves. Hypotension, bradycardia, and peripheral vasodilation result from spinal shock and associated loss of vasomotor tone.*†

*Barker, E. (2008). *Neuroscience nursing: A spectrum of care*. St. Louis: Elsevier Mosby.
†Spinal Injury Network. (2010). *Spinal shock fact sheet*. Retrieved from www.spinal-injury.net/spinal-cord-shock.htm.

consequence of injury to the spinal cord related to anatomic differences in the structure of the spinal column and cord during childhood (Sidram, Tripathy, Ghorai, & Ghosh, 2009). It is more frequently seen in children younger than 10 years old and is caused by the spinal cord stretching beyond its normal range (Lee et al., 2009).

Therapeutic Management

Current treatment of spinal cord injury includes immobilization and steroid therapy. If used, steroids must be given within 8 hours of the injury as a bolus of 30 mg/kg followed by a continuous infusion of 5.4 mg/kg/hr for 23 hours. Because of the adverse effects associated with steroid administration, their use is controversial. More research is needed to evaluate the effectiveness of steroid therapy for cervical spine injuries and to determine protocols for steroid administration times after spinal injury (Bracken, 2009). Until permanent surgical stabilization can be performed, other treatments—such as halo traction (Figure 28-6) and Gardner-Wells tongs—may be used as a temporary stabilization method.

Autonomic dysreflexia (AD) is characterized by severe peripheral hypertension. AD can occur in a child after a spinal cord injury at or above the T6 (thoracic vertebrae 6) level. Early signs are sudden, significant rise in systolic and diastolic blood pressure, usually with bradycardia; flushing of the face, neck and shoulders; goose bumps above the T6 level; blurred vision; spots in the child's visual field; and nasal congestion. It is essential to recognize these signs and initiate emergency treatment to lower the blood pressure to prevent cerebral and retinal hemorrhage, seizures, and myocardial infarction (Campagnolo, 2011).

NURSING CARE OF THE CHILD WITH A SPINAL CORD INJURY

■ Assessment

The spine must be immobilized before any attempt is made to move the child. The airway is assessed immediately, and if intubation is necessary it is done without hyperextending the neck (see Chapter 10). Circulation is then assessed; hypotension may be a result of either

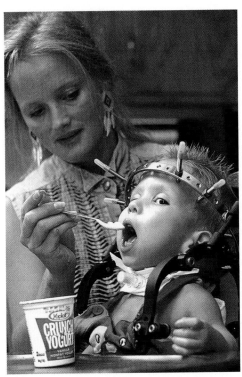

FIG 28-6 Children who have injuries or birth defects that involve the upper spine may be placed in halo traction to stabilize the spine and prevent added nerve damage. Spinal cord injury is a catastrophic event for the child and family; intense nursing support and education as well as referral to support groups, will be needed. (Courtesy Cook Children's Medical Center, Fort Worth, TX.)

hypovolemia or neurologic shock. Bradycardia and hypothermia may occur. The nurse closely monitors the child's body temperature and oxygenation status.

The neurologic assessment by the nurse includes evaluating mobility, sensation, and reflexes. The nurse considers the suspected level of spinal cord injury and whether the injury is thought to be complete or incomplete. The neurologic assessment is ongoing and carefully documented so that changes can be promptly reported. The child is also assessed for other areas of trauma and the impact of the spinal cord injury on other systems including genitourinary, gastrointestinal, and integumentary.

■ Nursing Diagnosis and Planning

The following nursing diagnoses and expected outcomes may be appropriate after assessment of the child with spinal cord injury:
- Ineffective Breathing Pattern related to weakness or paralysis of respiratory muscles after spinal cord injury.

Expected Outcome. The child will not have respiratory distress, as evidenced by arterial blood gas (ABG) values within normal limits, stable vital signs, and adequate motor and sensory function.
- Risk for Impaired Skin Integrity related to immobility.

Expected Outcome. The child will maintain skin integrity, as evidenced by intact skin and absence of breakdown.
- Anxiety related to having a child with an acute condition.

Expected Outcome. The child and parents will have decreased anxiety, as evidenced by an ability to verbalize the impact the child's spinal cord injury will have on their lives.
- Interrupted Family Processes related to having a child with an acute and chronic injury.

Expected Outcome. The parents will show signs of adapting to their child's injury, as evidenced by participating in the child's care and seeking appropriate support within the community.
- Impaired Physical Mobility related to neuromuscular impairment.

Expected Outcome. The child will maximize potential for improvement of mobility, as evidenced by involvement in physical therapy and occupational therapy.

■ Interventions

The goals of nursing care are to minimize the potential for further injury, prevent the sequelae of immobility, and promote maximal spinal cord recovery. The spinal cord is first immobilized with the use of tongs or halo traction. The child remains in traction for several weeks (see Chapter 26). The nurse is responsible for maintaining proper alignment by monitoring the status of the traction every 1 to 2 hours. Towels and rolls can be useful to help position the child. The nurse should perform a motor and sensory assessment after each change of position (see Chapter 9).

If the child's condition becomes unstable, surgical stabilization may be necessary. Progressive neurologic deterioration is the major indicator for surgery.

The child who is immobilized and neurologically impaired is at risk for respiratory complications as a result of muscle weakness and immobility. Respiratory status and pulse oximetry readings are assessed and recorded every 1 to 2 hours. Supplemental oxygen may be indicated. Nebulizer, incentive spirometry, and intermittent positive-pressure breathing (IPPB) are administered as ordered. Some children need a tracheostomy for prolonged mechanical ventilation if the respiratory muscles are involved.

The nurse evaluates perfusion and neurologic integrity by continuously monitoring circulation, sensation, and motion. In addition, the nurse assesses hourly vital signs, color, core body temperature, skin, and intake and output. If alterations in perfusion occur, the child receives crystalloids by bolus infusion. Vasopressors can also be used and are often required for cervical spinal injuries. However, more research is needed to determine which vasopressors are most effective so that protocols can be developed (Ploumis, Yadlapalli, Fehlings et al., 2010).

Children with spinal cord injuries often have difficulty with body temperature control. Some are unable to maintain body heat because of dermal vasodilation (*poikilothermia*) (Walker, 2009). These children will need to be gradually warmed or cooled as indicated. If the child has an elevated temperature, samples of wound material and blood are obtained for culture. Sputum cultures may be ordered. Antipyretic and broad-spectrum antibiotic therapies are initiated after the specimens are sent to the laboratory.

Each time the child is repositioned (every 1 to 2 hours); the nurse thoroughly inspects the child's skin and administers skin care. Pressure on the bony prominences is minimized with the use of special mattresses and padding. Because of bladder muscle weakness or paralysis, an indwelling urinary catheter is often used to facilitate bladder emptying and permit accurate measurement of intake and output on an hourly basis. While the indwelling catheter is in place, care is taken to prevent infection. Intermittent catheterization may eventually be initiated.

The child may have a nasogastric tube in place with gravity drainage or low, intermittent suction. The nurse maintains tube patency, and observes and records the characteristics and quantity of the drainage. Since these children are at risk for stress ulcers and gastrointestinal hemorrhage, the pH of the gastric fluid is tested and the child treated with antacids or histamine blockers as indicated. A bowel regimen is initiated and maintained to prevent impaction. Bowel training includes ingestion of a high-fiber diet (when the child is able to eat), the use of stool softeners, and increased water intake. Adequate nutrition is essential to the healing process. Caloric intake is monitored, and the child may receive nutrition by oral intake, tube feeding, or total parenteral nutrition. A good indicator of a favorable response to the nutrition is timely healing of wounds.

Spinal cord injury is a catastrophic event. The lives of the child and family have been suddenly and permanently altered. They will need intense assistance and support. These nursing care goals can be achieved through therapeutic play, promotion of independent functioning, referral to a multidisciplinary rehabilitation team, referral to support groups, psychological counseling, and thorough discharge planning. Following stabilization, most children are transferred to a rehabilitation unit for ongoing interdisciplinary care, therapy, and teaching in preparation for returning home.

▪ Evaluation

- Are body functions (respiration, elimination, muscle strength) maintained as normally as possible?
- Is the child's skin intact and free from breakdown?
- Do the child and parents verbalize feelings and emotions about the injury and the prognosis?
- Do the parents demonstrate ability to provide physical and emotional support for the child?
- Has the child's neurologic function improved?

SEIZURE DISORDERS

A seizure consists of brief paroxysmal behavior caused by excessive abnormal discharge of neurons. Epilepsy is marked by recurrent seizure activity that does not occur in association with an acute illness. The three types of seizures are focal, generalized, and unknown. Focal seizures occur in one part of the brain and may or may not alter consciousness. Generalized seizures occur over the entire brain and do alter consciousness. A seizure of the unknown type cannot be characterized as focal or generalized; epileptic and infantile spasms are examples (Berg, Berkovic, Brodie et al., 2010).

Etiology

Seizures are symptomatic of altered neuronal activity in the CNS. Seizures can occur for many reasons and are categorized by etiology: *genetic, structural/metabolic,* or *unknown* (Berg & Scheffer, 2011). Genetic seizures occur as a direct result of a genetic defect (known or presumed). Structural/metabolic seizures are associated with specific conditions or diseases, including strokes, trauma, and infection. If the cause is not known, the seizure etiology is categorized as unknown. This category accounts for a third of all epilepsies (Berg et al., 2010).

Incidence

Approximately 180,000 new cases of epilepsy are diagnosed each year, and 30% of these cases are children. Most of the newly diagnosed cases in pediatrics occur in early childhood and adolescence. An estimated 2% to 4% of all children will have a febrile seizure, and the majority outgrow the tendency for this type of seizure by age 5 (Epilepsy Foundation of America, 2010b).

Because of the subtlety of neonatal seizures the incidence is difficult to determine. Seizure manifestations may be easily confused with normal infant behavior. Infants who have neonatal seizures in the first few days after delivery have poorer outcomes than those who develop seizures later in the neonatal period (Epilepsy Foundation of America, 2010c).

Pathophysiology

During a seizure, excessive, self-limiting neuronal discharges occur. The result of these discharges is activation of associated motor or sensory organs. The extent of the seizure depends on the location and extent of the abnormal neuronal discharges. The brain consists of millions of nerve cells; electrical impulses are sent through many of these cells by neurotransmitters. When numerous nerve cells fire abnormally at the same time, a seizure may result.

Manifestations

Many types of seizures exist. The International Classification of Seizures is used to divide seizures into the three major groups (Box 28-5).

Febrile seizures are generally seen in young children. Febrile seizures alone are not diagnosed as epilepsy (Berg et al., 2010). However, even though the risk of having a nonfebrile seizure is very low in a child who had a febrile seizure, febrile seizures are considered a risk factor for the development of epilepsy (American Academy of Pediatrics, 2008). The height and rapidity of temperature elevation seem to be factors in precipitating febrile seizures. The temperature is usually elevated above 102° F (38.8° C). The seizure activity occurs during the temperature rise rather than after prolonged elevation. Simple febrile seizures are familial and previously thought to be transmitted by an autosomal dominant inheritance pattern. However, current research shows that the inheritance pattern may be polygenic (Kira, Ishizaki, Torisu et al., 2010). Most febrile seizures occur as a result of fever caused by otitis media, pharyngitis, and adenitis. The family of a child who has a febrile seizure should be given information about these seizures and instructed what to do if another seizure occurs.

Neonatal seizures are usually caused by an underlying pathologic process. The most frequent cause of neonatal seizures is perinatal asphyxia leading to hypoxic-ischemic encephalopathy. The second major contributing factor is intracranial hemorrhage. Other causes include metabolic disturbances, intrauterine and perinatal infectious disorders, cerebral infarcts, drug withdrawal, hyperthermia, hypoglycemia, sodium and potassium imbalances, congenital anomalies of the CNS, and inherited syndromes (Epilepsy Foundation of America, 2010a).

The mechanism of neonatal seizures is not clearly understood. Because of the overall anatomic and physiologic immaturity of the neonate's nervous system including a lack of myelinization of fiber tracts, generalized tonic-clonic seizures are rare. Seizures in neonates may produce subtle signs such as sustained eye opening, tonic horizontal deviation of the eyes, blinking or eyelid fluttering, sucking, smacking, drooling, tongue thrusting, pedaling movements of the legs, swimming movements of the arms, and apnea. These manifestations are more common in preterm infants and infants with hypoxic-ischemic encephalopathy. Neonatal seizures also can be focal, tonic, or myoclonic, with jerking movements of the extremities.

Diagnostic Evaluation

The child's health history and family history are important parts of the initial workup. A thorough description of the child's behavior before, during, and after the seizure activity is important to delineate the type of seizure. Video recording and EEG monitoring help identify the seizure. Serum electrolyte determinations, CBC, blood glucose determination, lumbar puncture, and other laboratory tests can help uncover metabolic causes. CT and MRI will indicate trauma, tumor,

BOX 28-5 INTERNATIONAL CLASSIFICATION OF SEIZURES

Generalized Seizures

Onset starts at any age. Clinical features indicate involvement of both cerebral hemispheres. Consciousness is impaired.

Tonic, Clonic, and Tonic-Clonic Seizures

Formerly called *grand mal seizures*, tonic-clonic seizures cause an abrupt arrest of activity and impairment of consciousness. The *tonic phase* consists of a sustained, generalized stiffening of muscles, including the diaphragm, lasting a few seconds. The *clonic phase* is symmetrical and rhythmic, consisting of alternating contraction and relaxation of major muscle groups. This phase usually ends spontaneously in less than 5 minutes. Respirations are irregular, and the child may have stridor. Sphincter incontinence (stool and/or urine) may or may not occur. The tonic-clonic seizure is followed by a variable period of confusion, lethargy, and sleep (postictal phase).

Atonic Seizures

Atonic seizures cause an abrupt loss of postural tone, impairment of consciousness, confusion, lethargy, and sleep. A child may have multiple episodes of sudden and brief head drop or the child may have a drop attack; fall to the ground, often face down, lose consciousness for a few seconds, and then get back up as if nothing happened.*

Myoclonic Seizures

Myoclonic seizures are brief, random contractions of a muscle group, followed by loss of muscle tone and forward falling. They can occur on both sides of the body and may occur singly or in clusters. Impairment of consciousness may occur during myoclonic seizures. Onset can occur as early as age 2 months, but myoclonic seizures are more frequently seen in school-age children or adolescents than in very young children.

Absence Seizures

Formerly called *petit mal seizures*, absence seizures are very brief episodes of altered consciousness. Typically, no muscle activity occurs except for upward rolling of the eyes. The child has a blank facial expression. Absence seizures last only 5 to 10 seconds or less, but they may occur up to hundreds of times a day. They are characterized by the child immediately returning to the activity involved in just prior to the seizure.* Children with atypical absence seizures may experience some myoclonic movements (eyelid fluttering) and muscle tone changes (head bobbing). The onset of absence seizures usually occurs between ages 5 to 8 years.

Focal Seizures

Onset starts at any age. The clinical features suggest that only a limited functional area in one hemisphere of the brain is involved, and therefore symptoms are seen on only one side of the body. Focal seizures are described according to the features exhibited by the child during the seizure. Types of features are awareness/responsiveness (altered or intact), sensory/psychic (aura), motor, and autonomic. Impairment in consciousness or awareness and decreased responsiveness occur with some but not all focal seizures. An aura, the sensation of an upcoming seizure, is actually part of a focal seizure. Other sensory symptoms include a rising abdominal feeling, an unexplained sense of fear, déjà vu feeling, an odd taste in the mouth or odd smell, and visual/auditory hallucinations. Children under age 7 years are less likely to report sensory symptoms, however, parents may observe them staring or looking around without purpose, being less responsive, and exhibiting automatisms.*

Motor features, which are commonly seen, include involuntary, brief movements (tonic, clonic, or atonic) that are localized to one area, and turning eyes and head away from the side of the seizure. During a focal seizure, children can exhibit automatisms, repetitive, nonpurposeful movements of mouth and extremities such as lip smacking, chewing, teeth grinding, scratching, pulling at clothing or sheets, and shuffling. Salivation, dilation of pupils, and skin flushing occur as well. The average duration of a focal seizure is 1 to 2 minutes. A variable period of confusion, lethargy, and sleep follows the event.

A focal seizure may become a bilateral, convulsive seizure when the electrical impulses pass across the corpus callosum to the other hemisphere. The child may experience bilateral tonic and clonic movements, urinary and stool incontinence, and loss of consciousness.

Unknown

This classification is for seizures that cannot be characterized as generalized or focal. These include epileptic spasms (Lennox-Gastaut syndrome) seen in older children as well as infantile spasms (West syndrome) seen in infants between ages 2 to 12 months. These infants exhibit brief contractions of the neck, arms, trunk, and legs (myoclonic spasms) and eventually suffer developmental regression.*

Data from Berg, A., Berkovic, S., Brodie, M., et al. (2010). Revised terminology and concepts for organization of seizures and epilepsies: Report of the ILAE commission on classifications and terminology, 2005-2009. *Epilepsia, 51*(4), 676-685. Retrieved from www.ilae-epilepsy.org/Visitors/Centre/ctf/documents/ClassificationReport_2010_000.pdf; Berg, A., & Scheffer, I. (2011). New concepts in classification of the epilepsies: Entering the 21st century. *Epilepsia, 52*(6), 1058-1062. Retrieved from www.ilae-epilepsy.org/Visitors/Centre/ctf/documents/NewConcepts-Classification_2011_000.pdf.
*Mikati, M. (2011). Seizures in childhood. In R. Kliegman, B. Stanton, J. St. Geme, et al. (Eds.), *Nelson textbook of pediatrics* (19th ed., pp. 2013-2039). Philadelphia: Elsevier Saunders.

or congenital malformation. In neonates, several other laboratory tests may be included—such as *t*oxoplasmosis, *o*ther agents, *r*ubella, *c*ytomegalovirus, and *h*erpes simplex virus (TORCH) titers—to exclude congenital viral infections, as well as amino acid and organic acid studies to exclude inborn errors of metabolism.

Therapeutic Management

The basic tenet of treatment for the child with seizures is to treat the whole child. Antiepileptic medications are commonly used to manage seizures. Treatment goals are to identify and correct the cause of the seizure, eliminate the seizure with a minimum of side effects and the least amount of medication, and normalize the lives of the child and the family (Table 28-3).

Vagus nerve stimulation (VNS) may significantly reduce the number and intensity of seizures in many children. A generator is implanted in the chest wall, and a wire is clipped to the vagus nerve to deliver electrical impulses to the brain. Side effects include a tickling sensation in the throat, change in voice tone during stimulation, slight coughing during stimulation, and rarely, shortness of breath, swallowing difficulties, and infection (Cyberonics, 2010). Positive side effects include increased cognition and improved mood and behavior (Grill & Ng, 2010). VNS therapy may decrease the need for pharmacologic intervention and emergency care.

A ketogenic diet is another treatment option for children with epilepsy. The diet is essentially carbohydrate-free, composed mostly of fat, and produces a state of ketosis that is thought to control seizures.

TABLE 28-3 COMMON SEIZURE MEDICATIONS

DRUG NAME	SEIZURE TYPE	SIDE EFFECTS	NURSING IMPLICATIONS
Carbamazepine (Tegretol)	Focal or generalized	Sedation, cognitive deficits, behavior outbursts	Watch for change in behavior or decrease in school performance. Child should not be given erythromycin, which will cause an increase in drug level. Monitor blood tests for therapeutic levels
Rufinamide (Banzel)	Lennox-Gastaut (multiple seizure types)	Headache, tremor, dizziness, fatigue, sleepiness, double vision	May be crushed and taken with food.
Felbamate (Felbatol)	Focal or generalized	Nausea and vomiting, weight loss, anorexia, agitation and aggression, aplastic anemia, liver failure	Shake oral suspension well. Monitor liver enzymes and CBC.
Ethosuximide (Zarontin)	Generalized	Nausea and vomiting, lethargy	Observe for excessive drowsiness; take with food.
Lamotrigine (Lamictal)	Generalized or focal	Rash (increased risk of severe rash exists in children with previous reaction to any drug or to another antiepileptic drug), dizziness, headache, double vision, nausea and vomiting, ataxia	Not affected by food absorption. Instruct parents to report any signs of rash immediately.
Gabapentin (Neurontin)	Generalized or focal	Drowsiness, dizziness, nystagmus, nausea and vomiting, ataxia	Dosage must be adjusted relative to renal function.
Levetiracetam (Keppra)	Focal, myoclonic, and generalized	Sleepiness, weakness, headache, infection	Monitor for side effects and frequency of seizures and renal dysfunction.
Phenobarbital	Generalized or focal	Sedation, cognitive deficits, behavior outbursts	Watch for excessive drowsiness, changes in school performance, and respiratory depression. Monitor blood tests for therapeutic levels
Phenytoin (Dilantin)	Focal, generalized, or status	Lethargy, nystagmus, ataxia, allergic reactions, hypertrophic gums, hirsutism	Teach meticulous oral care to decrease gum hypertrophy. IV form must be given in normal saline and filtered. Monitor blood tests for therapeutic levels
Topiramate (Topamax)	Focal or generalized tonic-clonic	Fatigue, nervousness, decreased attention, anorexia, renal stones, tremor	Affects levels of other antiepileptic drugs. Keep children well hydrated to decrease chances of renal stones.
Tiagabine (Gabitril)	Complex and focal	Lethargy, sedation, double vision, ataxia	Monitor for generalized weakness.
Valproic acid (Depakene)	Generalized, focal, absence, myoclonic	Nausea and vomiting, tremor, weight gain, hair loss, thrombocytopenia, liver failure	Do not crush or cut pills/sprinkles. Can cause stomach ulcers. Take with food. Monitor blood tests for therapeutic levels
Oxcarbazepine (Trileptal)	Focal	Fatigue, headache, dizziness, double vision, unsteadiness, nausea and vomiting	Interacts with other antiepileptic drugs; levels should be monitored.

This diet is very strict and considered mainly for children with epilepsy that is refractory to conventional treatment. It may be more readily accepted by children who have not developed taste preferences, those who are developmentally delayed, and those who are fed through gastrostomy tubes. Side effects include electrolyte imbalances, vitamin deficiency, altered growth patterns, constipation, and hypoglycemia (The Charlie Foundation, 2009).

Both the ketogenic diet and VNS therapy are considered adjunctive therapies for treatment of epilepsy. Antiepileptic medications will typically be continued for most children to achieve the best degree of seizure control.

STATUS EPILEPTICUS

Status epilepticus is a medical emergency. It is marked by prolonged seizure activity, in the form of either a single seizure lasting 30 minutes or more or recurrent seizures lasting more than 30 minutes with no return to a normal level of consciousness between seizures. Any seizure lasting 10 minutes or more can suggest pending status epilepticus and should be treated as such. The most common form of status epilepticus is generalized status, which has the highest potential for complications and possible death.

Etiology

The causes of status epilepticus are many. Acute CNS injury from head trauma, meningitis, or electrolyte imbalance frequently precipitates status epilepticus. The condition can also be caused by toxins, specific medications, chronic CNS injury, and sudden withdrawal from antiepileptic medications.

Incidence

Status epilepticus occurs in 5% to 10% of children with epilepsy. The most common form in children younger than 3 years is febrile status epilepticus.

NURSING CARE PLAN

The Child with a Seizure Disorder in the Community Setting

Focused Assessment

- Obtain a detailed prenatal, perinatal, and neonatal history to determine factors that may have caused the child's seizures
  - Pathologic factors include hypoxia, cerebral trauma, high fever, lead poisoning, metabolic disorders, brain tumors, birth trauma, and CNS infections
  - Nonpathologic factors include overhydration, oversedation, drug abuse, alcohol intoxication, sleep deprivation, antihistamine drug use, and family history
- Ask parents for detailed description of child's seizures
  - Age at onset of child's seizure activity
  - Time of day when seizures occur
  - Precipitating event(s)
  - Child's behavior before, during, and after a seizure
  - How the child looks during the seizure
  - How the seizure progresses
  - How long the seizure lasts
- Perform comprehensive physical exam with emphasis on the neurologic system
  - Assess behavior, motor skills, and developmental level
  - Assess emotional responses of the child and of the family to the child's seizure disorder
- For the school-age child with a known seizure history, the school nurse maintains pertinent information in the child's record and communicates appropriate information to teachers, if needed
- During a seizure, first provide for the child's safety. Observe the child closely and document findings; observations may assist with seizure management

Planning

Nursing Diagnosis

Risk for Injury related to seizure activity.

Expected Outcomes

The child will remain free from injury through the use of appropriate injury prevention strategies.

The parents and older child will discuss seizure prevention and demonstrate appropriate safety interventions for seizures.

Intervention/Rationale

1. If the child is hospitalized, institute seizure precautions including padded side rails, bed in low position, suction and airway at bedside. At home during a seizure, instruct the parents to place the child on a soft surface or keep in bed. Remove sharp objects and keep furniture out of the way.
   These actions make the environment safer for the child during the seizure.
2. Do not put anything into the child's mouth during a seizure.
   Forcing something into the child's mouth may injure the child's mouth, gums, or teeth or cause gagging and vomiting.
3. During a seizure, advise the parent or teacher to place the child on the side in a lateral position. Do not restrain the child. Loosen clothing around the child's neck.
   Positioning the child on the side prevents aspiration because saliva or vomit will drain out the corner of the child's mouth. Restraints could cause injury to the child. The nurse or family may gently guide or protect the child's movements and may suction the child's mouth after the seizure is over if suction is available.
4. Stay with the child who is having a seizure.
   Staying with the child reduces the risk of injury and allows observation and documentation of the seizure.

5. Record and instruct parents to record the time of seizures, precipitating factors, types of behavior including level of consciousness observed during and after the seizure, bladder or bowel incontinence, and frequency of seizures.
   These observations help pinpoint the focus of the seizure and help the physician treat the seizure correctly.
6. If a seizure lasts longer than 5 minutes, instruct parents to notify the physician immediately and administer rescue medications as ordered.
   Medication may need to be administered to stop prolonged seizures. The main side effect of diazepam (Valium) and lorazepam (Ativan) is respiratory depression.

Evaluation

Does the child remain injury free?

Do the child and family implement injury prevention strategies?

Do the parents monitor the seizure and record vital information?

Can the parents demonstrate safety interventions for seizures?

Can parents administer rescue medications as ordered?

Planning

Nursing Diagnosis

Deficient Knowledge related to the need for information about how to manage a child with a seizure disorder.

Expected Outcomes

The child and parents will seek information about the child's management and describe how to meet the child's physical, emotional, and educational needs.

Intervention/Rationale

1. Determine the educational needs of the child and parents.
   Determining educational needs provides baseline information to develop a teaching plan.
2. Provide an individual teaching plan for the child and parents for managing seizures.
   An individualized teaching plan ensures that what is needed by the child and parents will be taught.
3. Explore actual and potential problems that may arise and interfere with treatment.
   Exploring possible problems facilitates adjustment and normalizes life; it also provides anticipatory guidance.
4. Measure outcomes of education to ensure that learning has taken place and is facilitating acceptance of the child's condition.
   Evaluation of teaching is an ongoing process to ensure continued learning.
5. Refer to an epilepsy support group (see Evolve website for a list of resource organizations).
   Social support is helpful for some families and may promote adjustment to lifestyle changes.
6. Educate the child and parents about the medication regimen. Emphasize the importance of adhering to medical treatment and administering medications on time.
   The goal of pharmacologic management is to raise the seizure threshold, thus preventing seizures from occurring.
7. Identify the side effects of the medication and when medical attention should be sought.
   Knowledge of what is expected and normal will facilitate proper use of and adherence to the medication regimen.

Continued

◎ NURSING CARE PLAN

The Child with a Seizure Disorder in the Community Setting—cont'd

8. Identify the hazards of nonadherence to the medication regimen. Encourage the parents and child not to discontinue medications even if the child is seizure free.

   Nonadherence will affect the serum levels of anticonvulsant drugs and may cause a seizure to occur.

9. Emphasize to the child and parents the importance of regular medical evaluation and follow-up, including measurement of blood levels of the medication and evaluating for toxicity or side effects.

   Regular medical follow-up facilitates maintenance of appropriate therapeutic blood levels of antiepileptics and identification of side effects of medication.

10. Inform the parent about the need for a medical alert bracelet for the child.

    Medical alert bracelets alert others to the child's condition in an emergency. If the child has a seizure in a public place, the bracelet will inform other people about appropriate actions to take on behalf of the child.

11. Educate the parents about possible seizure triggers and avoidance of stressors. Many children are susceptible to having seizures when subjected to stress.

    Lack of sleep, illness, and other stressors may increase the likelihood of seizures occurring.

12. Encourage the family to find alternative activities besides contact sports for the child. The child should avoid swimming or climbing alone. Identify the child's strengths—**not the child's limitations.**

    Appropriate activities reduce the risk of injury while promoting a positive self-image.

13. Encourage verbalization of fears and concerns about having seizures.

    Therapeutic communication may identify issues that need to be addressed.

14. Teach the child and parent to educate other family members, friends, and teachers about seizures. Advise the family to provide necessary information to the school nurse.

    Accurate information reduces the stigma associated with epilepsy and helps inform others of the seizure rescue plan.

Evaluation

Does the child discuss having seizures, fears and concerns about seizures, and life with the condition?

Does the child participate in the medical regimen by discussing medication side effects and dosage?

Does the child demonstrate a positive self-image?

Does the family administer antiepileptic medications safely and appropriately and know when to call the physician?

PATIENT-CENTERED TEACHING

Guidelines for the Child or Adolescent Taking Seizure Medication

- Oral care is very important for children taking phenytoin (Dilantin) because phenytoin can cause gum problems. Your child should brush with a soft brush and floss after every meal. Take your child to the dentist every 3 to 6 months for a checkup and teeth cleaning.
- Once your child has started taking the medication, blood levels should be monitored to determine that the medication has reached and maintained a therapeutic level and to monitor for a toxic level. In addition, other blood tests may be needed to ensure that the medication is not harming the liver or blood cells. Blood levels should be measured periodically as your physician recommends, if a seizure occurs, or if side effects are noticed.
- If your child is taking valproic acid, be alert for any signs of unusual bleeding or bruising. Valproic acid can affect the platelets (cells that help the blood clot) and cause the platelet counts to drop. Valproic acid may also cause increased appetite. Offer healthy snacks and small meal portions.
- Be sure your child does not suddenly stop taking antiepileptic medications without discussing it with a physician or nurse. Suddenly stopping medications can cause the child to have a seizure or status epilepticus.
- Some states require a driver to be seizure free for a time ranging from a few months to a few years to obtain a driver's license. If your child is of driving age, discuss this with your health care provider.*
- Birth control pills may be less effective while taking antiepileptic medications. If sexually active, your adolescent should consult a nurse or physician

  for additional forms of birth control. Folic acid supplementation may be advised for teen females taking antiepileptic medications.
- Cognitive and behavior changes may be seen with some of the antiepileptic medications. Attention span, memory, and interpersonal interactions may become impaired.
- Alcohol, marijuana, and street drugs will lower the seizure threshold. These drugs should be avoided.
- Contact sports such as football and wrestling are not advised.
- Showers are preferred over baths for children who are concerned about privacy. Younger children with epilepsy should never be left alone in a tub of water. Swimming activities should be supervised by a strong swimmer who can rescue a child who has a seizure in the water.
- Depression is a diagnosis that often accompanies epilepsy and may be associated with antiepileptic medications. Report any symptoms of depression to the physician.
- Maintaining a seizure diary that lists seizure frequency, associated triggers, and details of seizure activity is a good way for parents to collaborate with the health care team in determining the effectiveness of the treatment plan.
- Call 911 if your child has a seizure that does not resolve after 5 minutes.
- Your child should wear a medical alert bracelet to alert others of potential problems if they appear.†

*Krumholz, A. (2009). Driving issues in epilepsy: Past, present, and future. *Epilepsy Currents, 9*(2), 31-35. Retrieved from http://onlinelibrary.wiley.com/doi/10.1111/j.1535-7511.2008.01283.x/full.

†Flower, D. (2009). Epilepsy part 3: Planning for emergencies. *British Journal of School Nursing, 4*(5), 164-168. Retrieved from www.internurse.com/cgi-bin/go.pl/library/contents.html?uid=2744;journal_uid=29.

! NURSING QUALITY ALERT

Observations and Nursing Care during a Seizure

- As the seizure begins, look at your watch or a clock. You should be able to describe how long seizure activity lasts.
- Protect the child from injury by loosening clothing at the neck and turning the child gently onto the side, removing any obstacles in the child's environment. *Do not* restrain the child or insert any object into the child's mouth.
- Carefully observe in which body part the seizure begins, its progression, and how it ends.
- Be able to describe any preceding or accompanying sensory or motor manifestations.
- When the seizure is over, allow the child to rest if she or he desires. Record the child's behavior before, during, and after the seizure and the approximate duration of the seizure.
- In neonates, if the movement can be initiated by a stimulus, such as touch, it is probably a tremor. If the movement cannot be stopped or controlled with gentle restraint or passive flexion, it is probably a seizure.

Pathophysiology

Status epilepticus is caused by the random discharge of large numbers of neurons firing abnormally. The discharges cause abnormal repetitive motor activity. In the CNS, the metabolic rate increases, glucose stores are depleted, and oxygen consumption increases. If cerebral metabolic demands are not met, these changes cause neuronal injury. Prolonged seizures cause lactic acidosis, an altered blood-brain barrier, and increased ICP.

Manifestations

See the International Classification of Seizures in Box 28-5.

Diagnostic Evaluation

Diagnostic laboratory tests should include blood glucose, arterial blood gases, electrolytes, anticonvulsant drug levels, a toxicology screen, and possibly lumbar puncture. Results may be similar to those of the child with increased ICP. An MRI may also be performed.

Therapeutic Management

Generalized tonic-clonic status epilepticus is a medical emergency. Treatment consists of maintaining optimal respiratory and hemodynamic function and identifying and treating the causes of the seizure activity. Diazepam (Valium), lorazepam (Ativan), or midazolam (Versed) is given IV. If IV access cannot be obtained, medication can be given orally or rectally. Fosphenytoin (Cerebyx) or phenobarbital may be given IV as a second round of drugs if diazepam or lorazepam does not stop the seizures. The intramuscular route is not used because absorption of the medication is unpredictable.

NURSING CARE OF THE CHILD WITH STATUS EPILEPTICUS

■ Assessment

On arrival at the hospital, the child will exhibit seizure activity and have unstable vital signs. Along with general seizure precautions, this child requires rapid assessment and vigorous supportive therapy. Supportive measures include assessing and maintaining a patent airway and administering oxygen. IV hydration and drug therapy are initiated to arrest the seizure activity.

■ Nursing Diagnosis and Planning

The following nursing diagnoses and expected outcomes may apply to the child with status epilepticus:

- Impaired Gas Exchange related to decreased respirations associated with seizures.

Expected Outcome. The child will remain free from respiratory distress, as evidenced by pulse oxygen saturation remaining at or above 95%.

- Ineffective Breathing Pattern related to loss of muscle control associated with seizures.

Expected Outcome. The child will maintain a normal breathing pattern, as evidenced by pulse oxygen saturation remaining at or above 95% and respiratory rate within normal range.

- Ineffective Airway Clearance related to possible aspiration during seizure.

Expected Outcome. The child's airways will be clear, as evidenced by clear breath sounds.

- Risk for Ineffective Cerebral Tissue Perfusion related to lactic acidosis with prolonged seizure activity.

Expected Outcome. The child will reestablish cerebral tissue perfusion, as evidenced by a return to normal levels of consciousness.

■ Interventions and Evaluation

The child will initially require establishment and maintenance of a patent airway. The nurse assesses vital signs and performs neurologic checks frequently. Once the child is stable, nursing interventions and evaluation are similar to those described for the child with epilepsy.

⚡ SAFETY ALERT

Drug Therapy for Generalized Tonic-Clonic Status Epilepticus

Generalized tonic-clonic status epilepticus is a medical emergency. IV diazepam (Valium) or lorazepam (Ativan) is given. IV diazepam must be given directly into the vein (not the tubing, because it interacts with plastic) at a rate no greater than 2 mg/min. It should not be mixed with other drugs or solutions, and it can be diluted only with normal saline. Diazepam rectal gel can be administered in a community or hospital setting and is useful when the child does not have a readily accessible IV. Other pharmaceutical options for emergency treatment include buccal administration of midazolam and intranasal lorazepam.* Research is ongoing regarding the use of newer antiepileptic drugs such as valproate and levetiracetam for the treatment of status epilepticus.† Resuscitation equipment should be at the bedside and the child's respirations closely monitored during IV antiepileptic drug administration.

*Sofou, K., Kristjánsdóttir, R., Papachatzakis, N., et al. (2009). Management of prolonged seizures and status epilepticus in childhood: A systematic review. *Journal of Child Neurology, 24*(8), 918-926. Retrieved from http://jcn.sagepub.com/content/24/8/918.abstract.

†Wheless, J., & Treiman, D. (2008). The role of the newer antiepileptic drugs in the treatment of generalized convulsive status epilepticus. *Epilepsia (Series 4), 49*, 74-78. Retrieved from http://onlinelibrary.wiley.com/doi/10.1111/j.1528-1167.2008.01929.x/full.

MENINGITIS

Meningitis is the most common infectious process affecting the CNS. It can occur as a primary disease or as a result of complications of neurosurgery, trauma, systemic infection, or sinus or ear infections. A wide variety of bacteria and viruses can be responsible for the primary infection. Earlier diagnosis and prompt antibiotic therapy reduce mortality rates and the incidence of complications from bacterial meningitis.

Etiology

The primary organisms responsible for causing bacterial meningitis vary according to age. The organisms primarily responsible for neonatal meningitis are group B streptococci and *Escherichia coli*. Among children ages 2 months to 12 years, three pathogens seem to be the most prevalent. *Haemophilus influenzae* type B, *Neisseria meningitidis*, and *Streptococcus pneumoniae* cause 95% of cases of purulent meningitis in this age-group. Tuberculous and *Borrelia burgdorferi* (Lyme disease) meningitis are becoming more common. These types of meningitis usually result from extension of a localized infection, such as otitis media, sinusitis, pharyngitis, or pneumonia, into the CSF.

Organisms also may be introduced directly after an injury in which the skin is broken and communication between skin, sinuses, and CSF occurs. Entry may occur in association with a lumbar puncture, skull fracture, or surgery.

Meningococcal meningitis caused by *Neisseria meningitidis* usually occurs in older children and adolescents. Because it is transmitted primarily by droplet infection, the risk increases as the number of contacts increases. Viral meningitis is associated with the mumps virus, paramyxovirus, herpesvirus, and enterovirus. In rare cases, protozoa or fungi can cause meningitis; usually in children with acquired immunodeficiency syndrome (AIDS).

Incidence

Meningitis most commonly affects children between ages 1 month and 5 years, but it can occur at any age. Boys are affected more frequently than girls, and the incidence is higher among African-American children than among white children. The incidence of *Haemophilus influenzae* type B meningitis has declined rapidly since the institution of routine immunization of infants.

Manifestations

Signs and symptoms of meningitis vary according to the age of the child and the duration of the preceding illness. No single hallmark sign or symptom exists. In the neonate, infant, and young child, the symptoms of meningitis are frequently vague and nonspecific.

Clinical signs of meningitis in the neonate include poor feeding; poor sucking; vomiting; diarrhea; poor muscle tone; weak cry; hypothermia or hyperthermia; apnea; seizures; sepsis; disseminated intravascular coagulation (DIC); a full, tense, and bulging fontanel; and lethargy.

Clinical signs of meningitis in the infant and preschool-age child include fever, poor feeding, vomiting, irritability, seizures, a high-pitched cry, a bulging anterior fontanel, and lethargy. Early clinical signs of meningitis in children and adolescents include severe headache, photophobia, nuchal rigidity, fever, altered level of consciousness (lethargy, irritability), decreased appetite, vomiting, diarrhea, agitation, and drowsiness. Muscle or joint pain and purpura may be noted. Kernig sign (pain with extension of leg and knee) (Figure 28-7) and Brudzinski sign (flexion of head causing flexion of hips and knees) are often exhibited. In the case of a meningococcal infection, a petechial or purpuric rash may be observed. Late signs include a decreased level of consciousness and seizures.

Diagnostic Evaluation

The diagnosis is made by testing CSF obtained by lumbar puncture. Findings usually include increased CSF pressure, cloudy CSF (in the case of bacterial meningitis), high protein concentration, and low glucose level. Blood cultures are obtained; nose and throat cultures may be done, particularly if the CSF culture is negative.

Therapeutic Management

Acute bacterial meningitis is a medical emergency requiring early recognition and prompt, aggressive management. The child is placed in a private room on Droplet Transmission Precautions, and these are maintained for at least 24 hours after antibiotics are initiated. Immediate initiation and uninterrupted IV administration of appropriate antibiotics are essential in cases of suspected bacterial meningitis; a delay could be fatal. Treatment is started before the causative organism is identified because cultures may take up to 3 days to yield results. Selection of the broad-spectrum antibiotics initially used is based on the age of the child, the suspected pathogens most frequently encountered in the child's age-group, and the initial appearance of the CSF. If IV access is difficult to achieve, the first dose of antibiotics should be administered intramuscularly.

PATHOPHYSIOLOGY

Meningitis

Meningitis is an inflammation of the meninges of the brain that results from a pathogen entering the CNS and causing a toxic response. As the process continues, increased ICP develops along with subdural empyema. If the infection spreads to the ventricles, edema and tissue scarring around the ventricle cause obstruction of the CSF and subsequent hydrocephalus.

This process can happen quite rapidly; CSF is an excellent growth medium for bacteria because it contains nutrient substances such as protein and glucose. Leukocytes are unable to function as a defense mechanism in the fluid environment of the CSF. Leukocytes require a tissue surface to destroy bacteria, so there is little defense to stop the growth of bacteria, and they can multiply quickly.

As the infection spreads further into brain tissue, changes occur in the permeability of capillaries and blood vessels in the dura mater. These changes lead to increased passage of albumin and water into the subdural space, with a subsequent accumulation of protein and fluid. This results in an additional increase in ICP.

The most common neurologic sequelae of meningitis are hearing loss, intellectual impairment, seizures, visual impairment, and behavioral problems. Other complications include cranial nerve dysfunction, brain abscess, and SIADH. Meningococcemia, a fulminating manifestation of *Neisseria meningitides* infection that manifests with petechiae and purpura and signs of viral-type illness, can proceed in a matter of a few hours to adrenal insufficiency, bilateral adrenal hemorrhage (Waterhouse-Friderichsen syndrome), and septic shock.*

*Bornstein, S. (2009). Predisposing factors for adrenal insufficiency. *New England Journal of Medicine, 360*(22), 2328-2339.

Treatment for neonatal bacterial meningitis consists of ampicillin and an aminoglycoside or a third-generation cephalosporin antibiotic. It is essential to monitor peak and trough antibiotic levels to prevent ototoxicity and nephrotoxicity from aminoglycosides. For older children and adolescents, the treatment of choice is ampicillin, penicillin G, or a third-generation cephalosporin. When the culture and sensitivity test results are available, treatment regimens may be refined. Morbidity and mortality associated with bacterial meningitis may also be reduced by adjunctive treatment with dexamethasone therapy

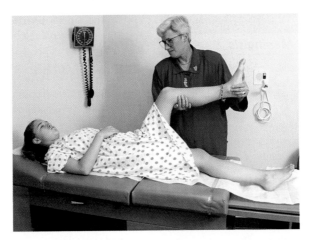

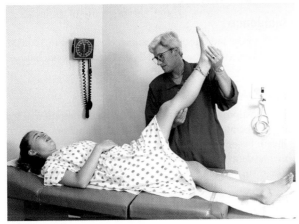

Kernig sign

The child can easily extend the leg when in the supine position. However, when the thigh is flexed toward the abdomen, pain prevents complete extension of the leg.

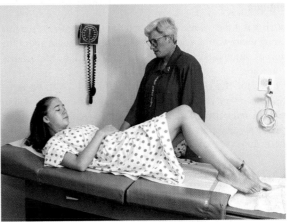

Brudzinski sign

In the supine position, the child bends her head toward her chest (in a younger child, the nurse can bend the child's head). This action usually produces involuntary hip and knee flexion in the child with meningitis.

FIG 28-7 As part of the assessment for meningitis, the nurse can attempt to elicit Kernig sign and Brudzinski sign. Both are early indicators of meningitis in children and adolescents. (Courtesy Parkland Health and Hospital System, Dallas, TX.)

(Nudelman & Tunkel, 2009). The treatment for viral meningitis is symptomatic and supportive, usually with complete recovery.

Current recommendations are that children be vaccinated with meningococcal vaccine at age 11 to 12 years, or by age 18 years, if previously unvaccinated. It is important that prospective college students receive meningococcal vaccine before college entry to prevent meningococcal meningitis and that children receive *Haemophilus influenzae* type B (Hib) vaccine as part of their routine immunization schedule during infancy and early childhood (Centers for Disease Control and Prevention, 2010b).

NURSING CARE OF THE CHILD WITH MENINGITIS

■ Assessment

Baseline data are obtained from the history and physical examination and a complete neurologic assessment that evaluates headaches, photophobia, hearing loss, seizure activity, changes in level of consciousness, changes in pupil reactions and size, nuchal rigidity, and muscle flaccidity. Personality changes, irritability, changes in food and fluid intake, nausea, vomiting, or loss of appetite are also addressed. The nurse should review the history for past immunizations, recent illnesses including upper respiratory tract infection, otitis media, and skull fracture, and recent surgery or lumbar punctures.

■ Nursing Diagnosis and Planning

Nursing diagnoses that apply to the child with meningitis include those common to other neurologic disorders (see Nursing Care Plan: The Child with a Neurologic System Disorder). The following nursing diagnosis is specific to the child with meningitis and the child's family:

- Deficient Knowledge related to seriousness of meningitis, possible residual neurologic deficits, home management, and prophylaxis.

Expected Outcome. The parents' level of understanding of meningitis will increase, as evidenced by an ability to discuss the disease process and possible sequelae, treatment, home management, and possible implications for spread of the disease.

> **! NURSING QUALITY ALERT**
>
> ### Guidelines for the Child with Meningitis
>
> - The close contacts of the child with *Haemophilus influenzae* infection need prophylactic treatment with rifampin.
> - Anyone who spent at least 4 hours with the child in the 5 to 7 days preceding the child's hospitalization with *H. influenzae* needs prophylactic treatment if not already immunized.
> - All close contacts of children with *Neisseria meningitidis* need prophylactic treatment regardless of age or immunization status.
> - Rifampin colors the urine and sweat red-orange and will stain contact lenses.

■ Interventions

The nurse discusses the disease process and prognosis with the parents after assessing their existing knowledge. The family is taught about the possible complications and sequelae of meningitis and the importance of follow-up care.

Prophylaxis for the close contacts of the ill child with bacterial meningitis is necessary. Parents are asked to identify others exposed to meningitis and refer them for treatment. Close contacts must seek prompt medical attention because they may be incubating the infection.

> **? CRITICAL THINKING EXERCISE 28-1**
>
> Pediatric nurses in the community often are in a position to answer questions about childhood illnesses. Recently, parents of high school children received a notice from the school nurse that a male student had been diagnosed with meningococcal meningitis. Close contacts of the student had been identified and treated appropriately. The nurse recommended that parents of children not in close contact with the student should be watchful but not overly concerned. Her letter advised parents to watch their children for 2 weeks and call the physician at any sign of illness.
>
> 1. Is this course of action prudent?
> 2. If so, why? If not, why not?

The nurse educates the child, if the age is appropriate, and parents about prescribed medications and treatments and provides written instructions. Parents must provide a return demonstration of all procedures they will perform at home, allowing the nurse to determine if further education is needed. The nurse is aware that parents are often anxious about the child's illness and outcome so learning may be difficult. It is important to repeat information and allow time for practice in order to reinforce learning. Complications of meningitis can include hydrocephalus, vision and hearing loss, delayed growth and development, seizures, subdural effusions, and cranial nerve palsy. Vigilant assessment by the nurse and prompt notification of the physician can facilitate initiation of effective interventions if complications do occur. Early recognition and treatment of meningitis and its complications can substantially reduce morbidity and mortality rates.

■ Evaluation

- Can the parents demonstrate the ability to administer the child's treatments and medications?
- Do the parents discuss the disease and treatments?
- Have the parents referred close contacts for treatment?

GUILLAIN-BARRÉ SYNDROME

Guillain-Barré syndrome (GBS) is an autoimmune neurologic disorder of the peripheral nervous system characterized by rapidly progressing limb weakness and the loss of deep tendon reflexes. In rare cases, the motor and cranial nerves may also be affected. Symptoms result from acute demyelinization of the nerves. The illness may originate as an upper respiratory or gastrointestinal viral infection. Associated viruses include rubella, enterovirus, Epstein-Barr virus, cytomegalovirus (CMV), mycoplasma, and varicella. *Campylobacter jejuni* is the most commonly identified pathogen linked to Guillain-Barré. The syndrome may also occur as a toxic response to seasonal influenza vaccines.

Incidence

GBS is rare and affects approximately 1 person in 100,000 each year worldwide (NINDS, 2010a). It affects all ages, including infants. It occurs moderately more often in males.

Pathophysiology

The most prominent feature of GBS is the infiltration of lymphocytes in peripheral nerves and subsequent inflammation. Initially, the myelin sheath becomes edematous; as further inflammation takes place, segmental demyelinization occurs. This process takes place along the membrane surrounding the Schwann cells. As the inflammatory process continues, myelin loss increases and results in axonal degeneration.

Manifestations

- *Limb paresthesia and/or pain,* including numbness, tingling, and weakness of the lower extremities with an ascending loss of deep tendon reflexes leading to a flaccid paralysis.
- *Autonomic instability,* including blood pressure fluctuations, cardiac arrhythmias, postural hypotension, and urinary and bowel incontinence.
- *Cranial nerve dysfunction,* with facial nerve paralysis, dysphagia, and inadequate cough, gag, and swallow reflexes. If this occurs, respiratory function will be impaired.
- *Respiratory failure* resulting from the progressive motor paralysis of the intercostal and phrenic nerves. Respiratory failure may occur in 15% to 25% of children with GBS.
- *Neuromuscular impairment* (bilateral ascending weakness or paralysis) usually progresses upward from the feet to the head. (As healing takes place, neuromuscular function returns gradually in reverse order—head to feet.)

Diagnostic Evaluation

Bilateral ascending weakness or paralysis occurring 1 to 2 weeks after an upper respiratory infection or gastric illness is a diagnostic indication. The paralysis can affect the respiratory muscles quickly. The CSF may demonstrate high protein levels.

Therapeutic Management

Children with rapidly progressing paralysis are treated with high-dose IV immune globulin (IVIG) for several days. A recent study showed that some children may benefit from a second course of IVIG due to patient differences in pharmacokinetics (Kuitwaard, Bos-Eyssen, Blomkwist-Markens, & van Doorn, 2009). Medical management of the

Animation—Guillain-Barré Syndrome

child with GBS is supportive, with attention given to the neurologic, respiratory, and cardiovascular systems. Respiratory support is of critical importance because most deaths are attributed to respiratory failure. Plasmapheresis may be beneficial, as may steroids or immunosuppressive medications (Lee, Sung, & Rew, 2008).

NURSING CARE OF THE CHILD WITH GUILLAIN-BARRÉ SYNDROME

■ Assessment

A complete history and physical examination are important to determine the presence of an antecedent viral illness and establish baseline clinical status. Special emphasis is given to evaluating the respiratory and neurologic systems. Respiratory assessment should be done hourly or more frequently in some cases because of the risk of respiratory compromise and the need for prompt action, including intubation and ventilator support, if the child's respiratory status deteriorates. Major assessment parameters include respiratory rate, chest excursion, energy expended to breathe, and breath sounds. Pulse oximetry assesses the effectiveness of gas exchange. Daily pulmonary function testing may be ordered. A thorough neurologic assessment is generally performed every 1 to 2 hours, though this may be done more frequently depending on the child's clinical condition. Neurologic parameters to address include cranial nerve function, motor capabilities, sensory perception, and deep tendon reflexes.

■ Nursing Diagnosis and Planning

The following nursing diagnoses and expected outcomes may be appropriate after assessment of the child with GBS:

- Ineffective Breathing Pattern related to neuromuscular impairment.

Expected Outcome. The child will remain free from respiratory distress, as evidenced by clear bilateral breath sounds, good chest expansion, and normal tidal volume.

- Decreased Cardiac Output related to autonomic instability.

Expected Outcome. The child will maintain cardiac output, as evidenced by brisk capillary refill, normal urine output, good pulses in all extremities, and no arrhythmias.

- Risk for Impaired Skin Integrity related to immobility with paralysis.

Expected Outcome. The child will maintain skin integrity, as evidenced by absence of skin breakdown or pressure ulcers.

- Impaired Verbal Communication related to neuromuscular impairment.

Expected Outcome. The child will maintain the ability to communicate, as evidenced by demonstration of new ways to communicate with available muscles, such as eye blinks or eye movements.

- Impaired Urinary Elimination related to paralysis.

Expected Outcome. The child will have acceptable urinary elimination, as evidenced by an empty bladder, no urinary tract infection or distention of the abdomen, and urine output within normal limits for age (see Chapter 20).

- Anxiety related to increasing ascending paralysis.

Expected Outcome. The child will display decreased anxiety, as evidenced by an ability to interact calmly with parents and health care providers and have decreased fretful periods and increased restful periods.

- Deficient Knowledge related to unfamiliarity with disease progression, treatment, and home care.

Expected Outcome. The child and parents will have increased knowledge of the disease and treatment, as evidenced by an ability to make plans about discharge care and discuss the illness and possible complications.

- Interrupted Family Processes related to having a child with a prolonged illness.

Expected Outcome. The parents will use coping strategies to adjust to their child's illness, as evidenced by discussing support systems and changes in the family.

■ Interventions

The goals of nursing care for the child with GBS are to achieve optimal neurologic function with an emphasis on maintaining independence in activities of daily living and to facilitate a recovery without complications.

Treatment of GBS is largely supportive, with a focus on assessing and monitoring the child's clinical status and preventing or minimizing complications. The nurse must be able to recognize any change in the child's condition and intervene in a timely and effective manner.

The nurse must anticipate possible deterioration in the child's respiratory status because of progressive muscle weakness leading to flaccidity. Resuscitation and ventilatory support may be urgently needed; appropriate emergency equipment and personnel should be available. Equipment, such as a bag-valve-mask device, oxygen, suction, endotracheal tubes with stylets, and a laryngoscope with a variety of blades, should be at the bedside for immediate access. To prevent infection, chest physiotherapy should be performed every 2 to 4 hours.

Interruption in the autonomic nervous system reflexes can cause circulatory changes, resulting in arrhythmias, hypotension, dizziness, and night sweats. Early detection of neurologic changes is made by serial assessments, and prompt action should be taken to correct problems and prevent complications.

The child with GBS is at an increased risk for developing complications associated with immobility. Maintaining skin integrity is a priority. Turning, repositioning, passive range of motion, and monitoring pressure points are performed by the nurse at least every 2 hours. Use of special mattresses and managing incontinence will help prevent skin breakdown. To prevent contractures, daily physical and occupational therapy are included in the child's treatment plan. Range of motion, active exercises, correct alignment, and application of splints and braces are all part of the child's daily care.

The risk of pulmonary embolus as a result of deep vein thrombosis is always a threat. Frequent turning and repositioning, with special attention to positioning the child's legs to alleviate pressure on the dorsal aspect of the knees, are essential. Anticoagulant therapy may be initiated; if so, the nurse should monitor clotting times and watch for any signs of bleeding.

As cranial nerve function is altered and interference with gag and swallow occurs, nutrition becomes a vitally important issue. Adequate caloric intake is essential to prevent catabolism. Alternative methods of providing nutrition must be used. The physician may order nasogastric, nasojejunostomy, or gastrostomy feedings. The nurse monitors the type and amount of feeding, tube placement and patency, tolerance of feedings (residuals, abdominal distention, stools), and weight gain. Total parenteral nutrition is provided to the child during the acute phase of the illness or if alternative methods of nutritional support are not tolerated.

The progression of GBS is unpredictable, the loss of function is frightening, and the recovery time varies from months to years.

These factors can result in considerable anxiety for the child and family. The nurse provides educational and emotional support to the child and family, reassuring them that a full recovery from GBS is possible. It is essential to keep them well informed and answer their questions. The nurse encourages the child and family members to verbalize feelings concerning the illness and hospitalization, and then supports and validates these feelings. Referrals to other health care providers, child life therapists, and counselors are often indicated.

Facilitating the child's development during the illness by normalizing the situation as much as possible is a key nursing intervention. As the child's clinical condition worsens and dependency on the parents and health care providers increases, the child is offered choices and encouraged to make decisions whenever possible. Communication is maintained with the child's teacher, classmates, and friends, and involvement in school work is continued.

The nurse supports the role of the parents as the primary caregivers by facilitating parental participation in the child's care. This helps the parents support their child. If the child's clinical condition requires transfer to a critical care unit, the nurse ensures that the child and family are prepared and takes other actions to lessen the family's anxiety. Compassionate and competent health care team members can optimize the child's recovery.

■ Evaluation

- Does the child demonstrate normal respiratory function?
- Is the child able to communicate needs?
- Has the child's neurologic status returned to normal?
- Is the child's skin intact?
- Do the parents participate in and discuss the child's care?

NEUROLOGIC CONDITIONS REQUIRING CRITICAL CARE

A number of neurologic conditions, including encephalitis, Reye syndrome, botulism, and tetanus, require critical nursing care. Children with these conditions are frequently admitted to hospital critical care units where the care is specialized (Table 28-4).

HEADACHES

Headaches are a common disorder in children of all ages, and their prevalence has significantly increased in western countries and in Asia over the past 30 years. Up to 70% of children and adolescents complain of occasional headaches, with 20% of these children being affected by chronic tension and migraine headaches (Gerber, Petermann, Müller et al., 2010).

Etiology

The three primary sources of recurrent headache are vascular, tension (stress), and increased ICP. Vascular headaches include migraines and headaches that occur as a result of arteriovenous malformations. Tension headaches frequently are the result of stress. Contributing factors to increased ICP are space-occupying lesions and hydrocephalus. Other causes of headache include lead or carbon monoxide poisoning, caffeine or alcohol withdrawal, sinusitis, eye disease, malocclusion of the teeth, and other systemic diseases (Abend, Younkin, & Lewis, 2010).

Incidence

Migraine (vascular) headaches occur in approximately 5% of children and adolescents (National Headache Foundation, 2009). Migraines in preadolescents are equally prevalent in males and females, but for adolescents, the incidence greatly increases for females. A family history of headaches is noted in a majority of these cases, and the frequency of children's headaches may be predicted by how often the mother complains of headaches (Arruda, Guidetti, Galli et al., 2010). Other frequent causes of headaches in children include tension-type headaches and nonmigrainous headaches.

Manifestations
Migraine

Symptoms range from mild episodes, in which case the child may continue with daily activities, to episodes that force the child to go to a quiet, dark room for relief. An aura may occur before the headache begins. The aura may include seeing flashing lights; smelling specific odors; blurry, double, or lost vision; and tingling in the arms or legs. Once the headache begins, the most common symptoms include throbbing pain, often on both sides of the head, nausea and vomiting, irritability, abdominal pain, photophobia, and phonophobia. The pain of a typical migraine lasts from 1 hour to more than 24 hours.

Tension-Type Headaches

The pain associated with tension-type headaches is usually more generalized than that of a migraine. The child may describe the pain as a bandlike tightness or pressure, tight neck muscles, or soreness of the scalp. Nausea is rare, but fatigue and dizziness are common. These headaches may last for days or weeks but usually do not interfere with the child's regular activities.

Diagnostic Evaluation

The International Headache Society published revised clinical criteria for classifying and diagnosing headaches in 2004 (International Headache Classification, 2nd ed. [ICHD-2]). Clinical manifestations and diagnostic criteria are more precisely identified, allowing for the development of targeted treatment plans (International Headache Society, 2010). In addition to addressing the signs and symptoms of headache as described in the ICHD-2, the child's blood pressure is evaluated and head size is measured, looking for evidence of chronically increased ICP. A detailed neurologic examination should be performed, with special attention given to auscultating for a bruit in the head (suggesting an arteriovenous malformation), assessing mental status, and examining both optic disks for papilledema. CT or MRI may be performed in children with chronic headaches or those with abnormalities found on the neurologic examination. A thorough assessment also includes obtaining a medication history, since daily use of analgesics may cause rebound headaches (National Headache Foundation, 2009).

┃ NURSING CARE OF THE CHILD WITH HEADACHES

■ Assessment

A detailed history of the child's headache and preheadache events is important to determine precipitating factors (e.g., poor diet, poor hydration, food sensitivities, altered sleep patterns, flashing lights). A social history of the child and family may identify

TABLE 28-4 NEUROLOGIC CONDITIONS REQUIRING CRITICAL CARE

PATHOPHYSIOLOGY, ETIOLOGY, AND INCIDENCE	MANIFESTATIONS	THERAPEUTIC MANAGEMENT	NURSING CONSIDERATIONS
Encephalitis Inflammation caused by infection or toxin, resulting in cerebral edema and neurologic dysfunction. Numerous agents are causative, such as St. Louis encephalitis and West Nile virus. Peak incidence is in middle to late childhood.	Headache, irritability, lethargy, altered level of consciousness, nuchal rigidity, seizures, fever, malaise, dizziness, nausea and vomiting, ataxia, sensory disturbances.	Diagnosed by lumbar puncture and CSF culture; EEG alterations are not unusual. Care includes hospitalization and monitoring for increased ICP. Medication: cephalosporin or acyclovir (depending on causative agent), antiepileptics.	Care is similar to that for any child with increased ICP. Care includes fever management with antipyretics; pharmacologic and nonpharmacologic headache relief measures; maintenance of fluid and electrolyte balance; support for anxious family members; assistance to the family with management of any long-term neurologic deficits; and facilitation of grieving for the family of a child with a poor prognosis.
Reye Syndrome Exposure to viral agent or toxin in at risk children leads to liver cell damage with rising serum ammonia levels. The toxic serum ammonia levels result in cerebral dysfunction (encephalopathy, cerebral edema), fluid and electrolyte and acid-base imbalances, and coagulopathies. The average age at onset is 6-7 yr. Reye syndrome may be related to administration of aspirin to children with a viral disease.	Antecedent viral infection; malaise, nausea and vomiting, progressive neurologic deterioration. Elevated serum ammonia levels, liver dysfunction on biopsy, hypoglycemia, altered coagulation times, increased ICP with respiratory dysfunction. Reye syndrome is clinically staged from I (lethargy) to V (coma with flaccidity/extension posturing).	Care includes hospitalization for monitoring of neurologic status, increasing ICP, hydration and acid-base balance, and cardiorespiratory status.	Care is similar to that for any child with increasing ICP, with the potential addition of mechanical respiratory support. Accurate, continuous monitoring of neurologic and cardiorespiratory status is essential because the child's condition can deteriorate suddenly. Fluid replacement is achieved with IV hypertonic solutions if ICP is not increased. Protect the child from coagulopathy-related injury.
Botulism Food poisoning caused by *Clostridium botulinum* toxin. The source is honey (in infants) or improperly sterilized canned foods.	CNS symptoms 12-36 hr after ingestion include weakness, headache, double vision, vomiting, difficulty talking, respiratory paralysis, decreased deep tendon reflexes, impaired gag reflex.	Care is supportive and includes respiratory support and administering antitoxin. Recovery after treatment takes an average of 1 mo.	Advise parents not to give infants honey or syrup in their milk or water. Educate the public about proper food preparation techniques.
Tetanus (Lockjaw) Caused by endotoxin produced by the anaerobic, spore-forming, gram-positive bacillus *Clostridium tetani*. Entry sites include puncture wounds, burns, lacerations, and compound fractures. The incubation period is 3 days to 3 wk.	Painful muscular rigidity of masseter and neck muscles, facial spasms, dysphagia, laryngospasm, severe pain, respiratory arrest.	Care includes ventilatory and respiratory support. Medication: diazepam (Valium) or lorazepam (Ativan) for seizures; tetanus immune globulin.	Assess the child's ventilatory and neurologic status and provide respiratory support as needed. Provide fluids and electrolytes, seizure precautions, quiet environment. Educate the child and family about immunizations.

triggering stressors (e.g., divorce; move to a new school; loss of a family member, friend, or pet). The child should receive a comprehensive physical examination with emphasis on the neurologic system.

■ Nursing Diagnosis and Planning

Nursing diagnoses that may apply to a child with a headache and the child's family include those common to other neurologic disorders, such as the following:

- Acute Pain or Chronic Pain related to underlying contributing factors.

Expected Outcome. The child will have decreased pain related to headaches, as evidenced by an ability to identify triggering factors and demonstrate appropriate nonpharmacologic approaches.

- Deficient Knowledge related to unfamiliarity with the management of a child with headaches and the medication regimen.

Expected Outcome. The child and parents will discuss the plan for managing the child's headaches including a description of the medication regimen.

- Risk for Injury related to headache symptoms (change in vision, dizziness).

Expected Outcome. The child will have risk for injury reduced, as evidenced by parents verbalizing a safety plan for the child during a headache and when receiving medication for treatment of a headache.

■ Interventions

The nurse educates the child and family about factors that can trigger the onset of a headache (e.g., stress, food, menstruation, visual stimuli, fatigue, certain medications), and how to make lifestyle changes that will lower stress and avoid triggers. Keeping a diary of the child's headaches and preheadache events will help identify specific triggers.

For mild or infrequent migraines and tension headaches, common analgesics, such as ibuprofen or acetaminophen, may be effective. For more severe migraine in adolescents over 12 years of age, or those with persistent symptoms, recommended treatment is nasal sumatriptan (Walker & Teach, 2008). If children have two or more severe migraine headaches per month, they may need daily prophylactic medication; commonly amitriptyline and propranolol are used. Psychological evaluation followed by relaxation therapy, counseling, and biofeedback therapy may help some children.

The nursing care for a child with headaches is both acute and long term. Acute management includes placing the child in a dark, quiet environment and administering medication. Long-term management focuses on education about and elimination of trigger factors, stress relief measures, and medication administration.

■ Evaluation

- Can the child and parents describe the management of headache and the medication regimen?
- Do the child and parents understand the need for following a safety plan to prevent injury during headache and when receiving treatment with medication?
- Are the child and parents learning to eliminate headache trigger factors?
- Can the child demonstrate and benefit from relaxation therapy and biofeedback?

KEY CONCEPTS

- The CNS is composed of the brain and spinal cord. The bones of the skull do not become fused until 12 to 18 months of life. The brain and spinal cord are covered by a fibrous connective structure containing many blood vessels known as meninges.
- CSF surrounds the brain and spinal cord. The brain consists of the cerebrum, cerebellum, and brainstem.
- The peripheral nervous system consists of 12 pairs of cranial nerves and 31 pairs of spinal nerves. The autonomic nervous system consists of the sympathetic and parasympathetic systems.
- The physiologic process of autoregulation helps the body regulate blood flow. When autoregulation fails to change vascular diameter in response to changes in cerebral perfusion pressure, cerebrovascular dilation is impaired and cerebral blood flow decreases.
- Hypercapnia or hypoxia leads to cerebral dilation and increased ICP. Hypocapnia leads to cerebral arterial constriction and decreased ICP.
- An infant's brain is two thirds the size of an adult's brain. The brain grows to 80% of adult size by age 1 year.
- Head circumference can change in the infant and young child, but the head of the adolescent and adult is unyielding. This change has implications for head circumference measurement for growth and development in the infant and young child.
- The spinal cord, cranial nerves, and peripheral nerves become longer during childhood; the spinal cord terminates at L3 in the newborn and L1 to L2 in the adult.
- Myelinization of nerves begins in the 3rd month of gestation and is completed in adolescence, as demonstrated by progressive development and coordination.

- Neurologic changes may be more subtle in the infant or child than in the adult and may be indicated by irritability or poor feeding behaviors.
- The neurologic examination assesses level of consciousness, pupil size and reaction to light, cranial nerve function, motor and sensory functions, respiratory status and function, vital signs, and head circumference.
- Different seizure types are treated with specific antiepileptic medications to achieve optimal seizure control. These medications have many side effects. The CBC, liver enzyme levels, and medication levels should be determined routinely.
- When antiepileptics are given IV, the most common side effect is respiratory depression.
- Mannitol and furosemide (Lasix) are diuretics that are used to help decrease ICP. Their effect is monitored with serum electrolyte levels and serum osmolality.
- Cerebral edema is decreased by maintaining adequate oxygenation and perfusion of the brain, administering diuretics, elevating the head of the bed 30 to 45 degrees, keeping the child in good alignment so that venous drainage is not impaired, and reducing agitation and noxious stimuli.
- Abnormal posturing (decorticate or decerebrate) is an ominous neurologic sign.
- Hydrocephalus may be communicating or noncommunicating. Enlarged ventricles and increased ICP may result. If the cranial sutures are not ossified, the head circumference will be abnormally large.

KEY CONCEPTS—cont'd

- Teaching for the child with a neurologic deficit and the child's family is begun after the child's and family's needs have been assessed. The family's grieving may be verbalized; emotions and fears should be expressed and validated. The nurse reinforces information that has been supplied by other members of the health care team.
- The nurse encourages parents in their caregiving efforts when appropriate, assists the family in setting realistic goals for the

child, and identifies support systems and refers to community agencies.
- The nurse has family members demonstrate skills necessary for home care and encourages therapeutic play and peer contact. The nurse provides incentives for accomplishments and identifies the child's positive qualities and coping mechanisms.

REFERENCES

Abend, N., Younkin, D., & Lewis, D. (2010). Secondary headaches in children and adolescents. *Seminars in Pediatric Neurology, 17*(2), 123-133.

American Academy of Pediatrics. (2008). Febrile seizures: clinical practice guideline for the long-term management of the child with simple febrile seizures. *Pediatrics, 121*(6), 1281-1286.

Arruda, M., Guidetti, V., Galli, F., et al. (2010). Frequency of headaches in children is influenced by headache status in the mother. *Headache: The Journal of Head & Face Pain, 50*(6), 973-980.

Atabaki, S. M. (2007). Pediatric head injury. *Pediatrics in Review, 28*(6), 215-224.

Berg, A., & Scheffer, I. (2011). New concepts in classification of the epilepsies: Entering the 21st century. *Epilepsia, 52*(6), 1058-1062. Retrieved from www.ilae-epilepsy.org/Visitors/Centre/ctf/documents/NewConcepts-Classification_2011_000.pdf.

Berg, A., Berkovic, S., Brodie, M., et al. (2010). Revised terminology and concepts for organization of seizures and epilepsies: Report of the ILAE commission on classifications and terminology, 2005-2009. *Epilepsia, 51*(4), 676-685. Retrieved from www.ilae-epilepsy.org/Visitors/Centre//ctf/documents/ClassificationReport_2010_000.pdf.

Bhatia, R., Tahir, M., & Chandler, C. (2009). The management of hydrocephalus in children with posterior fossa tumors: The role of pre-resectional endoscopic third ventriculostomy. *Pediatric Neurosurgery, 45*(3), 186-191.

Bracken, M. B. (2009). Steroids for acute spinal cord injury: A review. *Cochrane Library 2009, 1*. Retrieved from http://info.onlinelibrary.wiley.com/userfiles/ccoch/file/CD001046.pdf.

Campagnolo, D. (2011). *Autonomic dysreflexia in spinal cord injury.* Retrieved from http://emedicine.medscape.com/article/322809-overview.

Centers for Disease Control and Prevention. (2010a). *Injury prevention and control: Traumatic brain injury.* Retrieved from www.cdc.gov/TraumaticBrainInjury/statistics.html#A.

Centers for Disease Control and Prevention. (2010b). *Meningococcal: Who needs to be vaccinated?* Retrieved from www.cdc.gov/vaccines/vpd-vac/mening/who-vaccinate.htm.

The Charlie Foundation. (2009). *Ketogenic diet.* Retrieved from www.charliefoundation.org/content/ketogenic-diet.

Cyberonics. (2010). *What are the potential side effects with VNS therapy?* Retrieved from http://us.cyberonics.com/en/vns-therapy-for-epilepsy/patients-and-families/basics/what-are-the-potential-side-effects-with-vns-therapy.

Danzer, E., Gerdes, M., Bebbington, M., et al. (2009). Lower extremity neuromotor function and short-term ambulatory potential following in utero myelomeningocele surgery. *Fetal Diagnosis & Therapy, 25*(1), 47-53. Retrieved from http://content.karger.com/ProdukteDB/produkte.asp?Aktion=ShowAbstract&ArtikelNr=197359&Ausgabe=243502&ProduktNr=224239.

Dawodu, S. T. (2008). *Spinal cord injury—definition, epidemiology, pathophysiology.* Retrieved from http://emedicine.medscape.com/article/322480-overview.

Dumont, T. M., Visioni, A. J., Rughani, A. I., et al. (2010). Inappropriate prehospital ventilation in severe traumatic brain injury increases in-hospital mortality. *Journal of Neurotrauma, 27*(7), 1233-1241. Retrieved from www.liebertonline.com/doi/abs/10.1089/neu.2009.1216.

Epilepsy Foundation of America. (2010a). *Causes.* Retrieved from www.epilepsyfoundation.org/answerplace/medical/seizures/causes.

Epilepsy Foundation of America. (2010b). *Febrile convulsions.* Retrieved from www.epilepsyfoundation.org/infants/febrileconvulsions.html.

Epilepsy Foundation of America. (2010c). *Infants and epilepsy.* Retrieved from www.epilepsyfoundation.org/answerplace/medical/infants/neonatalonset.html.

Fanconi, M., & Lips, U. (2010). Shaken baby syndrome in Switzerland: Results of a prospective follow-up study, 2002-2007. *European Journal of Pediatrics, 169*(8), 1023-1028. Retrieved from www.springerlink.com/content/p574204x54v2873k/fulltext.html.

Fichter, M., Dornseifer, U., Henke, J., et al. (2008). Fetal spina bifida repair—current trends and prospects of intrauterine neurosurgery. *Fetal Diagnosis & Therapy, 23*(4), 271-286. Retrieved from http://content.karger.com/ProdukteDB/produkte.asp?Aktion=ShowAbstract&ArtikelNr=123614&Ausgabe=236416&ProduktNr=224239.

Fukuda, S., Yokoi, K., Kitajima, K., et al. (2009). Influence of premature rupture of membrane on the cerebral blood flow in low-birth-weight infant after the delivery. *Brain and Development, 32*(8), 631-635. Retrieved from www.brainanddevelopment.com/article/S0387-7604(09)00285-X/abstract.

Gerber, W., Petermann, F., Müller, G., et al. (2010). MIPAS-family-evaluation of a new multi-modal behavioral training program for pediatric headaches: Clinical effects and the impact on quality of life. *Journal of Headache & Pain, 11*(3), 215-225.

Grill, M., & Ng, Y. (2010). Dramatic first words spoken in 2 children after vagus nerve stimulation. *Seminars in Pediatric Neurology, 17*(1), 54-57.

Halstead, M., & Walter, K. (2010). Sport-related concussion in children and adolescents. *Pediatrics, 126*(3), 597-615.

International Headache Society. (2010). *IHS classification: ICHD II.* Retrieved from http://ihs-classification.org/en/02_klassifikation.

Keenan, E. (2010). Spasticity management, part 3: Surgery and the use of intrathecal baclofen. *British Journal of Neuroscience Nursing, 6*(1), 12-18. Retrieved from www.internurse.com/cgi-bin/go.pl/library/abstract.html?uid=46053.

Kira, R., Ishizaki, Y., Torisu, H., et al. (2010). Genetic susceptibility to febrile seizures: Case-control association studies. *Brain & Development, 32*(1), 57-63. Retrieved from www.brainanddevelopment.com/article/S0387-7604(09)00261-7/abstract.

Kirkham, F. J., Newton, C., & Whitehouse, W. (2008). Paediatric coma scales. *Developmental Medicine & Child*

Neurology, 50(4), 267-274. Retrieved from http://onlinelibrary.wiley.com/doi/10.1111/j.1469-8749.2008.02042.x/full.

Kuitwaard, K., Bos-Eyssen, M., Blomkwist-Markens, P., & van Doorn, P. (2009). Recurrences, vaccinations and long-term symptoms in GBS and CIDP. *Journal of the Peripheral Nervous System, 14*(4), 310-315.

Kunisaki, S. M., & Jennings, R. W. (2008). Fetal surgery. *Journal of Intensive Care Medicine, 23*(1), 33-51. Retrieved from http://jic.sagepub.com/content/23/1/33.abstract.

Lee, J., Sung, I., & Rew, I. (2008). Clinical presentation and prognosis of childhood Guillain-Barré syndrome. *Journal of Paediatrics & Child Health, 44*(7-8), 449-454.

Lee, J., Sung, I., Kang, J., & Park, S. (2009). Characteristics of pediatric-onset spinal cord injury. *Pediatrics International, 51*(2), 254-257. Retrieved from http://onlinelibrary.wiley.com/doi/10.1111/j.1442-200X.2008.02684.x/abstract.

Marsal, K. (2009). One year survival and extremely preterm infants after active perinatal care in Sweden. *Journal of the American Medical Association, 301*(21), 2225-2233.

Matschke, J., Voss, J., Obi, N., et al. (2009). Nonaccidental head injury is the most common cause of subdural bleeding in infants <1 year of age. *Pediatrics, 124*(6), 1587-1594. Retrieved from http://pediatrics.aappublications.org/cgi/content/abstract/124/6/1587.

May, K. (2009). The pathophysiology and causes of raised intracranial pressure. *British Journal of Nursing, 18*(15), 911-914.

National Headache Foundation. (2009). *Children and headaches.* Retrieved from www.headaches.org/blog/?p=65.

National Institute of Neurological Disorders and Stroke. (2010a). *Guillain-Barré syndrome fact sheet.* Retrieved from www.ninds.nih.gov/disorders/gbs/detail_gbs.htm.

National Institute of Neurological Disorders and Stroke. (2010b). *Hydrocephalus fact sheet.* Retrieved from www.ninds.nih.gov/disorders/hydrocephalus/detail_hydrocephalus.htm.

National Institute of Neurological Disorders and Stroke. (2011). *Spinal cord injury: Hope through research.* Retrieved from www.ninds.nih.gov/disorders/sci/detail_sci.htm.

Neumann, J. O., Chambers, I. R., Citerio, G., et al. (2008). The use of hyperventilation therapy after traumatic brain injury in Europe: an analysis of the BrainIT database. *Intensive Care Medicine, 34*(9), 1676-1682. Retrieved from https://springerlink3.metapress.com/content/v81rjq5p55n00327/resource-secured/?target=fulltext.html&sid=mypppaqvod3gme454bh3byzw&sh=www.springerlink.com.

Nudelman, Y., & Tunkel, A. (2009). Bacterial meningitis: Epidemiology, pathogenesis and management update. *Drugs, 69*(18), 2577-2596.

Ogiwara, H., Dipatri, A., Alden, T., et al. (2010). Endoscopic third ventriculostomy for obstructive hydrocephalus in children younger than 6 months of age. *Child's Nervous System, 26*(3), 343-347.

O'Shea, T. M. (2008). Diagnosis, treatment, and prevention of cerebral palsy. *Clinical Obstetrics & Gynecology, 51*(4), 816-828. Retrieved from http://journals.lww.com/clinicalobgyn/toc/2008/12000.

Ploumis, A., Yadlapalli, N., Fehlings, M., et al. (2010). A systematic review of the evidence supporting a role for vasopressor support in acute SCI. *Spinal Cord, 48*(5), 356-362.

Rosenbaum, P. L., Palisano, R. J., Bartlett, D. J., et al. (2008). Development of the gross motor classification system for cerebral palsy. *Developmental Medicine and Child Neurology, 50*(4), 249-253.

Shankaran, S. (2008). Prevention, diagnosis, and treatment of cerebral palsy in near-term and term infants. *Clinical Obstetrics & Gynecology, 51*(4), 829-839. Retrieved from http://journals.lww.com/clinicalobgyn/toc/2008/12000.

Sidram, V., Tripathy, P., Ghorai, M., & Ghosh, S.N. (2009). Spinal cord injury without radiographic abnormality (SCIWORA) in children: A Kolkata experience. *Indian Journal of Neurotrauma, 6*(2), 133-136.

Spina Bifida Association. (2009a). *Latex (natural rubber) allergy in spina bifida fact sheet.* Retrieved from www.spinabifidaassocation.org/site/c.liKWL7PLLrF/b.2642343/k.8D2D/Fact_Sheets.htm.

Spina Bifida Association. (2009b). *Precocious puberty in children who have spina bifida with hydrocephalus.* Retrieved from www.spinabifidaassociation.org/site/c.liKWL7PLLrF/b.2664425/apps/s/content.asp?ct=3822593.

Straub, K., & Obrzut, J. E. (2009). Effects of cerebral palsy on neuropsychological function. *Journal of Developmental and Physical Disability, 21*(2), 153-167. Retrieved from www.springerlink.com/content/y17473n16t397602.

Swaminathan, A., Levy, P., & Legome, E. (2009). Evaluation and management of moderate to severe pediatric head trauma. *Journal of Emergency Medicine, 37*(1), 63-68. Retrieved from www.jem-journal.com/article/S0736-4679(09)00089-4/abstract.

Tang, M. E., & Lobel, D. A. (2009). Severe traumatic brain injury: Maximizing outcomes. *Mount Sinai Journal of Medicine, 76*(2), 119-128.

Walker, D., & Teach, S. (2008). Emergency department treatment of primary headaches in children and adolescents. *Current Opinion in Pediatrics, 20*(3), 248-254.

Walker, J. (2009). Spinal cord injuries: Acute care management and rehabilitation. *Nursing Standard, 23*(42), 47-56.

Ward, A., Hayden, S., Dexter, M., & Scheinberg, A. (2009). Continuous intrathecal baclofen for children with spasticity and/or dystonia: Goal attainment and complications associated with treatment. *Journal of Paediatrics & Child Health, 45*(12), 720-726. Retrieved from http://onlinelibrary.wiley.com/doi/10.1111/j.1440-1754.2009.01601.x/abstract.

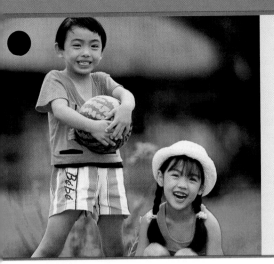

Psychosocial Problems in Children and Families

evolve WEBSITE

http://evolve.elsevier.com/James/ncoc

LEARNING OBJECTIVES

After studying this chapter, you should be able to:
- Identify risk factors for emotional and behavioral disorders that emerge in childhood and during adolescence.
- Recognize symptoms, behaviors, and characteristics for emotional and behavioral disorders.
- Identify the individual and familial factors and behaviors that correlate to childhood depression, suicide, or suicide attempts.
- Develop a nursing care plan for a child at risk for suicide and the child's family, as well as for the support of a family with a child who has committed suicide.
- Discuss the incidence, risk factors, symptoms, and nursing interventions for children with eating disorders and their families and describe their nursing care.

- Identify the primary symptoms and manifestations of children with attention deficit–hyperactivity disorder and describe their nursing care.
- Identify signs and symptoms of substance abuse disorders and develop a nursing care plan.
- Describe the major types of abuse and neglect seen in children, their contributing factors, and nursing care for abused children and their families.

CLINICAL REFERENCE

OVERVIEW OF PSYCHOSOCIAL DISORDERS OF CHILDHOOD

Psychosocial or mental illness refers to disorders that affect personal and social functioning or cause acute distress. Psychosocial disorders are disturbances in mood, emotion, cognition, or behavior. In order to be considered disorders, these disturbances must be of sufficient intensity and duration to disrupt or impair the ability to engage in developmental life tasks and to impair social and emotional functioning. In this sense, the concept of "mental health" is partially culturally defined; it includes the ability to engage in activities of daily living, to manage normal levels of stress, and to have meaningful interpersonal relationships. Disorders that impair mental health are characterized by disruption or alteration in thinking, mood, or behavior.

Mental health and mental illness are not mutually exclusive states, but rather a continuum. Mental health disorders may result from biologic, neurologic, cultural, societal, or psychological causes. Disorders may be triggered by trauma or stressful events. A child without underlying mental illness may experience life events that trigger mental health disruptions, and these may require treatment. Likewise, a child who has a mental illness may exhibit areas of psychological dysfunction, while at the same time showing areas of good or outstanding functioning.

Psychosocial disorders disrupt normal functioning for the affected child and the family. Children may lose interest in play and school activities, and relationships with family and friends are usually impaired. Children may exhibit learning deficits related to behavior in school or inability to concentrate on learning. Some disorders manifest through somatic complaints, such as recurrent abdominal pain, or headaches with no physical cause. Recurrent thoughts of death or suicide are sometimes reported. Hospitalization may be required. All of these occurrences have a powerful impact on parents, siblings, friends, and the child's school environment.

The first section of this chapter provides an overview of the emotional and behavioral disorders that may emerge during childhood and adolescence. It also discusses issues pertaining to suicide, because these emotional and behavioral disorders present a risk for the emergence of suicidal impulses or thoughts. The second section of this chapter surveys substance abuse and eating disorders. Finally, nursing care related to the child and family in which child abuse or neglect is occurring is described.

PSYCHOSOCIAL DISORDERS TYPICALLY MANIFESTED IN CHILDHOOD

- *Mood disorders:* Depression, dysthymia, adjustment disorder, bipolar disorder
- *Anxiety disorders:* Social anxiety disorder, separation anxiety disorder, posttraumatic stress disorder, phobias, obsessive-compulsive disorder
- *Attention deficit–hyperactivity disorder*
- *Eating disorders:* Anorexia nervosa, bulimia nervosa

Data from American Psychiatric Association. (2000). *Diagnostic and statistical manual of mental disorders* (4th ed., Text revision). Washington, DC: Author.

Precipitating Factors

Neuroscientists have identified complex interactions among inherited predispositions, emotional and behavioral factors, life stressors, and environmental events (Weissman, Wickramaratne, Nomura et al., 2006). Emotional and behavioral disorders may be manifested as disturbances in feeling (e.g., depression, anxiety), in body function (e.g., constipation, encopresis, enuresis), in somatic symptoms (e.g., headaches, stomachaches), in behavior (e.g., conduct disturbance, school avoidance, passive-aggressive behaviors), or in performance (concentration problems, test-taking difficulties). The manner in which a child responds to stress depends on multiple factors within these interactions (American Academy of Child and Adolescent Psychiatry [AACAP], 2007b).

Factors that influence the development of psychosocial disorders include genetic predisposition, age, developmental level, temperament, parental mental health, coping and adaptive abilities within the family, precipitating traumatic experiences, duration of stressors in the environment, stability and support within the family, and social supports outside the immediate family. Exposures to trauma, and posttraumatic stress disorder (PTSD), have been correlated to the development of anxiety and mood disorders (U.S. Department of Veterans Affairs, 2010).

Diagnostic Evaluation

When a child presents with symptoms that may be indicative of a psychosocial disorder, the nurse, as part of a multispecialty team, will gather information about physical condition, developmental level, cognitive ability and specific symptoms. In addition to the overall assessment, a structured mental status examination of the child is usually indicated. Laboratory and diagnostic tests may also help provide some insight into differential diagnosis and determine whether pharmacologic and psychological interventions are likely to be effective.

Accurate diagnosis is complicated by the fact that wide ranges of emotional, cognitive and social ability are normal because the brain develops at a different pace for each child. This means that emotional and behavioral responses can be inconsistent and unpredictable. For this reason, the nurse needs to attend to the environment where the child will be interviewed. The nurse should plan time to establish a relationship as a caregiver and to establish a level of trust and comfort. Repeated assessments in a variety of situations and across time will provide the most accurate sense of what is "normal" for an individual child.

Screening questionnaires and assessment tools are increasingly used as part of a developmental and psychosocial evaluation, and some have demonstrated reliability with children. A frequently used test that has demonstrated reliability is the Child Behavior Checklist (CBCL), which is given to parents to complete. This test assesses a variety of emotional and behavioral problems (Beers, 2010). In addition, a structured mental status examination conducted by a skilled child interviewer will provide important information for planning nursing care.

MENTAL STATUS EXAMINATION OF CHILDREN

- *Appearance:* This includes noting appropriateness of dress and grooming; ability to engage in greeting behaviors, eye contact, dress, gestures, posture, tics, other repetitive movements; physical presentation, such as age, stature, race, age-appropriate behaviors
- *Speech:* Fluency, tone, volume, vocabulary, age appropriateness, ability to articulate feelings
- Ability to sit and talk, attend to the interview or to tasks
- *Mood or affect:* Predominant feelings, mood fluctuations, congruence between observed mood and verbalization of mood state
- *Manner of relating to the examiner:* Exploration of the child's understanding of the purpose of the interview, approach or avoidance behaviors, use of play materials available, verbalizations
- *Intellectual skills:* Problem-solving abilities, conceptualization of causality, body image, memory, judgment, general fund of knowledge, insight (findings are compared with developmental norms)
- Capacity for imaginative thinking and play, ability to interact during play
- *Sensory and motor development:* Fine and gross motor skills, symmetry and coordination of movement, hand and eye dominance, right-left discrimination
- *Perceptions and thought content:* Presence or absence of suicidal-homicidal ideation, intent, plan; delusions or illusions; hallucinations

Recent research conducted and reported by the Institute of Medicine (2009) promotes a shift in the approach to childhood mental health issues from identification and treatment to an overall mental health promotion and illness preventive approach. Although this chapter is organized according to mental, emotional, and behavioral disorders, nurses need to think about facilitating preventive measures and mental health promotion for all children beginning in infancy.

The Future of Mental Health Care for Children: Focus on Prevention

Level I

In 2009 the Institute of Medicine (IOM), with the National Research Council, issued a consensus report that strongly called for health care providers and clinicians to address primary prevention approaches in regard to mental health disorders in children.* The report recognizes that half of all mental, emotional, and behavioral (MEB) disorders are recognizable by age 14, and three quarters are evident by age 24 (p. 15). The report suggests that a prevention focus requires a shift to implementing mental health promotion and illness prevention strategies before the onset of illness, and before the child shows signs or symptoms. Identification of populations at risk, early recognition of emerging signs (thought to occur up to 2 years before diagnosis), and interventions with families as well as children have the potential to decrease severity of illness.

The IOM report (2009) is a Level 1 systematic review that not only looked at randomized controlled trials and other evidence-based literature, but also solicited evidence from experts in the care of children with MEB problems. Levels of prevention for the mental health of all children are defined in this report to include the following:

1. *Mental health promotion:* Population-based interventions designed to enhance children's interactive competencies and self-esteem with the goal of achieving appropriate developmental milestones
2. *Universal prevention:* Interventions, such as school-based programs about mental health issues, that are available to all children
3. *Selective prevention:* Interventions targeted to children at risk (e.g., those with dysfunctional family situations, or family history of mental health problems)
4. *Indicated prevention:* Strategies that address issues with children who are beginning to exhibit signs of concern

Interventions for the prevention of mental, emotional, and behavioral disorders include such approaches as parenting programs for parents of young children, prevention of depression, and the use of psychoeducation, cognitive-behavioral strategies, and family or community-based interventions (IOM, 2009).

This report has enormous implications for the role of the professional nurse. As a nurse, think about specific strategies you could implement that will recognize and encourage the developmental competencies of children, support the mental health and parenting abilities of parents, promote prevention and health promotion in schools, and advocate for social justice in protecting populations from poverty and violence.

Data from Institute of Medicine. (2009). *Preventing mental, emotional, and behavioral disorders among young people: Progress and possibilities.* Retrieved from www.iom.edu.
*National Research Council and Institute of Medicine. (2009). Preventing mental, emotional, and behavioral disorders among young people: Progress and possibilities. In E. O. Connell, T. Boat, & K. Warner (Eds.), *Board on Children, Youth, and Families, Division of Behavioral and Social Sciences and Education.* Washington, DC: National Academies Press.

EMOTIONAL DISORDERS

Nurses caring for children frequently encounter moods or behaviors that compromise a child's ability to function at appropriate developmental levels and successfully establish interpersonal relationships. Research consistently shows that most psychosocial disorders are caused by a combination of predisposing or inherent factors and environmental factors that trigger symptoms.

Psychosocial disorders often occur in children who have a familial or genetic predisposition toward the disease. This predisposition may become apparent if physical or emotional stressors create a vulnerability for manifestation of the disorder. In addition to genetic and familial traits, contributors to a psychosocial disorder include physical problems, such as head injuries, sleep disorders, birth defects, physical injuries, and chronic illness. Environmental stressors, such as inconsistent or contradictory child-rearing practices, marital conflict, neglect, or traumatic events may also precipitate the development of a psychosocial disorder. Some cognitive, emotional, and behavioral manifestations are associated with genetic syndromes, such as fragile X syndrome. Other disorders, such as fetal alcohol syndrome (FAS), are associated with prenatal or infancy deficiencies or substance abuse by pregnant women (O'Donnell, Nassar, Leonard et al., 2009). Still other disorders are related primarily to an inaccurate or inappropriate relationship between the child and significant others in the social environment.

Psychosocial disorders, for many years, have been generally classified into two broad categories: emotional disorders and behavioral disorders. Emotional disorders are characterized by fear, sadness, depression, worry, and somatic complaints. The emotional disorders in the discussion that follows include anxiety, mood, and posttraumatic stress disorders. Behavioral disorders refer to problems with attention and behavior, such as attention deficit–hyperactivity disorder, and are discussed later in this chapter.

Anxiety Disorders

Anxiety is a normal human emotion, the body's adaptive response to change or challenges. Anxiety can be expected during times of transition or times of achieving developmental milestones. Most people can identify anxiety as an uncomfortable feeling of worry, dread, fear, or apprehension that occurs in response to external or internal stimuli. Symptoms and displays of anxiety are expected and normal in children at specific times in development. For example, infants and children up to preschool age often show intense distress at times of separation from their parents or family members (see Chapter 12). In addition, it is common for young children to have short-lived fears related to darkness, storms, animals, and imaginary situations (see Chapters 6 and 7).

Anxiety is generally considered to occur in two subtypes: state and trait. *State* anxiety refers to transitory feelings of apprehension, tension, or worry. These feelings vary in intensity and often have an identifiable event contributing to them, and the anxiety fluctuates over time. *Trait* anxiety describes a condition of anxiety that is prevalent, stable over time, and less likely to be associated with a specific triggering event.

Predispositions to anxiety result from a confluence of genetic factors, petrochemical and hormonal imbalances, parental patterns of coping with stress, and societal influences (AACAP, 2007a). The amygdala has a central role in the physical response to stress and fear, and some disorders may relate to amygdala activity (Stein & Stein, 2008).

Nurses caring for children often must differentiate normal or expected anxiety from the chronic conditions of anxiety, which should be treated. The identification, treatment, and management of an anxiety disorder can have a positive impact on children's enjoyment of their lives, their social and educational success, and their adjustment to adult life.

Exposures to trauma and PTSD have been linked to the development of anxiety disorders (U.S. Department of Veterans Affairs, 2010). Differentiation of normal anxiety from anxiety disorders is made when worry and distress become overwhelming or interfere with the child's ability to attend to tasks of daily functioning such as work, school, or home life. Symptoms such as muscle tension, increased respiratory rates, headaches, heightened startle reflex, tremors, and increased perspiration can be identified during the history and physical examination. Although school-age children typically express anxiety or fear of body harm or potentially real worries (e.g., thunder, lightning), adolescents may exhibit anxiety regarding social situations and acceptance (see Chapter 8).

Social Anxiety Disorder

Social anxiety disorder (social phobia) is the most common of the anxiety disorders and usually shows its first symptoms in childhood or early adolescence. It is also a disorder that, untreated, has wide-reaching effects on the child's ability to make friends, successfully transition to school, play sports, be part of a peer group during adolescence, and make the transitions to dating and to college. Research on adult populations has correlated the diagnosis with lower educational level, increased workplace difficulties, and difficulty engaging in intimate relationships such as marriage. Some research indicates that anxiety disorders may create social isolation that precedes depression and predisposes to substance abuse (Stein & Stein, 2008).

Social anxiety disorder generally responds well to treatment, and several different treatment approaches have been shown to be effective. Symptoms of social anxiety may be generalized or may be focused on specific triggers. Generalized social anxiety disorder is characterized by fearfulness or discomfort in many social situations. Nongeneralized social disorder (also called performance anxiety) is characterized by severe anxiety about discrete situations or tasks, such as public speaking and socializing at parties, that people without social anxiety disorder can manage (Stein & Stein, 2008).

Social anxiety can be misinterpreted as shyness. The child may seem aloof from groups of children, or uninvolved in social situations. Children may avoid social or performance situations to such a degree that their daily routine is affected (e.g., by refusing to participate in physical education exercises or by failing to raise their hands to ask a question in class). Social phobia can result in social isolation for the child who has difficulty establishing and maintaining peer relationships.

Separation Anxiety

The essential hallmark of separation anxiety is disabling anxiety about being apart from one's parents or another significant person to whom the child is attached, or anxiety about being away from home. It may develop spontaneously or under stress (e.g., in temporary relation to a move or a death in the family) and may last for several years, with symptoms developing and remitting in a cyclical pattern. Children with separation anxiety frequently fear that if they are apart from their parents, harm will come to the parent or themselves. Separation anxiety occurs in approximately 4% to 5% of children and young adults (Rosenberg, Vandana, & Chiriboga, 2011). Separation anxiety disorders in childhood are associated with increased risk for the subsequent development of panic disorders and depression (Rosenberg et al., 2011).

School refusal is related to separation anxiety disorder (AACAP, 2007a) and may also be related to a social anxiety disorder. Persistent reluctance or refusal to go to school or elsewhere may be the primary reason families seek intervention for separation anxiety disorder. Unlike truants, who are relatively fearless and avoid school to pursue other interests, children with separation anxiety stay home or attempt to remain with their parents. The child may complain of physical symptoms, cry, bargain, plead, or even exhibit panic symptoms as school time approaches. Symptoms resolve quickly if the child is allowed to stay home, but will reappear the next morning. Sometimes the child may simply refuse to leave the home. Consideration of this diagnosis should rule out precipitating factors such as fear of bullying, fatigue, boredom, learning challenges, upsetting incidents that occur in the school setting, or upsets that are occurring in the home.

Panic Disorder

Panic disorder (panic attacks) is distinguished from other anxiety disorders by the rapid onset of physical, cognitive, and emotional symptoms. The child's ability to cope may be quickly overwhelmed by the marked discomfort that includes physical symptoms such as cardiovascular (palpitations, chest pain) and respiratory (shortness of breath) distress, and psychological symptoms characterized by a strong feeling of impending doom or fear that the child is dying (Rosenberg et al., 2011).

Before considering panic disorder, organic causes should be ruled out. These include hyperthyroidism, hyperglycemia, temporal lobe epilepsy, and extreme caffeine intake, as well as other disorders. However, the presence of mitral valve prolapse does not exclude the diagnosis of panic disorder (Kaplan & Sadock, 2007) and both should be noted. The diagnosis of panic disorder is more frequently seen in adolescents than in children (Queen, 2010).

Posttraumatic Stress Disorder

PTSD is a disabling psychosocial disorder that follows a traumatic or overwhelming experience. Population studies estimate that exposure to at least one traumatic event is experienced by 14% to 43% of children and adolescents (U.S. Department of Veterans Affairs, 2010). The development of PTSD is correlated to severity of trauma, proximity, repeated experience of trauma, and social supports. PTSD affects approximately 6% of children younger than 18 years but less than 1% of preschoolers (U.S. Department of Veterans Affairs, 2010). A number of studies have linked the development of PTSD to sexual or physical abuse (Cutajar, Mullen, Ogloff et al., 2010), but PTSD also occurs as a sequel to other traumatic events, such as experience of a natural disaster, life-threatening accidents, loss of a parent, or severe injury.

PTSD is characterized by three main clusters of symptoms: intrusive symptoms, arousal symptoms, and avoidance symptoms (Cutajar et al., 2010). Intrusive symptoms include nightmares, flashbacks (terrifying memories), and a feeling of depersonalization. Arousal symptoms include trouble sleeping, agitation, exaggerated startle response, or regressive behavior. Avoidance symptoms are characterized by avoidance of people, places, or triggers that remind the child of the perpetuating traumatic event. Other symptoms of PTSD include intense fear, helplessness, or horror, along with physiologic symptoms of increased arousal. For example, the child may demonstrate determined avoidance of stimuli associated with the traumatic event but may have persistent nightmares or flashbacks. Children may reenact the event during play. Adolescents may exhibit antisocial or aggressive behaviors and may be at risk for using substances that they perceive will alleviate their feelings of distress (U.S. Department of Veterans Affairs, 2010). PTSD interferes with the child's developing brain and ability to concentrate, may contribute to sleep problems, and may cause the child to be hypervigilant or agitated.

Obsessive-Compulsive Disorder

Affecting approximately 1% of children (Massachusetts General Hospital, School Psychiatry Program, 2010), obsessive-compulsive disorder (OCD) manifests as repetitive unwanted thoughts (obsessions) or ritualistic actions (compulsions), or both. Obsessions are recurrent intrusive thoughts, feelings, and ideas. Compulsions are behaviors or actions that are repetitive and recurrent. Compulsions are designed to relieve the anxiety that the child usually realizes is irrational. Because young children cannot adequately describe their uncomfortable thoughts or concerns, severe temper tantrums, particularly when a ritual has been interrupted, may be the predominant symptom (Massachusetts General Hospital, School Psychiatry Program, 2010).

Children often go through transient stages of obsessive thinking or compulsive behavior, usually at times of anxiety or stress, and these transient symptoms do not warrant the diagnosis. This is usually manifested by the need to count, or to check and recheck locks on doors.

OCD is considered when obsessions and compulsions are intractable, disturbing to the child, and interfere with activities and relationships. Several studies link OCD to depressive disorders, with the prefrontal cortex, the basal ganglia, and the limbic system as areas that are affected (Kaplan & Saddock, 2007).

Pediatric autoimmune neuropsychological disorders (PANDAS) refer to the abrupt onset of OCD symptoms or tic disorder symptoms (see Chapter 30) following a group A beta-hemolytic streptococcal infection. Research suggests that the disease is not caused by the bacteria, but rather by the antibodies that respond to the infection (Schrag, Gilbert, Giovannoni et al., 2009). Some researchers speculate that PANDAS may be an element in subsequent development of other psychosocial disorders (Kerbeshian, Burd, & Tait, 2007).

Although the relationship between streptococcal infection and OCD has been described in several studies, recent evidence varies as to the strength of the relationship and what factors contribute to the development of the disorder following exposure to strep (Shulman, 2009).

Mood Disorders

Mood disorders are characterized by lowering of mood, or cycling between low mood and mania. Mood disorders are classified on the basis of severity of symptoms, the course of the illness, and the presence or absence of mania. The mood disorders include major depressive disorder (MDD), dysthymic disorder (DD), bipolar disorder, and adjustment disorder.

Major Depressive Disorder and Dysthymic Disorder

Major depressive disorder (MDD) and dysthymic disorder (DD) are diagnoses that have become increasingly prevalent in the adolescent age-group. Recent estimates for both disorders combined indicate a prevalence rate of 14% of 13- to 18-year-olds. Among that age-group, severe depression is estimated to have a prevalence of 4.7% (Merikangas, He, Burstein et al., 2010). The prevalence rate of depression among girls shows nearly three times the rate of depression in boys. In addition, the depression rates appear to increase with age; approximately 4% of children younger than 13 years are considered to be depressed, with a rate increase of 11.6% among 16-year-olds (Merikangas et al., 2010).

There appear to be numerous possible contributors to depression. These include genetic predisposition, familial situation, life events, physical or psychological trauma, or head injury components. In young children, depression may be related to abuse or neglect or other situational triggers. An episode of MDD increases the risk for subsequent episodes. Depression often manifests as a co-morbidity with substance abuse, so children who report depression should be assessed for substance abuse as well. The distinction between MDD and DD is based on the level of depression and the impact on the adolescent's functioning.

DD is considered to be a chronic lowered level of mood that is persistent. Children or adolescents who exhibit a less severe but depressed or irritable mood for at least 1 year meet the criteria for DD. Children with DD are generally able to continue overall functioning, but energy and motivation may be low (National Institute of Mental Health [NIMH], 2010d).

By contrast, MDD is a debilitating and severe depression, creating significant risk factors. Clinical signs and indicators include angry outbursts, irritability, loss of interest and enjoyment in usual activities, decreased energy, altered appetite, altered sleep patterns, decreased self-esteem, disengagement from family and friends, and thoughts of suicide. If the clinical presentation lasts at least 2 weeks (or longer), the child meets the criteria for MDD. Children and adolescents who are diagnosed with MDD should be carefully assessed for risk of self-harm, suicide, or aggression toward others.

Adjustment Disorder

Adjustment disorders are maladaptive reactions to identifiable traumas or stressors. The *Diagnostic and Statistical Manual of Mental Disorders* (4th ed., Text revision) (DSM-IV-TR) (American Psychiatric Association [APA], 2000) sets two conditions that are considered to be essential for the consideration of the diagnosis: The response to the stress or trauma must be "abnormal" (that is, beyond the level of stress that most children would display), and in addition, the child must experience significant impairment in social and developmental functioning (APA, 2000). In the case of adjustment disorders, the stressors act as precipitating events.

Adjustment disorders are characterized by less severe mood disturbance, fewer overall symptoms, and a self-limiting course (generally 3 months or less). Manifestations of adjustment disorder include depression, anxiety, mixed depression and anxiety, and disturbance of conduct.

The incidence of adjustment disorders is difficult to estimate, because other diagnoses are frequently co-morbid. Caretakers should be alert for signs of social isolation, withdrawal from socialization or affection, and suicidal thinking. Early identification, support, and intervention can be a powerful resource in minimizing the length and severity of mood disruption.

Bipolar Disorder

Onset for bipolar disorder occurs most often in late adolescence or early adulthood (NIMH, 2010b). Bipolar disorder is characterized by chronic, fluctuating, and extreme mood disturbances. Depression and lowered mood alternate with episodes of elation, irritability, anger, and aggression. The child or adolescent experiencing a manic mood state may be overly elated, grandiose, easily distracted, irritable, and aggressive, and may also demonstrate increased risk-taking behavior, talk rapidly, and not be able to sleep (NIMH, 2010b). Impaired social relationships are common.

When these mood fluctuations have been present for 1 year and are not related to a physical or developmental condition, bipolar mood disorder may be diagnosed. However, normal mood swings that accompany some developmental stages, particularly early adolescence, may confound the ability to make an accurate diagnosis. Recent findings indicate that most children with rapidly shifting moods are experiencing normal developmental or personality states. This means that the diagnosis of bipolar disorder has been incorrectly assigned to children who are "difficult" (Findling, Youngstrom, Fristad et al., 2010).

In young children, bipolar disorder most often manifests in a rapid cycling form, with swiftly changing and extreme mood swings (NIMH, 2010a). Other signs include irritability, anger, aggressive behavior, rapid speech, sleep disturbances, psychosomatic complaints, sadness, decreased energy, and suicidal ideation (NIMH, 2010a). Bipolar mood disorders affect approximately 1% to 5% of adolescents (NIMH, 2010b).

Parents of children who have bipolar disorder are more likely to have bipolar disorder themselves. A recent National Institutes of Mental Health study (NIMH, 2010b) found that 33% of such parents had the disorder.

Etiology and Physiology of Emotional Disorders

The contributing factors to emotional disorders include biologic, environmental, and traumatic.

Biologic Factors

Research supports the view that emotional disorders have biologic components that affect both brain structure and function; it is also possible that some overwhelming events may interrupt brain development (Kerbeshian et al., 2007). Biologic factors that contribute to mental disorders include genetic determinants, genetic predispositions (risk factors), traumatic brain injury, and disease states that affect brain function (Fay, Yeates, Drotar et al., 2009). Other factors can influence behavior by affecting a child's physiologic processes. Stress perception, such as posttraumatic stress disorder, and certain mood disorders, such as depression, are associated with increased cortisol levels over time, with emerging evidence that these increased cortisol levels may contribute to alteration in structural brain development (Fay et al., 2009).

One focus of exploration in the etiology of emotional disorders relates to the role of neurotransmitters. Neurotransmitters are chemical molecules that facilitate communication among neurons. Neurotransmitters conduct electrical impulses across nerve synapses. Normally, these neurotransmitters are synthesized in a presynaptic nerve, are released into the synaptic space, and bind to receptors in the postsynaptic nerve, where they excite, inhibit, or modify nerve action. The neurotransmitters are then released again by the postsynaptic nerve back into the synaptic space, where they are either destroyed or taken back into the presynaptic nerve for future use (reuptake) (Takashi, 2010). A deficit in some neurotransmitters in the synaptic space, particularly the monoamines norepinephrine and serotonin, has been implicated in the etiology of emotional disorders. In children with mood or anxiety disorders, available serotonin is decreased, either from decreased release or increased reuptake (Takashi, 2010); this particularly affects neurotransmitters in areas of the brain that regulate cognition, feelings and emotions, and motivation (prefrontal cortex and limbic system).

One other important area of exploration is into the hypothalamic-pituitary-adrenal axis, which regulates stress hormones. Theoretically, stress early in life can contribute to an exaggerated level of stress hormones with subsequent excessive stress response. The increase in stress hormones contributes to the symptoms seen particularly in children with anxiety disorders. In addition, children with OCD have heightened metabolic activity in areas of the brain associated with strong emotions (Takashi, 2010).

Environmental Factors

A family history of depression (particularly parental) is a significant risk factor for depression in children or adolescents, which increases the risk for suicide (NIMH, 2010e). Emotional and behavioral theories emphasize the importance of the interaction within the family system and quality of relationships with siblings (Waldinger, Vaillant, & Orav,

2007). There is evidence that children with a history of verbal, physical, or sexual abuse; frequent separation from or loss of loved ones; drug use; incarceration; lower socioeconomic status; homosexuality; chronic illness; behavioral disorders; and dysfunctional families are more likely than peers with healthy family patterns to have anxiety or depressive disorders (NIMH, 2010b).

Traumatic Brain Injury

Growing evidence points to the secondary development of mood disorders in children and adolescents who have sustained traumatic brain injury (TBI), including concussion. The impact of damage resulting from brain injury depends on a number of factors, including the extent, location, and treatment of the injury (Fay et al., 2009). One significant factor is the maturational stage of the brain at the time the damage occurs. Another physiologic factor is the length of time the brain tissue is impaired (as a result of swelling, hemorrhage, or tissue destruction). Finally, the specific area of the brain that is damaged may determine the precise areas of deficit.

The range of severity of TBI may be mild, with only a brief change in mental status, or it may be severe, causing functional long-term changes that can affect emotions, sensations, memory, or cognition. Damage may be cumulative over consecutive injuries (Centers for Disease Control and Prevention [CDC], 2010a).

Manifestations

Disruption in emotional state, including sadness, worry, fear, and somatic complaints, is often prominent in the clinical presentation of emotional disorders, which include both anxiety disorders and mood (depressive) disorders. In addition, suicide risk is increased, particularly with mood disorders.

Anxiety disorders and mood disorders may present with mixed features (i.e., depression and anxiety are both present), which complicates establishing an accurate diagnosis. For example, the child who is anxious may be withdrawn, tearful, unwilling to engage in play, or prone to acting aggressively toward others. These same symptoms typically occur in children who are depressed. Moreover, it is often difficult to differentiate between normal mood changes that are the result of normal developmental maturation and adaptation and abnormal, persistent mood disturbances.

Generally, however, mood disturbance is more intense and persistent and interferes with social relations and daily functioning. Finally, the child or adolescent can have both anxiety and a mood disorder. Mood disorders are also varied and are specified according to the intensity or duration of depressive symptoms or the particular behaviors displayed by the child. For these reasons, careful assessment by a specialist in psychosocial disorders and the use of screening tools is essential.

Therapeutic Management of Children with Emotional Disorders

The management of depression and anxiety in the pediatric population is focused toward providing immediate symptom relief, stabilizing the family situation, and planning for supports that will help mitigate the intensity and frequency of recurrences. Interventions will vary based on the age, developmental level, and social support available to the child.

Recurrence of symptoms is common, with every recurrence increasing the likelihood of future events. For this reason, accurate identification, appropriate intervention, and long-term follow-up are essential to protect the child's physical, intellectual, and social development, because poor health behaviors and social isolation accompany the disorders.

NURSING CARE OF THE CHILD WITH AN EMOTIONAL DISORDER

■ Assessment

In addition to the diagnostic methods described earlier in this chapter (see Diagnostic Evaluation) a thorough physical and developmental history should be obtained from the child and/or the family, with attention paid to previous episodes of the presenting problem. Children may initially be most comfortable having parents present, but when the child is comfortable with the nurse, a private interview should also be offered. Presenting emotional symptoms, physical symptoms (e.g., headaches, stomachaches), and precipitating events should be identified. Initial assessment should also include descriptions of the child's moods, patterns of daily activity, stressors, and coping style (Briggs-Gowan & Carter, 2008).

It is important to gain information regarding risk for self-harm or suicide, particularly if the child shows symptoms of depression. Assessment of risk for self-harm and suicide includes questions about ideation (thoughts), impulses, or plans. Assessment of previous suicide attempts is essential because this raises the risk of future attempts (Wintersteen, Diamond, & Fein, 2007).

Family history provides a contextual framework for understanding the child's symptoms. This should include identification of extended family members who may share living arrangements, and questions about the family interaction patterns. Family (particularly parental) history of psychosocial disorder, mood or anxiety disorder, or substance abuse are all risk factors for a child's development of a psychosocial disturbance. Parents or caregivers should be asked to describe changes in the child's behaviors and when these changes began. Other areas of inquiry include the child's ability to engage in routine activities or play and to interact with friends, and school performance (Wintersteen, Diamond, & Fein, 2007).

For a child who presents with symptoms of OCD or tic disorder, history of sore throats related to strep infection should be noted, along with whether OCD symptom onset was sudden or occurred after an illness (see PANDAS, this chapter).

Screening instruments and self-reporting instruments are increasingly used as part of outcomes measurement and are useful for differential diagnosis of depression and anxiety. As retest measures, they have shown some reliability in assessing treatment effectiveness (Briggs-Gowan & Carter, 2008; Queen, 2010).

■ Nursing Diagnosis and Planning

The nursing diagnoses and expected outcomes that apply for children who are experiencing depression and anxiety include:

- Ineffective Coping related to loss of energy, sleep disturbance, biochemical imbalance, loss of control, or side effects of medication.

Expected Outcome. The child will display adaptive ability, as evidenced by participation in and enjoyment of regular activities. The parent will describe any expected or unexpected side effects from the prescribed medication.

- Situational Low Self-Esteem related to cognitive distortions, inability to manage daily events, and a sense of hopelessness or guilt.

Expected Outcome. The child will display increased self-esteem, as evidenced by verbalization of an increase in self-confidence and an increase in positive feelings about self.

- Risk for Self-Directed Violence related to suicidal ideation, guilt, or hopelessness.

Expected Outcomes. The child will demonstrate more positive moods and reduced anxiety levels and will talk to a responsible family member or professional about any thoughts of self-directed violence.

- Disturbed Sleep Pattern related to anxiety, depression, and inactivity.

Expected Outcome. The child will exhibit appropriate sleep patterns, as evidenced by expressing feelings of being well rested, showing no signs of sleep deprivation (e.g., irritability, lethargy, restlessness), and showing no signs of excessive sleeping.

- Risk for Delayed Development related to poor concentration, fatigue, inability to participate in school

Expected Outcomes. The child will engage in appropriate play for developmental level, attend school, maintain educational progress, and continue positive relationship with peers.

■ Interventions

Social skills training or group therapy may be most helpful for social anxiety. Children will often try to avoid anxiety by limiting social interactions. This creates a cycle of avoidance and associated shame. Behavioral interventions with school phobias are directed toward keeping the child attending school, while offering interventions during school time to reduce anxiety symptoms, such as refusing to pick up the child from school, even if the child insists. This form of intervention is a type of desensitization therapy.

Controversy has surrounded the use of antidepressants. Most antidepressants were studied in adult populations, and evidence is emerging that children may not metabolize these substances in the same manner as adults. A black box warning about the potential for increased risk of suicidal ideation and behavior in children, adolescents, and young adults appears on all dispensed prescription antidepressants. Schneeweiss et al. (2010) conducted an extensive study of antidepressant use and suicidal thoughts or acts in over 20,000 children and adolescents and found that increased suicide risk does not differ among various classes of antidepressants. Therefore the decision on prescribing a particular antidepressant should be based on its potential for therapeutic effect and not on its relative risk for suicide (Schneeweiss et al., 2010). It is not prohibited to use antidepressants to treat these disorders in children or adolescents; however, it is advised to keep a close watch on initiating any type of medication treatment in this population. Use of selective serotonin reuptake inhibitors (SSRIs) for medication management is still an appropriate and widely used treatment for depression and anxiety in children, with careful monitoring when drugs are introduced (Tishler, Reiss, & Rhodes, 2008; Walter & Damaso, 2011).

Children, parents, and clinicians may prefer to initiate psychotherapy before, and perhaps in lieu of, medications; however, the most effective treatment combines medication and the child's and family's exploration of situations and environmental factors that are related to the child's symptoms (March & Vitiello, 2009). Individual therapy and family counseling are essential for children with suicidal ideation or persistent mood disturbances, and in these cases consideration for hospitalization is paramount to protect the child from harmful impulses. Additionally, severe and disabling anxiety warrants serious intervention (Connolly & Bernstein, 2007) and may require day treatment or hospitalization. If the child needs hospitalization, admission will generally be to a psychosocial unit where specialized nursing is available (AACAP, 2007b).

Day treatment programs have increasingly become an alternative to hospitalization. Hospital and day treatment settings utilize cognitive-behavioral therapies (CBTs) to increase coping skills and social skills and to provide tools that can be used to manage stress. The underlying principle of CBT is that individuals, by consciously becoming aware of stressful thoughts and feelings associated with various events or situations, can learn to analyze behaviors related to these thoughts or feelings and begin to think and behave in more positive ways. Cognitive behavioral therapies have shown benefit for all of the emotional disorders. They can be done individually or in groups. Other behavioral strategies for managing depression and anxiety include relaxation therapy, distraction strategies, self-talk, or cognitive strategies, as well as support from adults or friends who are safe and reassuring (Pull, 2007).

■ Evaluation

- Does the child exhibit an energy level that allows for interactions, play, and school?
- Does the child seem interested in people and events?
- Does the child communicate positive statements about self?
- Does the parent report that the child appears happier and more engaged?
- Does the child exhibit normal patterns of eating and sleeping?
- Can the parent describe the medication effects and side effects?

SUICIDE

Suicide is a major public health problem, the third leading cause of death among adolescents between 15 and 24 years old and the fifth among children 5 to 14 years old (National Center for Health Statistics, 2011). Suicide rates among adolescents in the United States have risen dramatically. Estimates of the prevalence of suicidal ideation are 10.5% in males and 17.4% in females. The prevalence of suicide attempts is 4.6% in males and 8.1% in females (CDC, 2010c).

Among young people, suicide incidence rises with age. Suicide by children under 10 is uncommon. Children between the ages of 5 and 14 died by suicide at the rate of 0.7 per 100,000, and adolescents between ages 15 and 24 at the rate of 10.1 per 100,000. This compares to an overall rate of 11.9 per 100,000 people (National Center for Health Statistics, 2011). Other differences are also noted. For example, males are more likely to die by suicide than females, at a ratio of 4:1. Methods appear to vary by gender, with girls using poisons and boys using firearms most frequently (CDC, 2009).

Risk for suicide should be assessed by ascertaining prior suicide attempts, family history of suicide, history of depression, substance abuse, alcohol abuse, an overwhelming life stressor, access to methods, and history of arrest or incarceration (CDC, 2010b). Presence of risk factors does not mean that a suicide attempt is inevitable, but should raise the awareness of anyone who interacts with the child or adolescent.

! NURSING QUALITY ALERT

Resources for People with Thoughts of Suicide

Resources for anyone who is having thoughts of suicide are available through the National Suicide Prevention Lifeline (1-800-273-8255), through their website (www.suicidepreventionlifeline.org), or from the American Association of Suicidology at www.suicidology.org/web/guest/home.

Of significant importance, gay, lesbian, bisexual, and possibly transgender adolescents are two to seven times more likely to attempt suicide than are their heterosexual peers (Suicide Prevention Resource Center, 2008). This appears to be linked to social stigma, feelings of isolation, and level of vulnerability and stress, such as lack of social and family support (Suicide Prevention Resource Center, 2008). Suicide ideation is also significantly higher in lesbian, gay and, bisexual (LGB) adolescents (Suicide Prevention Resource Center, 2008).

Suicide potential should always be assessed for a child with symptoms of a mood disorder, or multiple disorders (comorbidity), or history of previous suicide attempts. Family history of psychosocial disorders (especially depression or a parent who has died by suicide) creates increased risk. Other significant risk factors are chronic medical illness, family violence, substance abuse, poor impulse control, poor school performance, homosexuality, and access to firearms in the household (Moscicki, 2009).

Underlying major depression, poor self-concept, and hopelessness appear to be the most significant factors contributing to suicide, regardless of age or sex. Long-standing family dysfunction is often present, with emotional detachment and isolation among family members. The suicide victim is typically a vulnerable individual who, under stress and unable to envision a solution, seeks and finds a way to die. In the case of children, risks are greatest when there is not adequate adult support to identify and intervene in the escalation of symptoms.

Most adolescent suicide attempts are impulsive: motivated by a desire to influence others, gain attention, communicate love or anger, or escape a difficult or painful situation. Suicide hotlines or drop-in centers can often serve to keep the young person safe until the impulse passes.

However, any verbalization or gesture of suicide should be taken very seriously and should never be ignored. The young person should be encouraged to discuss the thought specifically to determine whether there is a plan and the lethality of the plan (Wintersteen, 2010). Help should be obtained from qualified health professionals.

Suicide remains a rare phenomenon for young children, although a child who has lost a parent before the age of 13 has increased risk for mood disorder and suicide. Until about the age of 6 most children do not have a realistic concept of death, although they may express thoughts about harming themselves. However, children as young as 3 have tried to commit suicide and apparently understood what they were doing.

Knowledge regarding prevention of suicide is an essential role for the community health nurse and the school nurse, especially for nurses at the middle or high school level. It is imperative that school nurses educate school personnel about recognizing the subtle signs of an impending suicide attempt so intervention can occur. Considerations included in continuing education should be whom to contact if a teacher or other school worker suspects a child is considering suicide, who will interview and evaluate the child, and what personnel will notify the family. Often, schools have professional teams that perform the evaluation and make appropriate referrals. Suicide prevention and incidence reduction are two of the national goals described in *Healthy People 2020* (U.S. Department of Health and Human Services [USDHHS], 2010).

Manifestations and Risk Factors

The risk for suicide should be considered if the following are present:
- Previous suicide attempts
- Past psychosocial hospitalization; overt signs of mental illness manifested as delusions or hallucinations
- A family member or friend who has committed suicide; exposure to violence in the home or social environment
- Death of a parent before the child reached 13 years of age

- Recent losses, such as the death of a relative, a family divorce, a breakup, or any significant change or life event that disrupts the emotional status quo
- Preoccupation with death; statements about suicide or self-harm; suicidal clues, such as cryptic verbal messages, giving away personal items, and changes in expected patterns of behaviors (e.g., sudden calmness in a normally anxious teenager)
- History of risk-taking or self-abusive behaviors; use of alcohol or drugs to cope with emotions
- Overwhelming sense of guilt or shame; obsessional self-doubt
- Social isolation—the individual does not have social alternatives or the skills to find alternatives to suicide
- Handguns in the home, especially if accessible or loaded
- History of physical or sexual abuse
- Homosexuality, especially if the teen discovers same-sex orientation early in adolescence, experiences violence because of homosexual identity, or is rejected by family members as a result of sexual orientation

Therapeutic Management
Prevention

Recognition of risk factors for suicidal feelings by health care providers and at schools is one of the most significant prevention strategies. Children or adolescents who commit suicide have usually offered at least veiled information about their suicidal ideation or feelings of despair to classmates, teachers, or health care providers. Children or adolescents with suicidal ideation should undergo a thorough psychosocial evaluation by a mental health professional. The child may need pharmacotherapeutic agents, such as antidepressants or antipsychotic medications. The use of medications in children at risk for suicide requires close monitoring, and medications should be distributed in small doses because they could be used in a suicide attempt or act (AACAP, 2007b). The decision to discharge a child for observation or to hospitalize is based on the nature of the ideation, the access to methods, and the ability of the family to provide a supportive and safe environment (Tishler et al., 2008).

When Prevention and Intervention Fail

A suicide attempt or a death by suicide is a crisis event for all family members and friends. Counseling by a mental health specialist who is experienced in the area of suicide should be provided to all family members and the child's immediate friends. It is important that these services be offered quickly, preferably within the first 24 hours. In the event of a death by suicide, counselors should remain available for at least 1 year after the event. Grieving and emotional adjustments often take several months and may peak around the anniversary of the suicide event. The experience of losing someone by suicide creates an increased risk that others may act on similar impulses.

NURSING CARE OF THE CHILD OR ADOLESCENT AT RISK FOR SUICIDE

■ Assessment

The risk of suicide is best assessed by a systematic approach to behaviors, attitudes, and risk factors, as described previously. Several instruments have been developed to assess lethality and potentiality, which lessens the likelihood of overlooking contributing factors. The instruments are similar and explore risk factors, stressors, lethality of method, coping mechanisms, and support systems. Subtle symptoms of depression or anxiety, such as decreased energy, persistent restlessness, or

---

BOX 29-1 QUESTIONS TO ASSESS SUICIDE POTENTIAL

1. Have you ever thought of trying to hurt yourself? How might you do this?
2. Have you ever thought of killing yourself? How might you do this?
3. Have you known anyone who has committed suicide? When did this occur? What was it like for you?
4. Do you have access to firearms or knives?
5. Do you ever do things to deliberately place yourself in danger, such as driving when you are drunk or playing Russian roulette with a gun?
6. Have you ever told anyone about wanting to kill yourself?
7. Have you ever been hospitalized for suicidal behavior?
8. Can you describe how you feel right now?

---

anger, should also be considered. It is important to explore thought content and organization, awareness and expression of feelings, perceived level and types of stress, perceived availability of support resources, prior suicidal behaviors, and medical status (Box 29-1).

■ Nursing Diagnosis and Planning

The nursing diagnoses and expected outcomes that apply to the child or adolescent at risk for suicide and the family are as follows:
- Risk for Self-Directed Violence related to a desire to end emotional pain, to solicit the attention of others, or to avoid responsibility.

Expected Outcome. The child or adolescent will indicate a decrease in the risk for self-directed violence, as evidenced by an ability to use effective communication techniques to express needs and feelings and to verbalize alternative solutions to problems.
- Situational Low Self-Esteem or Chronic Low Self-Esteem related to a perception of failure and hopelessness about the ability to change self or circumstances.

Expected Outcome. The child or adolescent will demonstrate increased self-esteem, as evidenced by verbalization of ability to change self or circumstances.
- Anxiety related to current or anticipated events.

Expected Outcome. The child or adolescent will have decreased anxiety, as evidenced by recognizing and expressing anxiety and use of effective coping mechanisms to decrease anxiety.
- Interrupted Family Processes related to relational disturbance or possible abuse or neglect.

Expected Outcome. The child or adolescent and family will access and mobilize appropriate support systems in an effective manner.
- Ineffective Coping related to a sense of despair or limited availability of support.

Expected Outcome. The child or adolescent and family will work with professionals to begin to identify and express feelings and identify strengths, and to discuss appropriate actions when feelings become overwhelming.

■ Interventions

Adolescents who are experiencing suicidal ideation and impulses are generally depressed, experiencing themselves as isolated and rejected. Caregivers should be empathic and nonjudgmental; voice and demeanor should be clear, direct, and supportive. At the same time, the ability to create a safe environment is the first priority if suicidal impulses are present. The nurse should ensure that potentially harmful objects are removed, to prevent self-injury. It is important for the nurse to assess how closely a child needs to be monitored throughout the day, realizing that the potential for self-harm fluctuates. If the adolescent is not hospitalized, the nurse should ensure that the family has removed weapons from the home.

Recent results from the Treatment for Adolescents with Depression Study (March & Vitiello, 2009) have demonstrated that CBT alone or, even more effective, combined with medication therapy reduced the risk of suicide in adolescents with a history of a mood disorder. CBT can help individuals learn to consider alternative actions when thoughts of self-harm arise. The identification of trigger events and strategies to avoid or manage these events is important. Nursing interventions include exploration of coping strategies to be used when impulses arise. Planning alternative activities, avoiding isolation, and talking to the treatment team are all effective ways to manage thoughts of self-harm.

Families are also affected when a member harms or kills him- or herself. Individual as well as family meetings provide an opportunity to explore the issues raised and to learn to effectively provide emotional and social support to grieving family members. Grieving will occur even if the suicide attempt was unsuccessful. Individual and family therapy will also provide an opportunity to explore contributory factors that can be altered to reduce the suicide potential. Nurses, as members of the treatment team, work to help the parents regain their ability to assist their child and manage the home environment.

■ Evaluation

- Is the child able to identify situations, events, or times when ideas or impulses are likely to occur? Does the child have a strategy for seeking help during these times?
- Does the child participate in activities that reduce feelings of despair and hopelessness?
- Does the child display evidence of positive self-esteem through positive self-statements or ability to describe how circumstances can be changed?
- Has the child or adolescent verbalized a decrease in anxiety?
- Is the family able to identify warning signs of suicidal risk?
- Do family members support one another, and can the family identify community resources to assist?
- Has the child or adolescent developed coping mechanisms and effective problem solving?
- Has the family developed a suicide prevention plan?

BEHAVIORAL DISORDERS

All children misbehave at times; this is a normal feature of childhood development. Incidents of unacceptable or risky behavior are common, particularly among adolescents. These are not considered to be behavior disorders. Behavioral disorders are not incidents or stages of difficulty in behavior. Instead, behavioral disorders represent a chronic pattern of aggression, hostility, or disruption that is persistent, is unresponsive to parental controls, and has lasted for more than 6 months.

Children with behavioral disorders typically exhibit clusters of signs and symptoms that are primarily inattentive (attention deficit disorder [AD]), primarily impulsive/hyperactive (hyperactivity disorder [HD]), or a combination of both types of symptoms (ADHD).

Warning signs for behavioral disorders include (AACAP, 2011):
- Impulsive or overly aggressive behavior
- Harm, or threats of harm, directed at themselves or others
- Stealing, damaging or destroying property, or other violation of the rights of others
- Lying (sometimes compulsive lying)
- Poor school performance, avoiding school

- Early smoking, drinking, or drug use
- Early sexual activity
- Frequent tantrums and arguments
- Consistent hostility toward authority figures

Behavioral disorders include conduct disorders (aggressive and oppositional disorders), attention deficit disorders, and hyperactivity disorders. A mental health specialist with experience in the area should make the diagnosis of a behavioral disorder.

Attention deficit–hyperactivity disorder (ADHD) is the most common chronic behavioral disorder that emerges during childhood. ADHD is associated with significant problems in three areas: (1) attention and concentration, (2) impulse control, and (3) hyperactivity. In the past, a number of terms have been used, including postencephalitic behavior disorder, restlessness syndrome, hyperkinetic impulse disorder, minimal brain dysfunction, and hyperactive child syndrome. In recent years, however, the descriptive term ADHD has subsumed these other diagnoses.

Estimates of the prevalence of ADHD in children ages 4 to 17 years old in the United States is 9.5% (CDC, 2010a). In epidemiologic studies, the male-to-female ratio is approximately 2:1 among referred children displaying ADHD symptoms (CDC, 2010a). Aggressive, oppositional, and antisocial behaviors are thought to explain the higher rate of referrals of boys.

The DSM-IV-TR lists symptoms related to attention and concentration, including trouble sustaining attention, trouble organizing tasks, appearing to not hear when spoken to, and losing items necessary to complete tasks, such as losing assignments, pencils, or books. Symptoms related to impulsivity include difficulty waiting, blurting out comments, interruptions, or intruding. Symptoms related to hyperactivity include fidgeting, excessive talking, excessive running, and an inability to engage in quiet activities (APA, 2000). Symptoms generally emerge early in childhood, with the mean age at onset 3 or 4 years; however, medication treatment may not be started until the child is in a structured school setting. Parents, teachers, or pediatric caregivers may make referrals for ADHD. Of concern are not only the primary symptoms, which often result in frequent injuries, poor scholastic performance, and low performance motivation, but also the associated symptoms, which may include depression or anxiety, aggressiveness toward peers, and antisocial or oppositional defiance toward authority figures.

A child affected with ADHD may have exceptional sensitivity to noises or disruptions in the environment. For example, ambient sounds such as an air conditioner switching on may disrupt attention to tasks. Rigid controls on physical activity or talking are likely to trigger symptoms. For this reason, the classroom setting is often the place where the disorder is identified. Teachers describe their frustration with having children call out answers (instead of raising their hand), or talking to other children. In situations where structure is rigid or if behavior is severely restricted, the child with ADHD becomes increasingly frustrated and symptoms increase.

Etiology

ADHD occurs more commonly in first-degree biologic relatives of people with the disorder than in the general population, which suggests a genetic predisposition for the disorder. Other central nervous system (CNS) abnormalities, such as the presence of neurotoxins and epilepsy or other neurologic disorders are thought to be predisposing factors, along with prenatal factors, such as maternal substance use, and complications related to labor or delivery (Raishevich Cunningham & Jensen, 2011). Chaotic or abusive environments may predispose to the appearance of ADHD.

Inconclusive but consistent evidence indicates that the basis of ADHD is a sluggish or underreactive neurologic, electrophysiologic response to stimulation. Prefrontal and limbic system connections in the brain are viewed as the likely locations for neurologic functional abnormalities. Hypotheses have been made that dopaminergic and noradrenergic function plays a central role because medications addressing these neurotransmitters are effective for treatment. This information suggests that higher levels of norepinephrine and lower levels of epinephrine activity seen in children with ADHD may play a role.

Manifestations

According to the *DSM-IV-TR* (APA, 2000), a diagnosis of ADHD requires the exhibition of symptoms of inattention and symptoms of impulsivity/hyperactivity.

- *Inattention:* Carelessness, inattention to details, difficulty attending to work or games, does not listen, poor follow-through with instructions or does not complete tasks, difficulty with organization skills, avoidance of tasks that require mental effort, misplaces equipment or supplies necessary to complete tasks, easily distracted, forgetful
- *Impulsivity/hyperactivity:* Fidgets with hands, feet, or hair; unable to remain in a seat for extended periods; runs and climbs excessively in inappropriate settings; difficulty in engaging in quiet activities; mostly "on the go"; talks excessively; blurts out questions or answers; cannot await a turn; interrupts conversations

Signs usually must be present for at least 6 months, have occurred before the age of 7 years, be present in two or more settings (e.g., home, school, recreation, church), not be associated with another mental or developmental disorder, and significantly impair at least one level of functioning (academic, social, occupational) (APA, 2000).

Although the American Psychosocial Association calls this disorder ADHD, not all children with the disorder exhibit hyperactivity, although most demonstrate a degree of impulsivity. ADHD is frequently co-morbid with other disorders, such as motor disorders, oppositional defiant disorder, mood disorders, and anxiety disorders. Therefore, children with ADHD should be screened for co-morbid depression, anxiety, and social impairment. Children with ADHD often have a diagnosed learning disability (Yoshimasu, Barbaresi, Colligan et al., 2010).

Diagnostic Evaluation

Although high-resolution magnetic resonance imaging and blood and urine studies of metabolites of brain neurotransmitters have been performed in individuals with ADHD, none of these tests have provided consistent diagnostic information. The behaviors and symptoms of ADHD must be present in two of three areas—home, school, or social situations—to support the diagnosis. These reports are coupled with psychological assessments conducted while the child is completing tasks requiring vigilance, attention, and concentration and those involving delayed gratification. Clinical interviews may be coupled with clinical trials of psychopharmacologic agents to determine the child's behavioral response. In addition, standardized questionnaires for parents and teachers allow in-depth information to be collected.

Therapeutic Management

The goal of therapeutic management is to reduce the frequency and intensity of unsocialized behaviors. This requires achieving a balance between the child's temperament and environmental demands,

expectancies, and supports. Therefore, treatment interventions must be targeted at enhancing the child's capabilities and self-esteem. Expectations that may be appropriate for a child without ADHD—"he should be able to sit still in school for 40 minutes," or "she should be able to handle 1 hour of homework"—may need to be modified for the child with ADHD. In every case, the nurse should work with the parents to modify the environment and to develop strategies that foster competencies in the child.

Most clinicians combine pharmacotherapy with behavior-oriented family therapy to achieve alterations in the child's internal functioning and external environment. Stimulant medications commonly used as part of the treatment plan include methylphenidate (Ritalin), dextroamphetamine (Dexedrine), and amphetamine/dextroamphetamine (Adderall). Newer timed-released formulas of methylphenidate (Concerta, Ritalin LA, and Metadate ER) and amphetamine/dextroamphetamine (Adderall XR) are advantageous for once-a-day dosing, thereby eliminating mid-day trips to the nurse's office. Atomoxetine (Strattera), a nonstimulant medication, has also been used with success in the treatment of ADHD. Medication treatment is most effective when it is used in conjunction with behavior and emotional and behavioral therapy. It is important to individually tailor the child's medication dosage to achieve maximum results with the fewest side effects. For this reason, medications usually are titrated over several weeks (McDonnell & Moffett, 2010).

NURSING CARE OF THE CHILD WITH ATTENTION DEFICIT–HYPERACTIVITY DISORDER

■ Assessment

The nurse documents the parent's description of the child's typical behavior playing alone and with other children, during mealtimes, and while the parent is on the telephone or occupied with chores. The length of time it takes the child to bathe or dress and how often the child becomes distracted during these tasks are also explored. These behaviors are then compared with those exhibited when the child is engaged in highly stimulating activities and activities with frequent feedback, such as video and computer games. The child's behavior is also compared during novel versus routine activities.

The child's developmental and family history are explored in detail, with the nurse noting the age at which the child began to exhibit independent behaviors, such as walking, getting out of bed alone, and exploring the environment. It is not uncommon for children with ADHD to explore the environment at an early age, with only limited need to return to the caregiver for support or approval. Family members diagnosed with ADHD or who exhibit similar behaviors are noted. Parents should be given self-report inventories, such as the CBCL, Conner's Teacher Rating Scale—Revised, or the Attention-Deficit/Hyperactivity Disorder Rating Scale, to complete and return to the appropriate professional.

Observation within the home or school setting is likely to generate the most valid information because the clinic environment may be unfamiliar and, by the nature of the disorder, may inhibit the child's natural tendency to explore, become distracted, or display limited motivation in task completion.

■ Nursing Diagnosis and Planning

The nursing diagnoses and expected outcomes that apply to the child with ADHD and the child's family are as follows:

- Impaired Social Interaction related to impulsivity, poor self-management skills, and aggressive behaviors.

Expected Outcomes. The child will demonstrate an improvement in social interactions, as evidenced by improvement in impulse control and an ability to sustain attention on tasks. The child will relate in a more positive way with peers.

- Risk for Injury related to impulsivity, limited judgment skills, or excessive need for mobility and stimulation.

Expected Outcome. The child will remain safe from injury, as evidenced by a decrease in injuries and implementation of a plan to prevent injuries.

- Compromised Family Coping or Disabled Family Coping related to the need for consistent and close supervision of the child, the child's hyperactivity, or social stigma of having a child with impulsive or aggressive behaviors.

Expected Outcome. The family will mobilize coping strategies, as evidenced by an ability to discuss the child's needs and a plan to provide the needed support.

- Deficient Knowledge related to perceptions that the child is willfully defiant or disobedient in following directions or in testing limits.

Expected Outcome. The family will increase knowledge related to their child's condition, as evidenced by a willingness to discuss the child's condition and display an understanding of the condition and its treatment.

▪ Interventions

Living with a child who has ADHD can be challenging for parents and other family members on a daily basis. Because of their sometimes disruptive or oppositional behavior, children with ADHD often interact in provocative or intrusive manners. Social and family conflicts are common. Often, parents of children with ADHD have difficulties because their child's behavior offers fewer positive parenting experiences, decreases parenting self-confidence, and increases stress. These parenting outcomes can contribute to negative social, emotional, and educational outcomes in the child. One nursing goal is to teach the family about the disorder. Emphasis is placed on reducing the parents' feelings of blame and guilt about the child's problems and altering their perceptions that the child intentionally misbehaves or lacks motivation to learn or achieve. Demonstrate ways to provide frequent positive reinforcement. Also important for parents and the child is instruction about medications and the adaptations in environment that are needed to allow the child to practice new skills.

The nurse may facilitate communication between the family and the school about ways to accommodate the child's shortened attention span and increased need for mobility and frequent breaks. Often cognitive-behavioral therapy, provided by a specially trained professional, is helpful in identifying specific exercises that can reduce bothersome traits. Support groups for parents can help families cope with the child with ADHD and modify their interactions with and expectations of the child. Ordinarily, positive effects of medication on the child's behavior are seen immediately; however, it may take several weeks to titrate the medication to the point that symptoms are controlled with the fewest side effects.

Children with ADHD who are treated with medication are likely to increase their academic achievement (Yan, 2009). It is common for the family to observe a rapid change in the child's behavior and to feel relief as manifestations subside. Continuing support is required, because this disorder is lifelong and progress in self-control and behavioral patterns is usually slow. Parents and school nurses need to be actively involved in dispensing medication, even through adolescence, because children fluctuate in their willingness to adhere to therapy. Affected children also may have difficulty remembering to take the

medication because of the attention deficits characteristic of the disorder.

Nutritional management is also an issue with children taking medication for the treatment of ADHD. Many of the medications suppress appetite, and the children may begin to refuse meals or snacks. Maintaining appropriate developmental weight gain is an issue of concern. The nurse advises the parent to encourage high-calorie breakfasts and more frequent but smaller meals. Some children prefer to eat a large snack after arrival home from school in the afternoon. Providing high-nutrient meals and snacks is preferred; referral to a nutritionist may be advisable.

Some parents and professionals prefer more conservative approaches, such as dietary changes, to the treatment of ADHD. Although researchers continue to debate whether food additives and sugars have significant clinical influences on most children with ADHD, the general consensus is that they do not. Medication is typically administered during the school day, but it has become increasingly recognized that attention, concentration, and alertness are needed for any learning task, such as learning to play baseball or learning to drive a car. The side effects and potency of the medications used to treat ADHD often make parents and physicians hesitant to administer medications other than during critical learning periods.

▪ Evaluation

- Does the child adhere to the cognitive and pharmacologic strategies designed to increase self-control, as evidenced by a decrease in impulsivity and an increase in attention to task?
- Does the child complete school assignments in less time than formerly, with less distractibility?
- Does the child demonstrate increased skill in peer relations, as evidenced by fewer conflicts and more frequent positive statements to and about peers?
- Does the family provide a safe and supportive environment within the home, as evidenced by adequate supervision and opportunities for meeting the child's mobility needs in a safe manner?
- Is the child maintaining developmentally appropriate weight gain?
- Does the family demonstrate acceptance of the child and the child's special needs?
- Does the family demonstrate an increased acceptance of the child's condition as a medical problem rather than a social or behavioral problem?
- Does the family adhere to the medication regimen?

EATING DISORDERS: ANOREXIA NERVOSA AND BULIMIA NERVOSA

Eating disorders include anorexia nervosa, bulimia nervosa, pica, and binge eating disorder. Anorexia nervosa and bulimia nervosa are the two most frequently seen eating disorders in children. Anorexia and bulimia have overlapping features and similar underlying mechanisms, which supports viewing these disorders as a continuum. Females are more likely to be affected by the eating disorders. For example, prevalence of bulimia nervosa is approximately 3% to 5%; the prevalence of anorexia nervosa in girls is 0.5% to 1% (Kreipe, 2011). Eating disorders are less common in males; however, males comprise 5% to 10% of children or adolescents with an eating disorder (Rosen, 2010). Comorbidities are common with all types of eating disorders, including depression or anxiety (Rosen, 2010). Eating disorders are also comorbid for obsessive-compulsive disorder.

Anorexia nervosa is characterized by a deliberate refusal to maintain adequate body weight, a distorted body image, and amenorrhea (in females). Weight loss can be rapid, extreme, or dramatic. Bulimia nervosa is characterized by recurrent episodes of binge eating; a sense of lack of control over eating binges; self-induced vomiting or excessive use of laxatives, diuretics, or emetics to prevent weight gain; excessive exercise to prevent weight gain; and a persistent concern with body image, although body image is usually not distorted.

Children with eating disorders typically report shame and guilt about many life experiences, especially eating. Individuals with severe eating disorders, particularly anorexia nervosa, have a mortality rate up to 20% from complications of the disorder or from suicide (Nielsen, 2010).

Treatment resistance is common because of the cognitive distortions that support the inaccurate body image. Secondary gains for the disorders include a heightened sense of self-esteem, attention from family and caregivers, cultural admiration given to thin people, envy, and control over others through eating patterns. Ritualistic behaviors are seen frequently, particularly around issues of food. For example, the child may eat only at a particular time of day, eat foods only in a certain order, of a single color, or insist on washing all foods before eating them. The rituals are often an attempt to control the portions, fat content, or nutrients ingested. The rituals also serve to enhance the individual's sense of control over food or dietary intake.

Children or adolescents with anorexia will go to extreme measures to prevent others from becoming aware of the weight loss or lack of food intake. For example, they may ingest large amounts of water or insert heavy objects in the vaginal cavity before weighing to give the impression of weight gain. The child or adolescent with either anorexia or bulimia may eat in front of people and then go to the bathroom to purge after the meal.

Etiology

Disordered eating emerges from multiple risk factors including biologic, social, cultural, and psychological contributors. Children or adolescents with eating disorders often have a family history of emotional disorders, such as major depression. The disorder is more common among sisters and mothers of those with the disorder than in the general population, suggesting some genetic predisposition.

Neurobiologic research has demonstrated that levels of brain serotonin contribute to dysregulation of appetite, dysphoric mood, and difficulties with impulse control (Kaye, 2007). Community-based studies indicate that gene abnormalities may create a predisposition toward eating disorders (Klump, Suisman, Burt et al., 2009).

The development and severity of the risk for eating disorders appear to be related to the child's response to biologic, psychological, and social demands of maturation. Other significant risk factors are earlier pubertal development and higher body fat, depressive tendencies, concurrent stressors, alterations in brain neurotransmitters, history of eating problems, cultural expectations to be thin, and the individual's pervasive sense of ineffective control of the environment (Kaye, 2007).

Manifestations
Anorexia Nervosa

The hallmark of anorexia nervosa is the refusal to maintain a body weight that exceeds the minimal weight recommended for height (15% below expected weight). Intense preoccupation with and unrelenting fear of obesity and a disturbed body image (weight, size, or shape) that is obviously contrary to reality are also observed. Children who look in a mirror report seeing themselves as fat and are repulsed by the sight (Figure 29-1).

Other clinical manifestations in females include at least three missed menstrual periods (primary or secondary amenorrhea); a misperception of internal and external stimuli, particularly food-related cues such as hunger; overwhelming feelings of ineffectiveness and inadequacy; lanugo, dry or flaky skin, and dull, brittle hair; and fatigue and muscle wasting (Kaye, 2007).

Boys with eating disorders demonstrate many behavior patterns similar to girls' behavior patterns, including weight loss through excessive dieting, compulsive activities, and purging, to get strong or to become more muscular (rather than to be thin, as reported by females) (NIMH, 2010c).

Bulimia Nervosa

The clinical manifestations associated with bulimia nervosa include recurrent episodes of rapid, compulsive, uncontrolled (binge) eating linked to purging; a sense of lack of control over eating behaviors during binges; and use of strategies to prevent weight gain (self-induced vomiting; use of laxatives, diuretics, or emetics; fasting; vigorous and excessive exercise). A minimum of two binge eating episodes per week for at least 3 months and persistent irrational concern with body shape and weight are also common factors. These children are also at increased risk for tooth erosion because of the effects of the acidic stomach contents on the teeth from induced vomiting. Some children with bulimia also use excessive exercise to control weight. Unlike children with anorexia, those with bulimia are mostly within normal weight percentiles.

Diagnostic Evaluation

The medical history and physical assessment should be comprehensive, focusing on any medically based illness that mimics an eating disorder or exists concomitantly. Assessment of body image and identification of problems, substance abuse, and social support systems used by the child or adolescent are important components of the evaluation and treatment planning. A family history of eating disorders or other psychosocial illnesses should be noted. Family dynamics, including the level or quality of interaction, support, discipline, and individuation, should be explored in depth. Previous treatment attempts and successful coping strategies should be identified.

An electrocardiogram and a chest radiograph are typically obtained if symptoms of bradycardia, hypotension, or hypothermia are noted. Complete liver and renal function tests, thyroid function tests, and serum electrolyte studies are usually included in the medical workup.

Therapeutic Management

Children with severe eating disorders may need to be hospitalized to achieve physiologic stability. Priority for care is to stabilize body weight and protect from life-threatening complications (e.g., dysrhythmias, depression, or electrolyte imbalance).

One risk during this time is refeeding syndrome, which can be fatal if not recognized quickly and treated promptly. Refeeding syndrome is a fluid and metabolic disturbance that results from introducing nutrition too rapidly to someone who has been starving (Yantis & Velender, 2008). It occurs most commonly in people who have lost weight rapidly. Starvation can drastically alter fluid and electrolyte and metabolic balances; replacing fluids and foods too rapidly can result in fluid volume excess, deficiency in electrolytes and vitamins, and multisystem derangements (e.g., cardiac, neurologic, muscular, and endocrine) (Yantis & Velender, 2008). A high index of suspicion for this syndrome is warranted, because electrolyte and fluid balances can strain the cardiac and respiratory systems. This syndrome can occur at the beginning of treatment when patients are reintroduced to a healthy diet.

Once stabilized, the child or adolescent is generally transferred to a day treatment program. Care focuses on restructuring cognitive

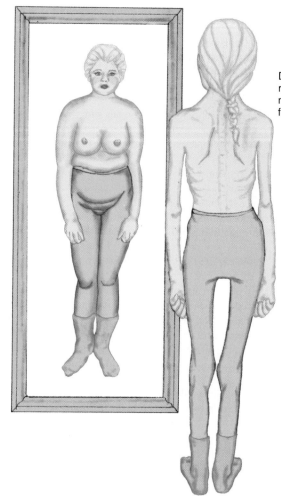

Distorted body image results in extreme need to control food intake.

Amenorrhea
Lanugo
Fatigue
Constipation
Dry, flaky skin
Severe caries
Dull, brittle hair
Muscle wasting

FIG 29-1 In anorexia nervosa, the adolescent refuses to maintain adequate body weight, partly because of a distorted body image: she perceives herself as overweight when in fact she is below minimum weight.

perceptions, reducing opportunities to engage in ritualistic and self-injurious behaviors, and reestablishing physiologic homeostasis. The programs typically include interventions that enlist the adolescent's cooperation in a refeeding program. Nutritional consultation is provided to facilitate gradual weight gain. Intake and output, weight gain, vital signs, laboratory values, electrolyte status, and cardiac status are carefully monitored.

NURSING CARE OF THE CHILD OR ADOLESCENT WITH AN EATING DISORDER

■ Assessment

School nurses or nurses in community settings are in an optimal position for recognizing children with eating disorders. They become familiar with students they see on a regular basis and can assess changes in weight, emotional status, or behaviors. Once considered an adolescent problem, eating disorders are now observed in much younger children, so nurses in elementary schools need to be alert for early signs of the disorders. Awareness programs organized by school nurses offer opportunities for inquiries from children who might not normally speak about their eating problems or concerns about weight. Short and reliable screening tools are available to assist school nurses in identifying children who may be at risk for the disorder.

Children with eating disorders typically convey mistrust, ambivalence, and denial. It is generally better if the assessment is conducted in a structured and concrete manner (rather than as an open-ended exploration), with an emphasis placed on alliance building and periodic review.

Determining motivations for changing behaviors is crucial, and motives should be assessed for each specific behavior (i.e., weight gain, induced vomiting, altered self-perception of body). A mental status examination should also be included because the side effects of restrictive dieting can impair cognitive functioning and perpetuate emotional disturbances. Any history of self-injury should be noted. The nurse should assist the child or adolescent in gaining an understanding of impulse control problems and ritualistic and compulsive behaviors.

Before beginning a refeeding program, the nurse must assess baseline weight, electrolyte status, blood glucose, and vital signs. Assessment of intake and output is essential.

■ Nursing Diagnosis and Planning

The nursing diagnoses and expected outcomes that apply to the child or adolescent with an eating disorder follow:

* Imbalanced Nutrition: Less Than Body Requirements related to inadequate intake, malabsorption from extended periods of starvation, or distorted body image.

Expected Outcome. The child or adolescent will meet daily nutritional requirements, as evidenced by sufficient weight gain or maintenance of an adequate weight to sustain systemic homeostasis and physiologic health.

- Anxiety, Fear, or Powerlessness related to weight gain, sense of inadequacy, and lack of control over body and self.

Expected Outcome. The child or adolescent will display decreased anxiety, fear, and powerlessness, as evidenced by demonstration of the ability to seek help with anxiety management and demonstration of improved coping strategies, including open expression of feelings.

- Risk for Activity Intolerance or Disturbed Sleep Pattern related to fatigue, depression, and an excessive drive to exercise and expend energy.

Expected Outcome. The child or adolescent will have adequate rest, as evidenced by an ability to establish improved sleeping and activity patterns with a corresponding improvement in affect, energy, and sense of well-being.

- Deficient Fluid Volume related to excessive use of diuretics or laxatives or inadequate fiber and fluid intake.

Expected Outcome. The child or adolescent will maintain fluid and electrolyte balance, as evidenced by electrolyte levels within normal limits, normal skin turgor, and moist mucous membranes.

■ Interventions

The treatment of eating disorders initially focuses on disrupting the cycle of the eating disorder and addressing the secondary effects of self-induced vomiting, excessive use of diuretics and laxatives, and insufficient nutrients to sustain the function of body systems. Treatment may take place in an outpatient setting or an inpatient setting if the child's physical and emotional status requires more intensive treatment and monitoring (APA, 2006). Electrolyte levels and body chemistry values should be stabilized to prevent sustained damage to body systems, especially the cardiac, respiratory, and gastrointestinal systems. Adequate caloric intake is the next major goal of treatment and often requires strict monitoring to prevent sabotage of medical treatment. Fluids and foods are introduced gradually in order to reduce the risk of refeeding syndrome. Continuing intensive and highly individualized therapy helps the adolescent cope with complex issues. Family intervention usually is necessary. Finally, alteration of misperceptions about body image and a reorientation to issues of control and self-management are necessary. Follow-up therapy for the individual and family is indicated for a period of several months to 3 years. A long-term consequence related to eating disorders is osteoporosis from interruption to bone density formation during adolescence (APA, 2006). Psychopharmacologic treatment of children with anorexia nervosa has not been generally effective, although use of SSRIs has shown benefit for adolescents with bulimia (National Institute of Mental Health, 2010c).

Support in exploring refeeding, sensations of fullness, bloating, and delayed gastric emptying and help in tolerating these feelings and body sensations are important. The nurse and child or adolescent jointly participate in monitoring affect, mood, and potential for suicide. They also agree to a contract specifying necessary interventions to ensure safety and to monitor daily food intake and feelings. These interventions may take the form of interacting with the staff at regular intervals or agreeing to approach the staff if suicidal ideation is present. The nurse will need to validate the adolescent's feelings of ambivalence, fear, and powerlessness. If hyperalimentation or nasogastric tube feedings are required to ensure adequate nutritional intake, the nurse should offer support regarding the discomfort and education about the importance of the interventions and should closely monitor

feedings. As the child begins to show physical and cognitive gains, the nurse should provide educational information about the short-term and long-term effects of starvation.

The nurse is likely to participate in providing or supporting treatments, such as individual, group, and family therapy sessions. Especially in the early phase of treatment, the child or adolescent may be very resistant to efforts to increase nutritional intake and may resort to denial, trickery, or manipulation to prevent a weight increase or thwart adherence to dietary regimens. It may be necessary to observe the child or adolescent after meals to prevent episodes of purging.

Families are informed and involved in treatment goals and apprised of progress toward these goals. Participation in family therapy is generally a required part of the treatment plan for eating disorders, because family patterns of communication and interaction can be contributory factors in success or relapse. The nurse supports the family in voicing concern for the child's health and well-being, while encouraging the view that the child needs an independent identity and sense of control.

■ Evaluation

- Does the child or adolescent demonstrate an increase in food consumption adequate to sustain growth and developmental needs?
- Has the child or adolescent controlled impulses to overeat and purge?
- Can the child or adolescent demonstrate a positive alteration in self-perceptions and body image, as evidenced by verbalizing an increased sense of self-control and decreased anxiety about the present and the future?
- Does the child or adolescent demonstrate a decrease in ambivalence and mistrust about self and significant others?
- Does the child or adolescent show increased energy and display appropriate affect?
- Are electrolyte levels within normal limits, and are mucous membranes moist?

SUBSTANCE ABUSE

Chemical agents that are typically abused by children and adolescents include alcohol, hallucinogens, sedatives, analgesics, anxiolytics, steroids, inhalants, and stimulants. The substance chosen depends on its availability and cost as well as social influences and parental behaviors or tolerance of drug use. Most professionals differentiate between substance abuse and substance addiction. However, the basic treatment concerns are similar. Substance abuse is generally considered to increase over time.

Great variation exists in the types of substances abused across sexes and ages (Table 29-1). Typically, boys consume alcohol more than girls do. Female junior high school students are increasing their use of tobacco, whereas tobacco use by their male counterparts has remained consistent.

The National Institute on Drug Abuse (NIDA) (USDHHS & NIDA, 2010) has tracked illicit drug use and attitudes toward drug, alcohol, and cigarette use among middle school and high school students nationwide since 1975. Each fall, the updated results of the *Monitoring the Future (MTF) Survey* are released. According to the 2009 survey, marijuana use has continued to decline over the past decade (USDHHS & NIDA, 2010). However, there are continued rates of nonmedical use of prescription medications, particularly opiates (USDHHS & NIDA, 2010). The greatest concern in current trends of illicit use of drugs by teenagers is the increase in use of painkillers. In its 2009 report NIDA reported a prevalence of Vicodin (hydrocodone and acetaminophen) use as 2.5% of 8th graders, 8.1% of 10th graders, and 9.7% of 12th

TABLE 29-1 COMMONLY ABUSED DRUGS AND THEIR EFFECTS

DRUG	EXPECTED BEHAVIORS AND EFFECTS	SPECIAL CONSIDERATIONS
Tobacco	Chronic cough, wheezing, increased phlegm production, atherosclerosis	Considered a gateway drug; initial use usually begins in elementary school
Alcohol	Amount-related effects include euphoria followed by depression or hostility, decreased inhibitions, impaired judgment, lack of coordination, and slurred speech	Considered a gateway drug; easily accessible
Marijuana	Relaxation, mild euphoria, loss of inhibition, decreased motivation, red eyes, dry mouth	Considered a gateway drug
Opiates	Euphoria, elation, pain relief, detachment and apathy, drowsiness, constricted pupils, constipation, slurred speech, impaired judgment	Long-term apathy about self, often leading to physical malnutrition and dehydration; criminal behaviors associated with obtaining drugs likely to occur; infections at injection sites common
Barbiturates	Similar to those associated with alcohol	Often used in conjunction with stimulants; may have a paradoxical effect of hyperactivity in children
Amphetamines	Euphoria, hyperactivity, agitation, irritability, insomnia, weight loss, tachycardia, hypertension	May have a paradoxical effect of depression in children
Cocaine	Euphoria, elation, agitation, hyperactivity, irritability, pressured speech, grandiosity, tachycardia, hypertension, diaphoresis, anorexia, weight loss, insomnia	Psychotic behavior possible if the dose is large; can be fatal if combined with other drugs
Hallucinogens Lysergic acid diethylamide (LSD) Methylenediooxy-methamphetamine ("ecstasy")	Distorted perceptions, heightened awareness, hallucinations, illusions, depersonalization, dilated pupils, hypertension, increased salivation	Psychotic behaviors, panic flashbacks long after drug use ceases, self-destructive behaviors
Phencyclidine hydrochloride (PCP)	Euphoria, distorted perceptions, agitation, violence, antisocial behaviors, hypertension, increased salivation, increased pain response	Panic, irrational behaviors, psychosis

graders; use prevalence of OxyContin (oxycodone) was similar, but slightly lower. Alcohol use ranged from 15% in 8th graders to 44% in 12th graders.

In addition to the use of prescription drugs, the abuse of over-the-counter (OTC) drugs has increased in recent years, especially by 10th graders (USDHHS & NIDA, 2010). Abuse of OTC drugs is most common in adolescents 12 to 17 years old. Unlike alcohol, which is regulated for minors, OTC drugs are readily available. The most common OTC drugs that are abused are antitussives, central nervous system stimulants, and antihistamines (Johnston, O'Malley, Bachman, & Schulenberg, 2010).

It is estimated that 72% of adolescents have tried alcohol by the time they reach adulthood (USDHHS & NIDA, 2010). Experimentation with marijuana, the most widely used illicit drug, is reported to be on a slight increase after several years of decline (USDHHS & NIDA, 2010). Research consistently supports the hypothesis that drug use progresses from beer or wine to cigarettes or hard liquor and then marijuana, followed by other illicit drugs. These substances are sometimes referred to as gateway substances. Substance abuse is strongly associated with other high-risk behaviors in adolescence, such as unintentional injuries and unprotected sexual encounters (Box 29-2).

Public awareness and emphasis on treatment and prevention seem to be working. Although these factors had very limited impact on teenagers in the 1990s, there is a promising indication of an increase in the belief that illicit drugs are harmful and increased numbers of teenagers disapprove of their use. Reducing substance abuse is a national health goal identified in *Healthy People 2020* (USDHHS,

BOX 29-2 PHASES OF SUBSTANCE ABUSE

Phase 1: Experimentation
The drug is taken to see what it does or to appease peers.

Phase 2: Early Drug Use
A specific drug or various drugs are used with some regularity for their pleasurable effects or to reduce anxiety. Social use of drugs typically falls into this category.

Phase 3: True Drug Addiction
Drugs are used regularly, and physical dependence begins if it is characteristic of the drug. Social functioning revolves around a drug focus.

Phase 4: Severe Drug Addiction
The physical condition of the addicted child or adolescent deteriorates. All activities are related to obtaining or using the drug, with isolation from nondrug culture.

2010), and by the Surgeon General of the United States (USDHHS & Office of the Surgeon General, 2007). An awareness of the possibility of substance abuse is the responsibility of the parent, teacher, and health professional. Knowing the clinical behavioral manifestations of substance abuse is essential, and much information is readily available to adults interested in prevention and early identification.

Etiology

Drugs affect the brain by altering the biochemical pathways in the CNS. The brain regions most affected in substance abuse are located within the mesocorticolimbic system and include the hippocampus, ventral segmental area, nucleus accumbens, and medial prefrontal cortex. Biochemical alteration results in a complex interplay among dopamine, serotonin, norepinephrine, and gamma-aminobutyric acid. Some drugs mimic natural neurotransmitters, which enable the drugs to activate neurons. Other drugs, such as amphetamines and cocaine, cause the nerve cells to flood the synaptic space, greatly amplifying the normal effect. All drugs of abuse directly or indirectly target dopamine, the neurotransmitter present in areas of the brain that regulate emotion, cognition, movement, and pleasure. This overstimulation creates the euphoric, energized feeling sought by users (USDHHS & Office of the Surgeon General, 2007).

Substance abuse and substance dependence tend to cluster in families, with clinical evidence of genetic influences. For alcohol, as for most other drugs, there also is some evidence that substance abuse often represents the child's or adolescent's attempt to cope with anxiety generated by impaired social skills, low self-esteem, poor interpersonal relationships, or lack of adaptive behaviors. Emotional and behavioral disorders, such as anxiety disorders, ADHD, depression, and conduct disorder, are associated with an increased risk of substance abuse.

Manifestations

The clinical manifestations of substance abuse are marked by increased antisocial behavior as the desire for social conformity and acceptance decreases and the need for the substance increases. Behaviors that may indicate substance abuse problems include irregular school attendance, low grades or poor school performance, aggressive or rebellious behavior, excessive dependence on peer influence, and deterioration of relationships with family members or former friends. Rapid or extreme changes in behavior or mood and loss of interest in hobbies, sports, or other favorite activities are often observed. Lack of parental support and supervision and changes in eating or sleeping patterns that increase as manipulative behaviors increase, especially those that are related to the need to acquire desired substances, may also be involved.

! NURSING QUALITY ALERT

Relapse among Substance Abusers

Substance abusers' rates of refusal to adhere to therapeutic recommendations, together with resulting relapses, are quite high. More than 60% of those completing a course of treatment continue to abuse substances throughout their lifetimes.

Therapeutic Management

Treatment in a center specifically designed for substance abuse is recommended and includes individual, group, and family therapy. Participation in Alcoholics Anonymous or Narcotics Anonymous is advocated. These organizations also offer support groups geared toward helping family members with programs that promote alterations in the family system to decrease the likelihood of relapse.

The relapse rate among youthful substance abusers is extremely high, and success in a short-term treatment program is not necessarily an indicator of long-term control. The incidence of relapse is generally reduced if the child and family maintain active, long-term involvement in support groups, such as Alcoholics Anonymous, Alateen, Alatot, and Narcotics Anonymous. Parenting groups may also be beneficial in providing counsel and support as parents navigate the numerous and often painful decisions they must make.

NURSING CARE OF THE CHILD OR ADOLESCENT WITH A SUBSTANCE ABUSE PROBLEM

■ Assessment

Physical assessment should include evaluation of respiratory rate, heart rate, blood pressure, activity level (hyperactive, hypoactive), mood, affect, judgment, speech, sensory responses, and memory. A thorough history of current and past drug use should be obtained. A family and social history, a medical history, and a legal history (e.g., past and current charges related to substance abuse) should be obtained as well. The possibility of pregnancy should also be considered, since drugs taken during pregnancy will also affect the neonate (American Academy of Pediatrics [AAP], 2009).

■ Nursing Diagnosis and Planning

The nursing diagnoses and expected outcomes that apply to the child or adolescent with a substance abuse problem follow:

- Acute Confusion (Disturbed Thought Processes) related to the specific effects of the particular substance involved.

Expected Outcome. The child or adolescent will exhibit behaviors indicative of the absence of substance abuse, as evidenced by the ability to maintain orientation to time, place, and person.

- Disturbed Sensory Perception related to the specific effects of the particular substance involved.

Expected Outcome. The child or adolescent will remain free from sensory changes, as evidenced by the absence of falls or other injuries.

- Anxiety related to a decrease in sense of control over self or the environment.

Expected Outcome. The child or adolescent will display decreased anxiety, as evidenced by verbalization of increased feelings of self-worth and the ability to change behavior.

- Ineffective Coping related to limited development of effective social interactions and problem-solving skills.

Expected Outcome. The child or adolescent will increase ability to interact socially and to problem solve, as evidenced by an ability to identify current stressors leading to substance use or abuse.

- Impaired Social Interaction related to anxiety or limited social skills.

Expected Outcome. The child or adolescent will begin to develop healthy social skills, as evidenced by an ability to identify alternative activities, people, and social situations that discourage substance abuse.

- Situational Low Self-Esteem or Chronic Low Self-Esteem related to limited social skills, ineffective coping skills, or a poor sense of self-management.

Expected Outcome. The child or adolescent will increase self-esteem, as evidenced by replacing substance abuse with more appropriate social skills and developing meaningful relationships with nonabusing peers and family members.

■ Interventions

The nurse's responsibilities in caring for children or adolescents with substance abuse problems depend on the care setting, the severity of the abuse, and the treatment goals. Often, other students report a child's use or abuse of substances to the school nurse. In this instance, appropriate care and referral begin in the school setting and may include a thorough assessment and parent notification. The nurse can be a resource for parents and community members as to agencies within the community that can assist the child and family. Many school districts have a zero-tolerance policy for tobacco, drugs, and alcohol; in some instances, the school resource officer or local police may need to be called. Often a crisis team within the school that includes the school nurse as a participating member makes this decision. Most school districts actively incorporate alcohol and drug prevention programs in their curricula for students at various grade levels.

If the youth has been identified as a substance abuser and referred to a treatment facility, the nurse's primary responsibility will be to stabilize the physiologic status and support recommendations for treatment. Explaining the expectations and the types of services offered is important because most treatment programs increase child or adolescent and family responsibilities over time.

Initially, maintaining safety and an optimal level of physical comfort is necessary, especially if detoxification is required. This includes close observation, removal of any potentially dangerous items, and monitoring vital signs. Being readily available to discuss thoughts, concerns, and perceptions is important to create an emotional sense of safety. Additional interventions include educating the child or adolescent and family members about necessary laboratory tests and providing information about the nature of substance abuse.

Another significant nursing intervention is to assist the child or adolescent and family in developing social support systems and refer them to appropriate resources that can offer additional support as they make long-term changes in their social and emotional patterns of relating. It is also essential to help the youth assume responsibility for the substance abuse problem, rather than passing the blame on to others. Providing emotional support for the youth and family as they develop insight into their behaviors and the need for changes is important because these changes are often difficult to effect.

■ Evaluation

- Has the child or adolescent remained substance free and been oriented to time and place?
- Has the child or adolescent remained injury free as a result of sensory or perceptual changes?
- Is the child or adolescent able to identify stressors and use appropriate coping mechanisms?
- Has the child or adolescent assumed responsibility for changing behaviors related to the substance abuse?
- Is the child or adolescent participating in daily activities?
- Does the child or adolescent show improvement in peer and family relationships?
- Does the child or adolescent demonstrate an increased sense of self-confidence?

INFANT WITH NEONATAL ABSTINENCE SYNDROME

Infants born to women who abuse drugs during their pregnancy may have withdrawal symptoms after birth and require nursing care on a pediatric unit or in a children's hospital. Neonatal abstinence syndrome refers to withdrawal symptoms in neonates caused by heroin or other opiates to which they have been exposed. Methadone exposure is a frequent cause of neonatal abstinence syndrome.

Incidence

Chemical dependence is one of the most frequently missed diagnoses in the management of pregnant women, increasing the risk for substance dependence in the neonate. Approximately 4.5% of pregnant women use illicit drugs at some time during their pregnancies (USDHHS, Substance Abuse and Mental Health Services Administration, 2010). Six percent of pregnant women continue to use alcohol, and 14% of pregnant women use tobacco (USDHHS, Substance Abuse and Mental Health Services Administration, 2009). The true incidence of perinatal substance abuse is unknown because self-reporting of use is unreliable and toxicology screens usually detect use over only a short time frame. Approximately 10% to 11% of infants have prenatal substance exposure, and many of these display symptoms after birth (Hamdan, 2010).

Manifestations

The onset of withdrawal symptoms is variable. Symptoms may be present at birth or may not occur until 4 to 10 days after delivery. Infants born addicted to narcotics may exhibit withdrawal symptoms for 4 to 12 months. The majority of affected infants exhibit signs and symptoms as follows: wakefulness, irritability with high-pitched and persistent cry, tremulousness, temperature variation, hyperactivity, hyperreflexia (exaggerated Moro reflex), hypertonus, gastroenteritis with dehydration, diaphoresis, uncoordinated and constant suck, weight loss, respiratory signs (rhinorrhea, tachypnea, respiratory distress, apnea, respiratory alkalosis), autonomic dysfunction, and excessive tearing,

In addition, the infant might exhibit seizures.

Diagnostic Evaluation

When drug withdrawal has been identified or is suspected, obtaining urine and blood toxicology and drug screens on the mother and obtaining urine, blood, and meconium toxicology and drug screens on the infant can help confirm the diagnosis. There are several types of screening/scoring systems that assess the severity of withdrawal symptoms; these include the Lipsitz and Finnegan systems. These scoring systems are easy to use; however, they are most appropriate for use in infants who have been exposed to opiates (Hamdan, 2010).

Therapeutic Management

Many infants undergoing withdrawal respond well to supportive measures. Sensory stimulation can be decreased by swaddling; a quiet, darkened environment; and comfort measures to prevent excessive crying. Early breastfeeding decreases the intensity of symptoms and should be encouraged in mothers who are not HIV positive (Schub & Davidson, 2010). In formula-fed infants, small feedings of high-calorie formula help supply the additional caloric requirements.

More specific therapy may be required when withdrawal symptoms are severe and known exposure can be documented (Carlo, 2011). Therapy is related to the type of substance to which the newborn has been exposed. Depending on the drug exposure involved, pharmacologic agents used in the treatment of withdrawal include tincture of opium, morphine, methadone, clonidine, diazepam (Valium), chlorpromazine (Thorazine), and phenobarbital. Sublingual buprenorphine is a newer medication that has been used with success in treating these infants; it appears to have a safer profile with fewer side effects than other conventional treatments (Hamdan, 2010). Polydrug exposure may require a combination of drugs.

Medication doses can be stabilized and then tapered once the infant sleeps well, eats effectively, and gains weight for 3 to 5 days. Failure to taper the dose may result in prolonged hospitalization. Treatment may last a few days or several weeks, depending on the severity of symptoms and the infant's response to treatment. Long-term follow-up of the infant's physical and mental development should be supervised by a physician who is knowledgeable about the symptoms and treatment of addicted infants and who is willing to communicate effectively with the parents. Although residual physical and psychosocial problems may persist in these infants, these are thought to result from a combination of the effects of the exposure and the child's subsequent social environment (Carlo, 2011). Social workers are essential in determining the parents' ability to care for the infant after discharge.

Nursing Considerations

The nurse can help identify infants who are at risk for withdrawal by obtaining a social history from the parents and a detailed maternal drug history, including prescription and nonprescription drugs. The nurse should assess infants who are at risk for the presence of signs and symptoms of withdrawal. When drug withdrawal has been identified or is suspected, obtaining urine and blood toxicology and drug screens on the mother and urine, blood, and meconium toxicology and drug screens on the infant can help confirm the diagnosis. Nursing care is aimed at decreasing environmental stimuli, meeting the infant's nutritional needs, and promoting healthy parent-infant interaction. The infant's care is coordinated to limit the number of times the infant is disturbed. Noise and light levels in the nursery or home, especially in the infant's immediate vicinity, are maintained at minimal necessary levels. A light blanket can be placed over the top of the incubator to darken the area. Appropriate comfort measures are provided immediately when the infant exhibits irritability. These may include offering a pacifier, swaddling the infant, or rocking. The infant's ability to breastfeed or bottle feed is assessed, and the infant is gavage fed if necessary to provide adequate fluid and caloric intake. Weight gain is monitored daily, and length and head circumferences are monitored weekly to ensure that nutritional intake is sufficient for growth. Because these infants are usually irritable, providing their nursing care can be challenging and stressful. Parent-infant interaction is at an especially high risk in these cases, and special effort is made to involve the parents in the infant's care. Contact between parents and social services, such as child protection and community health agencies, is made before discharge in an effort to optimize the functioning of the family unit and the child's long-term psychological outcome.

CHILDHOOD PHYSICAL AND EMOTIONAL ABUSE AND CHILD NEGLECT

Child abuse includes emotional abuse, physical abuse, and sexual exploitation or molestation by caretakers or other individuals. Deliberate failure to provide for a child's physical, educational, or emotional needs is considered to be neglect (Shipman & Taussig, 2009). Although the federal definition of child abuse includes neglect, some states separately define neglect and each major type of abuse (USDHHS Child Welfare Information Gateway, 2010).

Etiology

Family dysfunction underlies most forms of child abuse or neglect. The family profile varies with the type of abuse, although it is not uncommon for multiple types of abuse to exist in a single family. Generally, the dysfunctional family dynamics are multigenerational and involve both parents (Copeland, Keeler, Angold, & Costello, 2007) (Box 29-3).

Socioeconomic factors also appear to influence the incidence and etiology of child abuse, with increased physical abuse observed during

---

BOX 29-3 CHARACTERISTICS OF THE ABUSIVE FAMILY

- Isolation from community and social groups
- Intense competition for emotional resources within the family, such as affection, attention, and nurturing
- Low levels of differentiation among family members
- Low trust for outsiders and family members
- Unpredictable and unstable family environment
- Conflict resolution generally achieved through aggression or power struggle between family members
- Current focus and crisis-oriented actions for immediate gratification
- Communication often characterized by mixed or double messages, threats, or a focus on nonverbal communication rather than direct verbalization
- Family roles that are typically fixed and traditional, with rigid rules
- Frequent domination by a single family member who maintains control through manipulation, intimidation, deceit, and aggression

---

periods of economic hardship or external stress. The typical perpetrator is a direct relative of the child, usually the mother (40%) or father (20%), or both parents (18%) (USDHHS Child Welfare Information Gateway, 2010).

In sexual abuse, the perpetrator is more likely to be a family friend or neighbor (75.9%) compared with a parent (2.7%) (Jouriles, McDonald, & Slep et al., 2008). Perpetrators are most often males who may have mental health issues, cognitive distortions (rationalizing behavior), social skills and empathy deficits, and decreased coping skills; many were abused during childhood or adolescence (Center for Sex Offenders Management, 2011). The typical profile of an abused child is more difficult to determine. A substantial percentage of children (33%) who have been maltreated are younger than 4 years, with girls being abused more often than boys (USDHHS Child Welfare Information Gateway, 2010). Some research indicates that the child who is maltreated often has mild physical abnormalities, is developmentally or physically delayed, or has behavior problems.

Incidence

Child abuse reports to child protective services have increased. This increase has been attributed to public awareness, as well as increased awareness and willingness to report on the part of teachers and health care providers. In 2009, 60% of reports to child protective services nationwide were made by professionals (USDHHS Child Welfare Information Gateway, 2010).

In 2009, approximately 700,000 children were identified as victims of substantiated physical, sexual, or emotional abuse or neglect. Of those identified, 78.3% suffered from neglect, 17.8% were physically abused, 9.5% were sexually abused, and 7.6% were emotionally maltreated (USDHHS Child Welfare Information Gateway, 2010). The national rate of victimization is 12.4 in 1000 children (Shipman & Taussig, 2009).

Approximately 1500 children died from maltreatment in 2009. Eighty percent of children killed were younger than 4 years and 46.2% were younger than 1 year when they died (USDHHS Child Welfare Information Gateway, 2010).

Manifestations

Indicators of specific types of child abuse can be both physical and behavioral. The health provider needs to be aware that there may be more than one type of abuse occurring simultaneously in a given child.

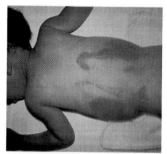
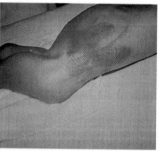

Nonaccidental distribution of bruises: All four surfaces of the torso are involved, but there are no bruises on arms and legs.

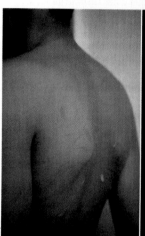
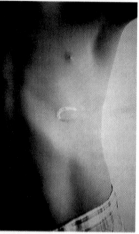
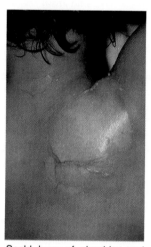

Pattern of injury: Linear scars of various ages indicate repeated abuse with a switch or a whip. The loop pattern on the boy's anterior torso is consistent with a looped electrical cord used as a whip.

Scald burn of shoulder and neck: The typical distribution of a scald burn in a toddler. This type of injury occurs when a toddler pulls a cup of coffee or pan of water off a stove.

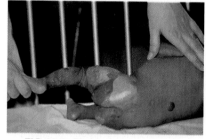

Nonaccidental immersion scald: Involvement of virtually the entire posterior surface of the legs indicates that the legs were held under scalding water; even an infant this young would flex the knees to avoid the hot water.

FIG 29-2 Physical signs of child abuse. The nurse should be alert for the typical behavioral indicators of abuse. (Courtesy Barbara Tenney, MD. From Henry, M. C., & Stapleton, E. R. [1992]. *EMT: Prehospital care* [p. 675]. Philadelphia: Saunders.)

Indicators of Physical Abuse

The physical signs that raise suspicion of physical abuse include the appearance of bruises, especially bruises in various stages of healing, bite marks, burns in unusual locations (e.g., back, palms of the hands) (Figure 29-2), or signs and symptoms of skeletal injury (e.g., multiple bone fractures). The child may be unwilling, unable, or too frightened to explain the origin of the injuries. The child's behavior might demonstrate wariness or fear of adults and, if in school, the child may resist going home. In some cases, the child may report an inflicted injury. Interview with the child's parents may reveal an inconsistent story about how the child sustained the injuries. Parents may demonstrate inconsistent or overly harsh discipline when interacting with the child (USDHHS Child Welfare Information Gateway, 2007). Adolescents who are physically abused may cope by running away.

Indicators of Neglect

Children experiencing neglect will most often show inadequate weight gain for age, poor growth pattern, and failure to thrive. Teachers may notice that the child comes to school inappropriately dressed for the weather (e.g., wearing shorts in winter, without shoes) or has signs of inadequate hygiene. The child may be lacking routine health care, such as immunizations or needed eyewear. Truancy may be a problem with neglected children. Children who are neglected may beg for money or steal food. The child may report being home alone for long periods of time unsupervised. Observation of parent-child interaction may reveal a parent who appears indifferent or unaware of the child's needs, or who demonstrates behaviors that indicate a possible emotional or substance disorder (USDHHS Child Welfare Information Gateway, 2007).

Indicators of Emotional Abuse

Signs of emotional abuse may include delays in both physical and emotional development. One hallmark of a child who is emotionally abused is that the child may behave in ways that are too adult in relation to the child's age (e.g., being protective of others), or too immature for age. Behavioral extremes (e.g., overly aggressive or overly compliant) are not unusual. The child may demonstrate repetitive habits, such as head banging, rocking, biting, and sucking. The parent-child relationship appears to lack warmth or attachment, and parents may demonstrate an overly critical approach. Children who are emotionally abused are at high risk for suicide (USDHHS Child Welfare Information Gateway, 2007).

Indicators of Sexual Abuse

The sexually abused child may exhibit difficulty walking or sitting and complain of pain on urination or in the genital area. Examination may reveal physical signs of bruising or laceration of perineal tissue (e.g., vaginal, anal) or the diagnosis of a sexually transmitted infection. Previously toilet-trained children may experience urinary accidents. Nightmares or other sleep disturbances, decreased appetite, sudden refusal to participate in gym or other physical activities, and overt aggression are also behavioral indicators. The child may exhibit signs of emotional distress or self-destructive behaviors. Sexually abused children may use sexual language and innuendo that is not appropriate for age; sexually abused adolescents may be promiscuous. Behavioral indicators in the parents include being overly protective, isolating the child from other children, or overly controlling behavior toward family members (USDHHS Child Welfare Information Gateway, 2007).

Children who are sexually abused may or may not report the abuse or may deny the abuse happened, even with direct questioning. Sometimes memories of childhood abuse surface years later. The manner in which disclosure of sexual abuse occurs has important legal implications because in the absence of physical signs, reliance is on the child's report. In 1983, Summit (as cited in London, Bruck, Wright, & Ceci, 2008) described how children often cope with sexual victimization through an accommodation syndrome in which the coping mechanisms become the child's normal behaviors in response to an abnormal event. There is nothing the child can do to prevent the abuse. The child may be reluctant to reveal the abuse because of shame or embarrassment or fear of alienation from family and others. In some cases, lack of or delayed disclosure or denial of abuse is directly related to fear that the child or a loved one will be punished (Summit as cited in London et al., 2008). Summit describes an initial strategy of secrecy, followed by assuming self-blame for the abuse, denial, delayed disclosure, or recantation after disclosure.

To empirically confirm Summit's theory, London et al. (2008) analyzed published studies of adults who had been abused as children and children who were undergoing forensic interviews about abuse. Their analysis confirms Summit's theories about denial and delayed disclosure, but not recantation. They found that children were more likely to delay disclosure if they were younger than 7 years old, were boys, or the abuse occurred within the family, but not necessarily because of the child's relationship with the perpetrator. The incidence of recantation was found to be low and more likely to be associated with accusations that were found to be unsubstantiated (London et al., 2008).

In addition to the preceding description of how the child may accommodate to sexual abuse, many sexually abused children, like other victims of severe child abuse, dissociate during the abuse to avoid feelings of physical pain, dissociation similar to that associated with posttraumatic stress syndrome (Cutajar et al., 2010).

Other Specific Abusive Situations

Shaken Infant Syndrome. Shaken infant, or shaken baby, syndrome is a widely recognized form of physical child abuse that is caused by vigorous shaking of the infant while the child is held by the extremities or shoulders. This type of physical abuse leads to whiplash-induced intracranial and retinal bleeding. There is generally no external sign of head trauma, which makes this syndrome difficult to detect (Mraz, 2009). Although there might not be any overt sign of head trauma, shaken infant syndrome should be considered in any infant with signs of increased intracranial pressure, with retinal hemorrhage, seizures, subtle hydrocephalus, and papilledema. Inconsistent caregiver report of the development of signs and symptoms, along with other signs of abuse, such as skeletal fracture should raise suspicion (Mraz, 2009). The most common trigger of severe shaking is crying, especially if the child is colicky.

Munchausen Syndrome by Proxy. Munchausen syndrome is a psychiatric disorder considered to be a factious disorder, a condition where people feign illness to gain attention. Munchausen syndrome by proxy occurs when a person with Munchausen syndrome falsifies illness in a child. Although considered to be a rare disorder, it may be the most difficult form of child abuse to diagnose. Most victims are children who are younger than school age.

The caretaker falsifies illness in the child through simulation or production of illness and then takes the child for medical care, claiming no knowledge of how the child became ill. The most common reasons these caretakers give for seeking medical treatment for the child are bleeding, seizures, CNS depression, apnea, diarrhea, vomiting, fever, and rash.

Some clinicians suggest that the syndrome be considered a form of medical abuse. Mortality rates are hard to estimate, but the long-term mortality rate in these cases is as high as 10% to 15%. Under the supervision of other adults, the child exhibits no symptoms and may appear normal and healthy. The parent's behavior reflects a serious disturbance that requires specialized psychiatric treatment and removal of the child from the parent's care. A multidisciplinary team is the best approach to diagnosing this disorder (Elder, Coletsos, & Bursztajn, 2010).

> ### ❓ CRITICAL THINKING EXERCISE 29-1
>
> Matthew, age 2 years, is brought to the emergency department by his mother, Ms. Jackson, and her boyfriend. Ms. Jackson tells the nurse that Matthew has been crying and holding his arm since she picked him up at the babysitter's earlier in the evening. On further questioning, Ms. Jackson states "Matthew is all boy. You have to watch him every minute or he is into something. He is constantly climbing and falling."
>
> On examination, the nurse notes several bruises on Matthew's right leg and right arm. He also has a small abrasion on his nose. Ms. Jackson is holding Matthew and seems concerned, as does her boyfriend. Matthew quiets when his mother holds him and drifts off to sleep. Ms. Jackson's boyfriend leaves the room and returns with a snack for both Matthew and Ms. Jackson. He offers to hold Matthew.
>
> 1. What are some of the possible reasons Matthew is crying and holding his arm? Support your assumptions with rationales.
> 2. If the nurse suspects child abuse, what added assessments should be performed?
> 3. What legal responsibility does the nurse have in cases of suspected child abuse?

◎ NURSING CARE PLAN

The Abused Child

Focused Assessment

- Examine the skin for any impaired integrity or bruising, especially of the scalp, bottoms of the hands and feet, front and back of the trunk, and genitalia.
- Obtain a baseline measurement of height and weight; document infant birth weight.
- Assess the child's anxiety level, ability to relate to the examiner, and emotional tone.
- Assess family supports: Patterns of interaction, belief systems, and social support systems.
- Unemotionally request information about bruises, injuries, and sexual abuse with particular attention to the child's need for privacy and dignity.
- Record the child's comments verbatim; these may be needed for legal proceedings later.
- Encourage the child to make self-care decisions and to discuss thoughts and feelings that might possibly have been repressed to survive the trauma (Figure 29-3); facilitate a supportive environment for the child and family.
- Recognize that the child may have low self-esteem, feelings of inadequacy, fear, and a possible desire to protect the perpetrator.
- Use an appropriate assessment tool to identify behaviors typical of a sexually abused child.
- Report any suspected abuse to the appropriate authorities.

Planning

Nursing Diagnosis

Impaired Parenting related to immaturity, lack of knowledge, apathy on the part of parental caregivers, or limited or negative past parenting experience.

Expected Outcome

The family will exhibit appropriate parenting skills, as evidenced by describing the aspects of positive parenting models and responding to the child's needs in a timely and appropriate manner.

Intervention/*Rationale*

1. Elicit information about the parents' strengths and weaknesses, normal coping mechanisms, and the presence or absence of support systems. Special attention should be paid to:
   a. Expectations with regard to the child
   b. Comforting behaviors
   c. Response to the child
   d. General knowledge about the child
   To provide optimal care for the child, involvement of the family is crucial. By understanding the needs of the family, the nurse can develop a plan of care, including referral to appropriate supportive agencies.
2. Discuss with the parents the parenting they received as children.
   Parenting is a learned behavior.
3. Observe the parents' interactions with the child.
   Although parents may verbalize a positive relationship with their child, observation of actual interactions provides a more realistic view of the parent-child relationship.
4. Provide an accepting environment.
   Communication is encouraged by demonstrating acceptance.
5. Provide information for parents regarding normal growth and development.
   Parents who are abusers often have unrealistic expectations of their children, in part because of their lack of knowledge regarding growth and development.
6. Include role modeling as a method of teaching parenting.

By observing the way the nurse touches and talks to the child in an affirming manner, the parents can observe firsthand the child's response to positive parenting-type skills.

7. Devote part of the time spent with the child and family to focusing on the child's positive attributes. For example:
   You might say "I appreciate how quietly you have played with your toys while I have been talking with mommy," or "Look at how nicely you are talking to your doll."
   Parents' negative perceptions of the child, which may be based on their own life experiences, can be altered by viewing the child through another's eyes.
8. Encourage the parents to participate in the child's care. Reinforce positive behaviors.
   Strategies that encourage and reinforce positive parental participation in child care build self-esteem and confidence in parenting skills.

Evaluation

Do the parents interact appropriately with the child through verbal, physical, and visual contact?
Have the parents described features of normal growth and development?
Do the parents make positive statements about the child?
Do the parents bring the child in for follow-up visits?

Planning

Nursing Diagnosis

Fear and/or Powerlessness related to the possible outcomes of disclosure, sense of shame, and possible loss of family.

Expected Outcomes

The child will verbalize the source of fear.
The child will express feelings related to shame and fear of loss of family.

Intervention/*Rationale*

1. Reassure the child in regard to personal safety.
   Verbal reassurance can provide a sense of security.
2. Identify specific strategies the child can use to maintain a sense of stability (i.e., stay with a trusted adult, refuse to answer intrusive questions, limit exposure to adults who are not trusted).
   By providing some viable options, the nurse can help the child begin to gain a sense of control over the experience.
3. Acknowledge the child's fear.
   Acknowledgment helps the child identify feelings and opens up new areas of communication.
4. Spend time with the child. Use both verbal and nonverbal forms of communication.
   Actions of support provide comfort and encourage verbalization of feelings.
5. Offer choices, when available, regarding activities of daily living, recreation time, and time with other children and adults.
   Being offered choices gives the child a sense of control and diminishes feelings of powerlessness.

Evaluation

Does the child participate in play activities?
Has the child verbalized specific fears related to abuse and disclosure?
Has the child verbalized fears related to being removed from the family?

NURSING CARE PLAN

The Abused Child—cont'd

Planning

Nursing Diagnosis

Deficient Knowledge about the child's realistic developmental abilities, how to access external support resources, or ways to manage internal and external stressors related to past inexperience with parenting.

Expected Outcomes

The family will increase knowledge related to growth and development, as evidenced by verbalization of an understanding of the child's developmental and emotional needs in a framework that is oriented to the child's welfare. The family will identify support systems.

Intervention/Rationale

1. Determine the parents' knowledge of child growth and development.
   A baseline assessment must be done to develop a plan of care.
2. Serve as a role model for positive parenting skills.
   Learning can be enhanced through observing the application of parenting skills, which is more effective than listening to a lecture.
3. Assist the family in identifying stressors and the support systems and resources that may help decrease the parents' stress level.
   If the parents' level of stress is decreased, the risk of abuse is decreased.
4. Refer the family to pertinent support groups, such as Parents Anonymous.
   Lack of support and isolation are common among abusive families. A support group may decrease isolation.
5. Involve the parents in the care of the child.
   Participation in care will provide opportunities for positive reinforcement, teaching, and increased emotional attachment to the child.
6. Provide education in the following areas: Growth and development, nutrition, care related to activities of daily living, routine well-child care, manifestations of illness, and need for care and loving.
   Education in parenting skills may decrease unrealistic expectations, increase awareness of the needs of children, and increase the chances of positive parenting. Parents may not have had positive parenting role models as children.
7. Provide a consistent caregiver from among the nursing staff.
   Consistency of care increases the child's feelings of trust and security and provides increased opportunities for the child to verbalize feelings.

Evaluation

Can the parents describe normal child growth and development and developmental expectations?

Have the parents joined a support group?

Planning

Nursing Diagnosis

Risk for Injury related to a family with a history of physical abuse, physical neglect, emotional abuse, or sexual abuse.

Expected Outcome

Injury related to abuse will cease, as evidenced by the child remaining free from physical or psychological injury and neglect.

Intervention/Rationale

1. Describe the child's physical and mental status.
   All children should undergo a thorough physical assessment on presentation to the health care setting and should be assessed for bruises, burns, scars, and other signs of abuse. Children may enter the health care system for reasons other than injury.
2. Observe the interactions between child and family.
   Subtle signs of abuse may be detected in the way the child interacts with the abuser and other adults.
3. Obtain a thorough history.
   Frequent presentation of the child for injuries or signs of healed injuries may indicate a pattern of abuse.
4. Use a nonthreatening, nonjudgmental manner when interacting with the child's parents.
   By building a trusting relationship with the parents, the nurse can help the child. If the parents become suspicious or alienated, they may deny the child access to health care. They will become defensive and will not be open to teaching.
5. Report all cases in which abuse is suspected.
   All 50 states require health care professionals to report all cases of suspected abuse.
6. Assist in removing children from an unsafe environment.
   Suspected abuse should be evaluated immediately so that the child can be removed to an environment that is safe, thereby preventing further injury.
7. Document the following: Results of the child's physical assessment, observations of interactions between the child and family and between the child and other adults and the child's reaction to hospitalization or the health care setting, direct comments made by the child and the family that pertain to the child or the child's injury, and child's developmental level.
   Objective documentation is essential in all cases of suspected abuse.
8. If the child is removed from the home, provide the child and family with support and opportunities to verbalize feelings. Play therapy may be used effectively with children.
   Children who are removed from the custody of their parents will grieve their loss. Parents will need support in dealing with guilt and loss.

Evaluation

Does the child remain free of inflicted injury?

Has the child been placed in a safe environment?

Has the child verbalized feelings regarding placement outside the home?

Has the family sought psychological counseling?

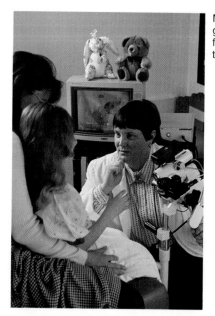

Note the communication techniques designed to reassure the child and give the child some power. The little girl is not immediately positioned for a genital examination. The health care provider first sits to talk with the child at her eye level and makes eye contact with her.

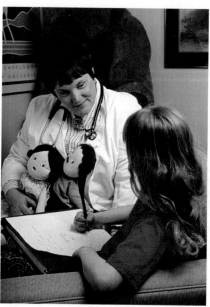

Drawings may help to identify the abused child and assist in therapy. Art can also help the child express what cannot be expressed in words.

FIG 29-3 Disclosure of abuse may be slow because the child often has difficulty trusting any adult. Physical examination and interview of children who may be victims of sexual abuse require particular sensitivity because physical inspection of the child's genitalia to detect signs of injury or sexually transmissible infection may frighten the child, who associates handling of the genitalia with pain or shame. Anatomically correct dolls are often used in the assessment of abuse within a family. These dolls help children express what they cannot express in words; young children in particular have a limited vocabulary to use when describing the events that have occurred. (Courtesy Cook Children's Medical Center, Fort Worth, TX.)

KEY CONCEPTS

- Childhood psychosocial disorders include emotional and behavioral disorders. It is sometimes difficult to differentiate between normal developmental behaviors and behaviors that precipitate a concern.
- Emotional disorders include anxiety disorders, such as social or separation anxiety, posttraumatic stress disorder, and obsessive-compulsive disorder; and disorders of mood that include depression, bipolar disorder, and adjustment disorder.
- Nursing care for a child with an emotional disorder and the child's family include facilitating coping, encouraging participation in regular activities, promoting self-esteem, facilitating sleep, and referral for counseling.
- Nurses should act quickly to assist any child who threatens to commit suicide. Support for grieving families of suicidal or potentially suicidal children or adolescents is best provided on both an individual and a group basis to allow exploration of personal issues and social support.
- Behavioral disorders of childhood include attention deficit–hyperactivity disorder and conduct disorder; nursing care for children with these disorders and their families includes promoting positive social interactions, protection from injury, and enhancing coping strategies.
- The focus of care for an adolescent with an eating disorder involves restructuring cognitive perceptions, reducing opportunities for engaging in ritualistic and self-injurious behaviors, and reestablishing physiologic homeostasis.
- Low grades, irregular school attendance, aggressive or rebellious behavior, deteriorating relationships with family members or former friends, rapid or extreme changes in behaviors or mood, and loss of interest in hobbies, sports, or other activities are some common signs of substance abuse.
- A child or adolescent with a substance abuse problem, together with the family, should receive help in developing social support systems, with referral to appropriate resources that can offer additional support as they attempt to make long-term changes in their social and emotional patterns of relating.
- Child abuse is categorized as physical, psychological, or sexual; child neglect is a form of maltreatment. All suspected cases of child abuse or neglect must be reported to the appropriate authorities.
- Child abuse often occurs when families are isolated with lack of supports, when parents have unrealistic expectations of child development, when families exhibit low levels of trust, and when they resolve conflicts through aggression.
- Role modeling positive parenting skills is an effective intervention in the care of the child who has been abused.

REFERENCES

American Academy of Child and Adolescent Psychiatry. (2007a). Practice parameters for the assessment and treatment of children and adolescents with anxiety disorders. *Journal of the American Academy of Child and Adolescent Psychiatry, 46*(2), 267-283.

American Academy of Child and Adolescent Psychiatry. (2007b). Practice parameters for the assessment and treatment of children and adolescents with depressive disorders. *Journal of the American Academy of Child and Adolescent Psychiatry, 46*(11), 1503-1525.

American Academy of Child and Adolescent Psychiatry. (2011). *Facts for families: When to seek help for your child.* Retrieved from www.aacap.org.

American Academy of Pediatrics. (2009). Increasing prevalence of neonatal withdrawal syndrome: Population study of maternal factors and child protection involvement. *Pediatrics, 123*(4), e614-e621.

American Psychiatric Association. (2000). *Diagnostic and statistical manual of mental disorders* (4th ed., Text revision). Washington, DC: Author.

American Psychiatric Association. (2006). *Practice guidelines for the treatment of patients with eating disorders* (3rd ed.). Washington, DC: Author.

Beers, N. (2010). *Developmental screens in the office setting.* Retrieved from www.aap.org.

Briggs-Gowan, M., & Carter, A. (2008). Social-emotional screening status in early childhood predicts elementary school outcomes. *Pediatrics, 121*, 957-962.

Carlo, W. (2011). Metabolic disturbances. In R. Kliegman, B. Stanton, J. St. Geme, et al. (Eds.), *Nelson textbook of pediatrics* (19th ed., pp. 823-825). Philadelphia: Elsevier Saunders.

Center for Sex Offenders Management. (2011). *Common characteristics of sex offenders.* Retrieved from www.csom.org.

Centers for Disease Control and Prevention. (2009). *Suicide: Facts at a glance.* Retrieved from www.cdc.gov.

Centers for Disease Control and Prevention. (2010a). *Attention-deficit/hyperactivity disorder (ADHD).* Retrieved from www.cdc.gov.

Centers for Disease Control and Prevention. (2010b). *Traumatic brain injury.* Retrieved from www.cdc.gov/TraumaticBrainInjury/index.html.

Centers for Disease Control and Prevention. (2010c). Youth risk behavior surveillance—United States, 2009. *MMWR, 59*(SS-5). Retrieved from www.cdc.gov.

Connolly, S., & Bernstein, G. (2007). Practice parameters for the assessment and treatment of children with anxiety disorders. *Journal of the American Academy of Child and Adolescent Psychiatry, 46*(2), 267-283.

Copeland, W. E., Keeler, G., Angold, A., & Costello, E. J. (2007). Traumatic events and posttraumatic stress in childhood. *Archives of General Psychiatry, 64*, 577-584.

Cutajar, M., Mullen, P., Ogloff, J., et al. (2010). Suicide and fatal drug overdose in child sexual abuse victims: A historical cohort study. *Medical Journal of Australia, 192*(4), 184-187.

Elder, W., Coletsos, I., & Bursztajn, H. (2010). Factitious disorder/Munchhausen syndrome. In F. Domino (Ed.), *The 5-minute clinical consult* (18th ed.). Philadelphia: Wolters Kluwer/Lippincott Williams & Wilkins.

Fay, T., Yeates, K., Drotar, D., et al. (2009). Predicting longitudinal patterns of functional deficits in children with traumatic brain injury. *Neuropsychology, 23*(3), 271-282.

Findling, R., Youngstrom, E., Fristad, M., et al. (2010). Characteristics of children with elevated symptoms of mania: The Longitudinal Assessment of Manic Symptoms (LAMS) study. *Journal of Clinical Psychiatry, 71*(12), 1664-1672.

Hamdan, A. (2010). *Neonatal abstinence syndrome.* Retrieved from http://emedicine.medscape.com.

Institute of Medicine (2009). *Preventing mental, emotional, and behavioral disorders among young people: Progress and possibilities.* Retrieved from www.iom.edu/Reports/2009/Preventing-Mental-Emotional-and-Behavioral-Disorders-Among-Young-People-Progress-and-Possibilities.aspx.

Johnston, L. D., O'Malley, P. M., Bachman, J. G., & Schulenberg, J. E. (2010). *Monitoring the future national results on adolescent drug use: Overview of key findings* (NIH Publication No. 10-7583). Bethesda, MD: National Institute on Drug Abuse.

Jouriles, E., McDonald, R., Slep, A., et al. (2008). Child abuse in the context of domestic violence. *Violence & Victims, 23*(2), 221-235.

Kaplan, H. I., & Sadock, B. I. (2007). *Synopsis of psychiatry: Behavioral sciences/clinical psychiatry* (10th ed.). Baltimore, MD: Wolters Kluwer/Lippincott Williams & Wilkins.

Kaye, W. (2007). Neurobiology of anorexia and bulimia nervosa. *Physiology & Behavior, 94*, 112-135.

Kerbeshian, J., Burd, L., & Tait, A. (2007). Chain reaction or time bomb: A neuropsychiatric-developmental/neurodevelopmental formulation of tourettisms. Pervasive developmental disorder, and schizophreniform symptomatology associated with PANDAS. *World Journal of Biological Psychiatry, 8*(3), 201-207.

Klump, K., Suisman, J., Burt, S. A., et al. (2009). Genetic and environmental influences on eating disorders: An adoption study. *Journal of Abnormal Psychology, 118*(4), 797-805.

Kreipe, R. (2011). Eating disorders. In R. Kliegman, B. Stanton, J. St. Geme, et al. (Eds.), *Nelson textbook of pediatrics* (19th ed., pp.90-98). Philadelphia: Elsevier Saunders.

London, K., Bruck, M., Wright, D., & Ceci, S. (2008). Review of the contemporary literature on how children report sexual abuse to others: Findings, methodological issues, and implications for forensic interviewers. *Memory, 16*(1), 29-47.

March, J., & Vitiello, B. (2009). Clinical messages from the Treatment for Adolescents with Depression Study (TADS). *American Journal of Psychiatry, 166*(10), 1118-1123.

Massachusetts General Hospital, School Psychiatry Program. (2010). Retrieved from http://www2.massgeneral.org/schoolpsychiatry/info_ocd.asp.

McDonnell, M., & Moffett, C. (2010). Coming into focus. Pharmacologic treatment for ADHD. *Advance for NPs and PAs, 1*(14), 16-23.

Merikangas, K., He, T., Burstein, M., et al. (2010). Lifetime prevalence of mental disorders in U.S. adolescents: Results from the National Comorbidity Survey Replication—Adolescent Supplement (NCS-A). *Journal of the American Academy of Child and Adolescent Psychiatry, 49*(10), 980-989.

Moscicki, E. (2009). Identification of suicide risk factors using epidemiologic studies. *Psychiatric Clinics of North America, 20*(3), 499-517.

Mraz, M. (2009). The physical manifestations of shaken baby syndrome. *Journal of Forensic Nursing, 5*(1), 26-30.

National Center for Health Statistics. (2011). Deaths and death rates for the 10 leading causes of death in specified age groups: United States preliminary 2009. *National Vital Statistics Reports, 59*(4), 52. Retrieved from www.cdc.gov/nchs.

National Children's Advocacy Center. (n.d.). *Physical and behavioral indicators of abuse.* Retrieved from www.nationalcac.org.

National Institute on Drug Abuse (2009). *Monitoring the future: National results on adolescent drug use.* National Institute of Health, Department of Health and Human Services. Retrieved from www.drugabuse.gov.

National Institute of Mental Health. (2010a). *Bipolar disorder in children and teens.* Retrieved from www.nimh.nih.gov.

National Institute of Mental Health. (2010b). *Child and adolescent bipolar disorder: An update from the National Institute of Mental Health.* Retrieved from www.nimh.nih.gov/statistics/1BIPOLAR_CHILD.

National Institute of Mental Health. (2010c). *Eating disorders.* Retrieved from www.nimh.hih.gov.

National Institute of Mental Health. (2010d). *Major depressive disorder in children.* Retrieved from www.nimh.nih.gov/statistics/1MDD_CHILD.

National Institute of Mental Health. (2010e). *Suicide in the U.S., statistics and prevention.* Retrieved from www.mentalhealth.gov.

National Research Council and Institute of Medicine. (2009). Preventing mental, emotional, and behavioral disorders among young people: Progress and possibilities. In E. O. Connell, T. Boat, & K. Warner (Eds.), *Board on Children, Youth, and Families, Division of Behavioral and Social Sciences and Education.* Washington, DC: National Academies Press.

Nielsen, S. (2010). Epidemiology and mortality of eating disorders. *Psychiatric Clinics of North America, 24*(2), 201-214.

O'Donnell, M., Nassar, N., Leonard, H., et al. (2009). Increasing prevalence of neonatal withdrawal syndrome: Population study of maternal factors and child protection involvement. *Pediatrics, 123*(4), 614-621.

Pull, C. B. (2007). Combined pharmacotherapy and cognitive-behavioral therapy for anxiety disorders. *Current Opinions in Psychiatry, 20*(1), 30-35.

Queen, A. (2010). *Screening for adolescent panic disorder in pediatrics settings* (Master's thesis). Retrieved from http://scholarlyrepository.miami.edu/oa_theses/68.

Raishevich Cunningham, N., & Jensen, P. (2011). Attention-deficit/hyperactivity disorder. In R. Kliegman, B. Stanton, J. St. Geme, et al. (Eds.), *Nelson textbook of pediatrics* (19th ed., pp.108-112). Philadelphia: Elsevier Saunders.

Rosen, D. (2010). Identification and management of eating disorders in children and adolescents. *Pediatrics, 125*(6), 1240-1253.

Rosenberg, D., Vandana, P., & Chiriboga, J. (2011). Anxiety disorders. In R. Kliegman, B. Stanton, J. St. Geme, et al. (Eds.). *Nelson textbook of pediatrics* (19th ed., pp. 77-82). Philadelphia: Elsevier Saunders.

Schneeweiss, S. Patrick, A. R., Solomon, D. H., et al. (2010). Comparative safety of antidepressant agents for children and adolescents regarding suicidal acts. *Pediatrics, 125*, 876-888.

Schrag, A., Gilbert, R., Giovannoni, G., et al. (2009). Streptococcal infection, Tourette syndrome and OCD, is there a connection? *Neurology, 73*(16), 1256-1263.

Schub, E., & Davidson, H. (2010). *Evidence-based care sheet: Neonatal abstinence syndrome.* Glendale, CA: CINAHL Information Systems.

Shipman, K., & Taussig, H. (2009). Treatment of child abuse and neglect: The promise of evidence-based practice. *Pediatric Clinics of North America, 56*, 417-428.

Shulman, S. (2009). Pediatric autoimmune neuropsychiatric disorders associated with streptococci (PANDAS): Update. *Current Opinion in Pediatrics, 21*(1), 127-130.

Stein, M., & Stein, D. (2008). Social anxiety disorder. *Lancet, 371*(9618), 1115-1125.

Suicide Prevention Resource Center. (2008). *Suicide risk and prevention for lesbian, gay, bisexual, and transgender youth.* Newton, MA: Educational Development Center Inc.

Takashi, L. (2010). Neurobiology of schizophrenia, mood disorders, and anxiety disorders. In K. McCance, S. Huether, V. Brashers, & N. Rote (Eds.), *Pathophysiology* (6th ed., pp. 646-664). St. Louis: Elsevier Mosby.

Tishler, C., Reiss, N., & Rhodes, A. (2008). Suicidal behavior in children younger than twelve: A diagnostic challenge for emergency department personnel. *Academic Emergency Medicine, 14*(9), 810-818.

U.S. Department of Health and Human Services. (2010). *Healthy People 2020: Mental health and mental disorders.* Retrieved from www.healthypeople.gov.

U.S. Department of Health and Human Services Child Welfare Information Gateway. (2007). *Recognizing child abuse and neglect: Signs and symptoms.* Retrieved from http://www.childwelfare.gov/pubs/factsheets/signs.cfm.

U.S. Department of Health and Human Services Child Welfare Information Gateway. (2010). *Child maltreatment 2009.* Retrieved from www.acf.hhs.gov/programs/cb/pubs/cm09/cm09.pdf.

U.S. Department of Health and Human Services & National Institute on Drug Abuse. (2010). *Monitoring the future: National results on adolescent drug use. Overview of key findings 2009.* Retrieved from www.drugabuse.gov.

U.S. Department of Health and Human Services & Office of the Surgeon General. (2007). *The Surgeon General's call to action to prevent and reduce underage drinking.* Retrieved from www.surgeongeneral.gov/topics/underagedrinking/calltoaction.pdf.

U.S. Department of Health and Human Services & Substance Abuse and Mental Health Services Administration. (2009, May 21). *The NSDUH Report: Substance use among women during pregnancy and following childbirth.* Retrieved from www.oas.samhsa.gov.

U.S. Department of Health and Human Services & Substance Abuse and Mental Health Services Administration. (2010). *Report from the 2009 National Survey on Drug Use and Health. Volume I: Summary of national findings.* Retrieved from www.oas.samhsa.gov.

U.S. Department of Veterans Affairs. (2010). *National Center for PTSD.* Retrieved from www.ptsd.va.gov.

Waldinger, R., Vaillant, G., & Orav, E. (2007). Childhood sibling relationships as a predictor of major depression in adulthood: A 30 year prospective study. *American Journal of Psychiatry, 164*(6), 949-954.

Walter, H., & Damaso, D. (2011). Mood disorders. In R. Kliegman, B. Stanton, J. St. Geme, et al. (Eds.), *Nelson textbook of pediatrics* (19th ed., pp. 82-85). Philadelphia: Elsevier Saunders.

Weissman, M., Wickramaratne, P., Nomura, Y., et al. (2006). Offspring of depressed parents: 20 years later. *American Journal of Psychiatry, 163*, 1001-1008.

Wintersteen, M. (2010). Standardized screening for suicidal adolescents in primary care. *Pediatrics, 125*, 938-944.

Wintersteen, M., Diamond, G., & Fein, J. (2007). Screening for suicide risk in the pediatric emergency and acute care setting. *Current Opinions in Pediatrics, 19*(4), 398-404.

Yan, J. (2009). Children taking ADHD medication do better on math, reading tests. *Clinical & Research News, American Psychiatric Association, 44*(12), 2.

Yantis, M. A., & Velender, R. (2008). How to recognize and respond to refeeding syndrome. *Nursing, 38*(5), 34-39.

Yoshimasu, K., Barbaresi, W., Colligan, R., et al. (2010). Gender, attention-deficit/hyperactivity disorder, and reading disability in a population-based birth cohort. *Pediatrics, 126*(4), e788-e795.

The Child with a Developmental Disability

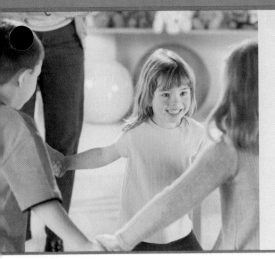

⊖volve WEBSITE

http://evolve.elsevier.com/James/ncoc

LEARNING OBJECTIVES

After studying this chapter, you should be able to:
- Define the concepts of maturational and developmental disorders, including intellectual disability, developmental disorders, and autism spectrum disorders.
- Develop understanding of the use of the terms *intellectual disability* versus *mental retardation.*
- Identify the various causes of intellectual and developmental disabilities.
- Identify educational and support resources for families with a child who has an intellectual disability or developmental delay.
- Develop appropriate nursing strategies for supporting the family and child with an intellectual disability or developmental delay.
- Develop nursing strategies for families caring for a child with Down syndrome.

- Identify behavioral characteristics and appropriate nursing actions when working with a child with fragile X syndrome.
- Identify characteristics and appropriate nursing interventions for an infant with fetal alcohol syndrome, and appropriate family assessment and intervention.
- Identify the basic diagnostic criteria for the autism spectrum disorders.
- Identify genetic aspects of intellectual and developmental disorders.
- Identify the major considerations in working with the family of a child with an intellectual or developmental disorder or disability.
- Develop home care interventions appropriate to the family's abilities and to the developmental needs of a child with an intellectual or developmental disorder or disability.

CLINICAL REFERENCE

GENETICS AND GENOMICS

The sequencing of the human genome opened a new window in our understanding of human traits, skills, and disabilities. Genetic breakthroughs will require nurses to be active participants in using genetic information in all aspects of providing patient care (American Association of Colleges of Nursing, 2008). Some nursing activities will include assessment of genotypes, identification of signs of developmental or intellectual disorders, referral for care, and education of patients and families with the goal of maximizing individual development (Goldberg, Jenkins, & Spahis, 2010). A number of resources are

available for nurses to gain essential knowledge and skill in the area of genetics (De Sevo, 2010) (see Chapter 4).

Various aspects of genetics influence the discussion of most of the disorders covered in this chapter. The human genome is the full set of DNA instructions that creates the characteristics of a human. However, the human genome has innumerable small variations, called genotypes. Genotypes are small variations in specific parts of the genome's DNA sequences. These small changes account for the phenotype—the visible differences in eye color, skin color, height, and every other observable physical characteristic. The term genotype may describe large groups of people who share common physical characteristics,

CLINICAL REFERENCE

COMMON DIAGNOSTIC TESTS FOR INTELLECTUAL AND DEVELOPMENTAL DISORDERS

DESCRIPTION/PURPOSE	NORMAL FINDINGS	INDICATIONS	NURSING IMPLICATIONS
Vision Test Assessment of vision, ocular pressure, and structural defects	Normal vision, normal structures	Children with Down syndrome; 40%-45% have refractive errors, cataracts, or other visual problems.	Explain pupil dilation. Provide protective eyewear after examinations.
Hearing Test Assessment of perception of sound frequency and volume	Normal hearing range	Children with Down syndrome; 70%-80% have hearing defects. Children with autism and PDD often appear to have defective hearing despite normal hearing function, so hearing tests should be conducted.	Explain the test in simple terms. The test may require that the child wear a headphone, which may be difficult to tolerate.
Thyroid Studies Blood serum tests to determine thyroid levels—serum thyroxine	Ages 1-3 yr: 6.8-13.5 µg/dL Ages 3-10 yr: 5.5-12.8 µg/dL Puberty to adulthood: 4.2-13.0 µg/dL	Children with Down syndrome; slowed growth rates are common.	These studies should not be performed within 7 days of a radionuclide scan.
Adaptive Behavior Scales* Assessment of language, motor, social, and self-care skills	Age-expected skills within 1 SD from mean	Children with suspected developmental delays.	Explain the test and how results will be interpreted.
IQ Tests† Assessment of intellectual abilities	Age-normal skills within 1½ SD from the mean	Children with suspected developmental delays.	Explain the test and how results will be interpreted.
Bone Roentgenography Assessment of bone plates and joint spaces	Age-expected bone age	Children with Down syndrome; decreased growth rate is common; children with Down syndrome have atlantoaxial instability.	The child must be motionless during the study; cervical spine radiographs should be done for all children with Down syndrome at a young age and before they participate in athletics.
Brain Sonography Ultrasonogram of cranium	Normal position of brain's midline structures and normal blood flow velocity, no hemorrhages	Microcephaly or macrocephaly, misshapen cranium, family history of hydrocephaly.	The child must be supine. Any jewelry or metal objects should be removed from the child's head. The child may need sedation or may need to be restrained, because this procedure takes 1 hr to complete. Explain to the child that the test is not painful. Keep the child warm during the procedure.
Genetic Analysis Cytogenic bonding, culture media analysis	Normal findings for gene product analysis	Suspected genetic or neoplastic disorders.	Allow the child and family an opportunity to ask questions and express concerns about the possible results and implications of the testing.
Computed Tomography Special noninvasive radiographic technique that images brain tissue in very thin sections	No blood clots, tumors, or infections	Impaired development, such as microcephaly; family history of CNS malformations; possible tumors or subdural hematomas.	The child may need to be sedated or restrained and will need to assume supine position. Scans require the use of contrast medium so require informed consent.
Magnetic Resonance Imaging Noninvasive method used to create images corresponding to density of tissue	Normal anatomy and physiology of the brain and spinal column	Same as for computed tomography.	The test requires informed consent. Remove metal or magnetic objects from the child before the study. Sedation of the child is usually required.

COMMON DIAGNOSTIC TESTS FOR INTELLECTUAL AND DEVELOPMENTAL DISORDERS—cont'd

DESCRIPTION/PURPOSE	NORMAL FINDINGS	INDICATIONS	NURSING IMPLICATIONS
Positron Emission Tomography			
Noninvasive means of comparing cerebral brain flow and metabolic changes; used to localize seizure foci, visualize brain hemodynamics, and study brain pharmacology using radioisotopes	Normal metabolism of glucose in brain, normal blood flow and electrical activity	Seizures, hydrocephaly, evidence of cerebral dysfunction.	The test requires informed consent. The child will need to be sedated. Liquids may be limited before the procedure. If not in diapers, the child will need to void before the procedure. Parents may be able to remain with the child during the procedure.

CNS, Central nervous system; *PDD,* pervasive developmental disorder; *SD,* standard deviation.
*Adaptive behavior scales include the AAMR test, the Minnesota Child Development Inventory Profile, the DDST-II, the Wechsler Preschool and Primary Scale of Intelligence (WPPSI), the Wechsler Intelligence Scale for Children (WISC-III), and the Wechsler Adult Intelligence Scale—Revised (WAIS-R).
†IQ tests include the Bayley Scales (birth to 3 yr), the Stanford-Binet Scale (2 yr and older), the WPPSI (3-6 yr), the WISC-III (6-16 yr), and the WAIS-R (16 yr and older).

or phenotypes. The phenotype is the visible representation of the genotype.

Changes *(mutations)* in a specific stretch of DNA occur through deletion, addition, or recopying. Some of these mutations do not result in any change in the individual's appearance or functioning. However, some small mutations create enormous negative effects in cell and individual development. These small mutations are the underlying cause of the intellectual and developmental disabilities that will be discussed in this chapter. Some of these genetic changes affect intellectual ability; some affect physical development.

INTELLECTUAL AND DEVELOPMENTAL DISORDERS

Children who have intellectual or developmental disorders experience genetic or external influences that may limit their potential abilities. However, these potential limits will be minimized or maximized by their interaction with the environment. Many intellectual or developmental disorders will respond to early and intensive intervention and close attention. However, children and families face lifelong challenges that require assistance from both health care and educational professionals to maximize the child's developmental potential. The family of a child with an intellectual or developmental impairment copes with frequent and exceptionally high demands, often including chronic medical and educational challenges that require lifelong management. Independence and self-management should be emphasized throughout childhood and adolescence so that, as the individual reaches adulthood, the possibility of independent living and gainful employment can be maximized.

Developmental Disability and the Americans with Disabilities Act: The Impact of Public Policy

Historically, intellectual, sensory, and developmental disorders were considered to be distinct, although overlapping syndromes. In recent years the term *developmental disability* has become an umbrella term to encompass children with intellectual disability, sensory deficits (hearing, vision, and speech), orthopedic problems, and conditions such as cerebral palsy and autism spectrum disorders. Uniting these disorders under the term *developmental disability* has important legal and policy implications because it unites a number of people who have similar psychosocial and developmental disorders and similar needs for services. From a health policy perspective, united groups are more powerful in gaining legislative and policy recognition. This effort was successful in the passage and enactment of the Developmental Disabilities Assistance and Bill of Rights Act of 2000 (PL 106-402) (2000). The purpose of this act is to attempt to ensure equal rights and accessibilities for all disabled individuals.

In this bill, the United States Congress defined a developmental disability as having the following components (Developmental Disabilities Assistance and Bill of Rights Act of 2000):

- Severe and chronic disability that is attributable to mental or physical impairment or a combination of both
- The impairment must be present before the individual turns 22 years old
- The impairment is likely to continue, reflecting the need for lifelong individual services or support
- There must be substantial functional limitations in three or more areas, such as self-care, receptive and expressive language, learning, mobility, self-direction, capacity for independent living, or economic self-sufficiency

As a result of this bill, and also of earlier legislative efforts, such as the Individuals with Disabilities Education Act (IDEA) of 1997, every disabled child must have a written Individualized Education Plan (IEP) that outlines specialized instruction and services the public school system will provide. The child's parents and school personnel design the plan following an educational assessment. School nurses often participate in IEP evaluations, providing expert advice about classroom adaptations or medical services needed for these children. When working with these children, teachers, families, and communities, the nurse may serve as a resource for identifying advocacy services.

Nursing goals when caring for children with an intellectual or developmental disorder or disability include accurate assessment of the specific cause and nature of the disorder or disability, and the identification of possible co-morbidities and risk factors. Complete information enables the nurse to plan interventions that will maximize the child's development and adaptive functioning. Nursing care in this specialty area always includes assessment, referral, education and follow-up, and advocacy for the child and family members.

Intellectual and developmental disorders are frequently co-morbid, with both occurring together. These children are also at risk for psychosocial disorders. For example, a child who is diagnosed with Asperger syndrome is at risk for symptoms of depression. In the same manner, children who are diagnosed with autism frequently also show symptoms of intellectual disability.

The nurse is an integral part of the multidisciplinary team that manages the care of a child with a developmental disorder. The nurse is involved in early assessment of the child, support of the family, assistance with self-care training and behavioral training, referral to support services, and providing the necessary nursing care for other disabilities the child may have. School and community nurses need a broad range of knowledge to support children who have multiple intellectual and physical disabilities.

The first section of this chapter reviews intellectual impairment disorders (formerly referred to as disorders associated with mental retardation). The considerations in the care of a child with Down syndrome will illustrate nursing care for children with intellectual disabilities. The second section of the chapter gives an overview of developmental disorders that have clear genetic causes (fragile X syndrome, Rett syndrome). The third section looks at developmental disorders where the cause is related to environmental or prenatal toxins (fetal alcohol syndrome). The last section examines the autism spectrum disorders. The nursing care for a child with autism will demonstrate considerations in planning care that promotes maximal development for all children with developmental disorders and their capability to move through the expected stages of childhood development.

Terminology
Mental Age, Functional Age, Adaptive Functioning
Children with developmental disabilities have impairments in motor skills or sensory ability that may be minor and manageable, or they may demonstrate significant impairment in intellectual, functional, and adaptive development. *Mental age* and functional age are terms used to compare a child's current ability with children of the same chronologic age. These terms are generally more useful than references to the intelligent quotient (IQ), which can be misleading, especially for children with language disabilities. Mental age gives the caregiver information regarding level of intellectual understanding. For example, if an individual has a mental age of 5 years, the nurse's explanations should be simple and specific, regardless of chronologic age. However, if the individual has a mental age of 12 years, the nurse's explanations can be complex and use some abstractions. Functional age refers to the level of *adaptive function*, the level of coping that a child has developed that supports activities of daily living (ADLs), communication skills, and social skills (American Association on Intellectual and Developmental Disabilities [AAIDD], 2011). Maximizing the child's adaptive function by supporting identified strengths and supplementing weak

areas will allow the child to develop realistically to full potential (AAIDD, 2011). It is possible for a child with a low mental age to function well beyond what would be expected. This is an example of a high level of adaptive functioning.

Intellectual Impairment and Intellectual Disability
Intellectual impairment is a descriptive term that denotes a significant limitation in both intellectual and functional capacity. This means that the impairment manifests in measured intelligence (IQ) and also in adaptive behavior. Intellectual impairment distinguishes intellectual or cognitive deficits from specific, limited sensory deficits (e.g., vision, hearing). It also differentiates emotional or psychological disability. Specific intellectual impairments are considered through assessment of language, cognition, academic ability, self-help skills, social behaviors, and motor performance.

The term is used to describe conditions that originate before the age of 18, with significant evidence of below-average intellectual functioning and adaptive functioning in areas such as communication, ability to work, home living, community use, health and safety, leisure, self-care, social skills, self-direction, functional academics, or work abilities (AAIDD, 2011). The level of intellectual disability may be mild, moderate, severe, or profound. Intellectual impairment can result from genetic mutations that cause malformations of the brain and central nervous system (CNS), or it may result from injury, infection, anoxia, poisoning, prenatal alcohol use, brain trauma, accidents, Down syndrome, or other inherited disorders. In some cases the cause may be unknown.

Children with intellectual disabilities require support and interventions to acquire self-care and adaptive skills; however, many children are educated, hold a job, and independently accomplish some self-care activities (Centers for Disease Control and Prevention [CDC], 2009; National Dissemination Center for Children with Disabilities, 2011).

Intellectual Impairment versus Mental Retardation
Intellectual impairment has replaced the term *mental retardation* (MR) to describe people with below-average general intellectual functioning. Over time "mental retardation" has generally been removed as a clinical classification, and the term was formally removed from the Individuals with Disabilities Education Act in 2010 (National Dissemination Center for Children with Disabilities, 2011). This is a significant decision, and a number of rationales were cited for the change, including the scientific inaccuracy of the term *retardation* and the stigma associated with the term (AAIDD, 2011). As a result of this change in clinical classification, the American Association on Mental Retardation (AAMR) voted to change the name of its organization (and its publications) to the American Association on Intellectual and Developmental Disabilities (AAIDD, 2011).

Autism Spectrum Disorders versus Pervasive Developmental Disorders
Pervasive developmental disorders (PDD) vary widely in etiology and level or type of impairment. They are termed *spectrum disorders* because the range of impairment can be mild or severe.

Some of the PDDs are clear genetic disorders such as Rett syndrome, fragile X syndrome, and Down syndrome. These disorders are characterized by recognizable physical characteristics and usually by impairment in physical development and cognition, as well as by significant intellectual impairment.

The PDD classification also includes the autism spectrum disorders (ASDs), where genetic influence is likely, but less definitive. The ASDs include attention deficit disorder (ADD), attention deficit–hyperactivity disorder (ADHD), Asperger syndrome, and autism. A third group within the PDD classification represents disorders that result from toxins or prenatal influences, such as fetal alcohol syndrome.

Although these disorders are different in origin, they remain linked in the *Diagnostic and Statistical Manual of Mental Disorders* (4th ed., Text revision). The expected release of the DSM-V in 2013 may clarify some of these classifications (American Psychiatric Association [APA], 2000).

The PDDs discussed in this chapter include Rett syndrome, fragile X syndrome, fetal alcohol syndrome, failure to thrive, and the autism spectrum disorders of Asperger syndrome and autism. ADD and ADHD are discussed in Chapter 29.

Etiology of Intellectual Disabilities and Pervasive Developmental Disorders

These disorders may be the result of genetic mutations, prenatal environment, or congenital or early environmental factors such as maternal substance abuse or lack of stimulation in early childhood. They may also be the result of head injury, asphyxia, intracranial hemorrhage, infections, poisoning, or the presence or treatment of a brain tumor. Developmental disorders have more than 350 known causes, but a specific cause is unknown in nearly half of all diagnosed cases. New etiologies are being identified, and underlying mechanisms of known causes are becoming more clearly understood.

As medical technology advances, a medical basis for intellectual and adaptive impairments is found in an increasing proportion of intellectually impaired children. Often the cause is a subtle but nonetheless significant biologic factor, such as minor chromosomal abnormalities, rare genetic syndromes, subclinical lead intoxication, nutritional deficiencies, or exposure to numerous prenatal risks or trauma. Evidence suggests that early intervention programs that promote neurodevelopment can show benefit for later neurologic integrity and intellectual ability. Low socioeconomic status and related factors have also been consistently reported as influencing intellectual function (Box 30-1).

Incidence of Intellectual and Developmental Disorders

In the United States it is estimated that a PDD is diagnosed in approximately 1 of 150 children. Boys are more likely to be diagnosed with PDD than are girls (Cole, 2008; Rizzolo & Cerciello, 2009). Families with children or adolescents who are mildly or moderately impaired are likely to care for children at home. An increased incidence of intellectual disability is reported in the early school years, and then the incidence declines in late adolescence as the children leave the formal education setting and are assimilated into the adult world. Most intellectually impaired individuals are able to marry (often to individuals with normal intellectual functioning), maintain employment, and have satisfying relationships.

Psychiatric co-morbidity is common in people with both intellectual and developmental disorders, probably because underlying conditions that cause intellectual disabilities also affect areas of the brain that regulate emotional state. The most frequent accompanying diagnoses include disruptive behavioral disorders, depression, and atypical psychosis. Prevalence estimates for co-morbidity between psychosocial disorders and developmental disorders are up to 60% to 70%, but the incidence is lower in children and adolescents compared with adults with developmental disorders (Sadock & Sadock, 2008).

Developmental disorders may increase risk for child abuse. According to the Administration on Children, Youth, and Families, 11.1% of all reported child abuse cases involved children with disabilities, including developmental disabilities (U.S. Department of Health and Human Services [USDHHS], 2010a). Possible reasons for this strong

---

BOX 30-1 CAUSES OF INTELLECTUAL DISABILITY

Genetic
- *Inborn errors of metabolism:* Galactosemia, Tay-Sachs disease, phenylketonuria
- *Hereditary syndromes:* Muscular dystrophy, tuberous sclerosis, neurofibromatosis
- *Chromosomal aberrations:* Down syndrome, fragile X syndrome (leading cause of intellectual disability)

Alterations Occurring during Pregnancy
- *Sporadic chromosomal changes:* Down syndrome
- *Intrauterine infections:* Congenital rubella, toxoplasmosis, herpes
- *Exposure to environmental toxins:* Fetal alcohol syndrome, drug exposure
- *Fetal malnutrition:* Placental insufficiency, pregnancy-induced hypertension, maternal uterine cancer, multiple pregnancy

Neonatal Alterations
- *Prematurity*
- *Neonatal asphyxia*
- *Other conditions present at birth:* Hyperbilirubinemia, hypoglycemia, CNS hemorrhage, ABO incompatibilities

Acquired Childhood Conditions or Diseases
- *Complications of infections:* Meningitis, encephalitis, pertussis, varicella
- *Lead or other poisoning*
- *Central nervous system alterations:* Trauma, infection, tumors
- *Cardiac arrest*
- *Asphyxiation*

Environmental Problems
- *Psychosocial deprivation*
- *Poverty and inadequate health care*
- *Parental neurosis, psychosis, character disorder*
- *Childhood psychosis, autism, other pervasive developmental disorders*

Unknown Causes

Data from American Psychiatric Association. (2000). *Diagnostic and statistical manual of mental disorders* (4th ed., Text revision). Washington, DC: The Association; The Arc. (2009). *Causes and prevention of intellectual disabilities.* Retrieved from www.thearc.org; National Dissemination Center for Children with Disabilities. (2009). *Intellectual disability fact sheet.* Retrieved from www.nichcy.org.

---

relationship are the intense stress experienced by families of disabled children, parental isolation, and unrealistic expectations for the child's performance because of a lack of knowledge about normal growth and development. Despite available funding and support groups, families of children with developmental delays often feel isolated from supportive services and report that professionals have limited understanding of their children's needs. These factors further perpetuate the sense of helplessness and lack of control in these family systems, leading to a climate with a heightened potential for abusive behaviors.

Manifestations

The cardinal sign for the developmental disorders is delayed achievement of developmental milestones. Specific congenital malformations often result in specific clinical manifestations. Also, the severity of the impairment affects the types and frequency of problem behaviors (Box 30-2).

EVIDENCE-BASED PRACTICE

Supporting the Family of a Child with a Disability Evidence

Level VI

Having a child who has a physical, developmental, or intellectual disability is challenging for parents, particularly if the child will require lifelong care and support. Parents must adjust not only to the child's diagnosis but also to the long-term implications that their child's disability will have for social, emotional, and educational outcomes. Often referred to as the "burden of care," these parenting challenges involve generalized uncertainty about how to maximize the child's health and developmental outcomes within a climate of unpredictability.*

Nurses, in both community and acute-care settings, can assist parents in various ways, through care, advocacy, and provision of support. Lindblad, Rasmussen, and Sandman (2005) suggest that providing support is an essential nursing intervention; however, in assessing what would constitute meaningful support, the nurse must first determine types of support parents believe they need. To this end, Lindblad, Rasmussen, and Sandman conducted a qualitative research study whose purpose was explore how parents of disabled children perceive receiving support from health professionals.

Unlike quantitative research, qualitative phenomenologic research explores a specific phenomenon in depth to gain a better understanding of its meaning to the participants. Lindblad, Rasmussen, and Sandman (2005) interviewed parents in 10 families and asked them to describe their experiences of being supported by health professionals. The authors recorded the interviews and later analyzed transcripts to identify relevant themes of support.

Overall, parents described increased support as that which assisted them with their daily burden and resulted in increased self-confidence in parenting a disabled child. Conversely, they described decreased support as devaluing their child, minimizing their daily struggles, and decreasing their parenting self-confidence. Actions by health professionals that were seen by parents as disempowering included ignoring the parents' needs, minimizing their contributions to the child's care, focusing exclusively on the child's disability, viewing the child as being unworthy of assistance, and being unhelpful with the management of the daily burden.* The authors suggest that unsupportive professionals can provoke confrontational and oppositional parenting strategies as the parents attempt to protect themselves and their child from perceived lack of caring.

Parents in this study described affirming issues such as recognizing the parents as individuals with their own needs and methods of coping, not just as being a parent of a disabled child; taking the time to establish and continue a trusting relationship; acknowledging parents as the experts in their child's care; being available and open for questions; assisting with referrals and information about legal rights; recognizing and valuing the child as a unique individual through effective communication with the child; and focusing on the child and not the disability. These constituted effective strategies of support that increased parents' self-confidence and empowered them.

After reading about this research on how parents perceive support, think about how you can improve the support you can provide to parents, whether you will practice in an acute-care setting or in the community. What specific strategies might you use, for example, when admitting a child with a disability to a hospital unit or when communicating with parents in a school setting?

*Lindblad, B., Rasmussen, B., & Sandman, P. (2005). Being invigorated in parenthood: Parents' experiences of being supported by professionals when having a disabled child. *Journal of Pediatric Nursing, 20*, 288-297.

BOX 30-2 PROBLEMS RELATED TO INTELLECTUAL DISABILITY

Mild
- Self-esteem issues related to presence or absence of physical features, largely determined by the cause of the intellectual disability
- Social isolation and loneliness
- Depression

Severe
- Self-injury
- Fecal smearing
- Tearing of personal clothes and objects
- Severe temper tantrums
- Disrobing

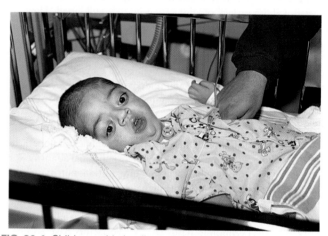

FIG 30-1 Children with intellectual impairments may have other dysfunctions as well. The family of a child with an intellectual impairment often feels continual grief because the child does not meet their expectations. This child has additional dysfunctions that require respiratory and nutritional support. (Courtesy Children's Medical Center, Dallas, TX.)

In addition to general clinical manifestations based on the degree of impairment, many syndromes are characterized by features that are helpful in determining the cause of the disability. Two genetic disorders in which intellectual disability is a central feature are Down syndrome and fragile X syndrome. An infant born with fetal alcohol syndrome (FAS) will show both intellectual and developmental disorders and also specific physical growth, facial, skeletal, and cardiac features.

Many disorders associated with intellectual disability can further limit a child's adaptive skills. These include cerebral palsy, visual deficits, seizure disorders, communication deficits, feeding problems, autism spectrum disorders, failure to thrive, and attention-deficit hyperactivity disorder. Speech and language development are often profoundly affected. Depending on the condition, seizure disorders frequently develop as the child matures.

Although children who are intellectually impaired can be generally physically healthy, the presence of associated disabilities may place these children at increased risk for illness (Figure 30-1). For example, if a child who is intellectually impaired also has cerebral palsy, the risk for gastroesophageal reflux and aspiration pneumonia is high. Motor or swallowing problems may result in inadequate oral intake or insufficient weight gain.

Diagnostic Evaluation

Diagnostic evaluations may be performed during pregnancy, during the neonatal period (based on risk factors), or after the child fails to achieve expected developmental milestones. Early identification is important so that early intervention treatment plans can be established. Tests may be general or specific for the neurologic or intellectual area in question. Several tests assess the child's current level of functioning and help the clinician anticipate persistent intellectual disabilities. These tests—which may involve pencil-and-paper tasks, motor tasks, sensory tasks, or some degree of intellectual processing—help determine both the severity and type of intellectual disability (Box 30-3). Learning disabilities are often identified by using some of these same instruments, and many are available through the school system. Nurses also can learn to administer developmental screening tools. The American Academy of Pediatrics recommends formal developmental screening and surveillance for all children at ages 9 months, 18 months, and 24 to 30 months (American Academy of Pediatrics, 2006/2010)

(see Chapter 4). Often, a diagnosis of developmental disorder is not made until the child begins school and has significant academic failure, prompting formal psychological and neurologic testing. Routine assessment of development during pediatric visits, however, is the best method of early detection.

New understandings of human behavior suggest that levels of functioning vary in every individual, and that a one-time test offers information only about that moment in time. Accurate scores are best obtained by repeated testing over a short period of time, giving a range of scores that may more accurately describe a child's potential.

Management

Both general strategies and strategies designed to keep children safe provide the basis for managing children with intellectual or developmental disorders or disabilities.

General Strategies

Therapeutic management depends largely on community and educational resources. Obtaining services for these children, however, requires multidisciplinary efforts and strong advocacy on the part of both parents and professionals. Reduction in the occurrence of developmental disorders is a national priority identified in *Healthy People 2020* (USDHHS, 2010b). Adequate prenatal care is of primary importance. An additional priority related to children with disabilities is increasing the percentage of time children with disabilities spend in regular school programs (USDHHS, 2010b).

For children with associated medical co-morbidities, medical strategies are directed toward preventing and treating infections, correcting structural deformities, and treating associated behaviors, such as aggressiveness. Corrective measures might include congenital heart surgery for malformations, inserting tympanostomy tubes, or placing splints on joints that are hypotonic and hyperextended. The treatment of behavioral difficulties and psychosocial disturbances may involve administration of medications.

Safety Challenges

Children who are intellectually impaired are less capable of managing environmental challenges than are their peers who are unimpaired. Because of impaired executive and motor functioning, injuries are generally more common when compared to same-age children. Among preschool-age children, however, injuries are less common in those with intellectual disability, perhaps due to parental oversight and less exposure to risk. Table 30-1 presents some safety issues to be taught in the home and in the community. Although the learning needs of children who are intellectually impaired are similar to those of children without disabilities, children with intellectual disabilities may need prolonged teaching, more demonstration during teaching, frequent verbal and visual reminders, and more practice. Resources for schools and teachers have been essential in helping children with intellectual or developmental disabilities integrate into classrooms (National Educational Psychological Service, 2011).

BOX 30-3 EXPECTED SKILLS ACCORDING TO INTELLIGENCE QUOTIENT SCORES

Normal Intelligence (IQ 85 to 115)
Age-normal skills across all domains

Borderline Intellectual Disability (IQ 71 to 84)
Early milestones achieved, including language and social skills
Likely to be noticed when school performance is monitored
Vocational skills adequate for competitive employment, can live independently as adults

Mild Intellectual Disability (IQ 50-55 to ~70)
Slight delay in achieving developmental milestones but can communicate well and demonstrate some social skills
May require special education services with an emphasis on vocational and self-maintenance skills
Able to form and maintain adult relationships and can care for themselves

Moderate Intellectual Disability (IQ 35-40 to 50-55)
Noticeable delay in motor and speech development by preschool age
Can communicate, although have less than adequate social skills
Usually can achieve cognitively at an elementary school level
Can live best as an adult in a supportive and supervised setting, such as a group home
Can perform unskilled work in a supervised setting, such as a sheltered workshop

Severe Intellectual Disability (IQ 20-25 to 35-40)
Early and marked delay in all motor skills
Limited expressive speech and self-help skills
Constant supervision required, with group home living possible as an adult

Profound Intellectual Disability (IQ <20 to 25)
May be able to walk
May have primitive speech
Usually requires complete provision of activities of daily living

Modified from American Psychiatric Association. (2000). *Diagnostic and statistical manual of mental disorders* (4th ed., Text revision). Washington, DC: The Association; Kerr, L. (2008). *Intellectual disability/mental retardation classification.* Retrieved from www.medicalhomeportal.org.

⚡ SAFETY ALERT

The Child with a Developmental Disorder

Safety is a persistent concern of parents, teachers, and health professionals, because the child's maturation in anticipating danger, in problem solving, and in judgment is delayed and remains generally impaired across the life span. Children with motor disabilities are often unable to perform skills in ways that foster safety.

◎ NURSING CARE PLAN

The Child with a Developmental Disorder or Disability in the Community Setting

Focused Assessment: The Child

- Assess intellectual skills and level of adaptive functioning, especially social interaction, competence in independent ADLs, and communication.
- Alternate between questions and demonstrations when conducting the assessment.
- Look directly at the child and speak in a direct and simple yet noncondescending manner in vocabulary appropriate for the child's developmental level, not the child's age.
- Ask the child for as much of the necessary information as possible, rather than relying solely on the parents to provide the information.

Focused Assessment: The Family

- Assess the family's level of functioning, particularly interaction patterns, available coping skills, and the family's awareness of and involvement in addressing the child's needs.
- Observe and elicit information about signs of grief or anxiety related to the child's condition or changes in the child's developmental status.
- Explore the family's social and financial resources in a manner that is informative but respectful of privacy.
- Assess the family's requirements for short- and long-term assistance in the child's comprehensive management.
- Assess the family's ability to identify and maximize the child's strengths.
- Identify the need for interdisciplinary services, including genetic counseling, respite care, in-home services, parent training, and support groups.

Planning

Nursing Diagnosis

Risk for Injury related to level of self-care skills and inability to anticipate danger.

Expected Outcome

The parent and child will describe and avoid unsafe situations that lead to self-injury or unintentional injury.

Intervention/*Rationale*

1. Provide anticipatory guidance relative to the child's specific developmental abilities.
   Parents may not be able to anticipate the child's intellectual or functional level accurately, particularly if the parents are inexperienced or have limited intellectual skills themselves.
2. Keep safety rails up on hospital beds and on the bed at home if the child is predisposed to falling or roaming at night. Provide child-size furniture, and select age- and skill-related play equipment.
   These strategies help prevent accidental falls.
3. Give simple explanations about unsafe areas in the environment. Use the child's intellectual level as a key to what the child can understand or the degree of unsupervised freedom that can safely be allowed.
   Young or intellectually delayed individuals can understand concrete explanations.

Evaluation

Can the parent or child describe unsafe situations?
Has the child remained safe and free from injury?

Planning

Nursing Diagnosis

Deficient Knowledge (family members) related to unfamiliarity with the cause and likely outcomes of the child's intellectual disabilities, available support

systems, or information about sexuality, vocational options, leisure skills, and so on.

Expected Outcomes

The family will describe and plan for the child's special needs.
The family will access and use personal and community resources to increase the child's ability to develop personal skills for appropriate social, leisure, and vocational abilities.

Intervention/*Rationale*

1. Provide information that is simple, concrete, and solution focused.
   Stress may impair the family's adaptive coping skills.
2. Explain any medical terms without assuming that the family knows the terminology. Give explanations to both the child and the parents. Use demonstrations and therapeutic play. If the child is hospitalized, communicate information about the child's intellectual and functional level to other team members.
   The child may have a limited capacity to understand words but may be able to understand a demonstration.
3. Select skills that enhance self-care and socially appropriate behaviors. As the child reaches puberty, provide simple information about sexuality and physical changes. Support training in leisure skills.
   Education that is practical and functional for the child's mental and chronologic age fosters self-esteem, compliance, and cooperation.
4. Identify for the parents local and national resources for care, education, and training of intellectually impaired children.
   Additional services will be needed as the child grows or needs more specialized training. Families may have to find out-of-home placement if the child's disability is severe or destructive to the family.
5. Provide parents with anticipatory guidance about developmental milestones and anticipated skills, including safety, sexuality, skills that can be expected, and behavioral changes throughout the developmental process.
   Parents may have unrealistic expectations or expect too little from the child.

Evaluation

Has the family made progress in describing and planning for the child's special needs?
Has the family used the resources available in the community to maximize the child's abilities?

Planning

Nursing Diagnosis

Impaired Social Interaction (child) related to an inability to initiate and maintain social relationships.

Expected Outcomes

The child will develop positive relationships with family and peers.
The child will have solitary leisure skills.

Intervention/*Rationale*

1. Encourage the parents to support the child in participating in group activities that promote peer interactions (e.g., Special Olympics, special camps) (Figure 30-2). The family will arrange social activities with other children (e.g., visiting the park with friends, inviting friends to the home to play).
   To accommodate to social expectations and demands, children who are intellectually impaired or developmentally disabled need to be exposed to children who are not impaired and to children with similar challenges.

NURSING CARE PLAN
The Child with a Developmental Disorder or Disability in the Community Setting—cont'd

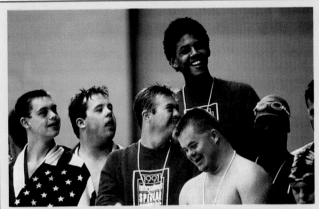

FIG 30-2 Special Olympics International is the largest recreational program in the world for people with mental retardation. With more than 1 million athletes in 125 countries, Special Olympics offers opportunities for social interaction with peers and assists children who are intellectually disabled in reaching their maximum potential. (Courtesy Special Olympics, Inc.)

Intervention/Rationale—cont'd

2. Encourage the parents to participate in interactive activities, such as reading books and playing, on a regular basis.
   Families are likely to limit interactions because the child offers reduced reinforcements in social situations.

Evaluation

Has the child demonstrated a sense of pleasure in social interactions with family members and with other individuals within the child's social sphere?

Planning
Nursing Diagnosis

Compromised Family Coping or Disabled Family Coping related to excessive emotional and financial strain on family members caring for a child who is intellectually impaired, lack of acceptance by society, or an extended grieving process associated with diagnosis of a child with a chronic disability.

Expected Outcomes

The family will integrate the child in the family system in a manner that facilitates maximum growth and maturity.
The family will express self-satisfaction in their family management.
The family will demonstrate social acceptance within the community.

Intervention/Rationale

1. Provide anticipatory and continuing support for the grieving process. Parents should be told the diagnosis and be given needed information as quickly as possible. This information should be given when both parents and supportive family members are available. Information may need to be explained in different ways (orally, in writing, with videos) to help parents grasp the meaning of the diagnosis.
   Families typically experience a cycle of grieving that is repeated when milestones are not reached or when the child has an illness or a change in behavior.
2. Assist in identifying appropriate resources for social interactions and social training (e.g., early intervention programs, special education programs, recreational programs for developmentally disabled children).
   Individuals who are mildly or moderately impaired often feel loneliness and depression as a result of insufficient stimulation and social contact. Such programs can assist the child in reaching maximum potential.
3. Identify and refer the family to appropriate community resources for both emotional support and family and child education. The nurse may need to act as an advocate and referral center (about support groups, education consultants, home health agencies).
   The grieving process and the need to accommodate to the child's skill level are continuous; families often feel isolated and helpless in locating necessary resources.
4. Assist family members to identify realistic short- and long-term goals for the child and themselves. Encourage the family to express feelings and concerns; provide hope when appropriate.
   Stress, grieving, and limited knowledge may impair the family's ability to set reasonable goals without assistance.
5. Educate the parents in monitoring the child for alterations in health status. Help the family recognize nonverbal signs of discomfort.
   The child may be unable to verbalize pain typically associated with ear infections, colds, or major illnesses.
6. Assist family members in exploring their choices for home care, a group home, or a residential facility.
   Families may hesitate to discuss care options out of fear of being perceived as uncaring or unable to provide home care.

Evaluation

Does the family integrate the child in the family system in a manner that facilitates growth and maturity to the greatest degree possible?
Does the family seek medical attention when needed and use several resources to meet the child's social, emotional, educational, and medical needs?
Is the family able to meet financial responsibilities?
Does the family participate in social activities outside the family?

DISORDERS RESULTING IN INTELLECTUAL OR DEVELOPMENTAL DISABILITY

Disorders that result in intellectual disability, developmental disability, or both can be classified and discussed according to any of a number of schemes. To facilitate understanding of their common features and specific differences, disorders are discussed in the following order:

- Disorder of intellectual impairment: Down syndrome
- Disorders of known genetic cause: Fragile X syndrome and Rett syndrome
- Disorders related to environmental alterations: Fetal alcohol syndrome, nonorganic failure to thrive
- Disorders with little understood genetic influence: Autism spectrum disorders

DOWN SYNDROME

Down syndrome (DS) is a syndrome, a collection of associated symptoms and disorders that tend to occur together; it is not a disease. It is the genetic disorder most frequently seen as causing moderate to severe

TABLE 30-1	SAFETY CONCERNS FOR DEVELOPMENTALLY DELAYED OR IMPAIRED CHILDREN	
SITE OF CONCERN	POSSIBLE INJURY	EDUCATION AND TRAINING ISSUES
Home		
Kitchen	Burns Poisoning	*Preschool age:* preventive education (i.e., instruct not to touch hot stove, not to ingest toxic substances) *Elementary school age:* safe use of equipment, basic safety *High school age:* cooking safety, emergency precautions
Bathroom	Falls Burns Cuts	*Elementary school age:* tub safety, precautions on wet floors *High school age:* safe use of hair care equipment, shaving utensils, and similar objects
General		Preschool and elementary school age: avoidance of electrical outlets, safe passage around objects
Outdoors		
Yard or playground	Animal bites Poisoning Abduction	*Preschool age:* staying within boundaries, appropriate response to strange animals and people, safe use of equipment, avoidance of ingestion of berries *Elementary school age:* stranger safety, bicycle safety, traffic safety, water safety
Vehicles	Cuts Falls Serious injury	*Preschool and elementary school age:* seatbelt use, keeping hands in car *High school age:* traffic safety

intellectual impairment. The assessment and nursing interventions for a child who is intellectually impaired are applicable to children with DS; however, additional issues need consideration.

Depending on the severity of the symptoms, most parents raise the child at home until early adulthood, after which group home placement is an option. Supported employment is encouraged, and parents are typically advised to initiate vocational training in elementary school. The partnership of parents and professionals is vital in managing the symptoms and in providing the comprehensive services that are needed. In the past 10 years advocacy groups have supported the integration and support for children and families with Down syndrome (National Down Syndrome Society [NDSS], 2011).

Services required throughout the life span include education and vocational training, transitional services, respite care, social services, financial supplements, psychotherapy, and preventive or corrective medical care (Box 30-4). This array of needed services may be overwhelming to the family, and the potential for frustration on the part of both the parents and the professional team is high. Communication and coordination of services are considered primary tasks for each team member (Figure 30-3).

Etiology

Several chromosomal alterations that result in Down syndrome have been identified. *Trisomy 21* accounts for approximately 95% of Down syndrome cases (NDSS, 2011). In trisomy 21, the gamete (e.g., an egg cell) is created that contains three copies of chromosome 21. This is termed *nondisjunction,* a failure of the chromosomes to separate normally during meiosis.

Most of the remaining 5% result from either of the following, with mosaicism being the most rare:
- *Translocation,* in which an adult who appears normal carries a chromosome that is partially fused to another chromosome (generally chromosomes 21 and 14) (Summar & Lee, 2011). This type of transmission is not associated with maternal age or parental gender.
- *Mosaic Down syndrome (mosaicism),* a condition in which some of the cells in the body are normal and some of the cells have

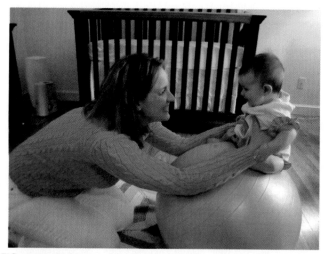

FIG 30-3 Children with delayed motor or cognitive function, whether temporary or pervasive, benefit from early and vigorous therapy to help them reach their maximum development.

trisomy 21. Children who have mosaic Down syndrome may have fewer signs of the condition (NDSS, 2011).

World Down Syndrome Day takes place on March 21 every year. The date is chosen to reflect the origin of the syndrome, the result of three copies of the 21st chromosome, the unique genetic feature of people with Down syndrome (World Down Syndrome Day, 2011).

Incidence

Down syndrome is the most common genetic cause of intellectual and developmental disability and occurs in one out of 800 births in the United States (National Institute on Child Health and Human Development, 2008). Overall, the CDC estimates the rate as 1 per 733 live births in the United States, or an incidence of approximately 5429 new cases per year (CDC, 2009). Down syndrome affects boys more often than girls and is highest in non-Hispanic white children (Shin, Besser, Kucik et al., 2009).

BOX 30-4   MEDICAL CONDITIONS ASSOCIATED WITH DOWN SYNDROME

Conditions Frequently Identified during the Neonatal Period

Cardiac conditions:
- Endocardial cushion defect
- Tetralogy of Fallot
- Atrial septal defects
- Patent ductus arteriosus
- Ventricular septal defects

Gastrointestinal conditions:
- Tracheoesophageal fistula
- Pyloric stenosis
- Imperforate anus
- Duodenal atresia
- Aganglionic megacolon (Hirschsprung disease)

Congenital cataracts
Hypothyroidism
Dysplastic hips
Leukemia-like conditions

Conditions Frequently Identified during Childhood

Endocrine disorders:
- Decreased growth
- Obesity resulting from overeating, insufficient exercise, or undetected hypothyroidism
- Thyroid dysfunction
- Infertility (male)
- Alopecia
- Thin hair

Sensitive skin and propensity for rashes
Ophthalmic problems, such as myopia, strabismus, nystagmus, cataracts, blepharitis, and keratoconus
Chronic serous otitis media

Hematologic abnormalities:
- Subtle immune deficiencies
- Acute nonlymphoblastic leukemia
- Acute lymphoblastic leukemia

Craniofacial defects:
- Malocclusions
- Delayed tooth eruption
- Periodontal disease and gingivitis
- Bruxism
- Sinusitis and rhinitis
- Sleep apnea as a result of cranial malformations

Musculoskeletal abnormalities:
- Hypotonia
- Joint laxity and dislocations
- Atlantoaxial subluxation or dislocation

Sensory deficits
Seizure disorders
Psychiatric disorders, particularly adjustment reaction disorders, anxiety disorders, depression, behavior disorders, dementia
ASDs

Maternal age has been consistently identified as one of the most significant risk factors associated with Down syndrome. The risk of a 35-year-old woman bearing a child with Down syndrome is 1 in 400; by age 40 years, the risk increases to 1 in 100. Most of these children are now born to women younger than 35 years (80% of affected children) (March of Dimes, 2011). This probably reflects the overall fertility of the age-group. Although maternal age is the greatest predictor of risk, some couples are at increased risk for producing multiple offspring with Down syndrome due to carrier genes.

Other than maternal age and genetic predispositions, no specific risk factors are known for Down syndrome, and no geographic or economic risks have been identified.

PATHOPHYSIOLOGY

Down Syndrome

Trisomy 21, or Down syndrome, occurs when three representatives of chromosome 21 are present instead of the usual two. There is some evidence that a particular region of chromosome 21 is responsible for the facial features, heart defects, intellectual impairment, and dermatologic changes. Many of the malformations in this disorder result from incomplete rather than abnormal embryogenesis. Examples include malformations of the atrioventricular canal, tracheoesophageal fistula, and imperforate anus. Alterations in neurotransmitters, particularly in the cholinergic system, are responsible for the premature aging and Alzheimer-type dementia that are common in individuals with Down syndrome.

A number of medical problems in the newborn period can seriously compromise health and survival. If the child survives these complications, a number of less serious difficulties are generally encountered in childhood.

Manifestations

The phenotype for Down syndrome is often identified at birth by characteristic facial and head features, such as brachycephaly (disproportionate shortness of the head); flat profile; inner epicanthal folds; wide, flat, nasal bridge; narrow, high-arched palate; protruding tongue; and small, short ears, which may be low set. In addition, children with Down syndrome may have other serious abnormalities that affect their development, including congenital cardiac defects, vision and hearing difficulties, and childhood leukemia.

In addition to facial and head features, certain body features also may be apparent in the child with Down syndrome. These include short stature; short, broad hands; singular transverse creases across the palm and the sole of the foot; wide gap between first and second toes; short, broad neck; increased likelihood of umbilical hernia; dry skin with a tendency to crack and fissure; hyperextensibility of joints with hypotonicity of muscles; and atlantoaxial instability (i.e., at the first and second cervical vertebrae).

Risks for associated medical conditions include malformations of the atrioventricular canal, tracheoesophageal fistula, and imperforate anus. Alterations in neurotransmitters, particularly in the cholinergic system, are responsible for premature aging and the concomitant increased risk for early development of Alzheimer disease.

Most children with Down syndrome have mild (IQ 50 to 70) to moderate (IQ 35 to 50) intellectual impairment. Children with the mosaic form of the syndrome typically show an IQ that is 10 to 54 points higher than the nonmosaic form. Down syndrome is associated with intellectual, language, and social dysfunctions; language development characterized by particular difficulty with grammar but general strength in social language (e.g., greeting others, carrying on a conversation in a give-and-take manner); social skills that exceed expected skills on the basis of intellectual capacity; limited ability to use the environmental cues available (i.e., infrequent scanning and use of only a few referential cues, such as eye contact with the primary caregiver); and blunted affect.

As they age, people with Down syndrome have declining intellectual abilities, reduced social and adaptive skills, and the onset of Alzheimer-type dementia. About 25% of people with Down syndrome who are over the age of 35 are estimated to show clinical signs of Alzheimer-type dementia (University of California, n.d.).

Diagnostic Evaluation

Prenatal testing includes amniocentesis or chorionic villus sampling. An abnormal triple maternal serum screen value (low alpha-fetoprotein, low unconjugated estriol, and increased human gonadotropin levels) may prompt additional testing. Down syndrome is usually evident at birth because of the characteristic phenotype facial features, although chromosomal analysis is conducted to confirm the diagnosis. Other diagnostic tests are conducted to identify associated medical conditions, such as nasopharyngeal abnormalities or cardiac defects.

To rule out associated disorders and to detect frequently encountered difficulties, clinicians recommend that the child be monitored frequently throughout the first 12 months of life, with an emphasis on gastrointestinal and cardiac symptoms. The diagnosis often requires a full cardiac workup initially and an electrocardiogram at the end of the first year. In the second to fourth years of life, the medical emphasis is on sleep and behavioral difficulties, along with annual thyroid screening and ophthalmologic assessment. Generally, the child is referred for dental assessments at 24 months; tooth development and alignment problems are common. Generally, children should be reevaluated medically and behaviorally on an annual basis.

Therapeutic Management

Regular screening, early intervention, and active management of identified problems are essential, because there is no cure for the disorders caused by the syndrome. Surgery to correct cardiac abnormalities, gastrointestinal malformations, and craniofacial deviations has been used to prolong life, alleviate discomfort, and decrease the likelihood of further medical complications. Neck radiography should be performed before the child participates in any sports because of the risk for children with Down syndrome to have atlantoaxial instability.

NURSING CARE OF THE CHILD WITH DOWN SYNDROME

■ Assessment

Neonatal assessment is crucial in diagnosing Down syndrome on the basis of physiologic characteristics. A thorough physical examination should be conducted, including hearing and vision examinations. Children with Down syndrome are at increased risk for hearing deficits and refractive errors or cataracts. When Down syndrome is suspected or already confirmed on the basis of prenatal genetic testing, serum alpha-fetoprotein levels, or amniotic fluid samples, an assessment is conducted to determine the severity of the manifestations and the family's ability to cope with and accommodate the needs of the infant. Assessment for intellectual disability is also appropriate for the child with Down syndrome.

If a child with Down syndrome is hospitalized for surgical repair, infections, or injury, assess the child's typical coping patterns to support strategies already in place. Children with Down syndrome prefer routine and consistency, so an assessment of their daily routine is important; include times and habits related to mealtimes, bathing, and order of dressing. Assessing the child's understanding of language and ability to communicate is important for providing information that the child can understand. Knowing the child's words for specific body functions, such as voiding, defecating, or sleeping, will allow for greater comfort for the hospitalized child. It is important to assess the child's learning abilities before initiating any education or procedure-related play.

The child's motor skills are assessed to determine what procedures will be necessary to ensure the child's safety. Sensory deficits, such as vision or hearing difficulties, should be identified as part of routine regular follow-up. Some deficits can be detected by closely observing as the child reaches for objects, by listening to conversation, or by speaking the child's name. The child with Down syndrome, however, may respond to sensory stimuli less noticeably than unimpaired children or may respond with dulled affect, even if hearing or vision deficits are not present. Developmental delays in balance and coordination increase the risks of injuries from falls. Self-stimulating behaviors (e.g., picking at the arm) need to be identified because they are often used as coping strategies but may also be self-injurious.

Identification of areas of good functioning and adaptive behavior is important, because families need reassurance about developmental gains and emotional support for their efforts at care. A child with Down syndrome is most often a beloved member of the family, viewed by parents and siblings as a valuable addition. Nurses, who can offer important support for the normalization of the syndrome, should support these attachments. Assessment of the family and living environment is critical to ensure that both physical safety and stimulation of development are present. Affected children frequently do not seek out stimulation and may need encouragement through colors, sound, and motion. An assessment of social behaviors is also important and should include play, social judgment skills, and social interest in the environment. The child may demonstrate inappropriate behaviors similar to those associated with severe intellectual disability. Moreover, the child's natural curiosity may be diminished as a result of fear or frustration. Nursing care of the child with Down syndrome is similar to that for any child with an intellectual disability with some specific additions.

■ Nursing Diagnosis and Planning

The nursing diagnoses and expected outcomes that are appropriate for the child with Down syndrome and the child's family are as follows:

- Impaired Parenting related to the child's delayed development, physical appearance, and medical complications.

Expected Outcome. The family will demonstrate satisfying and supportive relationships that meet the physical and emotional needs of each family member.

- Self-Care Deficit (Feeding, Toileting) related to intellectual immaturity.

Expected Outcome. The child will demonstrate the ability to independently meet needs related to bathing/ hygiene, dressing/grooming, feeding, and toileting.

- Delayed Growth and Development related to poor sucking abilities or mouth deformities, flaccid facial muscles, or other abnormalities.

Expected Outcomes. The child will maximize progress toward attaining developmental milestones and will demonstrate appropriate and measurable growth during childhood.

▪ Interventions

The stigma attached to Down syndrome can be pervasive and crippling, particularly for parents. and caregivers. Nurses should be aware of their personal response to the diagnosis. It is not uncommon for parents to describe delivery room scenes in which medical and nursing staff "become quiet" at a time when the parents expect congratulations on the birth of their child. This reaction sends the message that the birth of the child is a tragedy. This experience creates anger at health care professional prejudice and is viewed by the parents as both cruel and inaccurate. Children with Down syndrome are frequently welcomed by their parents, siblings, and extended family. The goal of all nursing interventions is directed toward the goal of benefiting the child and the family in adaptation and assimilation.

When the diagnosis is made at birth, parents greatly benefit from support in accepting the diagnosis and quick identification of resources available to teach them the special care needs for their children. The nurse can encourage bonding and attachment by identifying the positive features and behaviors in the child; looking at the child's strengths from the beginning reduces the likelihood that parents will see the child negatively when the child does not attain milestones along with others of the same chronologic age.

The nurse helps the parents explore options for fluid and calorie intake. Breastfeeding may not be possible if the child's muscle tone or sucking reflex is immature, although some children with Down syndrome can breastfeed adequately. As the child develops, special bottles or adaptive utensils may assist the child with feeding. Refer the parents for nutritional counseling as needed. Provide resources for behavioral training to encourage intake of new foods or the acquisition of new skills.

Children with Down syndrome benefit from regular schedules, and changes in the child's routine can cause frustration and decreased coping abilities. When the child is hospitalized, the nurse must try to keep the child's environment and routine as close to the home routine as possible; families can generally identify the important routines associated with waking, sleeping, eating, and conversation. An accurate and detailed description of these routines on the child's written care plan ensures consistency. Care plans are based on the child's unique personality, as well as the child's intellectual, developmental, and adaptive abilities. Chronologic age is generally not a good indicator, because the child's skills may be age appropriate in some areas but markedly delayed in others. Parents are encouraged to observe the child for signs of readiness to learn a new task (reaching for a cup, attempting to dress) and encourage self-care whenever possible. The child's level of coordination, muscle strength, and dexterity may not allow the child to zip, button, or feed himself or herself in the usual way, so adaptive tools may be needed.

As the child grows, advise the parents to encourage participation in recreational activities that the child can manage. Be sure to advise them that the child will need to have neck radiography before participating in any active sports program.

▪ Evaluation

- Have the child and family demonstrated positive and mutually satisfying interactions?
- Are the parents able to identify the child's strengths and positive attributes?
- Do the parents state an interest and willingness to help the child learn new skills through demonstration, repetition, and much positive feedback?
- Does the child demonstrate continued development and a sense of competence in self-care skills?

- Does the child demonstrate steady progress toward attaining developmental milestones and appropriate measurable growth?

FRAGILE X SYNDROME

Fragile X syndrome (FXS) is the most common inherited cause of cognitive impairment, and the most common known genetic cause of autism (Cornish, Turk, & Levitas, 2007), although the syndrome may present with or without autism. Males are generally more severely affected by the syndrome than females, who may be genetically protected from the most extreme manifestations of the disease by their double X chromosome. The majority of boys who inherit this disorder display significant cognitive and learning disabilities (Bacino & Lee, 2011). Fragile X syndrome in girls may present in a less severe form, which has led to underidentification of the syndrome. Females who are not affected by the syndrome may become carriers of the syndrome to their children, which presents an important opportunity for nurses to use educational approaches regarding risk of passing the syndrome to a child (Hagerman & Tranfaglia, 2009).

Etiology

The gene that causes fragile X syndrome *(FMR1)* is located on the X chromosome, and inheritance of the gene is through a sex-linked inheritance pattern (see Chapter 4). Because females carry doubles of the X chromosome, that doubling provides protection from full manifestation of the syndrome, which may be absent or present with only mild symptoms. A male child who inherits the X chromosome with a fragile site is not protected, because males carry XY chromosomes. These children will usually exhibit the full effects of the syndrome.

A female child can inherit the gene from either parent. A girl who inherits the X chromosome that has a fragile site may be a carrier and may continue to pass on the abnormal X chromosome. Transmission of the syndrome occurs only through carrier mothers, because the fragile site is located on the X chromosome. This means that males who are not affected by the syndrome will not be genetic carriers, whereas females who are not affected may still be carriers of the fragile site.

Incidence

Fragile X syndrome affects approximately 1 in 4000 male children and 1 in 8000 female children (CDC, 2010b). Both males and females can carry the fragile X gene. The gene can be carried either as a partial mutation or as a full mutation. In general, only males exhibit the full effects of this X-linked recessive disorder because their single X chromosome has the abnormal gene.

PATHOPHYSIOLOGY

Fragile X Syndrome

Fragile X syndrome is caused by an underlying single gene defect on the X chromosome that produces excessive repetitions of the nucleotide CGG deoxyribonucleic acid (DNA) sequences. This abnormality in the fragile X *(FMR1)* gene results in intellectual impairment in all affected individuals.

Manifestations

Fragile X syndrome, like the autism spectrum disorders, can show a number of different symptoms of varying levels of dysfunction. Overall, the areas of functioning that are affected span six categories:

- Intellectual functioning
- Physical characteristics
- Social and emotional relatedness

- Speech and language capability
- Sensory impairment
- Presence of co-morbid disorders that are commonly associated with the syndrome

Intellectual Functioning

Boys exhibit intellectual deficits in the moderate to severe range.

Physical Characteristics

Physical features associated with fragile X syndrome include facial dysmorphism, which may include large or prominent ears and a long, narrow face; a head circumference that may be disproportionate to height and weight; lowered epicanthal folds; and prominent nasal alae (cartilaginous flap on outer side of each nostril). In addition, the child may manifest enlarged testicles (postpubertal macro-orchidism), flat feet, lax ankles, hyperextensible fingers, soft and smooth skin, and mitral valve prolapse.

Social and Emotional Relatedness

FXS is also a disorder of social connectedness; decreased activity is seen in the prefrontal regions of the brain that are related to social connections (Holsen, Dalton, Johnstone, & Davidson, 2008). Characteristics include difficulty looking at people directly (gaze aversion) and difficulties with peer social relationships. This difficulty appears to be related to facial recognition, the ability to recognize a face that has been seen before (face encoding).

Speech and Language Capability and Sensory Impairment

Language and sensory impairments likely contribute to the social and behavioral dysfunctions associated with fragile X syndrome, which include disruptive behaviors, such as temper tantrums; self-injurious behaviors; extreme agitation; autism-like behaviors, such as gaze avoidance, hand flapping, echolalia, and abnormal speech patterns; hyperkinetic behaviors, including restlessness, agitation, and attention deficits; hand biting; and sensory motor integration deficits, such as poor coordination, motor planning deficits, and tactile defensiveness. The child may have strengths in visual memory but weaknesses in auditory processing abilities and abstract reasoning; improved performance with simultaneous, rather than sequential, processing; language delays; perseveration; tangential speech; and other communicative disorders. Girls manifest only mild intellectual deficits, but with many variations. People with fragile X syndrome experience worsening of symptoms across the life span, including high risk for progressive dementia.

Co-morbid Disorders

A variety of physical and emotional disorders can coexist with signs and symptoms of fragile X. Depression is not uncommon. Physical conditions include seizures, ear infections, and mitral valve prolapse (Hagerman & Tranfaglia, 2009).

Diagnostic Evaluation

Deoxyribonucleic acid testing is the definitive method of diagnosing fragile X syndrome. Identification of the *FMR1* gene mutation allows diagnosis in both carriers and those affected. Children with intellectual disability of unknown cause or learning disabilities, together with manifestations of fragile X syndrome, should be considered for fragile X testing.

Therapeutic Management

Treatment is provided through interventions that are targeted to the presenting symptoms, including various types of physical, learning, and psychological therapies (Hagerman & Tranfaglia, 2009). Special education, vocational programs, and behavioral management classes are important to overall development. Speech and language evaluation and therapy are generally prescribed during the first year of life and are made available on a continuing basis. Sensorimotor integration therapy may be offered to enhance motor planning, joint stability, coordination, and integration of visual, auditory, and tactile information. Sensorimotor therapy is considered to be the intervention of choice for these children with learning disabilities.

Nursing Considerations

The nursing care of children with fragile X syndrome is similar to care for any child with an intellectual disability, with specific attention to the behavioral and intellectual difficulties presented by the individual child. The plan should include a multidisciplinary team approach to assessment. Anticipatory guidance should be provided, with a review of the support groups and services available. Special education services will be necessary to address the child's specific intellectual and academic difficulties, to foster continued skill development, and to reduce the stress created in the typical educational setting. Remediation services should include behavioral interventions specific to the child's needs, speech and language assistance, and possibly occupational and physical therapy to address visual-motor and motor skill deficits. Family members of children with fragile X syndrome should receive genetic counseling and testing, because unaffected females may be carriers (Hagerman & Tranfaglia, 2009).

RETT SYNDROME

Unlike fragile X syndrome, which affects primarily males, Rett syndrome (RS) is almost exclusively linked to female gender, with an estimated 1:10,000 to 1:15,000 females affected (National Institute of Mental Health [NIMH], 2007). However, both disorders are related to the X chromosome. The syndrome is characterized by an initial period of normal development, with symptoms emerging between the ages of 6 and 18 months. Social and intellectual development stops, and seizures and physical disabilities emerge (Krivoshik, 2007). The emergence of symptoms in a child who was developing normally is devastating for the families of children with Fragile X or Rett syndrome.

RS is considered to be a developmental disorder, as opposed to a degenerative disorder, because neurons are not destroyed (International Rett Syndrome Foundation, 2008). RS has been characterized as an autism spectrum disorder, which means that it is the only ASD for which the cause is known. Diagnosis is made by presence of mutations on the X chromosome, gene *MECP2*, combined with clinical evaluation for the characteristic clinical signs. These signs include stereotyped hand movements, gait disturbances, slowing of normal rate of head growth, seizures, and disorganized breathing patterns (International Rett Syndrome Foundation, 2008).

Research into RS has taken different directions, looking at the genetics, the neurobiologic issues, and animal studies to gain a more in-depth understanding of the syndrome, its causes, and its progression. For example, Guy and colleagues (Guy, Gan, Selfridge et al., 2007) reported on a study that showed that tamoxifen reversed some symptoms of RS in mice. Although high toxicity rates resulted in the deaths of 9 of 17 mice, the mice that survived saw regression of the symptoms. This study is unlikely to be a breakthrough in treatment, but it does demonstrate that symptoms may be reversible (Guy et al., 2007).

Nursing considerations for the child with Rett syndrome are similar to those for the child with fragile X syndrome or other child with an intellectual or developmental disability.

FETAL ALCOHOL SPECTRUM DISORDER

As with other spectrum disorders, signs and symptoms related to prenatal alcohol exposure can range in effect from mild to severe (CDC, 2010a). Fetal alcohol syndrome is the most severe form of fetal alcohol spectrum disorder experienced by the infant exposed to alcohol in utero. FAS refers to the classic defects of persistent symmetrical growth retardation, malformations of the face and skull, skeletal and cardiac malformation, and central nervous system deficits, including intellectual and developmental disabilities.

Etiology and Incidence

Maternal alcohol consumption is the cause of FAS. No safe level of alcohol consumption during pregnancy has been established. The incidence of FAS is believed to be grossly underestimated because of lack of awareness in diagnosis and underreporting of alcohol intake during pregnancy. The incidence of FAS varies by country and ethnic group, but it is estimated to be 0.3 to 1.5 per 1000 live births in the United States (CDC, 2010a).

PATHOPHYSIOLOGY

Fetal Alcohol Syndrome

Alcohol and its metabolite (acetaldehyde) cross the placenta rapidly; therefore, the fetus has blood levels of alcohol equivalent to the maternal levels. Prenatal alcohol exposure is thought to affect protein synthesis, influencing growth and development of the brain and other tissues. This can result in a decreased number of brain cells, diminished intelligence, and brain malformation.

Assessment for other related abnormalities, such as cleft palate, foot deformities, hip dislocations and other conditions involving joint hyperextensibility, hernias, and hypertonia, should also be performed. These children may have seizures, so medications and educating the family about seizure disorders may be warranted.

Manifestations

The infant with FAS exhibits prenatal and postnatal growth deficiency, microcephaly, joint anomalies, mild to moderate intellectual disability, tremulousness in the neonatal period, and irritability; the child with FAS exhibits hyperactivity. Infants may have characteristic facial features, including short palpebral fissures, smooth philtrum (the vertical groove in the median portion of the upper lip), and a thin upper lip (Figure 30-4). Other abnormalities, including altered palmar crease patterns, short distal phalanges, cervical vertebral malformations, ear anomalies, cleft lip and palate, severe cardiac defects, renal anomalies, strawberry hemangiomas, and genital anomalies, are associated with this syndrome.

Diagnostic Evaluation

Diagnostic features of FAS include the following criteria developed by the CDC (2010a). Alcohol exposure during pregnancy is established by self-report, reports by other reliable individuals, documented elevated blood alcohol level, alcohol treatment, or documentation of other known alcohol-related problems. The use of alcohol is not totally necessary, however, for a diagnosis of FAS (CDC, 2010a). An infant or child can be diagnosed with FAS if the following criteria are present (CDC, 2010a):

- *Three facial abnormalities:* Smooth philtrum, thin vermilion border, small palpebral fissures
- *Growth deficit:* ≤10th percentile for height, weight, or both

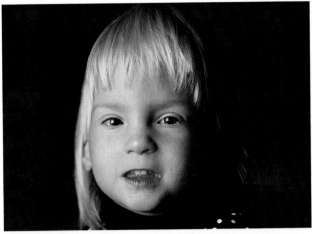

FIG 30-4 Toddler with fetal alcohol syndrome. Subtle indicators are flat mid-face, indistinct philtrum, and low-set ears. (From Fortinash, K. M., & Holoday Worret, P. A. [2012]. *Psychiatric Mental Health Nursing* [5th ed.]. St. Louis, MO: Mosby.)

- *CNS abnormalities:* Head circumference ≤10th percentile; brain abnormalities identified by imaging studies; motor deficits or seizures from no other identified cause
- *Developmental milestones* below the expected range for the child's age and physical or psychosocial circumstances in at least three of the following: cognitive function, executive function, attention, motor function, and social skills. Associated problems, such as abnormal sensitivities to taste and touch or inability to appropriately respond to facial expression or parenting techniques, comprise the final criteria.

FAS is diagnosed through physical examination and perinatal history, and a referral is often made to a geneticist. Families require counseling to help them cope with the diagnosis and to help them understand the risks involved in future pregnancies if lifestyle changes are not made.

NURSING CARE OF THE INFANT WITH FETAL ALCOHOL SYNDROME

■ Assessment

When FAS is suspected, an extensive diagnostic workup is required. Microcephaly, hypotonia, tremulousness, and irritability can raise levels of suspicion. Feeding difficulties may be encountered as well.

The family requires assistance in coping with the diagnosis and the inherent difficulties associated with caring for a child who may be difficult to soothe or who may have feeding problems. Special attention must be given to involving the parents in the care of the infant. As with other developmental disorders, there is evidence that early intervention will maximize the developmental potential of the nervous system.

■ Nursing Diagnosis and Planning

The nursing diagnoses and expected outcomes that apply to the infant with FAS and the family are as follows:

- Ineffective Infant Feeding Pattern related to congenital anomaly.
  Expected Outcome. The infant will establish appropriate sleep-wake and feeding patterns, as evidenced by appropriate weight gain and growth.
- Delayed Growth and Development related to FAS.

Expected Outcome. The infant will develop to maximum potential, as evidenced by growth and development behaviors relative to age and potential.

- Deficient Knowledge (infant's anomalies and potential sequelae) related to lack of exposure to accurate information.

Expected Outcome. Parents will increase knowledge related to the child's disorder, as evidenced by recognition of FAS and acknowledgment of the potential for future problems.

- Interrupted Family Processes related to birth of a disabled child.

Expected Outcome. The family will use coping strategies to care for the child, as evidenced by an ability to mobilize their energies toward caring for the infant with FAS.

■ **Interventions**

Daily weight gain is monitored, and intake and output are measured and documented. Various feeding strategies (e.g., varying the positioning of the infant; trying smaller, more frequent feedings; using different nipples) should be attempted until the infant is successful with nipple feedings or breastfeeding. Because parents may become frustrated or feel inadequate in dealing with a difficult feeder, it is important to assist the parents with feeding in a supportive manner. Promoting early parent-infant attachment will support the child's well-being. Encourage the family to visit frequently and involve parents in caretaking activities.

The infant with FAS is likely to have severe permanent neurologic and developmental consequences. Discuss the infant's recognizable anomalies and the possible sequelae. Allow the parents to verbalize their concerns about their infant's future. Avoid encouraging unrealistic expectations; rather, acknowledge the infant's existing problems and suggest coping strategies.

The family is in a crisis situation, and the mother may feel guilt or may be blamed by other family members for the infant's disability. Encourage family members to verbalize their feelings. Initiate referrals to appropriate community resources. The needs of the high-risk family are significant and require long-term follow-up.

■ **Evaluation**

- Are the infant's sleep patterns appropriate for age?
- Is the infant gaining weight at a rate that is appropriate for age?
- Is the child able to attain appropriate growth and development milestones?
- Are the parents discussing the cause and prevention of FAS?
- Is the family able to identify its own strengths and weaknesses, coping skills, and support systems?
- Have referrals to community resources been made and implemented?

NONORGANIC FAILURE TO THRIVE

The term *failure to thrive* is used to describe children whose weight or rate of weight gain is significantly below that of comparably aged children. These children appear dramatically smaller than their peers. Failure to thrive can result from numerous organic or medical causes, including chromosomal abnormalities, defects in the heart or lung, central nervous system damage, or exposure to toxins. It can result also from nonorganic causes related to the psychosocial environment, such as with child neglect, inadequate or underdeveloped parenting skills, or history of parental mental health problems (McLean & Price, 2011). Most clinicians agree that failure to thrive is not an actual diagnosis but rather a term that describes a cluster of concurrent symptoms. In practice, if a child is considered to be

significantly smaller than peers or if a child fails to gain appropriate weight over time, the child is considered to be at risk for failure to thrive, and a more thorough evaluation is warranted (McLean & Price, 2011).

Etiology

Failure to thrive can be organic, caused by an underlying physical problem, or nonorganic. The contributing factors to and interventions for physical growth delay have been described in detail in previous chapters. Nonorganic failure to thrive is thought to be caused by multiple factors, including poverty, maternal depression, poor social support systems, poor bonding or maladaptive interactions between the child and mother, and an irritable, resistant-to-touch infant. Nonorganic failure to thrive can result in both intellectual and developmental delays.

Incidence

It is estimated that 10% of children seen in the primary care setting have symptoms of failure to thrive (Rabinowitz, Katturupalli, & Rogers, 2010). Although failure to thrive occurs in children of all social classes, a disproportionate number of these children are from low-income families.

Manifestations and Risk Factors

Physical indicators of nonorganic failure to thrive include weight below the 5th percentile, a sudden or rapid deceleration in the growth curve, delay in reaching developmental milestones, and decreased muscle mass. Muscle hypotonia, abdominal distention, generalized weakness, and cachexia (general ill health and malnutrition) are additional signs.

Behavioral indicators of failure to thrive include avoidance of eye contact, avoidance of physical touch, intense watchfulness, and sleep disturbances. Lack of age-appropriate stranger anxiety, inappropriate lack of preference for one's own parents, and disturbed affect (e.g., apathy, extreme irritability, extreme compliance) may also be observed. Repetitive self-stimulating behaviors, such as rocking, head banging, intense sucking, intense chewing on fingers or hands, and head rolling, are also seen.

Diagnostic Evaluation

The differential diagnosis is generally made by a multidisciplinary team whose initial task is to search for an organic cause of the growth failure. If no cause is identified, the approach is to diagnose by response. Nutrition and nurturing are provided in a consistent manner, and if the infant gains the expected weight, nonorganic failure to thrive is considered to be the appropriate diagnosis.

Therapeutic Management

Children with nonorganic failure to thrive should be managed primarily in an outpatient setting using a multidisciplinary team approach (Cincinnati Children's Medical Center, 2009). Treatment provides nutritional therapy to increase the child's caloric intake. The goal is for the child to grow at two to three times the average rate for age. Daily multivitamin supplements with minerals are often prescribed to ensure that specific nutritional deficiencies do not occur in the course of rapid growth. Caloric enrichment of food is essential, and formula may be concentrated in titrated amounts up to 24 calories per ounce. Greater concentrations can lead to diarrhea and dehydration.

Family therapy may be indicated. Effective parenting classes can assist the parent to identify psychological and physical factors that have contributed to the child's condition.

Nursing Considerations

In addition to assessing contributing factors that would suggest organic failure to thrive (e.g., age at onset, history of illness, especially gastrointestinal illness, and dietary patterns), the nurse should complete a thorough psychosocial history that focuses on income, family disorganization, social isolation, stress factors, support systems, and family psychopathologic conditions, such as maternal depression, family violence, or alcoholism. It is important to ask about the availability of food, especially around the time of arrival of a paycheck or other forms of income. Finally, the psychosocial history should include questions about facilities for storing and preparing food.

Assessment of infant-parent interactions should focus on the ways in which the child is held and fed, how eye contact is initiated and maintained, and the facial expressions of both the child and the caregiver during interactions. Observations of various kinds of interactions are also important and should include play, talk, and touch by both the child and caregiver and the other's reaction to these attempts to engage in interaction. The nurse should note the responses of the caregiver to the child's cues, such as when the child cries, reaches out, or looks toward the caregiver. A feeling of synchrony or harmony should be sensed in the interaction.

The focus for nursing intervention is to facilitate improvement in the child's physical and developmental status as well as enhancing positive parenting. If the child is hospitalized, providing a consistent caregiver from the nursing staff increases trust and provides the child with an adult who anticipates needs and who is able to role model child care to the parent. Role modeling and teaching appropriate adult-child interactions (including holding, touching, and feeding the child) will facilitate appropriate parent-child relationships and enhance parents' confidence in caring for their child and expression by the parents of realistic expectations based on the child's developmental needs.

AUTISM SPECTRUM DISORDERS

Autism spectrum disorders (ASDs) (also considered to be a subset of pervasive developmental disorders) range in severity from severe (autism disorder), to a milder form (Asperger syndrome). A child who has symptoms of either of these disorders, but does not meet the criteria for either diagnosis, is generally diagnosed with the classification pervasive developmental disorder—not otherwise specified (APA, 2000). Two other rare genetic manifestations of autism spectrum disorders are Rett syndrome and fragile X syndrome, which were discussed earlier (NIMH, 2007).

All forms of ASD are characterized by atypical patterns of development and clusters of developmental problems and deficits. These include difficulty developing and maintaining social relationships, disordered communication, and stereotyped interests and behaviors (APA, 2000). Symptoms are usually noticeable by 3 years of age and may be gradual or sudden in onset. Diagnosis of an ASD has been made as early as 1 year of age (Autism Society of America, 2009b). Occasionally the disorder is not identified until the child reaches school age, particularly in cases where gross motor skills show normal progression. ASDs are frequently linked to co-morbidity with intellectual, emotional, and behavioral disorders or other medical conditions (Sadock & Sadock, 2008).

Indicators of autism spectrum disorders include lack of social ability (e.g., poor eye contact), lack of verbalization (such as babbling), little interest in verbal interaction, inability to use toys, lack of smiling, excessive preoccupation with creating order, and lack of response to verbal interactions. Parents often express concern that their child does not appear to be attaching to them and does not seek comfort or cuddling. Social cues and gestures have little meaning to children with ASD.

Asperger Syndrome

Historically, Asperger syndrome was classified as "high-functioning autism." New understandings of the disorder have led to the classification of Asperger syndrome as a distinct subcategory within the autism spectrum. Children with Asperger syndrome do not show the level of disability seen in autism, and these children typically show normal and often high levels of intellectual and language development. Symptoms are primarily social and emotional. Children with Asperger syndrome display an impaired ability to understand common social cues and an inability to behave according to social norms. They will often be fluent in language, but the content of conversations is fixated on the topic of interest to the child, with no regard for the reaction of the listener. They also frequently display rigidity regarding schedules, motor clumsiness, trouble handwriting, and organizational skill problems. Children with Asperger syndrome are often friendly and would like to establish peer relationships, but their inability to understand social cues creates difficulty in establishing and maintaining relationships (Autism Society of America, 2009a).

Autism

Autism is the most severe form of the ASDs (NIMH, 2007). It is a complex disorder, with many potential causes, one of which may be genetic. To date, there is no evidence that autism can be cured, so treatment is generally lifelong and is characterized by varying degrees of success. Early diagnosis, with comprehensive and ongoing intervention targeted to presenting symptoms, appears to offer the best prognosis for educational and psychosocial outcomes (Table 30-2).

TABLE 30-2	**DIFFERENTIAL DIAGNOSIS OF AUTISM, INTELLECTUAL DISABILITY, AND SCHIZOPHRENIA**
AUTISM	**INTELLECTUAL DISABILITY**
Peaked skill profile	Flat skill profile
Lack of imitative skills	Imitation skills and gesturing
Nonsocial behaviors with little initiation	Social behavior, initiation of social contact
Abnormal communication and language	Limited language ability but sufficient for communication
Development of seizures possible during adolescence	Usually no seizures, Alzheimer-type dementia in adulthood
AUTISM	**SCHIZOPHRENIA**
Onset before age 54 mo	Onset during pubescence or adolescence
No remissions	Remissions and relapses
Hallucinations and delusions rare	Hallucinations and delusions common
Absence of thought disorder	Thought disorder
No family history of schizophrenia	Family history of schizophrenia
Self-stimulating behaviors	Odd behavior but no self-stimulating behaviors
Medications of limited use	Medications often helpful in reducing symptoms

Etiology

Researchers theorize that the disorder can be caused by a wide range of prenatal, perinatal, and postnatal conditions, including maternal rubella, untreated phenylketonuria, tuberous sclerosis, anoxia during birth, encephalitis, seizures, and fragile X syndrome (Sadock & Sadock, 2008). There have also been theories of possible connections between autism and hazardous chemical exposures, including chemicals, such as thimerosal, in vaccines administered during infancy and childhood. Epidemiologic studies have examined the relationship between the occurrence of autism and either the measles, mumps, rubella (MMR) vaccine or vaccines preserved with thimerosal. Price, Thompson, Goodson et al. (2010) conducted a case control study that examined a sample of 256 children diagnosed with autism spectrum disorders matched to a random sample of 752 children without ASD. Researchers looked at prenatal and postnatal exposures to thimerosal to determine whether children exposed to thimerosal-containing vaccines during infancy and early childhood increased their risk for developing ASD. Statistical analysis of data revealed no increased risk for ASD related to thimerosal (Price et al., 2010).

It was once believed that family child-rearing practices and parental personality characteristics influenced the development of autism, but no controlled studies confirm this view, and the view of autism as having a psychogenic origin in family dysfunction is largely discounted.

There is a growing body of research directed toward identifying genetic mutations related to autism. The American Recovery and Reinvestment Act of 2009 has allocated a significant amount of funding to address contributing factors to autism, including genetic and genomic factors (National Institute of Environmental Health Sciences [NIEHS], 2011).

Inherited genetic mutations have been thought to be contributory, particularly in families where multiple siblings have been affected by the disorder. However, researchers have identified tiny rare mutations that appear unpredictably across the genome; these mutations may be related to autism in families where only one child is affected (Sebat, Lakshmi, Malhotra, & Wigler, 2007). This has led to the proposition that two subtypes of genetic disorders exist. The first, spontaneous mutation, is linked to families with single cases of autism (sporadic autism); the second subtype, inheritance, is linked to families with multiple members affected by the disorder (familial autism). Sebat and colleagues found spontaneous deletions and duplications that were 10 times more prevalent when healthy control subjects were compared to children with the sporadic subtype. The mutations were only twice as prevalent when control subjects were compared to children from families with multiple children affected by autism (Sebat et al., 2007). This implies that autism may share common neurobiologic aspects with a variety of biologic and emotional disorders (Raviola, Gosselin, Walter, & DeMarco, 2011).

Incidence

Prevalence rates for autism have been difficult to establish. Most recent data looking at 8-year-old children reveals an overall prevalence of ASDs to be 9 per 1000 children, or 1 in every 110, in the United States (Autism and Developmental Disabilities Monitoring Network [ADDMN], 2009). This is a substantial increase over the past several years. Autism is more common in boys than in girls and is highest in the white, non-Hispanic population of children (ADDMN, 2009).

Manifestations

Autism can be a severely incapacitating, lifelong developmental disability that is characterized by a qualitative impairment in four developmental areas: disturbance in the acquisition of physical, social, and language skills (although has evidence of cognitive capacity); abnormal responses to normal body sensations; evidence of cognitive capacity, but with absence or delay in language; abnormal ways of relating to people, objects, or events; and difficulty regulating emotions (APA, 2000; NIMH, 2007).

The variety of forms that autism can take makes planning care difficult, because it must be individually targeted. A child may have a large vocabulary yet have no comprehension of the meaning of the words. Another child may be able to solve intricate mathematical problems but not be able to make change from a dollar. Children may be unresponsive to the sound of their own names, but come running into the room at the sound of a truck. Generally, children with autism show a fixed, unchanging response to a particular stimulus. Self-stimulation is common and generally involves repetition of a particularly pleasing sensory stimulus, such as twirling a toy or rubbing the top of the head.

Apparently, interest is limited by nature, rather than by choice, to an extremely narrow range. The child with autism generally overreacts to any change within the environment. Often, autistic children do not have a typical sense of personal space and so may touch others on the face or stand face to face, with noses touching, even when encountering a total stranger.

Landa, Holman, and Garrett-Mayer (2007) indicate that about half of children with autism spectrum disorders manifest signs soon after their first birthday; others with these disorders may appear to develop normally until that age and then falter or regress during their second year. This prospective study of children at risk is the first to identify two distinct patterns of illness onset (Landa et al., 2007). The later-diagnosis group was not easily distinguished from healthy children at 14 months; however, their functioning deteriorated by age 2 years.

Impairment secondary to autism covers a wide range, with 75% of autistic children considered intellectually impaired. A few children with autism also have an extremely developed skill in a particular area, such as music or mathematics. These individuals are sometimes known as *autistic savants* because they have both a severe intellectual disability and an extraordinary intellectual skill or expertise. High-functioning autistic children were once considered to have Asperger syndrome, but these are now considered distinct disorders.

The child with autism exhibits the following behaviors and characteristics (American Psychiatric Association, 2000).

Social

- Marked lack of awareness of the existence or feelings of others (e.g., child ignores emotions of others)
- Lack of or abnormal amount of comfort-seeking at times of distress (e.g., child does not show pain when hurt)
- Lack of or abnormal imitation of others' actions
- Lack of or abnormal social play (generally plays alone or involves others only as mere objects)
- Gross impairment in social peer relationships (appears not to want or need friends)

Language

- Lack of or impaired verbal communication and abnormalities in the production of speech (inappropriate volume, pitch, rate, rhythm, or intonation, such as a monotone voice or echolalia)
- Markedly abnormal nonverbal communication (e.g., the child uses no gestures or behavioral cues)
- Absence of imaginative play (no imitative or dramatic role playing)
- Impaired interactive speech and communication (the child does not allow for the normal give and take of conversation and tends

to become preoccupied with a given subject or word out of context with the conversation)

Restricted Behavioral Repertoire

- Stereotyped body movements (e.g., spinning around, head banging, "flapping," rocking)
- Persistent preoccupation with characteristics of objects (smell, taste, texture) or an abnormal attachment to objects (e.g., piece of string, picture of a whale)
- Marked distress over a minor change in the environment (e.g., exhibiting tantrums when a light is turned on, refusing to look at a teacher who is wearing a new dress)
- Unreasonable insistence on routine (e.g., following a schedule exactly to the minute or second, refusal to attend an assembly during a scheduled mathematics class)
- Self-injurious behaviors (e.g., biting, picking at skin, scratching eyes)
- Marked restriction in range of interests (e.g., may repeatedly align objects and cannot be diverted from doing so)

Diagnostic Evaluation

A diagnosis of autism is usually established on the basis of specific behavioral manifestations, with evidence gained through parental consultation, patient history, and direct observation. Often, the family is interviewed initially, followed by observation of the child alone, with the parent, and interacting with the examiner or others in the environment. Interviews are coupled with observations and the clinician's rating scales. The onset of characteristic delays or of abnormal functioning must occur before age 3 years.

The American Academy of Pediatrics (2006/2010) strongly recommends formal developmental screening for all children at well visits when the child is 9 months, 18 months, and 24 to 30 months old, and autism-specific screening at 18 and 24 months. The use of screening tests that are sensitive and specific for developmental alterations should be used. Sensitive and specific screening tests include, but are not limited to, the Ages and Stages Questionnaires (ASQ) for children 4 to 60 months, Communication and Symbolic Behavior Scales—Developmental Profile (CSBS-DP) (ages 6 to 24 months), Pervasive Developmental Disorders Screening Test-II (PDDST-II) (12 to 48 months), and the Modified Checklist for Autism in Toddlers (M-CHAT) (AAP, 2006/2010). These, along with parental concern about the child's development, and clinical observation, can assist with early diagnosis (Cole, 2008).

A more complete diagnostic workup for a child with autism involves intelligence testing, although the ability to test intelligence levels is limited, because traditional tests such as the Wechsler Intelligence Scale for Children (WISC) rely heavily on language ability. Another test, the Raven's Progressive Matrices (RPM), is used to test "fluid intelligence" which is the ability to infer rules, set goals, and use high-level abstractions. Matrix tests do not rely on language, but rather on memory, attention, and executive functioning capacity. Although the WISC test is most commonly used with autistic children, Bolte, Dziobek, and Poustka (2009) report that the RPM may be a more accurate measure of intellectual capability in children with more severe manifestations of autism.

Therapeutic Management

Early identification of autism is essential. Treatment generally entails creating an environment that facilitates interaction and promotes replacement of stereotypical behaviors with more normal behaviors. Behavioral methods are typically used. Autistic people have a normal life span; consequently, they require significant financial resources for treatment and supervision.

Because of the severity of the social impairment and the ineffectiveness of normal environmental interventions, affected children are usually referred to special programs designed to offer stimulation, modify stereotypical behaviors, or establish routines for teaching as soon as the disorder has been identified. Programs usually focus on safety precautions for self-injurious behaviors, such as head banging, and the promotion of communication. Facilitative communication through the use of picture boards or keyboards is controversial but has been used in many educational settings to help autistic children interact with the environment.

? CRITICAL THINKING EXERCISE 30-1

You are a nurse working in a clinic and conducting a health assessment on a 9-month-old infant. As you provide the parent with information about the MMR vaccine, which would be given to the infant at the 1-year well visit, the parent expresses concern that he has heard that the MMR vaccine causes autism.

1. What will be your response to this parent?
2. What kind of information can you give the parent to assist him in evaluating information he reads or hears about through the lay media?

NURSING CARE OF THE CHILD WITH AUTISM

■ Assessment

Because there are no classic physical features that highlight autism, the nurse must assess the child with possible autism as if no physical or intellectual disabilities are present. This is done before establishing a diagnosis. The primary characteristic of autism is lack of social interaction and awareness. For this reason, if the child is very young, the nurse who interacts only with the child's parents is unlikely to be aware of the child's degree of social disengagement. If the child has already been diagnosed as having autism and the purpose of assessment is to determine the severity of the disorder—or the assessment occurs before a procedure or hospitalization—it is performed in the same manner as with any normally developing child. The nurse, however, will quickly become aware of the child's social detachment or lack of language as the assessment continues.

A systematic exploration of the child's skills and comparison with developmental norms are essential. For the staff nurse or school nurse, this process may include evaluating the child's ability to feed self, dress, and toilet. The assessment should include the child's interactive patterns and verbalization skills. It is also important to note the child's motor skills, because these have major implications for safety and self-care. For initial, generalized screening, using a reliable and valid developmental screening instrument may be helpful (see Chapter 4). A family history of autism or other mental disorders, family coping skills, and available social support systems should also be included in the assessment.

■ Nursing Diagnosis and Planning

The nursing diagnoses and expected outcomes that may be appropriate after assessment of the child with autism are as follows:

- Risk for Injury related to an inability to anticipate danger, a tendency for self-mutilation, and sensory perceptual deficits.

Expected Outcome. The child's safety will be ensured, as evidenced by maintaining integrity of skin and avoiding self-injury or accidental injury.

- Impaired Social Interaction related to an inability to initiate and maintain social relationships and limited verbal skills.

Expected Outcomes. The child will demonstrate improvement in communication skills and will begin to show appropriate interaction with others.

- Risk for Delayed Development related to an inability to perceive self or others accurately and to intellectual and perceptual dysfunction.

Expected Outcomes. The child will show progress in developing an interest in surroundings and the ability to acknowledge others in the environment; will demonstrate orientation to person, place, and time; and will perform activities of daily living appropriate to this orientation.

■ Interventions

When working with autistic children in the hospital setting, the nurse needs to work closely with the family to determine the child's routines, habits, and preferences. The nurse should write down any specific cues that will help the child remain oriented to the environment and that will facilitate tolerance to change. For example, the nursing staff should be limited to as few individuals as possible. The child may need to perform toileting and self-care activities in a particular order. The child may need an environmental cue, such as stroking a favorite blanket, before being able to move from one activity to the next. The nurse can generally evaluate the child's tolerance of the situation by monitoring signs of anxiety or emotional comfort, as evidenced by such behaviors as attending or observing the nurse in the room or demonstrating a willingness to participate in self-care.

! NURSING QUALITY ALERT

Maintaining Routine for the Child with Autism

Children with autism often are unable to tolerate even the slightest change in routine and may become withdrawn, self-abusive, or violent if their routines are altered.

The nurse must work closely with the family to determine the specific ways in which the child communicates. The child may use sign language or pictures to specify needs if no verbal skills are developed. Children with autism are often reluctant to initiate or sustain direct eye contact, so the nurse may interpret this behavior as meaning that the child is not listening or is unaware of what is being said. In addition, the child may answer questions after several minutes' delay. The nurse should identify these behaviors, allow extra time, and be alert to differences in communication styles. Children with autism generally understand much more language than they are able to use expressively.

The child who demonstrates a tendency for head banging may need a helmet or side rolls. Meticulous observation may be necessary if the child is unable to remain in the bed at night. The nurse should help the parents understand and explain to their child any safety precautions that are unfamiliar to the child. The presence of a parent or older sibling is almost always necessary when an autistic child is hospitalized. Evaluating the child for safety is a continuing nursing function. Reducing the adjustment demands for the child may be necessary if the nurse recognizes behaviors indicating stress or anxiety.

■ Evaluation

- Has the child remained free of injury?
- Has the child developed a way to communicate needs?
- Does the child demonstrate an interest in surroundings?
- Does the child acknowledge the presence of others in the environment?
- Has the child developed the ability to perform activities of daily living?

▮ KEY CONCEPTS

- The causes of intellectual disabilities and developmental disorders can be genetic or environmental.
- Children with an intellectual disability may have limitations in both intellectual and adaptive functioning, which include social interactions, use of language for self-expression, and self-care abilities. If these limitations are severe, the child will need lifelong care by mature, caring adults.
- Children with intellectual impairment have many normal needs, including the need for positive attention and opportunities for self-discovery and growth. Both children and families need to actively participate in care and planning for the child's future.
- Primary nursing responsibilities when caring for a child with an intellectual disability and the child's family include facilitating initial grief, assistance with coping, and identifying resources to help meet the child's lifelong needs.

- *Developmental disability* is a legal term that encompasses intellectual disability as well as disability as a result of a developmental disorder.
- Early screening to identify children who may have a developmental disorder is imperative for facilitating maximum development, and the American Academy of Pediatrics recommends routine screening at certain intervals during infancy and early childhood.
- Conditions that cause intellectual or developmental disability include: (1) disorder of intellectual impairment—Down syndrome, (2) disorders of known genetic cause—fragile X syndrome and Rett syndrome, (3) disorders related to environmental alterations—fetal alcohol syndrome, nonorganic failure to thrive, and (4) disorders with little understood genetic influence—autism spectrum disorders.

REFERENCES

American Academy of Pediatrics. (2006, reaffirmed 2010). Identifying infants and young children with developmental disorders in the medical home: An algorithm for developmental surveillance and screening. *Pediatrics, 118*(1), 405-419.

American Association of Colleges of Nursing. (2008). *The essentials of baccalaureate education for professional nursing practice.* Washington, DC: Author.

American Association on Intellectual and Developmental Disabilities. (2011). *FAQ on intellectual disability.* Retrieved from www.aaidd.org.

American Psychiatric Association. (2000). *Diagnostic and statistical manual of mental disorders* (4th ed., Text revision). Washington, DC: The Association.

Autism and Developmental Disabilities Monitoring Network. (2009). *Prevalence of autistic spectrum disorders (ASDs) in multiple areas of the United States, 2004 and 2006.* Retrieved from www.cdc.gov/ncbddd/autism/states/ADDMCommunityReport2009.pdf.

Autism Society of America. (2009a). *Asperger syndrome.* Retrieved from www.autism-society.org.

Autism Society of America. (2009b). *Autism statistics.* Retrieved from www.autism-society.org.

Bacino, C. & Lee, B. (2011). Fragile chromosome sites. In R. Kliegman, B. Stanton, J. St. Geme, et al. (Eds.), *Nelson textbook of pediatrics* (19th ed., pp. 411-412). Philadelphia: Elsevier Saunders.

Bolte, S., Dziobek, I., & Poustka, F. (2009). Brief report: The level and nature of autistic intelligence revisited. *Journal of Autism and Developmental Disorders, 39,* 678-682.

Centers for Disease Control and Prevention. (2009). *Intellectual disorders.* Retrieved from www.cdc.gov/nchddd/dd/ddmr.

Centers for Disease Control and Prevention. (2010a). *Fetal alcohol spectrum disorders (FASD).* Retrieved from www.cdc.gov

Centers for Disease Control and Prevention. (2010b). *Learn more about fragile X syndrome.* Retrieved from www.cdc.gov.

Centers for Disease Control and Prevention. (2010c). *Tracking fetal alcohol syndrome.* Retrieved from www.cdc.gov.

Cincinnati Children's Hospital Medical Center. (2009). *Best evidence statement (BESt) failure to thrive treatment protocol.* Retrieved from www.guidelines.gov.

Cole, L. (2008). Autism in school age children. *ADVANCE for Nurse Practitioners, 16*(3), 38.

Cornish, K., Turk, J., & Levitas, A. (2007). Fragile X syndrome and autism: Common developmental pathways? *Current Pediatric Reviews, 3,* 3-4.

De Sevo, M. (2010). Genetics and genomics resources for nurses. *Journal of Nursing Education, 49*(8), 470-474.

Developmental Disabilities Assistance and Bill of Rights Act of 2000 (PL 106-402). (2000). Passed by U.S. Congress on October 30, 2000.

Goldberg, P., Jenkins, J., & Spahis, J. (2010). *Genetics: Soon to be part of nursing practice.* Retrieved from www.nurse.com.

Guy, J., Gan, J., Selfridge, J., et al. (2007) Reversal of neurological defects in a mouse model of Rett syndrome. *Science, 315*(23), 1143-1147.

Hagerman, R., & Tranfaglia, M. (2009). Advances in the treatment of fragile X syndrome. *Pediatrics, 123*(1), 378-380.

Holsen, L., Dalton, K., Johnstone, T., & Davidson, R. (2008). Prefrontal social cognition network dysfunction underlying face encoding and social anxiety in fragile X syndrome. *NeuroImage, 43,* 592-604.

International Rett Syndrome Foundation. (2008). *About Rett syndrome.* Retrieved from www.rettsyndrome.org/about-rett-syndrome.html.

Kerr, L. (2008). *Intellectual disability/mental retardation classification.* Retrieved from www.medicalhomeportal.org.

Krivoshik, C. (2007). Silent angels. *ADVANCE for Nurses, 8*(1), 29-30.

Landa, R., Holman, K., & Garrett-Mayer, E. (2007). Social and communication development in toddlers with early and later diagnosis of autism spectrum disorders. *Archives of General Psychiatry, 64*(7), 853-864.

Leshin, L. (2011). *Mosaic Down syndrome.* Retrieved from www.imdsa.org/MDS.

Lindblad, B., Rasmussen, B., & Sandman, P. (2005). Being invigorated in parenthood: Parents' experiences of being supported by professionals when having a disabled child. *Journal of Pediatric Nursing, 20,* 288-297.

March of Dimes. (2011). *Down syndrome.* Retrieved from www.milesforbabies.org/professionals.

McLean, H., & Price, D. (2011). Failure to thrive. In R. Kliegman, B. Stanton, J. St. Geme, et al. (Eds.), *Nelson textbook of pediatrics* (19th ed., pp. 147-149). Philadelphia: Elsevier Saunders.

National Dissemination Center for Children with Disabilities. (2009). *Intellectual disability fact sheet.* Retrieved from www.nichcy.org.

National Dissemination Center for Children with Disabilities. (2011). *Intellectual disabilities.* Retrieved from www.nichcy.org.

National Down Syndrome Society. (2011). *What causes Down syndrome?* Retrieved from www.ndss.org.

National Educational Psychological Service. (2011). *Behavioural, emotional and social difficulties—A continuum of support: Guidelines for teachers.* [Ireland.] Retrieved from www.ncse.ie/uploads/1/Special_Schools_Guidelines_2011_2012.doc.

National Institute of Child Health and Human Development. (2008). *New NIH research plan on Down syndrome.* Retrieved from www.nichd.nih.gov/news/resources/spotlight/012208_research_plan_down_syndrome.cfm.

National Institute of Environmental Health Sciences. (2011). *AARA investments in autism.* Retrieved from www.niehs.nih.gov/recovery/critical/autism.cfm.

National Institute of Mental Health. (2007). *Autism spectrum disorders: Pervasive developmental disorders.* Retrieved from www.nimh.nih.gov/science-news/2007.

Price, C., Thompson, W., Goodson, B., et al. (2010). Prevalence of infant exposure to thimerosol from vaccines and immunoglobulins and risk of autism. *Pediatrics, 126,* 656-664.

Rabinowitz, S., Katturapalli, M., & Rogers, G. (2010). *Nutritional considerations in failure to thrive.* Retrieved from http://emedicine.medscape.com/article/985007.

Raviola, G., Gosselin, G., Walter, H., & DeMarco, D. (2011). Autistic disorder. In R. Kliegman, B. Stanton, J. St. Geme, et al. (Eds.), *Nelson textbook of pediatrics* (19th ed., pp. 100-106). Philadelphia: Elsevier Saunders.

Rizzolo, C., & Cerciello, R. (2009). Recognizing autism spectrum disorder. *Clinical Advisor, 12*(7), 45-46, 50-52.

Sadock, B., & Sadock, V. A. (2008). *Kaplan & Sadock's synopsis of psychiatry: Behavioral sciences/clinical psychiatry* (10th ed.). Philadelphia: Lippincott Williams & Wilkins.

Sebat, J., Lakshmi, B., Malhotra, D., & Wigler, M. (2007). Strong association of de novo copy number mutations with autism. *Science, 316,* 445-449.

Shin, M., Besser, L., Kucik, J., et al. (2009). Prevalence of Down syndrome among children and adolescents in 10 regions of the United States. *Pediatrics, 124*(6), 1565-1571.

Summar, K., & Lee, B. (2011). Down syndrome and other abnormalities of chromosome number. In R. Kliegman, B. Stanton, J. St. Geme, et al. (Eds.), *Nelson textbook of pediatrics* (19th ed., pp. 399-404). Philadelphia: Elsevier Saunders.

U.S. Department of Health and Human Services. (2010a). *Child maltreatment 2009.* Administration for Children and Families, Administration on Children, Youth and Families, Children's Bureau. Retrieved from www.acf.hhs.gov/programs/cb/stats_research/index.htm#can.

U.S. Department of Health and Human Services. (2010b). *Healthy people 2020.* Retrieved from http://healthypeople.gov.

University of California. (n.d.). *Basic research on the neurobiology of Down syndrome.* Retrieved from www.downsyndrome.ucsd.edu/2page.php?id=ds5.

World Down Syndrome Day. (2011). Retrieved from www.worlddownsyndromeday.org.

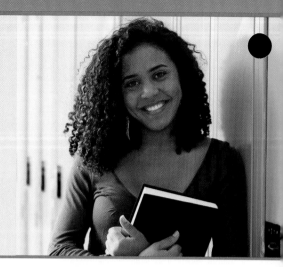

℮volve WEBSITE

http://evolve.elsevier.com/James/ncoc

LEARNING OBJECTIVES

After studying this chapter, you should be able to:

- Describe the structure and function of the eye and ear.
- Describe the specific information required in a health history for a child with potential sensory alterations.
- Define the nurse's role in assessing for sensory alterations.
- Describe specific nursing care for children with health problems affecting the eye and ear.

- Describe how alterations in the sensory organs affect the child's ability to communicate.
- Identify potential growth and development interruptions that may occur with problems affecting the sensory organs.

CLINICAL REFERENCE

REVIEW OF THE EYE

Structure and Function

The eye is attached to the skull by six accessory muscles. These are used to move the eye to achieve vision. Ciliary muscles function to alter the shape of the eye to provide focus and accommodation at various distances. Cranial nerves II, III, IV, V, and VI all affect the eye (see Chapter 9 for cranial nerve assessment).

The orb, or eye, is made up of several parts. The cornea is the clear area located in the front of the eye, where light enters the eye. The cornea and sclera (white outer covering) make up the eye's outer layer. The middle layer is composed of the choroid (vascular lining), the lens (a clear structure that changes shape to allow accommodation of light on the retina), and the iris (the colored muscular ring located behind the cornea that expands or contracts to control the amount of light entering the eye). The inner layer of the eye is known as the *retina*. This area contains the rods and cones. These receive light impulses and transmit them through the optic nerve (cranial nerve II) to the brain. The macula contains the greatest concentration of nerve endings. The cornea and lens focus light onto the macula. The optic disk is the area where the optic nerve enters the eye.

Neonatal Development

The eyes begin to develop at approximately 22 days of gestation. The critical period for development is considered to be 22 to 50 days. Congenital abnormalities appear to be caused by either genetic or environmental factors or a combination. The eye is especially sensitive to teratogens, in particular infections such as cytomegalovirus and rubella.

REVIEW OF THE EAR

Structure and Function

The ear is divided into three parts: the outer ear, the middle ear, and the inner ear. The outer ear includes the auricle and external ear canal. It is separated from the middle ear by the tympanic membrane (eardrum). The tympanic membrane vibrates to conduct sound waves to the middle ear. The middle ear contains the bones of hearing—the malleus (hammer), incus (anvil), and stapes (stirrup). These bones conduct sound waves from the tympanic membrane to the inner ear. The inner ear contains the nerve endings that conduct sound impulses to the brain. These are located in a snail-shaped chamber (the cochlea) that is filled with fluid. The inner ear also controls balance. The

Anatomy of the Eye

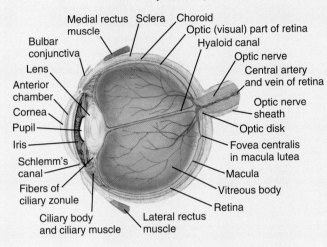

Medial rectus muscle — Sclera — Choroid — Optic (visual) part of retina — Hyaloid canal — Optic nerve — Central artery and vein of retina — Optic nerve sheath — Optic disk — Fovea centralis in macula lutea — Macula — Vitreous body — Retina — Lateral rectus muscle

Bulbar conjunctiva — Lens — Anterior chamber — Cornea — Pupil — Iris — Schlemm's canal — Fibers of ciliary zonule — Ciliary body and ciliary muscle

Anatomy of the Ear

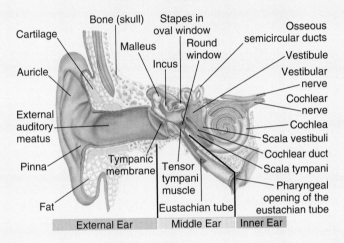

Cartilage — Bone (skull) — Stapes in oval window — Malleus — Incus — Round window — Osseous semicircular ducts — Vestibule — Vestibular nerve — Cochlear nerve — Cochlea — Scala vestibuli — Cochlear duct — Scala tympani — Pharyngeal opening of the eustachian tube

Auricle — External auditory meatus — Pinna — Tympanic membrane — Tensor tympani muscle — Fat — Eustachian tube

External Ear | Middle Ear | Inner Ear

eustachian tube connects the middle ear with the nasopharynx. It functions to allow fluids to drain into the nasopharynx and assists in equalizing pressure between the outer ear and the middle ear.

Neonatal Development

The ear begins to develop during the 3rd week of gestation. The critical period for the development of the ear is between 4 and 6 weeks of gestation. Like the eye, the ear is highly sensitive to teratogens. It is innervated by the acoustic nerve (cranial nerve VIII). Congenital deafness largely appears to be the result of genetic factors.

SPEECH DEVELOPMENT

Because the fetus is capable of hearing during the second trimester of pregnancy and is able to hear voices and the mother's heartbeat, the infant is born with a sensitivity to variations of speech. Adequate hearing is essential for the development of speech. The infant begins to coo and vocalize quite early (birth to 4 months). Babbling begins at approximately 4 to 6 months. Babbling is followed by receptive language development (understanding words) and expressive language development (saying words; see Chapters 5 through 8 for specifics of speech development). Any hearing impairment can interfere with speech development, as can any alteration affecting the oral cavity.

PEDIATRIC DIFFERENCES IN SENSORY FUNCTION

Vision

- Development of the eye is not complete at birth, but the newborn is able to fixate, follow an object to midline, and react to a change in intensity of light.
- By 3 months of age, the infant can follow moving objects; by 4 months of age, the infant can recognize familiar objects.
- Binocularity, the ability to fixate on one visual field with both eyes, is not present at birth but is established by 6 months of age. Frequent eye crossing after 6 months of age is abnormal and indicates strabismus.
- Visual acuity changes with age:

4 months:	20/50 to 20/80
1 year:	20/40 to 20/70
4 years:	20/30 to 20/40
5 years:	20/20 to 20/30

- Lacrimal glands are not fully developed at birth. Tears are not often present with crying until after 1 to 3 months. Temporary obstruction of lacrimal ducts may cause overflow of tears.
- The size of the orbits doubles by the time the child is 1 year of age and doubles again by age 6 years. Eye growth is completed at 10 to 12 years of age.

Hearing

- Development of the ear begins during the 3rd week of gestation and is complete by the 3rd month of embryonic life. Infection or other insult to the fetus during this time can cause irreparable damage to the ear. Ear development occurs at the same time as kidney development, so malformation in one system may indicate problems in the other.
- An infant as young as 3 days is able to distinguish between familiar and unfamiliar sounds and can recognize the mother's voice. The infant can distinguish between frequently heard words and other words (nonsense language) by 1 year.
- Basic auditory skills are in place by 3 years of age. Hearing can be evaluated by audiometry testing by this age.
- Infants and young children have shorter, more horizontal, and more flaccid eustachian tubes, predisposing them to otitis media.

Speech and Language

- Infants can imitate sounds heard by 3 to 5 months of age.
- Verbal dialogue similar to an adult's is noted by approximately 6 months of age.

Because a child learns so much through the senses, deficits in hearing and vision can have profound effects on development. Appropriate screening and early interventions are crucial. Early identification of vision and hearing deficits allows for early intervention—either correction or the provision of adaptive measures—so that the child's "normal" growth and development may be preserved. Because a child cannot report sensory deficits, nurses must carefully assess for alterations in vision or hearing.

U.S. legislation PL 94-142 (the Education for All Handicapped Children Act) was passed in 1975 and subsequently updated as the Individuals with Disabilities Education Act (see Chapter 30); it mandates special education services for children with severe sensory deficits. The identification of children who might be eligible for special educational services at a young age is important so that their education can be maximized.

The health history of a child with a potential sensory deficit is essentially the same as for any child (see Chapter 9) but should include the following additional pieces of information:

- Thorough prenatal history
- Growth and developmental history
- History of any infections (including treatment, because many medications can cause sensory deficits)
- Previous trauma to the eye or ear
- Changes noted in behavior (e.g., rubbing the eyes, turning up the volume on the television, decreased attention span)
- Changes in appearance (e.g., red, inflamed eyes; drainage from the eye or ear)
- Physical symptoms (e.g., reports of ear or eye pain, headache, nausea and vomiting)

After carefully reviewing the health history, the nurse performs a thorough physical examination with age-appropriate measures of vision and hearing acuity (see Chapter 9).

DISORDERS OF THE EYE

The nurse has an important role in the prevention and early detection of eye problems. All children should have sensitive and specific vision screening performed at well visits. The American Academy of Pediatrics (AAP), American Association of Certified Orthoptists, The American Academy of Ophthalmology, the American Association for Pediatric Ophthalmology and Strabismus, and the Children's Eye Foundation (Donahue & Ruben, 2011) recommend the following:

- *At birth:* External and internal appearance for structural abnormalities, red reflex, fixation.
- *Age 3 to 6 months:* Fixation and ability to follow, alignment (cover/uncover test, corneal light reflex, photo screening).
- *Birth to 3 years:* All of the above with ocular history.

The United States Preventive Services Task Force (USPSTF) (2011), along with the previously mentioned organizations (Donahue & Ruben, 2011) recommend the following for older children:

- *Age 3 years and older:* All of the above plus visual acuity using developmentally appropriate charts (HOTV, Lea symbols, "tumbling E") and ophthalmoscopy; stereopsis can be tested by using the random dot E test (see Chapter 9).

For children who are uncooperative or who are otherwise unable to participate in traditional vision screening photoscreening or autorefraction may be used. Photoscreening (photo refractive screening), a process of photographing images of eye light reflexes, can easily detect a variety of eye problems in young children. Photoscreening is particularly useful for detecting refractive errors, strabismus, and other conditions that contribute to amblyopia (USPSTF, 2011). Autorefraction is

> ## BOX 31-1   SIGNS AND SYMPTOMS OF POTENTIAL VISION PROBLEMS
>
> - Inability to fix both eyes on an object and follow the track of a moving object with both eyes
> - Persistent discharge from one or both eyes, especially accompanied by redness of the sclera
> - Excessive tearing, especially when accompanied by itchiness or pain
> - Cloudiness or white areas in the pupil
> - Deviation of the iris in an inward or outward direction (crossing)
> - Head tilting or closing one eye to see
> - Squinting
> - Reports of headache or blurred or double vision
> - The need to sit close to a television or blackboard to see
> - Holding reading material close to the eyes
> - Excessive fatigue with visual concentration

the process for estimating refractive error in order to predict actual refractive problems in children (Children's Eye Foundation, 2011). Through use of equipment that uses ultrasound measurements, refracted error can be estimated (Children's Eye Foundation, 2011). Refer children who do not pass structural or vision screening for complete ophthalmologic evaluation. Careful attention to behavior and appearance changes, as well as physical symptoms, assists in the early detection and treatment of eye disorders (Box 31-1). Children who have any symptoms should be referred for further evaluation.

Nursing Considerations for the Child with Color Deficiency

Colorblindness, or color deficiency, occurs in approximately 8% of the population and primarily affects males. It interferes with the ability to distinguish between colors within certain groups, such as red, blue, and green.

Testing should be done if the clinician suspects a problem (i.e., a suspected optic nerve or retinal dysfunction) or the family has a history of color deficiency. Testing is routine in preschool boys. The most common detection test is the pseudoisochromatic (color confusion) test, in which color plates include patterns that are hidden to a person with a color deficit. Pseudoisochromatic plates are also available for children who cannot yet read. If a problem is detected, more sophisticated testing may be necessary to determine the exact type of color deficiency. Although color deficiency has no cure, certain types of tints used in contact lenses and glasses can help the child discriminate color differences.

Because color deficiency cannot be cured, nursing care focuses on adaptive and supportive measures. Encourage parents to have children tested if the family has a history of color deficiency or if the nurse suspects the child is having trouble distinguishing colors.

Parent and child education are important for the child with color deficiency. Teaching should focus on alternative ways to discriminate the deficient colors. For the older child who can dress without assistance, clothes can be labeled or organized so that items can be easily coordinated.

Safety is a major concern for the color-deficient child. For example, the child who cannot distinguish red and green must learn another way to distinguish traffic signals and other warning lights. Finally, anticipatory guidance is sometimes related to appropriate career choices. For example, color deficiency might prohibit an adult from becoming a pilot, police officer, or firefighter.

SAFETY ALERT

Vision Screening

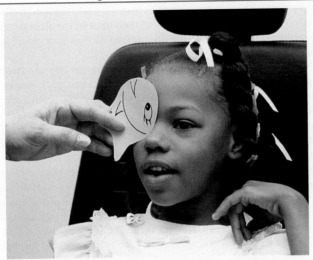

- Thoroughly explain the procedure to the child before beginning. If using a symbol (HOTV, Lea) chart, show the child the symbols and ask the child to identify or match them. If using a machine to test the child's vision, demonstrate in advance how it works.
- Take the child to a quiet, nondistracting area that has been marked for the appropriate distance from the chart.
- Have the child cover one eye. Use a colorful, opaque cover that completely blocks the child's vision. The parent can help hold the cover in place.
- Point to a symbol on a line that the child can probably see readily, and move to smaller lines. Vary the direction (left to right, right to left) to reduce the likelihood that the child is memorizing the symbols.
- Give positive feedback. Perform the test as quickly as possible because small children lose interest quickly.
- Test both eyes. Refer for further evaluation if a discrepancy of two lines exists or if the child tests in the abnormal range on two successive screenings.

Nursing Considerations for the Child with a Blocked Lacrimal Duct

A blocked lacrimal (tear) duct is characterized by excessive tearing (epiphora) and crusting on the eyelids on awakening. Parents may also note a small mass just below the inner aspect of the eye. Treatment usually consists of massaging the duct. If the duct remains blocked despite massaging or remains blocked after 1 year of age, surgical opening of the duct is indicated.

The nurse should carefully assess the mucoid drainage. In a noninfected duct, the drainage is usually white or clear. If the duct has become infected, however, the drainage may be green or yellow. If the drainage suggests an infected duct, treatment with antibiotic eyedrops or ointment is indicated.

The nurse teaches the parent about the proper technique for lacrimal massage. This process involves washing hands thoroughly and placing the index finger over the lacrimal duct (at the inner aspect of the eye by the bridge of the nose) and "milking," or gently massaging, the duct in an upward motion. Emphasize that massaging down the nasal bone has very little effect on the duct because the lacrimal system is intraosseous and unaffected by massage over bone. Other teaching includes monitoring for signs and symptoms of infection.

Nursing Considerations for the Child with a Refractive Error

Refractive errors cause vision disturbances from alterations in the path of light rays through the eye. They usually result from an abnormally shaped orb; the orb may be flattened or elongated (Table 31-1). Refractive errors are often discovered when a child squints, frowns, or moves objects so they are more easily seen. Reports from the child or a teacher may also alert parents. *Legal blindness* is defined as a correction of 20/200 or worse in the better eye or a visual field of 20 degrees or less.

Nurses should assess children's vision at every well-child visit, particularly during the preschool years. Visual acuity can be reliably tested in a cooperative child as young as 3 years. When testing visual acuity, the nurse needs to remember that a vision discrepancy of two lines or more on the vision chart, even if one eye tests normal, is cause for referral. A child with this discrepancy could have *anisometropia*, or a

TABLE 31-1 TYPES OF REFRACTIVE DISORDERS

DESCRIPTION	CLINICAL MANIFESTATIONS	TREATMENT
Myopia Nearsightedness Ability to see close objects more clearly than those at a distance Caused by the image focusing in front of the retina	Difficulty seeing the blackboard or television clearly Decreased interest in activities requiring distance vision Squinting, head tilting, holding books close to eyes Decreased attention span, poor school performance	Treated with biconcave lenses New lenses may be required every 1-2 yr as the child grows
Hyperopia Farsightedness Ability to see distant objects more clearly than those close up Caused by the image focusing beyond the retina	Most children are normally hyperopic until approximately 7 yr of age but are able to accommodate to see clearly Strabismus or amblyopia may develop from prolonged hyperopia	Most young children with hyperopia need no correction If correction is required, convex lenses are used
Astigmatism Unequal curvature of the cornea or the lens causing light rays to bend in different directions May coexist with myopia or hyperopia	Mild astigmatism may be asymptomatic Manifestations may be similar to myopia	Treated with special lenses to compensate for the unequal curvature of the cornea

large refractive discrepancy between eyes. If not corrected, this condition can lead to amblyopia.

School nurses routinely test children's vision and, in fact, annual vision screening is offered to children throughout the United States. The USPSTF (2011) has recommended that vision screening begin early in the preschool years (at 3 years of age) to identify amblyopia and other associated vision alterations Several states in the United States mandate that a child have an approved vision screening test (administered by a trained examiner) within the year prior to entering kindergarten. HOTV, Lea symbols and the "tumbling E" test are comparatively effective as screening measures for preschool-age children (Chou, Dana, & Bougatsos, 2011). Evidence suggests that vision screening tests, which can include photoscreening or autorefraction testing, can accurately identify vision problems in young children (Chou et al., 2011). School nurses have used various methods of notifying families of children who do not pass a school vision screening (e.g., telephone call to parents, letter brought home by the child, letter mailed home). However, the parent is responsible for follow-through with a visit to a specialist. Nurses need to be aware that some parents, for a variety of reasons, do not take the child for a follow-up comprehensive eye examination; for this reason, nurses in other settings must ask for details about the child's vision and previous vision testing.

Corrective lenses are used to improve the child's vision. Encourage the parent to look for impact-resistant eyeglasses with spring-loaded frames, which are less likely to bend or warp. Fitting glasses to an infant or young child can be challenging; the goal is to choose shatter-resistant lenses in a type of frame that can be closely fitted to prevent easy dislodging during activity. Infant frames often have elasticized straps to keep them properly positioned. Teach the parent, and child if appropriate, to always store the glasses in a case when not being used. Special directions for cleaning must be followed to avoid scratching the lenses.

Both gas-permeable and soft contact lenses provide an alternative for children old enough and responsible enough to care for contact lenses independently. The nurse needs to teach parents and children about appropriate care of corrective lenses and should educate parents and children about recognizing and intervening with vision problems early.

Protective eyeware made of shatterproof polycarbonate, should be worn by all who participate in sports that have risk for eye injury. A variety of prescription sports glasses are available for athletes. Protective eyewear should be selected according to the sport and the relative risk for injury (American Academy of Ophthalmology, 2011).

Nursing Considerations for the Child with Amblyopia

Amblyopia, or "lazy eye," one of the most common causes of diminished vision in children, results from a variety of eye alterations seen in children whose visual acuity is impaired. Various reports state that the prevalence of amblyopia is between 2% and 4% of children (USPSTF, 2011).When both eyes are unable to focus simultaneously, the brain suppresses the image from the deviating eye to avoid double vision (diplopia). Amblyopia frequently accompanies strabismus, as well as other eye conditions such as congenital cataract and severe refractive error. If the underlying eye condition is untreated in a child younger than 4 years (the critical period for development of the visual cortex), permanent loss of vision from amblyopia can result; amblyopia can be treated in the older child but it is more resistant to treatment approaches at that time (Olitsky, Hug, Plummer, & Stass-Isern, 2011). Because the child loses binocular vision, depth perception may also be impaired. Early detection and treatment of strabismus or other underlying causes of amblyopia are essential to prevent loss of vision.

Two primary approaches, penalization (blurring) and occlusion, are used to correct amblyopia, and each is designed to alter or obscure vision in the stronger eye to force the child to use the amblyopic eye. Atropine, which is a cycloplegic (paralyzes the ciliary muscles to dilate the eye), most often is used to blur the vision in the stronger eye. Wearing eyeglasses in which the lens over the stronger eye creates blurring has a similar effect (Doshi & Rodriguez, 2007).

Wearing lenses corrective for refraction error can improve amblyopia in some children (Stewart, Moseley, & Fielder, 2011). Patching, combined with use of corrective lenses, has been demonstrated to have better outcomes than wearing corrective lenses alone for treatment of amblyopia caused by strabismus (Taylor & Elliott, 2011). Patching is used primarily to correct amblyopia and is used mostly during the preschool years when the visual cortex is developing. In this treatment, the normal eye is patched so that the child is forced to use the weaker eye. The schedule for patching is individualized. Recent evidence suggests that some children will respond well to a patching regimen that does not require 24 hour occlusion, but as little as 2 to 4 hours of daily use (Olitsky et al., 2011; Stewart et al., 2011).The patching regimen is prescribed by the ophthalmologist. Cooperation with the patching regimen is essential. Teaching should explain the reasons for patching or corrective lenses, the expected results of wearing the patch or lens, correct placement of the patch, the number of hours per day the patch or lens is to be worn, and the expected length of treatment (see Patient-Centered Teaching: Information about Eye Patching box). The child needs to understand that wearing the patch or lens is not negotiable. The nurse often must teach parents strategies for dealing with resistant behaviors.

PATIENT-CENTERED TEACHING

Information about Eye Patching

- Your child will need to wear the eye patch for the exact time your physician has prescribed. Not adhering to the full wearing time could interfere with the treatment.
- Prescribed patching will not harm your child's stronger eye but will force the muscles of the weaker eye to be used.
- Apply the patch directly to your child's face, being sure to cover the whole eye. Do not leave any openings through which the child can peek.
- If your child wears eyeglasses as well, put the glasses on over the patch.
- It can be frustrating for the child to have to wear the patch. Try to be patient, understanding, and supportive. Patching must be nonnegotiable. Find decorative patches or put your own decoration on the patch. Praise your child frequently for cooperating with the treatment.

Nursing Considerations for the Child with Strabismus

Strabismus is a condition in which the eyes are not aligned because of lack of coordination of the extraocular muscles. It is present in approximately 4% of children younger than 6 years of age (Olitsky et al., 2011). Strabismus is most often caused by muscle imbalance or paralysis of the extraocular muscles but may also result from conditions such as a brain tumor, myasthenia gravis, or infection. Infants and children with strabismus often have a close relative with the condition. Other contributing factors include genetic abnormalities, neuromuscular disease, exposure to teratogens, and trauma; the prevalence is higher in children who were born prematurely or who were of low birth weight (Pathai, Cumberland, & Rahi, 2010). The type of deviation noted defines strabismus (Box 31-2). When assessing infants for strabismus, the nurse needs to remember that strabismus is normal in the young infant but should not be present after approximately 3 months of age.

BOX 31-2   TYPES OF STRABISMUS

- *Comitant strabismus:* Most common type of strabismus in children. Constant deviation in all fields of gaze; not associated with eye muscle paralysis. All extraocular muscles function but are not coordinated. Child has difficulty seeing at close range and often squints. Accommodative nonparalytic strabismus may develop between 2 and 4 years of age as a result of a large refractive error.
- *Paralytic strabismus:* Caused by a weakness or paralysis of one or more of the extraocular muscles. Usually involves dysfunction of one or more cranial nerves involved with ocular movement. The eye appears crossed when turned in the direction of the affected muscle. May cause headache and poor coordination. Diplopia may cause child to close one eye or tilt the head.
- *Esotropia (convergent):* The eye turns inward; most common type of strabismus in infants. May occur with hyperopia as the eyes compensate for the refractive error by overconvergence.

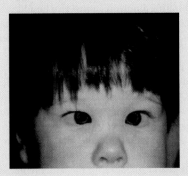

Child with early-onset esotropia. The deviation may not be apparent until age 3 or 4 months.

- *Exotropia (divergent):* The eyes turn away from the midline; occurs most often when the child attempts to focus on a distant object. May be present at birth.

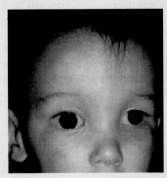

Child with left exotropia. Most exodeviations in childhood are intermittent.

- *Pseudostrabismus:* Not true strabismus. The eyes appear to deviate inward but are actually in alignment. Facial features, such as epicanthal folds and a broad, flat nasal bridge, can give the appearance of misalignment.
- *Phoria:* A tendency for the eye to deviate. More evident during times of stress, fatigue, or illness.
- *Tropia:* A continuous or intermittent misalignment of the eye.

Photographs from Albert, D. M., & Jakobiec, F. A. (Eds.). (1994). *Principles and practice of ophthalmology* (pp. 2731, 2733). Philadelphia: Saunders.

The corneal light reflex test, simultaneous red reflex test, cover-uncover test, and alternate-cover test (see Chapter 9) are used in the diagnosis of strabismus. The nurse may suspect strabismus when the child reports frequent headaches, squints, or tilts the head to see. The parent may suspect something is wrong when a flash photograph of the child reveals unequal "red eye." Children who have family members with strabismus should be regularly assessed for development of the condition. Strabismus can contribute to amblyopia in the infant or young child.

Treatment of strabismus may include special corrective lenses, vision therapy, surgery, or pharmacologic therapy. If the deviation is caused by hyperopia, corrective lenses are indicated to correct vision. Eyeglasses with specially ground prism power may also be indicated. These glasses correct vision in the affected eye so that the brain receives the same image from both eyes.

Botulinum toxin (Botox) was approved in 1989 by the U.S. Food and Drug Administration as an alternative to surgery in some cases. The toxin is injected into the eye muscle and produces temporary paralysis. This condition allows the muscles opposite the paralyzed muscle to straighten the eye. With successful treatment, the correction remains after the medication wears off (in approximately 2 months). The most common side effect is a drooping eyelid (ptosis), which usually resolves spontaneously.

Surgery may be indicated to realign the weakened muscles in a child with strabismus. It is most often indicated when amblyopia is present and should be performed before the child is 2 years of age. The stronger eye may be patched before surgery to treat any existing amblyopia. Surgery may be required only on the weakened eye or on both eyes. More than one surgery may be necessary. During the surgery, small incisions are made and the weakened muscles are tightened or the stronger muscles are weakened and lengthened (Modi & Jones, 2008).

If the child is to have a surgical correction, the nurse should prepare the child and parents before surgery for what to expect after surgery and provide information about dressing changes, eyedrops, corrective lenses, and any other postoperative treatments that may be required. Interventions are similar to those for any child having eye surgery (see pp. 822-823).

Nursing Considerations for the Child with Glaucoma

Glaucoma is a condition in which the intraocular fluid pressure of the eye is increased. This pressure increase, if left untreated, leads to atrophy of the optic disk and, ultimately, blindness. Glaucoma is a significant cause of blindness in children (Aponte, Diehl, & Mohney, 2010).

Several types of glaucoma occur in children. Congenital glaucoma and infantile glaucoma occur during the first 3 years of life and are caused by a defect in the drainage network of the eye. Primary congenital glaucoma has a genetic origin, with an autosomal recessive inheritance pattern. Secondary glaucoma, which may be associated with other ocular anomalies, refers to disease that occurs after 3 years of age and may be the result of inherited disease (juvenile glaucoma) or may be acquired from infection, trauma, or cataract removal (acquired glaucoma) (Olitsky et al., 2011).

Clinical signs of glaucoma include excessive tearing, light sensitivity, blepharospasm (muscle spasm causing involuntary closing of the eyelid), and enlargement of the globe and cornea. Parents often note excessive tearing or corneal haziness caused by edema and bring the child in for clinical evaluation. The child may also be brought to the practitioner for what appears to be conjunctivitis ("pink eye").

Physical examination includes an assessment of visual acuity, measurement of intraocular pressure (tonometry), assessment of corneal diameter and clarity, and an examination of the retina to assess for optic nerve cupping. Any infant with a visible iris diameter greater than 10.5 mm should be evaluated. If retinal edema is present, the light reflex is diffuse. Because young children may not be able to cooperate during an examination, they are often sedated. Intraocular pressure should be measured only under light sedation, however, because deeper sedation may alter readings (either high or low, depending on the agent used).

The preferred treatment for childhood glaucoma is surgery. Medications to clear the cornea may be used before surgery to allow better visibility. Surgery should be performed as soon as possible after diagnosis to prevent loss (or further loss) of vision. The goals of surgery are to increase the outflow of the aqueous humor from the anterior chamber by correcting the structural abnormality that is causing the decreased outflow, create a different route for the outflow (trabeculotomy), or decrease production of aqueous fluid (Olitsky et al., 2011). Medications such as cholinergic agents, beta-adrenergic blocking agents, or adrenergic agents may be indicated after surgery to maintain low intraocular pressure.

Prognosis varies from child to child. The earlier the glaucoma develops, the poorer the prognosis, because infants and children with early-onset glaucoma usually have defects in the development of the anterior chamber of the eye that occurred during fetal development (Olitsky et al., 2011). In general, with prompt treatment most children attain appropriate vision. Decreased vision may result from damage to the optic nerve, opacity of the cornea or lens, or amblyopia resulting from refractive errors. Children with glaucoma must be followed closely over the long term to identify any rise in intraocular pressure quickly.

Nursing interventions are similar to those for any child having eye surgery. Postoperative nursing care includes monitoring for signs and symptoms of increased intraocular pressure (pain, nausea and vomiting, increased inflammation) and administering any ordered medications, such as miotic eyedrops (used to constrict the pupils) and antibiotic ointments or eyedrops. If the child's eyes are patched, the nurse pays special attention to the resulting sensory deficits. The nurse also considers safety to be an issue when eyes are patched.

Parental education is essential to maintain the appropriate intraocular pressure and prevent complications (including blindness). Education includes the use of any prescribed medications, patching, and any other measures designed to correct refractive errors. The importance of returning for follow-up care should be emphasized. The child and caregivers should also be taught signs and symptoms of increasing intraocular pressure. Any signs of increasing intraocular pressure or infection should be immediately reported to the ophthalmologist. Because certain types of glaucoma can be related to genetic abnormalities, referral for genetic counseling may be indicated.

Nursing Considerations for the Child with a Cataract

A cataract is an opacity, or loss of transparency, of the lens. Causes include an inherited tendency (usually an autosomal dominant trait), infection (e.g., rubella), trauma, or a metabolic imbalance; the cause of congenital cataracts is unknown (Davenport & Patel, 2011). Cloudiness of the lens may be noted during examination in the newborn nursery (indicated by a white instead of red reflex) or by the parents. Ophthalmoscopy may reveal a dark spot in the lens. Parents may note that the infant exhibits visual inattentiveness and come in for an evaluation. Other clinical signs include nystagmus and strabismus. The cataract alters vision because it does not allow a sharp, clear image to be formed on the retina.

Treatment for cataracts in most instances is the surgical removal of the opaque lens as soon as possible and optimally within 6 to 10 weeks of age (Davenport & Patel, 2011). The resultant hyperopia is then dealt with by using a contact lens or, in older children, an intraocular lens implant. Any resulting amblyopia must also be addressed. Glasses may also be used to correct the resultant vision problem, although these may be difficult to manage in infants and small children (Olitsky et al., 2011).

Amblyopia may be a consequence of congenital cataract. In this case, the normal eye may be patched after surgery to develop the weakened eye.

Postoperative interventions are directed toward avoiding increased intraocular pressure. Measures include preventing coughing, straining, vomiting, and touching the operative site. A patch and "hard shield" are usually in place after surgery to prevent injury to the operative site. To prevent edema and pressure on the site, the nurse should elevate the head of the bed slightly and position the child so that the affected eye is not in a dependent position. Monitor the child for signs and symptoms of infection (fever, drainage, redness). Medications, including antibiotics, mydriatics, and steroids, may be used after surgery.

Postoperative teaching includes how to insert, remove, and care for the child's contact lens. Parents need to be taught the signs and symptoms of infection and increasing intraocular pressure. To provide visual stimulation to the affected eye and prevent further loss of vision, the importance of adhering to any prescribed patching regimen should also be emphasized. Finally, the nurse teaches the importance of returning for follow-up visits to ensure that the lens fits correctly, the vision correction is appropriate, and no signs and symptoms of complications are present. As with glaucoma, the occurrence of some cataracts has a genetic component, so referral for genetic counseling may be indicated.

◎ NURSING CARE PLAN

The Child Having Eye Surgery

Focused Assessment
- Determine the child's and family's understanding of the planned surgical procedure and why surgery is necessary; include assessment of their knowledge of postsurgical and discharge care.
- Assess the child's and family's knowledge of strategies to maintain safety for a child who has a visual deficit.
- Assess potential discharge teaching needs.

Planning
Nursing Diagnosis
Acute Confusion related to visual impairment from eye patching or surgical procedure.

Expected Outcomes
The child and family will describe any anticipated temporary vision changes.
The child and family will demonstrate familiarity with the surroundings and associated sights and sounds.
The child will remain alert and oriented to time and place.

Intervention/*Rationale*
1. Prepare the child and family before surgery for any changes expected in vision, including blurred vision or patched eyes.
   Preoperative preparation allows the child and family to know what to expect, thus lessening anxiety.

The Child Having Eye Surgery—cont'd

Intervention/*Rationale*—cont'd

2. Before surgery, orient the child and family to the surroundings, including the recovery room and hospital room. Describe any unfamiliar sounds the child may hear; have the child close his or her eyes and listen.
Preoperative orientation to surroundings allows the child a feeling of familiarity during the postoperative period.

3. Provide reality orientation (time, day) for the child during the postoperative period, especially if vision is impaired or eyes are patched.
Providing a sense of time passage and orienting to day and night prevent the child from becoming disoriented and confused.

4. Provide emotional support and allow expression of feelings of anger and frustration, possibly through play therapy and therapeutic communication.
Allowing the child and family to express their fears and frustrations provides an appropriate outlet and encourages the use of other senses.

Evaluation

Can the child and family describe expected temporary postoperative vision changes?

Can the child describe the hospital and room environment and its associated sounds?

Does the child remain alert and oriented to time and place?

Planning
Nursing Diagnosis

Risk for Injury related to increased intraocular pressure resulting from bleeding, edema, hematoma, postoperative vomiting.

Expected Outcome

The child will remain free from injury (increased intraocular pressure, bleeding) through appropriate management of postoperative eye care, crying, nausea, and vomiting.

Intervention/*Rationale*

1. Fully orient the child to surroundings and ensure that unsafe objects are removed from the environment.
Orienting the child to the environment and ensuring that the environment is safe prevents falls and other injuries when the child is out of bed.

2. Ensure that the child wears eye patches or shields as ordered. *Eye patches and shields are often prescribed to prevent any further injury to the eye.*

3. Encourage the parents to remain with the child and prevent the child from rubbing the eyes. Restraints are used as a last resort to prevent injury. Encourage the parent to keep side rails up at all times.
Rubbing the eyes can damage the surgical site. If restraints are needed, elbow restraints provide protection without total restriction.

4. Monitor for signs and symptoms of increased intraocular pressure. Give ordered antiemetics if the child is nauseated. Administer intravenous fluids until the child is stable.
Increasing intraocular pressure can damage the eye and seriously impair vision. Vomiting can increase intraocular pressure.

5. Approach the child in a calm and soothing manner. Assign personnel whom the child has met and trusts. Encourage the parent to soothe the child who is crying.
Avoidance of crying postoperatively reduces the risk for increasing intraocular pressure. Assigning the child to a familiar nurse reduces fear and anxiety that may lead to crying.

Evaluation

Does the child remain free of physical injury?

Is the child's intraocular pressure within normal limits?

Is the child free from crying, nausea, and vomiting?

Planning
Nursing Diagnosis

Risk for Infection related to surgical incision.

Expected Outcome

The child will remain free from infection, as evidenced by normal temperature and absence of discharge and excessive tearing or edema.

Intervention/*Rationale*

1. Monitor the child for signs and symptoms of infection, including redness, drainage, fever, and excessive tearing or edema.
These are physical signs that a postoperative infection is developing in the eye.

2. Administer antibiotic therapy as ordered.
Antibiotics may be used as prophylaxis against infection.

Evaluation

Is the child free from fever, redness, edema, or excessive eye drainage?

Planning
Nursing Diagnosis

Acute Pain related to surgical procedure.

Expected Outcome

The child will experience minimal discomfort during the postoperative period, as evidenced by acceptable pain scale rating, normal vital signs, and participation in approved quiet activities.

Intervention/*Rationale*

1. Monitor the child frequently (every 2 to 4 hours while awake) for pain by using a verbal age-appropriate pain scale. Use a preverbal pain scale, in addition to self-reported pain, to assess pain level in infants and young children whose eyes are occluded. Monitor physiologic signs of pain in the young child (increased pulse, restlessness, inability to sleep, inability to play).
Pain can increase anxiety and restlessness that could lead to increased intraocular pressure. The young child who would ordinarily use a visual scale to rate pain is unable to do so if eyes are patched.

2. Administer pain medications as ordered.
Pain control decreases the child's need to rub or touch the eyes, which can cause trauma to the surgical site.

3. Provide nonpharmacologic pain-relief measures, such as ice pack and moist heat, as indicated. Use distraction techniques frequently (music, stories).
Nonpharmacologic pain-relief measures can replace or augment pharmacologic measures. Verbal distraction techniques can decrease pain and take the child's mind off the bandages.

Evaluation

Does the child express relief of pain with an age-appropriate pain scale?

Are the child's vital signs within normal limits, and can the child participate appropriately in approved quiet activities?

EYE SURGERY

Several eye disorders, as mentioned previously, that are seen in infancy and childhood require surgical correction. Any surgical procedure is stressful for the child and family. Eye surgery is particularly stressful because the child's visual fields or acuity may be greatly reduced or absent for a period. If both eyes are affected, the child's ability to maneuver and perform activities of daily living independently is also affected.

The nurse should pay special attention to education. If the child is going home with patches, drops, or any other procedure that must be performed, the family needs to know how to perform this care and should also know the safety precautions involved.

EYE INFECTIONS

Nursing Considerations for the Child with Conjunctivitis

Conjunctivitis ("pink eye") is an inflammation of the conjunctiva (the clear, membranous lining of the lid and sclera). Signs and symptoms of conjunctivitis may include itching, burning, light sensitivity (photophobia), "scratchy" eyelids, redness, edema, and discharge. It is caused usually by either allergy or infection. Accurate diagnosis before treatment is important because inappropriate treatment can lead to complications.

Conjunctivitis noted in the first few weeks of life is called ophthalmia neonatorum. In infants, conjunctivitis occurring in the first 24 hours of life is usually caused by chemical irritation from infection prophylaxis administered soon after birth. Either infection or a blocked lacrimal duct can cause conjunctivitis that occurs after the first 24 hours. Infants acquire infection during birth (from passing through the birth canal) or after birth. *Chlamydia* is responsible for most eye infections noted in infants (Palafox, Smitha, Tauber, & Foster, 2011). Medical treatment should be directed at the cause of the infection. Antibiotic or antiviral eyedrops or ointments are most often used to treat infectious conjunctivitis. If *Chlamydia* is the cause, however, systemic antibiotics (e.g., erythromycin) are also used to prevent pneumonia.

Conjunctivitis in older children may have a variety of causes, including bacteria, viruses, allergy, infection, and trauma. Organisms most frequently implicated in bacterial conjunctivitis include *Haemophilus influenzae* and *Streptococcus pneumoniae,* although with the introduction of *H. influenzae* type B (Hib) vaccine, *H. influenzae* has decreased as a major cause. As with the infant, treatment depends on the cause. The nurse obtains a detailed history to help determine the cause. Infection should be suspected if the child has recently been exposed to another person with conjunctivitis or has had an upper respiratory infection. Itching often identifies the cause as an allergic response. Although children with allergic conjunctivitis exhibit redness of the conjunctiva, they usually do not manifest the type of thick discharge seen in bacterial conjunctivitis.

Chlamydial conjunctivitis is rare in children older than 3 years. It may be suspected, however, in a sexually active adolescent with persistent conjunctivitis. A diagnosis of chlamydial conjunctivitis in an older child who is not sexually active should signal the health care provider to assess the child for possible sexual abuse.

Medical management depends on the cause of the conjunctivitis. If the cause is infection, antibiotic or antiviral eyedrops or ointment may be prescribed. If allergies are suspected, antihistamines, either oral or in the form of eyedrops, may be indicated. In severe cases of allergic conjunctivitis, steroid eyedrops and cromolyn sodium eyedrops may be helpful. The steroid eyedrops are tapered over an approximately 7-day period. Because steroids can worsen the severity of many infections, they are used with caution and only for a short time. Used over

the long term, steroids can exacerbate glaucoma and contribute to cataract development.

Teach parents to keep the child's eye clean and administer any prescribed medications (see Chapter 14). The parent can gently remove crusted material from the eye with a cotton ball soaked in warm water. Teach the parent to wipe the eye from the inner to the outer aspect and wash the hands and use a new cotton ball for the other eye. Because bacterial or viral conjunctivitis is extremely contagious, the nurse should teach infection control measures. These include good handwashing and not sharing towels and washcloths. Bottles of eye medication should never be shared with another person. The tip of the dropper or ointment tube should not touch the child's eye or eyelid during administration. The child with purulent conjunctivitis should also be kept home from school or daycare until 24 hours after antibiotics are started (American Academy of Pediatrics [AAP], 2009b).

Preventing injury from rubbing the eye is also important. Mittens may be used for infants. These may be fashioned from bootie-type socks or may be commercially made. Distraction and constant reminding are recommended for toddlers and older children. If the child wears contact lenses, advise discontinuing them until the infection has completely cleared. Securing new contact lenses eliminates the chance of reinfection from contaminated contact lenses and also lessens the risk of a corneal ulceration. Eye makeup should also be discarded and replaced because the chance of reinfecting eyes from contaminated makeup is high. Mascara should be replaced routinely at least every 3 months.

If the conjunctivitis is allergic in origin, cool compresses and dark glasses may also help lessen the irritation and photophobia. If cromolyn sodium eyedrops are prescribed, parents should be taught to begin using them *before* the allergy season because they need several weeks to reach full effectiveness. Ophthalmic nonsteroidal antiinflammatory preparations may also be helpful.

Nursing Considerations for the Child with Orbital Cellulitis

Orbital cellulitis is caused by an infection of the soft tissues of the orbit. It may occur as a result of trauma or, more commonly, an infection of the ethmoid sinus (Seltz, Smith, Durairaj, & Enzenauer, 2011). The usual infecting organisms are *Staphylococcus aureus* and *Streptococcus pneumoniae.* Clinical signs and symptoms include severe eyelid edema, erythema, and an anteriorly displaced eye. Decreased or absent vision, increased intraocular pressure, and pain can complicate the child's condition. The child is febrile and has an elevated white blood cell count. Orbital cellulitis is distinguished from periorbital cellulitis in that periorbital cellulitis is inflammation and infection of the superficial skin tissues that surround the eye (e.g., eyelids) and not the tissue of the eye itself.

Computed tomography (CT) scanning of the eye and brain confirms the diagnosis, assesses complications, and assists with developing the treatment plan (Olitsky et al., 2011). After cultures have been taken, the child is treated with intravenous administration of an antibiotic designed to act on the major causative organisms; the treatment is individualized when the culture results are available. If the area is painful, analgesics may also be prescribed. Children with orbital cellulitis need to be admitted to the hospital for observation and treatment because of the potential for rapid progression to systemic disease. Left untreated, the infection causing the orbital cellulitis can spread to the optic nerve and then directly to the brain, causing meningitis and blindness. Affected children need frequent vision assessments during treatment. Surgical intervention may be required.

Nursing care involves administering prescribed medications and monitoring the child receiving intravenous therapy. The child also should be carefully monitored for signs and symptoms that the infection is spreading. This includes a thorough neurologic assessment. Finally, the nurse frequently assesses the child's pain status. Heat application four times a day and prescribed analgesics can relieve pain.

Nursing Considerations for the Child with a Corneal Ulcer

Corneal ulcers are usually caused by ocular infection as a result of trauma. Signs and symptoms include pain, tearing, purulent discharge, and blurred vision. Besides trauma, risk factors for corneal ulceration include extended wearing of soft contact lenses, surgical procedures, and viral infection in the eye (usually herpesvirus type 1). Corneal ulcerations may be a sign of underlying systemic disease. If not properly and aggressively treated, corneal ulcerations can cause corneal scarring and blindness.

Treatment includes aggressive topical antibiotic therapy with a broad-spectrum antibiotic until cultures return. Treatment is started with a potent new generation of fluoroquinolones: ciprofloxacin, ofloxacin, and norfloxacin. Topical antiviral preparations are used for ulcers caused by viral infection. Systemic acyclovir may be prescribed by the ophthalmologist to treat ocular herpesvirus infection. The nurse teaches the parent about administration of any prescribed medications and the cause and prevention of future ulcerations. The parent needs to discourage the child from rubbing the eyes (which can worsen the injury). The child who wears contact lenses should avoid wearing them until the ulceration and infection are completely healed. Any lenses worn during the episode should be discarded.

EYE TRAUMA

Nursing Considerations for the Child with a Corneal Abrasion

Corneal abrasions usually result from a scraping or tearing of the cornea by foreign bodies, contact lenses, paper, or fingernails. The child may have light sensitivity, pain, excessive tearing, and decreased vision. The abrasion is diagnosed by instilling a fluorescein dye in the eye and examining the eye under a blue-filtered light (Wood lamp) to highlight the injury. If foreign bodies remain in the eye, they should be removed.

If the abrasion is small, treatment consists only of the instillation of an appropriate antibiotic ointment or drops four times a day for 1 to 2 days with a follow-up evaluation to check healing. Referral to an ophthalmologist should be considered with any eye injury, but particularly for a large abrasion or with the suspicion of a penetrating injury. Many authorities now recommend no patching unless the wound is large. When large abrasions are patched, the patch remains in place for 24 hours and the eye is reexamined at the end of the 24-hour period. Failure to treat an abrasion can result in loss of visual acuity or permanent scarring and opacity of the cornea.

Parent education is important in caring for the child with a corneal abrasion. Because an abrasion increases the risk of infection, parents should be taught the importance of administering ophthalmic antibiotics as prescribed. The child should not rub the eye because rubbing can worsen an abrasion. If the eye is patched, advise the parents not to remove the patch for 24 hours, even to instill ointment. Keeping the patch in place prevents further damage to the eye from blinking. The nurse also reinforces injury prevention, especially wearing safety goggles during sports and other activities, such as woodworking.

Nursing Considerations for the Child with Hemorrhage

Subconjunctival hemorrhages manifest as red areas beneath the conjunctiva. They are often the result of Valsalva maneuvers, such as coughing, vomiting, or straining. Subconjunctival hemorrhages resolve on their own within 2 to 3 weeks and require no treatment. Although they often appear worse than they are, they may be associated with other ocular or physical problems and should be evaluated.

Because these hemorrhages resolve spontaneously, care is aimed at reassurance. Parents should be told that the hemorrhage will appear to grow larger in the first few days because of the effects of gravity.

Hemorrhages can occur with nonaccidental eye injury as well. In a child suspected of having shaken baby syndrome, for example, retinal hemorrhaging of various types can occur. The child will manifest abnormal findings on funduscopic examination and may exhibit retinal detachment (Olitsky et al., 2011). The infant or child who receives a direct blow to the eye will usually demonstrate bruising around the eye. Hyphema and damage to the eye structures are a consequence of this type of trauma.

Nursing Considerations for the Child with Hyphema

A hyphema is a hemorrhage resulting from a blow or penetrating injury to the eye. Symptoms include a recent history of injury, pain, light sensitivity, decreased vision, the presence of floaters, and excessive tearing. The child is usually sleepy. If the child has no known history of injury, the child should be assessed for a bleeding disorder, anticoagulant therapy, renal or hepatic disease, retinoblastoma, or child abuse. Children with sickle cell disease are prone to hyphema. An examination of the eye reveals blood in the anterior chamber (between the cornea and iris) of the eye. Traumatic hyphema usually fills less than one third of the anterior chamber.

Hyphema usually results from blunt trauma to the eye (Pons, 2011), but can result also from penetrating eye trauma (Olitsky et al., 2011). Any penetrating eye injury is an emergency, requiring rapid referral to an ophthalmologist and treatment to prevent blindness. At the scene of the injury, the eye should be immediately covered with a sterile dressing and an eye shield (manufactured rigid eye shield, Styrofoam or plastic cup). Keep the child's head as still as possible until emergency services arrive. Treatment for hyphema includes bed rest with the head elevated 30 to 40 degrees, sedation, and protective shielding of the eye. Treatment can be managed at home if the child is cooperative with bed rest; otherwise, hospitalization is indicated (Bord & Linden, 2008). There is a risk of a rebleed between the third and fifth days after the trauma; children who experience a rebleed should be hospitalized (Bord & Linden, 2008).

Medications such as steroid eyedrops, antifibrinolytic eyedrops (tranexamic acid is best for pediatric use), antiglaucoma medications, and cycloplegic eye drops (atropine) may also be used. The child should be closely monitored for side effects of medications, which will vary according to the prescribed therapy.

Careful assessment is required for the child with a hyphema. Assess the eye frequently for a secondary hemorrhage, or rebleed. This condition is characterized by an increase in the size of the hyphema, with bright-red "new" blood noted over the existing clot. Children who rebleed have a poorer long-term prognosis for vision because acute or chronic glaucoma can be a consequence. The child should also be monitored for signs and symptoms of increasing intraocular pressure (pain, nausea and vomiting, increased inflammation). The child is usually restricted to bed rest with bathroom privileges. Elevating the head of the bed 30 to 40 degrees helps settle the hyphema in the inferior anterior chamber angle. Television viewing may or may not be allowed, and reading and other close-up activities are usually forbidden. Therefore, boredom is a problem for most children. Offer diversional activities that do not involve reading or straining the eyes, such as music and books on tape. If both eyes are patched, the nurse orients the child to the environment and provides for safety.

Discharge teaching includes use of prescribed home medications, patching regimen (the eye is usually patched at night for 2 weeks after discharge), and prevention of further injury. The child's eye should be protected with a shield if an eye patch is worn at night. The child can usually return to all normal activities several weeks after the injury. Eye protection is recommended for all children who participate in sports or other high-risk activities, but lifelong use of protective eyewear is recommended for the child who has had hyphema. The nurse should also emphasize the importance of follow-up because the child is at risk for complications such as glaucoma and cataracts.

Teaching to prevent eye injury is an important nursing intervention (see Patient-Centered Teaching: How to Prevent Eye Injuries While Participating in Sports box). Many school and recreational athletic organizations have policies regarding eye protection during sports activities. Teens who attend vocational schools must wear protective eye covering in shops where eye injury is a risk. Of more concern is the potential for eye injury occurring during unsupervised play.

PATIENT-CENTERED TEACHING

How to Prevent Eye Injuries While Participating in Sports

- High-risk sports include those in which no eye protection is worn, such as basketball, baseball/softball, tennis and other racquet sports, paintball, martial arts, and boxing.
- The highest percentage of injuries is seen in basketball and baseball.
- Wear certified protective eyewear—such as goggles or eyewear made of hard polycarbonate lenses, helmets, and face shields—when possible.
- Wear sports goggles under helmets and with hockey masks.

Data from American Academy of Ophthalmology. (2011). *Eye health in sports and recreation*. Retrieved from www.aao.org.

Nursing Considerations for the Child with a Chemical Splash Injury

Splash injury can occur any time infective, hot, or corrosive liquid splashes into a child's eye; burns of the eye constitute an ocular emergency. Burns may occur from any number of common household items, such as bleach, ammonia, drain opener, and oven cleaner.

Initial care of the child with a splash injury to the eyes focuses on immediate irrigation with water or saline to prevent further injury. In a chemical splash, if the chemical is alkaline, the irrigation may continue for several hours because the damaging action of alkaloids may be prolonged. Irrigation of a frightened child's eyes can be difficult and painful for the child. Pre-irrigation anesthetizing of the eye may facilitate irrigation (Pons, 2011).

If the burn is mild, irrigate for at least 30 minutes, using at least 2 L of irrigant; if the burn is severe, continue irrigating for 2 to 4 hours or with at least 10 L of irrigant (Olitsky et al., 2011). Periodically check the eye pH with litmus paper until the results are within normal range (Olitsky et al., 2011). The cornea may appear cloudy after an alkali burn. Further treatment may include referral to an ophthalmologist for topical steroids, medications to dilate the pupils and decrease the risk of adhesions, antibiotic ointment, and patching. Oral antibiotics and analgesics may also be indicated. Nursing care focuses on prescribed medical treatments, comfort measures, and injury prevention (particularly if both of the child's eyes are patched).

Discharge teaching focuses on the prescribed medical treatments and the importance of adherence with long-term follow-up and injury

prevention. Follow-up care includes monitoring visual acuity and for side effects such as increased intraocular pressure and cataracts.

⚡ SAFETY ALERT

Working with a Child Who Has a Visual Impairment

- Orient the child to the hospital environment on admission. Orientation can be done by walking the child around the room and identifying objects such as the bed, bathroom, doorways, windows, and chairs.
- Never touch the child without identifying yourself and explaining what you plan to do.
- When describing objects or the environment to a child who is blind or visually impaired, use familiar terms. For example, if the child is older and recently blinded, you may be able to use color when describing objects. If the child has been blind since birth, color has no meaning. Describing how many steps away something is or the placement of eating utensils on a tray are both useful tactics. Remember that parents are often the best source for communication.
- Identify noises for the child because children who are visually impaired or blind often have difficulty establishing the source of a noise.
- Orient the child frequently to time and place. Confusion can be frightening.
- Keep all items in the room in the same location and order. Changing the order or spacing of objects may cause confusion or lead to injury.
- Provide detailed explanations and allow the child to progress through care in steps to learn the order.
- As with any child, allow as much control over the situation as possible.
- Supervise the child and counsel parents to supervise the child as needed.

HEARING LOSS IN CHILDREN

Etiology

Damage to, or impairment of, any part of the ear can cause hearing loss. Four types of hearing loss have been identified: conductive, sensorineural, mixed, and central. Each has a different treatment regimen and response to intervention (Box 31-3). Hearing loss can be congenital or acquired. In infants with sensorineural hearing loss, an autosomal recessive inheritance pattern is the cause in more than 80% of cases (Haddad, 2011). Infection, damage from ototoxic medications, head injury, and trauma from noise exposure are the major causes of acquired hearing loss in children (American Speech-Language-Hearing Association, 2011).

Incidence

The reported prevalence of hearing loss in infants ranges from 1 to 3 per 1000 (Ross, Holstrum, & Gaffney et al., 2008). It is difficult to estimate the true prevalence of hearing loss in infants and children because most newborn screening tools identify only those newborns with moderate to severe hearing loss. Children with mild or unilateral hearing loss may not be identified until they reach school age and encounter difficulties with their academic performance (Tharpe, 2008).

Because evidence suggests that many preschool and school-age children experience hearing loss to the extent that their academic performance is affected when they begin school (American Academy of Audiology, 2011), the American Academy of Pediatrics (AAP) (2009a) has taken the position that pediatric providers must be proactive in assessing risk for hearing loss throughout childhood and refer as necessary. Box 31-4 lists criteria used to assess infants and children who may

BOX 31-3 TYPES AND ETIOLOGY OF HEARING LOSS

- *Conductive:* Outer or middle ear affected by damage, inflammation, or obstruction. Sound conduction is prevented from progressing from the outer ear to the inner ear. May be the result of excessive cerumen (wax), foreign bodies, perforated tympanic membrane, or otitis media (with or without effusion). Hearing loss is often temporary and reversible.
- *Sensorineural:* Result of damage or malformation of structures of the inner ear and/or auditory nerve. May be the result of heredity or environmental factors, such as infection (meningitis or intrauterine), exposure to loud noise, ototoxic medications, or prematurity. Meningitis is a significant cause of acquired sensorineural hearing loss in children. Hearing loss is usually permanent.
- *Mixed:* Combination of conductive and sensorineural loss. Conductive loss is often reversible, whereas sensorineural loss is not.
- *Central:* Result of damage to the conduction system between the auditory nervous system and cerebral cortex. May be the result of trauma, neurovascular changes, or brain tumors. May cause difficulty in differentiation of sounds, auditory memory.

BOX 31-4 RISK FACTORS INDICATING THE NEED FOR HEARING SCREENING

Neonates (Birth to 28 Days)
- Family history of inherited permanent sensorineural hearing loss
- Exposure to intrauterine infections such as rubella, cytomegalovirus, and toxoplasmosis
- Presence of craniofacial abnormalities, including those of the outer ear
- Neonatal intensive care unit (NICU) admission lasting more than 5 days
- Any findings associated with a syndrome that includes hearing loss

Infants (29 Days to 2 Years) Developing Certain Conditions Associated with Hearing Loss
- Regardless of passing the newborn hearing screen, presence of parental concern about hearing, speech, language, or developmental delay
- History of exposure to intrauterine infection
- Acquired infections associated with sensorineural hearing loss (e.g., meningitis)
- Head trauma resulting in loss of consciousness or skull fracture
- Any findings associated with a syndrome or disorder that includes hearing loss, or syndromes that result in progressive hearing loss
- History of neonatal problems requiring intensive intervention
- Recurrent otitis media with effusion lasting at least 3 months
- Chemotherapy treatment

Data from Joint Committee on Infant Hearing. (2000). Year 2000 position statement: Principles and guidelines for early hearing detection and intervention programs. *Pediatrics, 106*(4), 798-817; AAP Joint Committee on Infant Hearing. (2007). Year 2007 position statement: Principles and guidelines for early hearing detection and intervention programs. *Pediatrics, 120*(4), 898-921.

be at risk for hearing loss. The AAP (2009a) recommends assessing for hearing loss risk at all well visits during infancy and early childhood, with objective hearing screening routinely initiated when the child reaches 4 years of age. Furthermore, any child who demonstrates one or more risk factors by routine assessment should be referred to an audiologist by the time the child is 2 years old (AAP, 2009a).

BOX 31-5 HEARING TESTS USED FOR INFANTS

Auditory Brainstem Response
- Electrodes, which record brain wave activity, are placed on the infant's head.
- Foam-padded earphones are placed over the ears.
- The earphones sound a click at a 35-dB volume.
- The resulting brain wave measurement is compared with the brain wave measurement from a normal infant.
- The test takes 10 to 60 minutes to administer, depending on the underlying testing objective.

Evoked Otoacoustic Emissions
- This test assesses the integrity of the inner ear structures by recording sounds (otoacoustic emissions) generated by the inner ear. It cannot assess the degree of hearing loss but can assess whether hearing is present.
- An ear probe, which contains a sound transmitter and microphone, is attached to a computer and placed in the ear.
- Click sounds evoke the emissions, which are displayed on the computer screen.
- Emissions are present in infants who can hear at 20 dB but not present in infants who hear only at 30 dB or higher.*
- The test takes approximately 5 minutes to administer.

*American Speech-Language-Hearing Association. (n.d.). *Hearing screening*. Retrieved from www.asha.org.

Diagnostic Evaluation

Evidence demonstrates that infants with hearing loss who have been identified and treated before 6 months of age have a better prognosis than those for whom treatment has been delayed. The use of risk criteria for screening infants for hearing loss helps identify only approximately 50% of infants affected (see Box 31-4). The AAP Joint Committee on Infant Hearing (2007) has recommended that all infants be screened before 1 month of age, that hearing loss be identified before 3 months of age, and that intervention occur before 6 months of age. Many states have passed legislation making newborn hearing screening mandatory, and more than 95% of infants born in hospitals are screened before discharge (American Academy of Audiology, 2011).

Hearing screening for infants is challenging because of their inability to give accurate behavioral cues indicating intact hearing. Historically, assessing hearing in the newborn or young infant often relied on eliciting a startle reflex with a loud noise. However, being certain that the response is actually caused by the sound itself is difficult. Two hearing screening tests can accurately identify infants with hearing deficits: the auditory brainstem response and the evoked otoacoustic emissions test (Box 31-5). Newer equipment has allowed these tests to be completed quickly and accurately in the hospital nursery. Both tests have a pass/refer option. If the infant does not pass after two tries (2 weeks apart), referral to an audiologist for more accurate testing is required. More sophisticated testing, such as visual reinforcement audiometry or conditioned-play audiometry, is performed by audiologists.

Hearing testing in the older child (ages 3 years and older) is done by play audiometry (e.g., the child performs a play activity when the sound is heard) or conventional audiometry (Haddad, 2011). The child is presented tones of varying frequencies at a standard volume (usually 20 decibels [dB]). A quick screening test performed in a physician's office with a hand-held audiometer tests frequencies of 500, 1000, 2000, and 4000 hertz (Hz). If the child does not pass the screening,

PATHOPHYSIOLOGY

Hearing Loss

Adequate hearing depends on intact auditory structures and quality of sound. Sound is described in terms that combine volume (expressed in decibels [dB]) and pitch, or frequencies (expressed in hertz [Hz]). Normal speech ranges in volume between 10 and 60 dB. Normal hearing ranges from −10 to +15 dB at a variety of frequencies. Most people can hear frequencies between 10 and 20,000 Hz. Hearing loss is categorized as follows:

Slight: Failure to hear at 16 to 25 dB

Mild: Failure to hear at 26 to 40 dB

Moderate: Failure to hear at 41 to 55 dB

Moderately severe: Failure to hear at 56 to 70 dB

Severe: Failure to hear at 71 to 90 dB

Profound: Failure to hear at more than 90 dB

A child with mild hearing loss may have difficulty hearing speech in a classroom setting. This deficit obviously poses academic problems for children who have not been identified as having a hearing loss and miss most of what a teacher says in a classroom.

Data from Smith, W., Bale, J., & White, K. (2005). Sensorineural hearing loss in children. *Lancet, 365,* 880.

particularly at lower frequencies and lower volume, a tympanogram may indicate middle ear effusion (see Chapter 21) . The problem with office audiometric screening is that it can miss hearing loss at higher frequencies, which is usually sensorineural. When doing audiometric screening of children, the nurse should therefore perform the test in a quiet environment and determine ahead of time what signal the child will use to indicate hearing the tone. All infants and young children should be assessed regularly at well visits for any communication delay or academic difficulty that might be related to decreased hearing. Should problems arise, referral for complete audiologic examination is warranted (AAP, 2009a).

Therapeutic Management

The goals of identification and management of infants and children with hearing loss are directed toward maximizing language development and preventing later problems with school performance and social interaction. Treatment of hearing loss depends on the type of loss. Conductive hearing loss is managed by medical or surgical correction of the underlying problem (otitis, cerumen).

Sensorineural hearing loss, which is seldom reversible, requires a different approach. Hearing aids are often recommended for these children. The type of aid chosen depends on the specific needs of the child. The aid should provide the best acoustics and be cosmetically appropriate. For example, an adolescent seldom chooses a body-type hearing aid if an ear-level aid (one inserted into the ear canal) suffices. The four types of hearing aids most commonly used for pediatric patients are behind-the-ear, ear-level (in the ear), eyeglass (aids attached to the temples of eyeglass frames), and body (a box with wires connected to an ear mold). Infants and young children often do better with ear-level hearing aids. Infants diagnosed with hearing loss need to begin wearing hearing aids as soon as possible to help facilitate language development.

Cochlear implants offer new options for children with sensorineural hearing loss, even those with some residual hearing. The implant is a small electronic device surgically implanted in the cochlea. It delivers electrical stimulation to the inner ear, causing nerve impulses to travel to the brain, where they are interpreted as normal sound. The implant improves communication, but commitment to rehabilitative efforts and proper use and maintenance of the device by the family and child are essential for success (National Institute on Deafness and Other Communication Disorders, 2007). Cochlear implants are being used more frequently and successfully in infants younger than 12 months; the goal is to maximize hearing during the critical time for speech and language development (Miyamoto, Hay-McCutcheon, Kirk et al., 2008).

Nursing Considerations for the Child with Hearing Loss

Assess the child's hearing at each well-child visit and at other times when warranted (e.g., with chronic otitis media [see Chapter 21]). Note an infant's response to bells, rattles, clapping of hands, or horns held approximately 12 inches from the ear. Older children can be asked to repeat whispered words or phrases or listen for a ticking watch. Begin audiometry testing at 3 years of age or younger in a cooperative child.

Assess language skill development. Infants who are deaf babble like hearing infants until approximately 5 to 6 months of age, at which time babbling is noted to cease. The nurse also questions parents about the child's attention span, disruptive behavior, and other behaviors, such as increasing the volume on the television. If the child appears to have hearing loss or is lagging behind in developmental milestones, refer for further evaluation by an audiologist and ear, nose, and throat specialist.

When caring for a child who is hearing impaired, the nurse should do the following:

- If the child has a hearing aid, encourage its use. Make sure it is in place before beginning to speak.
- Look directly into the child's face. To enhance lip reading, have the child's complete attention before beginning to speak.
- Speak clearly. Slow speech slightly. Do not speak loudly.
- Eliminate background noise.
- Use visual aids to assist communication. These include pictures, hands, and written messages for older children.
- If the child uses American Sign Language to communicate, have a diagram of commonly used words readily available. Use an interpreter for more complex discussions.

An important nursing responsibility is to educate parents about preventable hearing loss. Mild sensorineural hearing loss can occur from exposure to loud noises, such as from firecrackers, firearms, loud infant squeak toys, outdoor yard equipment, boat and snowmobile motors, and rock music. People exposed to loud sounds over long periods need to wear protective ear coverings (e.g., ear plugs, mufflers). Advise teens to decrease exposure to loud rock music and to turn music volume down, especially when listening through earphones. Referral for genetic counseling, if the child has congenital sensorineural hearing loss, is important. Prevention also includes appropriate prevention and treatment of prenatal infection and infection during infancy and early childhood. Children with hearing loss may need speech therapy; referral to a speech therapist or early intervention program should occur as soon as possible.

? CRITICAL THINKING EXERCISE 31-1

At the recommendation of the Joint Committee on Infant Hearing, most U.S. states and many areas of Canada have implemented mandatory newborn infant hearing screening programs. As part of these programs, newborns are screened before hospital discharge. Consider the advantages and disadvantages of this issue. Why should nurses advocate that their states implement similar programs if they do not already exist?

LANGUAGE DISORDERS

Until 10 to 12 months of age, a child is considered prelingual. The sounds the child makes have no direct meaning or connection to future language. They are, instead, practice of a learned skill. Before approximately 6 months of age, infants make few sounds other than crying. At approximately 4 to 6 months of age, however, they enter the babbling phase. These are the cooing, happy sounds that an infant makes when content. The first words appear at approximately 10 to 12 months of age. First sentences appear at approximately 18 months of age. By 2 years of age, most children have at least a 50-word spoken vocabulary.

Girls have more rapid language development until approximately 3 years of age, when the difference disappears. By adolescence, however, girls again show superior verbal skills. Although a correlation exists between developmental delay and verbal skills, the relation between language development and intelligence is unclear. No scientific evidence seems to suggest that a child who talks early is brighter than one who does not. Children who talk quite early do appear, however, to be bright, whereas those who talk extremely late appear to have some developmental delay.

Language disorders in the child are usually of two types, receptive or expressive. A receptive disorder is when the child has decreased ability to comprehend language, and an expressive disorder is when the child cannot express thoughts through speech. Some children have a combination of both expressive and receptive language difficulty. Language disorders can result from genetic influences, infection, trauma, autism, or hearing loss, among other etiologies (Simms & Schum, 2011).

Expressive disorders are most often of three types. The first is a disorder of the voice. This is an alteration in the pitch and intonation that may result from a medical condition, such as a cleft palate. The second is a defect of articulation, or the way in which words are pronounced. This is the most common type of speech defect and may be related to neuromuscular disease or structural abnormalities of the nose, throat, and mouth. It may also be idiopathic. Finally, fluency disorders interrupt the flow of normal speech. Included in this category are lisping and stuttering. If stuttering persists after 5 years of age, the child should receive appropriate referrals for speech evaluation (Figure 31-1).

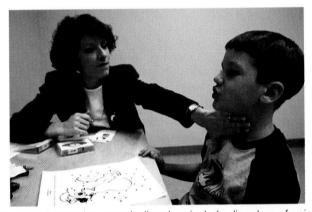

FIG 31-1 Expressive speech disorders include disorders of voice, articulation, and fluency. A speech therapist works with the child to help the child speak more clearly and be better understood. Early intervention is important to correct speech disorders. The nurse should therefore assess speech patterns during each health screening. Referrals should be made for any problems noted. (Courtesy Cook Children's Medical Center, Fort Worth, TX.)

PATIENT-CENTERED TEACHING
How to Encourage Language Development

Talk
Talking to your child is necessary for language development. Because children usually imitate what they hear, how much you talk to your child, what you say, and how you say it affect how much and how well your child talks.

Look
Look directly at your child's face and wait until your child pays attention before you begin talking.

Control Distance
Be sure you are close to your child when you talk (no farther than 5 feet). The younger the child, the closer you should be.

Loudness
Talk slightly louder than you normally do. Remove background noise (e.g., turn off the radio, television, dishwasher).

Be a Good Speech Model
- Describe daily activities to your child as they occur.
- Expand what your child says. For example, if your child points and says "car," you say, "Oh, you want the car."
- Add new information. You might add, "That car is little."
- Build vocabulary. Make teaching new words and concepts a natural part of everyday activities. For example, use new words while shopping, taking a walk, or washing dishes.
- Repeat your child's words with adult pronunciation.

Play and Talk
Set aside times throughout each day for play time for just you and your child. Play can be looking at books, exploring toys, singing songs, coloring, and so on. Talk to your child during these activities, keeping the conversation at your child's level.

Read
Begin reading to your child at a young age (younger than 12 months). Ask a librarian for books that are right for your child's age. Reading can be a calming activity that promotes closeness between you and your child. Reading provides another opportunity to teach and review words and ideas. Some children enjoy looking at pictures in magazines and catalogs.

Do Not Wait
Your child should have the following skills by these ages:
- *18 months:* Three-word vocabulary
- *2 years:* 25- to 30-word vocabulary and several two-word sentences
- *2½ years:* At least a 50-word vocabulary and two-word sentences consistently

If your child does not have these skills, tell your physician. A referral to an audiologist and a speech pathologist may be indicated. Hearing and language testing may lead to a better understanding of your child's language development.

From Northern, J. L., & Downs, M. P. (1991). *Hearing in children* (4th ed., pp. 26-27). Baltimore: Williams & Wilkins.

As with screens for hearing loss, the nurse should assess the child's communication patterns with each well-child visit. Any problems should be noted and referrals made to provide appropriate intervention as soon as possible. Encourage parents to take measures to encourage speech and prevent speech problems (see Chapters 5 to 8 for specific information about language development).

KEY CONCEPTS

- Anything that alters a child's sensory perception can adversely affect growth and development.
- Sense organs develop quite early and are sensitive to teratogens. Any interference with development can result in later sensory alteration.
- Special care should be taken when caring for the child with sensory alterations. Orientation to a new environment is critical in preventing stress and possible injury.

- Most screenings for sensory alterations are noninvasive and relatively painless.
- Parent education and support are critical in assisting the child with sensory alterations to develop as normally as possible.
- Early intervention and special school supports for the child with sensory alterations allow for more normal growth and development.
- Health teaching should include injury prevention.

REFERENCES

American Academy of Audiology. (2011). *Childhood hearing screening guidelines.* Retrieved from www.audiology.org.

American Academy of Ophthalmology. (2011). *Eye health in sports and recreation.* Retrieved from www.aao.org.

American Academy of Pediatrics. (2009a). Hearing assessment in infants and children: Recommendations beyond neonatal screening. *Pediatrics, 124,* 1252-1263.

American Academy of Pediatrics. (2009b). *Red book: Report of the Committee on Infectious Diseases* (28th ed.). Elk Grove Village, IL: Author.

American Academy of Pediatrics Joint Committee on Infant Hearing. (2007). Year 2007 position statement: Principles and guidelines for early hearing detection and intervention programs. *Pediatrics, 120*(4), 898-921.

American Speech-Language-Hearing Association. (n.d.). *Hearing screening.* Retrieved from www.asha.org.

American Speech-Language-Hearing Association. (2011). *Causes of hearing loss in children.* Retrieved from www.asha.org.

Aponte, E., Diehl, N., & Mohney, B. (2010). Incidence and clinical characteristics of childhood glaucoma: A population-based study. *Archives of Ophthalmology, 128*(4), 478-482.

Bord, S., & Linden, J. (2008). Trauma to the globe and orbit. *Emergency Medical Clinics of North America, 26,* 97-123.

Children's Eye Foundation. (2011). *Types of vision screening devices.* Retrieved from www.childrenseyefoundation.org.

Chou, R., Dana, T., & Bougatsos, C. (2011). *Screening for visual impairment in children ages 1 to 5 years: Systematic review to update the 2004 U.S. Preventive Services Task Force recommendations.* Rockville, MD: Agency for Healthcare Research and Quality.

Davenport, K., & Patel, A. (2011). Cataracts. *Pediatrics in Review, 32,* 82-83.

Donahue, S., & Ruben, J. (2011). U.S. Preventive Services Task Force vision screening recommendations. *Pediatrics, 127,* 569-570.

Doshi, N., & Rodriguez, M. (2007). Amblyopia. *American Family Physician, 75,* 361-367.

Haddad, J. (2011). Hearing loss. In R. Kliegman, B. Stanton, J. St. Geme, et al. (Eds.), *Nelson textbook of pediatrics* (19th ed., pp. 2188-2196). Philadelphia: Elsevier Saunders.

Miyamoto, R., Hay-McCutcheon, M., Kirk, K., et al. (2008). Language skills of profoundly deaf children who received cochlear implants under 12-months of age: A preliminary study. *Acta Otolaryngology, 128*(4), 373-381.

Modi, N., & Jones, D. (2008). Strabismus: Background and surgical techniques. *Journal of Perioperative Practice, 18*(12), 532-535.

National Institute on Deafness and Other Communication Disorders. (2007). *Cochlear implants.* Retrieved from www.nidcd.nih.gov/health/hearing/coch.asp.

Olitsky, S., Hug, D., Plummer, L., & Stass-Isern, M. (2011). Disorders of the eye. In R. Kliegman, B. Stanton, J. St. Geme, et al. (Eds.), *Nelson textbook of pediatrics* (19th ed., pp. 2148-2187). Philadelphia: Elsevier Saunders.

Palafox, K., Smitha, J., Tauber, A., & Foster, C. (2011). Ophthalmia neonatorum. *Journal of Clinical & Experimental Ophthalmology, 2*(1). doi:10.4172/2155-9570.1000119.

Pathai, S., Cumberland, P., & Rahi, J. (2010). Prevalence and early-life influences on childhood strabismus. *Archives of Pediatric and Adolescent Medicine, 164*(3), 250-257.

Pons, J. (2011). Eye trauma. *CME, 29*(2), 66-68.

Ross, D. S., Holstrum, W. J., Gaffney, M., et al. (2008). Hearing screening and diagnostic evaluation of children with unilateral and mild bilateral hearing loss. *Trends in Amplification, 12*(1), 27-34.

Seltz, L., Smith, J., Durairaj, V., & Enzenauer, T. (2011). Orbital cellulitis in children. *Pediatrics, 127*(3), e566-e572.

Simms,, M. & Schum, R. (2011). Language development and communication disorders. In R. Kliegman, B. Stanton, J. St. Geme, et al. (Eds.), *Nelson textbook of pediatrics* (19th ed., pp. 114-121). Philadelphia: Elsevier Saunders.

Smith, R., Bale, J., & White, K. (2005). Sensorineural hearing loss in children. *Lancet, 365,* 879-890.

Stewart, C., Moseley, M., & Fielder, A. (2011). Amblyopia therapy: An update. *Strabismus, 19*(3), 91-98.

Taylor, K., & Elliott, S. (2011). Interventions for strabismic amblyopia. *Cochrane Database of Systematic Reviews* (8), CD006461.

Tharpe, A. (2008). Unilateral and bilateral hearing loss in children: Past and current perspectives. *Trends in Amplification, 12*(1), 7-15.

United States Preventive Services Task Force. (2011). Screening for visual impairment in children ages 1 to 5: Recommendation statement. *Pediatrics, 127,* 340-346.

ABCDEs Airway, breathing, circulation, disability, and exposure; critical components of the primary assessment that require assessment and interventions in the stabilization of a critically ill or injured child. (*Ch. 10*)

abduction Movement of a limb away from the midline of the body. (*Ch. 26*)

ablation Destruction of diseased tissue. (*Ch. 22*)

achalasia Failure of smooth muscle fibers of the gastrointestinal tract to relax, resulting in a functional obstruction and difficulty in passage of food and chyme along the tract. (*Ch. 19*)

acidosis Abnormal accumulation of acid in, or loss of base from, the body, with serum pH less than 7.35. (*Ch. 16*)

active immunity Protection that forms in response to exposure to natural antigens or vaccines; protection can last months, years, or a lifetime. (*Ch. 18*)

active listening Listening empathically to gain a better understanding of both the actual and the implied message. (*Ch. 3*)

addiction A neurobiologic disease state influenced by genetic, psychological, and environmental factors characterized by impaired control over drug use, compulsive use, continued use despite harm, and cravings. (*Ch. 15*)

adduction Movement of a limb toward the midline of the body. (*Ch. 26*)

adjuvant A pharmacologic or nonpharmacologic intervention with additive effects on pain management; designed to assist the primary pain management intervention. (*Ch. 15*)

adolescence Period between the onset of puberty and the cessation of physical growth; the passage from childhood to adulthood. (*Ch. 8*)

afterload The amount of force against which the ventricles contract. (*Ch. 22*)

airway management Correct positioning of the airway, appropriate interventions used to ensure patency of the airway, and adequate oxygenation and ventilation. (*Ch. 10*)

alkalosis Abnormal accumulation of base in, or loss of acid from, the body, with serum pH more than 7.45. (*Ch. 16*)

allergy A hypersensitivity reaction in various body systems resulting from the immune system's response to exposure to an irritant (allergen). (*Ch. 18*)

alopecia Hair loss; a common side effect of chemotherapy. (*Chs. 24, 25*)

amblyopia Reduced visual acuity not correctable by refractive means and not attributable to structural or pathologic ocular anomalies. (*Ch. 31*)

anastomosis Surgical connection of separate tubular hollow organs to form a continuous channel, as between two parts of the intestine or esophagus. (*Ch. 19*)

angioplasty Procedure that dilates vessels. (*Ch. 22*)

anorexia Loss of appetite. (*Ch. 24*)

antibody A protein that the immune system produces to bind to specific antigens and eliminate them from the body. (*Ch. 18*)

anticipatory grief The processes of mourning, coping, interacting, planning, and psychosocial reorganizing that occur as part of the response to the impending death of a loved one. (*Ch. 12*)

anticipatory guidance Providing the family with information on what to expect regarding a future event, a potential problem or issue, or a child's next developmental phase. (*Ch. 2*)

antigen A substance that possesses unique configurations enabling the immune system to recognize it as foreign. (*Ch. 18*)

antipyretic An agent that reduces or relieves fever. (*Ch. 13*)

apical pulse rate Heart rate determined by placing the stethoscope over the point of maximal intensity and counting for 1 minute. (*Ch. 13*)

Arnold-Chiari malformation Abnormalities of the fourth ventricle, lower cerebellum, and brainstem characterized by herniation of the cerebellum through the foramen magnum into the spinal canal; often associated with myelomeningocele. (*Ch. 28*)

arrhythmia Disturbance of rhythm. (*Ch. 22*)

arteriovenous fistula A connection between an artery and a vein, usually for the purpose of hemodialysis. (*Ch. 20*)

asphyxiation A state of suffocation that severely compromises oxygen delivery to the body. (*Ch. 5*)

associative play Group play without group goals. (*Chs. 4, 6*)

astigmatism Abnormal curvature of the cornea or the lens. (*Ch. 31*)

atelectasis A collapsed or airless state of the lung that may involve all or part of the lung. (*Ch. 21*)

atresia Absence or abnormal closure of a normal body orifice or passage. (*Ch. 19*)

auscultate To listen to body sounds (e.g., heart sounds, breath sounds) using a stethoscope. (*Ch. 13*)

auscultation Elicitation and evaluation of sounds produced by the body, frequently by using a stethoscope to magnify body sounds. (*Ch. 9*)

autism spectrum disorders Developmental disorders characterized by impairment in communication skills, social interaction, repetitive and stereotyped patterns of behavior; one group of pervasive developmental disorders. (*Ch. 30*)

autoimmune disease and disorder Disease that occurs when the immune system produces antibodies—called autoantibodies—against cells of the body. (*Ch. 18*)

autonomy The ability to function independently without the control of others. (*Chs. 6, 8*)

autoregulation The unique ability of the cerebral arteries to maintain a steady blood flow during changes in blood pressure and perfusion by adjusting their diameter in response to alterations in cerebral perfusion pressure. (*Ch. 28*)

avascular necrosis Tissue damage caused by inadequate blood supply. (*Ch. 26*)

azotemia The presence of urea and other nitrogenous bodies in the blood; an elevated blood urea nitrogen or creatinine level. (*Ch. 20*)

basal ganglia A major communication and sorting area for messages to and from the cerebral hemispheres composed of masses of gray matter; controls movement and participates in emotion and cognition. (*Ch. 28*)

Battle sign Bruising or hemorrhage over the mastoid which may be indicative of a basilar skull fracture. (*Ch. 28*)

behavioral disorders Disorder of conduct or attention. (*Ch. 29*)

benign Slow-growing cells, often almost normal in appearance, forming a tumor with distinct borders. (*Ch. 24*)

beta cells Specialized cells in the pancreas that manufacture and secrete insulin; thought to be the target of the autoimmune destructive process of type 1 diabetes mellitus. (*Ch. 27*)

bioethics Rules or principles that govern right conduct, specifically those that relate to health care. (*Ch. 1*)

blast cells Immature white blood cells, such as lymphoblasts, myeloblasts, or monoblasts. (*Ch. 24*)

blood-brain barrier Selective anatomic or physiologic capillary obstruction that prevents potentially harmful substances, such as certain medications, radioactive ions, and viruses, from entering the parenchyma of the brain. (*Chs. 14, 28*)

brainstem Structure connected to the cerebral hemispheres by thick bunches of nerve fibers; all nerve fibers traverse through the brainstem from the hemispheres to the cerebellum and spinal cord. (*Ch. 28*)

callus Tissue that joins fractured bone ends or repairs damaged bone; begins as cartilaginous tissue and becomes hardened through osteoblastic activity. (*Ch. 26*)

cardiomegaly An enlarged heart. (*Ch. 22*)

cardiopulmonary resuscitation Protocol performed when an individual's respiratory and cardiovascular systems require support to maintain vital functions; airway management, ventilation, and chest compressions are provided to improve tissue perfusion until definitive care is available. (*Ch. 10*)

caries Tooth decay. (*Chs. 6, 7*)

case management A practice model that uses a systematic approach to identify specific client needs and to manage client care to ensure optimal outcomes. (*Ch. 1*)

cataract A loss of transparency of the crystalline lens or its capsule. (*Ch. 31*)

central venous access device Venous access device in which the catheter is placed centrally rather than peripherally, usually in the superior vena cava or jugular vein; used for long-term intravenous therapy. (*Ch. 14*)

cephalocaudal Progression from head to toe. (*Ch. 4*)

831

cerebral cortex Gray matter of the cerebrum where the higher functions of thinking occur. *(Ch. 28)*

cerebral perfusion pressure The difference between mean arterial blood pressure and intracranial pressure. *(Ch. 28)*

chelation Binding of a metallic ion with a structure so that the ion is inactivated. *(Ch. 23)*

chronic grief Mourning after the death of an individual that is of excessive duration and interferes with the person's ability to return to normal living. *(Ch. 12)*

chronic illness or condition A condition or illness that is long term and either is without cure or has a residual effect that limits activities of daily living. *(Ch. 12)*

chronic sorrow Recurrent feelings of grief, loss, and fear related to the child's illness and loss of the ideal, healthy child. *(Ch. 12)*

chronologic age Age in years. *(Ch. 4)*

circumduction Circular movement of a limb or an eye. *(Ch. 9)*

clean margins Evidence of normal, disease-free tissue in the outermost layer of cells of a surgical sample. *(Ch. 24)*

comorbidity The occurrence of two or more different disorders in the same individual; children with intellectual disabilities often have coexisting psychiatric disorders. *(Chs. 29, 30)*

compensation Maintenance of an adequate blood flow without distressing symptoms; accomplished by cardiac and circulatory adjustments, such as tachycardia, cardiac hypertrophy, and increased blood volume from sodium and water retention. *(Ch. 22)*

complement An accessory system to a humoral response that is composed of serum proteins that facilitate enzyme action and antigen death. *(Ch. 18)*

conductive hearing loss Reversible loss caused by damage, inflammation, or obstruction to outer or middle ear; sound is prevented from progressing across middle ear. *(Ch. 31)*

congenital (infantile) glaucoma Increased intraocular fluid pressure that occurs during the first 3 years of life because of a defect in the drainage network of the eye. *(Ch. 31)*

conservation Ability to understand that certain properties of objects do not change simply because their order, form, or appearance has changed. *(Ch. 7)*

contractility The ability of muscle tissue to contract when its thick (myosin) and thin (actin) filaments slide past each other. *(Ch. 22)*

cooperative play Organized play with group goals. *(Chs. 4, 6)*

coping Efforts directed toward managing and solving various problems, events, and stressors. *(Ch. 2)*

crackles Abnormal, discontinuous, nonmusical sounds heard on auscultation, primarily during inhalation; also called rales. *(Ch. 21)*

crepitation A dry, crackling sound or sensation. *(Ch. 9)*

crepitus May be felt or heard at a fracture site when the ends of a broken bone move against each other. Used to describe the grating, crack-ling or popping sounds and sensations experienced under the skin and joints. *(Ch. 26)*

critical milestones Developmental milestones that, if not reached appropriately, would initiate a full developmental assessment. Critical milestones are based on the Denver Developmental Screening Test II milestones (see Chapter 4) and appear in the Growth and Development boxes. *(Chs. 5, 6)*

culture The sum of values, beliefs, and practices of a group of people that are transmitted from one generation to the next. *(Ch. 2)*

Cushing's response Late sign of increased intracranial pressure; includes increased blood pressure, widened pulse pressure, decreased heart rate, and decreased or irregular respiratory rate. *(Ch. 28)*

débridement Removal of foreign material and devitalized or contaminated tissue from a traumatic or infected lesion to expose healthy tissue. *(Ch. 25)*

debulking The surgical removal of as much of a tumor as possible. *(Ch. 24)*

decompensation Inability of the heart to maintain adequate circulation; may be marked by dyspnea, venous engorgement, cyanosis, and edema. *(Ch. 22)*

denial A defense mechanism in which unpleasant realities are kept out of conscious awareness. *(Ch. 11)*

dental emergencies Injuries or infections of a tooth or teeth occurring when the period of time to definitive care is critical for the survival of the tooth or to alleviate pain. *(Ch. 10)*

development Changes that occur over time in function and psychosocial and cognitive behavior. *(Ch. 9)*

developmental age Age based on functional behavior and ability to adapt to the environment; does not necessarily correspond to chronologic age. *(Ch. 4)*

developmental disability Disorders of childhood that are characterized by delays and impairments of expected developmental level. These can be intellectual, motor, or sensory disorders. *(Ch. 30)*

developmental milestones Benchmarks of development that indicate whether the infant is developing normally; not achieving milestones within a certain time frame might be cause for concern. *(Ch. 5)*

diabetic ketoacidosis Metabolic consequence of severe insulin deficiency; marked by hyperglycemia, acidosis, and ketosis. *(Ch. 27)*

diplopia Double vision. *(Ch. 31)*

discipline The structure an adult sets for a child's life, designed to allow the child to interact socially in the real world in an appropriate manner; the training expected to produce a specific type or pattern of behavior. *(Ch. 2)*

dislocation Displacement of a bone from its normal articulation within a joint. *(Ch. 26)*

dramatic play Play in which children act out roles and experiences that may have happened to them, that they fear will happen to them, or that they have observed happening to someone else. *(Ch. 4)*

dysfluency Disorders in the rhythm of speech in which individuals know precisely what they wish to say but are unable to do so because of an involuntary, repetitive prolongation or cessation of sound. *(Ch. 6)*

dysphagia Inability to swallow or difficulty in swallowing. *(Chs. 19, 21)*

dysplasia Abnormal development of tissue. *(Ch. 26)*

dyspnea Difficulty breathing. *(Ch. 21)*

dysuria Pain on urination. *(Ch. 20)*

echolalia Stereotyped repetition of another person's words or phrases. *(Ch. 30)*

edema Presence of abnormally large amounts of fluid in the intercellular tissue spaces of the body. *(Ch. 20)*

egocentric Preoccupied with one's own interests and needs. *(Ch. 11)*

egocentrism Complete absorption with self; an inability to understand that others have a different point of view. *(Chs. 5, 6, 8)*

emergency Psychological, medical, or traumatic condition that requires immediate care or care within 1 hour to prevent further deterioration. *(Ch. 10)*

emotional disorders Disorder of mood (depression) and anxiety disorders. *(Ch. 29)*

empathy Seeing from another's perspective while remaining objective. *(Ch. 3)*

empowerment Provision of appropriate tools (education, information, support) to individuals that enable them to participate fully in decision making. *(Ch. 3)*

encopresis Incontinence of feces. *(Ch. 19)*

enteral By way of the digestive system (e.g., enteral feeding). *(Ch. 13)*

envenomation Injection of venom by an animal (e.g., usually snakes, lizards, spiders, scorpions) into a human body. *(Ch. 10)*

environmental injuries injuries occurring as a result of outside or environmental factors. *(Ch. 10)*

epidemiology The study of health, illness, and the factors that determine health and illness in a selected population. *(Ch. 17)*

epidural Potential space that surrounds the spinal cord and lies outside the dura mater. *(Ch. 15)*

epiglottitis Inflammation of the epiglottis. *(Ch. 13)*

erythema Redness of the skin. *(Ch. 25)*

erythropoiesis Production of erythrocytes (red blood cells [RBCs]). *(Ch. 23)*

eschar Dark plaque associated with tissue necrosis, which can form an inelastic shell over wounds. *(Ch. 25)*

ethical dilemma A situation in which no solution seems completely satisfactory. *(Ch. 1)*

ethics Rules or principles that govern right conduct and distinctions between right and wrong. *(Ch. 1)*

ethnic Pertaining to religious, racial, national, or cultural group characteristics, especially speech patterns, social customs, and physical characteristics. *(Ch. 2)*

ethnicity Condition of belonging to a particular ethnic group; also refers to ethnic pride. *(Ch. 2)*

ethnocentrism The opinion that the beliefs and customs of one's own ethnic group are superior to those of others. *(Ch. 2)*

eutectic mixture of local anesthetics (EMLA) Cream used to numb the skin at a depth of 0.5 mm; used before needle punctures. *(Ch. 14)*

euthyroid Normal thyroid function. *(Ch. 27)*

exanthema An eruption or rash on the skin. *(Ch. 17)*

excoriation Scratch or abrasion of the skin. *(Ch. 25)*

extension (decerebrate) posture Abnormal extension of the upper extremities with internal rotation of the upper arms and wrists; lower extremities will extend with some internal rotation. *(Ch. 28)*

external fixation Placement of pins, screws, or bars through bone and soft tissue to immobilize or correct a deformity. *(Ch. 26)*

external rotation Turning outward, or laterally, within a joint. *(Ch. 26)*

extracellular fluid Fluid found outside the cell, comprising approximately one third of the body's fluid in older children and about one half of the body's fluid in infants. *(Ch. 16)*

extracorporeal life support Temporary method of providing cardiovascular, pulmonary, and circulatory support for children for whom other methods of treatment are not effective. *(Ch. 10)*

extramedullary Outside the bone marrow. *(Chs. 23, 24)*

extrapyramidal motor system (tract) Descending pathway of the motor neurons concerned with involuntary or unconscious skeletal muscle coordination and reflex control of coordination. *(Ch. 28)*

familiarization play Use of materials that are commonly associated with health care situations in creative and playful activities. *(Ch. 4)*

family Two or more people who are joined together by bonds of sharing and emotional closeness and who identify themselves as being part of the family (Friedman, Bowden, & Jones, 2003). *(Ch. 2)*

fasciculation A small, local, involuntary muscular contraction visible under the skin. *(Ch. 9)*

fatalism The belief that events are predestined. *(Ch. 2)*

fistula Abnormal passage or communication between two organs or tissues. *(Ch. 19)*

flexion (decorticate) posture Abnormal flexion of the upper extremities and extension of the lower extremities. *(Ch. 28)*

fracture A break or disruption in a bone's continuity. *(Ch. 26)*

fremitus A vibration perceptible on palpation or auscultation. *(Ch. 9)*

frequency Urination at short time intervals. *(Ch. 20)*

functional age The age equivalent at which the child is actually able to perform specific self-care or relational tasks; for example, the child may be 6 years old chronologically but only able to perform skills representative of children 4 years old, and thus the child's functional age is 4 years old. *(Ch. 30)*

fundoplication A 270- to 360-degree wrap of the stomach fundus around the distal esophagus to tighten the lower esophageal sphincter and prevent gastric reflux. *(Ch. 19)*

genetic mutation A variation (deletion, addition or recopy of a stretch of DNA) in a gene that affects its function. *(Ch. 30)*

genome (human) The DNA (genetic sequence) structure that is unique to humans. *(Ch. 30)*

genotype Genetic makeup of an individual, determines specific traits or conditions; the blueprint for the phenotype. *(Ch. 30)*

gland An organ or structure that secretes a substance or hormone to be used in another part of the body. *(Ch. 27)*

glucagon A hormone produced by the alpha cells of the pancreas; counteracts the action of insulin by converting liver stores of glycogen to blood glucose, resulting in an elevation of the blood glucose concentration. *(Ch. 27)*

glucose The substrate of choice for cellular energy; the breakdown product of stored glycogen or dietary carbohydrate. *(Ch. 27)*

glycosuria Glucose in urine that occurs when the blood glucose level exceeds the renal threshold and glucose "spills" into the urine. *(Ch. 27)*

glycosylated hemoglobin A laboratory test used to evaluate long term blood glucose control by measuring glycosylation (glucose attachment to a protein) of a portion of the hemoglobin molecule in red blood cells; offers a 3-month average of blood glucose control. *(Ch. 27)*

gradient Difference. *(Ch. 22)*

granulocytes Polymorphonuclear leukocytes (neutrophils, eosinophils, basophils). *(Ch. 23)*

growth Measurable physical and physiologic changes that occur over time. *(Ch. 9)*

growth spurts Brief periods of a rapid increase in growth rate. *(Ch. 4)*

hand hygiene Cleansing of the hands with soap and water, antiseptic hand wash, alcohol-based hand rub, or surgical hand antisepsis. *(Ch. 13)*

hematemesis Vomiting of bright red blood or of denatured blood that looks like coffee grounds; usually represents a bleeding source proximal to the jejunum. *(Ch. 19)*

hematopoiesis Production of all types of blood cells (red blood cells, white blood cells, and platelets); normally occurs in the bone marrow but may occur in extramedullary sites. *(Chs. 23, 24)*

hemolysis Breakdown of red blood cells. *(Ch. 23)*

hemosiderosis Focal or general increase in tissue iron stores without associated tissue damage. *(Ch. 23)*

hemostasis Process of vasoconstriction and coagulation to stop bleeding. *(Ch. 23)*

hepatosplenomegaly Enlargement of the liver and spleen detected by palpation of the abdomen. *(Ch. 24)*

heredity Transmission of genetic characteristics from parent to offspring. *(Ch. 4)*

herniation Shift of brain tissue sideways, under the falx cerebri, or downward, causing severe neurologic dysfunction. *(Ch. 28)*

history The aggregate of subjective data that describes past and present health status. *(Ch. 9)*

honeymoon phase An early stage of diabetes characterized by residual endogenous insulin production that results in a lower need for exogenous insulin to maintain normal blood glucose. *(Ch. 27)*

hormone A chemical substance produced by one gland or tissue and transported by the blood to other tissues or organs, where it causes a specific effect. *(Ch. 27)*

hospice care A system of comprehensive care that provides support and assistance to clients and families affected by terminal illness; the purpose is to humanize the dying experience while providing the means for living as comfortably and as fully as possible. *(Ch. 12)*

host The organism from which a parasite obtains its nourishment. *(Ch. 17)*

hydrotherapy Therapy entailing water soaks to clean wounds, which removes old dressings and softens dead tissue for easier removal. *(Ch. 25)*

hypercapnia Increased levels of carbon dioxide in the blood, as indicated by an elevated $PaCO_2$ as determined by blood gas analysis. *(Ch. 21)*

hyperglycemia Blood glucose in a diabetic child above the target range; in a nondiabetic child, fasting blood glucose of 110 mg/dL or higher. *(Ch. 27)*

hyperkalemia Elevated serum potassium level above the range for age. *(Ch. 27)*

hypernatremic (hypertonic) dehydration State in which the sodium concentration is above that of normal body fluids (i.e., 150 mEq/L). *(Ch. 16)*

hyperopia Farsightedness; abnormal close vision. *(Ch. 31)*

hyphema A hemorrhage or sanguineous exudate in the anterior chamber of the eye. *(Ch. 31)*

hypoalbuminemia Low albumin levels in the blood. *(Ch. 20)*

hypocapnia Decreased levels of carbon dioxide in the blood. *(Ch. 21)*

hypoglycemia Blood glucose levels less than 70 mg/dL. *(Ch. 27)*

hyponatremic (hypotonic) dehydration State in which the sodium concentration is below that of normal body fluids (i.e., 130 mEq/L). *(Ch. 16)*

hypothalamus Portion of the brain that secretes releasing factors to the pituitary gland for the maintenance of endocrine and metabolic activities. *(Ch. 27)*

hypothermia Cooling of body temperature to subnormal levels; temperature levels considered dangerous to infants and children are core body temperatures less than 96° F (35.6° C). *(Ch. 10)*

hypoxemia Decreased levels of oxygen in the blood. *(Ch. 21)*

hypoxia Decreased oxygenation of cells and tissues. *(Ch. 21)*

identity formation The acquisition of psychosocial, sexual, and vocational identity. *(Ch. 8)*

idiopathic For unknown reasons. *(Ch. 27)*

illness trajectory The course of a chronic illness, including the work for and impact on the lives of all those involved. *(Ch. 12)*

immune (lymphoreticular) system The body's internal defense against foreign substances, such as bacteria, viruses, parasites, and fungi. (*Ch. 18*)

immunity Resistance of the body to the effects of a harmful organism or its toxin. (*Ch. 17*)

immunodeficiency A defect in the immune system leading to increased susceptibility to multiple and repeated infections. (*Ch. 18*)

immunosuppression A weakening or cessation of the body's normal immune response. (*Ch. 24*)

implanted venous access device Surgically implanted port or reservoir in which the catheter tip is placed in the superior vena cava; used for long-term intravenous therapy. (*Ch. 14*)

infant mortality rate Number of deaths per 1000 live births that occur within the first 12 months of life. (*Ch. 1*)

infection Condition resulting from invasion of the body by pathogenic or nonpathogenic organisms, such as bacteria, viruses, protozoa, helminths, or fungi. (*Ch. 17*)

inflammation A tissue response to injury or destruction of cells. (*Ch. 17*)

informed consent A requirement, both legal and ethical, that the child and the parent or guardian completely understand proposed procedures or treatments, including their benefits and risks. (*Ch. 13*)

ingestion Swallowing of a potentially toxic substance, such as inappropriate amounts or types of medication, petroleum products, insecticides, or toxic plants. (*Ch. 10*)

inotropic Affects the force of muscular contractions; can cause a positive or negative effect. (*Ch. 22*)

inspection Careful observation to identify physical findings. (*Ch. 9*)

intellectual disability Term adopted by learning specialists to describe disabilities of learning, thinking, and problem solving; replaces "mental retardation" as a descriptor unless specific criteria are present. (*Ch. 30*)

intelligence The innate capacity of the individual; what individuals can do relative to learning, thinking, and problem solving; results obtained on intelligence tests that measure specific skills, such as verbal, nonverbal, or mechanical abilities. (*Ch. 30*)

intermittent infusion port Intravenous catheter used to administer intermittent medications or fluids; remains clamped when not in use. (*Ch. 14*)

internal fixation Placement of instruments (wires, pins, rods, screws) inside the body to immobilize bone parts. (*Ch. 26*)

interstitial fluid Extracellular fluid surrounding the cell, including lymph fluid. (*Ch. 16*)

intracellular fluid Fluid found within the cells, composing approximately two thirds of the body's fluid in older children and about one half of the body's fluid in infants. (*Ch. 16*)

intrathecal Within the spinal canal. (*Ch. 24*)

irreversibility The inability to understand a process in reverse or mentally undo an action that has been performed. (*Ch. 6*)

isonatremic (isotonic) dehydration State in which the sodium concentration is practically identical to that of body fluids (i.e., between 135 and 145 mEq/L). (*Ch. 16*)

ketone, ketoacid An acid produced in response to starvation (in the diabetic child, a result of insulin deficiency); produced from fat stores, which can be used for energy by some tissues when glucose is unavailable. (*Ch. 27*)

Kussmaul respiration Deep, rapid respiration seen with diabetic ketoacidosis in which carbon dioxide is expelled as a respiratory compensation for acidosis; also described as "air hunger." (*Ch. 27*)

lavage Wash. (*Ch. 13*)

learning Behavior changes that occur as a result of both maturation and experience with the environment. (*Ch. 4*)

leukocoria Appearance of a whitish reflex or mass in the pupillary area behind the lens of the eye. (*Ch. 24*)

leukocytes White blood cells, whose chief function is to protect the body against foreign substances; includes five types: lymphocytes, monocytes, neutrophils, eosinophils, and basophils. (*Ch. 18*)

lichenification Thickening and hardening of the skin with accentuation of skin markings; often the result of chronic scratching. (*Ch. 25*)

lymphadenopathy Swelling of the lymph nodes detected by palpation. (*Ch. 24*)

lymphocytes The primary white blood cells of the immune system (e.g., B lymphocytes, or B cells; and T lymphocytes, or T cells). (*Ch. 18*)

malignant Abnormal cells that have invasive and unregulated growth and the potential to spread to distant locations in the body; life-threatening. (*Ch. 24*)

malocclusion Misalignment of the teeth or dental arches; teeth may be crowded, crooked, or out of alignment. (*Ch. 7*)

malpractice Negligence by a professional person. (*Ch. 1*)

melena Rectal passage of black, tarry stools, indicating denatured blood from the upper gastrointestinal tract. (*Ch. 19*)

menarche Onset of menstruation. (*Ch. 7*)

mental retardation A type of developmental disorder that has early onset, pervasive decrease in intellectual functioning, and deficits in at least two areas of functional ability. (*Ch. 30*)

metered-dose inhaler Hand-held device that delivers "puffs" of medication for inhalation. (*Ch. 14*)

mistrust The negative resolution of the first developmental task, according to Erikson's theory; results in acute emotional tension and behavioral signs of unmet needs. (*Ch. 5*)

Monro-Kellie doctrine Theory describing the compensatory mechanism of the cranial contents to maintain a steady volume and pressure. (*Ch. 28*)

mood A pervasive and sustained emotion. (*Ch. 29*)

mood disorder Recurrent disturbances or alterations in mood that inhibit functioning or cause distress. (*Ch. 29*)

morbidity Ratio of sick to well persons in a defined population. (*Ch. 1*)

myelinization Formation of the proteolipid coating of the nerves that facilitates conduction of impulses. (*Ch. 28*)

myocardial contractility Ability of myocardial cells and tissues to shorten in response to an appropriate stimulus; force of contraction of the myocardium. (*Ch. 22*)

myopia Nearsightedness; abnormal distance vision. (*Ch. 31*)

nasal flaring A serious sign of air hunger demonstrated by widening of the nares to enable an infant or a young child to take in more oxygen. (*Ch. 21*)

nasal polyps Semitransparent herniations of respiratory epithelium. (*Ch. 21*)

negativism The attitude of opposing or resisting the directions of others. (*Ch. 6*)

negligence Failure to act in the way a reasonable, prudent person of similar background would act in similar circumstances. (*Ch. 1*)

neurons Structural units (cells) of the nervous system that function to initiate and conduct impulses. (*Ch. 28*)

neuropathic pain Pain resulting from trauma or disease that damages the peripheral nerves or the central nervous system. (*Ch. 15*)

neutropenia Decrease in the number of circulating neutrophils that results in a decreased ability of the body to fight infection. (*Ch. 24*)

nociceptive Impulse from a specific body area that gives rise to the sensation of pain. (*Ch. 15*)

nonspecific immune functions Protective barriers, such as chemicals, interferon, inflammation, and phagocytosis, that are activated in the presence of an antigen but are not specific to that antigen. (*Ch. 18*)

normalization Responses used to counteract an illness or abnormal behavior to maintain appropriate and valued social roles. (*Ch. 12*)

nurse practice acts Laws that determine the scope of nursing practice in each state. (*Ch. 1*)

nutrients Foods that supply the body with elements necessary for metabolism. (*Ch. 4*)

nystagmus Involuntary eye movements that make the eyes appear to be darting back and forth. (*Ch. 31*)

object permanence The realization that objects continue to exist even though they are out of sight. (*Ch. 5*)

obtund To render dull or blunt. (*Ch. 9*)

occult blood Blood in such minute quantity that it can be recognized only by microscopic or chemical means. (*Ch. 19*)

oliguria Diminished urine output. (*Ch. 16*)

ophthalmia neonatorum Conjunctivitis noted in the first few weeks of life; usually gonococcal or chlamydial. (*Ch. 31*)

opioid Natural and synthetic agonists and antagonist with morphine-like activity. (*Ch. 15*)

opportunistic infection An infection that occurs as a result of a weakened immune system. (*Ch. 24*)

orthopnea Difficulty breathing except in an upright position. (*Ch. 21*)

ossification The process of forming bone from osseous tissue or cartilage. (*Ch. 26*)

osteoblasts Mesodermal cells whose activity produces bone. (*Ch. 26*)

osteotomy Surgical cutting of bone. *(Ch. 26)*

pain "An unpleasant sensory and emotional experience associated with actual or potential tissue damage or described in terms of such damage" (International Association for the Study of Pain, 1979). Pain is whatever the person experiencing the pain says it is (Paseo & McCaffery, 2011). *(Ch. 15)*

pain threshold Level of intensity at which pain becomes appreciable or perceptible as painful. *(Ch. 15)*

palliative care Medical treatments or procedures that aim to promote comfort and quality of life rather than cure the underlying disease. *(Ch. 12)*

palliative therapy Medical and nursing care that either slows the progression of disease or increases the patient's comfort, but is not curative. *(Ch. 24)*

palpation The use of touch to determine factors such as texture, temperature, moisture, and organ size and location. *(Ch. 9)*

palpitations Sensation of rapid or irregular heartbeat. *(Ch. 22)*

pancytopenia A reduction in all types of blood cells. *(Ch. 23)*

papilledema Edema of the optic disk. *(Ch. 28)*

parallel play Playing alongside but not with other children. *(Chs. 4, 6)*

parent-infant attachment A sense of belonging to or connection between a parent and an infant. *(Ch. 5)*

paresthesia Sensation of numbness and tingling. *(Ch. 26)*

passive immunity Protection that occurs when serum containing an antibody is given or transmitted to a person who does not have that antibody. *(Ch. 18)*

pathogen A disease-producing microorganism. *(Ch. 17)*

pediculocide An agent used to destroy lice. *(Ch. 25)*

percussion Tapping of the body to determine the density, location, and size of organs. *(Ch. 9)*

peripherally inserted central catheter (PICC) Central line that is inserted peripherally (usually through a vein of the upper arm) into the superior vena cava. *(Ch. 14)*

peristalsis Progressive, wavelike movements caused by contraction and relaxation of the longitudinal and circular muscles of the gastrointestinal tract; propels a bolus of food or fluid forward. *(Ch. 19)*

pervasive developmental disorders (PDD) A group of disorders including autistic disorder, Rett disorder, childhood disintegrative disorder, Asperger syndrome, and fetal alchol syndrome. *(Ch. 30)*

petechiae Tiny (less than 3 mm), nonblanching red spots that are the result of intradermal hemorrhage, often associated with a low platelet count. *(Ch. 24)*

pharmacodynamics Behavior of medications at the cellular level. *(Ch. 14)*

pharmacokinetics The time and movement relationships of medications. *(Ch. 14)*

phenotype Physical manifestation of the individual genotype (genetic code), determines eye color, height, facial features, and genetic conditions (special skills or developmental disabilities). *(Ch. 30)*

physiologic anorexia Decreased appetite because of relatively decreased caloric need. *(Ch. 6)*

pincer grasp The use of index finger and thumb to grip objects. *(Ch. 5)*

pituitary An endocrine gland attached to the base of the brain that secretes numerous hormones, including thyroid-stimulating hormone, growth hormone, adrenocorticotropic hormone, antidiuretic hormone, prolactin, luteinizing hormone, and follicle-stimulating hormone. *(Ch. 27)*

polydactyly Extra fingers or toes. *(Ch. 26)*

posttraumatic stress disorder Emotional, psychological and cognitive disorders that result from exposure to an overwhelming traumatic event, or to repeated traumatic experiences. *(Ch. 29)*

preload Amount of stretch of the myocardial fibers before contraction; most easily measured by determining central venous pressure. *(Ch. 22)*

preparation Provision of information before procedures, treatments, or events; facilitates coping. *(Ch. 3)*

primary sexual characteristics Internal and external reproductive organs in males and females (i.e., uterus, fallopian tubes, ovaries, vagina, vulva, penis, testes, spermatic cord). *(Ch. 8)*

prodrome The initial stage of a disease; symptoms indicating an approaching disease. *(Ch. 17)*

projectile vomiting Vomiting that is projected with force, perhaps 2 to 4 feet away from the mouth; may be preceded by deep gastric left to right peristaltic waves characteristic of pyloric stenosis. *(Ch. 19)*

prosthetic Artificial limb(s). *(Ch. 26)*

proteinuria Protein in the urine. *(Ch. 20)*

protocol A systematic plan of care outlining drug therapy and follow up care based on research in cancer treatment. *(Ch. 24)*

proximodistal Progression from the center outward or from the midline to the periphery. *(Ch. 4)*

pruritus Itching. *(Ch. 25)*

puberty Period of time during which adolescents experience a growth spurt, develop secondary sexual characteristics, and achieve reproductive maturity. *(Ch. 8)*

pulmonary edema Collection of excessive fluid in the alveoli of the lungs. *(Ch. 22)*

pulmonary hypertension Increased pressure in the pulmonary arteries and arterioles. *(Ch. 22)*

pulmonary vascular resistance Amount of resistance in the pulmonary vascular bed against which the right ventricle must pump to achieve blood flow to the lungs. *(Ch. 22)*

purpura Larger (greater than 3 mm) areas of nonblanching red, blue, or purplish spots that are the result of intradermal hemorrhage (bruising), often a result of a low platelet count. *(Ch. 24)*

pylorus The distal opening of the stomach where the stomach contents pass into the duodenum; the pylorus is surrounded by muscle bands. *(Ch. 19)*

pyramidal motor system (tract) Descending pathway of the upper motor neuron concerned with voluntary movement. *(Ch. 28)*

pyrogens Substances that cause fever. *(Ch. 13)*

reduction Repositioning of bone fragments into normal alignment. *(Ch. 26)*

refeeding syndrome A life-threatening metabolic complication that can emerge when a starving person is reintroduced to food. *(Ch. 29)*

refractive error Light rays passing through eye structures come into focus at an inappropriate location relative to the retina. *(Ch. 31)*

regression Appearance of behavior more appropriate to an earlier stage of development; often used to cope with stress or anxiety. Defense mechanism in which conflict or frustration is resolved by returning to a behavior that was successful in an earlier stage of development. *(Chs. 4, 6, 11)*

reproductive maturity The establishment of menstruation and ovulation in females and the development of spermatogenesis in males. *(Ch. 8)*

respite care The provision of temporary relief of care responsibility to people who are caring for a family member at home who might otherwise need permanent hospital or residential care. *(Ch. 30)*

retention Application of a device or mechanism that maintains alignment until healing occurs. *(Ch. 26)*

reticulocyte Immature red blood cell. *(Ch. 23)*

reticuloendothelial system The collection of cells, throughout the body, that are capable of phagocytosis. *(Ch. 23)*

retractions Abnormal movements of the chest wall during inspiration; may be subcostal, intercostal, substernal, suprasternal, or supraclavicular. *(Ch. 21)*

rhonchi Abnormal breath sounds caused by the passage of air through an airway obstructed by thick secretions; sounds usually clear with coughing. *(Ch. 21)*

risk-taking behaviors Behaviors that predispose the adolescent to physical or psychosocial harm. *(Ch. 8)*

ritualism The need to maintain sameness and reliability. *(Ch. 6)*

secondary glaucoma Increased intraocular fluid pressure that occurs after 3 years of age and may be the result of disease or surgery. *(Ch. 31)*

secondary sexual characteristics Physical characteristics of males and females influenced by reproductive hormones but having no direct role in reproduction (i.e., voice, body shape, pubic hair distribution, breasts). *(Ch. 8)*

self-care children Children who care for themselves at home after school; formerly called latch-key children. *(Ch. 7)*

self-esteem Personal value that individuals place on themselves. *(Ch. 3)*

sensorimotor stage Piaget's first stage of cognitive development, in which infants and young toddlers use mainly senses and movement to begin to understand and control their environment. (*Ch. 5*)

sensorineural hearing loss Result of damage or malformation of the middle ear or auditory nerve; hearing loss is usually permanent. (*Ch. 31*)

sensory information Information gained from sight, taste, touch, smell, and hearing. (*Ch. 3*)

separation anxiety Distress and apprehension caused by being removed from parents, home, or familiar surroundings. (*Ch. 11*)

sexual maturity rating Stages of sexual maturation based on pubic hair and breast development in girls and pubic hair and genital development in boys. (*Ch. 8*)

shock Inadequate tissue perfusion, usually caused by illness or injury that results in respiratory or cardiovascular compromise. (*Ch. 10*)

shunt Abnormal blood flow from one part of the circulation to another. (*Ch. 22*)

situational crisis Unanticipated event that poses a threat to an individual's psychosocial or psychological well-being. (*Ch. 11*)

specific immune functions Humoral (B cell and antibody production) and cell-mediated (T cell) responses that are activated in a highly discriminatory way to antigens that survive in the body. (*Ch. 18*)

standard of care Level of care that can be expected of a professional. This level is determined by laws, professional organizations, and health care agencies. (*Ch. 1*)

Standard Precautions Infection control guidelines developed by the National Center for Infectious Disease and the Hospital Control Practices Advisory Committee to prevent the spread of infectious organisms from blood, body fluids, secretions and excretions, mucous membranes, and nonintact skin. (*Ch. 13*)

stereopsis Ability to see dimensions and perceive depth that results from convergence of visual images received by each eye. (*Ch. 31*)

stomatitis Painful inflammation of the mucous membranes lining the mouth often associated with oral ulcerations, as a result of chemotherapy. (*Ch. 24*)

strabismus "Squint," "cross-eyes"; a condition in which the eyes are not straight because of lack of coordination of the extraocular muscles; most often caused by muscle imbalance or paralysis of the extraocular muscles but may also result from conditions such as a brain tumor, myasthenia gravis, or infection. (*Ch. 31*)

stranger anxiety The infant's ability to distinguish between caregivers and others, to prefer parents to other caregivers, and to become distressed when separation occurs. (*Ch. 5*)

stress Any situation or condition, positive or negative, requiring adjustment on the part of the individual, family, or group. (*Ch. 2*)

stridor A shrill, harsh sound that can be heard during inspiration, expiration, or both; produced by the flow of air through a narrowed segment of the respiratory tract. (*Ch. 21*)

subconjunctival hemorrhages Bleeding situated beneath the conjunctiva; in children, the most frequent cause is trauma or severe coughing or sneezing episodes (Valsalva maneuvers); also caused by infection with *Streptococcus pneumoniae* or *Haemophilus influenzae*. (*Ch. 31*)

subluxation Partial dislocation of a joint. (*Ch. 26*)

submersion injury Injury resulting from a near-drowning incident; may be immediately apparent or appear up to 48 hours after the submersion incident. (*Ch. 10*)

substance abuse Use of medications, drugs, or other substances beyond their intended or prescribed purpose. Use of substances for the purposes of intoxication, mood modification, or behavior change. (*Ch. 29*)

suicide potential Assessment of the individual's risk toward self-harm to end life. Includes suicidal ideation, gestures, threats, impulses, attempts and self-termination of life. (*Ch. 29*)

symbolic play The use of games and interactions that represent an issue or concern to be addressed. (*Chs. 4, 6*)

symbolic thought The ability to allow a mental image (word or object) to represent something that is not present. (*Ch. 6*)

syndactyly Fusion or webbing of two or more fingers or toes. (*Ch. 26*)

systematic approach Organized method of collecting data. (*Ch. 9*)

systemic vascular resistance Amount of resistance in the systemic vascular bed against which the left ventricle must pump to achieve cardiac output. (*Ch. 22*)

tachypnea Increased respiratory rate. (*Ch. 21*)

tenesmus Ineffective, painful, or continuous urge to defecate. (*Ch. 19*)

therapeutic play Guided play that promotes the child's psychophysiologic well-being. (*Ch. 11*)

therapeutic relationship A balance between appropriate involvement and professional separation in relating to child/family interactions. (*Ch. 3*)

thrombocytopenia A reduction in platelet count; places the individual at risk for increased bruising and bleeding. (*Ch. 24*)

time-release medication Medication taken in a single dose but designed to dissolve slowly, releasing medication into the bloodstream over a specified period of time (usually 12 to 24 hours). (*Ch. 14*)

toxin A poison produced by pathogenic microorganisms. (*Ch. 17*)

transductive reasoning Reasoning from the particular to the particular rather than from the general to the particular. (*Ch. 6*)

trauma Injury from an external cause, such as a motor vehicle collision, fall, gunshot wound, or stabbing; may be self-inflicted, may be deliberately inflicted or accidental, and may be psychological in nature. (*Ch. 10*)

trauma score Numeric score assessed by health care providers to determine the extent of trauma; usually results from adding, subtracting, dividing, or multiplying numbers representing physiologic parameters or specific types of injuries; used for field triage and assessment; correlates to survivability. (*Ch. 10*)

traumatic brain injury One of the leading causes of death or permanent disability; severity of injury may range from mild to severe; can result in short term and long term disabilities. (*Ch. 10*)

triage Sorting process used to decide the urgency of an individual's illness or injury and allocate appropriate resources effectively; purpose is to ensure that the most seriously ill or injured people receive the appropriate level of care before those with less urgent or emergent conditions. (*Ch. 10*)

trust The basic emotion established during infancy as a result of satisfying interactions between child and caregiver; provides the foundation on which a healthy personality is built. (*Ch. 5*)

tunneled central line A surgically placed central line that is held in place by a Dacron polyester cuff located in a subcutaneous tunnel; most commonly placed in the external jugular vein. (*Ch. 14*)

urgency Sudden urge to urinate. (*Ch. 20*)

valgum Abnormal position of a limb in which it is bent away from the midline of the body. (*Ch. 26*)

valvuloplasty Mechanical procedure to open a valve. (*Ch. 22*)

valvulotomy An opening surgically created in a valve. (*Ch. 22*)

varum Abnormal position of the limb in which it is bent toward the midline of the body. (*Ch. 26*)

vector A carrier that transfers an infective agent from one host to another. (*Ch. 17*)

violence The use of force or a destructive action that results in injury, discordance, shame or outrage; engaging in sudden intense activity to the point of loss of control. (*Ch. 29*)

virulence Strength of effect produced by a pathogenic organism. (*Ch. 17*)

visual acuity Clarity of vision; tested through use of vision charts, with results compared with what a person with normal vision can see at a distance of 10 or 20 feet. (*Ch. 31*)

wheezing High-pitched, musical sounds that can be heard with or without a stethoscope; may be inspiratory or expiratory; caused by bronchial constriction or obstruction of the airway and commonly occurs in asthma. (*Ch. 21*)

WIC A Special Supplemental Food Program for Women, Infants, and Children that provides nutritious food and nutrition education to low-income pregnant and postpartum women and their children. (*Ch. 1*)

win-win solution Solution to a problem, such as the resolution of a conflict, which both parties can support as a common goal. (*Ch. 3*)

Wood light Ultraviolet light used to help diagnose fluorescent skin lesions, including some superficial fungal infections. (*Ch. 25*)